OBESITY

OBESITY

Per Björntorp, M.D., Ph.D.
Professor of Medicine
Sahlgren's Hospital
University of Göteborg
Göteborg, Sweden

Bernard N. Brodoff, M.D.
Adjunct Professor of Physiology
Clinical Professor of Medicine
New York Medical College
Valhalla, New York

With 93 additional contributors

J. B. Lippincott Company Philadelphia
New York • London • Hagerstown

Acquisitions Editor: Charles McCormick, Jr.
Developmental Editor: Kimberley Cox
Production Manager: Janet Greenwood
Production: P. M. Gordon Associates
Compositor: Achorn Graphic Services
Printer/Binder: R. R. Donnelley & Sons

1 3 5 6 4 2

Library of Congress Cataloging-in-Publication Data

Obesity / [editors] Per Björntorp, Bernard N. Brodoff.
   p. cm.
  ISBN 0–397–50999–5
  1. Obesity. I. Björntorp, Per. II. Brodoff, Bernard N.
  [DNLM: 1. Obesity. WD 210 021]
 RC628.0215 1992
 616.3′98—dc20
 DNLM/LC
 for Library of Congress   91–17315
                                     CIP

This book is dedicated to the memory of
Professor Albert E. Renold, M.D., Ph.D. (1923–1988)

Contributors

Jonathan Alexander, MD
Associate Clinical Professor of Medicine
Yale University School of Medicine
New Haven, Connecticut
Director, Cardiac Rehabilitation Program
Medical Director, Nuclear Cardiology Division
Danbury Hospital
Danbury, Connecticut

Keaven M. Anderson, PhD
Statistician
National Heart, Lung and Blood Institute
Framingham, Massachusetts

Gerd Assmann, MD
Professor of Medicine
Institute of Clinical Chemistry and Laboratory
    Medicine
Vast-Tyskland

William A. Bauman, MD
Clinical Director
Spinal Damage Research Center
    and Associate Professor of Medicine
Mount Sinai Medical Center
State University of New York
New York, New York

Richard N. Baumgartner, PhD
Research Associate Professor
Department of Biochemistry
University of New Mexico
School of Medicine
Albuquerque, New Mexico

Jerrold G. Bernstein, MD
Assistant Clinical Professor of Psychiatry
Harvard Medical School
Visiting Scientist, Clinical Research Center
Massachusetts Institute of Technology
Assistant Psychiatrist
Massachusetts General Hospital
Boston, Massachusetts

Edwin L. Bierman, MD
Professor of Medicine
Head, Division of Metabolism, Endocrinology
    and Nutrition
University of Washington
Seattle, Washington

Per Björntorp, MD, PhD
Department of Medicine
Sahlgren's Hospital
University of Göteborg
Göteborg, Sweden

Alexander Blau, MBBS
Instructor in Medicine
Sackler School of Medicine
University of Tel-Aviv
Ramat Aviv, Israel
Nephrologist
Department of Nephrology
The Chaim Sheba Medical Center
Tel-Hashomer, Israel

Vicki Sara Blumberg, MD
Assistant Attending Physician
Danbury Hospital
Danbury, Connecticut

Alfred Jay Bollet, MD
Clinical Professor of Medicine
Yale University School of Medicine
New Haven, Connecticut
Chairman, Department of Medicine
Danbury Hospital
Danbury, Connecticut

Riccardo Bonadonna, MD
University of Piza School of Medicine
CNR Institute of Physiology
Piza, Italy

Claude Bouchard, PhD
Professor of Exercise Physiology
Physical Activity Sciences Laboratory
Laval University
Ste-Foy
Quebec, Canada

George A. Bray, MD
Professor of Medicine
Executive Director
Pennington Biomedical Research Center of
    Louisiana State University
Baton Rouge, Louisiana

Bernard N. Brodoff, MD
Adjunct Professor of Physiology
Clinical Professor of Medicine
New York Medical College
Valhalla, New York

Peter J. Brown, PhD
Associate Professor and Chair
Department of Anthropology
Emory University
Atlanta, Georgia

Kelly D. Brownell, PhD
Professor, Department of Psychiatry
University of Pennsylvania School of Medicine
Co-Director
Obesity Research Clinic
Philadelphia, Pennsylvania

John D. Brunzell, MD
Professor of Medicine
University of Washington
Seattle, Washington

M. A. Cawthorne, PhD
Diabetes Research Group
SmithKline Beecham Pharmaceuticals
Epsom, Surrey, England

R. A. John Challiss, BSc, DPhil
Wellcome Lecturer in Biochemical
    Pharmacology
Department of Pharmacology and Therapeutics
University of Leicester
Leicester, United Kingdom

Wm. Cameron Chumlea, PhD
Fels Professor of Community Health
Fels Professor of Pediatrics
Wright State University
School of Medicine
Yellow Springs, Ohio

Veronica R. Collins, BSc, Dip Ed
Epidemiologist
International Diabetes Institute
Victoria, Australia

Eain Cornford, PhD
Associate Professor
Department of Neurology
University of California School of Medicine
Brain Research Institute
Chief, Neuropharmacology Laboratory
Southwest Regional Veterans Administration
    Epilepsy Center
Research and Neurology Services
Veterans Administration West Los Angeles
    Medical Center
Los Angeles, California

Marcia E. Cornford, MD, PhD
Neuropathology Fellow
Department of Pathology
University of California, Los Angeles
Center for Health Sciences
Los Angeles, California

Isabelle Cusin
Geneva University
Laboratoires de Recherches
    Metaboliques
Geneva, Switzerland

Ralph A. DeFronzo, MD
Professor of Medicine
Chief, Diabetes Division
University of Texas Health Science Center
San Antonio, Texas

Michael J. Devlin, MD
Assistant Clinical Professor of Psychiatry
Columbia University College of Physicians and
   Surgeons
Assistant Attending Physician in Psychiatry
The Presbyterian Hospital
New York, New York

William H. Dietz, MD, PhD
Associate Professor of Medicine
Tufts University School of Medicine
Director of Clinical Nutrition
New England Medical Center
Division of Pediatric GI/Nutrition
Boston Floating Hospital
Boston, Massachusetts

F. Avraham Dilmanian, PhD
Associate Scientist, Medical Department
Brookhaven National Laboratory
Upton, New York
Health Sciences Center
State University of New York at Stony Brook
New York, New York

Gary K. Dowse, BMedSc, MBBS, MSc
Epidemiologist
International Diabetes Institute
Victoria, Australia

Andrea Dunaif, MD
Associate Professor of Medicine
Mount Sinai School of Medicine
New York, New York

Johanna T. Dwyer, DSc, RD
Professor of Medicine and Community Health
Tufts University Medical School
Professor
Tufts School of Nutrition
Director
Frances Stein Nutrition Center
New England Medical Center Hospital
Senior Scientist
US Department of Agriculture
Human Nutrition Research Center at Tufts
   University
Boston, Massachusetts

Björn Ekblom, MD
Professor in Physiology
Department of Physiology III
Karolinska Institutet
Stockholm, Sweden

Haskel E. Eliahou, MD
Professor of Medicine
Sackler School of Medicine
Tel-Aviv University School of Medicine
Tel-Aviv, Israel
Head, Department of Nephrology
Chaim Sheba Medical Center
Tel-Hashomer, Israel

Frederick H. Epstein, MD, FRCP (London)
Professor of Preventive Medicine
Institute of Social and Preventive Medicine
University of Zurich
Zurich, Switzerland

John D. Fernstrom, PhD
Professor of Psychiatry and Behavioral
   Neuroscience
University of Pittsburgh School of Medicine
Director, Basic Neuroendocrine Program
Western Psychiatric Institute and Clinic
Pittsburgh, Pennsylvania

Caroline F. Finch, BSc, MSc
Medical Statistician
International Diabetes Institute
Victoria, Australia

Jean-Pierre Flatt, PhD
Professor of Biochemistry
University of Massachusetts Medical School
Worcester, Massachusetts

James Gibbs, MD
Professor of Psychiatry
Cornell University Medical College
White Plains, New York

James R. Givens, MD
Professor Emeritus, Medicine
Professor Emeritus, Obstetrics and Gynecology
University of Tennessee College of Medicine
Memphis, Tennessee

Barbara C. Hansen, PhD
Professor, Department of Physiology
Director, Obesity and Diabetes Research Center
University of Maryland School of Medicine
Baltimore, Maryland

Gail G. Harrison, PhD
Professor
Department of Family and Community
    Medicine
College of Medicine
University of Arizona
Tucson, Arizona

Rosa Hendler, MD
Research Associate
Yale University School of Medicine
Director
Yale University Weight Control Unit
New Haven, Connecticut

Luis Hernandez, MD
Professor
Facultad de Medicina
Universidad de Los Andes
Mérida, Venezuela

Steven B. Heymsfield, MD
Associate Professor of Medicine
Columbia University
College of Physicians and Surgeons
Director, Weight Control Unit
St. Lukes-Roosevelt Hospital Center
New York, New York

Millicent Higgins, MD, DPH
Associate Director for Epidemiology and
    Biometry
National Heart, Lung, and Blood Institute
Bethesda, Maryland
Professor Emeritus, Epidemiology and Internal
    Medicine
University of Michigan
Ann Arbor, Michigan

Jean Himms-Hagen, DPhil
Professor, Department of Biochemistry
University of Ottawa
Ottawa, Ontario
Canada

Bartley G. Hoebel, PhD
Professor
Department of Psychology
Princeton University
Princeton, New Jersey

Shuji Inoue, MD
Associate Professor
The Third Department of Internal Medicine
Yokohama City University School of Medicine
Yokohama City, Japan

Bernard Jeanrenaud, MD
Professor at the Faculty of Medicine
Geneva University
Professor and Head of the Laboratoires de
    Recherches Metaboliques
Geneva, Switzerland

Eric Jéquier, MD
Professor of Physiology
University of Lausanne
Chairman of the Institute of Physiology
Lausanne, Switzerland

Ronald K. Kalkhoff, MD
Professor of Medicine
Medical College of Wisconsin
Senior Attending Staff
Froedtert Hospital
Milwaukee, Wisconsin

Yakov Kamen, MS
Applied Physics and Nuclear Engineering
  Department
Columbia University
New York, New York
Research Collaborator
Brookhaven National Labs
Upton, New York

William B. Kannel, MD, MPH
Professor of Medicine and Public Health
Boston University School of Medicine
Attending Physician
University Hospital
Boston, Massachusetts

Peter Kopelman, MD, MRCP
Senior Lecturer in Medicine
The London Hospital Medical College
Consultant Physician
Newborn General Hospital
London, England

John G. Kral, MD, PhD
Professor of Surgery
State University of New York
HSC Brooklyn
Director of Surgery
Kings County Hospital Center
Brooklyn, New York

M. E. J. Lean, MD, FRCP
Senior Lecturer, Department of Human
  Nutrition
University of Glasgow
Consultant Physician
Glasgow Royal Infirmary
Glasgow, Scotland

Anthony R. Leeds, MB, BS, MSc
Lecturer, Department of Food and Nutritional
  Sciences
King's College London
Clinical Assistant, Lipid and Obesity Clinic
Parkside North Health District
London, England

Sarah F. Leibowitz, PhD
Associate Professor
Rockefeller University
New York, New York

Steven Lichtman, MEd
Columbia University
College of Physicians and Surgeons
Research Coordinator, Weight Control Unit
St. Lukes-Roosevelt Hospital Center
New York, New York

Lauren Lissner, PhD
Visiting Scientist
University of Göteborg
Göteborg, Sweden

Peter Lönnroth, MD, PhD
Associate Professor
Department of Medicine II
Sahlgren's Hospital
University of Göteborg
Göteborg, Sweden

Walter M. Lovenberg, PhD
President
Merrill Dow Research Institute
Cincinnati, Ohio

Henry C. Lukaski, PhD
Research Physiologist
USDA-ARS
Grand Forks Human Nutrition Research Center
Grand Forks, North Dakota

Edward J. Masoro, PhD
Professor and Chairman
Department of Physiology
University of Texas Health Science Center at
  San Antonio
San Antonio, Texas

John Forbes Munro, MBChB, FRCPE
Part-time Senior Lecturer
Department of Medicine
Western General Hospital
University of Edinburgh
Consultant Physician
Eastern General Hospital, Edinburgh
Edenhall Hospital, Musselburgh
Edinburgh, Scotland

Euro Murzi, MD
Physiology Laboratory
Faculty of Medicine
Los Andes University
Mérida, Venezuela

Christine A. Nathan, MD
Institut de Recherches Internationales Servier
Courbevoie Cedex
France

Eric A. Newsholme, PhD, DSc
Reader in Cellular Nutrition
Department of Biochemistry
University of Oxford
Tutor and Fellow in Biochemistry
Merton College
Oxford, England

Dan A. Oren, MD
Senior Clinical Investigator
National Institute of Mental Health
Senior Staff Fellow
Clinical Center
National Institutes of Health
Bethesda, Maryland

F. Xavier Pi-Sunyer, MD
Professor of Clinical Medicine
Columbia University College of Physicians and
    Surgeons
Chief, Division of Endocrinology, Diabetes and
    Nutrition
Director, Obesity Research Center
St. Luke's-Roosevelt Hospital Center
New York, New York

Cheryl K. Ritenbaugh, PhD, MPH
Associate Professor, Department of Family and
    Community Medicine
University of Arizona
Tucson, Arizona

Alex F. Roche, MD, PhD, DSc
University Professor
Fels Professor of Community Health and of
    Pediatrics
Yellow Springs, Ohio

Judith Rodin, PhD
Chair and Philip R. Allen Professor of
    Psychology
Yale University
New Haven, Connecticut

Françoise Rohner-Jeanrenaud
Geneva University
Laboratoires de Recherches
    Metaboliques
Geneva, Switzerland

Norman E. Rosenthal, MD
Chief, Section on Outpatient Studies
Clinical Psychobiology Branch
National Institute of Mental Health
Bethesda, Maryland

Stephan Rössner, MD, PhD
Professor of Health Behavior Research
Karolinska Institute
Stockholm, Sweden

Christopher J. Schmidt, PhD
Senior Research Biochemist
Merrill Dow Research Institute
Cincinnati, Ohio

Dale A. Schoeller, PhD
Research Associate Professor
Committee on Human Nutrition and
    Nutritional Biology
University of Chicago
Chicago, Illinois

Helmut Schulte, MD
Dr. Rer. Medic
Institut fur Arterioskleroseforschung
Münster, Germany

David H. Schwartz, PhD
Department of Psychology
Princeton University
Princeton, New Jersey

Anthony Sclafani, PhD
Professor of Psychology
Brooklyn College of the City University of New
    York
Brooklyn, New York

Pagiel Shechter, MD
Instructor
Tel Aviv University
Sackler School of Medicine
Tel Aviv, Israel
Research Fellow
Division of Nephrology
Stanford University
Stanford, California

Artemis P. Simopoulos, MD
Director
The Center for Genetics, Nutrition, and Health
Washington, DC

Gerard P. Smith, MD
Professor of Psychiatry
Cornell University Medical College
Attending Psychiatrist
New York Hospital–Cornell Medical Center
White Plains, New York

Ulf Smith, MD, PhD
Professor and Chairman
Department of Medicine II
University of Göteborg
Physician-in-Chief
Sahlgren's Hospital
Göteborg, Sweden

I. H. Stolarek, MB, ChB, MRCP
University of Edinburgh
Registrar, Medical Unit
Eastern General Hospital
Edinburgh, Scotland

Albert Stunkard, MD
Professor of Psychiatry
University of Pennsylvania
Physician
Hospital of the University of Pennsylvania
Philadelphia, Pennsylvania

Theodore B. VanItallie, MD
Professor Emeritus of Medicine
Columbia University College of Physicians and
  Surgeons
Senior Attending Physician
St. Luke's-Roosevelt Hospital Center
New York, New York

Robert William Vaughan, MD
Professor and Chairman
Department of Anesthesiology
University of North Carolina
School of Medicine
Chairman, Department of Anesthesiology
University of North Carolina Hospitals
Chapel Hill, North Carolina

Thomas A. Wadden, PhD
Associate Professor
Department of Psychiatry
University of Pennsylvania School of Medicine
Philadelphia, Pennsylvania

B. Timothy Walsh, MD
Professor of Clinical Psychiatry
Columbia University
College of Physicians and Surgeons
Research Psychiatrist
New York State Psychiatric Institute
New York, New York

Paul Webb, MD
Clinical Professor
Department of Community Health
Wright State University School of Medicine
Dayton, Ohio

David A. York, BSc, PhD
Professor and Chief of Experimental Obesity
  Research
Pennington Biomedical Research Center
Louisiana State University
Baton Rouge, Louisiana

Paul Z. Zimmet, MD, PhD, FRACP
Director
International Diabetes Institute
Professor of Diabetes
Monash University
Consultant Physician
Caulfield General Medical Centre
Victoria, Australia

Preface

Rapid progress in our understanding of adipose tissue and energy metabolism has led to a deeper understanding of the complexities underlying human obesity. Although obesity has long been considered a health hazard, only in 1985 was it officially designated so by the National Institutes of Health Consensus Development Conference on the health implications of obesity. Treatment of all individuals whose body weight exceeded desirable body weight (according to Metropolitan Life Insurance tables) by 20 percent or more was recommended. Weight reduction to lean body weight was also recommended at lower percentage increases in which hypertension, diabetes, or a familial predilection for obesity existed. When it is considered that over 35 million Americans, as well as a substantial number of individuals in Europe and elsewhere in the world, are overweight, obesity can be seen as one of the major nutritional disorders in our society and, when taken with its associated illnesses, one of the major health risks.

Treatment would appear to be a simple matter, because the patient merely has to reduce caloric intake below energy expenditure to lose weight. Successful treatment of the obese subject, however, is frustrating. While substantial research progress has been made, the molecular mechanisms of obesity are still obscure and the achievement of lasting weight reduction remains a baffling therapeutic dilemma.

Because of its complex nature and the interaction of diet, genetics, social, behavioral, medical, and economic factors, many disciplines are involved in fundamental and clinical research on obesity and its treatment. This book is directed to the following individuals: the basic researcher, medical clinician, nurse, dietician and nutritional expert, social worker, house staff officer, medical student, and medical educator. We have attempted to cover the field, experimental and clinical, in a comprehensive manner with clear and concisely written chapters that are authoritative and contemporary, with extensive bibliographies and references to primary sources. All the chapters in this book have been written by preeminent scientists and clinicians, each one an acknowledged authority in his or her field, and any success that this book has will be in large measure the result of their efforts.

Examination of the table of contents reveals just how extensively the subject matter of obesity is covered. The book is divided into 11 major subsections and 66 chapters. It begins with a treatise on Fat Metabolism, followed by an in-depth exploration of Body Composition, Energy Metabolism, Animal Models of Obesity, General Aspects of Human Obesity, Hunger Satiety and Mood, Associated Health Impairments, Health Impairments Associated with Abdominal Obesity, Special Forms of Obesity, and finally, Treatment—Nonpharmacologic and Pharmacologic. Any individual interested in or actively working in this field should find this book a valuable up-to-date source of factual information and stimulating ideas. It is our hope that the scientific material gathered in this book will contribute to real progress in the field and an improved understanding of the underlying mechanisms and treatment of this complex and important disease.

In closing, we wish to acknowledge with gratitude the help and support of the staff at J. B. Lippincott, in particular Beth Oram and Kimberley Cox, with a special thank you to the Medical Editor, Charles McCormick, for his devoted work and commitment to high quality throughout the production of this book.

Per Björntorp, M.D., Ph.D.   Bernard N. Brodoff, M.D.

Contents

PART ELEVEN

TREATMENT—PHARMACOLOGIC   743

OBESITY

PART ONE

FAT METABOLISM

Intermediary Metabolism with an Emphasis on Lipid Metabolism, Adipose Tissue, and Fat Cell Metabolism: A Review

PETER LÖNNROTH and ULF SMITH

Fat cells are uniquely adapted for their main function—to store and release energy. Surplus energy is assimilated by the fat cells and stored as triglycerides in lipid droplets. To accommodate the lipids, the fat cells are capable of changing their diameters 20-fold and, consequently, their volumes by several thousandfold.

A normal person has 10 to 20 kg of body fat or 90,000 to 180,000 calories stored in the subcutaneous and intraperitoneal depots. In obese individuals, body fat may range from 40 to 100 kg or more. Clearly, the adipose tissue is the major energy store in the body, capable of satisfying the energy requirements for several months.

Under situations of energy need, the triglycerides are hydrolyzed and released as free fatty acids (FFA) and glycerol. Figure 1-1 shows a schematic picture of a fat cell and outlines the major pathways for lipid assimilation and degradation. Each metabolic pathway is addressed in greater detail later in this overview. The metabolic processes involved in lipid assimilation and degradation are precisely regulated by humoral, neural, and local factors. The cellular targets and intracellular mechanisms for this interplay are also discussed later.

HORMONAL REGULATION OF METABOLISM

The Insulin Signal

The exact mechanism by which insulin elicits its hormonal effects in target cells such as the adipocytes is not yet fully understood. However, it is well established that the first step in the hormonal signaling system is the coupling of insulin to specific cellular receptors situated at the surface of the plasma membrane. The insulin receptor is a heterodimer of two glycoproteins (the α- and β-subunits [Fig. 1-2]), joined by disulfide bonds. The α-subunits are directed toward the extracellular space, whereas the β-subunits transverse the plasma membrane and direct their distal part toward the cytoplasm. The nature of the transmembranous propagation of the insulin signal to the different effector systems situated in the plasma membrane (e.g., glucose and amino acid transport), the cytoplasm (intracellular glycolytic and antilipolytic effects), and the nucleus (regulation of protein synthesis and cell growth) is currently under intense investigation.[1] This research has in recent years resulted in two major observations, both of which separately or in combination may represent tentative pathways for the insulin signal. A summary of these hypothetical pathways is depicted in Figure 1-2.

Autophosphorylation of the Insulin Receptor

After coupling of insulin to the α-subunits, the receptor undergoes a conformational change associated with an increased receptor affinity, and the hormone-receptor complex becomes internalized by endocytosis.[2] In parallel with this, the β-subunits become autophosphorylated at probably five sites.[3] This autophosphorylation leads to the expression of a tyrosine kinase activity

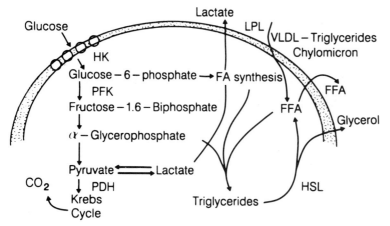

FIGURE 1-1

Metabolic pathways relevant for adipose cell metabolism. (HK, hexokinase; PFK, phosphofructokinase; PDH, pyruvatedehydrogenase; LPL, lipoprotein lipase; HSL, hormone-sensitive lipase)

within the β-subunit of the insulin receptor. Consequently, the insulin receptor is both a phosphoprotein and a phosphokinase. When activated, the β-subunit has the capacity to phosphorylate exogenous and endogenous substrates at tyrosine sites. It is likely that the phosphorylation cascade elicits insulin action by activation of the different effector systems.

The importance of the receptor autophosphorylation and activation of the tyrosine kinase activity for the insulin effect is supported by several findings. First, antibodies directed toward the insulin receptor may both activate the tyrosine kinase and exert insulin-like effects.[4] Antibodies against the β-subunit may both inhibit the tyrosine kinase activity and block the cellular response to insulin.[5] Second, the insulin effect is absent[6] in mutant cells in which the insulin receptors lack tyrosine kinase activity. Third, the

tyrosine kinase activity of the β-subunit is decreased in different insulin-resistant states.[1]

However, other observations are not consonant with the theory that the phosphorylation cascade can account for all the different metabolic effects of insulin. For example, it has been reported that some anti-insulin-receptor antibodies can stimulate glucose transport without activating the tyrosine kinase of the β-subunit.[1] Furthermore, the glucose-transporting protein (transporter) does not appear to become phosphorylated by insulin.[7]

Formation of a Second Messenger

After insulin binding to the receptor, a glucolipid in the plasma membrane becomes hydrolyzed, presumably by phospholipase C.[8-11] This glucolipid leads to the production of diacylglycerol and inositol, which may activate the protein ki-

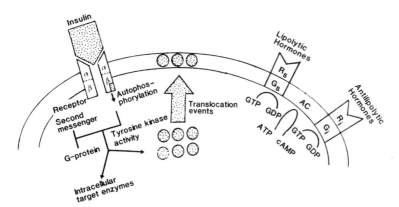

FIGURE 1-2

Structure and function of the insulin receptor and the adenylyl cyclase system. (R$_s$, stimulatory receptor; G$_s$, stimulatory nucleotide-binding protein; R$_i$, inhibitory receptor; G$_i$, inhibitory nucleotide-binding protein; AC, adenylyl cyclase)

nase C.[9] In accordance with this concept, it has repeatedly been shown that substances activating protein kinase C can exert an insulin-like effect, although this effect is usually not of the same magnitude as that of insulin.

The two models described earlier for the transmembranous propagation of the insulin signal may act in parallel on different intracellular targets but may also interact. In fact, recent evidence suggests that guanosine triphosphate (GTP)-binding protein(s) (G protein) may be important for insulin action.[1] Such a G protein may link the two putative signaling systems.

In summary, both autophosphorylation of the β-subunit of the insulin receptor and the formation of a glucolipid may play important roles for some of the insulin effects, but the relationship between these two systems is not yet clear.

Adenylate Cyclase and cAMP Formation

A schematic picture of the regulation of the adenylate cyclase activity and the generation of the second messenger 3'5' cyclic adenosine monophosphate (cAMP) is shown in Figure 1-2.

Cyclic AMP is produced from adenosine triphosphate (ATP) after activation of the adenylate cyclase by β-adrenergic agonists (epinephrine, norepinephrine) and, to a lesser extent, at least in human fat cells, by peptide hormones such as parathyroid hormone, thyroid-stimulating hormone, and adrenocorticotropic hormone. Hormones activating the adenylate cyclase bind to specific receptors, which in turn are coupled to a stimulatory GTP-binding protein (G_s). This protein is a heterotrimer consisting of α-, β-, and γ-subunits, which dissociate after GTP binding to the α-subunit. The free α-subunit activates the catalytic subunit of the adenylate cyclase, which forms cAMP from ATP.

Cyclic AMP production in human fat cells is decreased by exposing the adipocytes to α_2-adrenergic agonists as well as adenosine and prostaglandin E_2. Hormones inhibiting the adenylate cyclase activity bind to receptors that activate the inhibitory GTP-binding protein (G_i). This protein is also a heterotrimer and consists of an α-, β-, and γ-subunit. The α-subunit dissociates after hormonal coupling to the inhibitory receptor and subsequent GTP binding. The β-

subunit is capable of binding to the free α-subunit of the G_s, leading to a decrease in the adenylate cyclase activity and, in turn, an attenuation of the cAMP production.[12]

Regulation of Lipolysis

The cAMP produced by the adenylate cyclase after hormonal stimulation activates the cAMP-dependent protein kinase (protein kinase A). This kinase phosphorylates and activates the hormone-sensitive lipase, which in turn hydrolyzes the stored triglycerides to glycerol and FFA.[13] FFA are released from the cell through an energy-requiring transporting process also triggered by increased intracellular cAMP levels.[14]

Thus, hormones that generate cAMP also stimulate lipolysis. In adult humans, PTH and TSH only slightly stimulate lipolysis. In contrast, it has been suggested that TSH may have a more important role as a lipolytic agent in neonates.[15] However, it is quite clear that the most dramatic increase of cAMP production and lipolysis in human fat cells is exerted by β-adrenergic agonists.

Antilipolytic Hormones

Insulin is the major but not the only antilipolytic hormone. The hormone-sensitive lipase becomes dephosphorylated and inactivated by insulin action.[13] Research strongly suggests that the ability of insulin to dephosphorylate the lipase is the result of activation of the low-K_m phosphodiesterase (PDE) which hydrolyzes cAMP to 5'-AMP.[16,17] PDE is activated by both β-adrenergic stimulation and insulin and hence serves as a self-limiting enzymatically triggered process. The activation of PDE is presumably due to the phosphorylation of the enzymatic protein.

Lipolysis also seems to be regulated at the cellular level by antilipolytic agents that are released from the adipose tissue itself. Adenosine is released from adipocytes both in vitro[18] and in vivo following sympathetic nerve stimulation.[19] Adenosine binds to the inhibitory extracellular α_2-receptors, which inhibit the adenylate cyclase by activating the G_i. However, some studies have questioned the previous view that adenosine is released from adipocytes in vivo.[20] The intercellular concentration of adenosine in the subcutaneous tissue is similar to that in peripheral venous plasma (approximately 150 mmol/l).[21] This concentration is sufficient to exert an antilipolytic effect in both the basal and stimulated states. Thus adenosine does not appear to serve as an autoregulatory, antilipolytic agent but rather acts as a tonic regulator of lipolysis.

Prostaglandins are also released from adipocytes after β-adrenergic stimulation[22] and may exert an antilipolytic effect through specific receptors coupled to G_i. However, their potential importance as local regulators of lipolysis in vivo is not yet clear.

Other factors such as FFA and lactate may also have a role in the local regulation of lipolysis, presumably by lowering the local pH. In vivo, interstitial accumulation of these metabolites sufficient to lower the pH can probably occur only if the local blood flow is markedly decreased. Thus, their physiological importance as local regulators of lipolysis is conjectural at present.

GLUCOSE METABOLISM

Glucose metabolism is essential to the fat cells, not only for energy supply but also for maintaining a normal (re)esterification rate of FFA. FFA are continuously released from the fat cells and re-esterified with the α-glycerophosphate formed by the glycolytic process. Exogenous FFA, produced from hydrolysis of very low density lipoprotein (VLDL) triglycerides by the lipoprotein lipase (LPL) and, to a variable degree dependent on species, endogenous FFA formed in the pentose shunt are also esterified and stored as triglycerides in lipid droplets (see Fig. 1-1). These metabolic functions require only a small part of the total body glucose turnover in humans. By measuring the incorporation of a pulse of ^{14}C-glucose into the triglycerides in humans, it was calculated that the total body fat could account for only 1% to 2% of the glucose normally ingested.[23] Thus, adipose tissue has generally not been regarded as important for glucose homeostasis. Some studies, however, have shown that the adipose tissue seems to be a significant source of lactate production from glucose.[24,25] This metabolite has not previously been taken into account. Based on balance studies in vitro, it has been concluded that lactate is the major metabolite from glucose, exceeding the sum of both carbon dioxide and lipid formation.[24] When in vitro data are used to reassess the potential importance of the adipose tissue for glucose homeostasis in vivo, it becomes clear that fat cell glucose metabolism is not trivial. Also, in vivo data gathered with the microdialysis technique support the concept that the adipose tissue is an important source of lactate formation.[25] In fact, it may account for around 10% to 20% of the total glucose utilization during a glucose load in normal humans.[24] Interestingly, lactate formation by the fat cells may be enhanced in certain insulin-resistant conditions like diabetes.[26]

It is not clear at present which step is rate limiting for glucose metabolism in fat cells: glucose transport over the plasma membrane or a later step of intracellular glucose metabolism. However, in the presence of insulin, glucose transport is only rate limiting at low glucose concentrations (<1 mmol/l).[27] Because the intercellular glucose concentration in the adipose tissue is equal to that in the blood,[28,29] it seems likely that glucose metabolism may be the key regulatory step under most physiological conditions.

Characteristics of the Glucose Transporting System in Fat Cells

Glucose is taken up by the fat cells through a facilitated diffusion process that is energy requiring. Our current understanding of its regulation by hormones and other factors is mainly credited to the pioneering work by Cushman and Wardzala[30] and by Suzuki and Kono.[31] These investigators described independently and concurrently the "translocation hypothesis" of insulin action, which is today an accepted model. It was shown[30,31] that insulin increases the rate of glucose transport through a rapid and reversible translocation of specific glucose-transporting proteins from an intracellular, Golgi-associated reticulum to the plasma membrane. Following their fusion with the plasma membrane, the larger number of glucose carriers accounts for the enhanced transport rate. When insulin dissociates from its receptor, the glucose carriers are recycled to the intracellular pool. Figure 1-2 is a schematic representation of this process.

The size of the intracellular pool is a major regulatory step for the ability of insulin to stimulate glucose uptake by the fat cells.[32] Most insulin-resistant conditions have been shown to have a reduced number of glucose carriers, thus leading to an impaired insulin action on glucose uptake. However, it has also become clear during the past years not only that glucose transport in response to insulin is a function of the number of carriers but that the intrinsic activity of the individual carriers may also determine the glucose transport rate and the maximal insulin effect.[33] The intrinsic activity of the transporting proteins can also be modulated by cAMP-dependent and cAMP-independent processes.[34,35] Cyclic AMP exerts a potent insulin-antagonistic effect not only by influencing the intrinsic activity of the glucose transporters but also by inhibiting the insulin signaling process.[36,37]

Although insulin is the most important hormone for glucose transport in fat cells, it is by no means the only regulatory factor. Adenosine decreases the cellular cAMP content and thus modulates the activity of the glucose transporters. In addition, it exerts an insulin-like effect and increases insulin sensitivity.[34-36] In contrast, catecholamines and other hormones exerting their action through cAMP impair the intrinsic activity and thus exert an insulin-antagonistic effect at both the level of the glucose transporter and the insulin receptor.[34-37]

Intracellular Glucose Metabolism and Key Steps of Regulation

As pointed out earlier, it is likely that the intracellular enzymes involved in glucose metabolism constitute the rate-limiting step for glucose disposal under most physiological conditions. However, this should not be taken to indicate that glucose transport cannot be the key regulatory step in other organs.

In contrast to experimental animals, in humans, the pentose shunt for endogenous FFA synthesis from glucose is not important in fat cells.[38] Thus the glucose taken up by fat cells in humans enters the glycolytic pathway. A key step of regulation is the phosphorylation of glucose and its metabolites by hexokinase and phosphofructokinase (PFK). PFK is subject to regulation by endogenous metabolites like citrate and fatty acids, constituting the basis of the important glucose-fatty acid cycle described later.[39] Another key regulatory step for glucose metabolism is the balance between pyruvate and lactate formation. The accumulation of pyruvate and lactate is regulated by pyruvate metabolism through the pyruvate dehydrogenase (PDH) complex. This enzyme is activated by insulin.[40] Consequently, in insulin-resistant states like diabetes there appears to be an increase in lactate formation.[26] Because lactate is an important precursor for gluconeogenesis and, as discussed earlier, adipose tissue seems to be an important contributor to total body lactate production, the activity of PDH may influence not only glucose disposal but also glucose production by the liver.

Another key metabolite of glucose conversion is α-glycerophosphate. Uptake of exogenous FFA and re-esterification of endogenously formed FFA are dependent on an adequate formation of α-glycerophosphate. Thus, if glucose metabolism is impaired, FFA release increases even without an increase in lipolytic rate. Certain insulin-antagonistic hormones like cortisol primarily impair glucose metabolism through a reduction in glucose uptake.[41,42] As a consequence, α-glycerophosphate formation is impaired and FFA release increased through a reduction in the re-esterification process. It is likely that the increase in plasma FFA levels during treatment with cortisol is to a large extent due to this mechanism.

LIPOPROTEIN LIPASE ACTIVITY

LPL is the key enzyme for hydrolysis of triglyceride-rich lipoproteins into monoacylglycerol and FFA. These FFA are the major source of substrate for triglyceride formation in human fat cells, because endogenous FFA synthesis de novo is very low.[38] LPL is synthesized in the adipocytes, secreted, and transported to the capillary endothelium, where triglyceride hydrolysis occurs. The gene for human LPL has been cloned, and the complete amino acid sequence is known.[43] Specific antibodies to human LPL have been raised; they give a molecular mass of around 53 kilo dalton on Western blot analysis.[44]

Glycosylation of the LPL protein is important for both activity and secretion.[45] LPL regulation seems to occur at at least two levels: stimulation of LPL synthesis as a proenzyme and activation of this proenzyme. Various nutritional and humoral factors activate LPL at different levels. Specific antibodies to the LPL protein, mRNA probes, and activity measurements have provided tools for clarifying the mechanisms involved in regulating LPL activity.[44]

A number of studies have shown that LPL activity increases after a meal. This increase is functionally important both to facilitate lipid clearance and to promote storage of the excess energy as triglycerides in the fat cells. Insulin stimulates LPL activity and plays an important part in the meal-stimulated increase. Detailed studies have shown that the increased LPL activity following a meal occurs through a posttranslational activation of a previously inactive LPL precursor.[44]

LPL activity per cell is increased in obesity.[46] In contrast to lean individuals, in obese persons, LPL activity remains essentially unchanged after a meal.[44] The changes in fat cell LPL activity after weight reduction has been a subject of controversy during the past years. Some studies have shown an increased activity,[47] whereas others have found a decrease or no change.[48,49] This is an important issue, considering the key role of LPL in fat cell lipid accumulation. In a detailed study of LPL responsiveness to both intravenous insulin and glucose infusion as well as a mixed meal, it was found that the LPL activity increased after weight loss.[50] This perturbation could be envisaged to increase the lipid assimilation of the fat cells when higher levels of calorie intake resume after a diet restriction.

A number of factors other than insulin and glucose are capable of altering LPL activity through different mechanisms. In general, factors stimulating lipolysis and FFA release, such as catecholamines, inhibit LPL activity whereas several antilipolytic agents enhance it. Surprisingly, cortisol enhances the effect of insulin to stimulate LPL activity, at least in fat cells from the abdominal subcutaneous tissue.[42] In contrast, cortisol alone tends to decrease LPL activity. Both adenosine and inosine stimulate LPL activity in human fat cells.[44] Thus, adenosine seems to influence most aspects of adipocyte metabolism and may have an important regulatory role.

INTEGRATED FUNCTION OF THE ADIPOSE TISSUE

Methods for Studying Adipose Tissue Metabolism

In Vivo Studies

Measurements of the plasma glycerol and FFA levels only indirectly reflect adipose tissue function. More specific techniques are required to follow the flow of substrates, such as measuring the rates of appearance and disappearance. This usually requires the use of isotopically labeled substances, which are given at a constant infusion rate. By calculating the dilution of the labeled substance, the net production or consumption of the substance can be estimated. However, this is only possible if the distribution volume of the substance is compatible with a one-compartment model and if no recycling of the substance takes place. A more precise method for measuring adipose tissue metabolism *in vivo* is badly needed.

A microdialysis technique enabling *in vivo* studies at the cellular level in the adipose tissue has been described.[51] The microdialysis measurements are performed with a thin (approximately 0.3 mm) dialysis tubing, allowing a continuous flow of the dialysis fluid at a low rate (1 to 5 μl/min). This technique was previously used in neurobiologic research and has now been applied to study adipose tissue metabolism *in vivo* in humans.[51] The microdialysis technique makes it possible to accurately determine the concentration of a substance in the interstitial water and, thus, to follow fat cell metabolism under various physiological conditions. Regional differences in adipose tissue metabolism can also be defined *in vivo* with this technique. In the following discussion, the microdialysis data so far obtained are used as a reference for evaluating the information available from various *in vitro* measurements of adipose cell metabolism.

In Vitro Studies

Traditionally, segments of adipose tissue may be studied in short-term or long-term incubation systems. Isolated adipocytes can be obtained after treating the tissue biopsy specimens with collagenase, and more detailed information about the cellular function made available.[52]

Measurements of glycerol release or FFA to the incubation medium give an estimate of lipolytic rate.

By including ^{14}C-U-glucose in the incubation medium at a low glucose concentration, an indirect measurement of glucose transport rate can be achieved.[53] Glucose transport is measured directly by "pulsing" the cells with ^{14}C-3-O-methylglucose for 2 to 5 seconds after preincubating the cells with insulin.[54] Glucose metabolism can be measured by following the rate of ^{14}C-glucose conversion into carbon dioxide, lipids, or lactate. The metabolic data obtained with isolated cells are then related to the mean cell size and corrected for differences in surface area. The reason for this correction is that fat cell size markedly influences the cellular rates of metabolism, as discussed later.[46] By relating the metabolic rates to unit cell surface area, meaningful information about the cellular functions can be obtained.

The correlation between data obtained in vitro with measurements in blood or plasma may in some instances be poor. However, a more meaningful intermediate correlate should be searched for at the tissue level. The microdialysis technique is a useful probe for this.

Function of Adipose Tissue in Obesity

Insulin Resistance

Obesity is often complicated by insulin resistance, particularly in subjects with abdominal obesity.[55,56] However, it is unclear to what extent this resistance is reflected in the adipose tissue itself. There is no doubt that insulin sensitivity for glucose transport and metabolism is decreased in isolated adipocytes from obese subjects.[53,57,58] However, insulin responsiveness is less consistently influenced.[53] The underlying mechanism for the decreased insulin sensitivity was previously thought to be a decreased number of insulin receptors per cell. Apart from the difficulties involved in interpreting these in vitro findings in terms of the in vivo situation, several studies have shown that the number of insulin receptors is not decreased in adipocytes from obese subjects.[53,59] However, because of the expanded cell size, the number of receptors per unit cell surface area is decreased. The implica-

tion of this is not clear, because the sensitivity for the antilipolytic effect of insulin has in most studies been found to be normal[60] or even increased[61] in large fat cells. Rarely, a decreased sensitivity to the antilipolytic effect of insulin has been reported.[57] In accordance with most findings, the tyrosine kinase activity per insulin receptor also seems to be normal in adipocytes from obese subjects.[62]

Regulation of Lipolysis—Effect of Cell Size

Basal lipolysis and the lipolytic response to hormonal stimulation are increased in large fat cells. If corrections are made for cell size, the responsiveness and the sensitivity to catecholamines are normal. Similarly, the antilipolytic response to insulin is increased in large fat cells but unchanged if the data are calculated per unit cell surface area or cell volume. It has also been shown that the glycerol content in the intercellular water of the adipose tissue is increased both in the postabsorbative state and after a glucose load in obese subjects, probably reflecting the increased lipolytic rate, whereas the net decrease in glycerol concentration following a glucose load is similar to that in lean subjects.[63]

Increased Lipid Turnover

As discussed earlier, it is clear that lipolysis, both in the nonstimulated and stimulated states, is increased in large adipocytes from obese individuals, whereas the antilipolytic effect of insulin seems to be normal. The net effect is an increased outflow of glycerol and FFA from the large adipocytes and a decrease in cell size, unless lipolysis is balanced by an increased lipid assimilation. As pointed out earlier, LPL activity is also increased in large fat cells.[46] The net result then is that the large adipocytes at steady state remain unchanged as the result of the increased turnover rate of lipids. This may explain why obese persons with large fat cells decrease more in cell size and body fat than lean subjects during fasting.[64] In addition, this finding clearly indicates that an enhanced antilipolytic effect of insulin cannot be implicated as an underlying mechanism in obesity.

An increased turnover rate of glycerol may result in enhanced gluconeogenesis.[65] Increased FFA levels in the portal blood, possibly due

TABLE 1-1

Regional Differences in Adipose Tissue Metabolism

Region	Fat Cell Size	Basal Lipolysis	Stimulated Lipolysis	Insulin Responsiveness	LPL Activity
Omental	+	+	+ + +	+	+
Abdominal	+ +	+ +	+ +	+ +	+ +
Femoral	+ +	+ +	+	+	+ +

to further enhanced lipolysis in the intra-abdominal depots, may reduce both insulin sensitivity[66] and insulin uptake and degradation by the liver.[67] Furthermore, increased FFA levels reduce glucose uptake by the muscles, resulting in a peripheral insulin resistance.[39,66] Taken together, the increased turnover rate of lipids in obesity may be of major importance for the development of the various metabolic complications of obesity, such as hypertriglyceridemia, insulin resistance, and type II diabetes. It is in this context of special interest to note that abdominal obesity (male type) is more strongly associated with insulin resistance and type II diabetes than the gluteofemoral (female type) obesity.[56] Furthermore, the importance of the adipose tissue *per se* is suggested by the observation that a relative abdominal preponderance is not associated with these metabolic perturbations in the absence of obesity.[68] These findings suggest that the relative importance of the adipose tissue may vary between different body regions and that such metabolic differences may be of pathogenetic importance for the development of both insulin resistance and type II diabetes. Consequently, regional differences in adipose tissue morphology and metabolism are undergoing extensive study.[69]

Regional Differences in Fat Cell Metabolism

The adipose tissue distribution is conspicuously different between normal males and females. The typical male obesity is a preponderant accumulation in the abdominal region, whereas in women it leads to the more peripheral gluteofemoral distribution. Currently, the most accepted way of characterizing the relative distribution of the adipose tissue in humans is the ratio between the waist and hip circumferences (waist/hip ratio

[WHR]). Jean Vague, who made important early observations on the different distribution patterns, constructed ratios between adipose tissue thickness at different sites and measurements of the apparent muscle thickness (adipomuscular circumference ratios).[70] Although these ratios may also be important for characterizing the individuals at risk for the metabolic perturbations of obesity, the epidemiologic studies showing the increased morbidity and mortality with an abdominal distribution have used WHR.[69] Although not conclusive, these findings support the concept that adipose tissue metabolism, notably lipolysis and FFA turnover, is different in various body regions and that an increased risk profile for cardiovascular morbidity and mortality is associated with high WHR.

The rates of all important metabolic pathways differ between fat cells from various body sites. The most important differences are summarized in Table 1-1. In general, triglyceride turnover is higher in the intra-abdominal and abdominal subcutaneous sites.[71] Glucose conversion to carbon dioxide, α-glycerophosphate, and lactate is enhanced in abdominal compared with femoral fat cells.[24] Lipolysis in response to catecholamines is also markedly increased in the intra-abdominal and abdominal subcutaneous sites, possibly as a result of a preponderance of the stimulatory β-adrenergic receptors over the inhibitory α_2-receptors.[72] Increased lipolysis in these sites as compared with the peripheral depots is still encountered in the presence of high insulin concentrations.[63] In fact, there is evidence that the antilipolytic effect of insulin is reduced in the intra-abdominal cells as a result of both receptor and postreceptor perturbations.[73] Taken together, the data indicate that an enlarged intra-abdominal or abdominal fat depot is associated with increased lipolytic activity and release of both glycerol and FFA.

As discussed earlier, elevated FFA levels and increased turnover have been implicated as the link between obesity on one hand and insulin resistance, diabetes type II, and hypertriglyceridemia on the other. However, it should clearly be emphasized that although the FFA hypothesis has a lot of credence, it cannot at this time be ruled out that the metabolic aberrations associated with obesity, particularly of the abdominal type, are caused by a common factor such as elevated free testosterone levels.[74] It may also be questioned whether the *in vitro* results of elevated lipolysis in the abdominal/intra-abdominal cells are at all relevant for the *in vivo* situation. Apart from the increased FFA flux in abdominal obesity discussed earlier, the best evidence comes from the studies with the microdialysis technique. We have found that adipose tissue lipolysis in the postabsorptive state is, in fact, increased in the abdominal compared with the femoral region.[63]

Regional differences have been shown not only for glucose metabolism and lipolysis but also for LPL activity. In males, no clear differences have been noted between the femoral and abdominal depots, although the intra-abdominal depots, in general, have lower LPL activity.[75] In premenopausal females, however, LPL activity is enhanced in the femoral compared with the abdominal region.[76] This regional difference does not remain in postmenopausal women, suggesting an important effect of the female sex steroid hormones, particularly progesterone. This is also underscored by the finding that LPL activity decreases in the femoral region after partus and during lactation.[76] During the same period, lipolysis increases, showing differential regional regulation of fat tissue metabolism. The fact that gluteofemoral fat distribution is typical for females and that metabolism in these depots tends to favor lipid accumulation during pregnancy, followed by increased lipolysis during lactation, has led to the suggestion that these depots may subserve a specialized function in women—that is, an energy reserve during pregnancy to be used as substrates during lactation.

References

1. Goldfine ID: The insulin receptor: Molecular biology and transmembrane signaling. Endocr Rev 8:235, 1987

2. Gorden P: Hormone receptor interactions. Diabetes (suppl) 28:8, 1979

3. Kasuga M, Karlsson FA, Kahn CR: Insulin stimulates the phosphorylation of the 95,000-dalton subunit of its own receptor. Science 215:185, 1982

4. Gerzi R, Russell DS, Taylor SI et al: Reevaluation of the evidence that an antibody to the insulin receptor is insulinmimetic without activating the protein kinase activity of the receptor. J Biol Chem 262:16900, 1987

5. Morgan DO, Ho L, Korn LJ et al: Insulin action is blocked by monoclonal antibody that inhibits the insulin receptor kinase. Proc Natl Acad Sci USA 83:328, 1986

6. Ellis L, Clauser E, Morgan DO et al: Replacement of insulin receptor tyrosine residues 1162 and 1163 compromises insulin-stimulated kinase activity and uptake of 2-deoxyglucose. Cell 45:721, 1986

7. Joost HG, Weber TM, Cushman SW et al: Activity and phosphorylation state of glucose transporters in plasma membranes from insulin-isoproterenol- and phorbol ester-treated rat adipose cells. J Biol Chem 262:11261, 1987

8. Saltiel AR, Fox JA, Sherline P et al: Insulin-stimulated hydrolysis of a novel glycolipid generates modulators of cAMP phosphodiesterase. Science 233:967, 1986

9. Saltiel AR, Sherline P, Fox JA: Insulin-stimulated diacylglycerol production results from the hydrolysis of a novel phosphatidylinositol glycan. J Biol Chem 262:1116, 1987

10. Jarett L, Seals JR: Pyruvate dehydrogenase activation in adipocyte mitochondria by an insulin-generated mediator from muscle. Science 206:1407, 1979

11. Farese RV, Kuo JY, Babinschkin JS et al: Insulin provokes a transient activation of phospholipase C in the rat epididymal fat pad. J Biol Chem 261:8589, 1986

12. Katada T, Northup JK, Bokoch GM et al: The inhibitory guanine nucleotide-binding regulatory component of adenylate cyclase. J Biol Chem 259:3578, 1984

13. Strålfors P, Björsell P, Belfrage P: Hormonal regulation of hormone-sensitive lipase in intact adipocytes: Identification of phosphorylated sites and effects on the phosphorylation by lipolytic hormones and insulin. Proc Natl Acad Sci USA 81:3317, 1984

14. Abumrad NA, Perry PR, Whitesell RR: Stimulation by epinephrine of the membrane transport of long chain fatty acid in the adipocyte. J Biol Chem 260:9969, 1985

15. Marcus C, Ehrén H, Bolme P et al: Regulation of lipolysis during the neonatal period: Importance of thyrotropin. J Clin Invest 82:1793, 1988

16. Beebe SJ, Redmon JB, Blackmore PF et al: Discriminative insulin antagonism of stimulatory effects of various cAMP analogues on adipocyte lipolysis and hepatocyte glycogenolysis. J Biol Chem 260: 15781, 1985

17. Lönnroth P, Smith U: The antilipolytic effect of insulin in human adipocytes requires activation of the phosphodiesterase. Biochem Biophys Res Commun 141:1157, 1986

18. Schwabe U, Ebert R, Erbler HC: Adenosine release from isolated fat cells and its significance for the effects of hormones on cyclic 3',5'-AMP levels and lipolysis. Naunyn Schmiedebergs Arch Pharmacol 273:133, 1973

19. Fredholm BB, Sollevi A: The release of adenosine and inosine from canine subcutaneous adipose tissue by nerve stimulation and noradrenalin. J Physiol (Lond) 313:351, 1981

20. Kather H: Purine accumulation in human fat cell suspensions: Evidence that human adipocytes release inosine and hypoxanthine rather than adenosine. J Biol Chem 263:8803, 1988

21. Lönnroth P, Jansson PA, Fredholm BB et al: Microdialysis of intercellular adenosine concentration in subcutaneous tissue in humans. Am J Physiol 256:E250, 1989

22. Axelrod L, Levine L: Prostacyclin production by isolated adipocytes. Diabetes 30:163, 1981

23. Björntorp P, Sjöström L: Carbohydrate storage in man: Speculations and some quantitative considerations. Metabolism (suppl) 27:1853, 1978

24. Mårin P, Rebuffé-Scrive M, Smith U et al: Glucose uptake in human adipose tissue. Metabolism 36: 1154, 1987

25. Jansson PA, Smith U, Lönnroth P: Evidence for lactate production by human adipose tissue in vivo. Diabetologia 33:253, 1990

26. Newby FD, Bayo F, Thacker SV et al: Effects of streptozotonin induced diabetes on glucose metabolism and lactate release by isolated fat cells from young lean and older moderately obese rats. Diabetes 38:237, 1989

27. Gliemann J, Rees WD, Foley JA: The fate of labelled glucose molecules in the rat adipocyte: Dependence on glucose concentration. Biochim Biophys Acta 804:68, 1984

28. Lönnroth P, Jansson PA, Smith U: A microdialysis method allowing characterization of intercellular water space in humans. Am J Physiol 253:E228, 1987

29. Jansson PA, Fowelin J, Smith U et al: Characterization by microdialysis of intercellular glucose level in subcutaneous tissue in humans. Am J Physiol 255:E218, 1988

30. Cushman SW, Wardzala LJ: Potential mechanism of insulin action on glucose transport in the isolated rat adipose cell. J Biol Chem 255:4758, 1980

31. Suzuki K, Kono T: Evidence that insulin causes translocation of glucose transport activity to the plasma membrane from an intracellular storage site. Proc Natl Acad Sci USA 77:2542, 1980

32. Karnieli E, Zarnowski MJ, Hissin PF et al: Insulin-stimulated translocation of glucose transport systems in the isolated rat adipose cell. J Biol Chem 256:4772, 1981

33. Kahn BB, Cushman SW: Mechanism for markedly hyperresponsive insulin-stimulated glucose transport activity in adipose cells from insulin-treated streptozotocin diabetic rats. J Biol Chem 262:5118, 1987

34. Smith U, Kuroda M, Simpson IA: Counterregulation of insulin-stimulated glucose transport by catecholamines in the isolated rat adipose cell. J Biol Chem 259:8758, 1984

35. Kuroda M, Honnor RC, Cushman SW et al: Regulation of insulin-stimulated glucose transport in the isolated rat adipocyte: cAMP-dependent effects of lipolytic and antilipolytic agents. J Biol Chem 262:245, 1987

36. Lönnroth P, Davies JI, Lönnroth I et al: The interaction between the adenylate cyclase system and insulin-stimulated glucose transport. Biochem J 243:789, 1987

37. Häring, H, Kirsch D, Obermaier B et al: Decreased tyrosine kinase activity of insulin receptor isolated from rat adipocytes rendered insulin-resistant by catecholamine treatment in vitro. Biochem J 234:59, 1986

38. Sjöström L: Adult human adipose tissue cellularity and metabolism. Acta Med Scand 544 (suppl): 1, 1972

39. Randle PJ, Garland PB, Hales CN et al: The glucose fatty-acid cycle: Its role in insulin sensitivity and the metabolic disturbances of diabetes mellitus. Lancet 1:785, 1963

40. Coore HG, Denton RM, Martin BR et al: Regulation of adipose tissue pyruvate dehydrogenase by insulin and other hormones. Biochem J 125:115, 1971

41. Fain JN, Czech MP: Glucocorticoid effects on lipid mobilization and adipose tissue metabolism. In Blaschko H, Sayers G, Smith AD (eds): Handbook of Physiology, Vol 4, pp 169–178. Baltimore, Waverly

42. Cigolini M, Smith U: Human adipose tissue in culture. VIII. Studies on the insulin-antagonistic effect of glucocorticoids. Metabolism 28:502, 1979

43. Kirchgessner TG, Svenson KL, Lusis AJ et al: The sequence of cDNA encoding lipoprotein lipase. A member of a lipase gene family. J Biol Chem 262:8463, 1987

44. Kern PA, Ong JM, Goers JWF et al: Regulation of lipoprotein lipase immunoreactive mass in isolated human adipocytes. J Clin Invest 81:398, 1988

45. Ong JM, Kern PA: The role of glucose and glycosylation in the regulation of lipoprotein lipase synthesis and secretion in rat adipocytes. J Biol Chem 264:3177, 1989

46. Björntorp P, Smith U: The effect of fat cell size on subcutaneous adipose tissue metabolism. Front Matrix Biol 2:37, 1976

47. Schwartz RS, Brunzell JD: Increase of adipose tissue lipoprotein lipase activity after weight loss. J Clin Invest 67:1425, 1981

48. Rebuffé-Scrive M, Basdevant A, Guy-Grand B: Nutritional induction of adipose tissue lipoprotein lipase in obese subjects. Am J Clin Nutr 37:974, 1983

49. Sörbris R, Petersson B-G, Nilsson-Ehle P: Effects of weight reduction on plasma lipoproteins and adipose tissue metabolism in obese subjects. Eur J Clin Invest 11:491, 1981

50. Eckel RH, Yost TJ: Weight reduction increases adipose tissue lipoprotein lipase responsiveness in obese women. J Clin Invest 80:992, 1987

51. Lönnroth P, Smith U: Microdialysis: A novel technique for clinical investigations. J Int Med 227:295, 1990

52. Rodbell M: Metabolism of isolated fat cells: Effects of hormones on glucose metabolism and lipolysis. J Biol Chem 239:375, 1964

53. Kashiwagi A, Verso MA, Andrews J et al: In vitro insulin resistance of human adipocytes isolated from subjects with noninsulin-dependent diabetes mellitus. J Clin Invest 72:1246, 1983

54. Whitesell RR, Gliemann J: Kinetic parameters of transport of 3-0-methylglucose and glucose in adipocytes. J Biol Chem 254:5276, 1979

55. Kissebah AH, Vydelingum N, Murray R et al: Relation of body fat distribution to metabolic complications of obesity. J Clin Endocrinol Metab 54:254, 1982

56. Krotkiewski M, Björntorp P, Sjöström L et al: Impact of obesity on metabolism in men and women: Importance of regional adipose tissue distribution. J Clin Invest 72:1150, 1983

57. Kashiwagi A, Bogardus C, Lillioja S et al: In vitro insensitivity of glucose transport and antilipolysis to insulin due to receptor and postreceptor abnormalities in obese Pima Indians with normal glucose tolerance. Metabolism 33:772, 1984

58. Ciaraldi TP, Kolterman OG, Olefsky JM: Mechanism of the postreceptor defect in insulin action in human obesity. J Clin Invest 68:875, 1981

59. Lönnroth P, Digirolamo M, Krotkiewski M et al: Insulin binding and responsiveness in fat cells from patients with reduced glucose tolerance and type II diabetes. Diabetes 32:748, 1983

60. Jacobsson B, Holm G, Björntorp P et al: Influence of cell size on the effects of insulin and noradrenaline on human adipose tissue. Diabetologia 12:69, 1976

61. Arner P, Bolinder J, Engfeldt P et al: Influence of obesity on the antilipolytic effect of insulin in isolated human fat cells obtained before and after glucose ingestion. J Clin Invest 73:673, 1984

62. Freidenberg GR, Henry RR, Klein HH et al: Decreased kinase activity of insulin receptors from adipocytes of non-insulin-dependent diabetic subjects. J Clin Invest 79:240, 1987

63. Lönnroth P, Jansson P-A, Smith U: Adipose tissue metabolism measured by microdialysis: Obesity in Europe 88. Proceedings of the 1st European Congress on Obesity. London, John Libbey, 1989

64. Björntorp P, Carlgren G, Isaksson B et al: Effect of an energy-reduced dietary regimen in relation to adipose tissue cellularity in obese women. Am J Clin Nutr 28:445, 1975

65. Bortz WM, Paul P, Haff AC et al: Glycerol turnover and oxidation in man. J Clin Invest 51:1537, 1972

66. Ferrannini E, Barrett EJ, Bevilacqua S et al: Effect of fatty acids on glucose production in man. J Clin Invest 72:1737, 1983

67. Rossell R, Gomis R, Casamitjana R et al: Reduced hepatic insulin extraction in obesity: Relationship with plasma insulin levels. J Clin Endocrinol Metab 56:608, 1983

68. Landin K, Krotkiewski M, Smith U: Importance of obesity for the metabolic abnormalities associated with an abdominal fat distribution. Metabolism 38:572, 1989

69. Björntorp P, Smith U, Lönnroth P: Health implications of regional obesity. Acta Med Scand Symposium Series Number 4. Stockholm, Sweden, Almqvist & Wiksell International, 1988

70. Vague J: La différenciation sexuelle-facteur déterminant des formes de l'óbésité. Presse Med 30:339, 1947

71. Rebuffé-Scrive M, Andersson B, Olbe L et al: Metabolism of adipose tissue in intraabdominal depots of nonobese men and women. Metabolism 38:453, 1989

72. Wahrenberg H, Lönnqvist F, Arner P: Mechanisms underlying regional differences in lipolysis in human adipose tissue. J Clin Invest 84:458, 1989

73. Bolinder J, Kager L, Östman J: Differences at the receptor and post-receptor levels between human omental and subcutaneous adipose tissue in the action of insulin on lipolysis. Diabetes 43:207, 1983

74. Evans PJ, Hoffman RG, Kalkhoff RK et al: Relationship of androgenic activity to body fat topography, fat cell morphology and metabolic aberrations in menopausal women. J Clin Endocrinol Metab 57:304, 1983

75. Rebuffé-Scrive M, Lönnroth P, Mårin P et al: Regional adipose tissue metabolism in men and postmenopausal women. Int J Obes 11:347, 1987

76. Rebuffé-Scrive M, Enk L, Crona N et al: Fat cell metabolism in different regions in women: Effects of menstrual cycle, pregnancy and lactation. J Clin Invest 75:1973, 1985

CHAPTER 2

Brown Adipose Tissue Metabolism

JEAN HIMMS-HAGEN

HISTORICAL INTRODUCTION

During the 300 years that have passed since brown adipose tissue (BAT) was first identified as a distinct organ, initially thought to exist only in hibernating animals, there has been much speculation about its function and its relationship to white adipose tissue. The first evidence for a physiological role of BAT was obtained in 1963, when it was found to produce heat in marmots that were rewarming after hibernation.[133] Since then it has become generally recognized as an entirely different tissue from white adipose tissue and as endowed with the unique function of producing heat in many mammalian species. During the past two decades, it has been the subject of extensive investigation by researchers in several of the biomedical sciences: physiologists and biologists interested in mammalian thermoregulation, biochemists interested in the unique functioning of its mitochondria, neuroscientists interested in the central control of energy intake and expenditure, endocrinologists interested in the neurohumoral regulation of metabolism, nutritionists and clinicians interested in energy balance and body weight regulation, and, most recently, pharmacologists striving to develop drugs that exploit the thermogenic activity of BAT for the treatment of obesity. Three distinct lines of investigation have contributed to the present surge of interest in BAT. First, after a decade of argument over the extent to which BAT thermogenesis can contribute to the body's heat production and hence to overall energy expenditure, the work by Foster in 1978–1979[37] demonstrated its major importance in the survival of rats in a cold environment. Second, at about the same time, the demonstration of activation of BAT thermogenesis by diet and of defective functioning of BAT in obese animals established a connection between BAT metabolism and energy balance.[48,49,52,54,55,115,117,119] Third, contrary to previous assumptions, activity of the sympathetic nervous system, known to control BAT thermogenesis, was shown to increase with feeding and to decrease with fasting.[72,73] The expansion of research in this field during the past decade has provided the outline of a picture of central hypothalamic control, by way of the sympathetic innervation, of BAT thermogenesis as a significant component of overall energy expenditure.

This chapter summarizes current concepts of the metabolism of BAT and its neurohumoral control and includes some newer information on the control of gene expression in BAT. Reviews are cited, as well as some more recent publications to enable the reader to gain access to the rapidly growing literature on this subject. One multiauthored book on BAT[137] provides an excellent source of relevant literature up to 1986. In addition, other reviews by the author provide more comprehensive coverage of the recent literature on BAT metabolism and its control in relation to energy balance and to thermoregulation.[53-57]

The Function of Brown Adipose Tissue Is Thermogenesis

Heat is a product of all metabolic reactions that take place in all organs of the body. *Obligatory thermogenesis*, a measure of the energy expenditure necessary to keep the body alive, encompasses both heat production in a basal postabsorptive state at a thermoneutral temperature and energy expenditure associated with the processing of the foodstuffs required for maintenance of the living state. Over and above this obligatory level of energy expenditure is *facultative thermogenesis*, which occurs primarily in two organs, skeletal muscle and BAT. In skeletal muscle, it is associated with voluntary activity (exercise) or with thermoregulatory thermogenesis at low environmental temperature (shivering). In BAT, it is associated with thermoregulatory thermogenesis (nonshivering thermogenesis) or with diet-induced thermogenesis, both brought about by activation of the sympathetic nervous system, the former by low environmental temperature and the latter by certain aspects of diet (composition, amount, or palatability).

Because thermogenesis is an indispensable part of thermal balance, as well as of energy balance, and because thermoregulation relies on control of both facultative thermogenesis as well as heat loss mechanisms (Table 2-1), thermoregulatory requirements can not only activate BAT thermogenesis, as noted earlier, but can also suppress BAT thermogenesis, just as they can suppress shivering in skeletal muscle. Thus, any heat load on the body, whether imposed by a high ambient temperature, by pregnancy or lactation, by exercise, by hyperthyroidism, or even by the presence of other animals in the near vicinity, is capable of suppressing BAT thermogenesis.[54,57]

In considering BAT function, the important concept to keep in mind is that the thermogenic state of BAT is a result of a balance between stimulatory and inhibitory influences of central origin, working through the hypothalamus and the sympathetic innervation of BAT.

Location, Morphology, and Innervation of Brown Adipose Tissue

BAT exists as relatively small, discrete deposits, located superficially in interscapular, subscapu-

lar, axillary, cervical, intercostal, and inguinal regions and internally within the thoracic cavity around the heart and aorta and within the abdominal cavity along the aorta and around the vessels supplying the kidneys. In rodents, the interscapular BAT deposit is usually a major one and for this reason the most studied, whereas in primates, including humans, this deposit is absent and axillary BAT is a major deposit (see Chapter 11).

BAT has a very rich vasculature and, when stimulated, is subject to extremely high rates of blood flow. Arteriovenous anastomoses are present, and when BAT is stimulated, they constrict and thereby shunt blood into the parenchymal capillary vasculature.[96] Only about 40% of the cells in BAT are mature brown adipocytes. Apart from endothelial cells and mast cells, the remainder are interstitial cells and preadipocytes, which, by appropriate stimulation, can be induced to differentiate into brown adipocytes.[19,38,92]

BAT receives a rich sympathetic innervation. Two types of nerves have been identified on the blood vessels of BAT: sympathetic nerves containing both noradrenaline (NA) and neuropeptide (NPY) and others containing both substance P (SP) and calcitonin gene-related peptide (CGRP).[77,97] Parenchymal cells are supplied by sympathetic noradrenergic axons that form a ground plexus, making synaptic contact with brown adipocytes along their length as well as at their endings; unlike the nerves on the blood vessels, these nerves do not contain NPY.[92,97] Parenchymal cells also receive a sparser innervation of SP and CGRP-containing fibers, presumed to be sensory nerves. NA from the sympathetic innervation is generally agreed to have the major role in controlling BAT thermogenesis (see the later section on noradrenaline control) and in promoting the growth of BAT that occurs in response to chronic stimulation (the trophic response; see the later section on BAT growth when stimulated). A role for the sensory nerves in the maintenance of BAT function has also been suggested.[56]

BAT cells usually contain many small triacylglycerol (TAG) droplets and are described as multilocular. They are usually readily distinguishable by light microscopy from unilocular white adipose tissue cells. However, when they

TABLE 2-1

Factors Influencing Thermoregulation, Energy Balance, and Thermogenesis in BAT

Factors Influencing Thermoregulation

Ambient temperature
"Set-point"
  Normal
  Fever
  Torpor
  Hibernation
  Lateral hypothalamic lesions (acute)
Insulation
  Clothing
  Body fat
  Housing conditions (number of animals per cage)
Other physiological or pathological sources of heat
  Food
  Exercise
  Growth
  Pregnancy
  Lactation
  Hyperthyroidism
  Tumors
Energy intake
  Amount of thermic effect of food (TEF)
  Composition

Heat Loss Mechanisms	*Thermogenic Mechanisms*
Sweating	Obligatory
Vasodilation or vasoconstriction	Essential and endothermic (all organs)
Piloerection	Thermic effect of food (gut, liver, muscle)
Salivation	Facultative (regulated)
	Shivering thermogenesis (muscle)
	Nonshivering thermogenesis (BAT)
	Exercise thermogenesis (muscle)
	Diet-induced thermogenesis (BAT)
	cephalic phase
	postprandial phase

are thermogenically quiescent, as in the adults of certain species and in obese animals, they become replete with lipid and unilocular. They are then difficult to distinguish from white adipose tissue cells. They can be restored to their more typical multilocular form by chronic stimulation. This restoration of BAT has been demonstrated in species often thought to be deficient in BAT when adult, such as cats, dogs, guinea pigs, and humans, and in several types of obese rodents.

BAT cells are packed with large mitochon-dria that contain numerous well-organized cristae. They also contain the usual complement of other organelles, such as rough and smooth endoplasmic reticulum, Golgi apparatus, free ribosomes, peroxisomes, lysosomes, and nucleus. The plasma membrane surface is often invaginated, with small vesicles beneath it.[92] BAT cells are electrically linked through gap junctions. Some of these features of BAT vasculature, cells, and nerves are shown diagrammatically in Figure 2-1.

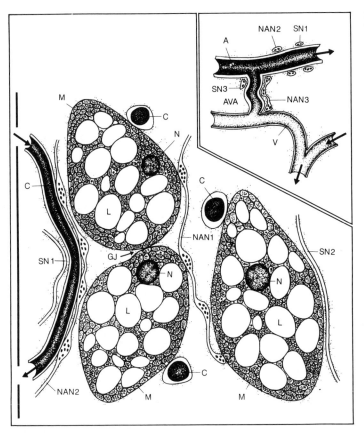

FIGURE 2-1

Diagrammatic representation of BAT cells with their vasculature and innervation. Three multilocular BAT cells are illustrated, with their nuclei (N), many lipid droplets (L), closely packed mitochondria (M), and gap junctions (GJ). Noradrenergic sympathetic nerves are shown close to the cells (NAN1) and vasculature (NAN2). The latter contain NPY as well as NA. The former are shown making synaptic contact with cells both *en passant* and at their endings. Sensory nerves are shown close to the cell (SN2) and to the vasculature (SN1). These contain substance P and CGRP. Capillaries (C) are illustrated in longitudinal- and cross section to emphasize their abundance among the parenchymal cells. The inset shows (on a different scale) a major artery (A) and vein (V) with a connecting arteriovenous anastomosis (AVA) and its sympathetic (NAN3) and sensory nerves (SN3). The representation is based on descriptions in several published reports[77,92,96,97] and illustrates only features important for thermogenesis in BAT and in maintenance of BAT in a functional state. Other cell types are also present in intact BAT (see text).

Brown Adipose Tissue Thermogenesis Needs the Mitochondrial Uncoupling Protein

In addition to the usual protein components of the electron transport system, of oxidative phosphorylation, and of various transporters, BAT mitochondria are unique in that they possess a protein known as the *uncoupling protein* (UCP). This UCP is responsible for their remarkable property of becoming reversibly uncoupled when BAT is stimulated by NA.[95] Some of the key features important for control of thermogenesis in BAT mitochondria are shown in diagrammatic form in Figure 2-2.

In order to understand how the UCP permits BAT mitochondria to vary the rate of thermogenesis in BAT, it must be recognized that the rate of heat production reflects the overall rate of fuel oxidation. For BAT, in which the major fuel is fatty acids, this is represented by the following equation:

$$C_{16}H_{32}O_2 + 23\,O_2 \rightarrow 16\,CO_2 + 16\,H_2O + heat$$

In most cells in which fatty acids are being oxidized and in which the mitochondria operate in a coupled manner, the rate of fatty acid oxidation depends on the rate of reoxidation by the mitochondrial electron transport system of the reduced coenzymes (nicotinamide adenine dinucleotide, reduced form [NADH] and flavin adenine dinucleotide, reduced form [FADH$_2$]). This rate, in turn, depends on the rate at which the proton gradient is used to drive the synthesis of adenosine 5′-triphosphate (ATP) by means of proton-translocating ATP synthetase (oxidative phosphorylation). The proton gradient is created by the pumping of protons out of the mitochondria as a consequence of and driven by the en-

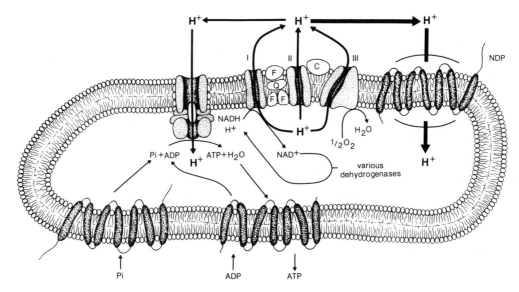

FIGURE 2-2

Components of BAT mitochondria that are important for the control of thermogenesis. Components of the inner membrane are, clockwise from top right, the proton-translocating UCP with the seven transmembrane domains and nucleoside diphosphate (NDP) binding site on the outer surface[1,31,68-70]; the adenine nucleotide translocase, showing marked homology to the UCP[1,31]; the phosphate carrier, also showing homology to the UCP[122]; the proton-translocating ATP synthetase; and, at top center, the electron transport system.[109,134] The three main components of the electron transport system, from left to right, are as follows: I, NADH-ubiquinone reductase; II, ubiquinone-cytochrome c reductase; and III, cytochrome oxidase. Ubiquinone (Q) links I and II, and cytochrome c (c) links II and III. Three flavoprotein dehydrogenases (F) (glycerol-3-phosphate dehydrogenase on the outer surface of the membrane, succinate and acyl CoA dehydrogenases on the inner surface of the membrane) are shown between I and II. The flavoprotein dehydrogenases use their substrates to supply $FADH_2$ to the electron transport system at the coenzyme Q level. Various mitochondrial dehydrogenases use their substrates to supply the mobile carrier, $NADH^+$, to the electron transport system at the complex I level. The operation of the electron transport system is restrained by having to pump protons against the proton gradient that it creates. The proton gradient is dissipated either to the left, by the proton-translocating ATP-synthetase, or to the right, by the proton-translocating UCP. The operation of the ATP synthetase depends on availability of ADP (by the translocase) and phosphate (by the phosphate transport protein) and is thus determined by the rate of utilization of ATP in the cytosol. The UCP operates only when switched on by fatty acids (not shown) or by removal of bound purine nucleotides (see text). The switch from the coupled to the uncoupled state thus changes proton entry from the ATP synthetase to the UCP. This functioning of the UCP replaces the functioning of its two homologues, the adenine nucleotide translocase and the phosphate transport protein. The binding of a purine nucleotide (guanosine diphosphate is usually used experimentally) to BAT mitochondria is a commonly used measure of BAT thermogenic state. The level of binding is not, however, directly related to the concentration of UCP in the membrane but rather to the functional state of the protein, for reasons that are not yet understood.[53,136]

ergy liberated during the oxidation of the reduced coenzymes. The extent to which this use of the driving force of the proton gradient occurs is itself, in turn, dependent on the availability of the substrates for the ATP synthetase, adenosine 5'-diphosphate (ADP) and phosphate. The availability of ADP depends on the rate at which the cell is using ATP (i.e., on the rate at which it is doing work of various kinds). In this type of cell, ATP synthesis is said to be coupled to electron transport, hence substrate oxidation (and heat production) is coupled to the rate at which ATP is being used. Only an increase in rate of ATP utilization (e.g., for biosynthetic reactions or for ion pumping) can bring about an overall increase in substrate oxidation and hence in heat production.

Unstimulated BAT cell mitochondria operate in a coupled way in the manner described earlier. However, when BAT is stimulated by NA, the UCP becomes functional and translocates protons from the exterior to the interior of the mitochondria (the way in which NA exerts this effect is discussed further in the next section).[69,95] Thus, an alternate means of using up the proton gradient is brought into play under the influence of NA, one in which no ATP is synthesized and in which the energy generated by oxidation of substrates and used to create a proton gradient is wasted. The consequence of invoking this alternate, uncoupling means of dissipating the proton gradient is that oxidation of reduced coenzymes by the electron transport system is no longer restrained by having to work against a proton gradient and so accelerates; the oxidation of substrates to supply more reduced coenzymes to the electron transport system likewise speeds up (because of increased availability of nicotinamide-adenine dinucleotide [NAD+] and flavin adenine dinucleotide [FAD], and overall heat production increases. The principal mitochondrial dehydrogenases involved are acyl CoA dehydrogenase and β-hydroxyacyl CoA dehydrogenase of the fatty acid β-oxidation cycle and isocitrate dehydrogenase, α-ketoglutarate dehydrogenase, succinate dehydrogenase, and malate dehydrogenase of the tricarboxylic acid cycle.

Control of the proton-translocating function of the UCP is probably brought about by varying the intracellular concentration of fatty acids. These interact with the UCP in such a way as to lower the membrane potential at which proton translocation occurs.[18,95] The concentration of fatty acids is regulated by the activity of hormone-sensitive lipase, itself activated by NA (see the next section). In addition, the binding of purine nucleotides (ATP and ADP) to UCP inhibits its proton-translocating function, and it is possible that removal of these nucleotides plays a part in initiating its function.[68,69] The binding of these nucleotides is extremely pH dependent; a high pH induces a reduced affinity and ready loss of the bound nucleotides. Thus, the slight alkalinization of BAT cells that follows stimulation by NA[40] may enhance the stimulation of UCP function by facilitating removal of the bound nucleotides.[65,68]

The UCP of BAT mitochondria has been purified and sequenced, and its gene has been cloned. It is a small protein of 306 amino acids and a molecular mass of about 32 kilodaltons (somewhat variable from one species to another because of minor variations in amino acid composition). The UCP has seven transmembrane domains, each coded for by a different exon on the Ucp gene,[15,71] and an extension on the cytosolic side that binds the regulatory purine nucleotides.[31] The UCP is highly homologous to two other proteins important in BAT mitochondrial function (see Fig. 2-2) but also present in mitochondria of other cells. These are ADP/ATP translocase[1] and phosphate carrier protein.[122] The two proteins have entirely different functions and modes of operation, however, the former acting as an exchanger, with a binding site for purine nucleotides that can switch from one side of the membrane to the other, the latter as a phosphate and proton cotransporter. Both are involved in the support of oxidative phosphorylation (see Fig. 2-2).

Noradrenaline Controls Brown Adipose Tissue Thermogenesis by Means of β- and α₁-Adrenergic Receptors

When NA from sympathetic nerves is released within BAT, the initial response is a very rapid increase in thermogenesis. This is mediated by the interaction of the NA with both β- and α_1-adrenergic receptors. The interaction of NA with BAT also produces a sequence of electrical changes that are propagated intercellularly through gap junctions. An initial brief and transient depolarization, associated with increased efflux of potassium, is mediated by α-adrenergic receptors. A delayed and extended depolarization is mediated by β-adrenergic receptors, and it, too, is associated with increased efflux of potassium.[127]

If the initial increase in sympathetic nervous system activity is followed by a persistent release of NA, there ensues an orderly and protracted sequence of events, termed the *trophic response*, which results in hypertrophy and hyperplasia of the BAT. This trophic response involves enhanced gene expression and an overall increase in protein synthesis, as well as selective increases in synthesis of certain proteins, so that the BAT has a greatly increased capacity for a thermogenic response to NA. This section describes the acute thermogenic response. The trophic response is discussed in more detail later.

Interaction of NA with β-adrenergic receptors results in activation of adenylate cyclase and consequent increased production of cyclic AMP (cAMP). As in other tissues, the activation of adenylate cyclase is mediated by a regulatory G protein. The principal effect of the cAMP is assumed to be activation of one or more protein kinases that phosphorylate other proteins. BAT contains several protein kinases as well as phosphoprotein phosphatases and phosphorylatable inhibitors of these phosphatases. When hormone-sensitive lipase is phosphorylated, its catalytic activity is increased and the rate of lipolysis increases. The fatty acids liberated within the BAT cell as a consequence of the increased rate of lipolysis serve both as the signal for increased operation of the proton-translocating UCP (see the previous section) and as the initial fuel for the increase in mitochondrial oxidation that occurs as a consequence of the activation of the UCP (see the next section).

The action of NA to activate adenylate cyclase is inhibited by adenosine.[125] Moreover, the stimulation by NA of uncoupled respiration results in large changes in relative concentrations of the adenine nucleotides such that ATP levels decline and AMP levels increase.[74,82] The active 5'-nucleotidase in BAT then converts some of the AMP to adenosine, thus restraining overstimulation of the tissue by NA.[125] Ion movements that occur as a result of the interaction of NA with the β-adrenergic receptor include increased sodium influx[23] and inhibition of calcium influx.[24]

Interaction of NA with α_1-adrenergic receptors in BAT enhances the operation of the phosphatidylinositolbisphosphate (PIP_2) cycle and thereby increases production of the two second messengers, inositol trisphosphate (IP_3) and diacylglycerol (DAG) as well as arachidonic acid.[91,124] There ensues a release of calcium from intracellular stores,[94] translocation of protein kinase C to the plasma membrane and its consequent activation.[7] The regulatory implications of most of these changes are not understood in detail. Many of them may be involved in the mitogenic and trophic responses to NA. Other ion movements include efflux of potassium[94,127] and an increase in sodium/proton exchange, with a resultant increase in sodium entry.[94]

NA thus alters the distribution of sodium and potassium through its actions on both α_1- and β-adrenergic receptors. The altered distribution of potassium and sodium in turn enhances sodium-potassium ATPase action. Hence, increased ATP utilization as a consequence of the increased pumping of ions could contribute to a small portion (about 20%) of the thermogenic effect of NA on BAT.[88] However, if BAT mitochondria are operating in an uncoupled fashion, one may question how BAT manages to generate any ATP to support such ion pumping. Indeed, other ATP-requiring processes are also stimulated in association with increased thermogenesis. These include fatty acid activation (by acyl CoA synthetase), lipogenesis (enzymes are citrate lyase and acetyl CoA carboxylase), generation of cAMP by adenylate cyclase, protein phosphorylation by protein kinases, as well as the extensive synthesis of mRNAs and proteins that supports the trophic response of BAT to chronic stimulation (see the later section on BAT growth). The answer lies in the remarkable acceleration of glycolysis and its attendant substrate-level phosphorylations, which appear to supply much of the ATP required for the described reaction and for other

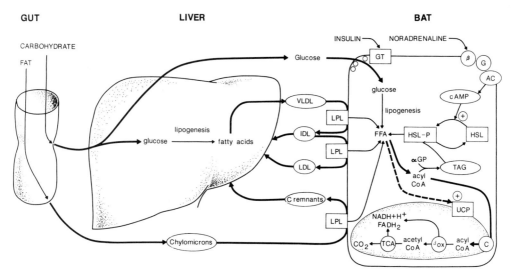

FIGURE 2-3

Sources of lipid for BAT thermogenesis. Sources of fatty acids (FFA) shown
are endogenous TAG stores in BAT itself, chylomicrons from dietary fat, very
low density lipoproteins (VLDL) made in the liver, and endogenous lipogenesis from glucose. Control is by NA acting on a β-adrenergic receptor (β), and
via a regulatory G protein (G) and adenylate cyclase (AC), increasing cAMP
levels. Cyclic AMP stimulates a protein kinase that phosphorylates hormone-
sensitive lipase (HSL), increasing the rate of hydrolysis of endogenous TAG
(lipolysis). Longer-term control is by synthesis of lipoprotein lipase (LPL) (see
also Fig. 2-5), which hydrolyzes TAG in VLDL and chylomicrons. The fatty
acids released are transported into the BAT cells, and the intermediate-density
lipoproteins (IDL) and chylomicron remnants (C remnants) return to liver.
(Further hydrolysis of TAG in IDL can also occur, forming low-density lipoproteins [LDL], which also eventually return to the liver.) Entry of glucose is
through glucose transporters (GT), location controlled by insulin (see Fig.
2.5). The FFA stimulate the proton-translocating function of the UCP (see
Fig. 2-2) and serve as fuel in the mitochondria for the dehydrogenases of the
β-oxidation cycle of fatty acid oxidation (β-OX) and the tricarboxylic acid
cycle (TCA), which provide the NADH and $FADH_2$ to the electron transport
system (see Fig. 2-2).

processes during the stimulation of BAT by NA
(see the later section on carbohydrate).

In intact animals, α_1-adrenergic receptor stimulation markedly potentiates the thermogenic
response to stimulation of β-adrenergic receptors.[81] The mechanism of this potentiation is not
entirely understood. However, the observation
that the α_1-adrenergic receptor stimulation can
enhance the release of cAMP that occurs in response to stimulation of β-adrenergic receptors[81]
suggests that the known effect of NA on α_1-adren-
ergic receptors to reduce the inhibitory effect of

adenosine on the β-adrenergic response[125] might
have been involved.

Lipid Is the Major Fuel for Brown Adipose Tissue Thermogenesis

Fatty acids are the immediate fuel for thermogenesis in BAT. Even when glucose is also available
and used rapidly by BAT, it appears to be only
a minor fuel for thermogenesis.[62,83,139] BAT can
derive the fatty acids from various sources (Fig.
2-3), depending on the nutritional state of the

animal and the extent to which previous stimulation of BAT has occurred. These sources include the TAG stores in BAT itself and TAG in blood chylomicrons or very low density lipoproteins (derived from dietary lipid and carbohydrate, respectively). *De novo* fatty acid synthesis from glucose can occur in BAT itself and can provide some fatty acids when glucose is plentiful. Finally, in the fasting state, it seems likely that plasma free fatty acids (derived from white adipose tissue TAG stores) can be used as an energy source for BAT thermogenesis.

NA-stimulated thermogenesis in BAT is totally dependent on fatty acid oxidation.[18] Although a minor pathway of fatty acid oxidation is present in peroxisomes, fatty acid oxidation for thermogenesis in BAT occurs almost entirely in mitochondria, the acyl groups entering by way of the carnitine-dependent transport system (see Fig. 2-2). The acetyl CoA produced in the mitochondrial β-oxidation pathway is oxidized by way of the tricarboxylic acid cycle (see Fig. 2-3). The reduced coenzymes produced, NADH and $FADH_2$, are reoxidized in the electron transport system. All the different long-chain fatty acids present in BAT appear to be equally effective as substrates for mitochondrial oxidations as they are in initiating the operation of the UCP.[17,21]

The action of NA on BAT elicits two changes important for the use of fatty acids as a fuel. The more rapid change occurs in minutes and involves activation of hormone-sensitive lipase as a consequence of phosphorylation of the enzyme.[59] This activation is mediated by the rise in cAMP levels caused by stimulation of adenylate cyclase after NA interacts with a β-adrenergic receptor and the consequent increase in activity of a cAMP-dependent protein kinase. When the rate of stimulated lipolysis keeps pace with the rate of stimulated fatty acid oxidation, there is no net export of fatty acid. However, the maximum capacity of BAT for lipolysis greatly exceeds its maximum capacity to oxidize the fatty acids produced during maximum thermogenesis. Thus, during intense stimulation, BAT becomes an exporter as well as a major user of fatty acids.[55]

The less rapid of the two changes induced by persistent stimulation by NA is an increased synthesis of the enzyme lipoprotein lipase, present on the capillary endothelium at the surface of

BAT cells and required for BAT to obtain fatty acids from blood lipoproteins. This increased synthesis is cAMP mediated, involves enhanced gene transcription and mRNA translation, and results in a selective increase in lipoprotein lipase activity several hours after the onset of stimulation.[22]

Lipogenesis is usually also enhanced when thermogenesis is stimulated in BAT of intact animals. However, these two processes are not obligatorily linked. For example, a high-fat diet suppresses lipogenesis but stimulates thermogenesis in BAT. Because in isolated cells the effect of NA on lipogenesis is inhibitory, the way in which lipogenesis is stimulated in intact animals remains unexplained.

Carbohydrate Is Required for Optimal Brown Adipose Tissue Thermogenesis

Glucose is not a major fuel for stimulated thermogenesis in BAT. Nevertheless, when BAT is stimulated, its glucose utilization increases markedly, and BAT may even be a major site of glucose utilization in the body under these conditions. The capacity of BAT for glucose utilization is very large.[26,39] The use of glucose is increased by both insulin and NA, usually acting in concert.

BAT contains glucose transporters, and as in other insulin-sensitive tissues, the translocation of these components to the plasma membrane, where they become functional, appears to be under the control of insulin.[45,46] The total amount of glucose transporters is increased in response to chronic stimulation, probably as a consequence of an action of NA.[45,46] Insulin resistance of BAT, as commonly occurs in most animal models of obesity (e.g., the ob/ob mouse,[86] the fa/fa rat,[34,105] and the gold thioglucose-obese mouse,[25]) is usually associated with defective sympathetic control of thermogenesis in BAT.

The paradoxical situation in which glucose utilization is great yet glucose is not a major fuel for thermogenesis is best explained by the operation of a BAT-liver cycle in which glucose is converted to lactate in BAT and lactate is converted to glucose in liver[55] (Fig. 2-4). Evidence from both *in vitro*[30,62] and *in vivo*[83] studies indicates

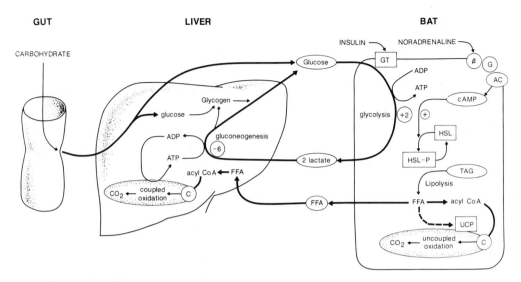

FIGURE 2-4

Carbohydrate metabolism in BAT during stimulated thermogenesis. The
BAT-liver cycle is shown, with blood glucose used through glycolysis to form
lactate in BAT and lactate used to form glucose again in liver. A net yield of 2
ATP per glucose used in BAT (substrate level phosphorylation in the cytosol)
requires the greater input of 6 ATP per glucose made through gluconeogenesis
in liver. This ATP is made in liver by oxidative phosphorylation, which requires oxidation of substrates, most probably fatty acids, in liver mitochondria. The BAT-liver cycle is in a sense a futile cycle because *coupled* oxidation of substrates in liver provides one third of its ATP yield to BAT, at the
time the latter is operating in the *uncoupled* mode, the remaining two thirds
being wasted. The actions of NA and insulin illustrated are the same as in
Figure 2-3.

that lactate (plus pyruvate) is a major end product of glucose metabolism in BAT. During maximal stimulation of thermogenesis, almost 90% of
the glucose used by BAT is exported as lactate
plus pyruvate.[83] The physiological function of
such a cycle would be similar to that of the Cori
cycle, involving exercising muscle and liver—
namely, to permit generation of ATP by substrate-level phosphorylations in a tissue in
which the generation of ATP by oxidative phosphorylation is hindered, by the operation of the
uncoupling protein in stimulated BAT, and by
the relative lack of oxygen in exercising muscle.
The ATP thus generated is required for various
purposes that must be increased during stimulation of BAT by NA (see the earlier section on
noradrenaline).

Because liver retains a capacity for gluconeogenesis in both fed and fasting states,[47] the BAT-

liver glucose-lactate cycle could operate whenever BAT was stimulated. A small proportion of
overall heat production based on fatty acid oxidation (about 3%) would be shifted to the liver
under conditions of maximally stimulated thermogenesis in BAT. In the liver, the coupled oxidation of the fatty acids would be needed for
synthesis of the ATP needed for resynthesis of
glucose from lactate. A role for the liver in diet-
induced thermogenesis in BAT has been suggested on other grounds.[84,85]

Another likely use for some of the glucose used
during stimulated thermogenesis is metabolism
in the pentose-phosphate pathway to provide the
reduced form of nicotinamide-adenine dinucleotide phosphate (NADPH) needed for stimulated
lipogenesis. In addition, pyruvate derived from
glucose is needed to maintain the level of tricarboxylic acid cycle intermediates by its conver-

sion to oxaloacetate through the pyruvate carboxylase reaction.

Brown Adipose Tissue Grows When Chronically Stimulated

Chronic sympathetic stimulation of BAT by cold or by diet induces hyperplasia. This is mediated by an action of NA on β-adrenergic receptors. New brown adipocytes are formed from preadipocytes and interstitial cells.[19,38] The vasculature also proliferates to supply the expanded mass of BAT cells.

Hypertrophy of BAT in response to chronic stimulation is not, however, simply production of more BAT cells of the same type. Rather, there are selective changes in gene expression such that certain components that are important in the thermogenic function of BAT increase to a greater extent than other components so that the capacity of BAT for NA-induced thermogenesis is enhanced (Fig. 2-5). Components that show such adaptive increases in response to chronic stimulation include the UCP, lipoprotein lipase, glucose transporters, gap junctions, thyroxine 5'-deiodinase (TD), and α_1-adrenergic receptors. The concentration of the vital hormone-sensitive lipase is not specifically increased, the activity of this enzyme being controlled by phosphorylation and dephosphorylation rather than by selective synthesis. It might be supposed that chronic stimulation for whatever reason would always produce the same pattern of growth of BAT. This is not the case. The pattern of adaptive changes differs according to the nature of the stimulus, and it is likely that factors other than NA from the sympathetic nerves are also involved. Glucagon may well be involved under some conditions, because this hormone is known to promote growth of BAT[14] and to increase TD activity in BAT.[132]

Increased synthesis of the mRNA for UCP is a very early event in the trophic response of BAT and occurs soon after the onset of the thermogenic response.[112] Increased synthesis of UCP and its insertion into the inner membrane of the mitochondria result in a marked increase in mitochondrial UCP concentration (relative to other mitochondrial proteins).[111] This aspect of the trophic response is best elicited by cold exposure; the response to diet is less marked.[33] Both β- and

α_1-adrenergic receptors are implicated in this response to cold in intact animals.[64]

Increased synthesis of TD in BAT can raise the level of the enzyme several hundred times during the initial phase of exposure to cold. This response is mediated by the sympathetic nerves to BAT[100] and can be mimicked by acute administration of NA.[131,132] It involves enhanced gene expression and increased protein synthesis.[12,13,130] NA is believed to exert this effect through an action on both α_1- and β-adrenergic receptors.[66] Paradoxically, activation of the sympathetic nervous system by diet does not alter the level of activity of this enzyme.[32,101,140]

The large burst in activity of TD in BAT during the initial stages of acclimation to cold leads to an increased production in BAT of 3,5,3'-triiodothyronine (T_3) from thyroxine (T_4) that is sufficient to virtually saturate the nuclear receptors for T_3.[13,130] This, in turn, is believed to amplify the effect of NA to increase the synthesis of mRNA for UCP.[12,13,103,130] T_3 alone is unable to induce the synthesis of mRNA for UCP in the absence of NA.[130] Because activation of the sympathetic nervous system by diet does not increase the activity of TD, the weaker effect of diet to increase UCP concentration in BAT mitochondria can be attributed to the lack of increase in T_3 production, which would otherwise facilitate the synthesis of UCP. The reason for the lack of increase in activity of TD in response to diet remains obscure.

Increased synthesis of lipoprotein lipase is another rapid response to chronic stimulation of BAT by NA. The increase is due to an action on β-adrenergic receptors and involves enhancement of gene expression and mRNA translation.[22,87] As with TD, the synthesis of lipoprotein lipase occurs rapidly in response to cold but not to the same extent in response to the sympathetic activation brought about by diet.[20] However, the pronounced circadian rhythm in lipoprotein lipase level in BAT[41] contrasts with the lack of any such rhythm in TD activity[101] and indicates a difference in control of these two adaptive enzymes of BAT.

Other adaptive changes that have been less studied but that presumably involve similar regulatory mechanisms to those outlined earlier include an increase in concentration of glucose transporters,[45,46] an increase in density of α_1-

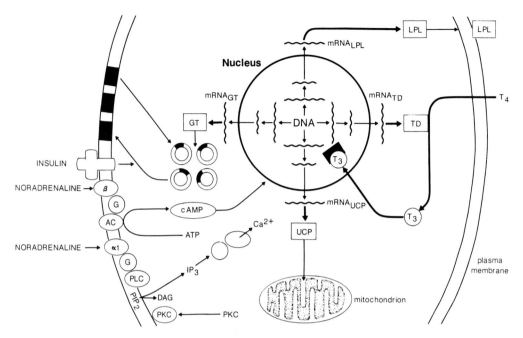

FIGURE 2-5

Some adaptive changes that occur in BAT in response to prolonged stimula-
tion. Increased synthesis of uncoupling protein (UCP), lipoprotein lipase
(LPL), thyroxine 5'-deiodinase (TD), and glucose transporters (GT) is illustrated. Only for UCP and for LPL is it established directly that stimulation by
NA, through a cAMP-mediated mechanism, results in increased transcription
of the appropriate gene.[22,111,112] For $mRNA_{UCP}$, the precursor mRNA is presumably much larger than the final form,[15,71] whereas this may not be true for the
$mRNA_{LPL}$.[67] Increased protein synthesis follows the increased abundance of
the mRNAs. Increased degradation of $mRNA_{UCP}$ also occurs during and after
chronic stimulation.[63,104,110] The UCP made is inserted into the inner mitochondrial membrane; it does not have an initial signal sequence, unlike most other
mitochondrial proteins that are made in the cytosol.[113] Increased transcription
and translation of the TD gene are inferred from studies with inhibitors.[132] The
increased conversion of T_4 to T_3 results in an increase in intracellular T_3 concentration and saturation of nuclear T_3 receptors. The T_3-receptor complex
(shown in the nucleus) amplifies the NA-induced increase in transcription of
Ucp gene.[12,130] Increased synthesis of glucose transporters is inferred only from
the increased concentration of this component in BAT that occurs in response
to chronic stimulation.[45,46] This diagram shows not only interactions of NA
with the β-adrenergic receptor (also shown in Figs. 2-3 and 2-4), but also the
interaction of NA with the $α_1$-adrenergic receptor (see text). The roles of IP_3,
DAG, calcium release (Ca^{2+}), and protein kinase C (PKC) translocation and activation in the trophic response have not been established.

adrenergic receptors,[107,108] and an increase in density of gap junctions.[126] The density of β-adrenergic receptors may decrease[123] or remain unaltered. However, the capacity of adenylate cyclase to respond to NA when it interacts with the β-adrenergic receptor is enhanced.[43,44] There is clearly a major reorganization of the plasma membrane of BAT cells during the trophic response to chronic stimulation by NA.

Brown Adipose Tissue Atrophies When Stimulation Is Weak or Absent

Whereas chronic stimulation promotes hypertrophy of BAT, chronic lack of stimulation renders BAT atrophic. Not only is BAT thermogenically quiescent when stimulation is weak or absent, but its capacity to respond to NA decreases because of loss of certain key adaptive components required for the thermogenic response.

Atrophy of BAT is seen at its most extreme after the surgical removal of sympathetic input to BAT. This reduces both its total metabolic mass and its mitochondrial mass. The change is most marked when previous hypertrophy has been brought about, for example, by acclimation to cold. Although there is a decrease in cellularity, there are selective reductions in mitochondrial UCP concentration, in TD, and in lipoprotein lipase activity.[53,55,56,100]

A similar atrophy of BAT, usually to a lesser extent and with a somewhat different pattern, occurs when sympathetic input to BAT is reduced by fasting, by acclimation to thermoneutrality, or by the increased heat load imposed by lactation or exercise.[53,55] Lack of insulin (as in streptozotocin-diabetic rats) likewise induces an atrophy of BAT that is in part mediated by reduced sympathetic nervous system activity in BAT.[8,9,128,132,141] BAT also tends to be in a relatively atrophic form in obese animals (see the next section), in aging animals, and even in adults of certain species; in all of these it can be reactivated by selective chronic stimulation.

Control of Brown Adipose Tissue Is Defective in Most Types of Obese Animals

In most types of obese animals, BAT is in a thermogenically quiescent and relatively atrophied state. This state is often associated with reduced sympathetic nervous system activity in BAT and is usually due to anomalous central regulation of the sympathetic input to BAT. BAT is usually also insulin resistant, thus exacerbating its hyporesponsive state. The inactivity of BAT results in a deficit in energy expenditure for thermogenesis and is believed to contribute to the high metabolic efficiency and obesity of these animals. The inactivity of BAT in most types of obese animals is improved by adrenalectomy, believed to work by removing a central suppressive effect of glucocorticoids on sympathetic nervous system activity in BAT.

Two major categories of obese animals in which BAT is deranged can be discerned among the many types studied. In the first category, thermogenesis in BAT cannot be induced by diet; such animals may or may not be hyperphagic. In the second category, the animals tend to thermoregulate at a low body temperature for all or part of the time, resulting in reduced energy expenditure in all organs (because of their lower than normal temperature) and suppressed thermogenesis in BAT. These animals may or may not also exhibit defective diet-induced thermogenesis in their BAT. A more complete review of BAT function in obese animals is presented elsewhere.[52,53,55]

Examples of the first category include rats with hypothalamic parasagittal knife cuts; rats with ventromedial hypothalamic lesions; adult, genetically obese, fa/fa, fatty rats; genetically obese, cp/cp, corpulent rats; and aging rats. All of these animals are capable of activating their BAT in the cold but not of activating their BAT in response to diet. When they live in a warm environment, the lack of diet-induced thermogenesis in their BAT contributes to their high metabolic efficiency.[52-55]

Examples of the second category include genetically obese, ob/ob, mice; genetically obese, diabetic, db/db, mice; gold thioglucose obese mice; newborn fatty, fa/fa, rats; and mice treated with glutamate in the neonatal period.

A third category of obese animals should also be noted, exemplified by rats with paraventricular hypothalamic lesions and by certain strains of rats that are susceptible to diet-induced obesity. Such animals do not exhibit abnormalities in their control of BAT thermogenesis.

The converse of a genetic propensity to obesity is seen in lean and obesity-resistant I-strain mice (I/Crgl), in which BAT is unusually active.[10] The converse of hypothalamic obesity also exists in lateral hypothalamic-lesioned rats, in which BAT is unusually reactive and may play a part in the very early stages of the febrile response to the lesion.[27,61,99,102]

The Hypothalamus and Control of Brown Adipose Tissue Thermogenesis

Both ambient temperature and diet can exert selective control over sympathetic nervous system activity in BAT, while leaving unaffected sympathetic nervous system activity in other organs.[29] The sensing of temperature involves both peripheral and central receptors, with signals being processed and integrated in various parts of the brain, particularly in the hypothalamus.[16] Food-derived chemicals implicated in control of diet-induced thermogenesis in BAT include glucose and ketone bodies. The hierarchical neural structures for chemical information processing[98] presumably mesh with those for thermal information processing at multiple levels. However, diet-induced thermogenesis in BAT appears to be much more dependent on hypothalamic structures than is cold-induced nonshivering thermogenesis.

Experiments involving electrical or chemical stimulation of specific hypothalamic or other sites have implicated the ventromedial hypothalamus and the lateral hypothalamus as well as a longitudinal inhibitory pathway that extends from the preoptic area of the hypothalamus to the lower brainstem.[56] A center that provides a thermogenic drive to BAT through its sympathetic innervation is located somewhere in the brainstem[11,121,129] and is controlled by inhibitory influences from higher brain structures. Of the various central neuropeptides that might be involved in control of BAT thermogenesis, corticotropin releasing factor (CRF) appears to be the most potent.[3,75] This peptide is believed to be involved in the normal control of BAT thermogenesis[42,60] as well as in the initiation of BAT thermogenesis during the rising phase of fever.[28,114]

The cephalic phase of food ingestion is also involved in activation of BAT thermogenesis, providing yet another central input from sight, smell, or taste of the food reaching the hypothalamus by way of other areas of the brain.[53,54,56] It is known that bypassing the cephalic phase of food ingestion by tube feeding attenuates diet-induced thermogenesis in BAT.[116]

Brown Adipose Tissue Thermogenesis as a Target for Antiobesity Drugs

During the past decade, the induction of thermogenesis in BAT by drugs has proved an attractive avenue of research into means of altering energy balance in the treatment of obesity. This idea is based on the evidence that many types of animal obesity are associated with relatively atrophic and thermogenically quiescent BAT. Because in many obese animal models the inactivity of the BAT is secondary to a reduction in the trophic influence of its sympathetic innervation, much attention has been given to the stimulation of BAT by sympathomimetic drugs.[5,58,135]

Research with sympathomimetic drugs to stimulate BAT has led to the development of compounds that promote BAT thermogenesis and weight loss in obese laboratory animals. Unfortunately, the cardiovascular effects of these compounds make them unsuitable for use in humans. The search for agents with a preferential action on BAT has promoted studies on the nature of the BAT β-adrenergic receptor. These studies have produced conflicting reports on its nature. Some have produced evidence for a third and unique type of BAT β-adrenergic receptor,[4-6,58] and others have revealed a mixture of β_1- and β_2-adrenergic receptors.[78,89,90,120,123] It is possible to interpret the results of this research as indicating either three types of adrenergic receptor in BAT, one being unique to BAT, or, on the other hand, a single type of receptor unique to BAT. It is entirely plausible that the family of highly homologous adrenergic receptors characteristic of many other tissues[76] could have an additional member unique to BAT. An analogous instance has already been discussed (see the earlier section on BAT thermogenesis)—namely, the presence in BAT of a unique protein, UCP, that is homologous to but not identical with a family of proteins found in all other tissues including BAT. Newer drugs are currently being developed. Some that have already been tested interact much more specifically with BAT[58] and are virtually devoid of cardiovascular activity. They provide additional support for the presence of a unique type of adrenergic receptor in BAT and may prove to be useful in the treatment of obesity.

An alternate approach in the search for drugs to stimulate thermogenesis in BAT is the search for compounds that act centrally to increase selectively activity of the sympathetic nervous system in BAT. Two currently available drugs not developed for this purpose, fenfluramine and mazindol, have been found to activate thermogenesis in BAT of rats through a central mechanism.[2,79,80,118]

PROSPECTS FOR THE FUTURE

A noninvasive method for the assessment of BAT function in intact conscious animals, including human beings, is needed in order to establish the quantitative contribution of BAT thermogenesis to overall energy expenditure and hence to energy balance.

A BAT cell culture system is needed in which BAT preadipocytes can differentiate and express the genes characteristic of BAT, such as those for UCP, for TD, and for lipoprotein lipase. Such a system is required in order to study the molecular mechanisms involved in the control of growth of BAT. So far there has been a disappointing lack of success in developing such a cell culture system.[35,36,93,106]

Most information about the function of BAT was previously derived from studies of laboratory rats. Even in this species, strain differences in BAT function can be discerned. Studies are needed with other species, such as mice, guinea pigs, and hamsters, to establish the various strategies adopted by different types of animals in the use of BAT.[50,51] An explanation of the way in which photoperiod influences BAT growth and function in certain species, such as the Syrian golden hamster,[138] might prove useful in discovering mechanisms for the switching on and off of BAT growth.

Because the ultimate control of BAT thermogenic function and growth resides in the central nervous system, it is clear that a fuller understanding of regulation of BAT metabolism requires a more detailed understanding of the way in which the hypothalamus and lower brain regions selectively control the sympathetic innervation and influence the sensory innervation of BAT.[56]

References

1. Aquila H, Link TA, Klingenberg M: The uncoupling protein from brown fat mitochondria is related to the mitochondrial ADP/ATP carrier. Analysis of sequence homologies and of folding of the protein in the membrane. EMBO J 4:2369, 1985
2. Arase K, Sakaguchi T, Bray GA: Effect of fenfluramine on sympathetic firing rate. Pharmacol Biochem Behav 29:675, 1988
3. Arase K, York DA, Shimizu H et al: Effects of corticotropin-releasing factor on food intake and brown adipose tissue thermogenesis in rats. Am J Physiol 255:E255, 1988
4. Arch JRS: The brown adipocyte β-adrenoceptor. Proc Nutr Soc 48:215, 1989
5. Arch JRS, Bywater RJ, Coney KA et al: Influences on body composition and mechanism of action of the β-adrenoceptor agonist BRL26830A. In Lardy HA, Stratman F (eds): Hormones, Thermogenesis, and Obesity, pp 465–476. New York, Elsevier, 1989
6. Arch JRS, Piercy V, Thurlby PL et al: Thermogenic and lipolytic drugs for the treatment of obesity: Old ideas and new possibilities. In Berry EM, Blondheim SH, Eliahou HE et al (eds): Recent Advances in Obesity Research, Vol V, pp 300–311. London, John Libbey & Co, 1987
7. Barge RM, Mills I, Silva JE et al: Phorbol esters, protein kinase C, and thyroxine 5'-deiodinase in brown adipocytes. Am J Physiol 254:E323, 1988
8. Bartness TJ, Billington CJ, Levine AS et al: Insulin and metabolic efficiency in rats. I. Effects of sucrose feeding and BAT axotomy. Am J Physiol 251:R1109, 1986
9. Bartness TJ, Billington CJ, Levine AS et al: Insulin and metabolic efficiency in rats. II. Effects of NE and cold exposure. Am J Physiol 251:R1118, 1986
10. Bazin R, Ricquier D, Dupuy F et al: Thermogenic and lipogenic activities in brown adipose tissue of I-strain mice. Biochem J 231:761, 1985
11. Benzi RH, Shibata M, Seydoux J et al: Prepontine knife cut-induced hyperthermia in the rat: Effect of chemical sympathectomy and surgical dener-

vation of brown adipose tissue. Pflügers Arch 411:593, 1988

12. Bianco AC, Sheng X, Silva JE: Triiodothyronine amplifies norepinephrine stimulation of uncoupling protein gene transcription by a mechanism not requiring protein synthesis. J Biol Chem 263:18168, 1988

13. Bianco AC, Silva JE: Cold exposure rapidly induces virtual saturation of brown adipose tissue nuclear T_3 receptors. Am J Physiol 255:E496, 1988

14. Billington CJ, Bartness TJ, Briggs J et al: Glucagon stimulation of brown adipose tissue growth and thermogenesis. Am J Physiol 252:R160, 1987

15. Bouillaud F, Raimbault S, Ricquier D: The gene for rat uncoupling protein: Complete sequence, structure of primary transcript and evolutionary relationship between exons. Biochem Biophys Res Commun 157:783, 1988

16. Brück K, Zeisberger E: Adaptive changes in thermoregulation and their neuropharmacological basis. Pharmacol Ther 35:163, 1987

17. Bukowiecki L: Mechanisms of stimulus-calorigenesis coupling in brown adipose tissue. Can J Biochem Cell Biol 62:623, 1984

18. Bukowiecki LJ: Lipid metabolism in brown adipose tissue. In Trayhurn P, Nicholls DG (eds): Brown Adipose Tissue, pp 105–121. London, Edward Arnold, 1986

19. Bukowiecki LJ, Géloën A, Collet AJ: Proliferation and differentiation of brown adipocytes from interstitial cells during cold acclimation. Am J Physiol 250:C880, 1986

20. Carneheim CMH, Alexson SEH: Refeeding and insulin increase lipoprotein lipase activity in brown adipose tissue. Am J Physiol 256:E645, 1989

21. Carneheim C, Cannon B, Nedergaard J: Rare fatty acids in brown fat are substrates for thermogenesis during arousal from hibernation. Am J Physiol 256:R146, 1989

22. Carneheim C, Nedergaard J, Cannon B: Cold-induced β-adrenergic recruitment of lipoprotein lipase in brown fat is due to increased transcription. Am J Physiol 254:E155, 1988

23. Connolly E, Nånberg E, Nedergaard J: Norepinephrine-induced Na^+ influx in brown adipocytes is cyclic AMP-mediated. J Biol Chem 261:14377, 1986

24. Connolly E, Nedergaard J: β-adrenergic modulation of Ca^{2+} uptake by isolated brown adipocytes. Possible involvement of mitochondria. J Biol Chem 263:10574, 1988

25. Cooney GJ, Astbury LD, Williams PF et al: Insulin response in individual tissues of control and gold

thioglucose-obese mice in vivo with [1-^{14}C] 2-deoxyglucose. Diabetes 36:152, 1987

26. Cooney G, Curi R, Mitchelson A et al: Activities of some key enzymes of carbohydrate, ketone body, adenosine and glutamine metabolism in liver, and brown and white adipose tissue of the rat. Biochem Biophys Res Comm 138:687, 1986

27. Corbett SW, Kaufman LN, Keesey RE: Thermogenesis after lateral hypothalamic lesions: Contributions of brown adipose tissue. Am J Physiol 255:E708, 1988

28. Dascombe MJ, Rothwell NJ, Sagay BO et al: Pyrogenic and thermogenic effects of interleukin 1β in the rat. Am J Physiol 256:E7, 1989

29. Dulloo AG, Young JB, Landsberg L: Sympathetic nervous system responses to cold exposure and diet in rat skeletal muscle. Am J Physiol 255: E180, 1988

30. Ebner S, Burnol A-F, Ferré P et al: Effects of insulin and norepinephrine on glucose transport and metabolism in rat brown adipocytes: Potentiation by insulin of norepinephrine-induced glucose oxidation. Eur J Biochem 170:469, 1987

31. Eckerskorn C, Klingenberg M: In the uncoupling protein from brown adipose tissue the C-terminus protrudes to the c-side of the membrane as shown by tryptic cleavage. FEBS Lett 226:166, 1987

32. Eley J, Himms-Hagen J: Brown adipose tissue of mice with gold thioglucose-induced obesity: Abnormal circadian control. Am J Physiol 256:E773, 1989

33. Falcou R, Bouillaud F, Mory G et al: Increase of uncoupling protein and its mRNA in brown adipose tissue of rats fed on "cafeteria diet." Biochem J 231:241, 1985

34. Ferré P, Burnol A-F, Leturque A et al: Glucose utilization in vivo and insulin-sensitivity of rat brown adipose tissue in various physiological and pathological conditions. Biochem J 233:249, 1986

35. Forest C, Doglio A, Casteilla L et al: Expression of the mitochondrial uncoupling protein in brown adipocytes: Absence in brown preadipocytes and BFC-1 cells. Modulation by isoproterenol in adipocytes. Exp Cell Res 168:233, 1987

36. Forest C, Doglio A, Ricquier D et al: A preadipocyte clonal line from mouse brown adipose tissue: Short- and long-term responses to insulin and β-adrenergics. Exp Cell Res 168:218, 1987

37. Foster DO: Quantitative role of brown adipose tissue in thermogenesis. In Trayhurn P, Nicholls DG (eds): Brown Adipose Tissue, pp 31–51. London, Edward Arnold, 1986

38. Géloën A, Collet AJ, Guay G et al: β-adrenergic stimulation of brown adipocyte proliferation. Am J Physiol 254:C175, 1988

39. Gibbins JM, Denton RM, McCormack JG: Evidence that noradrenaline increases pyruvate dehydrogenase activity and decreases acetyl-CoA carboxylase activity in rat interscapular brown adipose tissue in vivo. Biochem J 228:751, 1985

40. Giovannini P, Seydoux J, Girardier L: Evidence for a modulating effect of Na^+/H^+ exchange on the metabolic response of rat brown adipose tissue. Pflügers Arch 411:273, 1988

41. Goubern M, Portet R: Circadian rhythm and hormonal sensitivity of lipoprotein lipase activity in cold acclimated rats. Horm Metab Res 13:73, 1981

42. Goubern M, Laury MC, Zizine L et al: Brown adipose tissue in hypophysectomized rats: Involvement of sympathetic system. Experientia 44:508, 1988

43. Granneman JG: Norepinephrine infusions increase adenylate cyclase responsiveness in brown adipose tissue. J Pharmacol Exp Ther 245:1075, 1988

44. Granneman JG, MacKenzie RG: Neural modulation of the stimulatory regulatory protein of adenylate cyclase in rat brown adipose tissue. J Pharmacol Exp Ther 245:1068, 1988

45. Greco-Perotto R, Assimacopoulos-Jeannet F, Jeanrenaud B: Insulin modifies the properties of glucose transporters in rat brown adipose tissue. Biochem J 247:63, 1987

46. Greco-Perotto R, Zaninetti D, Assimacopoulos-Jeannet F et al: Stimulatory effect of cold adaptation on glucose utilization by brown adipose tissue: Relationship with changes in the glucose transporter system. J Biol Chem 262:7732, 1987

47. Hellerstein MK, Munro HN: Interaction of liver and muscle in the regulation of metabolism in response to nutritional and other factors. In Arias IM, Jakoby WB, Popper H (eds): The Liver: Biology and Pathobiology, pp 965–983. New York, Raven Press, 1988

48. Himms-Hagen J: Obesity may be due to a malfunctioning of brown fat. Can Med Assoc 121:1361, 1979

49. Himms-Hagen J: Brown adipose tissue thermogenesis as an energy buffer: Implications for obesity. N Engl J Med 311:1549, 1984

50. Himms-Hagen J: Brown adipose tissue and cold-acclimation. In Trayhurn P, Nicholls DG (eds): Brown Adipose Tissue, pp 214–268. London, Edward Arnold, 1986

51. Himms-Hagen J: Cold- versus diet-induced thermogenesis in brown adipose tissue: Different strategies in different species. In Heller HC, Musacchia XJ, Wang LCH (eds): Living in the Cold, pp 93–100. New York, Elsevier, 1986

52. Himms-Hagen J: Defective thermogenesis in obese animals. J Obes Weight Regul 6:179, 1987

53. Himms-Hagen J: Brown adipose tissue thermogenesis: Role in thermoregulation, energy regulation and obesity. Pharmacol Ther. In Schönbaum E, Lomax P (eds). Thermoregulation: Physiology and Biochemistry, pp 327–414. New York, Pergamon, 1990

54. Himms-Hagen J: Role of thermogenesis in regulation of energy balance in relation to obesity. Can J Physiol Pharmacol 67:394, 1989

55. Himms-Hagen J: Brown adipose tissue thermogenesis and obesity. In Holman R (ed): Progress in Lipid Research vol 28, pp 67–115. New York, Maxwell, Pergamon, Macmillan, 1989

56. Himms-Hagen J: Neural control of brown adipose tissue thermogenesis, hypertrophy, and atrophy. In Ganong WF, Martini L (eds): Frontiers in Neuroendocrinology, vol 12, pp 38–93. New York, Raven Press, 1991

57. Himms-Hagen J, Tokuyama K, Eley J et al: Hypothalamic regulation of brown adipose tissue in lean and obese rodents. In Lardy H, Stratman F (eds): Hormones, Thermogenesis and Obesity, pp 173–184. Proceedings of the 18th Steenbock Symposium. New York, Elsevier, 1989

58. Holloway BR: Selective β-agonists of brown fat and thermogenesis. In Lardy HA, Stratman F (eds): Hormones, Thermogenesis, and Obesity, pp 477–484. Proceedings of the 18th Steenbock Symposium. New York, Elsevier, 1989

59. Holm C, Fredrickson G, Cannon B et al: Hormone-sensitive lipase in brown adipose tissue: Identification and effect of cold exposure. Biosci Rep 7:897, 1987

60. Holt S, Rothwell NJ, Stock MJ et al: Effect of hypophysectomy on energy balance and brown fat activity in obese Zucker rats. Am J Physiol 254:E162, 1988

61. Holt SJ, York DA: Effect of lateral hypothalamic lesion on brown adipose tissue of Zucker lean and obese rats. Physiol Behav 43:293, 1988

62. Isler D, Hill H-P, Meier MK: Glucose metabolism in isolated brown adipocytes under β-adrenergic stimulation: Quantitative contribution of glucose to total thermogenesis. Biochem J 245:789, 1987

63. Jacobsson A, Cannon B, Nedergaard J: Physiological activation of brown adipose tissue destabilizes thermogenin mRNA. FEBS Lett 224:353, 1987

64. Jacobsson A, Nedergaard J, Cannon B: α- and β-adrenergic control of thermogenin mRNA expression in brown adipose tissue. Biosci Rep 6:621, 1986

65. Jezek P, Houstek J, Drahota Z: Alkaline pH, membrane potential, and magnesium cations are negative modulators of purine nucleotide inhibition of H^+ and Cl^- transport through the uncoupling

protein of brown adipose tissue mitochondria. J Bioenerg Biomembr 20:603, 1988

66. Jones R, Henschen L, Mohell N et al: Requirement of gene transcription and protein synthesis for cold- and norepinephrine-induced stimulation of thyroxine deiodinase in rat brown adipose tissue. Biochem Biophys Acta 889:366, 1986

67. Kirchgessner TG, Svenson KL, Lusis AJ et al: The sequence of cDNA encoding lipoprotein lipase: A member of lipase gene family. J Biol Chem 262:8463, 1987

68. Klingenberg M: Nucleotide binding to uncoupling protein. Mechanism of control by protonation. Biochemistry 27:781, 1988

69. Klingenberg M, Winkler E: The reconstituted isolated uncoupling protein is a membrane potential driven H^+ translocator. EMBO J 4:3087, 1985

70. Kopecky J, Jezek P, Drahota Z et al: Control of uncoupling protein in brown-fat mitochondria by purine nucleotides. Chemical modification by diazobenzenesulfonate. Eur J Biochem 164:687, 1987

71. Kozak LP, Britton JH, Kozak UC et al: The mitochondrial uncoupling protein gene: Correlation of exon structure to transmembrane domain. J Biol Chem 263:12274, 1988

72. Landsberg L, Young JB: Fasting, feeding and regulation of the sympathetic nervous system. N Engl J Med 298:1295, 1978

73. Landsberg L, Young JB: The role of the sympathoadrenal system in modulating energy expenditure. In James WPT (ed): Clinics in Endocrinology and Metabolism, Vol 13, pp 475–499. Philadelphia, WB Saunders, 1984

74. LaNoue KF, Strzelecki T, Strzelecka D et al: Regulation of the uncoupling protein in brown adipose tissue. J Biol Chem 261:298, 1986

75. LeFeuvre RA, Rothwell NJ, Stock MJ: Activation of brown fat thermogenesis in response to central injection of corticotropin releasing hormone in the rat. Neuropharmacology 26:1217, 1987

76. Lefkowitz RJ, Caron MG: Adrenergic receptors: Models for the study of receptors coupled to guanine nucleotide regulatory proteins. J Biol Chem 263:4993, 1988

77. Lever JD, Mukherjee S, Norman D et al: Neuropeptide and noradrenaline distributions in rat interscapular brown fat and in its intact and obstructed nerves of supply. J Auton Nerv Syst 25:15, 1988

78. Levin BE, Sullivan AC: Beta-1 receptor is the predominant beta-adrenoceptor on rat brown adipose tissue. J Pharmacol Exp Ther 236:681, 1986

79. Lupien JR, Bray GA: Effect of mazindol, d-amphetamine and diethylpropion on purine nucleo-

tide binding to brown adipose tissue. Pharmacol Biochem Behav 25:733, 1986

80. Lupien JR, Tokunaga K, Kemnitz JW et al: Lateral hypothalamic lesions and fenfluramine increase thermogenesis in brown adipose tissue. Physiol Behav 38:15, 1986

81. Ma SWY, Foster DO: Potentiation of in vivo thermogenesis in rat brown adipose tissue by stimulation of α_1-adrenoceptors is associated with increased release of cyclic AMP. Can J Physiol Pharmacol 62:943, 1984

82. Ma SWY, Foster DO: Redox state of brown adipose tissue as a possible determinant of its blood flow. Can J Physiol Pharmacol 62:949, 1984

83. Ma SWY, Foster DO: Uptake of glucose and release of fatty acids and glycerol by rat brown adipose tissue in vivo. Can J Physiol Pharmacol 64:609, 1986

84. Ma SWY, Foster DO, Nadeau BE et al: Absence of increased oxygen consumption in brown adipose tissue of rats exhibiting "cafeteria" diet-induced thermogenesis. Can J Physiol Pharmacol 66:1347, 1988

85. Ma SWY, Nadeau BE, Foster DO: Evidence for liver as the major site of the diet-induced thermogenesis of rats fed a "cafeteria" diet. Can J Physiol Pharmacol 65:1802, 1987

86. Mercer SW, Trayhurn P: Effects of ciglitazone on insulin resistance and thermogenic responsiveness to acute cold in brown adipose tissue of genetically obese (ob/ob) mice. FEBS Lett 195:12, 1986

87. Mitchell JR, Carneheim CMH, Jacobsson A et al: Regulation of expression of the lipoprotein lipase gene in brown adipose tissue. In Obesity in Europe 88, Björntorp P, Rössner S (eds), pp 235–239. London, John Libbey, 1989

88. Mohell N, Connolly E, Nedergaard J: Distinction between mechanisms underlying α_1- and β-adrenergic respiratory stimulation in brown fat cells. Am J Physiol 253:C301, 1987

89. Muzzin P, Colomb C, Giacobino J-P et al: Biochemical characterization of brown adipose tissue β-adrenergic receptor. J Recept Res 8:713, 1988

90. Muzzin P, Seydoux J, Giacobino J-P et al: Discrepancies between the affinities of binding and action of the novel β-adrenergic agonist BRL 37344 in rat brown adipose tissue. Biochem Biophys Res Comm 156:375, 1988

91. Nånberg E, Putney J Jr: α_1-adrenergic activation of brown adipocytes leads to an increased formation of inositol phosphates. FEBS Lett 195:319, 1986

92. Néchad M: Structure and development of brown adipose tissue. In Trayhurn P, Nicholls DG (eds):

Brown Adipose Tissue, pp 1–30. London, Edward Arnold, 1986

93. Néchad M, Nedergaard J, Cannon B: Noradrenergic stimulation of mitochondriogenesis in brown adipocytes differentiating in culture. Am J Physiol 253:C889, 1987

94. Nedergaard J, Mohell N, Nånberg E et al: α_1-adrenergic pathways in brown adipose tissue: Mode of action and recruitment pattern. In Heller HC, Musacchia XJ, Wang LCH (eds): Living in the Cold, pp 83–91. New York, Elsevier, 1986

95. Nicholls DG, Cunningham SA, Rial E: The bioenergetic mechanisms of brown adipose tissue thermogenesis. In Trayhurn P, Nicholls DG (eds): Brown Adipose Tissue, pp 52–85. London, Edward Arnold, 1986

96. Nnodim JO, Lever JD: Neural and vascular provisions of rat interscapular brown adipose tissue. Am J Anat 182:283, 1988

97. Norman D, Mukherjee S, Symons D et al: Neuropeptides in interscapular and perirenal brown adipose tissue in the rat: A plurality of innervation. J Neurocytol 17:305, 1988

98. Oomura Y: Control of food intake and hypothalamic activity by endogenous chemical substances. In Berry EM, Blondheim SH, Eliahou HE et al (eds): Recent Advances in Obesity Research, Vol 5, pp 229–239. London, John Libbey & Co, 1987

99. Park IRA, Coscina DV, Himms-Hagen J: Lateral and medial hypothalamic lesions do not acutely affect brown adipose tissue. Brain Res Bull 21:805, 1988

100. Park IRA, Himms-Hagen J: Neural influences on trophic changes in brown adipose tissue during cold acclimation. Am J Physiol 255:R874, 1988

101. Park IRA, Himms-Hagen J: A circadian study of the function of brown adipose tissue in the rat. FASEB J 2:A1612, 1988

102. Park IRA, Himms-Hagen J, Coscina DV: Long-term effects of lateral hypothalamic lesions on brown adipose tissue in rats. Brain Res Bull 17:643, 1986

103. Park IRA, Mount DB, Himms-Hagen J: Role of T_3 in thermogenic and trophic responses of brown adipose tissue to cold. Am J Physiol 257:E81, 1989

104. Patel HV, Freeman KB, Desautels M: Selective loss of uncoupling protein mRNA in brown adipose tissue on deacclimation of cold-acclimated mice. Biochem Cell Biol 65:955, 1987

105. Pénicaud L, Ferré P, Terretaz J et al: Development of obesity in Zucker rats: Early insulin resistance in muscles but normal sensitivity in white adipose tissue. Diabetes 36:626, 1987

106. Poissonnet CM, Ouagued M, Aron Y et al: Retrieval of precursors for white-type adipose conversion in brown adipose tissue. Biochem J 255:849, 1988

107. Raasmaja A, Mohell N, Nedergaard J: Increased α-1-adrenergic receptor density in brown adipose tissue of cold-acclimated rats and hamsters. Eur J Pharmacol 106:489, 1984

108. Raasmaja A, York DA: α_1- and β-adrenergic receptors in brown adipose tissue of lean (Fa/?) and obese (fa/fa) Zucker rats. Biochem J 249:831, 1988

109. Rawn JD: Biochemistry. Burlington, NC, Carolina Biological Supply, 1989

110. Reichling S, Ridley RG, Patel HV et al: Loss of brown adipose tissue uncoupling protein mRNA on deacclimation of cold-exposed rats. Biochem Biophys Res Commun 142:696, 1987

111. Ricquier D, Bouillaud F: The brown adipose tissue mitochondrial uncoupling protein. In Trayhurn P, Nicholls DG (eds): Brown Adipose Tissue, pp 86–104. London, Edward Arnold, 1986

112. Ricquier D, Bouillaud F, Toumelin P et al: Expression of uncoupling protein mRNA in thermogenic or weakly thermogenic brown adipose tissue: Evidence for a rapid β-adrenoceptor-mediated and transcriptionally regulated step during activation of thermogenesis. J Biol Chem 261:13905, 1986

113. Ridley RG, Patel HV, Gerber GE et al: Complete nucleotide and derived amino acid sequence of cDNA encoding the mitochondrial uncoupling protein of rat brown adipose tissue: Lack of a mitochondrial targeting presequence. Nucleic Acids Res 14:4025, 1986

114. Rothwell NJ: CRF is involved in the pyrogenic and thermogenic effects of interleukin 1β in the rat. Am J Physiol 256:E111, 1989

115. Rothwell NJ, Stock MJ: A role for brown adipose tissue in diet-induced thermogenesis. Nature 281:31, 1979

116. Rothwell NJ, Stock MJ: Energy balance, thermogenesis and brown adipose tissue activity in tube-fed rats. J Nutr 114:1965, 1984

117. Rothwell NJ, Stock MJ: Brown adipose tissue and diet-induced thermogenesis. In Trayhurn P, Nicholls DG (eds): Brown Adipose Tissue, pp 269–298. London, Edward Arnold, 1986

118. Rothwell NJ, Stock MJ: Effect of diet and fenfluramine on thermogenesis in the rat: Possible involvement of serotonergic mechanisms. Int J Obes 11:319, 1987

119. Rothwell NJ, Stock MJ: Brown adipose tissue: Does it play a role in the development of obesity? Diabetes Metab Rev 4:595, 1988

120. Rothwell NJ, Stock MJ, Sudera DK: β-adrenocep-

tors in rat brown adipose tissue: Proportions of β_1- and β_2-subtypes. Am J Physiol 248:E397, 1985

121. Rothwell NJ, Stock MJ, Thexton AJ: Decerebration activates thermogenesis in the rat. J Physiol (Lond) 342:15, 1983

122. Runswick MJ, Powell SJ, Nyren P et al: Sequence of the bovine mitochondrial phosphate carrier protein: Structural relationship to ADP/ATP translocase and the brown fat mitochondria uncoupling protein. EMBO J 6:1367, 1987

123. Scarpace PJ, Baresi LA, Morley JE: Modulation of receptors and adenylate cyclase activity during sucrose feeding, food deprivation, and cold exposure. Am J Physiol 253:E629, 1987

124. Schimmel RJ: The α_1-adrenergic transduction system in hamster brown adipocytes: Release of arachidonic acid accompanies activation of phospholipase C. Biochem J 253:93, 1988

125. Schimmel RJ, Elliott ME, Dehmel VC: Interactions between adenosine and α_1-adrenergic agonists in regulation of respiration in hamster brown adipocytes. Mol Pharmacol 32:26, 1987

126. Schneider-Picard G, Carpentier J-L, Girardier L: Quantitative evaluation of gap junctions in rat brown adipose tissue after cold acclimation. J Membr Biol 78:85, 1984

127. Schneider-Picard G, Coles JA, Girardier L: α- and β-adrenergic mediation of changes in metabolism and Na/K exchange in rat brown fat. J Gen Physiol 86:169, 1985

128. Shibata H, Pérusse F, Bukowiecki LJ: The role of insulin in nonshivering thermogenesis. Can J Physiol Pharmacol 65:152, 1987

129. Shibata M, Benzi RH, Seydoux J et al: Hyperthermia induced by pre-pontine knife-cut: Evidence for a tonic inhibition of nonshivering thermogenesis in anaesthetized rat. Brain Res 436:273, 1987

130. Silva JE: Full expression of uncoupling protein gene requires the concurrence of norepinephrine and triiodothyronine. Mol Endocrinol 2:706, 1988

131. Silva JE, Larsen PR: Interrelationships among thyroxine, growth hormone, and the sympathetic nervous system in the regulation of 5'-iodothyronine deiodinase in rat brown adipose tissue. J Clin Invest 77:1214, 1986

132. Silva JE, Larsen PR: Hormonal regulation of iodothyronine 5'-deiodinase in rat brown adipose tissue. Am J Physiol 251:E639, 1986

133. Smith RE, Horwitz BA: Brown fat and thermogenesis. Physiol Rev 49:330, 1969

134. Stryer L: Biochemistry, 3rd ed. New York, W.H. Freeman, 1988

135. Sullivan AC, Hogan S, Triscari J: New developments in pharmacological treatments for obesity. Ann NY Acad Sci 499:269, 1987

136. Swick AG, Swick RW: Changes in GDP binding to brown adipose tissue mitochondria and the uncoupling protein. Am J Physiol 255:E865, 1988

137. Trayhurn P, Nicholls DG (eds): Brown Adipose Tissue. London, Edward Arnold, 1986

138. Wade GN, Bartness TJ, Hamilton JM: Seasonal changes in body weight and brown adipose tissue in hamsters: Role of photoperiod and diet. In Lardy H, Stratman F (eds): Hormones, Thermogenesis and Obesity, pp 137–147. Proceedings of the 18th Steenbock Symposium. New York, Elsevier, 1989

139. Wilson S, Thurlby PL, Arch JRS: Substrate supply for thermogenesis induced by the β-adrenoceptor agonist BRL 26830A. Can J Physiol Pharmacol 65:113, 1987

140. Wu SY, Stern JS, Fisher DA et al: Cold induced increase in brown fat thyroxine 5'-monodeiodinase is attenuated in Zucker obese rat. Am J Physiol 252:E63, 1987

141. Yoshida T, Nishioka H, Nakamura Y et al: Reduced noradrenaline turnover in streptozotocin-induced diabetic rats. Diabetologia 28:692, 1985

PART TWO

ASSESSMENT OF BODY COMPOSITION

CHAPTER 3

Assessment of Body Composition: An Overview

STEVEN B. HEYMSFIELD, STEVEN LICHTMAN,
RICHARD N. BAUMGARTNER, F. AVRAHAM DILMANIAN,
and YAKOV KAMEN

Human tissues are composed of four major chemical species: water, protein, mineral, and lipid. Distributed in various proportions depending on cell type, these building blocks form the container and medium in which life processes are carried out. This overview focuses on the general concepts related to the study of human body composition.

CHEMICAL COMPONENTS

Water

Water constitutes the largest fraction of body weight.[1] As the primary solvent within tissues, water distribution can be partitioned into five categories (Table 3-1). The largest subcompartments of total body water (TBW) are found within cells (55%) and in the interstitial space (20%). Water binds to a varying extent with tissue proteins, glycogen, bone mineral, and other chemical compounds.

The amounts and distribution of water in the body are most commonly measured by the dilution of water isotopes and other substances that distribute differentially among the body water spaces. Bioelectric impedance, which is influenced by the concentration of electrolytes within water spaces, is a new method that is being explored.[2]

Protein

Proteins, which total 4 to 15 kg in healthy adults, are distributed in both the extracellular and intracellular compartments.[3] The major proteins consist of structural collagen in connective tissue and contractile actomyosin in muscle. Proteins undergo turnover at a total rate of about 0.3 kg/day, with half-lives differing markedly between protein species.[4]

There are no direct methods of measuring protein *in vivo*. At present the most suitable technique is to estimate total body nitrogen (TBN) by use of prompt-γ-neutron activation (PGNA) analysis.[5] In this regard, two assumptions are generally made—that TBN is almost entirely in the form of protein and that protein is 16% nitrogen. These assumptions are valid under most conditions, and the neutron activation approach is widely accepted.

A typical PGNA system is shown in Figure 3-1. Developed by Vartsky and his colleagues,[5] the present system uses 77 Ci of ^{238}PuBe as a neutron source. The neutron energy ranges between 0 and 11 MeV, with an average energy of 4.5 MeV. Because the reaction $^{14}N(n, \gamma)$ ^{15}N occurs chiefly with thermal neutrons, a 5-cm-thick heavy water (D_2O) moderator is used to slow neutrons as they emerge from the isotopic source. Two 15.24 × 15.24-cm NaI (Tl) crystals detect the 10.83-MeV and 2.23-MeV prompt (10^{-15}s) γ-rays from nitro-

TABLE 3-1

Distribution of Total Body Water

Intracellular fluid		55%
Extracellular fluid		45%
Plasma	7.5%	
Interstitial lymph	20.0%	
Transcellular	2.5%	
Dense connective tissue, cartilage, and bone	15.0%	
Total		100%

(From Edelman IS, Leibman J: Anatomy of body water and electrolytes. Am J Med 27:260, 1959)

gen and hydrogen, respectively. Hydrogen is then used as an internal standard, which allows calculation of absolute TBN. A patient's actual total body hydrogen is estimated based on an algorithm that includes the measured tritiated water dilution space.

Minerals

Eight tissue mineral fractions are present in amounts greater than 1 g (Table 3-2). These minerals are distributed between bone and soft tissues (Tables 3-3 and 3-4). The soft-tissue minerals are further partitioned into the extracellular and intracellular compartments (Table 3-5).

The osseous component of mineral is composed almost entirely of calcium hydroxyapatite $[Ca_{10}(PO_4)_6OH_2]$, which contributes to about 55% of skeletal weight (Fig. 3-2).[9] The remainder of bone mass is protein (organic + CO_2 fraction,

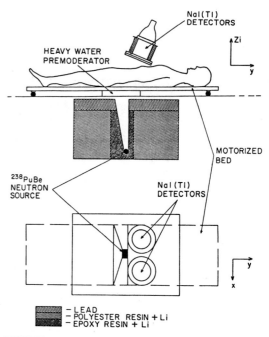

FIGURE 3-1

Brookhaven National Laboratory PGNA facility for total body nitrogen and hydrogen. Patient is scanned over a collimated neutron beam from a 77 Ci of $^{238}PuBe$. (Vartsky D, Ellis KJ, John SH: In vivo measurement of body nitrogen by analysis of prompt gamma ray analysis from neutron capture. J Nucl Med 20:1158, 1979)

TABLE 3-2

Minerals Present in Amounts Greater Than 1 g

Mineral	Amount (g)*	Major Distribution
Calcium (Ca^{++})	1000	Bone mineral
Phosphorus ($P^=$)	580	Bone mineral, body cell mass
Potassium (K^+)	140	Body cell mass
Sodium (Na^+)	100	Extracellular fluid, bone mineral
Chloride (Cl^-)	95	Extracellular fluid
Magnesium (Mg^{++})	19	Bone mineral, body cell mass
Iron (Fe^{++})	4.2	Hematopoietic system
Zinc (Zn^{++})	2.3	Soft fat-free tissues

*Based on 70-kg reference man.[6]

TABLE 3-3

Composition and Chemical Properties of Bone Mineral (g/100 g)

Calcium (Ca^{++})	34.1
Phosphorus ($PO_4^{=}$)	48.3
Sodium (Na^+)	0.9
Chloride (Cl^-)	*
Magnesium (Mg^{++})	0.6
Potassium (K^+)	*
Carbonate ($CO_3^{=}$)	7.4
Crystallization H_2O	3.6
Unaccounted	5.1
Density	2.982 g/ml

*Amounts of K and Cl in bone mineral are variable and small in quantity.

(From Brozek J, Grande F, Anderson JT et al: Densitometric analysis of body composition: Revision of some quantitative assumptions. Ann NY Acad Sci 110:113, 1963)

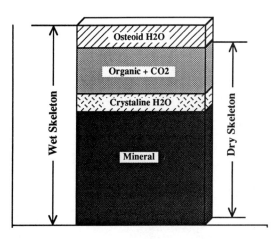

FIGURE 3-2

Composition of representative human bone. (From Heymsfield SB, Wang J, Funfar J et al: Dual photon absorptiometry: Accuracy of bone mineral and soft tissue mass measurement *in vivo*. Am J Clin Nutr 49:1283, 1953)

25.2%) and to a lesser extent osteoid and crystalline water (12.5%). Because of the ion exchange properties of bone, sodium, magnesium, and small amounts of other elements are tightly bound to the crystalline matrix (see Table 3-3).

Heating fresh bone at different specific temperatures results in fractions relevant to the study of body composition. Bone ash is the mineral portion that remains after prolonged heating (>24 hours) at temperatures greater than 500°C. Total bone mineral, which includes additional components such as crystalline water and carbonate, is 4% to 7% higher in mass than total bone ash.[7]

TABLE 3-4

Distribution of Total Body Mineral (g) into Osseous and Soft-tissue Components*

	Osseous	Soft Tissue	Total
Calcium (Ca^{++})	1000	†	1000
Phosphorus ($P^{=}$)	500	80	580
Potassium (K^+)	†	140	140
Sodium (Na^+)	27.5	72.5	100
Chloride (Cl^-)	†	95	95
Magnesium (Mg^{++})	16.2	4.7	20.9
Iron (Fe^{++})	†	4.2	4.2
Zinc (Zn^{++})	†	2.3	2.3

*Estimates based on 70-kg reference man.
†Not present in appreciable or consistent amounts.

(From Report of the Task Group on Reference Man: Int Comm Radiol Protection Report No 23. New York, Pergamon Press, 1975. Brozek J, Grande F, Anderson JT et al: Densitometric analysis of body composition: Revision of some quantitative assumptions. Ann NY Acad Sci 110:113, 1963)

TABLE 3-5

Electrolyte Concentration (mEq/kg) of Human Extracellular and Intracellular Fluids

	Extracellular Fluid		Intracellular Fluid
	Plasma	*Interstitial*	
Cation			
Na$^+$	150	144	5–10
K$^+$	4–5	4–5	150–160
Mg^{++}	2	1.5	25–35
Ca^{++}	5	3	3–5
H$^+$	4×10^{-5}	4×10^{-5}	1×10^{-4}
Total	161	153	
Anion			
Cl$^-$	110	114	5–10
HCO$_3^-$	27	28	10
HPO$_4^=$, H$_2$PO$_4^-$	2	2	
SO$_4^=$	1	1	
Proteinate	17	4	
Organic acids	4	4	
Total	161	153	

(From Maffly RH: The body fluids: volume, composition, and physical chemistry. In Brenner BM, Rector FC [eds]: The Kidney. Philadelphia, WB Saunders, 1976)

There are two primary approaches to estimating bone mineral mass *in vivo*. The first involves neutron activation analysis for total body calcium, because more than 99% of this divalent cation is within the mineral matrix of bone.[6] A typical system that uses a radioactive neutron source is the one described by Cohn.[10] The subject is first exposed bilaterally to an array of 14 50 Ci encapsulated ^{238}PuBe sources for 5 minutes (Fig. 3-3A). The subject is then removed from the irradiation facility and transported to the whole body counter (Fig. 3-3B). The decay products are then counted for 15 minutes, and results can be used to calculate total body calcium in grams. Because calcium occurs in a relatively fixed ratio to total bone mineral,[9] the measured amount of element can be easily converted to estimated bone ash or osseous mineral.[11]

The second method of evaluating bone mineral mass is dual photon absorptiometry, either through use of an isotope or dual energy x-ray (DEXA) source.[6,12,13] In both systems, the source provides photons at two discrete energy levels (approximately 40 to 44 and 70 to 100 keV). The photons are attenuated as they pass through soft and hard (skeletal) tissues, and the unattenuated radiation is recorded by the system's detectors.

A representative dual photon scanning system is illustrated in Figure 3-4.[12] A radioactive source emits photons, which are then collimated into a narrow beam that is turned on and off by a shutter. The collimated beam penetrates through the subject's soft tissues and bone and then continues upward and enters a photon detector. The system's components are mechanically connected to scan the photon beam across the subject's body. The transmitted single-energy photon beam intensity over soft tissue and bone is shown in Figure 3-4. Bone mineral content and soft-tissue mass are calculated from the attenuation of the two photon energies by solving a linear system of two simultaneous equations.

Both the neutron activation and dual energy methods of evaluating osseous mineral have been validated in phantoms, isolated skeletons, and intact cadavers.[6,12,14]

Minerals present in amounts greater than about 1 g can be estimated *in vivo* by the use of several different methods. Sodium, chloride, and phosphorus can be measured by delayed γ-neu-

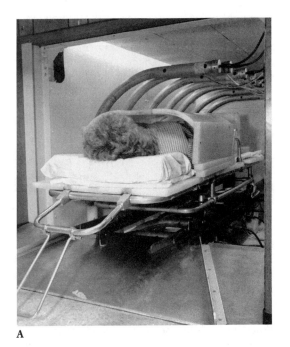

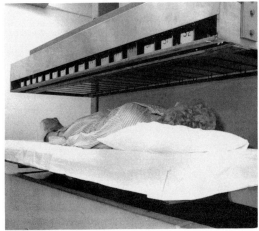

A   B

FIGURE 3-3

Total body neutron irradiator of the PGNA system at Brookhaven National
Laboratory. The system is used to measure total body calcium, phosphorus,
sodium, and chloride. **A:** The patient is placed as shown between upper and
lower source guide tubes, which are used to position 14 50-Ci sources of
^{238}PuBe. **B:** The induced activity is measured in the whole body counter.
(Cohn SH: Noninvasive techniques for measuring body elemental composition.
Biol Trace Elem Res 13:179, 1987)

tron activation methods in a system such as that
depicted in Figure 3-3. A portion of total body
sodium (approximately 80%), the exchangeable
fraction, can be estimated by administration of
the isotopes ^{22}Na ($t_{1/2}$ = 2.6 years, 1.275 MeV
γ-ray, 0.55 MeV β-ray) and ^{24}Na ($t_{1/2}$ = 15 hours,
1.37 and 2.75 MeV γ-ray, 1.39 MeV β-ray).[15] The
sodium contents of bone mineral and dense connective tissue are considered nonexchangeable.

Total body potassium (TBK) is measurable either by whole body counting[10] or by isotope dilution.[16,17] Potassium occurs naturally in three isotopic forms, ^{39}K (93.3%), ^{40}K (0.0117%), and ^{41}K
(6.7%). The isotope ^{40}K is radioactive ($t_{1/2}$ = 1.28
× 10^9 years), emitting a 1.46-MeV γ-photon in
its decay.[15] Detection and quantification are accomplished in a whole body counter. The general features of a good whole body counter are
adequate shielding from extrinsic sources of ra-

diation, γ-ray detectors with high energy resolution and high sensitivity, and data acquisition
and data processing systems. There are several
types of whole body counters, and these are reviewed in detail by Forbes and colleagues.[15] A
representative system used at Brookhaven National Laboratory is shown in Figure 3-3B. The
whole body counter is located within a very low
background chamber surrounded by 4 feet of
concrete, 4 inches of pre–World War II steel, $^1/_8$
inch of lead, and $^1/_{16}$ inch of aluminum. Sixteen
NaI detectors are positioned above and another
16 below the subject. Three ^{137}Cs sheets located
beneath the bed are used to provide a correction
in measured counts for the attenuation of γ-rays
in patients who differ in body size.

Another approach to estimating TBK is whole
body dilution of the radioactive isotope ^{42}K ($t_{1/2}$
= 12.4 hours, 1.52 MeV γ-ray, 3.5 MeV β-ray).

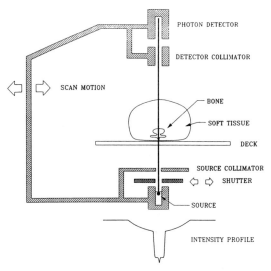

PHOTON DETECTOR

DETECTOR COLLIMATOR

SCAN MOTION

BONE

SOFT TISSUE

DECK

SOURCE COLLIMATOR

SHUTTER

SOURCE

INTENSITY PROFILE

FIGURE 3-4

A typical dual photon absorptiometry scanner show-ing essential components. Photon beam intensity for a single line scan is shown at the bottom. (Nord RH: Technical considerations in DPA. In Genant HK [ed]: Osteoporosis Update 1987.)

Although early body composition studies used ^{42}K to estimate the exchangeable potassium (K_e) pool,[17] the isotope is rarely used today because of its high energy β emission and its short half-life of 12.4 hours.

Although of great interest in other areas of clin-ical medicine, the minerals magnesium, iron, and zinc are not usually considered in relation to body composition and obesity.

Residual Fat-free Components

TBW, protein, and minerals (calcium, phospho-rus, potassium, sodium, and chloride) combined account for about 98% of nonlipid body mass. One half of the remaining chemical components consists of glycogen, the largely intracellular car-bohydrate fuel source. The body of a healthy adult contains 300 to 700 g of glycogen,[18] distrib-uted largely in the cytoplasm of skeletal muscle and liver. With fasting in one extreme and carbo-hydrate overfeeding in the other, total body gly-cogen can range between 100 and 1200 g.[18] Be-cause no established method of measuring whole body glycogen *in vivo* is available, most investi-

gators either ignore glycogen in their body com-position models or estimate total body glycogen to be about 1% of fat-free body mass (FFM).[19] Although other approaches are available, all share the potential for large errors.

The remaining 1% of FFM consists of unmeas-ured minerals and many other chemical com-pounds that occur in total body quantities of a few grams or less.

Fat

Fat represents the ether-soluble organic fraction of body weight. Largely in the form of triglycer-ide, fat is the body's primary source of stored fuel. There are four general approaches to es-timating total body fat: lipid-soluble gases; x-ray, magnetic resonance, and sound wave im-aging; body composition models; and prediction methods.

Fat-Soluble Gases

Both lipid-soluble gases and visualization meth-ods share direct analysis of the fat compartment. The gases cyclopropane, krypton, and xenon dis-solve in fat to a greater extent than in fat-free tissues.[15] For example, the fat-lean partition coef-ficient for cyclopropane is 34. When subjects are exposed to a fat-soluble gas either in a chamber or through a face mask, the rate of gas uptake is determined largely by total body fat. This ap-proach is currently of limited applicability be-cause of the long measurement intervals and the highly sensitive whole body counter needed for analysis of gas uptake curves.

X-ray, Magnetic Resonance, and Sound Wave Imaging

Direct visualization and quantification of fat are possible through application of electromagnetic or sound waves. These methods have in common the differing response between tissues interact-ing with electromagnetic waves (e.g., x-rays in computerized tomography [CT], radio frequency in magnetic resonance imaging [MRI] or sound waves in sonography). A selected region of the body is usually studied, although whole body analysis is possible in some cases.

The current radiographic technique of choice for direct visualization of fat is CT.[20] This method offers high image contrast and clear sep-

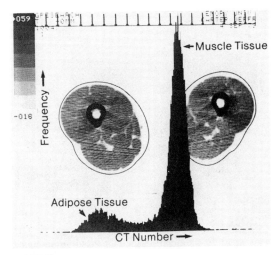

FIGURE 3-5

Cross-sectional CT image of the midthigh in a healthy subject and a histogram of the image pixels. (Heymsfield SB: Human body composition: Analysis by computerized axial tomography and nuclear magnetic resonance. AIN Symposium Proceedings. American Institute of Nutrition, 1987)

aration of fat from other soft tissues. As x-rays produced by an x-ray tube (0.1 to 0.2 A, 60 to 120 kVp) pass through tissue, they undergo attenuation as a result of coherent and incoherent scattering, photoelectric absorption, and Compton interactions.[20] The main determinants of these effects are atomic number, physical density, as well as mass electron density. The x-ray beam attenuation is quantitatively expressed as the CT number, which is calibrated relative to water (zero). Adipose tissue and skeletal muscle have average respective CT numbers of -70 and $+20$, expressed in Hounsfield units, in which air is -1000. The differing attenuation of adipose tissue and lean allows either visual or mathematical separation of image components. An example is presented in Figure 3-5, a cross-sectional image of the lower extremities in a young, healthy male. The adipose tissue, which is largely subcutaneous, can be isolated from muscle by means of an operator-directed cursor. Computer software then permits a delineation of adipose tissue area or a graphic display of total picture elements (pixels).[21] With the latter method, appropriate statistical techniques allow

quantitative estimates of the amount of adipose tissue, muscle, and bone by counting the pixels in each category.

Sequential scanning and the application of appropriate summing methods allow estimation of total body adipose tissue volume.[22] Alternatively, regional, subcutaneous, visceral, or other specific adipose tissue depots can be identified. Radiation exposure, expense, and unavailability restrict the epidemiologic use of CT.

A point worthy of emphasis is that CT adipose tissue represents a combination of intracellular stored triacylglycerol and adipocyte elements because of the overlap of lipid and cellular constituents within individual pixels, resulting in a weighted CT number that reflects this mixture. In contrast to this method, most other body composition techniques estimate fat, which chemically represents ether-extractable lipid. When adipose tissue derived by CT is subtracted from body weight, the remainder is referred to as *lean* or *adipose tissue-free body mass*.[22] In contrast, body weight minus fat results in the compartment termed *fat-free body mass*. A final point related to CT is that raw results are usually reported as the compartmental volumes. The volume estimate can be used directly in the study or converted to mass by assuming an average tissue density *in vivo*.[20-22]

Nuclear magnetic resonance (NMR), as with x-rays, can be used to compose MRI images.[20] Additionally, NMR is capable of spectral identification of tissue chemical compounds. This area of study is termed *NMR spectroscopy.*

The basic principle of NMR involves dipolar nuclei such as ^1H, ^{31}P, ^{13}C, and ^{23}Na. These nuclei have angular momentums or spins with dipole momentums arising from their inherent properties.[20] Because these nuclei are electrically charged, the spin generates a magnetic dipole. When placed in a magnetic field, these nuclei orient themselves parallel or antiparallel to the field's lines of induction. A resonant radio-frequency pulse can then be used to rotate these nuclei 90° with respect to the magnetic field. Equilibrium is restored through relaxation after the radio-frequency signal is discontinued. The absorbed energy is dissipated into the surrounding environment (lattice). In clinical instruments, a graded external magnetic field is applied while the subject is surrounded by a coil that carries a 5- to 30-mm wavelength (60 to 110 MHz) radio-frequency signal. The signal generated when nuclei relax is collected by the NMR receiver and stored for further analysis. These data are subsequently used to reconstruct the image and to evaluate body composition. At present, imaging is limited mainly to hydrogen protons (^{1}H) and to a lesser extent phosphorus (^{31}P) and sodium (^{23}Na).

The sharp image contrast of MRI allows clear separation of adipose tissue from surrounding nonlipid structures. Essentially the same information provided by CT is available from MRI, including total body and regional adipose tissue, subcutaneous adipose tissue, and estimates of various visceral adipose tissue components. The advantage of MRI is its lack of ionizing radiation and hence its presumed safety in children, younger adults, and pregnant women. The minimal present use of MRI in the study of human body composition can be attributed to the expense, limited access to instrumentation, and long scanning times (45 minutes for a limited body region) of this relatively new method.

NMR spectroscopy is a major new tool in the study of living organisms.[21] Initial studies of animals indicate the potential of NMR to accurately quantify tissue water[23] and other chemical components relevant to the study of body composition.[24,25] Studies using NMR spectroscopy in humans have been limited, although more research undoubtedly will follow.

Body Composition Models

Indirect estimates of fat and other compartments are made by use of body composition models. The term *model* is applied loosely to a given strategy, usually based on one or more assumptions, aimed at partitioning body weight into physiologically relevant compartments. Although there are many body composition models, four are relevant to this discussion.

The primary model is an elemental reconstruction of body weight. Eleven elements account for more than 99.5% of body mass (Fig. 3-6), with six (oxygen, carbon, hydrogen, nitrogen, calcium, phosphorus) representing 99% of all tissue chemical constituents.[6] An elemental reconstruction of body weight is now possible in living human subjects by combining neutron activation

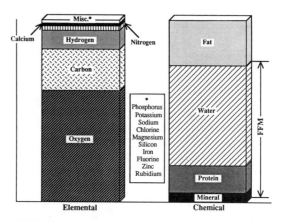

FIGURE 3-6

Human body composition models based on elemental (*left*) or chemical (*right*) models.

and other methodologies. Methods of measuring elements *in vivo* were described earlier. Total body hydrogen can be obtained from a prompt-γ measurement using a specially designed system.

The most recent addition to elemental analysis *in vivo* is quantification of total body carbon by inelastic neutron scattering. Because of the high carbon content of triglyceride, total body carbon measurements can provide a more direct evaluation of body fat in both normal and obese persons.[26-28] Total body carbon can be measured *in vivo* based on the reaction $C^{12}(n, n' \gamma)C^{12}$ by detecting the 4.44-MeV γ-rays resulting from inelastic scattering of fast neutrons by carbon nuclei.[27] Because the threshold energy for this reaction is 4.8 MeV, it cannot be accomplished using a standard source such as PuBe, which has an average energy of 4.5 MeV. A miniature 14-MeV generator is used in the Brookhaven National Laboratory system for this purpose (Fig. 3-7). Two (15.24 × 15.24 cm) NaI detect the 4.44-MeV γ-rays resulting from the inelastic neutron scattering reaction.

The chemical model divides body weight into five compartments: fat, protein, glycogen, water, and mineral (see Fig. 3-6). Mineral is usually further divided into osseous and nonosseous components, particularly in autopsy studies. The simplified chemical model is based on two compartments: fat and FFM (water + protein + mineral). The chemical model is fundamental to the study of human body composition, and much

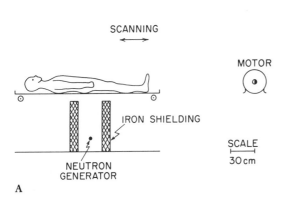

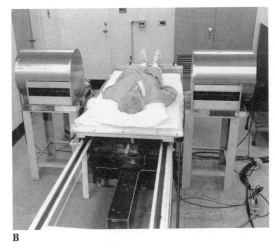

A　　　　　　　　　　　　　　　　**B**

FIGURE 3-7

The INS facility at Brookhaven National Laboratory. **A:** The neutron generator is positioned beneath a scanning bed. An iron shield, surrounded by a sheet of cadmium that absorbs thermal neutrons, provides a rectangular beam (61 × 4.8 cm) at the level of the bed. The bed is driven by a motor, with the shoulder-to-knee scan requiring about 15 minutes. **B:** The 4.44-MeV gamma rays resulting from the reaction $C^{12} (\eta,\eta'\gamma)C^{12}$ are recorded by two NaI detectors positioned laterally to the patient.

of the present knowledge of body fat and lean tissues is based either directly or indirectly on this approach.

Although early workers were limited to chemical analysis of cadavers,[7] the four major compartments can now be quantified *in vivo.* A representative approach is to estimate TBW by isotope dilution and to determine protein through measurement of TBN.[11] Whole body glycogen, which is highly variable and currently unmeasurable, is estimated. Minerals are quantified by neutron activation or dual energy techniques, and fat is estimated by carbon corrected for nonlipid sources of the element.[28] The growing capability of estimating chemical composition *in vivo* is revolutionizing the study of human body composition.

Three simplified two-compartment models are based on the classic chemical model and are widely applied in obesity research. The first model assumes that TBW is a fixed fraction (K) of FFM,[29] or

$$K = \frac{TBW}{FFM} \qquad (1)$$

Human cadaver and animal carcass analyses indicate that K averages 0.732.[30] The approach in humans is to measure an isotopic water dilution space and then correct the resulting volume for the overestimate related to hydrogen exchange. For D_2O and ^3H_2O, the volume overestimate is between 3% and 6%, whereas for H_2O_{18}, the dilution space overestimate is about 0.5%. Once TBW volume is known and it is assumed that K = 0.732, then

$$FFM = \frac{TBW}{0.732} \qquad (2)$$

and fat is the difference between body weight and FFM.

The second two-compartment model is based on TBK, which is entirely within FFM. As for the TBW method, this approach assumes that

$$C = \frac{TBK}{FFM} \qquad (3)$$

where C is the average potassium content of FFM. The potassium content of FFM is known from cadaver or *in vivo* studies.[15,29] For example, C for a 40-year-old man is 68.1 mmol/kg. Measurement of ^{40}K in a whole body counter then allows calculation of FFM as

$$\text{FFM} = \frac{\text{TBK}}{C} \qquad (4)$$

Total body fat is again considered the difference between body weight and FFM.

The third two-compartment chemical model is based on the assumed constant density of fat (0.900 g/ml) and FFM (1.100 g/ml). Extracted human lipid was used to develop the reference fat density, whereas chemically analyzed cadavers were used to estimate the fat-free density.[7] According to this model, body density (D) varies inversely as a function (f) of the fraction of body weight as fat (F):

$$D = f\frac{1}{F} \quad \text{or} \quad F = f\frac{1}{D} \qquad (5)$$

Alternatively, the specific volume of the body (1/D) can be considered the sum of the specific volumes of each of the primary components, such that

$$\frac{1}{D} = \frac{F}{d_F} + \frac{\text{FFM}}{d_{\text{FFM}}} \qquad (6)$$

where FFM is the fraction of body weight as fat-free mass. Given the reference densities for fat (d_f) and FFM (d_{FFM}), the solution for F (fraction of body weight as fat) in equation 6 becomes

$$F = 4.95\frac{1}{D} - 4.50 \qquad (7)$$

Body density can be measured in human subjects by several methods, although the most widely accepted and practical is hydrodensitometry. The subject's whole body density is calculated after appropriate corrections for water temperature and residual lung volume.[31]

Although the two-compartment hydrodensitometry model is well accepted, the assumption that water, protein, and mineral occur in constant proportions ($D = 1.100$ g/ml) in all subjects is acknowledged as an oversimplification. This assumption is considered to be invalid, especially in children,[32] who are chemically immature, in the elderly,[29] and in some patients with underlying disease. A three-compartment model, which includes an estimate of TBW, partitions

body weight into fat, water, and fat-free solids. Fat can be calculated in this approach[32] as

$$F = 2.118\frac{1}{D} - 0.780\,\text{TBW} - 1.354 \qquad (8)$$

In a four-compartment hydrodensitometry model,[33] the FFM is further subdivided into protein and mineral such that

$$\frac{1}{D} = \frac{F}{d_F} + \frac{\text{TBW}}{d\text{H}_2\text{O}_W} + \frac{M}{d_M} + \frac{P}{d_P} \qquad (9)$$

This model now accounts for all of the major chemical components of body weight presented in Figure 3-6. Because mineral may be more variable than protein, it is usually estimated from dual photon absorptiometry, and ($1 - F + W + M$) is substituted for P. The equation is then solved for F, assuming appropriate values for d_F, d_W, and d_M.

The third category of body composition models aims to derive fat and other compartments based on fluid and metabolic considerations. Fat, body cell mass, extracellular fluid (ECF), and extracellular solids are considered in this approach (Fig. 3-8).[17] Body cell mass represents the metabolically active tissue compartment and is assumed to have a hydration of 75% and an intracellular potassium concentration of 150 mEq/

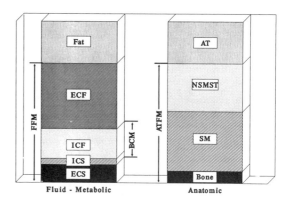

FIGURE 3-8

Human body composition models based on fluid-metabolic (*left*) and anatomical (*right*) models. (AT, adipose tissue; BCM, body cell mass; ECF and ECS, extracellular fluid and solids; FFM, fat-free body mass; ICF and ICS, intracellular fluid and solids; NSMST, nonskeletal muscle soft tissue; SM, skeletal muscle)

liter (Table 3-5). Because more than 99% of TBK is intracellular, estimation of potassium then allows calculation of intracellular fluid (ICF) volume and body cell mass.[17] The classic approach is to measure K_e using ^{42}K, but modern investigators prefer to estimate TBK based on whole body ^{40}K counting. In the absence of a whole body counter, K_e can be calculated from exchangeable sodium (Na_e) using the isotope ^{22}Na.[34] This method relies on the assumption that in normal individuals the ratio of sodium plus potassium to water is constant in all soft tissues. Accordingly,

$$K = \frac{Na_e + K_e}{TBW} \qquad (10)$$

and

$$K_e = (K)H_2O - Na_e \qquad (11)$$

The tritiated water dilution space is used to estimate TBW, and K_e is calculated as the whole blood level of potassium plus sodium divided by water.

ECF volume in the fluid-metabolic model is calculated as the difference between TBW and ICF volume. ECF can be estimated from the dilution space of bromide, sulfate, or other compounds[8] or by direct measurement of total body chloride using neutron activation analysis. Extracellular solids can be estimated from body weight, total body calcium (neutron activation),[35] or total body bone mineral (dual photon absorptiometry). FFM is then equal to the sum of body cell mass plus ECF plus extracellular solids, and fat is the difference between body weight and FFM. Thus, the fluid metabolic model can be approached using a combination of many different body composition methodologies.

The last model is based on the anatomical makeup of FFM as skeletal muscle, nonskeletal muscle or visceral soft tissues, and osseous mineral. Subjects evaluated using this model require measurement of TBN, potassium, calcium, and water.[35,36] Calcium and water are used to quantify FFM and fat as described earlier. Because the ratio of potassium to nitrogen differs between skeletal muscle and viscera, the proportion of FFM as skeletal muscle can be calculated using models based on direct tissue measurements *in vivo* or cadaver analyses.

Another approach to the anatomical model is to use CT scans at predefined intervals and then to integrate results for estimating adipose tissue, skeletal muscle, nonskeletal muscle soft tissue, and bone (see Fig. 3-8).[20-22] The CT approach also allows estimation of organ volumes[20] and examination of fat distribution.[20-22]

In vivo multicompartment analysis has expanded greatly during the past decade owing to advances in body composition technology. The four approaches presented illustrate the wide variety of techniques now available to investigators. All of these models have been used to study obesity in humans, and their clinical application is described in a later section.

Prediction Methods

The last approach to be considered estimates fat and other body compartments based on statistical techniques. These include anthropometry, bioelectric impedance, and total body conductivity.

Body circumferences, diameters, and subcutaneous fat thicknesses measured respectively with a flexible tape, blade calipers, and skin-fold calipers form the bases of anthropometry.[37] A close correlation exists between some of these anthropometric measures and body composition estimated by the methods described earlier. Therefore, predictions of body composition can be developed that relate anthropometric measurements to fat or FFM. A number of such equations are available, and several widely used ones are described elsewhere.[37-39] Anthropometry is also useful for quantifying fat distribution and frame size.

Bioelectric impedance and total body electrical conductivity methods rely on the association between body conductivity and tissue fluid and electrolyte content. The bioimpedance analysis (BIA) technique is reviewed in detail. Briefly, this method is based on the frequency-dependent impedance to the application of a high-frequency, low-amplitude alternating electrical current of biologic tissues. At low frequencies (1 to 5 kHz), the current passes primarily through ECF, but at frequencies equal to or greater than 50 kHz, the current passes through both ICF and ECF. Because of the high resistance of fat, the current is mostly conducted through the fat-free tissues. In general, the approach is to fasten electrodes at predefined anatomical sites and then to measure electrical resistance (e.g., 1/conductance) as an excitation current is introduced into the subject. From electrical theory, the resistance is proportional to the length/area of the conductor, or $R = PL/A$. Using simple algebra, the volume of the conductor can be derived as $V = PL^2/R$. The parameter P is estimated by regression of TBW, FFM, or L^2/R, where stature is used as an index of L. Alternatively, R may be used directly in equations including various anthropometric measurements. Reactance, or the reciprocal of capacitance produced in small amounts by cell membranes, may be considered also.

The total body electrical conductivity (TOBEC) technique is also based on the differences in electrical properties of fat and fat-free tissues.[40] The measurement chamber of the TOBEC instrument consists of a large cylindrical coil. An alternating electrical current is generated in the coil, inducing an electromagnetic field in the measurement chamber. A meter coupled to the system measures the change in coil impedance as the subject passes through the instrument's core. The change in impedance is related to the dielectric and conductive properties of the body, and as for BIA prediction, equations for water and FFM can be developed. In both BIA and TOBEC techniques, fat mass is usually derived as the difference between body weight and estimated FFM.[41]

The prediction methods thus have in common the incorporation of a measurable somatic physical property into a body composition prediction equation.

BODY COMPOSITION IN OBESITY

Chapters throughout the remainder of this book describe obesity and its linkages to body composition. A brief overview presented here organizes the previous discussion of human body composition in relation to obesity.

Excess accumulation of adipose tissue is the hallmark of obesity. Adipose tissue is divided into two major components, one extracellular and the other intracellular. The extracellular compartment includes fluid and electrolytes, collagen and other structural proteins, and blood vessels. The primary cellular component of adipose tissue is the adipocyte, which varies in size and number between individuals and with dif-

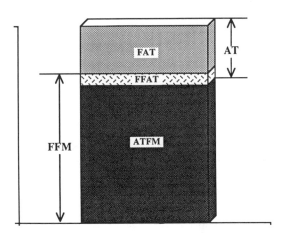

FIGURE 3-9

The two components of fat-free body, fat-free adipose tissue (FFAT), and adipose tissue free mass (ATFM). Adipose tissue (AT) = FFAT + FAT, and fat-free body mass (FFM) = FFAT + ATFM. The compartment proportions depicted in the figure are based on references 42–44.

ferent degrees of obesity. The intracellular compartment of adipose tissue consists of fluid, protein, and stored triglyceride.

In theory, fat-free adipose tissue has a chemical composition similar to that of other organs within FFM. Unfortunately, not much information is available on adipose tissue composition in very lean human subjects. As the adipocyte fills with triglyceride and more cells are formed, the overall compartmental proportions appear similar in normal weight and in obese subjects.[42,43] The limited information available allows reconstruction of a representative model of adipose tissue. About 80% of the total tissue weight is ether-extractable lipid, with the remainder fat-free adipose tissue (Fig. 3-9). The cell mass component of fat-free adipose tissue is relatively small, with ICF accounting for about 3% of excised adipose tissue weight. The extracellular space is three to four times larger, representing 12% of tissue mass. Hence, on average, adipose tissue is 80% lipid and 15% water (3% ICF + 12% ECF), and the remaining 5% is mainly protein.

Most body composition models as described earlier are based on estimates of fat rather than adipose tissue. Hence the nonlipid portion of adipose tissue is included in the FFM (see Fig. 3-9). In normal-weight individuals, the ECF compartment represents about 40% to 50% of TBW. Because the ratio of ECF to ICF is very high in adipose tissue (3 to 4:1), it would appear that obese subjects would have a higher proportion of total FFM as ECF. This issue remains unresolved, however, because studies indicate that FFM in obese subjects is either unchanged in compartmental proportions or relatively high in ECF compared with normal-weight controls.[42-44]

With severe obesity, many patients have clinically evident edema, which is secondary to venous stasis, congestive heart failure, and respiratory insufficiency. In addition to being technically difficult to study, as will be described in the next section, the traditional two-compartment body composition models are not applicable in severely obese subjects with clearly altered hydration. Not only is the ratio of TBW/FFM different from the assumed 0.73 (equation 2), but the K/FFM (equation 4) and density of FFM (equation 7) are altered from the constants developed in normal-weight subjects and on which the models are based. Similarly, calibration methods for estimating fat, which are usually referenced to fat derived by two-compartment methods, are inaccurate in the presence of edema.

The expanded FFM of obesity is in part related to the addition of fat-free adipose tissue. Cardiac and other organ hypertrophy,[45] an enlarged skeletal muscle mass, and an increased skeletal weight also contribute.[46] The result is that obese subjects have more TBW,[47] protein content,[46] and mineral mass[46] than their normal-weight counterparts.

The increase in FFM with accumulation of adipose tissue occurs in a systematic manner. Although complex mathematical functions may ultimately best describe these interrelations,[48] the generalization suggested by Webster and colleagues[49] provides useful guidelines for evaluating patients. Assume first that a hypothetical FFM exists devoid of adipose tissue fat. As fat mass then increases, there also occurs a corresponding enlargement of FFM. The combined fat and FFM are considered by Webster as excess body weight, which by regression analysis has a composition of about three fourths fat and one fourth lean. Although clearly an oversimplifica-

tion, this concept is useful in roughly estimating the composition of excess body weight (three parts fat to one part lean) and in providing guidelines for the composition of weight loss during dieting.

MEASUREMENT LIMITATIONS AND ERRORS

The following discussion provides a general overview of the limitations of body composition measurement methods.[1] Three categories of limitations are discussed: technical constraints of equipment, measurement reliability, and accuracy. Reliability is defined as the extent to which a measurement is reproducible.[50] Accuracy is a somewhat different concept and refers to the extent to which a measurement corresponds to a "true" value, or has "validity." The distinction between the two relates to the types of errors considered. In general, there are two types of errors: random and systematic. In the assessment of reliability, all errors are considered random. According to statistical theory, if all errors are random, the mean of a series of repeated measurements will approximate the "true" value. Reliability, therefore, considers the variation among the repeated measurements relative to their mean. For a sample of subjects, reliability considers the variation among repeated measurements within subjects relative to the variation between subjects. Accuracy also considers systematic errors. When systematic errors occur, the mean of a series of repeated measurements will not approximate the "true" value. The assessment of accuracy implicitly requires comparison of the values provided by a "test" method with those provided by some gold standard assumed to provide "true" values. In body composition analysis, the assessment of accuracy is hampered by the fact that there are no direct methods of exactly quantifying the primary variables of interest, the fat and FFM. The theory and mathematical principles of assessing accuracy and reliability have been described in detail by Fleiss,[51] and the application of these to anthropometry is discussed by Mueller and Martorell.[50]

Technical Limitations

The designs of many current methods of assessing body composition do not permit measurement of severely obese individuals. Patients heavier than 110 to 130 kg are simply too large to be accommodated in dual photon absorptiometry, TOBEC, CT, or MRI scanners. Obese individuals may have skin folds that are thicker than the 40- to 60-mm limits of currently available calipers. Special weight scales may be needed, and two or more observers may need to work together to obtain skin-fold and circumference measurements.

Many methods are difficult to apply to bed- or chair-fast elderly, handicapped, or ill patients. For example, stature cannot be measured in persons who are unable to stand and must be estimated from segment lengths. Edema may complicate skin-fold thickness measurements using calipers. Elderly or handicapped persons, infants, and small children may not be able to perform underwater weighing. Bioelectric resistance requires a minimum distance between electrodes and may not be applicable to infants and small children.

Reliability

The importance of assessing the reliability of body composition methods relates to the confidence that can be placed in the estimates, as well as the association of the estimates with other variables of interest. For example, if a certain method provides an unreliable estimate of percent body fat, the correlation of this estimate with another variable, for instance blood pressure, will be so attenuated that it may not be possible to detect an association when one exists.

In statistical measurement theory,[51] a measurement is considered an estimate (X) of a "true" value (T) such that $X = T \pm e$, where e is assumed to be a purely random error associated with measurement unreliability. For an individual, the mean of a series of repeated measurements provides an estimate of T, and the standard deviation provides information on the reliability of this estimate. For a sample of subjects, the total variance of X can be defined as $s_x^2 = s_T^2 + s_e^2$. The random measurement error variance, s_e^2, is estimated from the variation among repeated measurements for a sample of subjects, or the within-subject variance. The

value s_T^2 is considered the between-subject variance and theoretically represents the purely biologic variation between subjects. It can be estimated by subtracting the within-subject variance from the total variance or by averaging the deviations from the grand mean of the means of the repeated measurements for each individual of a sample. The reliability of X can be quantified as the intraclass correlation, $R = s_T^2/(s_T^2 + s_e^2)$, and the technical error of X as $\sqrt{s_e^2}$.[51] An intraclass correlation, or reliability coefficient, less than 0.50 indicates poor reliability because it implies that half the total variance among subjects is due to error in the method.

In practice, it may be very difficult to separate true biologic variability from technical errors of measurement. Mueller and Martorell[50] analyze within-subject error variance into two components: random measurement error and physiological variation over time. They call these components *precision* and *dependability*, respectively. This analysis is of more theoretical than practical value, because dependability cannot be directly quantified and methods for its inference are weak. The point is that some portion of the variation among repeated measurements within an individual is due to biologic factors rather than measurement error. The nature of the variable being measured should be considered. Some variables, such as stature, are more dependable than others, such as weight. Subsequently, reliability (or precision) will be underestimated for variables that have high degrees of undependability.

The cost of a reliability study may be high for certain methods such as neutron activation. If such costly methods are considered to have high degrees of precision, two replicate measurements for a sample of subjects may be sufficient to establish reliability. For other methods, for example, anthropometry, which require the skilled use of measuring instruments by observers or involve some aspect of active subject participation in the measuring process, as in underwater weighing, a design in which several repeated measurements are taken on a sample of subjects by at least two independent observers using at least two measuring instruments may be needed. Large sample sizes are usually not required for reliability studies: 15 to 20 subjects should be adequate for assessment of the reliability of quantitative body composition methods.[51]

Accuracy

The assessment of accuracy requires the comparison of the values provided by a method to those from some gold standard or criterion method believed to provide true values, or a validation study. The deviations of values provided by the test method from those of the criterion method may be random or systematic. If the deviations are purely random, accuracy is essentially equivalent to reliability. As noted earlier, the average of a series of repeated measurements that contain purely random errors will approach the true value. The number of repeated measurements needed to achieve equivalent levels of accuracy for two or more measurements can be calculated if an estimate of the reliability of a single measurement is available.[51] Himes[52] calculated the number of repeated measurements required to achieve equivalent levels of accuracy for various anthropometric measures. As many as five replicate skin-fold thickness measurements may be necessary to obtain the same degree of accuracy as two measurements of stature or weight.

If the deviations are systematic, the test method is considered inaccurate or biased. Corrections can be made if the magnitude and direction of the bias can be determined. This can be simple if the systematic error applies equally to all subjects and is additive. Such corrections may be tricky, however, when the magnitude of the systematic error changes with changes in the level of the measurement or estimates when derived from two or more measurements having multiplicative errors.

In practice, it is very difficult to assess the accuracy of body composition methods because all methods are more or less indirect and nearly all make assumptions that may not apply to all individuals. Variation among individuals in the relative amounts of basic constituents associated with sex, age, and physiological factors such as energy balance, physical fitness, and renal function affect the accuracy of indirect methods that assume constant relationships among these constituents. The accuracy of most body composition methods decreases in progressively fatter

patients, not only because of increasing body mass, but because of chemical changes secondary to fat accumulation. ECF expansion and altered hydration are typical of morbid obesity, and methods that assume a fixed fraction of FFM as water will be inaccurate. Changes in body composition with age occur in children and the elderly. Children are chemically immature in that they contain greater proportions of water and lower mineral densities than adults. In the elderly, TBW may decrease as a percent of FFM and the relative amount of water in extracellular space may increase. In elderly women, osteoporosis reduces bone mineral density. These changes affect the accuracy of estimates of body fat or FFM based on body density or TBW. Thus, there may be no single gold standard method applicable to all individuals.

The theoretical rationale for the use of multicompartmental models is that they should reduce errors associated with physiological factors to a minimum by incorporating measurements of the specific constituents that are presumed to be the most variable. In Mueller and Martorell's terminology, these constituents would be those that were the most "undependable." In body composition analysis, body water and mineral are the constituents of the FFM that vary the most with sex, age, and various physiological factors, and produce departures from the assumptions made when inferring fat and fat-free fractions of body weight. An important consideration in the application of multicompartmental models, however, is the propagation of the errors of the separate measurements of the constituents.

Propagation of Errors

For the sake of simplicity, we will consider a multicompartmental model in which the errors of the measurements of each of the constituents are random, independent, and additive. The law of propagation of errors[33] equates the error variance in a dependent variable to the error variances of a set of independent variables by the following formula:

$$e_Y^2 = \left(\frac{\partial Y}{\partial X_1}\right)^2 e_{X_1}^2 + \left(\frac{\partial Y}{\partial X_2}\right)^2 e_{X_2}^2 + \ldots \left(\frac{\partial Y}{\partial X_p}\right)^2 e_{X_p}^2$$

$$(12)$$

where e_Y^2 is the error variance in the dependent variable, and $e_{X_i}^2$, $i = 1, \ldots , p$, are the error variances of the measurements of each variable used to estimate Y. The terms $(\partial Y / \partial X_i)$ in the equation are partial differentials describing how Y changes with change in each variable X_i while holding the other variables constant and can be estimated from partial regression coefficients in this type of model.

Thus, when choosing multicompartmental over simpler models, one should be aware that the expected increase in accuracy is offset to some extent by decreases in reliability due to the propagation of the errors of the separate measurements. Theoretically, one may posit that there will be a "point of diminishing returns" in the elaboration of multicompartmental models at which increases in total error due to the propagation of measurement errors will balance or even exceed decreases gained from the reduction of physiological sources of undependability. The age, sex, ethnicity, and physiological condition of the patient or the members of a sample should be considered in selection of multicompartmental models. The choice of a multicompartmental model including measurements of body density, TBW, and bone mineral over one based on body density only may not be cost-effective for a sample of young white males. The propagation of the errors in the multicompartmental model may exceed any reduction gained, because the traditional assumption of a fat-free density of 1.10 g/ml is likely to be valid for all subjects in this sample.

CONCLUSION

Important technological developments during the past decade now make it possible to accomplish a nearly complete chemical analysis of human body composition *in vivo*. These developments have led to the rebirth and redefinition of constitutional medicine. Major advances in our understanding of body composition in health and disease are anticipated. Simple, inexpensive, and safe methodologies for estimating body fat and other compartments are now being introduced and are applicable in population studies, making the relation of body composition to disease epidemiology feasible.

These are timely developments, because the demand for practical but thoroughly evaluated body composition methodologies is rising as patients, now aware of the clear health implications of obesity, are increasingly seeking evaluation and treatment. At the population level, public health officials are focusing attention on data regarding the prevalences of obesity and its subtypes for planning preventive interventions. The future challenge is to refine body composition methodology so that it is safe, practical, and accurate in the evaluation of both individual patients and heterogeneous populations.

Acknowledgment: This work was supported by grants DK41000 and HO-12252 from the National Institutes of Health, Bethesda, MD.

References

1. Edelman IS, Leibman J: Anatomy of body water and electrolytes. Am J Med 27:256, 1959
2. Kushner RF, Schoeller DA: Estimation of total body water by bioelectrical impedance analysis. Am J Clin Nutr 44:417, 1986
3. Munro HN, Crim MC: The proteins and amino acids. In Shils ME, Young VR (eds): Modern Nutrition in Health and Disease. Philadelphia, Lea & Febiger, 1988
4. Waterlow JC, Garlick PJ, Millward DJ: Protein Turnover in Mammalian Tissues and in the Whole Body. Amsterdam, North-Holland, 1978
5. Vartsky D, Ellis KJ, Cohn SH: *In vivo* measurement of body nitrogen by analysis of prompt gamma-ray analysis from neutron capture. J Nucl Med 20:1158, 1979
6. Report of the Task Group on Reference Man: Int Comm Radiol Protection Report No 23. New York, Pergamon Press, 1975
7. Brozek J, Grande F, Anderson JT et al: Densitometric analysis of body composition: Revision of some quantitative assumptions. Ann NY Acad Sci 110:113, 1963
8. Maffly RH: The body fluids: Volume, composition, and physical chemistry. In Brenner BM, Rector FC (eds): The Kidney. Philadelphia, WB Saunders, 1976
9. Heymsfield SB, Wang J, Funfar J et al: Dual photon absorptiometry: Accuracy of bone mineral and soft tissue mass measurement *in vivo*. Am J Clin Nutr 49:1283, 1953
10. Cohn SH: Noninvasive techniques for measuring body elemental composition. Biol Trace Elem Res 13:179, 1987
11. Heymsfield SB, Wang J, Kehayias JJ et al: Chemical

determination of human body density *in vivo:* Relevance to hydrodensitometry. Am J Clin Nutr 50:1282, 1989

12. Nord RH: Technical considerations in DPA. In Genant HK (ed): Osteoporosis Update. San Francisco, Radiology Research and Education Foundation, 1987

13. Heymsfield SB, Wang J, Aulet M et al: Dual photon absorptiometry: Validation of mineral and fat measurements. In Yasumura S (ed): *In Vivo* Body Composition Studies. New York, Plenum Press, 1990, p 327

14. Mazess RB, Peppler WW, Gibbons M: Total body composition by dual-photon (153Gd) absorptiometry. Am J Clin Nutr 40:834, 1984

15. Forbes GB, Gallup J, Hursh JB. Estimation of total body fat from potassium-40 content. Science 133:101, 1961

16. Pierson RN Jr, Lin DHY, Phillips RA: Total body potassium in health: Effects of age, sex, height, and fat. Am J Physiol 226:206, 1974

17. Moore RD, Olesen KH, McMurrey JD et al: The Body Cell Mass and Its Supporting Environment: Body Composition in Health and Disease. Philadelphia, WB Saunders, 1963

18. Acheson KJ, Flatt JP, Jequier E: Glycogen synthesis versus lipogenesis after a 500 gram carbohydrate meal in man. Metabolism 31:1234, 1982

19. Knight GS, Beddoe AH, Streat SJ et al: Body composition of two human cadavers by neutron activation and chemical analysis. Am J Physiol 250:E179, 1986

20. Heymsfield SB, Noel RA: Radiographic analysis of body composition by computerized axial tomography. In Newell GR, Ellison NM (eds): Nutrition and Cancer, Vol 17, pp 161–172. New York, Raven Press, 1981

21. Heymsfield SB: Human body composition: Analysis by computerized axial tomography and nuclear magnetic resonance. *AIN Symposium Proceedings.* American Institute of Nutrition, Bethesda, MD, 1987.

22. Sjostrom L, Kvist H, Cederblad A et al: Determination of total adipose tissue and body fat in women by computed tomography, ^{40}K, and tritium. Am Physiol Soc 250: E736, 1986

23. Lewis DS, Rollwitz, WL, Bertrand HA et al: Use of NMR for measurement of total body water and estimation of body fat. J Appl Physiol 60:836, 1986

24. Gunby P: The new wave in medicine: Nuclear magnetic resonance. JAMA 247:151, 1982

25. Barrett EJ, Alger JR, Zaret BL: Nuclear magnetic resonance spectroscopy: Its evolving role in the study of myocardial metabolism. J Am Coll Cardiol 6:497, 1985

26. Kehayias JJ, Ellis KJ, Cohn SH et al: Use of a high repetition rate neutron generator for *in vivo* body composition measurements via neutron inelastic scattering. Nuclear Instruments and Methods in Physics Research B24/B25:1006, 1987

27. Kyere K, Oldroyd B, Oxby CB et al: The feasibility of measuring total body carbon by counting neutron inelastic scatter gamma rays. Phys Med Biol 27:805, 1982

28. Keyhayias JJ, Heymsfield SB, Dilmanian FA et al: Measurement of body fat by neutron inelastic scattering: Comments on installation, operation and error analysis. In Yasumura S et al (eds): *In Vivo* Body Composition Studies. New York, Plenum Press, 1990, p 339

29. Heymsfield SB, Wang J, Lichtman S et al: Body composition in elderly subjects: A critical appraisal of clinical methodology. Am J Clin Nutr 50:1167, 1989

30. Gundersen K, Shen G: Total body water in obesity. Am J Clin Nutr 19:77, 1966

31. Buskirk ER: Underwater weighing and body density: A review of procedures. In Brozek J, Henschel A (eds): Techniques for Measuring Body Composition, pp. 90–106. Washington, DC, National Academy of Sciences—National Research Council, 1961

32. Lohman TG: Skinfolds and body density and their relation to body fatness: A review. Hum Biol 25:181, 1981

33. Siri WE: Body composition from fluid spaces and density: Analysis of methods. In Brozek J, Henschel A (eds): Techniques for Measuring Body Composition, pp 223–244. Washington, DC, National Academy of Sciences, Natural Resources Council, 1961

34. Shizgal HM, Spanier AH, Humes J et al: Indirect measurement of total exchangeable potassium. Am J Physiol 233:F253, 1977

35. Cohn SH, Vaswani AN, Yasumura S et al: Improved models for determination of body fat by in vivo neutron activation. Am J Clin Nutr 40:255, 1984

36. Burkinshaw L, Hill GL, Morgan DB: Assessment of the distribution of protein in the human body by *in vivo* neutron activation analysis. IAEA-SM 227:39, 1978

37. Lohman TG, Roche AF, Martorell R: Anthropometric Standardization Reference Manual. Champaign, IL, Human Kinetics Books, 1988

38. Durnin JVGA, Womersley J: Body fat assessed from total body density and its estimation from skinfold thickness: Measurements on 481 men and women aged from 16–72 years. Br J Nutr 32:77, 1974

39. Steinkamp RC, Cohen NL, Siri WE et al: Measures of body fat and related factors in normal adults. J Chronic Dis 18:1279, 1965

40. Harrison GG, Van Itallie TB: Estimation of body composition: A new approach based on electromagnetic principles. Am J Clin Nutr 32:524, 1982

41. Presta E, Segal KR, Gutin B et al: Comparison in man of total electrical conductivity and lean body mass derived from body density: Validation of a new body composition method. Metabolism 32:524, 1983

42. Wang J, Pierson RN Jr: Disparate hydration of adipose and lean tissue require a new model for body water distribution in man. J Nutr 106:1687, 1976

43. Forbes G: Human Body Composition: Growth, Aging, Nutrition, and Activity, pp 209–247. New York, Springer-Verlag, 1987

44. Morse WI, Soeldner JS: Composition of adipose tissue and the non-adipose body of obese and nonobese men. Metabolism 12:99, 1963

45. Naeye RL, Roode P: The sizes and numbers of cells in visceral organs in human obesity. AJCP 54:251, 1970

46. Siwek RA, Wales JK, Swaminathan R et al: Body composition of fasting obese patients measured by *in vivo* neutron activation analysis and isotopic dilution. Clin Phys Physiol Meas 8:271, 1987

47. Hankin ME, Munz K, Steinbeck AW: Total body water content in normal and grossly obese women. Med J Aust 2:533, 1976

48. Forbes GB: Lean body mass-body fat interrelationships in humans. Nutr Rev 45:225, 1987

49. Webster JD, Hesp R, Garrow JS: The composition of excess weight in obese women estimated by body density, total body water, and total body potassium. Hum Nutr: Clin Nutr 38C:299, 1984

50. Mueller SH, Martorell R: Reliability and accuracy of measurement. In Lohman TB, Roche AF, Martorell R (eds): Human Kinetics, pp. 83–87, Champaign, IL, 1988

51. Fleiss JL: The Design and Analysis of Clinical Experiments. New York, John Wiley & Sons, 1986

52. Himes J: Reliability of anthropometric methods and replicate measurements. Am J Phys Anthropol 79:77, 1989

CHAPTER 4

New Approaches to the Clinical Assessment of Adipose Tissue

ALEX F. ROCHE and WM. CAMERON CHUMLEA

This chapter presents new ways in which established anthropometric procedures can be used clinically to obtain useful data about adipose tissue. Also, brief descriptions of more complex techniques are presented together with discussions of their advantages and limitations.

ANTHROPOMETRY

Anthropometry can be used as an indirect method to determine indices or the relative amount of adipose tissue in an individual. It is inexpensive, relatively simple, and noninvasive, and the equipment needed is portable. The clinical application of anthropometry is important to assess the degree of obesity in terms of percentile values for body fatness or to predict the amount of total body fat (TBF) or the percentage of body weight that is fat (%BF). Anthropometry is also necessary to help monitor any changes during treatment or nutritional therapy. The measurements that are important in an indirect assessment of adipose tissue are weight, skin-fold thicknesses of subcutaneous adipose tissue, and circumferences of the trunk and limbs. A list of recommended measurements is presented in Table 4-1. Ratios or indices using combinations of circumferences or skin folds are potentially useful to describe the patterns of adipose tissue distribution on the body. The possible associations between these patterns and risk of cardiovascular or metabolic diseases are an important area of research.

WEIGHT

Body weight is a gross measure of the body's composition; weight is highly correlated with levels of TBF and %BF in children, adults, and the elderly.[15,73] Weight should be measured with the subject nude and after voiding. If it is necessary for the subject to wear clothing, this should be minimal and recorded values should be adjusted for it. These adjustments will be more accurate if standardized garments are worn. Weight should be measured using a beam balance or electronic scale accurate to 0.1 kg. If measures of weight are collected at frequent intervals (i.e., daily or weekly) to monitor weight loss or treatment effects, the measurements should be made at approximately the same time of day.[51] This will help eliminate environmental effects or normal fluctuations in body weight, which can be large in obese persons.[93]

WEIGHT-STATURE INDICES

The use of combinations of weight and stature as indices of body fatness is controversial. This debate is understandable when this approach is compared with the others described in this chapter. Measures of weight and stature are familiar, and the equipment used is familiar also, but familiarity breeds contempt. Nevertheless, weight-stature indices have potential scientific value. This value is derived, in part, from the accuracy with which weight and stature can be measured. At the Fels Research Institute, the co-

TABLE 4-1

List of Recommended Measurements

Children (2 to 18 years)	Adults (18 + years)
Stature	Stature
Weight	Weight
Arm circumference	Arm circumference
	Abdominal circumference
	Hip circumference
Calf circumference	Calf circumference
Triceps skin-fold thickness	Triceps skin-fold thickness
Subscapular skin-fold thickness	Subscapular skin-fold thickness

efficients of reliability for these measures are 100% and 99.8%, respectively, and these measures are clearly valid. To these advantages can be added the possible retrospective calculation of weight-stature indices in serial studies and their derivation from data recorded in large surveys. This research has led to the establishment of longevity expectations in relation to values for these indices.[88] This approach provides a better basis for criteria of obesity than the distributions of values in the population.

Weight-stature indices have been criticized for failing to describe patterns of distribution of adipose tissue, but of course they were never intended for this purpose. More appropriately, they have been criticized for their inability to discriminate between individuals with an excess of adipose tissue and those with an excess of muscle. Despite the validity of this criticism, weight-stature indices are useful if interpreted with caution.

The usefulness of weight-stature indices is dependent on their associations with %BF or TBF; this is the basis on which a selection should be made from the many such indices that have been reported. The weight (W) -stature (S) indices that are easy to calculate and have been used commonly are relative W, W/S, W/S^2, and W/S^3. In this context, relative weight is 100 times the measured weight divided by the median reference weight for the measured stature. Relative weight has the disadvantage that the values depend on the choice of reference data. In children and adults, W/S^2 has higher correlations with %BF than do relative weight or W/S^3.[61,73] If used in combination with age, W/S^2 can predict %BF

with a standard error of the estimate (SEE) of 3.4%.[61,68,89] Either W/S^2 or W/S^3 could be chosen for adults if the interest is in %BF. W/S^2 is preferable if the interest is in TBF, and W/S^2 has the advantage of better reference data.[2,25]

Interest in weight-stature indices has led to the derivation of indices with fractional powers of stature or of both weight and stature. One set of these is usually written as W/S^P, where P is chosen so that the index is independent of stature.[6] The value of P can be determined mathematically in the absence of data for %BF. It is assumed that any weight-stature index that is independent of stature must be a good predictor of %BF, although some have reported negative correlations between these variables in adults,[94] and obese children tend to be tall before pubescence.[70]

Abdel-Malek and colleagues[1] constructed an index with fractional powers for weight and stature that maximized the relationship with %BF. Using the mathematical form %BF $= C(W^{1.2}/S^{3.3})$, in which C is an age-independent constant that differs between the sexes, they published nomograms that estimate %BF directly from weight and stature. In their study sample, the correlations between their index and %BF were considerably higher than those for W/S^2 in children, but not in adults. This index, in common with other weight-stature indices, should be validated for the population to be studied using data from a subset for which %BF is known.[71] In particular, the relationships of these indices to %BF may vary between populations that differ in relative leg length, as occurs between blacks and whites in the United States.[52]

SKIN FOLDS

A skin fold is a measure of the double thickness of the epidermis, underlying fascia, and subcutaneous adipose tissue. The fold should be formed with gentle pressure to avoid unwanted compression.[51] A skin-fold thickness can be measured wherever a fold can be formed, but specific body sites have been designated because of their higher correlations with TBF and %BF from more direct methods.[73] The triceps and the subscapular locations tend to have the highest correlations with TBF and %BF regardless of age or sex in whites, and these relationships are assumed applicable to other groups.[15,25,73] Other sites that are measured commonly include the suprailiac, midthigh, paraumbilical, and lateral or medial calf.[51] The choice of these sites is based in part on practicality in epidemiologic surveys and of the need to ensure high reliability. Other skin folds, such as the gonial skin fold, have been reported to have significant correlations with amounts of body fatness, but their utility has not been accepted as practical or tested in various samples. Skin folds cannot be used to describe amounts of adipose tissue or degrees of obesity in obese persons, because the calipers cannot measure beyond 50 mm and it is often impossible to grasp a skin fold.[9]

Different makes of skin-fold calipers give highly correlated but systematically different readings.[11,51,64,78] Some types of calipers are suitable for research, but others are suitable for clinical purposes only. Research skin-fold calipers should have a uniform jaw pressure of 10 g/cm^3,[10] but the intervals of measurement may vary from 0.1 to 0.5 mm. Clinical calipers can exert more variable pressures, and a scale readable to 2 mm is acceptable.

The distributions of skin-fold values differ by sex and race and change with age.[25] During the growth of normal children, the values increase for all skin folds, except for decreases in limb skin folds during pubescence in boys.[80] With adulthood, skin-fold values continue to increase with age, although not as rapidly as during growth.[25] After 60 years of age, however, skin-fold values decrease.[14,15] This decrease with old age is both real for an individual and artifactual for the sample. Some of the decrease on a samplewide basis in a cross-sectional study of the elderly is due to cohort effects and differential mortality with increasing old age.[31]

ULTRASOUND

Ultrasound is a possible alternative to skin-fold calipers for measuring subcutaneous adipose tissue thickness because it should be unaffected by compressibility or excessive thicknesses that limit caliper measurements.[49] To date, most studies have used A-mode ultrasound, but A-mode measurements are generally less reliable than caliper measurements of skin-fold thicknesses.[7,13,32,49] In a study of elderly men and women, the best interobserver reliability of A-mode ultrasound measurements of subcutaneous adipose tissue thickness was 68%, whereas the worst reliability for caliper measurements was 88%.[13] B-mode ultrasound, however, may be as reliable as skin-fold calipers.[90] B-mode ultrasound provides a real-time two-dimensional image in which the fat-muscle interface can be observed and confounding factors such as skin compression, fibrous tissue interfaces, and muscle contractions can be considered. The screen image can be frozen for measurement with electronic calipers or a hard copy obtained and measured using a digitizer. The use of B-mode ultrasound for measuring adipose tissue thicknesses in obese persons has not been tested. This method may be more informative for describing subcutaneous adipose tissue thickness in obese individuals than caliper measurements of skin-fold thicknesses or body circumferences.

CIRCUMFERENCES

Circumferences, like skin folds, can be measured at numerous body locations. In addition to providing information about subcutaneous adipose tissue, a circumference measurement also gives data about muscle tone, internal organs, and abdominal adipose tissue. Unlike skin folds, however, circumferences can be used to measure adipose tissue regardless of the amount of obesity, and circumferences are the only body measurements applicable to grossly obese individuals.[9] Various tape measures are available, but it is recommended that only nonelastic tapes be used.[51] The tape selected should have a leader of about 2 to 4 cm to facilitate taking the measurement.

Some tapes include a device that applies a preselected pressure, but this is not recommended. For circumference measures, it is important to apply minimal pressure so that as little compression of the adipose tissue occurs as possible. In general, reliability for circumferences is better than that for skin folds.[56]

The sites for circumference measurements that have been reported to be most important in describing amounts of adipose tissue and degrees of obesity are the upper arm, chest, abdomen, hips or buttocks, midthigh, and calf circumference. Several of these circumferences are at standard body locations determined by bony landmarks. Others are taken at the maximum circumference for that body dimension at that location, such as the hips, buttocks, and the calf. Of the body circumferences, the measurement at the abdomen or "waist" is the most variable in terms of its location or position, especially among obese and elderly persons.[14,51] For example, the abdominal circumference is correctly measured at the level of the umbilicus, but in many obese individuals, the umbilicus may be directed downward because of the excessive curvatures of the abdominal wall. Waist circumference is a clothing design measurement and can only be measured on someone who has a waist. As a result, waist circumference cannot generally be measured on obese or overweight individuals. Body circumferences are significantly correlated with TBF and %BF,[86,91] but the correlation coefficients are smaller than those between skin-fold thicknesses and either TBF or %BF, except in the elderly.[15]

Body circumferences and skin-fold thicknesses are useful in describing the patterns of adipose tissue deposition on the body.[47] Ratios of abdominal to hip circumferences or limb to trunk circumferences can partition groups of individuals into those with upper and those with lower body obesity. These differences can relate to the amount of adipose tissue that is internal or subcutaneous and to the risk for disease.[47] Measures of fat patterning, however, are not applicable to grossly obese persons.

REFERENCE DATA

A minimal list of recommended measurements for assessing the level of obesity is presented in Table 4-1. Self-reported values are not reliable. Recorded measurements must be compared with appropriate reference data to obtain a reliable interpretation of an assessment of body fatness. Selected sources of reference data are listed in Table 4-2. Percentiles or distribution statistics for weight and triceps skin-fold thicknesses can provide guides to the amount of TBF or %BF for individuals or groups.[73] The subscapular skin fold is not as highly correlated with TBF and %BF as the triceps skin fold in children, but it is included in the basic list of measurements because the correlations are high in adults. Calf circumference is needed to estimate TBF or fat-free mass (FFM) from bioelectric impedance.[38] For the other measurements such as abdominal, hip, and midthigh circumferences, suitable national reference data are not available, but some comparative data are available from military surveys.[17] Race- and sex-specific national reference data for abdominal, hip, and midthigh circumferences will be available on the completion of the Third U.S. National Health and Nutrition Examination Survey.[95]

Arm circumference and triceps skin-fold thickness can be used to estimate cross-sectional areas of adipose tissue and areas of "muscle plus bone" in the arm. The formulas applied in the past to calculate these areas are inaccurate, particularly in regard to muscle plus bone area,[40] but the available reference data were derived using the earlier formulas.[35] Arm adipose tissue area is only slightly more correlated with TBF than is triceps skin-fold thickness.[41] Consequently, the calculation of arm adipose tissue area is not recommended as a basic procedure.

Anthropometry is useful as an indirect method of assessing adipose tissue, but it is prone to significant errors when insufficient attention is given to training techniques and reliability. When used properly, it is a useful technique that can help to distinguish categories of obesity, to predict levels of body fatness, and to estimate relative risk for disease.[70]

ASSESSMENT OF TOTAL BODY COMPOSITION

Methods for the measurement and the prediction of TBF, %BF, and FFM (in kilograms) are discussed in the pages that follow. The meth-

TABLE 4-2

**Reference Data for Recommended
Measurements 6 Months to 74 Years**

Measures	Sources
Stature	Najjar and Rowland[59]; Tanner and Whitehouse[82]; Prader and Budliger[66]; Waaler[87]; Roede and Van Wieringen[74]; Sempé et al[76]
Weight	Najjar and Rowland[59]; Tanner and Whitehouse[82]; Prader and Budliger[66]; Waaler[87]; Roede and Van Wieringen[74]; Sempé et al[76]
Weight/stature^2	Najjar and Rowland[59]; Chumlea et al[16]
Triceps skin-fold thickness	Najjar and Rowland[59]; Tanner and Whitehouse[81]; Prader and Budliger[66]; Waaler[87]; Roede and Van Wieringen[74]; Sempé et al[76]
Subscapular skin-fold thickness	Najjar and Rowland[59]; Tanner and Whitehouse[81]; Prader and Budliger[66]; Waaler[87]; Roede and Van Wieringen[74]; Sempé et al[76]
Arm circumference	Najjar and Rowland[59]; Prader and Budliger[66]; Waaler[87]; Roede and Van Wieringen[74]; Sempé et al[76]

ods considered include densitometry, the measurement of total body electrical conductivity (TOBEC), total body potassium (^{40}K), dual photon absorptiometry, and infrared interactance. These methods are similar in replicability, but they differ in the extent to which they take account of systematic sex- and age-associated differences in FFM. The measurement of impedance and of total body water is excluded because these methods are considered in other chapters of this book. Many prediction equations use combinations of anthropometric variables and impedance to predict body composition values. These equations differ in the independent and dependent variables, in the statistical methods by which they were developed, and in the extent to which they have been cross-validated. Some consideration will be given to such equations, with particular reference to statistical methods.

Many readers might have hoped to find sets of reference data for body composition values in this chapter, but it was not practical to include them. The values differ by age, sex, and ethnic group, and they are dependent on the methods used. Some sources of reference data are listed in Table 4-3.

Densitometry

In its simplest conceptual form, densitometry involves the calculation of body density for an individual and the derivation of the amounts of fat and FFM in an individual's body from the known density of each of these components. Some workers refer to densitometry as the "gold standard." It is not. The measured body density will be inaccurate if the method is applied without close attention to detail, and erroneous body composition values will be derived if the densities of fat and of FFM are incorrect for the individual. Despite these limitations, densitometry is the best understood of the indirect methods, and when applied carefully, it is probably the best of the criterion methods.

The density of the human body can be calculated easily if body weight and volume are

TABLE 4-3

**Selected Sources of Reference Data
for Total Body Fat (TBF) and
Percent Body Fat (%BF)**

Sources	Samples
%BF	
Frerichs et al[34]	214 children
Parizkova[63]	40 boys, serially
Durnin and Womersley[29]	481 children, adults
Mukherjee and Roche[57]	399 children, adults
Slaughter et al[77]	310 children, adults
Hodgdon and Fitzgerald[42]	538 adults
VuTran and Weltman[86]	532 men
Jackson and Pollock[43]	308 men
Vickery et al[85]	319 men
Jackson et al[44]	249 women
TBF	
Burmeister and Bingert[12]	3292 children, adults
Noppa et al[60]	1300 women
Steen et al[79]	65 adults, serially

known. Body volume is usually obtained by measuring the weight of the water displaced when a person is underwater. With some corrections, this value is equal to the difference between weight in air and weight in water.[3] Weight in water is measured using a set of load cells that provide more accurate data than a spring scale or direct measurement of the displaced water.[54] For the measurement of weight in water, the subject submerges completely ten times; the mean of the final three values is used in the calculations.[5,45] Some perform densitometry with the subject's head out of the water and claim results very similar to those with complete immersion.[27,36]

Corrections are needed for residual volume, which should be measured using a washout method; errors are introduced if predicted or fixed values are used.[55] Residual volume can be measured "on land," with the subject in the same position that will be assumed underwater, or it can be measured underwater simultaneously with weight. The simultaneous measurement of residual volume and weight appears ideal because it avoids errors due to the effects of immersion on residual volume.[62] Unfortunately, immersion can cause the collapse of airways as

a result of increased extrathoracic pressure.[69] When this occurs, the dilution methods applied during immersion give erroneously low values. Ideally, corrections would be made for the amount of intestinal gas, but this is not practical.[30] Variability in intestinal gas can be reduced by obtaining data with the subjects fasting.

Replicability for densitometry is accurate. The standard error of a single measurement of body density for all sources of error combined is about 1% BF.[28] Variation in the water content of FFM can be reduced by not measuring body density during menstruation or the few days before it.

Densitometry requires considerable cooperation from the subjects. It is not applicable to children younger than 8 years or to those with impaired mobility or a history of cardiovascular disease or emphysema. Consequently, there have been attempts to measure body volume by gas displacement or acoustic resonance.[26,37] These promising methods are still experimental.

Body density values allow the calculation of %BF from which TBF and FFM can be calculated. The simple two-compartment model assumes that the body consists of fat, mostly in adipose tissue, and a remainder that is FFM. It further assumes that the density of each of these components is fixed. The density of fat is almost constant,[4] but the density of FFM varies with age, sex, ethnicity, and amount of physical activity. Acceptable age- and sex-specific constants for the density of FFM have been proposed for ages 7 to 25 years.[50] The use of these in place of a single value for all ages and both sexes causes large changes in the calculated values for body composition variables.[72] Ideally, the density of FFM would be calculated for each individual using measures of body density, skeletal mass, and total body water.[50]

Surrogate measures are commonly used instead of densitometry.[71] The best alternatives are prediction equations that include independent variables that are relatively easy to obtain. The ease of collecting the independent variables should not be exaggerated. Precision is necessary, and the procedures used should match those applied by the workers who developed the equation to be applied. Generally, the anthropometric procedures match those recommended by a recent Standardization Conference.[51]

There is some skepticism about the ability of

prediction equations to function well for groups other than those from which they were derived. This can be dispelled by cross-validation using an independent sample. Successful cross-validation is likely when the set of statistical methods applied is based on ridge regression and designed to produce robust equations.[72] The appropriate steps in the development of such equations are (1) selection of an outcome variable (e.g., %BF that has been obtained using age- and sex-specific values for the density of FFM); (2) selection of independent variables for testing that are logically related to the outcome variable; (3) use of all possible subsets of regression to select the best number and the best combination of independent variables; (4) calculation of variance inflation factors as indices of collinearity; (5) use of ridge regression to reduce collinearity, which makes the coefficients unstable; and (6) robust estimation using weighted least squares to reduce the influence of divergent values.

Total Body Electrical Conductivity

TOBEC is based on variations between various body components in their electrical conductivity and dielectric properties. The instrument is a large solenoidal coil with an oscillating 5-MHz radio-frequency current. The electromagnetic field associated with the coil induces an electrical current in any conductive material placed within the coil. The size of the induced current depends on the concentration and composition of the electrolytes in the material and the volume of the material.[48]

For a TOBEC measurement, the subject lies still on a carriage that moves through the coil. Clothes may be worn, but continuous metal bands must be removed. The procedure requires little cooperation from the subject and therefore is applicable to a larger group than densitometry.

In practice, the TOBEC instrument measures the difference between the coil impedance when empty and that when a subject is placed within the coil. When this difference is divided by the weight of the subject, it provides specific conductivity that is proportional to FFM.

The TOBEC-II instrument provides measurements at 64 equidistant levels along the carriage. These values produce a phase curve for a subject that reflects the convolutions of the field due to the conductive and dielectric masses. Fourier terms have been fitted to these curves and equations developed that predict FFM values obtained from densitometry. The best of these equations has an SEE of 1.53 kg, but they have not been cross-validated.[83]

TOBEC values are highly replicable,[67] and validation studies have been done using carcass analysis.[8,46,48] In addition, TOBEC findings have been compared with those from established methods,[18,67] resulting in rather large SEE (4.5 l for total body water, 430.7 mEq for total body potassium, and 5.8 kg for FFM from skin-fold thicknesses). The need for cross-validation is shown by the significant differences between prediction equations developed for two samples by Van Loan and colleagues.[84]

Some limitations of the TOBEC method result from effects of variations in body shape and, possibly, variations in the skeletal contribution to FFM.[39] Adjustments for these could be developed. The major limitation is the cost of the instrument and the large space required. Consequently, TOBEC is likely to remain a research instrument.

Total Body Potassium

Typically total body potassium is calculated by measuring the gamma radiation from ^{40}K, which is a naturally occurring isotope of potassium. The gamma radiation from ^{40}K can be measured by noninvasive external counting in a space shielded from contaminant radiation.[33] The shielding material is usually steel lined with lead. Because the radiation from this material must be low, most units use materials manufactured before World War II, when there was less radioactive contamination. A sensitive gamma-ray detector that can distinguish between the radiation from ^{40}K and that from other naturally occurring isotopes is placed near the subject.

The subject must remain in a small space for 40 minutes or more and may experience claustrophobia. The method is not applicable to children younger than 10 years because of the high ratio of background noise to the signal.[75] The within-individual variability is reduced by a controlled diet and by measuring at a fixed time of day.

The gamma counts are converted to potassium

(in grams) using a specific conversion factor for each instrument that is obtained experimentally. This value is adjusted for body size, which affects the measurement as a result of the inverse square law of radiation intensity and the absorption of radiation by body tissues.[19] In an alternative approach, it has been claimed that the effects of body size and shape were overcome by use of a set of 54 detectors.[20]

The weight of potassium is used to calculate FFM assuming that all the body potassium is in the FFM. An assigned value is used for the potassium concentration of FFM. Laboratories differ in these assigned values, but typically, each uses one sex-specific value for all ages, although age changes occur in the composition of FFM.[58,92] In addition, there are individual variations in the potassium content of FFM at any age as a result of differences in the relative size of various organs. A further complication is that the potassium content of FFM is low in obesity.[22] In an extension of the method, the muscle and non-muscle components of FFM can be calculated if total body potassium is known and total body nitrogen is measured by neutron activation.[21]

In summary, total body potassium can be measured with acceptable reliability in subjects who are older than 10 years and who are not claustrophobic. The limitations to the method result from variations in the potassium content of the FFM. These limitations are conceptually similar to those for densitometry. Although they have been largely overcome by the use of multicomponent densitometric models, there is a lack of such corresponding models for total body potassium content.

Dual Photon Absorptiometry

In dual photon absorptiometry, the body can be scanned with a rectilinear raster that has a transverse speed of 1 cm/sec and longitudinal steps of 2.5 cm.[65] The collinated isotope source is ^{153}Gd (1 Ci), which has two principal photopeaks at 44 and 100 keV. The first of these has energies that range from 40 to 48 keV. The photopeak at 100 keV is a composite of equal peaks at 97 and 103 keV. These variations in wavelength cause differential attenuation, for which adjustments are made in the computer program. The detector is a

NaI crystal coupled to a bialkali photomultiplier tube.

Because the delivery and attenuation of the photon beam are measured separately for the two principal photopeaks, the procedure allows the differentiation of two substances if their attenuation coefficients are known. The attenuation coefficients for fat and FFM are not well established. Various values have been used, and the differences between them would have large effects on the estimates.[53,65] The most common application has been to estimate total bone mineral mass, but dual photon absorptiometry can be used to estimate TBF and %BF. The sources of error include the effects of variations in soft-tissue thickness and effects of bone edges that cause variations in intensity across the finite beam.

The method has promise, particularly if the individual values can be adjusted for bone mineral content.[53] The disadvantages are whole body radiation, although the amount is only 1 mR, and the long time required for scanning while the subject lies on a hard table.

Infrared Interactance

The infrared interactance method employs a computerized spectrophotometer used in the transmittance mode, a single-beam rapid scanning monochromator, and a fiber-optic probe.[24] The probe conducts the radiation from the monochromator (source) to the measurement site, where it collects the interactive radiation and conducts it to the detector. The probe is surrounded by black felt to preclude other radiation from entering the site. By comparison with a reflectance standard, the instrument computes interactance (I) at 916 and 1026 mm; these wavelengths have been shown to be most useful for the prediction of %BF. The interactance data are transformed to log (1/I), and the ratio of the second derivatives at the two wavelengths is obtained to reduce the effects of particle size and temperature.

In 53 subjects, Conway and colleagues[24] measured five sites 20 times, averaged these data for each individual, and developed a prediction equation. In a validation study, the SEE for %BF was 3.2%, with a tendency to overpredict on cross-validation, especially in females. Later, Conway and Norris[23] developed a new equation for which the SEE was 4% and 3.1% for their validation and cross-validation groups, respectively. A wide-slit portable instrument is commercially available that measures interactance at the biceps site and uses this with sex, weight, stature, and self-reported categories of frame size and physical activity to predict %BF. The accuracy of these predictions has not been established.

The infrared method is interesting, but much more work is required before it can be recommended. It is important that the interactance characteristics of FFM be established. At present, the interactance of water is used as a surrogate, and it is assumed that the water content of FFM is fixed at 73%.

CONCLUSIONS

The preceding review does not lead to a single recommendation regarding the clinical assessment of adipose tissue. Much depends on the resources available. In general, selected anthropometric values, used with impedance in prediction equations, meet a need for estimated total body composition values. Indices of fat patterning should be derived from carefully measured skin-fold thicknesses.

Acknowledgment: This work was supported by grant HD-12252 from the National Institutes of Health.

References

1. Abdel-Malek AK, Mukherjee D, Roche AF: A method of constructing an index of obesity. Hum Biol 57:415, 1985
2. Abraham S, Carroll MD, Najjar MF et al: Obese and Overweight Adults in the United States. Vital and Health Statistics, Series 11, No. 230. DHHS publication (PHS) 83-1680. Washington, DC, US Govt Printing Office, 1983
3. Akers R, Buskirk ER: An underwater weighing system utilizing "force cube" transducers. J Appl Physiol 26:649, 1969
4. Allen TH, Krzywicki HJ, Roberts JE: Density, fat, water and solids in freshly isolated tissues. J Appl Physiol 14:1005, 1959
5. Behnke AR, Wilmore JH: Evaluation and Regula-

6. tion of Body Build and Composition. Englewood Cliffs, NJ, Prentice-Hall, 1974
6. Benn RT: Some mathematical properties of weight-for-height indices used as measure of adiposity. Br J Prev Soc Med 25:42, 1971
7. Borkan GA, Hults DE, Cardarelli J et al: Comparison of ultrasound and skinfold measurements in assessment of subcutaneous and total fatness. Am J Phys Anthropol 58:307, 1982
8. Bracco EF, Yang M-U, Segal K et al: Rapid communication: A new method for estimation of body composition in the live rat. Proc Soc Exp Biol Med 174:143, 1983
9. Bray GA, Greenway FL, Molitch ME et al: Use of anthropometric measures to assess weight loss. Am J Clin Nutr 31:769, 1978
10. Brozek J, Keys A: The evaluation of leanness, fatness in man: norms and interrelationships. Br J Nutr 5:194, 1950
11. Burgert SL, Anderson CF: A comparison of triceps skinfold values as measured by the plastic McGraw and the Lange calipers. Am J Clin Nutr 32:1531, 1979
12. Burmeister W, Bingert A: Die quantitativen Veranderungen der menschlichen Zellmasse zwischen dem 8. and 90. Lebensjahr. Klin Wochenschr 45:409, 1967
13. Chumlea WC, Roche AF: Ultrasonic and skinfold caliper measures of subcutaneous adipose tissue thickness in elderly men and women. Am J Phys Anthropol 71:351, 1986
14. Chumlea WC, Roche AF, Mukherjee D: Nutritional Assessment of the Elderly Through Anthropometry. Columbus, OH, Ross Laboratories, 1984
15. Chumlea WC, Roche AF, Webb P: Body size, subcutaneous fatness and total body fat in older adults. Int J Obes 8:311, 1984
16. Chumlea WC, Steinbaugh ML, Roche AF et al: Nutritional anthropometric assessment in elderly persons 65 to 90 years of age. J Nutr Elderly 4:39, 1985
17. Clauser CE, Tucker PE, McConville JT et al: Anthropometry of Air Force women Report No. AMRL-TR070-5, Dayton, OH, Wright-Patterson Air Force Base, 1972
18. Cochran WJ, Klish WJ, Wong WW et al: Fat, water and tissue solids of the whole body less its bone mineral. J Appl Physiol 14:1009, 1986
19. Cohn WH, Dombrowski CS: Absolute measurement of whole-body potassium by gamma-ray spectrometry. J Nucl Med 11:239, 1970
20. Cohn SH, Dombrowski CS, Pate HR et al: A whole-body counter with an invariant response to radionuclide distribution and body size. Phys Med Biol 14:645, 1969
21. Cohn SH, Vaswani AN, Vartsky D et al: *In vivo*

quantification of body nitrogen for nutritional assessment. Am J Clin Nutr 35:1186, 1982

22. Colt EW, Wang J, Stallone F et al: Possible low intracellular potassium in obesity. Am J Clin Nutr 34:367, 1981
23. Conway JM, Norris KH: Noninvasive body composition in humans by near infrared interactance. In Ellis KJ, Yasumura S, Morgan WD (eds): In Vivo Body Composition Studies. Proceedings of the International Symposium of Brookhaven National Laboratory. New York, September 28–October 1, 1986
24. Conway JM, Norris KH, Bodwell CE: A new approach for the estimation of body composition: Infrared interactance. Am J Clin Nutr 40:1123, 1984
25. Cronk CE, Roche AF: Race- and sex-specific reference data for biceps and subscapular skinfolds and weight/stature.[2] Am J Clin Nutr 35:347, 1982
26. Deskins WG, Winter DC, Sheng H et al: Use of a resonating cavity to measure body volume. J Acoust Soc Am 77:756, 1985
27. Donnelly JE, Brown TE, Israel RG et al: Hydrostatic weighing without head submersion: Description of a method. Med Sci Sports Exerc 20:66, 1988
28. Durnin JVGA, Satwanti: Variations in the assessment of the fat content of the human body due to experimental technique in measuring body density. Ann Hum Biol 9:221, 1982
29. Durnin JVGA, Womersley J: Body fat assessed from total body density and its estimation from skinfold thickness: Measurements on 481 men and women aged from 16 to 72 years. Br J Nutr 32:77, 1974
30. Edwards DK: Size of gas-filled bowel loops in infants. Am J Roentgenol 135:331, 1980
31. Exton-Smith AN: Epidemiological studies in the elderly: Methodological considerations. Am J Clin Nutr 35:1273, 1982
32. Fanelli MT, Kuczmarski RJ: Ultrasound as an approach to assessing body composition. Am J Clin Nutr 39:703, 1984
33. Forbes GB: Human Body Composition: Growth, Aging, Nutrition, and Activity. New York, Springer-Verlag, 1987
34. Frerichs RR, Harsha DW, Berenson GS: Equations for estimating percentage of body fat in children 10–14 years old. Pediatr Res 13:170, 1979
35. Frisancho AR: New norms of upper limb fat and muscle areas for assessment of nutritional status. Am J Clin Nutr 34:2540, 1981
36. Garrow JS, Stalley S, Diethelm R et al: A new method for measuring the body density of obese adults. Br J Nutr 42:173, 1979
37. Gundlach BL, Nijkrake HGM, Hautvast JGAJ: A rapid and simplified plethysmometric method for measuring body volume. Hum Biol 52:23, 1980

38. Guo S, Roche AF, Houtkooper L: Fat-free mass in children and young adults predicted from bioelectric impedance and anthropometric variables. Am J Clin Nutr 50:435, 1989
39. Harrison GG, Van Itallie TB: Estimation of body composition: A new approach based on electromagnetic principles. Am J Clin Nutr 35:1176, 1982
40. Heymsfield SB, McManus C, Smith J et al: Anthropometric measurement of muscle mass: Revised equations for calculating bone-free arm muscle area. Am J Clin Nutr 36:680, 1982
41. Himes JH, Roche AF, Webb P: Fat areas as estimates of total body fat. Am J Clin Nutr 33:2093, 1980
42. Hodgdon JA, Fitzgerald PI: Validity of impedance predictions at various levels of fatness. Hum Biol 59:281, 1987
43. Jackson AS, Pollock ML: Generalized equations for predicting body density of men. Br J Nutr 40:497, 1978
44. Jackson AS, Pollock ML, Ward A: Generalized equations for predicting body density of women. Med Sci Sports Exerc 12:175, 1980
45. Katch FI: Apparent body density and variability during underwater weighing. Res Quart 39:993, 1968
46. Keim NL, Mayclin PL, Taylor SJ et al: Total-body electrical conductivity method for estimating body composition: Validation by direct carcass analysis of pigs. Am J Clin Nutr 47:180, 1988
47. Kissebah AH, Vydelingum N, Murray R et al: Relation of body fat distribution to metabolic complications of obesity. J Clin Endocrinol Metab 54:254, 1982
48. Klish WJ, Forbes GB, Gordon A et al: New method for the estimation of lean body mass in infants (EMME Instrument): Validation in nonhuman models. J Pediatr Gastroenterol Nutr 3:199, 1984
49. Kuczmarski RK, Fanelli MT, Koch GG: Ultrasonic assessment of body composition in obese adults: Overcoming the limitations of the caliper. Am J Clin Nutr 45:717, 1987
50. Lohman TG: Applicability of body composition techniques and constants for children and youths. Exerc Sport Sci Rev 14:325, 1986
51. Lohman TG, Roche AF, Martorell R: Anthropometric Standardization Reference Manual. Champaign, IL, Human Kinetics Publishers, 1988
52. Martorell R, Malina RM, Castillo RO et al: Body proportions in three ethnic groups: Children and youths 2–17 years in NHANES II and HHANES. Hum Biol 60:205, 1988
53. Mazess RB, Peppler WW, Gibbons M: Total body composition by dual-photon (^{153}Gd) absorptiometry. Am J Clin Nutr 40:834, 1984

54. McClenaghan BA, Rocchio L: Design and validation of an automated hydrostatic weighing system. Med Sci Sports Exerc 18:479, 1986

55. Morrow JR Jr, Jackson AS, Bradley PW et al: Accuracy of measured and predicted residual lung volume on body density measurement. Med Sci Sports Exerc 18:647, 1986

56. Mueller WH, Malina RM: Relative reliability of circumference and skinfolds as measures of body fat distribution. Am J Phys Anthropol 72:437, 1987

57. Mukherjee D, Roche AF: The estimation of percent body fat, body density and total body fat by maximum R^2 regression equations. Hum Biol 56:79, 1984

58. Myhre LG, Kessler WV: Body density and potassium-40 measurements of body composition as related to age. J Appl Physiol 21:1251, 1966

59. Najjar MF, Rowland M: Anthropometric Reference Data and Prevalence of Overweight. Vital and Health Statistics, Series 11, No. 238. DHEW publication (PHS) 87-1688. Washington DC, US Govt Printing Office, 1987

60. Noppa H, Anderson M, Bengtsson C et al: Longitudinal studies of anthropometric data and body composition: The population study of women in Goteborg, Sweden. Am J Clin Nutr 33:155, 1980

61. Norgan NG, Ferro-Luzzi A: Weight-height indices as estimators of fatness in men. Hum Nutr Clin Nutr 36C:363, 1982

62. Ostrove SM, Vaccaro P: Effect of immersion on RV in young women: implications for measurement of body density. Int J Sports Med 3:220, 1982

63. Parizkova J: Growth and growth velocity of lean body mass and fat in adolescent boys. Pediatr Res 10:647, 1976

64. Parizkova J, Goldstein H: A comparison of skinfold measurements using the Bert and Harpenden calipers. Hum Biol 42:436, 1970

65. Peppler WW, Mazess RB: Total body bone mineral and lean body mass by dual-photon absorptiometry. I: theory and measurement procedure. Calcif Tissue Int 33:353, 1981

66. Prader A, Budliger H: Körpermasse, Wachstumsgischwindigkeit und Knochenalter gesunder Kinder in den usten Zwölf jaharen (Longitudinale Wachstumsstudie Zürich). Helv Paediatr Acta (Suppl) 37:1, 1977

67. Presta E, Casullo AM, Costa R et al: Body composition in adolescents: Estimation by total body electrical conductivity. J Appl Physiol 63:937, 1987

68. Revicki DA, Israel RG: Relationship between body mass indices and measures of body adiposity. Am J Public Health 76:992, 1986

69. Robertson CH, Engle CM, Bradley ME: Lung volumes in man immersed to the neck: Dilution and plethysmographic techniques. J Appl Physiol 44:679, 1978

70. Roche AF: Anthropometric methods: New and old, what they tell us. Int J Obes 8:509, 1984

71. Roche AF, Baumgartner RN, Guo S: Population methods: Anthropometry or estimation. In Norgan NG (ed): Human Body Composition and Fat Distribution. Report of an E C Workshop, December 10–12, 1985. London, England. Euro-Nut Report Series

72. Roche AF, Guo S, Houtkooper L: Biased estimation of fat-free mass. Proceedings of the 148th Annual Meeting of the American Statistics Association. New Orleans, LA, August 22–25, 1988

73. Roche AF, Siervogel RM, Chumlea WC et al: Grading body fatness from limited anthropometric data. Am J Clin Nutr 34:2831, 1981

74. Roede MJ, Van Wieringen JC: Growth diagrams 1980 Netherlands Third Nationwide Survey. Tijd Social Geyond (Suppl) 63:1, 1985

75. Rutledge MM, Clark J, Woodruff C et al: A longitudinal study of total body potassium in normal breastfed and bottle-fed infants. Pediatr Res 10:114, 1976

76. Sempe M, Pedron G, Roy-Pernot M-P: Auxologie: Méthods et Séquences, Paris. Paris, Laboratoire Théraplix, 1979

77. Slaughter MH, Lohman TG, Boileau RA et al: Skinfold equations for estimation of body fatness in children and youth. Hum Biol 60:709, 1988

78. Sloan AW, Shapiro M: A comparison of skinfold measurements with three standard calipers. Hum Biol 44:29, 1972

79. Steen GB, Isaksson B, Svanberg A: A body composition at 70 and 75 years of age: A longitudinal population study. J Clin Exp Gerontol 1:185, 1979

80. Tanner JM: Growth at adolescence. New York, Blackwell Scientific Publications, 1962

81. Tanner JM, Whitehouse RH: Revised standards for triceps and subscapular skinfolds in British children. Arch Dis Child 50:142, 1975

82. Tanner JM, Whitehouse RH: Clinical longitudinal standards for height, weight, height velocity, weight velocity and the stages of puberty. Arch Dis Child 51:170, 1976

83. Van Loan M, Mayclin P: A new TOBEC instrument and procedure for the assessment of body composition: Use of Fourier coefficients to predict lean body mass and total body water. Am J Clin Nutr 45:131, 1987

84. Van Loan MD, Segal KR, Bracco EF et al: TOBEC methodology for body composition assessment: A cross-validation study. Am J Clin Nutr 46:9, 1987

85. Vickery SR, Cureton KJ, Collins MA: Prediction of

body density from skinfolds in black and white young men. Hum Biol 60:135, 1988

86. VuTran Z, Weltman A: Predicting body composition of men from girth measurements. Hum Biol 60:167, 1988

87. Waaler PE: Anthropometric studies in Norwegian children. Acta Paediatr Scand (Suppl) 308:1, 1983

88. Waaler TH: Height, weight, and mortality: The Norwegian experience. Acta Med Scand 679:1, 1984

89. Watson PE, Watson ID, Batt RD: Obesity indices. Am J Clin Nutr 32:736, 1979

90. Weits T, Van Der Beek EJ, Wedel M: Comparison of ultrasound and skinfold caliper measurement of subcutaneous fat tissue. Int J Obes 10:161, 1986

91. Weltman A, Levine S, Seip RL et al: Accurate assessment of body composition in obese females. Am J Clin Nutr 48:1179, 1988

92. Widdowson EM, Dickerson JWT: Chemical composition of the body. In Comar CL, Bronner F (eds): Mineral Metabolism, Vol 2. New York, Academic Press, 1964

93. Williamson PS, Levy BT: Long-term body weight fluctuations in an overweight population. Int J Obes 12:579, 1988

94. Womersley J, Durnin JVGA: A comparison of the skinfold method with extent of "overweight" and various weight-height relationships in the assessment of obesity. Br J Nutr 38:271, 1977

95. Woteki CE, Briefel RR, Kuczmarski RM: Contributions of the National Center for Health Statistics. Am J Clin Nutr 47:320, 1988

CHAPTER 5

Body Composition Assessment Using Impedance Methods

HENRY C. LUKASKI

Various methods are currently available for the assessment of human body composition.[1] The majority of these methods are widely available and are based on anthropometric dimensions of the body, whole body density, or determination of total body water (TBW) using stable isotopes as tracers. Alternatively, more sophisticated methods using *in vitro* nuclear reactions or radiologic techniques are costly and not generally available. Two relatively new methods, tetrapolar bioelectrical impedance analysis (TBIA) and electromagnetic scanning (EMSCAN), the latter also known as total body electrical conductivity (TOBEC), which are based on specific electrical characteristics of biologic tissues, have been developed and applied to the estimation of body composition.

The TBIA and EMSCAN methods are dependent on the fact that water and electrolytes, which are located solely in the fat-free tissues, are effective conductors of electricity. In contrast, the triglyceride or the fat component of adipose tissue is relatively nonconductive because it is anhydrous and generally free of ions.[2] Thus, these electrical impedance methods have the potential to estimate fat-free mass (FFM), which then can be used to calculate body fat mass by difference from body mass and body fatness as a percentage of body mass.

The purpose of this review is to describe the general principles of the TBIA and EMSCAN methods and their applications for the assessment of human body composition. In addition,

an evaluation of current application of these methods is included.

TETRAPOLAR BIOELECTRICAL IMPEDANCE ANALYSIS

Theory and Model

The TBIA method is based on the conduction of an applied electrical current in the body. Introduction of a constant, low-level, alternating current results in a frequency-dependent opposition or resistance to the flow of the current in the body. In general, at low frequencies, the current passes through the extracellular fluids, whereas at higher frequencies it penetrates all fluid compartments.[2,3] The frequency-dependent conductive pathways are depicted in Figure 5-1.

Conduction of an applied electrical current is dependent on the volume and distribution of fluid and electrolytes in the conductor. Nyboer[4] described preliminary trials showing that resistive impedance was related to both water volume and electrolyte concentration. Meguid and colleagues[5] used an *in vitro* single-cell system to confirm that resistance was linearly related to fluid volume and electrolyte content.

The hypothesis that TBIA measurements can be related to conductive tissue volume and thus to FFM is based on the principle that the impedance of an isotropic conductor is related to some specific factors (Fig. 5-2). Using a constant signal frequency and assuming a relatively constant

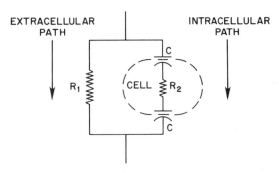

EXTRACELLULAR   INTRACELLULAR
PATH   PATH

FIGURE 5-1

Representation of the influence of signal frequency on extracellular and intracellular electrical conduction.

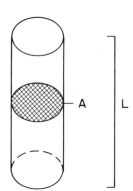

1. length (L)
2. configuration
3. cross-sectional area (A)
4. signal frequency

FIGURE 5-2

Factors affecting the impedance of a conductor.

conductor configuration, the bioelectrical impedance to the flow of current can be related to the volume of the biologic conductor[6]: $Z = \rho L^2 / V$, where Z is impedance in ohm, ρ is volume-resistivity in ohm · cm, L is conductor length (which is assumed to be stature) in centimeters, and V is volume in cubic centimeters or liters. Although difficulties may be encountered in applying this general relationship to a system with complex geometry and characteristics, as in the human body, this model has been used to develop mathematical models relating impedance measurements to body composition variables.

Instrumentation and Measurement

Determination of body bioelectrical impedance is performed using a tetrapolar impedance plethysmograph and surface electrodes (Fig. 5-3). The four-electrode approach is used to minimize contact impedance or surface-electrode interactions.[7] For the bioelectrical impedance measurement, individuals wear clothes but no shoes or socks and lie supine in a horizontal position on a cot. Generally, measurements are performed on individuals 2 to 4 hours after they eat a light meal. Instructions are given to subjects to avoid alcohol and exercise for 24 hours before scheduled testing. Measurements are not performed on individuals with sweat accumulated on the skin.

Aluminum foil spot electrodes are placed in the middle of the dorsal surfaces of the hands and feet proximal to the metacarpophalan-

geal and metatarsophalangeal joints, respectively, and also medially between the distal prominences of the radius and the ulna and between the medial and lateral malleoli at the ankle. The current-introducing electrodes are placed a minimum distance of the diameter of the wrist or ankle beyond the paired detector electrode. A thin layer of electrolyte gel is applied to each electrode before application to the skin. An excitation of 800 μA alternating current at 50 kHz is introduced into the individual at the distal electrodes of the hand and foot, and the voltage drop is detected by the proximal electrodes. Using phase-sensitive electronics, the impedance (Z) is partitioned into its geometric components of resistance (R) and reactance (Xc), where $Z^2 = R^2 + Xc^2$.

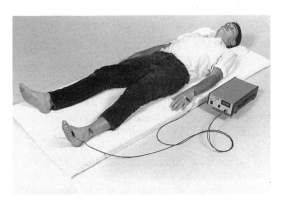

FIGURE 5-3

Measurement of bioelectrical impedance variables using an impedance plethysmograph (model 103, RJL Systems, Detroit, MI).

The technical reproducibility of the TBIA measurement determines its value in biologic applications. The error of repeated measurements of R using calibrated resistors ranging from 100 to 680 ohm measured twice daily for 11 days was 0.5 to 1.0%.[8]

Studies of biologic variability of R values among humans measured under similar conditions indicate small intraindividual deviation. Lukaski and colleagues[9] found a 2% (range: 0.9 to 3.4%) mean coefficient of variation in R values measured in 14 men during 5 days. Similar estimates of variability were reported by other investigators.[8,10]

Body Composition Assessment Using Tetrapolar Bioelectrical Impedance Measurements

Adults

Knowledge that water and electrolytes are located exclusively in fat-free tissues[11] stimulated investigators to develop mathematical relationships between FFM and impedance variables. Nyboer and colleagues[12] conducted a preliminary study that related height squared divided by resistance (Ht^2/R), where R was determined using electrodes placed on the right hand and foot, to body composition estimates in a sample of young men and women. Using densitometric data but lacking accurate residual lung volume data, the investigators developed preliminary statistical relationships between Ht^2/R and FFM. Using a similar impedance apparatus, Lukaski and associates[9] found that R, defined as the lowest R value observed along the four electrodes placement, was significantly correlated with FFM and total body potassium, an index of FFM ($r = -.86$ and $-.79$, respectively) in a sample of 37 young men whose FFM ranged from 44 to 98 kg and percent body fat (%BF) ranged from 8% to 43%. The best predictor of FFM, however, was Ht^2/R ($r = .98$). Other investigators[8,10,13,14] concluded that Ht^2/R was a significant predictor of FFM in their working models.

Although these preliminary findings suggested the potential of TBIA to estimate FFM, it was necessary to determine the validity of any proposed model using cross-validation studies. In a sample of 114 men and women who were between the ages of 18 and 50 years and whose %BF ranged from 4% to 41%, it was shown that the impedance equation developed in the men was capable of estimating FFM values in the women that were not statistically different than those determined using densitometry.[15] Similarly, the equation derived in the women predicted FFM values in the men that were not different from those estimated using densitometry. Also, the relationships between observed and predicted values in both groups were similar to the line of identity.

Another cross-validation study was conducted with a sample of 312 adults ages 18 to 73 years.[16] In this sample, FFM ranged from 31 to 99 kg and %BF was 7% to 55%. Individuals were randomly assigned to either a model or a validation group. Stepwise multiple regression analysis was used to develop the best FFM prediction equation in the model group; this equation then was tested in the validation group. This trial indicated that use of the derived model and the appropriate impedance variables resulted in compositional values not different from the densitometric reference values. Furthermore, measured and predicted values were distributed along a line similar to the line of identity (Fig. 5-4), indicating the validity of the impedance method to assess FFM in adults.

The TBIA method can also be used indirectly to assess %BF. Using impedance predictions of FFM and body mass, one can calculate %BF in the previously described study.[16] It is important to note that the relationship between the measured and predicted %BF values was not different from the line of identity (Fig. 5-5).

Comparisons of mean estimates of %BF derived using densitometry and anthropometry and calculated %BF using TBIA predictions of FFM indicated no statistical differences between these methods. However, the correlation coefficient relating densitometric and impedance-calculated %BF values was significantly greater than that observed between the densitometric and anthropometric values. The standard error of the estimate (SEE) of the relationship between densitometric estimates and impedance-derived predictions of %BF was 2.9%, which is similar to the theoretical precision of the densitometric method.[17] The SEE of the relationship between densitometric and anthropometric estimates of %BF was 3.7%.

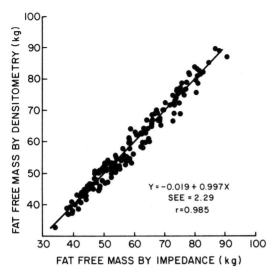

FIGURE 5-4

Relationship between FFM determined by densitometry and predicted by tetrapolar bioelectrical impedance analysis. (Lukaski HC, Bolonchuk, WW: Theory and validation of the tetrapolar bioelectrical impedance method to assess human body composition. In Ellis KJ, Yasumura S, Morgan WD [eds]: *In Vivo Body Composition Studies*, p 412. London, Institute of Physical Sciences in Medicine, 1987. Used with permission of Institute of Physical Sciences in Medicine)

Children

The TBIA method has been used to develop models for estimating FFM of children. Cordain and associates[18] studied 30 boys and girls ages 9 to 14 years and reported a significant correlation between FFM determined using densitometry and Ht^2/R, where R was measured along the right side of the body. Houtkooper and colleagues[19] developed an impedance model to predict FFM derived from measurements of body density and TBW in a group of 94 boys and girls. The prediction equation containing Ht^2/R, where R was determined using the electrodes placed on right hand and ankle, and body weight had a multiple correlation coefficient of 0.93. Stepwise multiple regression analysis identified the best equation as containing Ht^2/R, chest circumference, hip skeletal width, and Xc ($R^2 = 0.94$; SEE = 1.9 kg). Cross-validation using adult-based prediction equations[15] indicated statistical agreement between measured and predicted values.

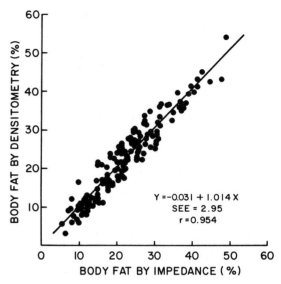

FIGURE 5-5

Relationship between percent body fat measured by densitometry and estimated by tetrapolar bioelectrical impedance analysis predictions of fat-free mass and body mass. (Lukaski HC, Bolonchuk, WW: Theory and validation of the tetrapolar bioelectrical impedance method to assess human body composition. In Ellis KJ, Yasumura S, Morgan WD [eds]: *In Vivo Body Composition Studies*, p 412. London, Institute of Physical Sciences in Medicine, 1987. Used with permission of Institute of Physical Sciences in Medicine)

Obesity

Several investigators[10,20,21] reported that the TBIA method overestimates %BF in lean individuals and underestimates it in obese people. Segal and colleagues[10] observed a significant relationship ($r = -.796$) between %BF residual FFM scores, calculated as the difference between measured and predicted FFM values derived from the impedance plethysmograph manufacturer's prediction equation. Subsequently, Segal and associates[21] reported a cross-validation study involving 1565 adults ages 17 to 62 years at four different centers. They confirmed the previous finding of an obesity-dependent error in predicting densitometrically determined FFM using TBIA. They also proposed and validated gender- and fatness-specific FFM prediction equations using Ht^2, R, weight, and age.

In contrast to these findings, only a minor in-

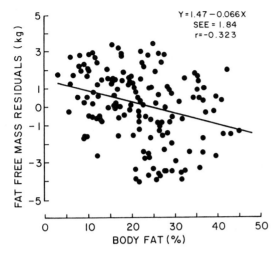

$$Y = 1.47 - 0.066X$$
$$SEE = 1.84$$
$$r = -0.323$$

FIGURE 5-6

Relationship between FFM residual scores and percent body fat. (Lukaski HC: Use of bioelectrical impedance analysis to assess human body composition: A review. In Livingston GA [ed]: Nutritional Status Assessment of the Individual. Trumbull, CT, Food and Nutrition Press, 1989. Used with permission of Food and Nutrition Press)

fluence of body fatness on the impedance prediction of FFM was reported elsewhere. Using data from a previous cross-validation study,[16] a weak relationship (Fig. 5-6) was observed between residual FFM scores and %BF in a sample of 161 adults.[22] These data indicate that body fatness accounts for a little more than 10% of the variance in the FFM residual scores in the sample studied. Thus, other factors are potentially more important than %BF in explaining the discrepancy between measured and predicted FFM.

Another cross-validation study was undertaken to further address this point.[23] An independent sample of 120 adults ages 18 to 60 years with a densitometrically determined FFM ranging from 30 to 85 kg and %BF ranging from 9% to 45% was studied. There was no difference between measured and impedance-predicted FFM values. The slope and intercept of the linear relationship between these values were similar to those of the line of identity. The correlation between FFM residuals and %BF was low (Fig. 5-7A). This observation confirms the previous findings of a minor influence of body fatness on the prediction of FFM using TBIA.

The %BF data were partitioned into quartiles, and the residual FFM values were calculated for each quartile to determine whether the magnitude of body fatness affected the errors in predicting FFM (Table 5-1). In each quartile, measured and predicted FFM values were related using regression analysis. The regression coefficients are summarized in Table 5-1. A significant difference was found between measured and predicted FFM in the group with the greatest %BF. With increasing fatness, the slopes of the regression lines relating the FFM values begin to deviate from unity. It is noteworthy that this divergence from unity is paralleled by an increase in the fraction of women in each quartile. Perhaps deviations from the assumptions of the two-compartment model of body composition[1] in these individuals are contributing to the residual scores. Thus, reference methods based on the two-compartment model may be inadequate for determining the validity of the TBIA method.

In a subsample of the individuals studied, deuterium dilution space was determined by standard methods.[24] When the FFM residual scores were plotted against deuterium space (Fig. 5-7B), the magnitude of the residual scores was relatively large in relation to the deuterium space. This observation supports the concept of a nonuniform water content in the FFM of these volunteers or the inconstancy of the chemical composition of the fat-free body.[25] Moreover, these data imply that an altered distribution of fluid—that is, an increased ratio of extracellular to intracellular water, which is present in obesity—may be responsible for the questionable TBIA predictions of FFM in the obese volunteers. This important point needs to be addressed further in future research.

Weight Loss

Some studies have addressed the potential of using TBIA to assess the composition of weight loss. Gray[26] reported a correlation coefficient of 0.94 between Ht^2/R and TBW determined before and after a 2-week fast in six obese women who experienced a 10-kg weight loss. Deurenberg and colleagues[14] found statistically similar values of change in FFM determined using densitometry and estimated using TBIA in 12 adults after 2 days on a very low calorie diet. In a second study, Deurenberg and associates[27] studied 13

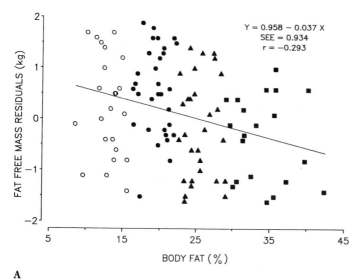

$$Y = 0.958 - 0.037 X$$
$$SEE = 0.934$$
$$r = -0.293$$

A

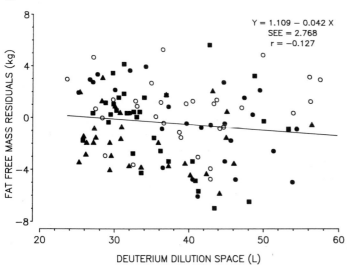

$$Y = 1.109 - 0.042 X$$
$$SEE = 2.768$$
$$r = -0.127$$

B

FIGURE 5-7

A: Distribution of FFM residuals by quartile of body fatness. *Open circles, closed circles, closed triangles, and closed squares* are first, second, third, and fourth quartile data, respectively. **B:** Distribution of FFM residuals in relationship to deuterium dilution space. Data are presented according to quartiles of body fatness. *Open circles, closed circles, closed triangles, and closed squares* are first, second, third, and fourth quartile data, respectively.

obese women whose body weight decreased 10 kg after an 8-week weight-reduction program. The TBIA estimates of FFM were significantly less than those determined by densitometry. The investigators concluded that disproportionate changes in TBW may have influenced the TBIA predictions of FFM.

Ross and colleagues[28] measured body composition using densitometry and TBIA[16] in a group of 20 obese adults before and after a 10-week program of supervised weight reduction through

caloric restriction and exercise. They reported no differences between measured and predicted FFM and %BF values.

Regional Impedance Measurements

The current practice of measuring body impedance using electrode placements at the wrist and ankle has been questioned because of possible error as the result of changes in the cross-sectional area between measurement sites.[29,30] It has been alternatively proposed that body seg-

TABLE 5-1

**Influence of Body Fatness on Prediction of Fat-Free Mass
Using Tetrapolar Bioelectrical Impedance Analysis**

	Percent Body Fat Quartiles			
	1	2	3	4
Number	31	27	31	31
Body fat, %	9–16	17–22	23–29	30–45
Mean fat-free mass residuals, kg	0.34	0.28	−0.38	−0.43*
Slope	0.99	0.98	1.03†	1.09†
Intercept	0.76	1.04	−1.03	0.17
F/M‡	4/27	12/15	22/9	25/6

*$p < .05$

†Significantly different than 1, $p < .05$

‡F/M = ratio of female to male volunteers

(From Lukaski HC: Applications of bioelectrical impedance analysis: A critical review. In Yasumura S, Harrison JE, McNeill KG, et al (eds): *In Vivo Body Composition Studies: Recent Advances*, p 365. New York, Plenum Press [in press])

ments be measured and mathematical models be developed for the prediction of whole body composition variables.

Some support of the use of regional or segmental TBIA measurements is available. Chumlea and colleagues[13] used anthropometric measurements, mathematical formulas, and regional impedance measurements to calculate the specific resistivities (e.g., ρ values) of the arms, trunk, and legs of 123 adults and children. They found that the specific resistivity of the trunk, including the thorax and abdomen, was significantly greater among those individuals with increased %BF, total fat mass, and subcutaneous adipose tissue mass estimated from skin-fold thicknesses. In another study, Baumgartner and colleagues[31] investigated the relationship between phase angle, calculated as the arctan Xc/R, determined for the whole body and body segments of 122 individuals ages 9 to 62 years. Phase angles for the trunk, leg, and body were inversely and significantly correlated with %BF. These preliminary findings indicate the potential of using regional impedance measurements to assess regional and total body composition in the population. Whether this approach can improve the predictive accuracy of the TBIA method remains to be determined.

ELECTROMAGNETIC SCANNING

General Principles and Model

In contrast to the TBIA method, in which the electrical signal is injected into the subject, the EMSCAN approach is based on the disruption that occurs when a conductor is placed in an electromagnetic field. The change in impedance predicts the conductor volume or mass placed in it. A high-frequency electromagnetic field is used to facilitate electrical conduction in all fluid compartments.

Figure 5-8 presents the general principle of the EMSCAN method.[32] When an oscillating electrical current is introduced into a large coil, an electromagnetic field is induced in the volume enclosed by the coil. An impedance meter attached to the system measures the change in the coil impedance when a sample is inserted into the coil. The change in impedance depends on the electrical properties of the inserted sample. In general, the electrical characteristics of the human body exert a net effect of decreasing the coil impedance relative to air.

When a biologic conductor is inserted in the electromagnetic field, electrical currents are induced because of the water and electrolytes present in the conductor. During this process, a small

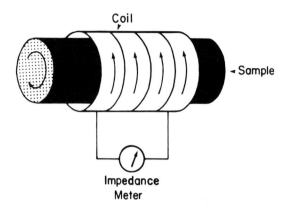

FIGURE 5-8

Noncontact whole body measurement principle of electromagnetic scanning. (Van Itallie TB, Segal KR, Funk RF: Measurements of total body electrical conductivity: A new method for the rapid estimation of human body composition. In Levander OE [ed]: Nutrition '87, p 82. Bethesda, MD, American Institute of Nutrition, 1987. Used with permission of American Institute of Nutrition)

portion of the energy generated by the coil is lost as heat. This loss is proportional to the conductive mass of the biologic sample and constitutes the change in the real part of the impedance of the coil. In an electromagnetic field such as that generated in the EMSCAN coil, the energy losses because of conductor mass in the sample are additive throughout the electromagnetic field.

In a definitive series of experiments, Klish and colleagues[33] demonstrated the validity of the EMSCAN method to predict water volume and sodium concentrations. Using an HA-1 instrument modified for pediatric use, they developed mathematical models to predict fluid volumes and electrolyte concentrations. These models were then tested in rabbits.

Instrumentation and Measurement

A prototype research instrument (HA-1) based on the work of Harker[34] (US Patent 3735247) was designed for human use (Dickey-John Medical Instrument Co, Auburn, IL). It contains a large solenoidal coil 12 feet in length with a rectangular configuration of 22 inches in width and 26 inches in height. A smaller, more recent version for pediatric use is shown in Figure 5-9. The coil

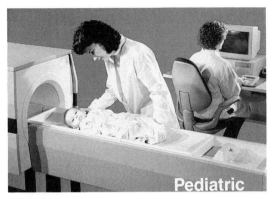

FIGURE 5-9

An electromagnetic instrument in a pediatric application. (Courtesy of EM-SCAN Inc, Springfield, IL)

is powered by a 5-MHz oscillating radio-frequency source and generates a focused magnetic field. This device exposes individuals placed in the coil to an energy field with a maximal energy flux of 0.01 mW/cm,[2] which is 1/1000 of the U.S. limit for microwave exposure during an 8-hour period.[35]

Subjects wear clothes but not shoes and lie on a stretcher or roller that is inserted into the device at the time of electromagnetic measurement. Each individual reading represents the mean of 10 determinations in a 10-second period. Ten successive readings are obtained for each subject, and the average is considered the individual's EMSCAN score. The total time required is less than 3 minutes.

The instrument is calibrated daily using a standard device to produce a constant signal. The calibration device is placed in the center of the magnetic field, and the instrument is adjusted to yield the appropriate calibration signal.[36]

Studies of the reliability of the HA-1 instrument show very good stability. Presta and colleagues[36] determined the intraclass correlation coefficient for ten repeated measurements of 32 adults to be .9999. Segal and associates[10] reported a 2% coefficient of variation for ten EMSCAN measurements in 75 adults.

The HA-1 instrument has been changed into a scanning device, the HA-2.[37] With this instrument (Fig. 5-10), the electromagnetic field is not a focused energy field, rather it encompasses an

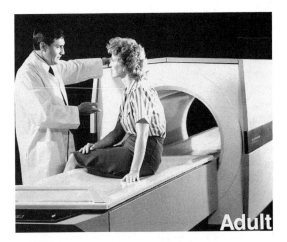

FIGURE 5-10

The HA-2 scanning electromagnetic device in an adult application. (Courtesy of EM-SCAM Inc, Springfield, IL)

area larger than that of the subject. Because the subject moves through the field, use of principles of convolution is necessary to assess the interaction between body geometry, including the distribution and volume of conductor, and the electromagnetic field.

Individuals are placed in the supine position and passed through the electromagnetic field head first. Each scan requires about 30 seconds. Individuals are scanned two to five times per trial. Using the scanning technique, the EM-

SCAN instrument measures 67 distinct conductive and dielectric points as the subject passes through the field. Each point is plotted to give the subject phase curve or waveform.

Figure 5-11 shows an example of an EMSCAN phase curve. The amount and distribution of the subject's FFM affect the shape of the phase curve. Because of convolution processing, the shape of the phase curve does not visually correspond to the geometry or shape of the subject or the FFM. Instead, the phase curve represents the sum of the convolution of the conductive mass and the dielectric mass of the subject moving through the electromagnetic field. The phase curve does not return to baseline because the subject does not pass completely through the magnetic field. Thus, the curve is extrapolated to the baseline within an abbreviated line using an algorithm dependent on the height of the subject. A simple numerical value, called *phase*, or phase average calculated for the area under the subject phase curve, is related to the subject's conductive mass.

The individual phase curve is subjected to Fourier analysis to describe the shape of the curve, which is dependent on the geometry or distribution of the conductive tissues, fluid, and electrolytes. This mathematical approach provides a means to correct for individual differences in subject geometry and enhance the predictive accuracy of the EMSCAN method.

The zero-order Fourier coefficient (FCO), as shown in Figure 5-11, represents the average

FIGURE 5-11

Typical subject phase curve generated during electromagnetic scanning in an adult application. (Van Loan M, Mayclin P: A new TOBEC instrument and procedure for the assessment of body composition: Use of Fourier coefficients to predict lean body mass and total body water. Am J Clin Nutr 45:131, 1987. Used with permission of American Society for Clinical Nutrition)

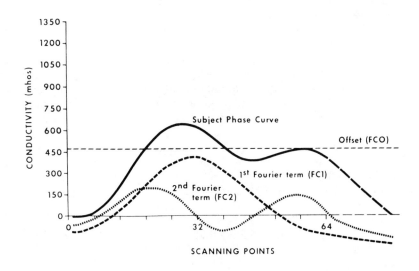

value of the extrapolated waveform. The higher-order coefficients (e.g., FC1 and FC2) represent the relative position of the individual components that, when added together, reconstruct the subject phase curve.

Calibration of this second-generation EMSCAN instrument also relies on an external standard.[37] The instrument is adjusted to a 1% tolerance of the 200-ohm calibration standard.

Body Composition Assessment

Adults

Presta and colleagues[36] developed a preliminary EMSCAN model to predict the FFM of adults. A sample of 32 adults ages 20 to 30 years underwent determinations of body composition by densitometry and EMSCAN using an HA-1 instrument. Body weight ranged from 45 to 155 kg, and percent body fat ranged from 10% to 53%. The EMSCAN number was significantly correlated with body weight and FFM (r = .942 and .903, respectively). A transformed EMSCAN score was calculated as height × EMSCAN number 0.5 to correct for interindividual differences in body geometry. This value was significantly correlated (r = .943) with FFM, but not different from the correlation between weight and EMSCAN number. A multiple regression equation for prediction of FFM was derived; it included the transformed EMSCAN score and gender (R^2 = 0.903; SEE = 3.76 kg).

Segal and colleagues[10] cross-validated this equation using an independent sample of 75 men and women ranging in body fatness from about 5% to 55%. They found a strong correlation between measured and predicted FFM values (r = .962; SEE = 2.99 kg); the relationship between these values was linear and similar to the line of identity. Also, the investigators reported that the slopes of the regression lines relating FFM by densitometry and the height × EMSCAN number$^{0.5}$ were significantly different between men and women. They found another transformation, height^2 × EMSCAN number$^{0.5}$, not gender dependent with measured FFM. Combining the raw data from the present study with that of Presta and colleagues,[36] Segal and associates[10] developed a predictive model of FFM that included gender and the new transformation of the EMSCAN number (R^2 = 0.947; SEE = 2.53 kg).

Using a scanning EMSCAN system, Van Loan and Mayclin[37] developed a model to predict densitometrically determined FFM in 40 adults with FFM of 36 to 78 kg and percent body fat of 6% to 30%. Correlations coefficients among FFM and FC0, FC1, and FC2 were significant (r = .97, .98, and .99, respectively). Each of the Fourier coefficients entered into the prediction model (R^2 = 0.983; See = 1.43 kg). Other multiple regression equations using the Fourier coefficients were developed for total body potassium (R^2 = 0.96; SEE = 294.5 mEq). In contrast to the prediction equations of Presta and colleagues[36] and Segal and associates,[10] which included height, the models of Van Loan and Mayclin[37] did not include an index of body geometry.

A cross-validation study was conducted using densitometric reference FFM data and HA-2 variables at two separate centers.[38] Adults were studied in California (n = 57) and New York (n = 103). Prediction models showed strong correlations between FFM and EMSCAN variables (r = .96 and .97). However, different prediction variables were identified in each sample. When the cross-validation method was applied to both data sets, it was determined that although the relationship between measured and predicted values was good (r = .94), there was a significant difference between the values. Regression analysis indicated that the relationships between these values were significantly different from the line of identity. Even with these differences, the authors combined data to yield another prediction model for FFM (R^2 = 0.96; SEE = 2.17 kg).

The second-generation EMSCAN was used to monitor changes in body composition during weight reduction.[37] Body composition was assessed using densitometry and EMSCAN variables in 11 overweight women before and after 3 and 6 weeks of supervised weight loss. After 6 weeks, an average of 6.6 kg of body weight, 1.7 kg FFM, and 4.9 kg of fat mass was lost. Significant correlations were observed among changes in phase, FC0, FC1, and FFM. A similar trend was noted between changes in FFM measured by densitometry and estimated by EMSCAN.

Infants

Reliable and accurate assessment of body composition of neonates and infants is a difficult challenge because most available methods are im-

TABLE 5-2

Characteristics of Impedance Methods for Assessment of Body Composition

Feature	Tetrapolar Bioelectrical Impedance Analysis	Electromagnetic Scanning
Safe	Yes	Yes
Noninvasive	Yes	Yes
Portable	Yes	No
Cost		
Purchase	Moderate	High
Operation	Low	Moderate
Ease of operation	Yes	Yes
Reproducibility		
Technical	Very high	Very high
Biologic	Very high	Very high
Accuracy	Acceptable	Acceptable

practical. The EMSCAN method is a reasonable alternative that may prove useful.

Cochran and associates[40] measured 16 infants, ranging in age from 2 days to about 10 months, in an HA-1 instrument and determined TBW using ^{18}O dilution. Estimates of FFM were calculated assuming a fixed fraction (82%) of the fat free body. They observed that the natural logarithm of the EMSCAN number was significantly correlated with TBW (r = .95). Also, a strong correlation (r = .96) was found between FFM calculated from TBW and the natural logarithm of FFM estimated from an equation derived in rabbits.[33] These preliminary findings indicated the potential of the EMSCAN method for assessing body composition of infants.

Subsequently, Fiorotto and colleagues[41] developed a more comprehensive equation to predict FFM based on direct chemical analysis of immature miniature pigs of size and weight approximating that of human infants. The independent variable in the derived model was the square root of the product of EMSCAN number × length. A very strong relationship was found between EMSCAN number corrected for length and chemically analyzed FFM (r = .998). Furthermore, the error of the prediction was 160 g, or less than 1% of the mean FFM value. Application of this model in a sample of 34 healthy infants ages 2 to 12 weeks yielded body composition estimates consistent with reference values.[42]

SUMMARY AND CONCLUSIONS

The ideal method for assessing human body composition should be safe, noninvasive, and inexpensive to purchase and operate. It should require limited technical skill for operation, be convenient for the subject, and yield highly reproducible and accurate results.[43] Unfortunately, no available method meets all of these stringent requirements.[1] In practice, investigators must reach a compromise between cost, ease of operation, reliability, and accuracy.

The TBIA and EMSCAN methods share many desirable functional traits for routine body composition assessment (Table 5-2). Some advantages of the TBIA include portability and reduced costs.

Both of these impedance methods have applications in population assessment of human body composition. The relatively large standard deviations observed in cross-validation studies indicate variability in within-subject predictive accuracy that may compromise the ability of these impedance methods to delineate small changes within individuals in a group. Whether this limitation is inherent in these methods or is an artifact of the problem of the generalizability of the two-compartment model of body composition assessment on which most human validation studies are based remains to be resolved.

References

1. Lukaski HC: Methods for the assessment of human body composition: traditional and new. Am J Clin Nutr 46:537, 1987

2. Pethig R: Dielectric properties of body tissues. Clin Phys Physiol Meas (Suppl A)8:5, 1987

3. Nyboer J: Workable volume and flow concepts of biosegments by electrical impedance plethysmography. T-I-T J Life Sci 2:1, 1972

4. Nyboer J: Electrical Impedance Plethysmography, 2nd ed. Springfield, IL, Charles C Thomas, 1970

5. Meguid MM, Campos ACL, Lukaski HC et al: A new single-cell in vitro model to determine volume and sodium concentration changes by bioelectrical impedance analysis. Nutrition 4:363, 1988

6. Hoffer EC, Meadow CK, Simpson DC: Correlation of whole body impedance with total body water. J Appl Physiol 27:531, 1969

7. Hoffer EC, Meador CK, Simpson DC: A relationship between whole body impedance and total body water volume. Ann NY Acad Sci 170:452, 1970

8. Van Loan M, Mayclin P: Bioelectrical impedance analysis: Is it a reliable estimator of lean body mass and total body water? Hum Biol 59:299, 1987

9. Lukaski HC, Johnson PE, Bolonchuk WW et al: Assessment of fat-free mass using bioelectrical impedance measurements of the human body. Am J Clin Nutr 41:810, 1985

10. Segal KR, Gutin B, Presta E et al: Estimation of human body composition by electrical impedance methods: A comparative study. J Appl Physiol 58:1565, 1985

11. Pace N, Rathburn EN: Studies of body composition. III. The body water and chemically-combined nitrogen content in relation to fat content. J Biol Chem 158:685, 1945

12. Nyboer J, Liedtke RJ, Reid KA et al: Nontraumatic electrical detection of total body water and density in man. Med Jadertina (Suppl)15:381, 1983

13. Chumlea WC, Baumgartner RN, Roche AF: Specific resistivity used to estimate fat free mass from segmental measures of bioelectrical impedance. Am J Clin Nutr 48:7, 1988

14. Deurenberg P, Weststrate JA, van der Kooy K: Body composition changes assessed by bioelectrical impedance measurements. Am J Clin Nutr 49:401, 1989

15. Lukaski HC, Bolonchuk WW, Hall CB et al: Validation of the tetrapolar bioelectrical impedance method to assess human body composition. J Appl Physiol 60:1327, 1986

16. Lukaski HC, Bolonchuk WW: Theory and validation of the tetrapolar bioelectrical impedance method to assess human body composition. In Ellis KJ, Yasumura S, Morgan WD (eds). In Vivo Body Composition Studies, p 410. London, Institute of Physical Sciences in Medicine, 1987

17. Lohman TG: Skinfolds and body density and their relationship to body fatness: a review. Hum Biol 53:181, 1981

18. Cordain L, Whicker RE, Johnson JE: Body composition determination in children using bioelectrical impedance. Growth Dev Aging 52:37, 1988

19. Houtkooper LB, Lohman TG, Going SB et al: Validity of bioelectrical impedance for body composition assessment of children. J Appl Physiol 66:814, 1989

20. Hodgdon JA, Fitzgerald PI: Validity of impedance predictions at various levels of fatness. Hum Biol 59:281, 1987

21. Segal KR, Van Loan M, Fitzgerald PI et al: Lean body mass estimation by bioelectrical impedance analysis: A four-site cross-validation. Am J Clin Nutr 47:7, 1988

22. Lukaski HC: Use of bioelectrical impedance analysis to assess human body composition: A review. In Livingston GA (ed): Nutritional Status Assessment of the Individual, p 189. Trumbull, CT, Food and Nutrition Press, 1989

23. Lukaski HC: Applications of bioelectrical impedance analysis: A critical review. In Yasumura S, McNeill KG, Harrison JE (eds). In Vivo Body Composition Studies: Recent Advances, p 365. New York, Plenum Press (in press)

24. Lukaski HC, Johnson PE: A simple, inexpensive method of determining total body water using a tracer dose of D_2O and infrared absorption of biological fluids. Am J Clin Nutr 41:363, 1985

25. Wedgewood RJ: Inconstancy of the lean body mass. Ann NY Acad Sci 110:141, 1963

26. Gray DS: Changes in bioelectrical impedance during fasting. Am J Clin Nutr 48:1184, 1988

27. Deurenberg P, Weststrate JA, Hautvaust GAJ: Changes in fat free mass during weight loss measured by bioelectrical impedance and by densitometry. Am J Clin Nutr 49:33, 1989

28. Ross R, Leger L, Martin P: Sensitivity of bioelectrical impedance to detect changes in human body composition. J Appl Physiol 67:1643, 1989

29. Settle RG, Foster KR, Epstein BR et al: Nutritional assessment: Whole body impedance and body fluid compartments. Nutr Cancer 2:72, 1980

30. Patterson R: Body fluid determinations using multiple impedance measurements. IEEE Eng Med Biol 8:16, 1989

31. Baumgartner RN, Chumlea WC, Roche AF: Bioelectric impedance phase angle and body composition. Am J Clin Nutr 48:16, 1988

32. Van Itallie TB, Segal KR, Funk RC: Measurements

of total body electrical conductivity: A new method for the rapid estimation of human body composition. In Levander OE (ed): Nutrition '87, p 82. Bethesda, MD, American Institute of Nutrition, 1987

33. Klish WJ, Forbes GB, Gordon A et al: New method for the estimation of lean body mass in infants (EMME instrument): Validation in non-human models. J Pediatr Gastroenterol Nutr 3:199, 1984

34. US Patent 3735247. Method and apparatus for measuring fat content in animal tissue either *in vivo* or in slaughtered and prepared form. May 22, 1973. Harker WH, inventor. The EMME Company, Assignee

35. Harrison GG, Van Itallie TB: Estimation of body composition: A new approach based upon electromagnetic principles. Am J Clin Nutr 35:1176, 1982

36. Presta E, Segal KR, Gutin B et al: Comparison in man of total body electrical conductivity and lean body mass derived from body density: Validation of a new body composition method. Metabolism 32:524, 1983

37. Van Loan M, Mayclin P: A new TOBEC instrument and procedure for the assessment of body composi-

tion: Use of Fourier coefficients to predict lean body mass and total body water. Am J Clin Nutr 45:131, 1987

38. Van Loan M, Segal KR, Bracco EF et al: TOBEC methodology for body composition assessment: A cross-validation study. Am J Clin Nutr 46:9, 1987

39. Van Loan M, Belko AZ, Mayclin P et al: Use of total body electrical conductivity for monitoring body composition changes during weight loss. Am J Clin Nutr 46:5, 1987

40. Cochran WJ, Klish WJ, Wong WW et al: Total body electrical conductivity used to determine body composition in infants. Pediatr Res 20:561, 1986

41. Fiorotto M, Cochran WJ, Funk RC et al: Total body electrical conductivity measurements: Effects of body composition and geometry. Am J Physiol 252:R794, 1987

42. Fiorotto M, Cochran WJ, Klish WJ: Fat free mass and total body water of infants estimated from total body electrical conductivity measurements. Pediatr Res 22:417, 1987

43. Garrow JS: New approaches to body composition. Am J Clin Nutr 35:1152, 1982

CHAPTER 6

Isotope Dilution Methods

DALE A. SCHOELLER

The principle of isotope dilution has been extensively applied to body composition analysis. Use has been extensive because isotope dilution analysis is ideally suited for measuring the mass of a chemical or element within the human body. Isotope dilution has been used to measure body potassium,[1] sodium,[2] and chloride,[3] but the vast majority of applications have been for the measurement of total body water.[4]

The principle of isotope dilution and many of the practical considerations are the same for each of these body components. These principles and considerations can therefore be discussed in a unified manner and illustrated with examples of total body water analysis.

ISOTOPE DILUTION PRINCIPLE

The principle of isotope dilution is that of mass balance. A known mass of tracer is administered and permitted to mix with body compartment. Because mass is conserved, the quantity of tracer in the compartment is equal to that in the dose. Thus, the size of the compartment is directly related to the dilution of the tracer in the body. For example, the measurement of total body water by isotope dilution is analogous to the addition of a known quantity of concentrated dye (isotope dose) to a larger beaker of water (body water). From the principle of mass balance, it can be calculated that

$$F_1 N_1 = F_2 N_2 \qquad (1)$$

where F is the mole fraction of the isotope in solution and N is the total number of moles of water. The subscripts refer to the dose (1) and the body water compartment (2). Typically, where F_1 and N_1 are known, F_2 is measured and N_2, the quantity of total body water, is calculated.

The major advantage of isotope dilution analysis is that not all the material being measured needs to be isolated and measured. Instead, only a representative aliquot of the material needs to be obtained and the concentration of tracer measured. Neither the shape of the container nor the addition of a second nonequilibrating material, such as triglycerides, to the beaker alters the measurement.

The analogy of measuring the amount of water in a beaker represents the ideal isotope dilution experiment. It is characterized by the tracer mixing almost instantaneously across the compartment to be measured, the tracer not being metabolized or excreted before reaching equilibrium, no new tracee being added to the system before equilibrium is reached, and the tracer exchanging totally and only with the tracee.

In vivo measurements are rarely made under the ideal conditions just listed. Unlike a beaker of water, water in the body is distributed among several anatomical compartments, and there is a finite delay from the time when the tracer is administered until it completely equilibrates with each of these compartments. Furthermore, water within the body does not exist in a static state because there is a continuous influx and efflux of water from the body. In addition, the tracer may not distribute equally into all compartments within the body. Alternatively, it may exchange with material other than the tracee.

These and other nonideal conditions pose some practical considerations for the application of isotope dilution analysis to human body composition analysis: determination of optimal time for tracer equilibration, demonstration of tracer equilibration and identification of the appropriate physiologic sample, correction for nonstatic conditions, and determination of the relationship between body composition and the measured tracer dilution space.

CALCULATION OF DILUTION SPACE

The influx and efflux of material from the body during the interval between administration of the tracer dose and final equilibration introduce a correction into the calculation of dilution space. The specific corrections to be applied to equation 1 depend on the protocol used for the administration of the dose and collection of physiologic samples.[5] These protocols are commonly referred to as the *plateau method*, the *overnight equilibration method*, and the *intercept method*.

Plateau Method

The plateau method is the most common protocol used in body composition analysis by *in vivo* isotope dilution. In this method, the tracer is administered at the instant in time at which the investigator wishes to measure body composition, and physiologic samples are collected serially until equilibrium is established. The important point is that the tracer is administered at the instant that body composition is being determined. Thus, in terms of the equality shown in equation 1, the amount of tracer in the body is by definition equal to the dose (F_1N_1), and tracer losses due to efflux of material from the body need not be considered because no time has elapsed between the administration of the dose and the time at which body composition is determined. There is, however, a delay between the time at which body composition is being determined and the time at which the equilibrated physiologic sample is collected. During this delay, new unlabeled material can enter the body and thus add to the size of the compartment being measured. This will result in a slightly lower tracer abundance at equilibrium than would be expected from only the material in the body at the time of the dose. Where this extra dilution is less than 5%, accurate corrections for the influx of new material can be made by following simple subtraction:

$$N_2 = (F_1N_1/F_2) - \text{new material} \qquad (2)$$

The size of this correction depends on the rate of material influx and the length of time to reach equilibration and thus is dependent on the body component being measured. Routes of influx include readily observed input (*i.e.*, sensible influx) as well as insensible influxes. For the example of body water, sensible routes of influx include food and drink and insensible routes of influx include metabolic water and environmental moisture.[6,7]

Food and drink can readily be controlled and measured during the period of equilibration. Under conditions in which the subject is not allowed to eat or drink, the only source of sensible water is the dose itself. The size of the dose varies from study to study, but a typical dose might include 50 ml of tracer and 50 ml of a chaser to wash out the container. For a 70-kg adult whose total body equals 57% of body weight, this 100-ml volume expands the body water pool by 0.25%.

Metabolic water cannot be readily measured. The influx can be estimated, however, from the rate of energy expenditure. For this same 70-kg adult, resting metabolic rate can be assumed to be 1 kcal/kg/hour. Assuming a respiratory quotient of 0.85, metabolic water production will be 0.25 g/kg/hour, which expands the body water pool by about 0.04%/hour.

The commonly overlooked insensible source of water is environmental water that enters through the skin and lungs. This influx occurs even under conditions of net evaporative water loss.[8] Because more than 99% of inspired water vapor exchanges with body water,[8] the rate of water influx from this source can be estimated from respiratory volume and ambient humidity.[6,7] For the example of the 70-kg adult with a resting energy expenditure of 1 kcal/kg and a relative humidity of 50% at 22°C, the estimated respiratory water influx is 0.06 g/kg/hour. Under the same conditions, influx of environmental water across the skin is estimated to occur at a rate of 4.9 g/m^2/hour.[8,9] Assuming that this rate is reduced by 50% in areas covered by clothing and that clothing covers about 50% of the body surface area, then transdermal water influx for a 70-kg adult with a body surface area of 1.8 m^2 is 0.1 g/kg/hour. Taken together, environmental water influx under temperate conditions is probably about 0.16 g/kg/hour, which would expand the total body water pool by about 0.03%/hour.

Overnight Equilibration

Overnight equilibration differs from the plateau method in that the tracer is not given at the time that body composition is measured but is instead given well before that time and allowed to equilibrate fully with the body compartment. Postequilibration physiologic samples are then collected at the time body composition is analyzed. Unlike the plateau method, then, there is no dilution between the time at which body composition is measured and the physiologic sample is collected, and thus there is no need to correct for dilution. There is, however, a delay between the time at which the tracer was administered and the time of the body composition measurement, and tracer can be lost from the body during this delay. Thus it is necessary to correct for tracer loss when using the overnight method:

$$N_2 = (F_1 N_1 - loss)/F_2 \qquad (3)$$

where loss is the sum of all the routes of tracer efflux.

The loss of tracer depends on the nature of the tracer and the length of time between dose administration and sampling. Again, turning to the measurement of total body water as the example for isotope dilution analysis, the routes of tracer efflux include urine production, respiratory gases, and transdermal losses.

The principal route of isotope loss is through urine production. Urine production averages 20 g/kg/day for an adult,[1] which is on average 0.8 g/kg/hour. Assuming that urine is fully equilibrated with body water, urination eliminates about 0.15% of the isotope dose per hour. In the absence of complete equilibration, which is most evident for the first urine produced after the dose, the exact loss can be measured by collecting the urine sample and measuring the volume and isotope abundance.

Loss of isotope through respiratory and dermal routes is rather difficult to quantitate. These losses can be estimated, but it should be noted that they are variable, depending on the ambient temperature and humidity.[11,12] Under temperate conditions, losses through these insensible routes account for about 40% of a typical water turnover of 7%/day. For a 70-kg adult with a total body water of 570 g/kg, this amounts to an average loss of 0.7 g/kg/hour or an isotope loss of about 0.12%/hour.

Isotope can also be lost in products other than the component of the body being measured. In the example of the measurement of total body water measured with ^{18}O, isotope can be lost as carbon dioxide (CO_2) in addition to the more obvious routes of water loss. For a typical 70-kg adult with a resting energy expenditure of 1 kcal/kg/hour and a respiratory quotient (RQ) of 0.85, this route eliminates about 0.05% of the ^{18}O tracer per hour.

In summary, the plateau and overnight methods differ in that the former measures body composition at the time of the dose and thus requires correction for excess dilution of the isotope during the interval between dose administration and equilibration, whereas the latter measures body composition at the time the equilibrated sample is collected and thus requires correction for isotope loss during the time between dose administration and sample collection. For the measurement of total body water by isotope dilution in a 70-kg adult, the dilution correction for the plateau method is on the order of 0.07%/hour of total body water plus the dilution of the dose itself. For a 4-hour equilibration, these add up to 0.5% correction. For the overnight method, isotope loss occurs at a rate of about 0.3%/hour, which can lead to 2% to 3% correction. These corrections are small, but not necessarily negligible. Moreover, the size of the correction increases with water turnover rate and thus can be two to three times larger in infants than in adults.

Intercept Method

Because the routes of isotope dilution and loss can often only be approximated, a third method of isotope dilution analysis has often been used. This method is the intercept method. Samples are collected during the initial portion of the isotope elimination period, and the isotope abundance versus time is plotted on semilog paper. The theoretical concentration at the instant of the dose is calculated by back extrapolation to the time of the dose. Because the time of the dose, the time of determining isotope abundance, and the time of measuring body composition all coincide, there is no need for corrections for either isotope loss or excess dilution. Equation 1 can be used directly to determine the isotope dilution space. Use of this method, however, is premised on two assumptions. First, the equilibration must be rapid relative to the elimination. If not, the isotope distribution phase displaces the curve to the right and alters the apparent initial isotope abundance. Second, the elimination rate must be constant over the period of sample collection. If not, the intercept is displaced from the true value.

TIME TO EQUILIBRATION

Application of any of the methods of isotope dilution requires knowledge of the period of equilibration. This period has been extensively evaluated for total body water analysis.[4,13,14] The time to equilibrate depends to some extent on the precision of the assay, because more sensitive assays can detect smaller differences from equilibration. It depends to a much larger extent on the nature of the tracer and the health of the subject. Under normal conditions, isotopic equilibrium in total body water is reached at 3 hours after the dose (Fig. 6-1). When large numbers of subjects are studied, there appears to be slight disequilibrium remaining at 3 hours. For example, when the ratio of isotopic abundances is compared for both ^{18}O (n = 20) and ^2H (n = 43), at 3 and 4 hours after the dose, the abundances average 0.3 ± 0.1% and 0.4 ± 0.1% greater at 3 hours than at 4 hours.[6] About one third of the change in isotopic abundance between 3 and 4 hours is due to the previously described dilution by metabolic and environmental water. The remaining 0.2% to 0.3% change is presumably due to a small continued mixing with compartments of body water that are slow to equilibrate.

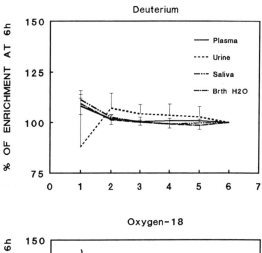

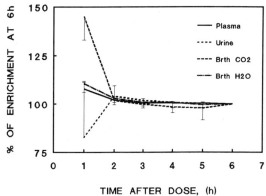

FIGURE 6-1

Time course for equilibration of deuterium (upper) and oxygen-18 (lower) labeled water in 20 adult men following oral administration. (From Wong WW, Cochran WJ, Klish WJ. *In vivo* isotope-fractionation factors and the measurement of deuterium- and oxygen-18-dilution spaces from plasma, urine, saliva, respiratory water vapor, and carbon dioxide. Am J Clin Nutr 47:1, 1988)

The shapes of the equilibration curves differ for various physiologic fluids. Plasma demonstrates a modest excess enrichment during the first hour after the dose. This results from the initial rapid influx of labeled water from the gastrointestinal tract and slightly slower mixing of plasma water with the remainder of total body water. This mixing, however, does not appear to represent a delay for equilibration with intracellular water in visceral tissues, because these tissues closely follow the isotopic abundance of plasma water.[15] Saliva, as does breath water, contains somewhat more tracer than plasma collected from the forearm during the first hour after the dose. This effect may be due to the higher relative blood perfusion of visceral organs at rest and thus a modestly greater delivery of rates absorbed tracer.

A much slower and more variable equilibration period is observed for urine samples than for saliva, blood, or breath water (see Fig. 6-1). Even at 6 hours after the dose, a larger coefficient of variation has been noted for the comparison of total body water volumes calculated from urine samples with that from sera samples (2.7%) than for saliva and sera (1.9%), indicating that urine equilibration may often be delayed several hours relative to other fluids.[13,14] The slower equilibration of urine is probably due to a mixing delay or "memory" within the bladder as a result of incomplete emptying. As such, the number of voids must be considered and is probably as important as time alone. In general, at least three voids need to be collected to ensure urinary equilibration with body water.

CHOICE OF PHYSIOLOGIC FLUID

As alluded in the previous section, the choice of the optimal physiologic fluid for sampling is predicated on the assumption that the isotope abundance in that fluid is representative of its abundance in the entire body pool. Thus, it must be shown that the isotopic abundance of the tracer in the physiologic fluid of choice is the same as in the body pool. This is obviously difficult in humans because the entire body pool cannot be sampled. Instead, the abundance of various physiologic fluids is compared with that in some central compartment after it has been demonstrated that the concentration of the isotope in that central compartment has reached a plateau abundance indicating complete equilibration. Demonstration of the same plateau abundance in various anatomical compartments is equally important, but this can usually only be done in animal models.

The choice of physiologic fluids for sampling has been carefully evaluated for total body water.[4,6,13,14] The study by Wong and colleagues[14] is one of the most complete. Recalculating isotopic

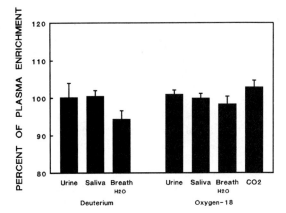

FIGURE 6-2

Comparison of apparent isotope dilution spaces of deuterium and oxygen in 20 adult men for samples collected 6 hours after the dose. Apparent dilution spaces are not corrected for isotope fractionation or exchange. (From Wong WW, Cochran WJ, Klish WJ. *In vivo* isotope-fractionation factors and the measurement of deuterium- and oxygen-18-dilution spaces from plasma, urine, saliva, respiratory water vapor, and carbon dioxide. Am J Clin Nutr 47:1, 1988)

abundances of both ^2H and ^{18}O in each of these physiologic fluids collected 6 hours after the dose demonstrates that urine and saliva do not differ from plasma (Fig. 6-2). In contrast, breath CO_2 is enriched in ^{18}O and breath water is depleted in both ^{18}O and ^2H relative to plasma. These differences amount to $+4\%$, -1%, and -6%, respectively, and are the result of isotope fractionation.[14] The isotopic fractionation arises as a result of isotope discrimination during the equilibration of oxygen between CO_2 and water and between water and water vapor, respectively. If breath CO_2 or breath water is used for sampling for the measurement of total body water without attention to the influences of isotope fractionation, the calculated total body water is in error in proportion to the isotope fractionation. This error can be eliminated by including a correction for isotope fractionation in the following calculation:

$$N_2 = \alpha F_1 N_1 / F_2 \qquad (4)$$

where α is the fractionation factor, which is equal to the isotope abundance of the tracer in physiologic fluid of interest divided by that in plasma.

RELATIONSHIP BETWEEN DILUTION SPACE AND BODY COMPOSITION

Isotope dilution analysis provides a measure of the dilution space of the tracer. Although this is related to body composition, the relationship is not necessarily one of equality. The dilution space can be either smaller or larger than the true body pool under investigation.

The isotope dilution space underestimates the body pool if not all of the material is exchangeable. For example, measurements of total body potassium by isotope dilution are slightly smaller than the true potassium pool, because not all potassium in the body is available for exchange.[1]

In contrast, measurement of total body water by isotope dilution overestimates the body pool because the isotopic tracers exchange with material other than water.[5,16] The degree of overestimation of the pool is subject to debate, but lies between 2% and 6% for deuterium or tritium isotope dilution and about 1% for ^{18}O isotope dilution.[5,13,16] The relationship between the isotope dilution space and the actual volume of total body water has been investigated by comparison of isotope dilution with total body water measured by desiccation. Most of these studies have involved hydrogen tracers. Individual results range from estimates of the dilution space being between 0 and 20% larger than body water, but the majority of the studies cite between 2% and 6%.[16] One of the difficulties in determining the exact relation from literature is that the measurement of the dilution space and the determination of water by desiccation are usually offset in time, and details needed to correct the dilution space for isotope loss or excess dilution by new water are not given. Moreover, obtaining desiccation results that are accurate to better than 1% or 2% is difficult.[16] Simultaneous measurements of deuterium and oxygen dilution spaces provide a much more accurate estimate of the minimal overestimate of total body water by deuterium because the measurements are not subject to the previously mentioned sources of error. These simultaneous estimates indicate that the deuterium space is 2% to 3% larger than the ^{18}O in neonates, who have a large ratio of body water to protein, and 3% to 4% larger than ^{18}O space in adolescents and adults.[17] A lively debate continues about whether the scatter of values about the mean in any one study represents real physiologic variation or measurement error.[17]

The expanded deuterium dilution space is evident soon after the dose and thus must be due to a rapid equilibration with nonaqueous sources of hydrogen. In eight subjects in whom we measured both the deuterium and ^{18}O dilution space and collected saliva samples at 3, 4, and 5 hours after the dose, the ratios of the deuterium to oxygen spaces were 1.032 ± 0.004 (standard error of the mean), 1.030 ± 0.005, and 1.027 ± 0.004. The trend in the dilution spaces is not significant with time, and the opposite trend has been noted in a second group of subjects.[6]

The likely sources of nonaqueous material with which the tracers can exchange are labile hydrogens in protein[18] and inorganic oxygen in minerals.[13] As indicated earlier, this exchange is quite rapid and appears to be relatively constant in a given population. As such, total body water can be calculated from the dilution space. Based on the difference between the deuterium and ^{18}O dilution spaces,[6,17] the observed relationships between the two dilution spaces and water by desiccation in small animals[18-20] and theoretical estimates of the amount of nonaqueous exchangeable material,[13,18] we have selected correction factors of 1.01 and 1.04 for the relationship between the deuterium and ^{18}O dilution spaces, respectively, with total body water.

ISOTOPE ELIMINATION METHODS

Elimination of the tracers from the body can provide valuable information in addition to that obtained about body composition. For example, the elimination rate of deuterium oxide provides a measure of water turnover.[7,20] Of even greater interest in the study of obesity, the simultaneous measurement of the elimination rates of deuterium oxide and $H_2^{18}O$ provides a measure of CO_2 production and hence energy expenditure. The use of the doubly labeled water method for measurement of CO_2 production and energy expenditure was pioneered by Lifson and McClintock.[21] They demonstrated that deuterium oxide was eliminated as water, whereas ^{18}O was eliminated as both water and CO_2. The difference between the elimination rates is therefore proportional to CO_2 production. The major advantage of the doubly labeled water method is that it can be easily applied in free-living individuals. Samples of physiologic fluids need to be taken only at the beginning and end of the elimination period. Between these times, subjects are free to perform their normal daily activities. Thus, CO_2 production and energy expenditure can be measured without the need to confine subjects to a metabolic ward or to be totally dependent on subjective diaries or logs.

The doubly labeled water method has been extensively reviewed.[17,20-22] As indicated earlier, the basic premise of the method is that deuterium is eliminated as water, whereas ^{18}O is eliminated as water and CO_2. Because the isotope elimination rates can be described by a single exponential function, the basic model can be easily described using the principles of mass balance:

$$Nk_H = r_{H_2O} \qquad (5)$$

and

$$Nk_O = r_{H_2O} + 2r_{CO_2} \qquad (6)$$

where N is total body water in moles, k_H and k_O are the elimination rates of deuterium and ^{18}O from body water, and r_{H_2O} and r_{CO_2} are the water and CO_2 production rates. Combining equations 5 and 6 and solving for r_{CO_2} yields the following:

$$r_{CO_2} = N(k_O - k_H)/2 \qquad (7)$$

As detailed earlier, neither deuterium nor ^{18}O is an ideal tracer. The isotope dilution spaces are larger than total body water, and evaporative water loss and CO_2 are subject to isotope fractionation. Incorporating these factors into the mass balance model yields a more complex but more accurate equation:

$$D_H = \alpha_1 r_{H_2Of} + r_{H_2Ol} \qquad (8)$$

and

$$D_O = \alpha_2 r_{H_2Of} + r_{H_2Ol} + \alpha_3 r_{CO_2} \qquad (9)$$

where D_O and D_H are the respective isotope dilution spaces, α_1 α_2, and α_3 are isotope fractionation factors between water and water vapor or CO_2, and the subscripts l and f refer to liquid and

fractionationed water, respectively. Combining equations 8 and 9 yields the following:

$$r_{CO_2} = (D_O k_O - D_H k_H)/2\alpha_3$$
$$- (\alpha_2 - \alpha_1)r_{H_2Of}/2\alpha_3 \qquad (10)$$

Thus, in addition to the isotope elimination, the isotope dilution spaces and the rate of fractionated water must be known. Investigators have used either individually measured isotope dilution spaces[22] or one measured space and the assumption that the deuterium space is 3% larger than the ^{18}O space.[17] Fractionated water losses include only breath and transdermal (nonsweat) water losses that have been estimated from CO_2 production[17] or a modified technique.[21] The best approaches to both of these corrections for nonideal tracer behavior is still controversial,[17,21] but the difference between the various correction techniques results in only small differences in average results for most individuals.[21] This may, however, prove more critical in subjects with large ratios of water output to CO_2 production.

The doubly labeled water method has been extensively validated in humans. Schoeller[17] has validated the method in 33 subjects including healthy adults, adults receiving parenteral nutrition, and postoperative infants. Validations were performed against both near-continuous respiratory gas exchange or measured dietary energy intake plus change in body energy stores. The mean difference between doubly labeled water and the reference method was 0.6 ± 6.3%. Coward and colleagues[23] and Roberts and associates,[24] at the Dunn Nutrition Laboratory, have validated the method in premature infants and healthy adults. The differences between doubly labeled water and respiratory gas exchange were −1.4 ± 4.8 and 1.9 ± 2.0%, respectively. Westerterp and colleagues[25] validated the method in bicyclists during heavy exercise. The difference between doubly labeled water and respiratory gas exchange during heavy exercise was 1 ± 7%.

The doubly labeled water method is a promising technique for measuring energy expenditure in free-living subjects. It has been validated in humans with an accuracy of 1% and a one standard deviation uncertainty of 3% to 7% depending on the dose of administered isotope and the length of the metabolic period.[26] Because the method is new in human research and is dependent on moderately expensive and technically difficult stable isotope methodology, it has only recently been applied in human obesity research. Both Prentice and colleagues[27] and Bandini and associates[28] have compared daily energy expenditure in obese and nonobese subjects. In both studies, the obese subjects were found to have a higher energy expenditure than the nonobese subjects, with the increase being not quite proportional to the larger body size. Both studies also documented a significant underreporting of energy intake by the obese subjects, such that the obese groups reported nearly the same intake as the nonobese but expended approximately 30% more energy—an observation that has important implications for previous studies of obesity based on reported dietary intake. In a related study, Bandini and colleagues[29] overfed both obese and nonobese adolescents with a high-carbohydrate diet supplemented with excess energy equal to the preoverfeeding basal metabolic rate. During the 2-week overfeeding, no increase in daily energy expenditure was observed, and both groups gained weight similarly. Thus, no difference in the partitioning of surplus energy was observed between the obese and nonobese adolescents.

CONCLUSIONS

Isotopic dilution analysis is the most precise method for the determination of the pool sizes of body water and other readily exchangeable components. Maximum precision, however, requires careful attention to the details of the dynamics of the distribution and turnover of the tracer. Isotope loss or excess dilution due to influx of new material can reach several percent because of the inherent delays between the time that the tracer is administered and the time at which the tracer reaches equilibrium. This time to equilibrium may vary depending on the sampling medium. Furthermore, it must be known whether the tracer equilibrates with the total body pool and only with the total body pool to determine the ultimate accuracy of the isotope dilution technique. In addition to body composition information, the ensuing rates of tracer elimination can provide additional information about the turn-

over in these compartments and are thus valuable for in vivo studies of human metabolism.

References

1. Forbes GB: Methods for determining composition of the human body. Pediatrics 29:477, 1962
2. Shizgal HM, Spanier AH, Humes J et al: Indirect measurement of total exchangeable potassium. Am J Physiol 233:F253, 1977
3. Threefoot SA, Burch GE, Ray CT: Chloride space and total exchangeable chloride in man measured with long-life radiochloride (Cl^{36}). J Lab Clin Med 42:16, 1953
4. Schloerb PR, Friis-Hansen BJ, Edelman IS et al: The measurement of total body water in the human subject by deuterium oxide dilution. J Clin Invest 29:1296, 1950
5. Schoeller DA, Jones PJH: Measurement of total body water by isotope dilution: A unified approach to calculations. In Ellis KJ, Yasumara S, Morgan WD (eds): p 138. London, Institute of Physical Sciences in Medicine, 1987
6. Schoeller DA, Kushner RF, Taylor P et al: Measurement of total body water: Isotope dilution techniques. Presented at the Sixth Ross Conference on Body Composition Assessments in Youth and Adults, Ross Laboratories, Columbus, Ohio, 1986
7. Fjeld CR, Brown KH, Schoeller DA: Validation of the deuterium oxide method for measuring average daily milk intake in infants. Am J Clin Nutr 48:671, 1988
8. Pinson EA, Langham WH: Physiology and toxicology of tritium in man. J Appl Physiol 10:108, 1957
9. Kuno Y: Human Perspiration, p 30. Springfield, IL, Charles C Thomas, 1956
10. Altman PL, Dittmer DS (eds): Biology Data Book, p 1496. Bethesda, MD, Federation of American Societies for Experimental Biology, 1974
11. Wilson D, Berardesca E, Maibach HI: In vitro transepidermal water loss: Differences between black and white human skin. Br J Dermatol 119:647, 1988
12. Shapiro Y, Pandolf KB, Goldman RF: Predicting sweat loss response to exercise, environment, and clothing. Eur J Appl Physiol 48:83, 1982
13. Schoeller DA, van Santen E, Peterson DW et al: Total body water measurement in humans with ^{18}O and ^{2}H labeled water. Am J Clin Nutr 33:2686, 1980
14. Wong WW, Cochran WJ, Klish WJ et al: In vivo isotope-fractionation factors and the measurement of deuterium- and oxygen-18-dilution spaces from plasma, urine, saliva, respiratory water vapor, and carbon dioxide. Am J Clin Nutr 47:1, 1988

15. Jeske DJ, Dietschy JM: Regulation of rates of cholesterol synthesis *in vivo* in the liver and carcass of the rat measured using [³H]water. J Lipid Res 21: 364, 1980

16. Culebras JM, Fitzpatrick GF, Brennan MF et al: Total body water and the exchangeable hydrogen. II. A review of comparative data from animals based on isotope dilution and desiccation, with a report of new data from the rat. Am J Physiol 232:R60, 1977

17. Schoeller DA: Measurement of energy expenditure in free-living humans by using doubly labeled water. J Nutr 118:1278, 1988

18. Culebras JM, Moore FD: Total body water and the exchangeable hydrogen. I. Theoretical calculation of nonaqueous exchangeable hydrogen in man. Am J Physiol 232:R54, 1977

19. Nagy KA: CO_2 production in animals: Analysis of potential errors in the doubly labeled water method. Am J Physiol 238:R466, 1980

20. Nagy KA, Costa D: Water flux in animals: Analysis of potential errors in the tritiated water method. Am J Physiol 238:R454, 1980

21. Lifson N, McClintock R: Theory and use of the turnover rates of body water for measuring energy material balance. J Theor Biol 12:46, 1966

22. Coward WA: The doubly-labelled-water ($^2H_2{}^{18}O$) method: Principles and practice. Proc Nutr Soc 47:209, 1988

23. Coward WA, Prentice AM, Murgatroyd PR et al: Measurement of CO_2 and water production rates in man using ^2H, ^{18}O-labeled H_2O: Comparisons between calimeter and isotope values. In van Es AJH (ed): Human Energy Metabolism: Physical Activity and Energy Measurements in Epidemiological Research Based on Direct and Indirect Calorimetry, p 126. Wageningen, Stichting Nederlands Instituut voor de Voeding, 1984

24. Roberts SB, Coward WA, Schlingenseipen K-H et al: Comparison of the doubly labeled water ($^2H_2{}^{18}O$) method with indirect calorimetry and a nutrient balance study for simultaneous determination of energy expenditure, water intake, and metabolizable energy intake in preterm infants. Am J Clin Nutr 44:315, 1986

25. Westerterp KR, Brouns F, Saris WHM et al: Comparison of doubly labeled water with respirometry at low- and high-activity levels. J Appl Physiol 65: 53, 1988

26. Schoeller DA: Energy expenditure from doubly labeled water: Some fundamental considerations in humans. Am J Clin Nutr 38:999, 1983

27. Prentice AM, Black AE, Coward WA et al: High levels of energy expenditure in obese women. Br Med J 292:983, 1986

28. Bandini LG, Schoeller DA, Dietz WH: Energy expenditure in obese and nonobese adolescents. Pediatr Res 27:189, 1990

29. Bandini LG, Schoeller DA, Edwards J et al: Energy expenditure during carbohydrate overfeeding in obese and nonobese adolescents. Am J Physiol 256:E357, 1989

PART THREE

ENERGY METABOLISM

Regulation of Energy Output
  Chapters 7–12

Regulation of Energy Intake
  Chapters 13–17

CHAPTER 7

Calorimetry in the Study of Obesity

PAUL WEBB

Physiological mechanisms underlying the prevalence of obesity in Western countries are largely unknown. Obesity is excessive fat storage, which has biologic value only in famine, and fat storage results from energy imbalance. Therefore, the study of obesity is a study of energy balance, and its major terms deal with intake and expenditure; fat storage represents a cumulative account of continuing energy imbalance.

The concept of energy balance is based on the first law of thermodynamics: energy is conserved. In a defined system, which is open to the import and export of energy and material,

$$\text{Energy in} = \text{Energy out} \tag{1}$$

$$Q_{food} + Q_{stores} = Q_{heat} + Q_{work} + Q_{urine} + Q_{feces} \tag{2}$$

where Q stands for quantity of energy, body energy stores are considered a source, and heat includes both body heat loss and heat storage. The energy actually available from food is the gross energy from complete oxidation less that which is not absorbed and that which is not oxidized; known as metabolizable energy (ME), it is $Q_{food} - (Q_{urine} + Q_{feces})$. Because work (external work, mechanical work accomplished) is normally a negligibly small quantity in a person's daily energy budget, it can be omitted from the equation, which then becomes:

$$ME + Q_{stores} = Q_{heat} \tag{3}$$

Whether or not there is food intake, there is continuous oxidation of fuel—metabolism, measured from respiratory gas exchange—and the fuel metabolized can be considered to be drawn from stores; thus,

$$Q_{metabolism} = Q_{heat} \tag{4}$$

For many purposes, energy expenditure can be measured either by direct calorimetry or from respiratory gas exchange, from the equivalence shown in equation 4.

By tradition, calorimetry is described as direct and indirect. The word *calorimetry* means, literally, the measurement of heat (calories), which is *direct* calorimetry. A measurement of respiratory gas exchange—that is, oxygen (O_2) uptake and carbon dioxide (CO_2) output—can be converted to energy equivalents (kilocalories, kilojoules), hence the term *indirect* calorimetry. This sounds as if the measurement is somehow less valuable. It is not. The measurement of gas exchange is just as accurate and reliable as the measurement of body heat loss, and there are additional meanings in the data (e.g., the estimation of what fuels have been oxidized). The choice of which method to use depends on the experimental situation, and direct calorimetry and respiratory gas exchange are often measured simultaneously. In any case, current reports usually provide data on energy expenditure during 24-hour periods.

"How much food does man require?" asked four important British nutritionists in a letter to *Nature*.[27] They believed that "the energy requirements of man and his balance of intake and expenditure are not known." This was especially true for individuals, and one of several examples was "the well recognized fact that many fat people eat no more, and sometimes less, than those who are not obese." They issued an urgent call for a calorimeter suitable for humans. A decade later, several calorimeters and several respiration chambers were active in human research, and the number has grown. These devices and how they are being used are the main topics of this chapter.

Fundamental questions in the study of obesity concern the differences between people who gain weight easily and those who do not, or between obese persons, postobese persons, and lean controls. Do they differ in the components of daily energy expenditure—sedentary and sleeping metabolic levels, thermic effect of eating, response to cooling, activities of daily living, exercise, and physical work? Do easy gainers lose less gross energy in body waste, or are they somehow more efficient metabolically? Do obese individuals fidget less or use less energy in a given exercise? Many of these questions are being addressed in calorimetric research.

The best answers come from studies in which energy expenditure is measured in periods of 24 hours or longer. Daily expenditure, or 24-hour expenditure, has become standard in calorimetric reports, a welcome contrast to earlier studies that relied on basal metabolic rate (BMR) data or the measurement of resting energy expenditure at various times of the day. Although continuous measurement in 24-hour periods requires effort and although each laboratory reports on only a small number of individuals, there are enough such reports now that 24-hour expenditure can be considered the new standard. In this chapter, only calorimeters and methods of respiratory gas exchange that are capable of 24-hour measurements are considered, and the results to be reviewed are those based on 24-hour data.

Although all the terms of energy balance listed in equation 2 are of interest in obesity research, the measurement of expenditure is the primary concern here. Therefore, the techniques of calorimetry are reviewed first.

DIRECT CALORIMETRY

In current use are calorimeter rooms and suits. The rooms[18,40,48,62,75] are well-insulated spaces in a larger temperature-controlled space so that there is a zero gradient for heat flow across the walls; heat from the occupant is taken up in recirculated air, which is cooled in an air-water heat exchanger. The measurement of heat loss is the measurement of water flow and temperature change across the heat exchanger or, exactly equivalent, the measurement of temperature change across a fixed heater located in the water stream compared with the temperature change across the heat exchanger. The rooms have fixed flows of ventilating air, which are carefully measured for gas composition coming in and going out, thus allowing simultaneous measurement of respiratory gas exchange. The rooms are furnished to allow for comfortable stays in multiples of 24 hours. The Vienna calorimeter[62] differs in that it measures heat loss from the power in a compensating heater added to the heat from the occupant to create a fixed rise in the temperature of the air flushing the room; it was not originally equipped for measuring respiratory gas exchange.

Internal temperatures of the calorimeter rooms are controlled for comfort or can be controlled over a small temperature range for studying responses to warm and cool conditions.

The occupant of the calorimeter room is in a normal air environment, not attached to any measuring equipment, and has space enough to live comfortably for days at a time. Although the subject has contact with the observer through an intercommunication system and can look outside through a window, he or she is nevertheless isolated to a degree. Social isolation seems to cause some subjects to become passive, with a consequent reduction in sedentary energy expenditure that affects the data.

A direct calorimeter in the form of a water-cooled suit worn next to the skin under thick insulating garments[69,73] measures heat loss by measuring the change in water temperature across the suit and the water mass flow. The insulating layers keep the heat exchange primarily between the water in the tubing network and the skin; a small and measured heat exchange remains, because no insulation is perfect. Evaporative heat loss from skin and from respiration is measured by periodic weighing. Temperature control is usually managed so that the experimental subject is always thermally comfortable,[66] and subjects can exercise quite vigorously without sweating. Alternatively, exposures to heat and cold can be simulated by changing the temperature of the water, because the suit is closely coupled to the skin, thermally and physically.

The suit can be worn for 1 or 2 days at a time; it is usually combined with the simultaneous measurement of respiratory gas exchange through a ventilated mask. The subject is encumbered with the bulkiness and weight (8 kg) of the clothing and must also contend with hoses and instrumentation cables. On the other hand, he or she is able to visit with an observer, chat directly with visitors, and move about in spaces that are less confined than the calorimeter rooms. Many forms of exercise can be studied—for example, walking on a treadmill, an unfeasible activity in a room calorimeter because of the heat that the treadmill generates within the room. Another advantage in some situations is the fast response inherent in the suit calorimeter, because the transit time of water through the suit is less than 30 seconds.

In any calorimetric measurement, body heat storage is one component of Q_{heat}. In 24-hour data, it is a negligibly small term, because in healthy people the circadian rhythm of body temperature completes its cycle, and energy balance over 24 hours has been repeatedly demonstrated when heat storage is taken to be zero.

Direct calorimeters are made to measure the rate of heat loss with an accuracy of 0.5% or greater. Long-term stability of instruments combines with this high accuracy to enable 24-hour measurements, and computer controls and data handling ease the burdens of experimenters. Direct calorimetry has become feasible in a number of laboratories because of modern instrumentation and computers. No longer should it be considered a rare and expensive technique for the lucky few. It continues to be the "gold standard"[44] for the measurement of energy expenditure.

Further details about direct calorimeters may be found in the cited literature and in two books on the subject.[46,69]

RESPIRATORY GAS EXCHANGE (INDIRECT CALORIMETRY)

In common use for most of this century, the measurement of O_2 uptake and CO_2 output is usually thought of in its early form—a mouthpiece and nose clip or a tightly fitting oronasal mask, with one-way valves to collect exhaled air—and therefore not comfortable enough for 24-hour measurement or measurement during sleep. In two current forms, the method is indeed comfortable and accurate enough to give reliable 24-hour data. The two forms are the ventilated canopy (or hood or face mask) and the respiration chamber. In both forms, the subject breathes room air while the apparatus gathers exhaust air, which is diluted exhaled air, and analyzes it for flow and change in gas composition.

Representative of the ventilated hood, canopy, or mask approach are the descriptions given by Buskirk and colleagues,[10] Garrow and Webster,[36] Jéquier,[41] Long and associates,[45] Spencer and co-workers,[59] and Troutman and Webb.[61] The ventilating flow is fixed at a level suitable to the activity of the person being measured. The flow is measured by an accurate volume flowmeter or mass flowmeter. A small sample is taken from the main stream of diluted exhaled air, dried, and led through stable, sensitive, and accurate gas analyzers for O_2 and CO_2. Analog signals from the flowmeter and the two analyzers are converted to digital data, and a computer calculates O_2 uptake and CO_2 output in standard liters per minute. (Well-engineered commercial versions of this equipment with excellent gas analyzers and flow sensors are currently available.)

Calculations include the Haldane transformation to adjust for the volume difference between incoming and outgoing air when O_2 volume differs from CO_2 volume—that is, when the respiratory quotient (RQ) is not 1. Final equations, as derived by McLean and Tobin,[46] are as follows:

$$\dot{V}O_2 = \dot{V}E\,[\Delta fO_2 + 0.2561\,(\Delta fO_2 + \Delta fCO_2)] \quad (5)$$

$$\dot{V}CO_2 = \dot{V}E\,(\Delta fCO_2) \quad (6)$$

where $\dot{V}O_2$ is oxygen uptake in liters per minute, $\dot{V}E$ is the flow rate of exhaust air in liters per minute, Δf is change in fractional composition of the gas, and $\dot{V}CO_2$ is CO_2 output in liters per minute.

An additional computation provides a continuous record of energy expenditure (in kilocalories) from one of several possible equations, usually that derived by Weir[76]:

$$M = 3.941\,O_2 + 1.106\,CO_2 - 2.17\,N_{urine} \quad (7)$$

or, more correctly, by Brockway[7]:

$$M = 3.962O_2 + 1.0779CO_2 - 1.41N_{urine} \quad (8)$$

The correction for urinary nitrogen, which is the residue of the incomplete combustion of protein, is small and little is lost if a standard value like 11 g/day is used.

If only energy expenditure is to be evaluated and the investigator does not need information about the mixture of fuel being oxidized, O_2 uptake can be measured simply from downstream airflow and O_2 content; the calculation simplifies to

$$M = 5\dot{V}E(\Delta fO_2) \quad (9)$$

The error in this simplification, 1% or less, is small because the error in not correcting for volume change from incoming to outgoing gas is almost compensated for by an opposite correction for the calorific equivalent of O_2 as the CO_2:O_2 ratio varies.[7,46]

Respiration chambers operate on the same principle as the ventilated mask, canopy, or hood. A sealed room contains the subject. (This has led to the use of the inappropriate term *whole body calorimetry*. Gas exchange, not heat, is measured. There is little improvement over systems that attach to the airway, because gas exchange is through pulmonary respiration and hardly at all through the skin.) As air flows through, it is carefully measured for volume flow and change in gas composition, and the same calculations are made as those for the ventilated hood.

One difference is notable. The respiration chamber has a large volume, from 9 to 30 m³, compared with a ventilated mask with a volume of 2 or 3 liters or a canopy with a volume of about 40 liters. The gas composition inside the large chamber volume thus changes slowly until a new steady state results from the balance of respiratory exchange and ventilation. Ventilation is controlled so that the CO_2 concentration is held to between 0.5% and 1%, a level thought to have little effect on respiratory ventilation rate or gas exchange. Because of the large volume in the chamber, a rapid change in O_2 uptake is attenuated in time. To partially overcome this—that is, to quicken the response time of the system— mathematical methods that are based on the rates of change of the gas concentrations are used.[12,47]

Descriptions of respiration chambers are given by Dauncey and colleagues,[18] Jéquier,[41,42] Jéquier and Schutz,[43] McLean and Tobin,[46] and Ravussin and associates.[54] The electronic gas analyzers are sometimes checked by an independent system for gas sampling with chemical analysis.[56,63]

A simplified form of respiration chamber was described by Dulloo and colleagues,[24] who proposed that a respiration chamber can become almost a field measurement and therefore widely used. Any small room can be partially sealed, ventilated with a suction pump, and the flow and O_2 content of the downstream air measured. Calculation with equation 9 gives energy expenditure.

PROOF OF ACCURACY

Current apparatus for both direct calorimetry and respiratory gas exchange is sufficiently accurate for studies of energy balance in obesity. Calibrated electrical heat sources and heated mannequins show that heat loss can be measured with an accuracy of 0.1%.[18,40,62,73] Evaporative heat loss is separately tested,[18,40,48,62] with accuracies of 2% to 3%. The measurement of respiratory gas exchange can be shown to be accurate at about the 2% level by injecting into the ventilated space from which the subject normally breathes a flow of dry nitrogen or CO_2 or both.[45,46,59,61] This test checks not only the accuracy of the gas analyzers but also the flow measurement and the data handling; it is a complete system check.

A second method often used is the alcohol or butane burner.[36,42] With care, complete oxidation of the fuel occurs, and the resulting loss of O_2 and production of CO_2 are measured by the apparatus. When a space is used for measuring both heat loss and gas exchange, the alcohol or butane burner acts as a complete system check for both measurements simultaneously. Its use began with the first successful human calorimeter at the turn of the century.[3]

A number of comparisons between direct calorimetry and respiratory gas exchange, conducted simultaneously over 24-hour periods, have shown quite satisfactory agreement, usually within 1% of each other.[18,65,72] One must not expect exact agreement in shorter periods, however, or during periods of high activity, owing to the temporal dissociation of heat production at the tissue level and the loss of that heat at the surface.[74] Other conditions may cause an apparent disagreement, such as the level of energy intake not matching the day's expenditure level.[67] Biologic variability and conditions other than rest during long periods must be carefully evaluated when looking for accuracy in comparisons of this sort.

Measuring the other terms in energy balance requires similar accuracy in research into the important questions in obesity. Some parameters can be measured with reliable accuracy, such as the gross energy of foods. Others, such as the measurement of change in fat mass, have poor accuracy, so that controlled conditions must last for weeks before a change is reliably distinguished from measurement variability.

Studies in which there was a determined effort to measure all the terms in energy balance show that this is still difficult. For example, in studies of undereating and overeating, investigators demonstrate errors in energy balance ranging from 100 to 600 kcal/day.[14,33,63,71,72] Reasons for the failures include inability to keep subjects in the calorimeter for enough time, estimating rather than measuring some of the terms, and the inherent inaccuracy in measuring some of the terms.

TWO NEW STANDARDS

After more than a decade of research with modern calorimeters and respiration chambers, it is clear that investigators prefer to report expenditure data in periods of 24 hours. Many of the same investigators have reported that the best predictor of daily expenditure is the fat-free mass of the body, an index of metabolic size that is independent of age, sex, or, very probably, ethnic origin.

Twenty-four-hour collections of data began as long ago as the 1860s in Germany and were impressively extended by Atwater and Benedict.[2] They reappeared after World War II in a study of energy balance during weight loss by Buskirk and associates[11] then by Apfelbaum and colleagues,[1] who did a study of the effects of over- and undereating on 24-hour expenditure, and in a 24-hour metabolic heat balance study by Webb.[65] Since the studies by Dauncey and co-workers,[18] reports based on 24-hour measure-

ment have become increasingly frequent. To illustrate, baseline descriptive data in normal men and women have been published by de Boer and colleagues,[21,22] Brun and associates,[8,9] Garby and Lammert,[29] Garby and co-workers,[30] Geissler and colleagues,[37] Murgatroyd and associates,[49] Prentice and co-workers,[50] Ravussin and colleagues,[52,54] Spurr and associates,[60] van Es and co-workers,[63] Warwick and colleagues,[64] Webb,[68] and Wolfram and associates.[77]

Studies of overeating and undereating with 24-hour data include those by Dallosso and James,[13] Dauncey,[15] de Boer and colleagues,[19] Garby and associates,[33] Ravussin and co-workers,[53] Schutz and colleagues,[57] Webb and Abrams,[71] and Webb and Annis.[72]

Studies that distinguish between lean and obese or postobese persons are those by Blaza and Garrow,[6] de Boer and colleagues,[20] Dulloo and Miller,[23] Dulloo and associates,[25] Geissler and co-workers,[38] Irsigler and colleagues,[39] Jéquier and Schutz,[43] Shah and associates,[58] van Es and co-workers,[63] and Webb and Annis.[72]

Twenty-four-hour data have been used to study many conditions that affect daily expenditure, including cool and warm room temperatures,[6,16] frequency of eating,[14] food composition,[17] diet-induced thermogenesis,[5,6,15,57] effects of stimulating drugs,[23,25] clerical work,[75] the menstrual cycle,[70] and pregnancy.[51]

Because so many groups have based so many studies on 24-hour data, it is hard to avoid using them as standards against which studies with lesser periods of measurement are compared.

A second standard concerns the confident prediction of 24-hour expenditure at rest from the fat-free mass of the body. For many years, daily energy expenditure has been estimated from a measurement (or prediction) of the BMR, which is typically the O_2 uptake during 6 to 10 min. The Harris-Benedict equation for converting BMR into 24-hour energy requirement and the estimates of food requirements for world populations based on BMR estimates[28] are still in use, despite the evident imprecision of the estimate for individuals.

As 24-hour data began to appear, so too did a new standard for daily energy need. Webb[68] reported that in 15 men and women ages 22 to 55, the relationship between 24-hour sedentary expenditure and fat-free body mass had a correlation coefficient of 0.95 and that this was independent of age and sex. Ravussin and colleagues[52] added 30 more individuals, normal in weight, overweight, and obese, showing the same high correlation of daily expenditure with fat-free mass. Since then, similar correlations can be found in many reports.[5,6,13,22,32,34,53,54] Some find equally reliable correlations with body weight.[20]

The argument is that the fat mass of the body has very low metabolic activity, whereas the fat-free mass can be thought of as the active cell mass, a concept based on experimental observation for more than 25 years, such as by Behnke,[4] who originated the technique for determining fat mass and fat-free mass from density. The older methods of BMR measurement or of the measurement of resting energy expenditure had failed to show unequivocally that fat-free mass was the proper index of metabolic size. Twenty-four-hour data made clear this logical relationship.

No longer is it necessary to include age, sex, or surface area in the prediction of daily expenditure. Age effects are explained by the loss of skeletal muscle mass over time, gender effects by the increased fat tissue in women, and surface area is an illogical measure of metabolic size. The surface area law implies that body heat loss has to increase as surface area increases, but this obligatory relationship denies the well-defined ability of humans to regulate body heat loss to maintain a nearly constant body temperature. These arguments were well set forth by Durnin and Passmore[26] and echoed by Webb[68] when 24-hour data had solidified the argument. Furthermore, two reports[9,22] strongly imply that people of Asian, African, and Indian origins do not differ in this respect from Europeans and American Caucasians.

BIOLOGIC VARIABILITY

If the techniques for measuring energy expenditure are demonstrably accurate, people are not as unvarying. Whether from biologic variability or from our inability to control all the factors that affect energy expenditure, the reproducibility of a single person's daily expenditure rate is on the order of $\pm$ 100 kcal/day, or about 5% of a daily total of 2000 kcal/day.[15,21,29-31,49,54,63,64,68,70]

Note that this level of reproducibility (5%) can

be very useful. Before modern methods made it possible to measure 24-hour expenditure routinely, the variability in individuals of BMR (or resting metabolic rate [RMR]) was on the order of 15%. Thus it was impossible to distinguish small effects like the increase of expenditure in the luteal phase of a woman's ovulatory cycle, which is about 8% on average.[70]

SOME RESEARCH FINDINGS

Several questions about mechanisms in obesity have been addressed with current calorimetric techniques. A brief review follows.

Do people who gain weight easily metabolize more of the food they eat than those who are thin and never gain weight? The answer is no in the several studies in which food intake was carefully measured, the foods analyzed for gross energy by bomb calorimetry, and waste collected to determine metabolizable energy.[20,63,71,72]

Does an obese person need less food to maintain weight than a thin person of the same stature? No. It has been shown that daily energy requirement under standardized, largely sedentary conditions is related to fat-free body mass (see earlier discussion) and that an obese person has a higher fat-free mass for his or her height than a thin person[5,6,20] and therefore requires a higher food intake to maintain body weight.

Do easy gainers and obese persons show blunted responses to the many conditions that increase metabolic rate (thermogenesis), such as food intake, anxiety, fidgeting, cool room temperatures, caffeine, and smoking? Garrow and Webster[35] reviewed the studies on these "small stimuli," noting that although they variously increased resting metabolism by 4% to 20% for from one to several hours, the effect on 24-hour energy expenditure was much smaller. They concluded that any abnormalities in thermogenic response, such as a lesser diet-induced thermogenesis in obese persons, were not important in explaining abnormal fatness or thinness. They emphasized the importance of direct observation of 24-hour expenditure by accurate calorimetric techniques, a viewpoint that is strongly supported here.

Variations in activity level are very difficult to monitor, but there is evidence that obese persons fidget less than thin people.[54] There is argument over whether obese people spend less energy than thin people during physical exercise and other activities of normal daily life, an important question that is difficult to answer by accurate but restrictive calorimetry in the laboratory. The methods of monitoring both the activity and its physiological cost are subject to unidentifiable variations, at least in methods such as heart rate monitoring[44,60] and actometry, which are often chosen because they interfere least with normal living patterns. The newly developed technique of measuring metabolic cost in free-living subjects, using doubly labeled water, as reviewed by Schoeller,[55] may provide better answers in time.

CONCLUSION

The difficult questions about the energetics of obesity can be best explored by calorimetric measurements that last at least 24 hours. Although the use of room calorimeters may be limited because of their high cost, suit calorimeters and respiration chambers can be installed with more modest investments, and ventilated mask, canopy, or hood machines can be widely used. With effective tools, imaginative hypotheses, and innovative procedures, investigators can hope to solve the difficult questions.

References

1. Apfelbaum M, Bostsarron J, Lacatis D: Effect of caloric restriction and excessive caloric intake on energy expenditure. Am J Clin Nutr 24:1405, 1971
2. Atwater WO, Benedict FG: Experiments on the Metabolism of Matter and Energy in the Human Body, 1900–1902. US Dept of Agriculture, Office of Experiment Stations, Bulletin 136. Washington, DC, US Govt Printing Office, 1903
3. Atwater WO, Rosa EB: Description of a New Respiration Calorimeter and Experiments on the Conservation of Energy in the Human Body. US Dept of Agriculture, Office of Experiment Stations, Bulletin 63. Washington, DC, US Govt Printing Office, 1899
4. Behnke AR: Relationship between basal metabolism, lean body weight and surface area. Fed Proc 12:13, 1953
5. Bessard T, Schutz Y, Jéquier E: Energy expenditure and postprandial thermogenesis in obese women

before and after weight loss. Am J Clin Nutr 38:680, 1983
6. Blaza S, Garrow JS: Thermogenic response to temperature, exercise and food stimuli in lean and obese women, studied by 24 h direct calorimetry. Br J Nutr 49:171, 1983
7. Brockway JM: Derivation of formulae used to calculate energy expenditure in man. Hum Nutr Clin Nutr 41C:463, 1987
8. Brun T, Webb P, de Benoist B et al: Calorimetric evaluation of the diary-respirometer technique for the field measurement of the 24-hour energy expenditure. Hum Nutr Clin Nutr 39C:321, 1985
9. Brun T, Webb P, Blackwell F: Energy expenditure over 24 hours, thermal comfort and fat-free mass in Asian men. Eur J Clin Nutr 42:113, 1988
10. Buskirk ER, Thompson RH, Moore R et al: Human energy expenditure studies in the National Institute of Arthritis and Metabolic Diseases metabolic chamber. Am J Clin Nutr 8:602, 1960
11. Buskirk ER, Thompson RH, Lutwak L et al: Energy balance of obese patients during weight reduction: influence of diet restriction and exercise. Ann NY Acad Sci 110:918, 1963
12. Cole TJ, Murgatroyd PR, Brown D et al: A rigorous mathematical analysis of gaseous exchange in indirect open-circuit calorimetry. In van Es AJH (ed): Human Energy Metabolism: Physical Activity and Energy Expenditure Measurements in Epidemiological Research Based on Direct and Indirect Calorimetry, pp 37–39. Euro-Nut Report No. 5. Wageningen, Netherlands, Agricultural University, 1985
13. Dallosso HM, James WPT: Whole-body calorimetry studies in adult men. I. The effect of fat overfeeding on 24 h energy expenditure. Br J Nutr 52:49, 1984
14. Dallosso HM, Murgatroyd PR, James WPT: Feeding frequency and energy balance in adult males. Hum Nutr Clin Nutr 36C:25, 1982
15. Dauncey MJ: Metabolic effects of altering the 24 h energy intake in man, using direct and indirect calorimetry. Br J Nutr 43:257, 1980
16. Dauncey MJ: Influence of mild cold on 24 h energy expenditure, resting metabolism and diet-induced thermogenesis. Br J Nutr 45:257, 1981
17. Dauncey MJ, Bingham SA: Dependence of 24 h energy expenditure in man on the composition of the nutrient intake. Br J Nutr 50:1, 1983
18. Dauncey MJ, Murgatroyd PR, Cole TJ: A human calorimeter for the direct and indirect measurement of 24 h energy expenditure. Br J Nutr 39:557, 1978
19. de Boer JO, Van Es AJH, Roovers LCA et al: Adaptation of energy metabolism of overweight women

to low energy intake, studied with whole-body calorimeters. Am J Clin Nutr 44:585, 1986

20. de Boer JO, van Es AJH, van Raiij JMA et al: Energy requirements and energy expenditure of lean and overweight women, measured by indirect calorimetry. Am J Clin Nutr 46:13, 1987

21. de Boer JO, van Es AJH, Vogt JE et al: Reproducibility of 24 h expenditure measurements using a human whole body indirect calorimeter. Br J Nutr 57:201, 1987

22. de Boer JO, van Es AJH, Voorrips LE et al: Energy metabolism and requirements in different ethnic groups. Eur J Clin Nutr 42:983, 1988

23. Dulloo AG, Miller DS: The thermogenic properties of ephedrine methylxanthine mixtures: human studies. Int J Obes 10:467, 1986

24. Dulloo AG, Ismail MN, Ryall M et al: A low-budget and easy-to-operate room respirometer for measuring daily energy expenditure in man. Am J Clin Nutr 48:1367, 1988

25. Dulloo AG, Geissler CA, Horton T et al: Normal caffeine consumption: influence on thermogenesis and daily energy expenditure in lean and post obese human volunteers. Am J Clin Nutr 49:44, 1989

26. Durnin JVGA, Passmore R: Energy, Work and Leisure. New York, William Heinemann, 1967

27. Durnin JVGA, Edholm OG, Miller DS et al: How much food does man require? Nature 242:418, 1973

28. FAO-WHO-UNU: Energy and Protein Requirements. WHO Technical Report Series 724. Geneva, World Health Organization, 1985

29. Garby L, Lammert O: Within-subjects between-days-and-weeks variation in energy expenditure at rest. Hum Nutr Clin Nutr 38C:395, 1984

30. Garby L, Lammert O, Nielsen E: Within-subjects between-weeks variation in 24-hour energy expenditure for fixed physical activity. Hum Nutr Clin Nutr 38C:391, 1984

31. Garby L, Lammert O, Nielsen E: Energy expenditure over 24 hours on low physical activity programmes in human subjects. Hum Nutr Clin Nutr 40C:141, 1986

32. Garby L, Garrow JS, Jorgensen B et al: Relation between energy expenditure and body composition in man: specific energy expenditure in vivo of fat and fat-free tissue. Eur J Clin Nutr 42:301, 1988

33. Garby L, Kurzer MS, Lammert O et al: Effect of 12 weeks' light-moderate underfeeding on 24-hour energy expenditure in normal male and female subjects. Eur J Clin Nutr 42:295, 1988

34. Garrow JS, Stalley S, Diethelm R et al: A new method for measuring the body density of obese adults. Br J Nutr 42:173, 1979

35. Garrow JS, Webster JD: Thermogenesis to small stimuli. In van Es AJH (ed): Human Energy Metabolism: Physical Activity and Energy Expenditure Measurements in Epidemiological Research Based Upon Direct and Indirect Calorimetry, pp 215–224. Euro-Nut Report No. 5. Wageningen, Netherlands, Agricultural University, 1985

36. Garrow JS, Webster JD: A computer-controlled indirect calorimeter for the measurement of energy expenditure in one or two subjects simultaneously. Hum Nutr Clin Nutr 40C:315, 1986

37. Geissler CA, Dzumbira TMO, Noor MI: Validation of a field technique for the measurement of energy expenditure: factorial method versus continuous respirometry. Am J Clin Nutr 44:596, 1986

38. Geissler CA, Miller DS, Shah M: The daily metabolic rate of the post-obese and the lean. Am J Clin Nutr 45:914, 1987

39. Irsigler K, Veitl V, Sigmund A et al: Calorimetric results in man: energy output in normal and overweight subjects. Metabolism 28:1127, 1979

40. Jacobsen S, Johansen O, Garby L: A 24-m^3 direct heat-sink calorimeter with on-line data acquisition, processing, and control. Am J Physiol 249: E416, 1985

41. Jéquier E: Métabolism énergétique. Encycl Méd Chir Paris, Nutrition, 10371 A 10, pp 1–14, 1980

42. Jéquier E: Long-term measurement of energy expenditure in man: direct or indirect calorimetry? In Bjorntorp P, Cairella M, Howard AN (eds): Recent Advances in Obesity Research, Vol III, pp 130–135. London, John Libbey & Co, 1981

43. Jéquier E, Schutz Y: Long-term measurements of energy expenditure in humans using a respiration chamber. Am J Clin Nutr 38:989, 1983

44. Kalkwarf HJ, Haas JD, Belko AZ et al: Accuracy of heart rate monitoring and activity diaries for estimating energy expenditure. Am J Clin Nutr 49:37, 1989

45. Long CL, Carlo MA, Schaffel N et al: A continuous analyzer for monitoring respiratory gases and expired radioactivity in clinical studies. Metabolism 28:320, 1979

46. McLean JA, Tobin G: Animal and Human Calorimetry. Cambridge, Cambridge University Press, 1987

47. McLean JA, Watts PR: Analytical refinements in animal calorimetry. J Appl Physiol 40:827, 1976

48. Murgatroyd PR: A 30 m^3 direct and indirect calorimeter. In van Es AJH (ed): Human Energy Metabolism: Physical Activity and Energy Expenditure Measurements in Epidemiological Research Based Upon Direct and Indirect Calorimetry, pp 46–48. Euro-Nut Report No. 5. Wageningen, Netherlands, Agricultural University, 1985

49. Murgatroyd PR, Davies HL, Prentice AM: Intra-

individual variability and measurement noise in estimates of energy expenditure by whole body indirect calorimetry. Br J Nutr 58:347, 1987

50. Prentice AM, Davies HL, Black AE et al: Unexpectedly low levels of energy expenditure in healthy women. Lancet 1:1419, 1985

51. Prentice AM, Coward A, Murgatroyd P et al: Energy expenditure during pregnancy. In Berry EM, Blondheim SH, Eliahou HE et al (eds): Recent Advances in Obesity Research, Vol V, pp 251–256. London, John Libbey & Co, 1987

52. Ravussin E, Burnand B, Schutz Y et al: Twenty-four-hour energy expenditure and resting metabolic rate in obese, moderately obese, and control subjects. Am J Clin Nutr 35:566, 1982

53. Ravussin E, Burnand B, Schutz Y et al: Energy expenditure before and during energy restriction in obese patients. Am J Clin Nutr 41:753, 1985

54. Ravussin E, Lillioja S, Anderson TE et al: Determinants of 24-hour expenditure in man. J Clin Invest 78:1568, 1986

55. Schoeller DA: Measurement of energy expenditure in free-living humans using doubly-labeled water. J Nutr 118:1278, 1988

56. Schoffelen PFM, Saris WHM, Westerterp KR et al: Evaluation of an automated indirect calorimeter for measurement of energy balance in man. In van Es AJH (ed): Human Energy Metabolism: Physical Activity and Energy Expenditure Measurements in Epidemiological Research Based on Direct and Indirect Calorimetry, pp 51–56. Euro-Nut Report No. 5. Wageningen, Netherlands, Agricultural University, 1985

57. Schutz Y, Bessard T, Jéquier E: Diet-induced thermogenesis measured over a whole day in obese and nonobese women. Am J Clin Nutr 40:542, 1984

58. Shah M, Miller DS, Geissler CA: Lower metabolic rates of postobese versus lean women: thermogenesis, basal metabolic rate and genetics. Eur J Clin Nutr 42:741, 1988

59. Spencer JL, Zikria BA, Kinney JM et al: A system for continuous measurement of gas exchange and respiratory functions. J Appl Physiol 33:523, 1972

60. Spurr GB, Prentice AM, Murgatroyd PR et al: Energy expenditure from minute-by-minute heart-rate recording: comparison with indirect calorimetry. Am J Clin Nutr 48:552, 1988

61. Troutman SJ, Webb P: Instrument for continuous measurement of O_2 consumption and CO_2 production of men in hyperbaric chambers. J Biomech Eng 100:1, 1978

62. Tschegg E, Sigmund A, Veitl V et al: An iso-thermic, gradient-free, whole-body calorimeter for long-term investigations of energy balance in man. Metabolism 28:764, 1979

63. van Es AJH, Vogt JE, Niessen CH et al: Human energy metabolism below, near and above energy equilibrium. Br J Nutr 52:429, 1984

64. Warwick PM, Edmudson HM, Thomson ES: Prediction of energy expenditure: Simplified FAO/WHO/UNU factorial method vs continuous respirometry and habitual energy intake. Am J Clin Nutr 48:1188, 1988

65. Webb P: Metabolic heat balance data for 24-hour periods. Int J Biometeorol 15:151, 1971

66. Webb P: Continuous thermal comfort in a suit calorimeter. In Durand J, Raynaud J (eds): Thermal Comfort: Physiological and Psychological Bases, pp 177–185. Paris, INSERM, 1980

67. Webb P: The measurement of energy exchange in man: an analysis. Am J Clin Nutr 33:1299, 1980

68. Webb P: Energy expenditure and fat-free mass in men and women. Am J Clin Nutr 34:1816, 1981

69. Webb P: Human Calorimeters. New York, Praeger, 1985

70. Webb P: 24-hour energy expenditure and the menstrual cycle. Am J Clin Nutr 44:614, 1986

71. Webb P, Abrams T: Loss of fat stores and reduction in sedentary energy expenditure from undereating. Hum Nutr Clin Nutr 37C:271, 1983

72. Webb P, Annis JF: Adaptation to overeating in lean and overweight men and women. Hum Nutr Clin Nutr 37C:117, 1983

73. Webb P, Annis JF, Troutman SJ Jr: Human calorimetry with a water-cooled garment. J Appl Physiol 32:412, 1972

74. Webb P, Annis JF, Troutman SJ Jr: Energy balance in man measured by direct and indirect calorimetry. Am J Clin Nutr 33:1287, 1980

75. Webster JD, Welsh G, Pacy P et al: Description of a direct calorimeter, with a note on the energy cost of clerical work. Br J Nutr 55:1, 1986

76. Weir JBdeV: New methods for calculating metabolic rate with special reference to protein metabolism. J Physiol 109:1, 1949

77. Wolfram G, Kirchgessner M, Müller HL et al: Energiebalanzversuche mit fettreicher Diät beim Menschem (Energy balance trials with fat-rich diet in humans). Ann Nutr Metab 29:23, 1985

CHAPTER 8

The Biochemistry of Energy Expenditure

J. P. FLATT

In a resting adult, some 25 to 35 g of adenosine triphosphate (ATP) is used every minute to drive the life-sustaining reactions that serve to transport molecules, maintain concentration gradients and muscle tone, accomplish the synthesis and secretion of biologic molecules, and produce the mechanical work required for respiration and blood circulation. This amount represents about half of the body's ATP content. During physical exercise, ATP utilization can increase to several hundred grams per minute. It is thus essential that the resynthesis of ATP from adenosine diphosphate (ADP) adjust itself very promptly to the rate of ATP utilization. This is made possible by a network of intracellular regulatory phenomena that are poised for effectively maintaining high ATP/ADP ratios and by the fact that the cells' enzymatic "machinery" usually operates far below its maximal capacity. Given the availability of various intracellular substrates, notably glycogen, substrate oxidation is in effect limited by the rate at which ADP is formed. This explains why ATP hydrolysis and its resynthesis from ADP and inorganic phosphate (P_i) are so closely matched and why the words *energy expenditure* and *energy production* are often used interchangeably. These intracellular features of energy metabolism are complemented by systemic and local regulation of blood flow to maintain tissue oxygenation and by a hormonal regulatory system capable of controlling the mobilization, distribution, and storage of metabolic fuels.

As verified by the classic studies of calorimetry,[13,37,43] the stoichiometric relationships between oxygen consumption and heat release associated with biologic substrate oxidations are the same as those observed during chemical combustions. The rate of energy expenditure and substrate oxidation can therefore be determined by measuring heat losses (i.e., by direct calorimetry) or by measuring oxygen consumption and carbon dioxide (CO_2) production.[48] If urinary nitrogen excretion (and possible changes in the body's urea pool) is also established, the changes due to metabolism in the body's content of carbohydrates, fats, and proteins can be computed, and the amount of energy released by these processes can be calculated. (It is useful to understand that "indirect calorimetry" establishes "changes in content," rather than "oxidation" of these substances, a distinction that helps to resolve possible concerns about the validity of the method when lipogenesis and fat oxidation or gluconeogenesis and glucose oxidation occur concomitantly.[21,35]) It should be kept in mind that this approach involves assumptions about the nature of the carbohydrates, fats, and protein oxidized, including notably that CO_2, water, and urea are the only quantitatively significant end products.[42] Measurements of energy expenditure have contributed much important information to our current understanding of energy metabolism. Much better quantitative information is available about the increases in ATP turnover and energy expenditure elicited by exercise and food intake than about the factors that determine and modulate energy expenditure in the resting state.

BASAL AND RESTING ENERGY EXPENDITURE

The rate of energy expenditure measured after an overnight fast in the postabsorptive state reflects a subject's "endogenous" or "basal" metabolic rate, because the effects of previous nutrient intake (if not excessive) and of prior physical exertion have by then maximally decayed. If adequate amounts of a typical mixed diet are consumed, the respiratory quotient (RQ) is then in the range of 0.8 to 0.85, depending on the relative proportions of carbohydrate and fat in the diet. Energy expenditures can be calculated by assuming a caloric equivalent of 4.83 kcal/liter of oxygen consumed. Basal, as well as resting metabolic rates (BMR, RMR) have been traditionally normalized by expressing them in relation to body surface area (BSA),[64] but data now show that they are more closely (and more logically) correlated with lean body mass (LBM) or fat-free mass (FFM).[11,53,54,60] Furthermore, differences previously attributed to age and sex are thereby largely eliminated. It is important to be aware of the fact that the correlation includes a substantial intercept on the vertical axis; BMRs (or RMRs) are therefore not proportional to FFM, and it follows that BMRs expressed per kilogram of FFM must be expected to be lower in heavy subjects. Variations in BMR have been extensively studied. They are known to be influenced by variations in the endocrine state. For example, variations of 6% to 10% have been reported to occur in the course of the menstrual cycle.[7,69] In addition to such circumstantial effects as may be due to diet selection and environmental conditions,[10,13] as well as to differences in body composition, some of the variability in resting energy expenditure is hereditary, because variations in metabolic rates among members of the same family are smaller than between unrelated subjects.[11] Substantial increases in RMR are elicited by catecholamine release,[39] hyperthyroidism,[15] fever, and various forms of stress, notably cold exposure.[13,32] Increases in resting energy expenditures caused by injuries, sepsis, and burns usually vary in parallel with variations in urinary nitrogen excretion, reflecting the significant metabolic cost of protein metabolism.[31]

EFFECTS OF FOOD INTAKE AND NUTRITIONAL STATE ON ENERGY EXPENDITURE

Meals induce a transient increase in resting energy expenditure, whose intensity and duration are related to the amounts and nature of the nutrients consumed,[37,43] as well as to the sensory stimulation that they elicit.[40] To characterize the thermic effect of food (TEF), the postprandial increment in energy expenditure above the resting rate is expressed as a fraction of the energy content of the nutrients consumed. The fraction of energy dissipated postprandially (formerly also known as *specific dynamic action* [SDA] of food) typically ranges from 5% to 10% for carbohydrate, 3% to 5% for fat, and 20% to 30% for protein.[37,43] Because their postprandial influx is much greater than the amounts of circulating substrates, nutrients must be promptly removed from the circulation and "stored" to preserve homeostasis. A substantial part of the TEF (usually 50% to 75%) can be attributed to the need to regenerate the ATP used for nutrient uptake and storage[22]; this is commonly referred to as the *obligatory component* of the TEF. Carbohydrate intake,[74] as well as the sensory stimulations caused by eating (or even merely by being exposed to foods),[40] stimulate the sympathetic nervous system. The ensuing catecholamine-mediated increase in the postprandial metabolic rate is generally referred to as the *facultative* or *regulatory* component of the TEF.[39] It can be largely suppressed by administration of β-adrenergic inhibitors, such as propranolol.[2]

Although the TEF is the most readily observed effect of nutrient intake on energy expenditure, the postprandial rise in energy expenditure has a lesser effect on overall energy expenditure than the sustained influence of nutrition on the resting metabolic rate (Fig. 8-1). During the elaborate studies of starvation conducted by Keys and colleagues[36] in human volunteers, a 45% decrease in overall energy expenditure was observed after 6 months of food restriction to half of the subjects' initial energy intakes. Decreases in body size and in physical activity accounted for most

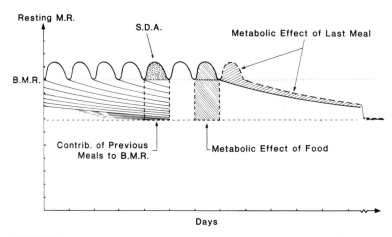

FIGURE 8-1

Effect of food intake on energy expenditure. The resting energy expenditure during successive days and the daily increases (TEF) due to food intake are shown schematically. A decline in the energy expenditure occurs on initiation of total starvation. (The rate of decline used in this drawing is somewhat steeper than it occurs in humans.) The dotted line shows the energy expenditure if food had been consumed for 1 more day. The difference between the two lines describes the metabolic effect of the last day's food intake. The surface of this band, being delineated by two pairs of parallel lines, is equivalent to that of a rectangle whose base has the length of 1 day. The delayed metabolic effects of previous food intake on energy expenditure during the fed period can thereby be inferred. The left half of the figure illustrates how the rate of energy expenditure in the basal, postabsorptive state is influenced by the food consumed on previous days. (From Flatt JP: Energetics of intermediary metabolism. In Garrow JS, Halliday D [eds]: Substrate and Energy Metabolism in Man, pp 58–69. London, John Libbey & Co, 1985)

of this decline in energy expenditure, complemented by a 15% decrease in the rate of energy expenditure per unit of body cell mass. On the other hand, BMRs are increased after a single day of excess consumption of a mixed diet,[16] but not if only excess fat is consumed.[66] During sustained overfeeding in humans, increases in body weight and body cell mass account for most of the increases in energy expenditure when mixed diet with a substantial fat content[52,60] or fat supplements are consumed.[14,66] Diet-induced thermogenesis (DIT) is generally considered to be the sum of the TEF plus whatever increase in the fasting metabolic rate may be induced by overeating. It should be appreciated, however, that a significant part of the RMR is diet related even in the absence of overeating (see Fig. 8-1). It is now increasingly recognized that increments in resting energy expenditures (i.e., DIT) caused by

overeating in humans[10,29,32,52,61] are a phenomenon of much smaller quantitative significance than the sometimes very substantial increases in DIT induced by overfeeding in many animals.[62] This type of nonshivering thermogenesis (NST) is mediated by activation of a special proton-conductive pathway in brown adipose tissue (BAT) that permits uncoupling of oxidative phosphorylation.[32,62]

EXERCISE-INDUCED INCREASE IN ENERGY EXPENDITURE

The increase in energy expenditure elicited by performing specific tasks under standardized conditions is highly reproducible and generally proportional to body weight.[13] Thus it is possible to predict more accurately the rate of energy expenditure of a walking individual (by taking into account body weight, speed of walking, slope of the track, weight that might be carried, and nature of the terrain) than that individual's RMR.[56] This indicates that the efficiency of metabolism in regenerating the ATP used up during muscle contractions is relatively constant. This ability to predict does not imply, however, that different individuals necessarily expend the same amount of energy to perform the same tasks, on account of differences in body weight and skill. At the end of a period of exertion, the rate of oxygen consumption decays rapidly but remains elevated above the resting rate.[5,6] This serves first to repay the "oxygen debt" (i.e., to restore myoglobin oxygenation, ATP, and creatine-phosphate to resting levels) and to reconvert to glucose some of the lactate, which may have accumulated by anaerobic energy production, though lactate is also readily oxidized by the heart. After vigorous exertion, a small increase in the metabolic rate can be noted even 24 hours later, possibly in part because of increased muscle protein synthesis.[6] It has been estimated that about 15% of the increase in energy expenditure induced by physical exertion occurs after the period of exertion itself.[5] Furthermore, the expansion of the muscle mass induced by regular physical activities also causes a long-term increase in the RMR.[70]

The actual impact of physical activities on overall energy expenditures is very difficult to assess accurately, because such activities vary so greatly among free-living subjects. This difficulty can now be overcome by assessing energy expenditure by the doubly labeled water method.[63] The application of this procedure has shown that daily energy expenditure in sedentary individuals may be less than 1.3 to 1.5 times their RMR, as often assumed,[58,59] whereas it is about twice the resting rate in young adults.[65] Furthermore, energy turnover can be substantially higher than one would infer from even carefully established food intake data.[75]

EFFICIENCY OF OXIDATIVE PHOSPHORYLATION AND P:O RATIO

The rate of ATP production is commonly calculated by multiplying observed rates of oxygen consumption by the P:O ratio, traditionally taken to be three high-energy bonds per atom of oxygen consumed when mitochondrial nicotinamide-adenine dinucleotide in the reduced form (NADH) is the source of the electrons fed into the mitochondrial electron-transmitter system. When the chemical theory of oxidative phosphorylation was replaced by the chemiosmotic theory,[50] the concept of a precise stoichiometry between oxygen consumption and high-energy bonds formed became less rigid. In fact there has been some debate about the number of protons pumped out of the mitochondrial membrane during the passage of two hydrogen atoms through the respiratory chain and about the number of proton translocations needed to induce the formation of one high-energy bond.[51] Furthermore, additional energy is required to transfer ATP from the mitochondrial to the cytoplasmic compartment, where the ATP:ADP ratio is higher. Finally, because some proton leakage always occurs, the number of high-energy bonds gained per oxygen consumed can be substantially less than three at low rates of substrate oxidation.[41]

In young men pedaling on a bicycle ergometer under "aerobic" steady-state conditions, 27% of the energy contained in the increment in substrate oxidation elicited by pedaling can be converted into mechanical energy[55] (i.e., the same value as that obtained for a horse on a treadmill).[37] By suddenly increasing the work load against which these subjects were pedaling, the transient use of preformed high-energy bonds (i.e., mostly creatine phosphate) could be induced, in addition to the amounts of ATP regenerated by oxidative phosphorylation. Comparing heat release and substrate oxidation rates during this transient phase and during steady-state pedaling, it was found that 41% of the energy content of preformed high-energy bonds was converted into mechanical energy (a value describing the "coupling coefficient" for the transformation of chemical into mechanical energy). The difference between 27% and 41% reflects the fact that only a fraction of the energy liberated by substrate oxidation is recovered in the form of ATP. In effect, the ratio of 27%:41% (i.e., 0.65) provides an in vivo estimate of the efficiency with which energy liberated by substrate oxidation is recovered in the form of ATP in working human muscles.[55] Of the 689 kcal/mol of free energy released by oxidation of 1 mol of glucose,[73] $689 \times 0.65 = 450$ kcal will accordingly be recovered in the form of high-energy bonds. Because the ΔG for ATP hydrolysis in muscle is about -14.3 kcal/mol[45] and because oxidative phosphorylation appears to be operating at near equilibrium conditions,[51] one can infer that 450/14.3, or some 31.5 mol of ATP are formed by oxidative phosphorylation during the complete oxidation of 1 mol of glucose. This corresponds to a P:O ratio of $31.5/(6 \text{ mol } O_2 \times 2) = 2.6$.[26] This *in vivo* estimate is in reasonable agreement with the limited number of situations in which evaluations of the P:O ratio in intact cells has been attempted.[26,41] Considering the number of assumptions and sources of possible errors inherent in these attempts, it is difficult to decide whether this value differs significantly from the traditional value of 3. In order to maintain consistency with common practices, a P:O ratio of 3 was used in subsequent calculations, even though it may be considered to be slightly high.[41] If the actual P:O ratio were lower than 3, the predicted costs of metabolic phenomena would be somewhat greater (i.e., by 15% to 20% for a P:O ratio of 2.6).

ATP UTILIZATION AND METABOLIC COSTS

When the stoichiometry of ATP consumption is known, it becomes possible to evaluate the costs of metabolic processes. Such costs should reflect the amount of substrate that needs to be oxidized to regenerate a given amount of ATP, rather than the energy liberated by ATP hydrolysis. Such estimates depend not only on the P:O ratio but also on the extent to which ATP is expended for the transport and handling of the metabolic fuels that provide the substrates for ATP regeneration.[25] For instance, 2 of the 38 mol of ATP produced during the oxidation of one glucose molecule are used for its "activation" to glucose-6-phosphate and fructose diphosphate, reducing the ATP yield to $36/38 = 95\%$. If one allows for the fact that perhaps 15% to 20% of the glucose released by the liver is recycled by way of the Cori and the glucose-alanine cycles (at a net cost of 4 mol of ATP/glucose recycled), only 90% of the ATP generated by oxidation of

glucose derived from liver glycogen becomes available to replace ATP used in peripheral tissues (Fig. 8-2). Significant portions of the carbohydrates supplied by the diet are now believed to be stored initially in the form of muscle glycogen,[17,38,44] so that a substantial part of the glucose released by the liver is in fact regenerated from lactate released by breakdown of muscle glycogen. The cost of gluconeogenesis would then consume additional ATP. Assuming that this cost applies to half of the glucose released by the liver, the net ATP yield during glycogen oxidation is reduced to about 82% (see Fig. 8-2). The heat of combustion (ΔH)[73] for glucose is 673 kcal/mol. It is numerically nearly equal to the ΔG for glucose oxidation $(-689$ kcal/mol), because changes in entropy associated with metabolic processes are relatively small. The turnover of 1 mol of ATP is thus indicated by the release of 685 kcal $(=$ estimated ΔH for fructose-1,6-diphosphate)/38 mol of ATP $=$ 18 kcal of heat. However, this amount would replace only 0.82 mol of ATP. It would require the oxidation of an amount of glucose containing $18/82\% = 22$ kcal to replace 1 mol of ATP consumed by a given metabolic process. To evaluate the energy expended in regenerating ATP by oxidation of fat, one has to consider that some of the free fatty acids (FFA) produced by triglyceride hydrolysis in adipose tissue are re-esterified (at a cost of 2.33 mol of ATP/FFA re-esterified) before leaving the adipocytes and that part of the FFA entering the circulation is removed and re-esterified by the liver and returned to adipose tissue in the form of lipoproteins (requiring 2×2.33 mol of ATP/FFA) (see Fig. 8-2). The rates at which lipolysis occurs relative to fat oxidation appear to be rather variable.[20] If one assumes that lipolysis proceeds at twice the rate of fat oxidation, that half of the nonoxidized fatty acids are re-esterified in adipose tissue and the other half return to adipose tissue through lipoproteins secreted by the liver, 3.5 mol of ATP are expended per mole of fatty acid oxidized. Oleate is the most common fatty acid in human triglycerides. During its oxidation, 146 mol of ATP/mol are generated, whereas 2 mol of ATP are expended for its activation to oleyl-CoA. The ATP yield for fat oxidation is thus approximately $140.5/146 = 96\%$. In view of the large amount of ATP gener-

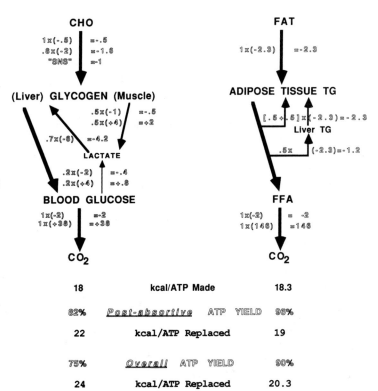

FIGURE 8-2

ATP expenditure during ATP generation by oxidation of carbohydrate and fat. The numbers in the schemes describe the product of substrate flux (in moles) multiplied by the number of moles of ATP consumed ($-$) or produced ($+$) per mole of substrate carried through various metabolic pathways. The fluxes are shown as they occur during the oxidation of 1 mol of glucose or 1 mol of oleic acid. The catecholamine-mediated increase in postprandial energy expenditure (assumed to account for one third of the thermic effect of carbohydrates) has been expressed in terms of an equivalent amount of ATP expenditure. (For further explanations, refer to the text.)

ated per mole of fatty acid oxidized, some variations in the rate of FFA re-esterification will not greatly modify this yield. The ΔH for oleyl-CoA oxidation is slightly higher than that for oleate (2657 kcal/mol), so that $2670/146 = 18.3$ kcal are produced per mole of ATP turned over, or $18.3/96\% = 19$ kcal per mole of ATP replaced by fatty acid oxidation (as compared to 22 by glycogen oxidation) (see Fig. 8-2). In the course of amino acid oxidation, 5.5 mol of ATP are expended for ureagenesis and gluconeogenesis per mole (110 g) of protein oxidized. This is equivalent to about 20% of the 28.8 mol of ATP generated by their oxidation.[22,47] During protein oxidation, a release of (110 g × 4.70 kcal/g[42] = 517 kcal)/28.8 mol of ATP = 18 thus indicates the turnover of 1 mol of ATP, but an expenditure of $18/0.8 = 22.5$ kcal of protein is required to replace 1 mol of ATP. Because only a fraction of the amino acids produced by protein breakdown is oxidized (possibly about one third[30]), amino acid oxidation is always accompanied by protein

resynthesis, a process requiring about 5 mol of ATP/amino acid incorporated into protein (i.e., 4 mol for the synthesis of the peptide bond plus an estimated additional mole for transport, mRNA synthesis, and so on). This would consume 10 mol of ATP in addition to the 5.5 used for glucose and urea synthesis per mole of amino acid oxidized. The net ATP yield for amino acid oxidation would accordingly be expected to be on the order of $(28.8 - 15.5)/28.8 = 45\%$.

It becomes evident from these considerations that the energy expenditure required to replace 1 mol of ATP can be expected to vary, depending on the mixture of endogenous metabolic fuels being oxidized. For example, when protein contributes 15% of the fuel mix oxidized, with carbohydrate and fat oxidized in proportions of 2:1 or 1:2 (RQ of 0.81 or 0.89), one would predict a heat release of 21.6 or 22.5 kcal/mol of ATP replaced, respectively, implying a 4% difference in the metabolic rate. This explains half of the 8% increase in the metabolic rate ($P < 0.005$)

during sleep observed in young adults when their diet was changed from a mixed to a high-carbohydrate diet.[34] If amino acids contribute 20% of the fuel mix oxidized and if this is considered to imply a commensurate increase in the rate of protein turnover as well, these values would increase to 22.2 and 23.1 kcal/mol of ATP replaced, respectively. Thus a 5% increment in the protein content of the fuel mix oxidized raises the metabolic rate by 3%.

The ATP yielded by different nutrients is further decreased when one takes into account the costs incurred for their initial transport and storage after ingestion. Assuming that in addition to the 2 mol of ATP used for the synthesis of glycogen, 0.5 mol of ATP are expended for active transport and intestinal enzyme synthesis and motility,[22] the energy expenditure would be equivalent to 2.5 × 22.5 kcal/mol of ATP replaced at a postprandial RQ of 0.89, or 56/673 = 8% for the storage of dietary carbohydrate as glycogen. The fact that some of the ingested glucose is used without prior conversion into glycogen (assumed to be 20% in Fig. 8-2) is more than offset by the stimulation of the sympathetic nervous system induced by carbohydrate intake.[39,74] In studies in which the amount of glycogen synthesis could be calculated from indirect calorimetry data, the energy expended for glucose storage was evaluated at 4% to 6% of the glucose energy infused, accounting for about two thirds of the observed increase in energy expenditure above the fasting rate, the remainder being attributable largely to increased catecholamine secretion.[2] When this latter component of the TEF was curtailed by administration of β adrenergic blocking agents, the thermic effect observed was consistent with the predicted metabolic expense for glucose storage.[2] Thus one can understand that the TEF for ingested carbohydrates is generally found to vary somewhat, being around 8% to 10%. Considering that one tenth or somewhat less of the energy provided by dietary carbohydrate is dissipated during the postprandial phase, the net ATP yield from carbohydrate is about 75% (i.e., 82% × 0.9). In the case of fat, the cost for the initial deposition of dietary fat would be predicted to reach about 3% of the energy provided by dietary fat,[22] but recent data indicate the TEF for fat in mixed meals to be near

5%.[14,27] The net ATP yield from dietary fat is thus reduced to about 90% (i.e., 96% × 0.95). These considerations suggest that the oxidation of 18/75% = 24 kcal of dietary carbohydrate, or the oxidation of 18.3/90% = 20.3 kcal of dietary fat is needed to replace 1 mol of ATP. This finding would indicate that 15% to 20% more energy may be required to sustain metabolism with dietary carbohydrate than with dietary fat, even in the absence of lipogenesis. The existence of such a difference is substantiated by data obtained during weight maintenance in *ad libitum* fed mice, where carbohydrate as a fuel, as compared with fat, was accompanied by a 9% to 12% increase in energy expenditure (Table 8-1). Such findings are consistent with Donato and Hegsted's[18] observation in growing rats that 35% of excess energy was retained when excess calories were provided in the form of fat, as compared with 28% with excess carbohydrate. In a group of 11 young adults studied by Hurni and colleagues,[34] the 24-hour energy expenditure measured in a respiratory chamber was 5% higher when they were consuming a high-carbohydrate, low-fat diet than when they ate a mixed diet (i.e., 2530 versus 2410 kcal/day). Carbohydrate intake and oxidation differed by 740 and 810 kcal/day, and fat intake and oxidation by 7.0 and 660 kcal/day, respectively. As shown in Figure 8-2, we estimated that 24 kcal have to be expended to replace 1 mol of ATP using dietary carbohydrate as the energy source, as compared with 20.3 kcal/ATP replaced (or 15% less) when fat is the substrate. Accordingly, one would expect daily energy expenditure to be some 810 × 15% = 120 kcal lower on the mixed as compared with the high-carbohydrate diet, in perfect agreement with the 120-kcal difference in daily energy expenditures that was observed. (It is important to appreciate, though, that a 10% shift in the energy provided by carbohydrate at the expense of fat, or *vice versa*, would be expected to alter overall energy expenditure by only 1.5% to 2%.)

The TEF elicited by protein usually falls into the 20% to 30% range. The ATP required to absorb and transport dietary amino acids into cells and then to convert them into protein may be estimated at about 5.5 mol of ATP per mole of amino acid mixture.[22] If the amino acids are oxi-

TABLE 8-1

Effect of Carbohydrate and Fat Content of Fuel Mix Oxidized on Energy Expenditure

$$\overbrace{\qquad\times 1.09\qquad}$$

(1) EnExp = 0.046 + 0.332 × 10^{-5} Rev/d + 1.10 CHOox + 1.01 FATox

$\pm$ .005 × 10^{-5}* $\pm$ .01* $\pm$ .01*

$[R^2 = 0.95*\qquad N = 1553]$

$$\overbrace{\qquad\times 1.12\qquad}$$

(2) EnExp = 0.02 + 0.338 × 10^{-5} Rev/d + 1.22 CHOox + 1.09 FATox

$\pm$ 0.005 × 10^{-5*} $\pm$ .01* $\pm$ .01*

$[R^2 = 0.96*\qquad N = 3225]$

(1) Daily energy expenditures, carbohydrate oxidations (CHOox) and fat oxidations (FATox) (in terms of kcal/g of body weight/day), and spontaneous running activities (number of running revolutions/day) observed in ten female CD1 mice during 160 consecutive days, on diets providing 18% of energy as protein, 13% or 45% as fat, and the remainder as sucrose and starch (1:1).

(2) Ten male CD1 mice studied during 345 consecutive days under similar conditions, except that the diets provided 13%, 27%, or 41% of dietary energy as fat.

*$P \leq$ .0001

dized instead, the ATP expenditure for transport, ureagenesis, and gluconeogenesis also equals about 5.5 mol of ATP.[22,47] Thus the TEF of protein is the same when either (or any combination) of these two processes is involved (i.e., 5.5 × 22.5 kcal/ATP replaced = 125 kcal/110 g of protein (contains 1 mol of amino acid mixture, whose energy content is 110 g × 4.70 kcal/g[42]) = 517 kcal of dietary protein ingested, or nearly 25%. However, depending on the proportion of amino acids initially converted into protein, subsequent costs for protein turnover vary, until an amount of amino acids equivalent to that initially incorporated into protein has in turn been degraded and converted into glucose and urea. Protein intake can thus be expected to influence energy expenditure beyond the postprandial phase. For instance, in patients receiving fixed amounts of energy by intravenous infusion but in whom 0.31 g of dextrose per kilogram of body weight per day was replaced by an equicaloric amount of amino acids (to provide 364 instead of 180 mg of amino acid nitrogen per kilogram

of body weight per day), an increase in energy expenditure of 2.2 kcal/kg/day was observed.[68] This is equivalent to 40% of the energy content of the additional dose of amino acids. Considering the concomitant decrease in the metabolic costs for handling glucose, dietary protein appears to raise the metabolic rate by an amount equivalent to about half of its energy content. On this basis, a 50 g/day difference in daily protein intake could be expected to alter energy expenditure by as much as 100 kcal/day.

METABOLIC COSTS OF LIPOGENESIS

Several reactions in the fatty acid synthesizing pathway require ATP, so that conversion of glucose into fat requires a substantial energy "investment," estimated at about 20% of the energy channeled into the lipogenic pathway.[22,23] If the costs for prior conversion of glucose into glycogen as well as for the transport of fatty acid synthesized in the liver to adipose tissue are also included, the cost for conversion of dietary carbohydrate into fat may be assessed at 25%.[4] In subjects consuming 1500 kcal/day of excess carbohydrate during 7 consecutive days, de novo fat synthesis reached 150 g/day. This was accompanied by a 35% increase in daily energy expenditure, equivalent to the dissipation of about 30% of the calories consumed in excess. About 25%/30%, or 83% of this increment can be attributed to the obligatory costs for de novo fat synthesis.[4] For humans, this is an uncommonly high rate of energy dissipation, manifesting itself only when lipogenesis is forcefully stimulated by deliberate and sustained overeating of large amounts of carbohydrate. In subjects consuming a Western diet, this process appears to be of minor quantitative significance,[57] because even the ingestion of an occasional carbohydrate load of 500 g can be accommodated by expansion of the glycogen reserves, without increases in body fat.[3] It can also be inferred from these results that glycogen reserves are spontaneously maintained in a range far below their maximal capacity, which implies that satiety occurs well before glycogen stores are full.[3,4,28]

Dissipation of dietary energy by conversion of glucose into fat is often considered to be a factor in explaining why high-carbohydrate diets are less conducive to obesity than high-fat diets. Given the limited quantitative significance of de novo lipogenesis when mixed diets are consumed, this is probably not a valid argument. Furthermore, the possible significance of lipogenesis for energy dissipation under conditions of energy balance is actually surprisingly small, when one considers that glucose energy channeled into fat, at a cost equivalent to 25% of its caloric content,[4] is followed by oxidation at the net ATP yield applicable to endogenous fat (i.e., 96%), for an overall net ATP yield of $0.75 \times 96\% = 72\%$, not much less than the 75% estimated in the absence of lipogenesis.

METABOLIC EFFICIENCY

The amount of energy retained during the development of obesity is quite small, when compared with daily energy turnover.[12] When averaged over a long period, the imbalance amounts to only a few percentage points between energy intake and energy expenditure. This observation

has elicited great interest in the possible role of even small differences in metabolic efficiency in the development or prevention of obesity. Relating energy deposited in the carcass to total amount of food energy consumed has for practical reasons long been important in judging "gross nutrient efficiency" in the production of meat. When defined in this manner, the apparent metabolic efficiency increases progressively as the amount of food consumed increases, simply because the energy dissipated to sustain metabolism thereby becomes relatively smaller. As shown in Figure 8-3, gross nutrient efficiencies are primarily a function of the rate of food overconsumption, next to which possible differences in efficiencies are obliterated. It also becomes obvious that gross nutrient efficiencies are lowered by physical activity, even if all metabolic processes proceed with unchanging efficiencies. Furthermore, in situations in which only small changes in body size occur, as is the case for adult humans, gross nutrient efficiencies calculated according to this definition are close to zero. They are thus quite useless in trying to judge the efficiency with which metabolic processes operate in the body.

A much more meaningful assessment of metabolic efficiency is possible by relating the amount of physical work produced to the change in metabolic rate that it involves, because in this situation the effect of the body's resting energy expenditure can be individually assessed and accurately subtracted. The impact of errors in correcting for resting energy expenditure are minimized by making observations under relatively high work load conditions. As mentioned earlier, typical values for aerobic exertion obtained in humans and animals are in the vicinity of 27%.[37,55] There appear to be no consistently detectable differences in work efficiency between normal and obese persons.[10,67] The idea to assess metabolic efficiency by establishing "net nutrient efficiencies" similarly involves making a suitable correction for maintenance energy expenditure. Accordingly, the amount of nutrient energy retained in the body is compared with the amount of food energy consumed in excess of maintenance requirements. This approach is made difficult, particularly in humans, because the required correction for maintenance energy

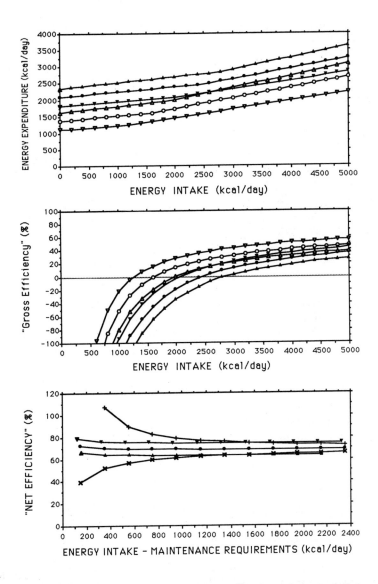

FIGURE 8-3

Conditions affecting the measurement of gross and net nutrient efficiency. The top panel shows how daily energy expenditure varies as a function of energy intake, assuming a basic metabolic rate of 1440 kcal/day (i.e., 1 kcal/min), a TEF of 10%, a decrease in metabolic rate attenuating energy deficits by 5%, and that 20% of the energy consumed in excess is dissipated (*open circles*). The effect of a ± 20% difference in resting and food-induced energy expenditure is shown by the *open triangles*. The *full symbols* are calculated for similar conditions except that physical activity is considered to raise energy expenditure by 720 kcal/day. The middle panel shows that the apparent gross nutrient efficiency is determined primarily by the level of energy intake and that differences in physical activity can have a greater impact on gross efficiency values than even large (i.e., ± 20%) differences in metabolic efficiency. The lower panel shows the apparent net nutrient efficiency for the case with exercise and the normal rate of energy dissipation (*full circles* in all panels). The two lines (*crosses*) show the impact of ± 5% errors in evaluating maintenance energy requirements. The lines identified by *full triangles* show net efficiencies when RMRs differ by ± 20%, assuming that maintenance energy requirements are based on actual measurements. The figure illustrates that errors in estimating maintenance requirements have an overwhelming impact when energy intake is less than 50% higher than maintenance requirements. Even at higher intakes, 5% errors have as great an impact on the apparent net nutrient efficiency as a ± 20% difference in metabolic efficiency.

requirements involves a rather large fraction of the energy turnover, and because these requirements keep changing as body weight and physical activities vary during the weeks needed to produce measurable changes in body composition. Because even small errors in estimating maintenance requirements have a considerable impact (see Fig. 8-3), the accuracy of such evaluations is quite uncertain and insufficient to reliably detect minor variations in metabolic efficiencies. Discussion of possible differences in metabolic efficiency in humans is thus generally based on comparisons of RMRs and of TEFs. Lower TEF has been reported for some but not all obese subjects, particularly following weight reduction.[71] Because the nonobligatory component of TEF dissipates no more than 3% to 5% of food energy, a partial reduction in this postprandial phenomenon has but a small effect on the overall resting energy expenditure, compared with the impact of changes in body size. Depending on the amount of physical activity, these may vary from 15 to 25 kcal/kg body weight change per day. Changes in body size must therefore be considered to be quantitatively the most significant variable in the adaptation of energy expenditure to energy intake.[72]

NUTRIENT BALANCE AND BODY WEIGHT MAINTENANCE

Maintenance of body weight requires not only that energy intake and energy expenditure vary about the same means, but also that the average composition of the fuel mix oxidized be equivalent to the nutrient distribution in the diet.[24,28] It has long been known from nitrogen balance studies that the body spontaneously maintains a nearly constant protein content (as long as the diet provides sufficient protein), irrespective of the proportions of carbohydrate and fat in the diet. The body's glycogen reserves (200 to 500 g)[9,33] are small compared with carbohydrate turnover (commonly 200 to 400 g/day).[12] Given the importance of maintaining blood glucose levels within a rather narrow range, the control of the carbohydrate economy is of critical physiological importance. This observation led Mayer and Thomas to develop the glucostatic theory of food intake regulation.[46] The endocrine and enzymatic regulatory phenomena developed in the course of biologic evolution indeed reflect that priority is given to the maintenance of carbohydrate balance, over the maintenance of fat or overall energy balance.[1,27,66] The adjustment of carbohydrate oxidation to carbohydrate intake is so well regulated that stable glycogen reserves can be maintained under widely different dietary situations.[9,33] It is noteworthy that the body's glycogen reserves are maintained in a range far below their maximal capacity (about 10 g/kg body weight in adults[4]), even when food intake is totally unrestricted.[3] This observation indicates that satiety signals exist that limit spontaneous food intake sufficiently to prevent the induction of rapid glucose conversion into fat, at least when mixed diets are consumed. If glucose does not escape from the carbohydrate pool by conversion into fat, carbohydrate oxidation and intake must be commensurate, just as is the case for amino acid intake and oxidation.

Maintenance of the fat balance assumes far less biologic importance, because the body's fat stores (commonly 50 to 200 times greater than its glycogen reserves) are too large to be markedly affected by daily errors in the fat balance.[12,14,66] Food intake leads to an increase in the carbohydrate content of the fuel mix oxidized, as evidenced by the postprandial increases in the RQ. This metabolic response is determined primarily by the carbohydrate and protein contents of a meal, but not by its fat content.[27] Thus carbohydrate intake promotes carbohydrate oxidation, whereas fat intake does not promote fat oxidation. On days of relatively high food intake, carbohydrate oxidation is enhanced to limit excessive accumulation of glycogen. The RQ is thus higher than the diet's Food Quotient (FQ) (i.e., the ratio of CO_2 produced to oxygen consumed during the oxidation of a representative sample of the diet) on days of high food intake and lower on days of less than average food intake.[28] As shown by data obtained in *ad libitum* fed mice (Fig. 8-4), carbohydrate oxidation is positively correlated with variations in food (and carbohydrate) intake, whereas fat oxidation is negatively correlated with food (and fat) intake.[24] As a consequence, the fat balance is least well regulated.[1,24] The failure of fat intake to promote fat oxidation is a circumstance that deserves special

FIGURE 8-4

Effect of variations in food intake on carbohydrate and fat oxidation in ten *ad libitum* fed female CD-1 mice. Individual cages were placed into separate 55-gallon drums hermetically sealed with Plexiglas lids. During 160 consecutive days, CO_2 accumulation and oxygen utilization were determined daily over 23 hours, and extrapolated to 24 hours. The animals had free access to a running wheel (whose use was recorded daily) and to one of two synthetic diets, containing 18% of energy as casein and either 13% or 45% of dietary energy as fat, with the balance as carbohydrate (half sucrose, half starch). Food intakes were measured daily, and individual corrections were applied for food spillage and incomplete nutrient absorption. Indirect calorimetry calculations were made assuming that the animals maintained nitrogen balance. Five of the mice were initially on the high-carbohydrate diet resembling laboratory chow in its macro nutrient distribution, and the other five were on the mixed diet. The diets were switched after 1 month; 2 months later, the animals were returned to their original diets. The bottom panel shows fat oxidation as a function of the difference between overall energy expenditure minus the energy consumed in the form of carbohydrate and protein. (For each correlation, N = 800.)

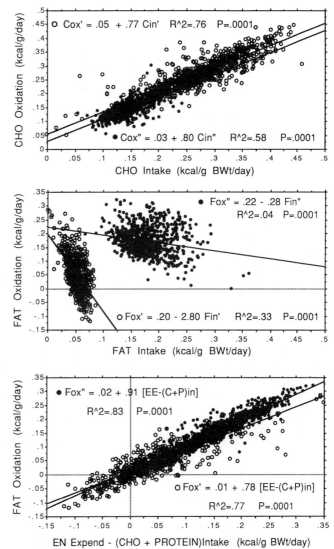

consideration, particularly in view of the impact of dietary fat on the incidence of obesity.[12,28,66] In effect, fat oxidation is determined by the difference between energy expenditure minus the energy consumed in the form of carbohydrate plus protein (see Fig. 8-4). Fat oxidation is thus limited by carbohydrate intake, promoted by depletion of the body's glycogen reserves and by exercise, and not much affected by the various phenom-ena involved in the metabolism of fat. Physical exertion increases energy expenditure

in skeletal muscle, the compartment of the body that most readily can burn fatty acids as well as glucose. Exercise is thus likely to increase fat oxidation to a greater extent than glucose oxidation, particularly during prolonged aerobic exertion of low to moderate intensity.[28,47] If spontaneous or deliberate restraint of food intake fails to maintain glycogen levels in a range sufficiently low to allow fat oxidation to proceed at a rate commensurate with fat intake and if aerobic exertion is too limited to substantially enhance fat

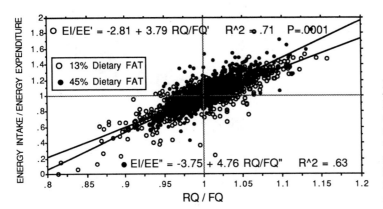

FIGURE 8-5

Relationship between energy balance and RQ, using the ratio of energy intake to energy expenditure versus the RQ:FQ ratio to make the relationship valid for diets of different composition. The data are those obtained during the study described in Figure 8-4.

oxidation, fat tends to accumulate in adipose tissue. Ultimately, weight maintenance tends to become established, albeit at high levels of adiposity, as is frequently the case among sedentary individuals consuming Western diets with a substantial fat content.[12] The increase in fat-free mass and in total body weight brought about by enlargement of the adipose tissue mass causes an increase in resting energy expenditure and raises the cost of physical activities.[10,56,60] If the composition of the fuel mix oxidized remained unchanged, it would need to be compensated by increments in food intake in order to maintain carbohydrate balance. There would be no reason to expect the establishment of a weight-maintenance plateau, unless total food intake were somehow restricted or limited. Expansion of the fat mass also leads to higher FFA levels[8] and tends to induce insulin resistance.[49] Both are susceptible to enhance the oxidation of fatty acids relative to that of glucose and thereby to bring about a decrease in the average RQ. The steady state of weight maintenance can only become established when average RQ equals average FQ (Fig. 8-5). In *ad libitum* fed mice, a progressive increase in adiposity appears to be required in most but not all animals to make fat oxidation commensurate with fat in the presence of gradual increments in dietary fat content.[24] This phenomenon has the appearance of a dose-response relationship over the fairly wide range of fat-to-carbohydrate ratios typical for mixed diets (Fig. 8-6). Remarkably wide individual variations in body weight are noted, and this variability appears to be enhanced as the fat content

of mixed diets increases (see Fig. 8-6), as seems to be the case for human populations. In humans, circumstantial, life-style, psychological, and socioeconomic factors exert influences that can readily override physiological cues regulating food intake. Thus it has been difficult to recognize short-term adjustment of food intake to variations in energy expenditure,[19] even though gains or losses of substrates are apparently able to influence food intake, given that stable body weights are maintained over long periods during the life of most individuals.

ROLES OF ENERGY EXPENDITURE AND ENERGY INTAKE IN BODY WEIGHT REGULATION

High rates of energy expenditure are not necessarily associated with low levels of adiposity. This is because of the fact that increases in energy expenditure, if they do not elicit some change in the average composition of the fuel mix oxidized, lead to equivalent increments in food intake, in order to maintain carbohydrate balance. However, if high energy expenditure is accompanied by a decline in the RQ, as during prolonged aerobic exercise, food needs to be consumed in lesser amounts. This is why high rates of energy expenditure lead to low body weights as a result of physical activity and why high rates of energy expenditure due to large body size are compatible with obesity.

Increases in energy expenditure may dissipate 10% to 20% of excess energy consumed by humans. (As mentioned, they can reach 30%, but

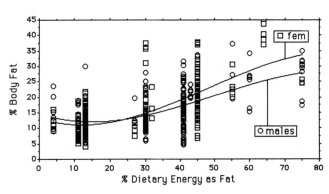

FIGURE 8-6

Effect of dietary fat content on body fat content (measured by carcass analysis) in 225 male and 198 female CD-1 mice (150 to 205 days old) maintained *ad libitum* on diets containing 18% of energy as casein, different proportions of fat (shown on the abscissa), and the balance as carbohydrate (half sucrose, half starch).

only under very exceptional circumstances in which rapid *de novo* lipogenesis is induced by deliberate and sustained ingestion of massive amounts of excess carbohydrate.[4]) Decreases in RMR (including a lower TEF) during days of food deprivation may attenuate an energy deficit by 5% to 10%. These quantitatively predictable responses to variations in food intake reduce the impact of energy imbalances, but only slightly. Daily variations in energy intake are considerably greater than those affecting energy expenditure, and substantial daily deviations from energy balance occur frequently.[19] Responses capable of correcting (rather than merely attenuating) such imbalances are needed to bring about appropriate compensation for such errors. Long-term weight maintenance must therefore be brought about primarily by adjustments of food intake, triggered by changes in the body's fuel reserves. Such responses are not readily detectable from data on the overall energy balance, because changes in glycogen content, which are much more likely to exert significant feedback on food intake regulation, are readily masked by errors in the fat balance. One might speculate that progress in research in this area will depend on the ability to assess the carbohydrate balance under conditions in which the physiological regulation of appetite/hunger have a chance to become manifest.

CONCLUSIONS AND IMPLICATIONS

Adjustment of metabolic rates cannot make energy expenditure equal to energy intake. The task of metabolic regulation in bringing about energy balance is therefore primarily in adjusting the composition of the fuel mix oxidized. The task of food intake regulation appears to be to influence food intake in such a manner that excessive depletion or accumulation of glycogen is avoided. An average RQ that is equal to the FQ also leads to energy balance (see Fig. 8-5). Because the average RQ is influenced by the degree of repletion of the body's glycogen reserves and by the size (and distribution) of its adipose tissue, weight maintenance occurs only when a particular body composition has been reached. The latter is determined by interactions between individual genetic traits and particular sets of circumstantial conditions. Because differences in the adipose tissue mass exert only a small impact on metabolism, the degree of adiposity for which the steady state of weight maintenance tends to become established can vary widely among different individuals.

Examination of the manner in which the body uses its fuels to regenerate the ATP expended thus suggests that all strategies for weight maintenance must succeed in making the average RQ equal to or less than the diet's FQ if correction of excess weight is desired (see Fig. 8-5). Because the organism by itself effectively strives to maintain carbohydrate and protein balances, the rule that ensues is simply *not to eat more fat than one burns, considering one's exercise habits.* This rule is obviously facilitated by selecting a diet with a relatively low fat content (and a relatively high FQ). Furthermore, physical activities that tend to decrease the RQ (i.e., sustained efforts of moderate intensity) can be expected to be more effective for the control of body weight than short bursts of vigorous exertion. Altogether, these observations suggest that weight-control measures can be based on considerations pertaining to the composition of the fuel mix oxidized relative to that of the diet, rather than on the overall amount of fuel oxidized, particularly when access to food is not a limiting factor.

Acknowledgment: This work was supported by NIH Grant DK 33214.

References

1. Abbott WGH, Howard BV, Christin L et al: Short-term energy balance: Relationship with protein, carbohydrate, and fat balances. Am J Physiol 255: E332, 1988
2. Acheson KJ, Ravussin E, Wahren J et al: Thermic effect of glucose in man, obligatory and facultative thermogenesis. J Clin Invest 74:1572, 1984
3. Acheson KJ, Schutz Y, Bessard T et al: Nutritional influences on lipogenesis and thermogenesis after a carbohydrate meal. Am J Physiol 246:E62, 1984
4. Acheson KJ, Schutz Y, Bessard T et al: Glycogen storage capacity and *de novo* lipogenesis during massive carbohydrate overfeeding in man. Am J Clin Nutr 48:240, 1988
5. Bahr R, Ingnes I, Vaage O et al: Effect of duration of exercise on excess postexercise O_2 consumption. J Appl Physiol 62:485, 1987
6. Bielinski R, Schutz Y, Jéquier E: Energy metabolism during the post-exercise recovery in man. Am J Clin Nutr 42:69, 1985
7. Bisdee JT, James WPT, Shaw MA: Changes in energy expenditure during the menstrual cycle. Br J Nutr 61:187, 1989
8. Bjorntorp P, Bergman H, Varnauskas E et al: Lipid mobilization in relation to body composition in man. Metabolism 18:840, 1969
9. Bjorntorp P, Sjostrom L: Carbohydrate storage in man: Speculations and some quantitative considerations. Metabolism 27:1853, 1978
10. Blaza S, Garrow JS: Thermogenic response to temperature, exercise and food stimuli in lean and obese women, studied by 24 h direct calorimetry. Br J Nutr 49:171, 1983
11. Bogardus C, Lillioja S, Ravussin E et al: Familial dependence of the resting metabolic rate. N Engl J Med 315:96, 1986
12. Bray GA: Obesity: A disease of nutrient or energy balance? Nutr Rev 45:33, 1987
13. Buskirk ER, Mendez J: Energy: Caloric requirements. In Alfin-Slater RB, Kritchevsky D (eds): Nutrition and the Adult: Macronutrients, Vol 3A, pp 49–95. New York, Plenum, 1980
14. Dallosso HM, James WPT: Whole-body calorimetry studies in adult men. I. The effect of fat overfeeding on 24 h energy expenditure. Br J Nutr 52:49, 1984
15. Danforth E Jr, Burger AF: The impact of nutrition on thyroid hormone physiology and action. Ann Rev Nutr 9:201, 1989
16. Dauncey MJ: Metabolic effects of altering the 24 h energy intake in man, using direct and indirect calorimetry. Br J Nutr 43:257, 1980
17. DeFronzo RA, Ferrannini E: Regulation of hepatic glucose metabolism in humans. Diabetes Metab Rev 3:415, 1987
18. Donato KA, Hegsted DM: Efficiency of utilization of various energy sources for growth. Proc Natl Acad Sci 82:4866, 1985
19. Edholm OG, Adam JM, Healy MJR et al: Food intake and energy expenditure of army recruits. Br J Nutr 24:1091, 1979
20. Elia M, Zed C, Neale G et al: The energy cost of triglyceride-fatty acid recycling in non-obese subjects after an overnight fast and four days of starvation. Metabolism 36:251, 1987
21. Elia M, Livesey G: The theory and validity of indirect calorimetry during net lipogenesis. Am J Clin Nutr 47:591, 1988
22. Flatt JP: The biochemistry of energy expenditure. In Bray G (ed): Recent Advances of Obesity Research, Vol II, pp 211–228. Westport, CT, Technomic, 1978
23. Flatt JP: Conversion of carbohydrate to fat in adipose tissue: An energy-yielding and, therefore, self-limiting process. J Lipid Res 11:131, 1970
24. Flatt JP: Dietary fat, carbohydrate balance, and weight maintenance: Effects of exercise. Am J Clin Nutr 45:296, 1987
25. Flatt JP: Energetics of intermediary metabolism. In Garrow JS, Halliday D (eds): Substrate and Energy Metabolism in Man, pp 58–69. London, John Libbey & Co, 1985
26. Flatt JP, Pahud P, Ravussin E et al: An estimate of the P:O ratio in man. TIBS 9:251, 1984
27. Flatt JP, Ravussin E, Acheson KJ et al: Effects of dietary fat on postprandial substrate oxidation and on carbohydrate and fat balances. J Clin Invest 76:1019, 1985
28. Flatt JP: Importance of nutrient balance in body weight regulation. Diabetes Metab Rev 4:571, 1988
29. Forbes GB: Energy intake and body weight: A reexamination of two "classic" studies. Am J Clin Nutr 39:349, 1984
30. Garlick PJ, Clugston GA, Swick RW et al: Diurnal pattern of protein and energy metabolism in man. Am J Clin Nutr 33:1983, 1980

31. Goldstein SA, Elwyn DH: The effects of injury and sepsis on fuel utilization. Ann Rev Nutr 9:445, 1989

32. Himms-Hagen J: Brown adipose tissue thermogenesis and obesity. Prog Lipid Res 28:65, 1989

33. Hultman E, Nilsson LH: Factors influencing carbohydrate metabolism in man. Nutr Metab (Suppl 1) 18:45, 1975

34. Hurni M, Burnand B, Pittet P et al: Metabolic effects of a mixed and a high-carbohydrate low-fat diet in man, measured over 24 h in a respiration chamber. Br J Nutr 47:33, 1982

35. Jéquier E, Acheson K, Schutz Y: Assessment of energy expenditure and fuel utilization in man. Ann Rev Nutr 7:187, 1987

36. Keys A, Brozek J, Henschel A et al: The Biology of Human Starvation. Minneapolis, University of Minnesota Press, 1950

37. Kleiber M: The Fire of Life, and Introduction to Animal Energetics. New York, Robert E. Krieger, 1975

38. Kurland IJ, Pilkis SJ: Indirect versus direct routes of hepatic glycogen synthesis. FASEB J 3:2277, 1989

39. Landsberg L, Saville ME, Young JB: Sympatho-adrenal system and regulation of thermogenesis. Am J Physiol 247:E181, 1984

40. LeBlanc J, Brondel L: Role of palatability on meal-induced thermogenesis in human subjects. Am J Physiol 248:E333, 1985

41. Livesey G: ATP yields from proteins, fats and carbohydrates and mitochondrial efficiency in vivo. In Blondheim J (ed): Recent Advances in Obesity Research, Vol V, pp 131–143

42. Livesey G, Elia M: The estimation of energy expenditure, net carbohydrate utilization and net fat oxidation and synthesis by indirect calorimetry: Evaluation of some errors with special reference to the detailed composition of fuels. Am J Clin Nutr 47:608, 1988

43. Lusk G: Science of Nutrition. New York, Johnson Reprint, 1976

44. Magnusson I, Chandramoulin V, Schumann WC et al: Quantitation of the pathways of hepatic glycogen formation on ingesting a glucose load. J Clin Invest 80:1748, 1987

45. Manchester KL: Muscle ATP and Creatine-P. Biochem Educ 8:70, 1980

46. Mayer J, Thomas DW: Regulation of food intake and obesity. Science 156:328, 1967

47. McGilvery RW, Goldstein G: Biochemistry: A Functional Approach. Philadelphia, WB Saunders, 1979

48. McLean JA, Tobin G: Animal and human calorimetry. Cambridge, Cambridge University Press, 1987

49. Meylan M, Henny C, Temler E et al: Metabolic factors in the insulin resistance in human obesity. Metabolism 36:256, 1987

50. Mitchell P: Keilin's respiratory chain concept and its chemiosmotic consequences. Science 206:1148, 1979

51. Murphy MP, Brand MD: Variable stoichiometry of proton pumping by the mitochondrial respiratory chain. Nature 329:170, 1987

52. Norgan NG, Durnin JVGA: The effect of 6 weeks of overfeeding on the body weight, body composition, and energy metabolism of young men. Am J Clin Nutr 33:978, 1988

53. Owen OE, Holup JL, D'Alessio DA et al: A reappraisal of the caloric requirements of men. Am J Clin Nutr 46:875, 1987

54. Owen OE, Kavle E, Owen RS et al: A reappraisal of caloric requirements in healthy women. Am J Clin Nutr 44:1, 1986

55. Pahud P, Ravussin E, Jéquier E: Energy expended during oxygen deficit period of submaximal exercise in man. J Appl Physiol 48:770, 1980

56. Pandolf KB, Givoni B, Goldman RF: Predicting energy expenditure with loads while standing or walking very slowly. J Appl Physiol 43:577, 1977

57. Passmore R, Swindells YE: Observations on the respiratory quotients and weight gains of man after eating large quantities of carbohydrate. Br J Nutr 17:331, 1963

58. Prentice AM, Coward WA, Davies HL et al: Unexpectedly low levels of energy expenditure in healthy women. Lancet i:1419, 1985

59. Prentice AM, Black AE, Coward WA et al: High levels of energy expenditure in obese women. Br Med J 292:983, 1986

60. Ravussin E, Burnand B, Schutz Y et al: Twenty-four-hour energy expenditure and resting metabolic rate in obese, moderately obese, and control subjects. Am J Clin Nutr 35:566, 1982

61. Ravussin E, Schutz Y, Acheson KJ et al: Short-term, mixed-diet overfeeding in man: No evidence for "Luxuskonsumption." Am J Physiol 249:E470, 1985

62. Rothwell NJ, Stock MJ: Regulation of energy balance. Ann Rev Nutr 1:235, 1981

63. Schoeller DA, Ravussin E, Schutz Y et al: Energy expenditure by doubly labeled water: Validation in humans and proposed calculation. Am J Physiol 250:R823, 1986

64. Schofield WN: Predicting basal metabolic rate, new standards and review of previous work. Hum Nutr Clin Nutr 39C:5, 1985

65. Schulz S, Westerterp KR, Bruck K: Comparison of energy expenditure by the doubly labeled water technique with energy intake, heart rate and activity recording in man. Am J Clin Nutr 49:1146, 1989

66. Schutz V, Flatt JP, Jéquier E: Failure of dietary fat

to promote fat oxidation: A factor favoring the development of obesity. Am J Clin Nutr 50:307, 1989

67. Segal K, Presta E, Gutin B: Thermic effect of food during graded exercise in normal weight and obese men. Am J Clin Nutr 40:995, 1984

68. Shaw SN, Elwyn DH, Askanazi J et al: Effects of increasing nitrogen intake on nitrogen balance and energy expenditure in nutritionally depleted adult patients receiving parenteral nutrition. Am J Clin Nutr 37:930, 1983

69. Solomon SJ, Kurzer MS, Calloway DH: Menstrual cycle and basal metabolic rate in women. Am J Clin Nutr 36:611, 1982

70. Tremblay A, Fontaine E, Poehlman ET et al: The effect of exercise-training on resting metabolic rate in lean and moderately obese individuals. Int J Obes 10:511, 1986

71. Tremblay A, Sauvé L, Després J-P et al: Metabolic characteristics of postobese individuals. Int J Obes 13:357, 1989

72. Waterlow JC: Metabolic adaptation to low intakes of energy and protein. Ann Rev Nutr 6:495, 1986

73. Weast RC: Handbook of Chemistry and Physics, 57th ed. Cleveland, CRC Press, 1976

74. Welle S, Lilavivat U, Campbell RG: Thermic effect of feeding in man: Increased plasma norepinephrine levels following glucose but not protein or fat consumption. Metabolism 30:953, 1981

75. Westerterp KR, Saris WHM, van EsM et al: Use of the doubly labelled water technique in humans during heavy sustained exercise. J Appl Physiol 61:2162, 1986

CHAPTER 9

Evidence for Brown Adipose Tissue in Humans

M. E. J. LEAN

The scientific and public excitement during the past decade about brown adipose tissue (BAT) and its relation to obesity arose out of initially speculative extrapolation from animal experiments described in detail elsewhere in this book.[27] In fact, it was as long ago as December of 1670 that it was first suggested that data on BAT might be useful in human therapeutics. This observation was made in a short letter from George Velschi of Augsburg[71] regarding the untimely death of his pet marmot and its hurried dissection by an assistant who had evidently allowed the animal to die while Velschi was out of town, but who had noted the remarkable abundance of BAT.

Recognition that variations in the metabolic activity of this tissue can determine the overall efficiency of energy utilization in experimental animals, strengthened by the demonstration of thermogenic responses to overfeeding, has directed interest toward the possibility that BAT could be of importance in energy balance and the etiology of obesity in humans. Perhaps more important, this concept has suggested a novel route for treatment.[26,32] For these ideas to have any substance, it needs to be demonstrated that BAT is present and functional in humans, capable not only of regulated heat production to maintain body temperature but also of physiological stimulation to remove unnecessary energy ingested as food. If BAT is potentially active in adults, then energy wastage might be inducible by therapeutic intervention for the treatment of obesity. Studies have explored some of the grounds for speculation about human BAT thermogenesis, to strengthen the analogies with animal models.

HUMAN THERMOGENESIS: WHY INVOKE BROWN ADIPOSE TISSUE?

Humans, as homeotherms, usually maintain a core temperature within the narrow limits of 36°C to 37.5°C. Even small changes outside this range are usually apparent to the individual, and temperature elevation above 41°C or hypothermia below 32°C can be lethal. Maintaining this degree of control requires sensitive systems to detect variations in the core and environmental temperatures, as well as regulable mechanisms for generating and for dispersing heat. The whole system must have the capacity to deal with both chronic exposure to ambient temperatures outside the thermoneutral range and also with acute exposure to extreme degrees of heat and cold. Feedback control must therefore be involved, and activation of thermoregulatory mechanisms should be possible without interfering with other biologic systems.

In adult humans, the need for these mechanisms has been largely obviated by the efficiency of behavioral responses and societal moves toward air-conditioning and central heating. Nevertheless, in physiological terms there remains a need for metabolic thermoregulation, and it is important in infants, in whom heat exchange is more rapid and shivering is not observed.[30] Nonshivering thermogenesis has been demonstrated[35] in response to cold exposure in men who had been treated with curare to abolish any possible contribution from shivering or muscle tone, and this observation contradicts earlier negative findings.[37] Fine control of body temperature on exposure to mild cold is mediated through nonshivering mechanisms.[8,19,44,45] Finally, it is only by nonshivering mechanisms that adaptive increases in thermogenic capacity can be achieved during acclimation to long-term low environmental temperatures, a well-known phenomenon in experimental animals[11] but one that has not yet been convincingly demonstrated in humans.

A number of mechanisms have been postulated to account for metabolic (nonshivering) thermogenesis. Those most likely to be quantitatively important are listed in Table 9-1.[36,60,62] All the so-called futile cycles in the first group probably have other regulatory functions, and all require secondary stimulation of sodium/potassium adenosine triphosphatase (Na/K ATPase). Thus it is difficult to be sure whether there can be a truly independent direct stimulation of sodium pump cycling, another postulated mechanism for thermogenesis. The uncoupled mitochondrial respiration of BAT is the only mechanism that is organ specific and whose specific activation does not potentially corrupt other biochemical pathways. The biochemistry of BAT thermogenesis is similar in all species examined.[27,70] From first principles, it would be curious if humans did not use the same very efficient process if BAT were indeed present.

There is a recurrent problem of scale when nonshivering thermogenesis is sought experimentally in humans, because the dominant physiological effect of cold acclimation in large animals is an improvement in thermal insulation, through peripheral blood flow changes.[34,48] This adaptation may obscure small alterations in thermogenic capacity. Interestingly, it appears that the increased subcutaneous adipose tissue of obese subjects does not in practice serve as an increased layer of thermal insulation, and obese subjects may in fact lose heat to a cold environment more rapidly than thin ones.[4] Certainly it is an important characteristic of congenitally obese

TABLE 9-1

Possible Biochemical Mechanisms for Regulatory Metabolic Thermogenesis

1. Intermediary metabolite cycling and structural macromolecule turnover leading to ATP utilization and resynthesis with tightly coupled respiration.

   Present in various tissues.

   Glycogen/glucose-1-phosphate
   Glucose/glucose-6-phosphate
   Fructose-6-phosphate/fructose-1,6-biphosphate
   Phosphoenolpyruvate/pyruvate
   Triglyceride/free fatty acids
   Glutamate/glutamine
   Acetate/acetyl CoA
   Adenosine/adenosine monophosphate
   Cori cycle
   Protein turnover
   RNA turnover
   Phosphoinositide turnover
   Arachidonate metabolism

2. Direct activation of Na/K ATPase with alterations in ionic gradients and membrane permeability.

   Present in all tissues.

3. Substrate oxidation without ATP generation (uncoupled respiration).

   Present and specifically regulated in BAT only.

(ob/ob) mice and probably an important element contributing to their weight gain that their metabolic rate does not increase in response to cold exposure: core temperature and, consequently, metabolic rate fall steadily. This is principally because of impaired BAT thermogenesis and is related to the development of insulin resistance.[27,70]

Some evidence from studies of Australian aboriginals,[66] Kalahari bushmen,[72] and Lapps[3] shows that overall energy expenditure may be reduced by a decline in core temperature at night. These ethnic groups are prone to obesity and diabetes when Western life-styles are adopted, leading to an analogy between the thermogenesis of congenitally obese animals and certain groups of obese humans. My colleagues and I investigated this possibility using whole body indirect calorimetry to seek supporting evidence for the view that BAT mediates human thermogenesis. Normal-weight human volunteers increase their overnight metabolic rate by about 8% when they sleep at a room temperature of 22°C, compared with a thermoneutral temperature of 28°C.[19,45] This adaptation occurs without any discomfort or shivering. Obese subjects in mild cold had a nonsignificant small reduction in the metabolic response.[8,45] Further studies[45] have shown significantly impaired metabolic responses to mild cold in overweight women (BMI > 27 kg/m^2) who had type II (maturity-onset) diabetes and were selected to explore certain clinical and biochemical similarities with the ob/ob mice. Whereas thin control subjects all had a higher sleeping metabolic rate at 22°C than 28°C (mean increase 3.8%), the diabetic obese women all had reduced energy expenditure at the lower temperature (mean fall 3.5%; $P < .001$) and defective thyroid responses to cold. An important subgroup of obese persons with a clear defect of nonshivering thermogenesis has thus been identified, and the similarity with the situation in congenitally obese animals (with defective BAT function to blame) is striking.

HISTOLOGY AND ANATOMY OF HUMAN BROWN FAT: STRUCTURAL INDICATIONS OF FUNCTION

The concept that these two types of adipose tissue exist in humans derives from embryological and anatomical considerations, now supported by biochemical evidence for functional differences. The crudest identification of BAT is on the grounds of its yellow-brown color—a result of its high vascularity and cytochrome content, reflecting high mitochondrial density. Its name is really very misleading, because the tissue is seldom brown, and in some circumstances it is as white (or yellow) as the subcutaneous "white" adipose tissue. Distinction between the two types of adipose tissue cannot be made by the unaided eye, and by histology only with confidence in infants.

The microscopic appearance of BAT in human neonates is similar to that in other species— cells characteristically containing multivesicular fat droplets and round nuclei (Fig. 9-1). It was first identified as analogous to the "hibernating

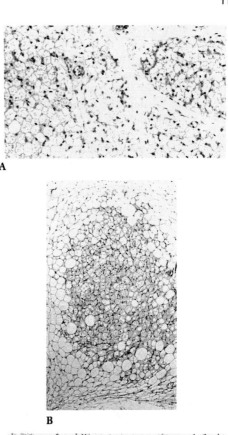

A

B

C

FIGURE 9-1

Hematoxylin and eosin stained sections of human BAT. **A:** Perirenal adipose tissue from a 6-month-old baby. ($\times$ 130) **B:** Perirenal adipose tissue from a 19-year-old man who died in a road traffic accident, showing an island of typical BAT histology among other lipid-replete cells. ($\times$ 52) **C:** Pockets of multilocular cells in the omentum of a 22-year-old woman. ($\times$ 52)

gland'' of animals in the cervical region of human embryos by Hatai in 1902.[23] Earlier anatomical descriptions had considered the tissue histology to be more related to that of endocrine glands and were confused by the proximity to lymph nodes. The widespread presence of histologically detectable BAT in human infants, and in adults at various locations in which it occurs in infancy, is now well established.[1,22,24] In common with other primates, in humans, the largest sites of BAT are the axillary/deep cervical and perirenal adipose tissues. The interscapular site is quantitatively unimportant in human infants, although readily detectable as a thin kite-shaped structure in most neonates. Human adults have essentially no histologically identifiable, typical, brown adipocytes in the interscapular region. The literature is consistent on this point, and our own findings from dissections in Cambridge, England, concur with those by Astrup and colleagues in Denmark[6] that the interscapular site cannot be quantitatively important for thermogenesis in adult humans.

Human superficial or subcutaneous adipose tissue shows typical white adipose histology at all ages, whereas virtually all internal sites of adipose tissue contain typical multilocular brown adipocytes in infancy. In adults, these internal sites contain at least isolated cells or islands of typical BAT adjacent to blood vessels[22,24] (see Fig. 9-1). Under the electron microscope, the BAT cytoplasm is seen to be densely packed with active mitochondria (Fig.

9-2). As in many other larger species, notably dogs,[29] the typical BAT histology of human infants is modified with age. Lipid accumulates so that the proportion of cells containing multivesicular droplets of lipid is reduced, and the tissue may ultimately become indistinguishable from subcutaneous white adipose tissue. Aherne and Hull[1] conducted large postmortem surveys of infant BAT and concluded that the histology reflected functional capacity. Lipid accumulation, with increased tissue bulk and unilocular histology, generally indicates *reduced* demands for thermogenesis. By comparison with histologic appearances in experimental animals whose BAT thermogenic activity is known, Hull[30] was able to conclude that the 30 g or so of BAT in a human infant (about 1% of body weight) is sufficient to account for total thermogenic capability in response to cold or noradrenaline, equivalent to a doubling of metabolic rate.[10]

BAT is found in humans in central and internal sites, in a distribution arranged such that heat generated there would warm the blood supply to vital organs.[41] Thus the cervical and axillary sites can warm the blood supply of the head, and the perirenal fat protects the kidneys. This concept is strengthened by the demonstration of direct vascular links between the perirenal BAT and the kidneys,[57] between the suprailiac BAT and the lumbar and azygos veins,[58] and between the interscapular site and the spinal cord.[1] Merklin[56] also demonstrated a vascular link between the

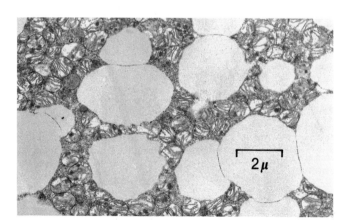

2μ

FIGURE 9-2

Electron micrograph of BAT from a 46-year-old woman with an adrenal pheochromocytoma. The cytoplasm between lipid droplets is packed with mitochondria.

anterior abdominal BAT and the liver, and the pericardial site is well placed to provide direct heating to the myocardium. Such anatomical observations certainly do not prove any BAT function in humans and would be consistent with a view that BAT is of phylogenetic interest only.

Under certain conditions, however, these sites of BAT show histologic changes to a more "active" histologic appearance, with reduced lipid content, increased multilocularity and mitochondrial density. These changes are more persuasive evidence for a functional thermogenic role. Heim and colleagues[25] observed lower BAT lipid content in infants kept at 22°C to 27°C than in others at 34°C to 35°C. Evidence also suggests that exposure to cold environments may lead to reduction in lipid content and reversion to typical BAT histology and histochemistry.[1,31] More convincing evidence for functional capability is that the noradrenaline-secreting tumor pheochromocytoma is associated with more abundant brown-type adipocytes in the perirenal fat.[55] Metabolic rate is known to be elevated by pheochromocytoma,[53] and BAT is thermogenically activated both in animal models[64] and in adult humans.[42] Tying these observations together, my colleagues and I used computed x-ray tomography to explore the hypothesis that if the intra-abdominal fat is a site of BAT in humans, then alterations in its lipid content, relative to that of subcutaneous (white) fat, might reflect changes in BAT function in relation to some of the pathophysiological influences (age, diabetes, Cushing's syndrome, and pheochromocytoma) that are known to affect BAT function in animal models.[44] Positive correlations were found between intra-abdominal lipid and age but not with BMI, and higher proportions of intra-abdominal fat were demonstrated in men than in women. Intra-abdominal fat was significantly increased in women with type II diabetes and in those with Cushing's syndrome, and it was reduced in subjects with pheochromocytoma (Fig. 9-3). If the subcutaneous fat is accepted to be white adipose tissue and the intra-abdominal fat is considered to be the brown compartment in a transverse abdominal cross section, then these alterations in its lipid content would indeed be those expected if its thermogenic capacity is decreased with age,

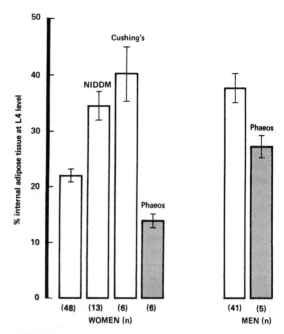

FIGURE 9-3

Abdominal CT fat distribution at L4 (umbilical) level and comparison with age- and sex-matched controls. Internal fat is expressed as a proportion of the total fat pixels at this level (L4, umbilical). Wilcoxon's test was used to demonstrate significant differences from age- and sex-matched controls, combining the data from the two sexes for pheochromocytomas.

type II diabetes, and Cushing's syndrome and increased with pheochromocytoma. In hypothyroidism, the lipid content of BAT (and thus its bulk) is increased,[17,67] suggesting a reduced thermogenic activity, which seems appropriate on clinical grounds. More formal examination of BAT in thyroid disease is awaited.

CLUES FROM TUMORS: HIBERNOMA AND PHEOCHROMOCYTOMA

Tumors of BAT (hibernomata) are rare. They tend to be misdiagnosed as lipomata (common and relatively uninteresting benign tumors of white adipose tissue) until after surgical removal but occur at sites of the BAT in infancy and contain typical BAT histology, hence the intriguing name *hibernoma*. Such benign tumors in other tissues are very often nonfunctional, but at least one case report[2] describes weight loss of 7 kg in a young man during a year before the removal of a hibernoma. It had a high cytochrome oxidase content and active-looking mitochondrial cristae on electron microscopy, and the amount of BAT in the tumor ($8 \times 11 \times 4$ cm) would be sufficient to account for that weight loss (about 50,000 kcal) by an increase in basal metabolism of about 5% (about 140 kcal/24 hours) if the thermogenic activity of BAT from a room temperature mouse is assumed. Other factors may have played a part in that case, and in practice it would be difficult to detect an increase in basal metabolism of only 5% in an individual patient. This issue is a fundamental problem in any attempt to quantify the role of BAT in humans.

Hibernomata have also been described in patients with pheochromocytoma, a catecholamine-secreting tumor from neural crest tissue, usually sited in an adrenal gland. In that situation, the hibernoma must result from prolonged trophic stimulation of the tissue by catecholamines. The biochemical evidence gathered by Bouillaud and colleagues[9] indicates that such hibernomata are almost certainly thermogenically active. They may be found in the periadrenal adipose tissue adjacent to the pheochromocytoma but can occur elsewhere, so pheochromocytoma should be ruled out in any patient with a hibernoma, particularly if there has been weight loss.

Prominent typical BAT histology in periadrenal adipose tissue removed at surgery for pheochromocytoma was first reported by Melicow in 1957,[55] in contrast to the usual "adult fat" at that site. Similar reports have followed, and the association seems established, although Medeiros and associates[54] argue that normal persons may have similar histologic appearances of BAT at this site and that firmer criteria are required. The work of Ricquier and colleagues[63] and my own work[42] (Table 9-2) have demonstrated that the periadrenal adipose tissue from patients with pheochromocytoma possesses the ultrastructural and biochemical features of BAT. My colleagues and I have also shown the content of mitochondrial uncoupling protein, unique to BAT and the best marker of thermogenic capacity, to be very significantly increased in the presence of pheo-

chromocytoma compared with cases of sudden death, and also that its concentration is elevated in sites of BAT distant from the tumor[42] (Fig. 9-4).

TEMPERATURE SENSING

Astrup and co-workers[6,7] have argued that if BAT in humans is indeed thermogenic, then its temperature should be higher than that of other, nonthermogenic, tissues. Several groups have approached this issue by measuring skin temperature with thermocouples or infrared thermography over regions where BAT was believed to exist.[15,49,50,65] Sadly, this literature must be dismissed as irrelevant to the BAT question and misleading. Most of these studies concentrated on the nape of the neck, confused with the interscapular region (which does not in any case contain a significant amount of BAT in human adults, as discussed earlier). The skin temperature over the lower neck tends to be higher for other reasons in both infants and adults,[65,68] and any differences in skin temperature in fact represent alterations in nonspecific heat loss, as a result of changing cutaneous blood circulation. Results are most dependent on the extent to which the experimental conditions provide insulation to other sites of regulatory heat loss.

More direct attempts to measure heat production have been attempted by placing thermocouples deeply in the intercostal[33] or perirenal adipose tissues.[7] Both these experiments did show an elevation in temperature, by reference to skeletal muscle or rectal temperature, in response to thermogenic treatment with noradrenaline or ephedrine. However, there is a general problem with the interpretation of temperature gradients because of alterations in local blood flow and countercurrent effects at both the test site and the reference site. When BAT is stimulated for heat production, the same sympathetic mechanisms tend to increase its blood supply, so the actual rise in tissue temperature is minimized, and the diffuse nature of the tissue makes accurate assessment of blood flow impossible except for on a very local basis. The assumption that a skeletal muscle temperature (let alone that of the fermenting large bowel) is a stable reference point may be incorrect, in view of redistributions of blood flow.

TABLE 9-2

Biochemical Findings in Brown Adipose Tissue from Three Cases of Pheochromocytoma and from Two Cases of Cot Death

	Cytochrome C Oxidase Activity	Uncoupling Protein	GDP Binding Activity	GDP Effect on Oxygen Uptake
	(μmol/min/g tissue)	(μg/mg mito protein)	(pmol/mg mito protein)	(% change)
Pheochromocytoma				
Female, 53 years, perirenal		24	157	
Male, 22 years, perirenal	9.7	50	43	−37.9
Female, 21 years, perirenal	6.8	26	616	−21.2
omental	4.5	22	103	−33.8
Cot deaths				
Baby A: 9 months				
Axillary	246	22	147	
Cervical	202	23	149	
Perirenal	94	11	133	
Interscapular	18	7	91	
Baby M: 5 months				
Axillary	66	10	129	−23%
Perirenal	23	9	104	−9%
Mice: 3 months (warm-cool)*				
33°C–22°C	40–178	9–43	69–200	

*Mean results obtained using the same methods on mitochondria from the interscapular BAT (the principal site) of mice housed at room temperatures of 33°C (warm) and 22°C (cool).[5]

GENERAL BIOCHEMICAL INDICATIONS OF HUMAN BROWN ADIPOSE TISSUE ACTIVITY

Various enzyme histochemical methods were used by Hassi[22] on human postmortem material to make an indirect assessment of thermogenic activity. Brown adipocytes had high contents of the enzymes necessary for fatty acid synthesis, lipolysis, β-oxidation of fatty acids, the citric acid cycle, and cytochrome oxidase production, which indicated a high oxidative capacity with lipid as an important substrate. High content of monoamine oxidase presumably reflected high noradrenaline turnover. Interestingly, the content of lactate dehydrogenase was also high, sug-

gesting considerable potential for carbohydrate oxidation. The enzyme activities all were greater in brown than in white adipocytes and, on a cellular basis, were not lower in older subjects. The results were considered indicative of thermogenic activity in BAT in humans.

On the negative side of the biochemical argument, Cunningham and colleagues[16] were vehement in concluding that human BAT was only minimally active. From human perirenal adipose tissue obtained from various subjects at postmortem examination or at surgery, they related cytochrome oxidase content to the *in vitro* rate of oxygen uptake of portions of tissue, and then whole body thermogenic potential was estimated by a series of extrapolations. This work is open

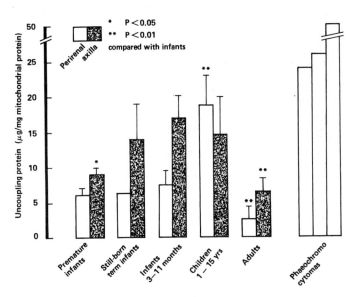

FIGURE 9-4

Uncoupling protein content of adipose tissue. Mean results ± standard error of the mean.

to some doubt, because the conclusion depended on *in vitro* estimations of tissue function, which always tend to underestimate maximal *in vivo* rates by perhaps fivefold to tenfold.[28] It also makes the assumption, which now seems incorrect, that the perirenal adipose tissue is representative of, and indeed contains, most of the BAT present in humans.

There is no other systematic study of general biochemistry of BAT in humans. However, most biochemists have failed to distinguish between the different types of human adipose tissues, presumably because they look alike to the unaided eye. Bearing in mind the confusion caused by the physical similarity between white adipose tissue and the lipid-replete BAT of humans, it is worth considering also the biochemical literature that has examined human adipose tissue from sites that are those of BAT in infancy. Hamosh and colleagues[21] compared the biochemistry of omental and subcutaneous adipose tissues and found enormously greater metabolic activity in the omental fat. The rate of *in vivo* fatty acid synthesis was up 20- to 70-fold higher in the omental adipose tissue. The omental adipose tissue is also more active than subcutaneous tissue in glucose metabolism by a factor of about five.[20,51] Omental fat has a threefold higher rate of lipolysis than subcutaneous fat and is markedly more responsive to noradrenaline.[61] Glycero-

kinase activity is high in human BAT[13] with increased lipogenesis in perirenal as compared with subcutaneous adipose tissue in children and some adults.[14] BAT is very active in lipolysis and lipogenesis in many species, the rate of lipogenesis correlating roughly with thermogenic activity,[52] so this literature provides some evidence to suggest continued BAT function in the intraabdominal adipose tissue of adult humans. Further support for this suggestion comes from the data of Nauman and colleagues,[59] showing much higher activity of type II thyroxine 5'-deiodinase in human omental compared with subcutaneous adipose tissue. Their study also indicated, intriguingly, reduced deiodinase activity in the omental adipocytes of obese subjects, expressed per unit of microsomal protein. If, as in experimental animals, locally generated triiodothyronine is important for thermogenesis in BAT,[27] then this work may be important evidence that the omental tissue under study was in fact behaving as BAT in humans.

A SPECIFIC BIOCHEMICAL MARKER FOR HUMAN BROWN ADIPOSE TISSUE: UNCOUPLING PROTEIN

The specific biochemical feature that uniquely characterizes BAT is the capacity for regulated uncoupling of mitochondrial respiration. This is achieved by virtue of a mitochondrial membrane protein of 32 kilodaltons, the uncoupling protein (sometimes referred to as *thermogenin*). The system is under regulation by catecholamines, acutely by activating the uncoupling protein to allow a proton leak across the mitochondrial membrane, chronically by increasing the numbers of mitochondria and their enrichment with uncoupling protein. Our studies on fresh BAT in humans have demonstrated uncoupled mitochondrial respiration with guanosine diphosphate (GDP) binding characteristics and uncoupling protein contents very similar to those found in experimental animals (Table 9-2).[47] Uncoupling protein content, indicating *thermogenic capacity*, of different BAT sites in infants correlated closely with tissue cytochrome oxidase activity as an index of *mitochondrial mass* ($r = .97$, $P < .001$) and also with mitochondrial GDP binding as an index of *thermogenic activity* ($r = .85$, $P < .02$).

In order to estimate the thermogenic capacity of human adipose tissue, we have established a solid-phase radioimmunoassay, using antisera generated against uncoupling protein purified from the mitochondria of human infant BAT,[40] to measure the uncoupling protein content of mitochondria.[43] Samples were obtained at routine autopsy from 48 subjects of all ages, all of whom had died suddenly in Cambridge, England, during the winter months. Uncoupling protein could not be detected in the mitochondria isolated from subcutaneous white adipose tissue, heart, or liver. The concentration was significantly higher in axillary than perirenal adipose tissue, and compared with infants there was significantly less in both adults and premature babies. The uncoupling protein contents of these human samples were quantitatively similar to those measured in young and adult experimental animals under normal environmental conditions. The different contents of uncoupling protein in the groups studied (see Fig. 9-4) would be consistent with known physiological changes in thermogenic capacity and requirement and support the view that BAT is an organ capable of regulated thermogenesis in humans. Low concentrations in premature infants are in keeping with their reduced thermogenic responses to cooling[10] and might also be expected in stillborn infants because synthesis of uncoupling protein will not

have been stimulated by exposure to cold temperatures.[69] The highest concentrations were found in older infants and children, who may have greater exposure to cold temperatures with relatively less clothing than is customary among young infants. There was no correlation between uncoupling protein content and age or weight/height[2] (BMI) as an index of fatness.

In three patients with pheochromocytoma, mitochondria isolated from intra-abdominal adipose tissue showed significantly uncoupled respiration, characteristic of BAT, which was inhibited by GDP.[42] Uncoupling protein content was high. Bouillaud and colleagues[9] have proceeded to demonstrate the presence of mRNA for human uncoupling protein in perirenal BAT in four cases of pheochromocytoma and from a hibernoma. Its structure indicates a close homology with rat uncoupling protein, thus strengthening our earlier findings of similarity in terms of antigenicity and GDP binding characteristics. Subcutaneous (white) adipose tissue does not contain the mRNA for uncoupling protein. All this research points to the conclusion that human uncoupling protein has the same function as that of the rat. Measurement of the uncoupling protein, as a structural part of the BAT mitochondrion, is probably still the most reliable indicator of thermogenic capacity, but it is possible that the more specific estimation of mRNA by Northern blot and complementary DNA probing will be of value in identifying BAT in unstimulated human adipose tissue, in which the uncoupling protein content may be below the limit of detection by immunoassay.[43]

PHARMACOLOGIC EVIDENCE FOR HUMAN BROWN ADIPOSE TISSUE

Physiological regulation of BAT thermogenesis involves sympathoadrenal and probably thyroidal function peripherally and a complex system of neuroendocrine mechanisms centrally.[70] Several drugs have been used to manipulate its function experimentally, some with rather specific actions on BAT. These provide tools to assess function in humans and have potential applications for the management of obesity and type II diabetes.

Noradrenaline itself[38] and its orally available isopropyl analogue[15] certainly stimulate thermogenesis. The less problematic sympathomimetic, ephedrine, has direct effects on animal BAT and produces thermogenesis of 15% to 25% above resting metabolism.[7] Our 6-week whole body calorimetry study of the noradrenaline-reuptake blocker, ciclazindol, were undertaken because this drug is concentrated in BAT and it stimulates BAT in animals. It had a significant effect on energy expenditure, equivalent to increasing metabolic rate by about 5% in young men, and there was also evidence of a sustained effect that would be compatible with a trophic action on thermogenic tissue.[18,39]

In all these studies, it has been difficult to attribute thermogenic effects in humans to BAT because of the possible contributions of mixed α- and β-adrenergic stimulation by the drugs tested in various tissues. Astrup and colleagues[7] have combined measurements of temperature gradients and ^{133}Xe clearance, to assess local blood flow. They estimate that the perirenal adipose tissue of young men is generally of low thermogenic importance, although in one case it produced up to 25% of the total thermic effects from oral ephedrine. This response is remarkable from a tissue that accounts for only 1% of body weight, considering that the entire muscle bulk at 50% of body weight provided only 50% of thermic effects. This study, despite its relatively imprecise methodology and small numbers, is important as the only quantitative information about BAT thermogenesis in humans.

Whether a thermogenic function is specific to BAT, or whether it applies to all adipose tissue but more markedly to tissue of BAT origin, is currently an interesting physiological problem. It is hoped that new scanning techniques may provide the answers. For the purposes of obesity management, it is more important that stimulant effects spare the cardiovascular and central nervous systems. The new class of lipolytic (β_3) β-agonists probably act on all adipose tissues.[12] It has not yet been shown to what degree the thermogenic effects in humans are attributable to the greater lipolytic activity of the deep adipose tissue in former sites of BAT.

CONCLUSIONS

It is now clear that BAT exists in humans and has the same thermogenic function as in experimental animals. The mitochondrial uncoupling protein, which is necessary for regulated nonshivering thermogenesis, can be demonstrated in the brown compartment of human adipose tissue. This is a specific tissue marker and is highly homologous with that in other species. The terminology brown adipose tissue is misleading, however, because the tissue is often quiescent and resembles white adipose tissue to the naked eye or light microscope.

In adults, the uncoupling protein content is generally low, although usually measurable in the axillary fat, but high levels of circulating noradrenaline from a pheochromocytoma stimulate thermogenic capacity in adipose tissue at sites of BAT. This finding raises two issues. First, adipose tissue in these sites retains in adulthood a biochemical distinction from the white subcutaneous adipose tissue (which does not contain uncoupling protein even in infancy). There is already evidence that intra-abdominal fat is more active than subcutaneous in lipolysis and lipogenesis and in its response to catecholamines: Such findings might be expected in BAT, which is relatively inactive and lipid replete. Second, the mechanism clearly exists for a possible therapeutic approach for obesity treatment if thermogenesis can be stimulated specifically.

The concept of a more metabolically active BAT compartment in human adults, as distinct from the subcutaneous white adipose tissue (even if there are regional variations in function within these compartments), is similar to that which is emerging in adult dogs, whose intra-abdominal adipose tissue can be shown to regain BAT characteristics after prolonged pharmacologic stimulation.[29] The intra-abdominal fat of adults may still show predictable responses to certain pathophysiological stimuli, analogous to experimental animal findings.

The role of BAT in thermogenesis and body weight control in adult humans is gradually becoming clearer, and it is possible that at least some important subgroups of obese persons have defects of BAT-type thermogenesis. It is an interesting and tenable hypothesis, in view of the studies on ephedrine, that BAT is able to increase metabolism by the 4% to 7% that would account for the calorimetric responses to mild cold. The abnormal responses in diabetes and Cushing's disease[44,45] would be expected if, as in experimental animal models, the regulation of their BAT function is impaired. There is no direct evidence for any involvement of BAT in physiological weight regulation, but responsibility for 1% to 2% of energy balance might be a reasonable possibility. Defects of this order, if not otherwise compensated, could lead to weight gain (without overeating, compared with others) of about 1 to 2 kg (2 to 4 pounds) per year. There is some evidence from whole body calorimetry studies that women prone to obesity may under some conditions have energetic defects of this size.[46]

References

1. Aherne W, Hull D: Brown adipose tissue and heat production in the newborn infant. J Pathol Bacteriol 91:223, 1966
2. Allegra SR, Gmuer C, O'Leary GP: Endocrine activity in a large hibernoma. Hum Pathol 14:1044, 1983
3. Andersen KL: Comparison of scandinavian Lapps, arctic fishermen and Canadian arctic indians. Fed Proc 22:834, 1963
4. Andrews F, Jackson F: Increasing fatness inversely related to increase in metabolic rate but directly related to decrease in deep body temperature in young men and women during cold exposure. Ir J Med Sci 147:329, 1978
5. Ashwell M, Jennings G, Richard D et al: Effect of acclimation temperature on the concent-ration of the "uncoupling" protein measured by radioimmunoassay in mouse brown adipose tissue. FEBS Lett 161:108, 1983
6. Astrup A, Bulow J, Christensen NJ et al: Ephedrine-induced thermogenesis in man: No role for interscapular brown adipose tissue. Clin Sci 66:179, 1984
7. Astrup A, Bulow J, Madsen J et al: Contribution of BAT and skeletal muscle to thermogenesis induced by ephedrine in man. Am J Physiol 248:(Endocrinol Metab 11), E507, 1985
8. Blaza S, Garrow JS: Thermogenic response to temperature, exercise and food stimuli in lean and obese women, studied by 24h direct calorimetry. Br J Nutr 49:171, 1983
9. Bouillaud F, Villarroya F, Hentz et al: Detection of brown adipose tissue uncoupling protein mRNA in adult patients by a human genomic probe. Clin Sci 75:21, 1988
10. Bruck K: Temperature regulation in the newborn infant. Biol Neonat 3:65, 1961
11. Cannon B, Nedergaard J: Biochemical aspects of acclimation to cold. J Therm Biol 8:85, 1983
12. Cawthorne MA, Carrol MJ, Levy AL et al: Effects of novel beta-adrenoceptor agonists on carbohydrate metabolism: Relevance for treatment of non-insulin-dependent diabetes. Int J Obes (Suppl 1) 8:93, 1984
13. Chakrabarty K, Chauduri B, Jeffay H: Glycerokinase activity in human brown adipose tissue. J Lipid Res 24:381, 1983
14. Chakrabarty K, Radhakrishnan J, Sharifi R et al: Lipogenic activity and brown fat content of human perirenal adipose tissue. Clin Biochem 21:249, 1988
15. Contaldo F, Presta E, di Biase G et al: Preliminary evidence for brown fat defect in human obesity. In Gioffi LA et al (eds): The Body Weight Regulatory System: Normal and Disturbed Mechanisms, pp 143-146. New York, Raven Press, 1981
16. Cunningham S, Leslie P, Hopwood D et al: The characterisation and energetic potential of brown adipose tissue in man. Clin Sci 69:343, 1985
17. Curling TB: Two cases of absence of the thyroid body, and symmetrical swellings of fat tissue at the sides of the neck, connected with defective cerebral development. Med Chir Trans 33:303, 1850
18. Dallosso HM, Davies HL, Lean MEJ et al: An assessment of ciclazindol in stimulating thermogenesis in human volunteers: A detailed metabolic study. Int J Obes 8:413, 1984
19. Dauncey MJ: Influence of mild cold on 24h energy expenditure, resting metabolism and diet-induced thermogenesis. Br J Nutr 45:257, 1981
20. Fessler A, Beck JC: The effect of insulin on the metabolism of human adipose tissue. Biochim Biophys Acta 106:199, 1965
21. Hamosh M, Hamosh P, Bar-Maur JA et al: Fatty acid metabolism by human adipose tissues. J Clin Invest 42:1648, 1963
22. Hassi J: The brown adipose tissue in man. Acta Universitatis Ouluensis D 21. Anatomy, Pathology and Microbiology 1:1, 1977
23. Hatai S: On the presence in human embryos of an interscapular gland corresponding to the so-called hibernating gland of lower mammals. Anat Anz 21:369, 1902
24. Heaton JM: The distribution of brown adipose tissue in the human. J Anat 112:35, 1972
25. Heim T, Kellermayer M, Dani M: Thermal conditions and the mobilisation of lipids from brown and white adipose tissue in the human neonate. Acta Paediatr Acad Sci Hungar 9:109, 1968
26. Himms-Hagen J: Obesity may be due to a malfunctioning of brown fat. Can Med Assoc J 121:1361, 1979
27. Himms-Hagen J: Brown fat metabolism. In Bjorntorp P, Brodoff B (eds): Obesity. Philadelphia, JB Lippincott, 1989

28. Hoffenberg R: Measurement of the synthesis of liver-produced plasma proteins with special reference to their regulation by dietary protein and aminoacid supply. Proc Nutr Soc 31:265, 1972

29. Holloway BR, Stribling D, Freeman S et al: The thermogenic role of adipose tissue in the dog. Int J Obes 9:423, 1985

30. Hull D: Brown adipose tissue and the newborn infant's response to cold. In Philipp EE, Barnes J, Newton M (eds): Scientific Foundation of Obstetrics and Gynaecology, 2nd ed, pp 545–550. London, William Heinemann, 1977

31. Huttunen PK, Hirvonen J, Kinnula V: The occurrence of brown adipose tissue in outdoor workers. Eur J Appl Physiol 46:339, 1981

32. James WPT: Energy requirements and obesity. Lancet 2:386, 1983

33. James WPT, Trayhurn P: Obesity in mice and men. In Beers RF, Bassett EG (eds): Nutritional Factors: Effects on Metabolic Processes. Thirteenth Miles International Symposium, pp 123–138. New York, Raven Press, 1981

34. Jequier E: Direct and indirect calorimetry in man. In Garrow JS, Halliday D (eds): Substrate and Energy Metabolism in Man, pp 82–92. London, John Libbey & Co, 1985

35. Jessen K, Rabol A, Winkler K: Total body and splanchnic thermogenesis in curarized man during short exposure to cold. Acta Anaesth Scand 24:339, 1980

36. Jessop NS, Smith GH, Crabtree B: Measurement of a substrate cycle between acetate and acetyl-CoA in rat hepatocytes. Biochem Soc Trans 14:146, 1986

37. Johnson RH, Smith AC, Spalding JMK: Oxygen consumption of paralysed men exposed to cold. J Physiol (Lond) 169:584, 1963

38. Jung RT, Shetty PS, James WPT et al: Reduced thermogenesis in obesity. Nature 279:322, 1979

39. Lean MEJ: Brown Adipose Tissue in Humans. MD Thesis, University of Cambridge, 1986

40. Lean MEJ, James WPT: Uncoupling protein in human brown adipose tissue mitochondria. Isolation and detection by specific antiserum. FEBS Lett 163:235, 1983

41. Lean MEJ, James WPT: Brown adipose tissue in humans. In Trayhurn P, Nicholls DG (eds): Brown Adipose Tissue, pp 339–365. London, Edward Arnold, 1986

42. Lean MEJ, James WPT, Jennings G et al: Brown adipose tissue in patients with phaeochromocytoma. Int J Obes 10:219, 1986

43. Lean MEJ, James WPT, Jennings G et al: Brown adipose tissue uncoupling protein content in infants, children and adult humans. Clin Sci 71:291, 1986

44. Lean MEJ, Trayhurn P, Murgatroyd PR et al: The case for brown adipose tissue function in humans: Biochemistry, physiology and computed tomography. In Berry EM, Blondheim SH, Eliahou HE et al (eds): Recent Advances in Obesity Research, Vol V, pp 109–119. London, John Libbey & Co, 1987

45. Lean MEJ, Murgatroyd PR, Reid IW et al: Thyroid involvement in metabolic responses to mild cold: Abnormality in obese diabetic women. Clin Endocrinol 28:665, 1988

46. Lean MEJ, James WPT, Garthwaite P: Obesity without overeating: Dependence of diet induced thermogenesis on carbohydrate intake, reduced in post-obese women. In Bjorntorp P, Rossner M (eds): Obesity in Europe, 88, pp 281–286. London, John Libbey & Co, 1988

47. Lean MEJ, Jennings G: Brown adipose tissue activity in pyrexial cases of cot-death. J Clin Pathol 42:1153, 1989

48. Leblanc J: Adaptation. In Leblanc J (ed): Man in the Cold, pp 90–145. Springfield, IL, Charles C Thomas, 1975

49. Leibel RL, Berry EM, Hirsch J: In-vivo evidence for catechol-responsive brown adipose tissue in obese patients. In Berry EM, Blondheim SH, Eliahou HE et al (eds): Recent Advances in Obesity Research, Vol V, pp 117–123. London, John Libbey & Co, 1987

50. Lev-Bari E, Horwitz C, Shilo R: Diet-induced thermogenesis visualised by thermography. Isr J Med Sci 18:889, 1982

51. McLean P, Brown J, Greenbaum AL: Hormonal control of carbohydrate metabolism in adipose tissue. In Randall PJ, Whelan WJ (eds): Carbohydrate Metabolism and Its Disorders, pp 397–425. New York, Academic Press, 1968

52. McCormack JG, Denton RM: Evidence that fatty acid synthesis in interscapular brown adipose tissue of cold-adapted rats is increased in vivo by insulin by mechanisms involving parallel activation of pyruvate dehydrogenase and acetyl CoA carboxylase. Biochem J 166:627, 1977

53. Mager WM, Gifford RW: Pheochromocytoma. New York, Springer-Verlag, 1977

54. Medeiros LT, Katsas GG, Balogh K: Brown fat and phaeochromocytoma: Association or coincidence? Hum Pathol 16:970, 1985

55. Melicow MM: Hibernating fat and pheochromocytoma. AMA Arch Pathol 63:367, 1957

56. Merklin RJ: The anterior abdominal fat body. Am J Anat 132:33, 1971

57. Merklin RJ: The fetal kidney and brown fat. Anat Rec 178:415, 1974

58. Merklin RJ: Growth and distribution of human fetal brown fat. Anat Rec 178:637, 1974

59. Nauman A, Nauman J, Sypniewska G et al: Thyrox-

ine 5'-deiodinase in human adipose tissue. In Bjorntorp P, Rossner M (eds): Obesity in Europe, 1989, pp 177–184. London, John Libbey & Co, 1988

60. Newsholme EA, Challis RAJ Crabtree B: Substrate cycles: Their role in improving sensitivity in metabolic control. Trends Biochem Sci 9:277, 1984

61. Ostman J, Arner P, Englefeldt P, Kager L: Regional differences in the control of lipolysis in human adipose tissue. Metabolism 28:1198, 1979

62. Reeds PJ, Fuller MF, Nicholson BA: Metabolic basis of energy expenditure with particular reference to protein. In Garrow JS, Halliday D (eds): Substrate and Energy Metabolism, pp 46–57. London, John Libbey & Co, 1985

63. Ricquier D, Nechad M, Mory G: Ultrastructural and biochemical characterization of human brown adipose tissue activity in phaeochromocytoma. J Clin Endocrinol Metab 54:803, 1982

64. Ricquier D, Mory G, Nechad M et al: Development and activation of brown fat in rats with pheochromocytoma PC 12 tumours. Am J Physiol 245:C172, 1983

65. Rothwell NJ, Stock MJ: A role for brown adipose tissue in diet-induced thermogenesis. Nature 281: 31, 1979

66. Scholander PF, Hammel HT, Hart JS et al: Cold adaptation in Australian aborigines. J Appl Physiol 13:211, 1958

67. Shattock SG: On the normal tumour-like formation of fat in man and the lower mammals. Proc R Soc Med 2:207, 1909

68. Silverman WA, Zamelis A, Sinclair JC et al: Warm nape of the newborn. Pediatrics 33:984, 1964

69. Stirling DM, Ashwell M: The effect of diet restriction on the development of pre-natal and post-natal brown adipose tissue thermogenesis in the guinea-pig. Proc Nutr Soc 47:75A, 1988

70. Trayhurn P, Nicholls DG: Brown Adipose Tissue. London, Edward Arnold, 1986

71. Velschi GH: Anatome muris alpini. Ephemerid Acad Nat Curr Ann (Obs. 160) I:338, 1670

72. Wyndham CH, Morrison JF: Adjustment to cold of bushmen in the Kalahari desert. J Appl Physiol 13:219, 1958

Regulation of Thermogenesis and Nutrient Metabolism in the Human: Relevance for Obesity

ERIC JÉQUIER

DEFINITION OF THERMOGENESIS

Thermogenesis is defined as the energy expenditure above basal metabolic rate due to food intake, cold exposure, thermogenic agents, and psychological influences resulting from anxiety or fear in a resting subject. The most important factor that stimulates thermogenesis is food intake; some developments in the field of nutrient-induced thermogenesis are presented in this short review. It is worth mentioning, however, that caffeine[3] and nicotine[19] are thermogenic agents that stimulate energy expenditure. Cold exposure, however, does not have any significant role in stimulating energy expenditure under usual life conditions.[20] Humans tend to avoid cold exposure by wearing clothes and by maintaining room temperature in the comfort zone.

NUTRIENT-INDUCED THERMOGENESIS OF CARBOHYDRATES, LIPIDS, AND PROTEINS

Nutrient-induced thermogenesis has been much studied during the past 10 years. In order to avoid problems due to the unknown rate of intestinal absorption, the thermogenic response to glucose and lipids has been measured by giving the nutrients by the parenteral route. With the glucose clamp technique,[28] it is possible to study glucose metabolism under steady-state plasma glucose and insulin levels. Throughout

the physiological and pharmacologic ranges of insulinemia, there is a highly significant relationship between the amount of glucose infused and the net increase in energy expenditure above the preinfusion baseline values. The slope of the regression line gives the glucose-induced thermogenesis (GIT). At physiologic plasma insulin levels (i.e., < 200 µU/ml), GIT was 6% of the energy content of glucose infused, whereas at supraphysiologic levels (i.e., > 400 µU/ml), GIT was increased up to 8% (Table 10-1). The rate of glucose storage can be obtained by subtracting the rate of glucose oxidation from the total rate of glucose infused.[30] If the individual values of glucose storage are plotted versus the increment in energy expenditure, a significant positive correlation is obtained.[30] The slope of the regression line represents the energetic cost of glucose storage; it was found to be 1.9 kJ/g of glucose stored. This cost amounts to 12% of the energy content of glucose infused (see Table 10-1). Most glucose storage occurs in skeletal muscles as glycogen. Because the energetic cost of glycogen synthesis represents 5.5% of the energy content of the glucose stored,[12] factors distinct from glucose storage contribute to the stimulation of energy expenditure.

These results support the concept of two components in the thermogenic response to glucose infusion: an "obligatory thermogenesis," which accounts for the energy costs of processing and storing the nutrient, and a "facultative thermo-

TABLE 10-1

Thermogenesis Induced by Nutrient in Humans and Cost of Nutrient Storage

Nutrient	Thermogenesis*	Cost of Nutrient† Storage
Glucose	6–8	12
Lipid	3	4
Amino acids	25–40	25–40

*In percent of the energy content of the infused nutrient.

†In percent of the energy content of the stored nutrient.

genesis," which is an energy dissipative process. Factors that may be involved in the facultative thermogenesis include stimulation of sympathetic activity,[27,32] increased recycling of three-carbon compounds such as lactate, and stimulation of protein synthesis. An acute increase in plasma noradrenaline levels follows glucose administration.[27,32] Because plasma noradrenaline levels mainly represent overflow of the neurotransmitter from sympathetic nerve endings, increased plasma levels of the transmitter are a reliable index of sympathetic nervous system activation. By contrast, ingestion of protein or fat did not significantly alter plasma noradrenaline levels.[33]

The role of sympathetic activity in eliciting a part of the thermogenic response after glucose administration in humans is further supported by the fact that infusion of propranolol significantly decreases the thermogenic response induced by glucose during euglycemic hyperinsulinemic glucose clamps[2] (Fig. 10-1). The residual increase in energy expenditure was fully accounted for by the obligatory thermogenesis. Thus, propranolol inhibits most of the facultative thermogenesis, suggesting that the latter is mediated by activation of the sympathetic nervous system. In addition, the β_1-selective antagonist metoprolol reduced the GIT by 64%,[31] showing that facultative thermogenesis was mediated by β_1-adrenoreceptors. Astrup and colleagues[4,5] have shown that the major part of thermogenesis elicited by exogenous β-agonists occurs in skeletal muscle and not in brown adipose tissue.

The thermogenic response to fat infusion was found to be 3% of the energy content of fat infused.[29] The energetic cost of lipid storage is 4% of the energy stored. This value corresponds to the predicted obligatory thermogenesis calculated from the adenosine triphosphate requirements for lipid storage.[12] The thermogenic response to protein ingestion or infusion of amino acids is about 25% to 40%[12] of the energy content of the nutrient load, depending on the metabolic fate of the amino acids.

WHAT IS THE RELEVANCE OF THESE FINDINGS FOR THE TREATMENT OF OBESITY?

These results show that a meal with a high ratio of carbohydrate to fat (CHO:FAT) is more thermogenic than a meal with a low ratio. For this reason, it is advisable to recommend that obese individuals increase the CHO:FAT ratio of the diet, particularly after a period of hypocaloric

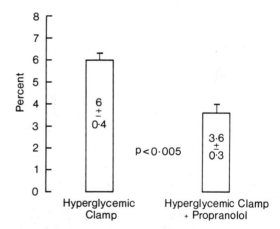

FIGURE 10-1

Thermogenesis induced by glucose infusion during a hyperinsulinemic clamp study (1 mU/kg/min) expressed in percent of the energy content of the glucose infused. After β-adrenergic blockade with propranolol, the thermogenic response to glucose infusion is reduced. The thermogenic response after β-adrenergic blockade is similar to the calculated cost of glucose storage as glycogen (i.e., it corresponds to the obligatory thermogenesis). The difference between the two thermogenic responses represents the facultative component of GIT.

diet when introducing a weight-maintenance diet.

Another important consideration is the marked limitation of lipogenesis from carbohydrate in humans[1]: The net synthesis of fat from a 500-g carbohydrate meal during a 10-hour period was found to be only 9 g. The same study also showed that carbohydrate balance was closely regulated in humans; even a large carbohydrate load is oxidized within a 24-hour period.[1] By contrast, fat balance is related to the amount of fat in the diet: We have found that during a 9-hour period, the same amount of carbohydrate, protein, and fat was oxidized, regardless of whether a 50-g fat supplement was included or not.[11] During overfeeding, the positive energy balance is closely related to the fat balance. These studies show that the body tends to maintain carbohydrate and protein balances, whereas fat balance is directly influenced by fat intake. The body's inability to regulate its fat balance contributes to explain why the incidence of obesity rises when the fat content of the diet increases.

ENERGY EXPENDITURE AND EFFICIENCY OF ENERGY UTILIZATION IN OBESITY

It is generally agreed that obesity results from a chronic imbalance between energy intake and energy expenditure. It is also well known that the energy expenditure of obese individuals is higher than that of sedentary lean persons.[9,25] The main reason for this elevated energy expenditure in obese subjects is the high basal metabolic rate that is due to the increased fat-free mass that accompanies the excessive development of the fat mass. Because basal metabolic rate is directly related to the size of the fat-free mass, obese individuals have an elevated basal metabolic rate. Another factor that contributes to increased energy expenditure in obese subjects is the energy cost of weight-bearing activities such as walking and standing: Greater energy is expended to move a heavy body than a light body. The practical consequence of the elevated energy expenditure of obese individuals is a corresponding elevated energy requirement to maintain constant body weight and body com-

position. This observation also suggests that excessive food intake is a cause of obesity.[14]

The question of an increased efficiency of energy utilization in obese subjects is controversial. The fact that obese individuals expend more energy than lean persons in the resting state has been considered as evidence that there is no increased efficiency of energy utilization in obesity.[14] It is questionable to consider the total energy expended without any reference to the mass of active tissues, however.

The metabolic rate per unit of fat-free mass is roughly similar in nondiabetic obese and in lean individuals.[7,9,25,26] However, the metabolic rate adjusted for fat-free mass, age, and sex, although similar, is not identical when one compares individual results.[26] Some subjects have a low resting metabolic rate per kilogram of fat-free mass; their energy expenditure is lower than that predicted on the basis of a large population study. Ravussin and colleagues[26] showed that the subjects with the lowest adjusted metabolic rate at rest, when studied 2 to 4 years later, had the highest incidence of weight gain. Not only the resting metabolic rate but also the adjusted 24-hour energy expenditure was found to be inversely related to the rate of change in body weight. In other words, low rates of energy expenditure adjusted for fat-free mass were significant predictors of gains in body weight. Subjects with a low 24-hour energy expenditure per unit of fat-free mass had a fourfold increase in the risk of gaining excessive body weight (more than 7.5 kg) during a 2-year period.[26]

IS NUTRIENT-INDUCED THERMOGENESIS REDUCED IN OBESITY?

After food ingestion, the total postprandial energy expenditure of obese subjects is higher than that of lean individuals,[9,25] mainly because the basal metabolic rate of the obese is larger than that of lean subjects. The relatively small component—the nutrient-induced thermogenesis—whether it is reduced or not, seems to have a limited role in energy balance.[6] This reasoning does not take into account the fact that most people, whether lean or obese, tend to remain at the same body weight for long periods.[18] Because in sedentary individuals the total 24-hour energy expenditure is proportional to the fat-free mass, lean or obese people must have a mean food intake that is related to their fat-free mass. The fate of any excess in food intake above the maintenance level depends on the importance of the nutrient-induced thermogenesis. Any difference in thermogenic responses to a caloric excess can be important to store or to oxidize part of the excessive energy intake.[21]

THE ROLE OF INSULIN RESISTANCE IN NUTRIENT-INDUCED THERMOGENESIS

The controversy about the existence and the role of a thermogenic defect in human obesity is due to the fact that different groups of patients have been studied.[21] The role of insulin resistance has been clearly established as a mechanism inducing a reduced thermogenic response to carbohydrate administration. It is likely that the divergent results previously published[6,10,22,34] are explained by the absence of insulin resistance in patients with normal diet-induced thermogenesis.

Golay and colleagues[17] found a decreased thermogenic response to glucose ingestion in obese subjects with insulin resistance, whereas the response was unaltered in young obese subjects without insulin resistance. During insulin/glucose infusions, obese persons with insulin resistance and non–insulin-dependent diabetic subjects demonstrate reduced glucose uptake. Studies by Ravussin and colleagues,[24] Bogardus and associates,[8] and Golay and co-workers[16] have shown that the thermic effect of infused insulin/glucose is reduced in insulin-resistant obese and non–insulin-dependent diabetic obese patients.

The thermic effect of insulin/glucose was found to be proportional to the rate of glucose storage. Thus the differences in the thermic effect of infusions of insulin/glucose between normal and insulin-resistant subjects largely appear to result from differences in rates of glucose storage. In other words, the thermogenic response is inversely related to the degree of insulin resistance. This observation is in agreement with the findings by Ravussin and colleagues[23] who showed similar thermic effect of glucose in lean and obese subjects when they were infused the rate

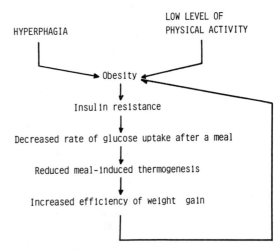

FIGURE 10-2

Reinforcement of weight gain due to a reduced meal-induced thermogenesis.

of insulin needed to obtain a predetermined glucose uptake. A given rate of glucose disposal was associated with the same thermogenic response in lean as in obese subjects. This observation indicates that under conditions in which insulin resistance is overcome (by a higher plasma insulin level), obese persons do not differ in their thermogenic response from normal individuals.

Insulin resistance induces impaired glucose uptake and a lower thermic effect of glucose in obese persons. After a meal, a fraction of the absorbed glucose remains in the extracellular space, and glycemia increases. This unstored glucose contributes to spare the energy that is needed in non–insulin-resistant subjects to synthesize glycogen. The thermic effect of glucose is therefore reduced in obese subjects with insulin resistance. This effect can increase the efficiency of weight gain (Fig. 10-2).

THE RELAPSE OF BODY WEIGHT GAIN AFTER WEIGHT LOSS

The major problem in the treatment of obesity is relapse and weight gain after a weight-reducing program: This occurs in the vast majority of patients. Body weight loss, induced by a hypocaloric diet, is accompanied by a decrease in 24-hour energy expenditure; a diminution in body weight influences both the resting metabolic rate and the energy cost of physical activity. The composition of the weight loss is approximately 75% fat and 25% fat-free mass, and the decrease in resting metabolic rate is related to the loss of fat-free mass. The total economy of energy induced by weight loss is about 85 to 100 kJ/kg weight loss per day.[21] Therefore, after a weight loss of 20 kg, the new maintenance energy requirement is 1700 to 2000 kJ/day less than before weight loss. Failure to decrease the everyday energy intake accordingly necessarily results in relapse of body weight gain.

The reduced thermogenic response to meals or to glucose ingestion in obese subjects remains lower than normal after weight loss (Fig. 10-3). Thus, the three components of energy expenditure—basal metabolic rate, the thermic effect of

food, and the energy cost of physical activity—contribute to an economy of the expended energy after weight loss. In formerly obese women who have reached a normal body weight after a prolonged hypocaloric diet, the overall energy expenditure was found to be lower by 1000 to 1200 kJ/day than that of control female volunteers of similar body weight.[15] If the formerly obese women were to consume the same amount of food energy as their matched lean controls, they would be in positive energy balance and gain weight until the rise in fat-free mass stimulates energy expenditure sufficiently to reach energy balance.

CONCLUSIONS

In sedentary individuals, total energy expenditure is related to the size of the fat-free mass, and it is likely that food intake is determined in part by the size of the fat-free mass. Some individuals, however, have a reduced metabolic rate per unit of fat-free mass, and they have an increased risk of gaining weight.[26] Studies have shown that heredity plays a role in determining the efficiency of metabolic rate.[13] Furthermore, a familial aggregation of the resting metabolic rate[7] suggests that a metabolic characteristic may predispose to obesity. The diet-induced thermogenesis could also be determined by the genotype. In addition, insulin resistance, which very often occurs in obese patients, is accompanied by a reduced meal-induced thermogenesis.[16,23,24]

More studies are needed to establish the role of the genotype in the regulation of the efficiency with which energy is utilized[13] and to determine whether impaired thermogenesis may be considered as an increased risk of subsequent gain in body weight.

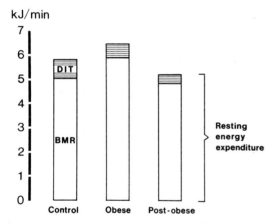

FIGURE 10-3

Basal metabolic rate (*open columns*) and dietary-induced thermogenesis (DIT) (*hatched columns*) measured in kilojoules per minute in a group of 17 control subjects (body weight 83 ± 1 kg). The same obese individuals were studied after a mean weight loss of 15 ± 2 kg consecutive to a 17 ± 3-week hypocaloric diet followed by 4 weeks of maintenance diet (*i.e.*, postobese). DIT was measured during 3 hours following a 100-g oral glucose load. The resting energy expenditure (BMR + DIT) was greater in the obese than in the control subjects (P<0.05), but the resting energy expenditure was lower in the post-obese group than in the control group (P<0.05). These results show that the resting energy expenditure of obese subjects after weight loss is markedly reduced. The require less energy to maintain their new body weight than before, when they were obese.

Acknowledgments: The participation of K. Acheson, J.P. Flatt, A. Golay, and Y. Schutz in a great number of studies summarized in this article is gratefully acknowledged.

References

1. Acheson KJ, Flatt JP, Jéquier E: Glycogen synthesis versus lipogenesis after a 500 gram carbohydrate meal in man. Metabolism 31:1234, 1982
2. Acheson KJ, Jéquier E, Wahren J: Influence of beta-adrenergic blockade on glucose-induced thermogenesis in man. J Clin Invest 72:981, 1983

3. Acheson KJ, Zahorska-Markiewicz B, Pittet PH et al: Caffeine and coffee: Their influence on metabolic rate and substrate utilization in normal weight and obese individuals. Am J Clin Nutr 33:989, 1980

4. Astrup A, Bulow J, Madsen J et al: Contribution of BAT and skeletal muscle to thermogenesis induced by ephedrine in man. Am J Physiol 248:E507, 1985

5. Astrup A, Bulow J, Christensen NJ et al: Ephedrine-induced thermogenesis in man: No role for intrascapular brown adipose tissue. Clin Sci 66:179, 1984

6. Blaza S, Garrow JS: Thermogenic response to temperature, exercise and food stimuli in lean and obese women, studied by 24 h direct calorimetry. Br J Nutr 49:171, 1983

7. Bogardus C, Lillioja S, Ravussin E et al: Familial dependence of the resting metabolic rate. N Engl J Med 315:96, 1986

8. Bogardus C, Lillioja S, Mott D et al: Evidence for reduced thermic effect of insulin and glucose infusions in Pima Indians. J Clin Invest 75:1264, 1985

9. de Boer JO, van Es JH, van Raaji JMA et al: Energy requirements and energy expenditure of lean and overweight women, measured by indirect calorimetry. Am J Clin Nutr 46:13, 1987

10. Felig P, Cunningham J, Levitt M et al: Energy expenditure in obesity in fasting and postprandial state. Am J Physiol 244:E45, 1983

11. Flatt JP, Ravussin E, Acheson KJ et al: Effects of dietary fat on post-prandial substrate oxidation and on carbohydrate and fat balances. J Clin Invest 76:1019, 1985

12. Flatt JP: The biochemistry of energy expenditure. In Bray G (ed): Recent Advances in Obesity Research II, pp 211–218. London, Newman, 1978

13. Fontaine E, Savard R, Tremblay D et al: Resting metabolic rate in monozygotic and dizygotic twins. Acta Genet Med Gemellol 34:41, 1985

14. Garrow JS, Blaza SE, Warwick PM et al: Predisposition to obesity. Lancet 1:1103, 1980

15. Geissler CA, Miller DS, Shah M: The daily metabolic rate of the post-obese and the lean. Am J Clin Nutr 45:914, 1987

16. Golay A, Schutz Y, Felber JP et al: Lack of thermogenic response to glucose/insulin infusion in diabetic obese subjects. Int J Obes 10:107, 1986

17. Golay A, Schutz Y, Meyer HU et al: Glucose-induced thermogenesis in nondiabetic and diabetic obese subjects. Diabetes 31:1023, 1982

18. Hirsch J, Leibel RL: New light on obesity. N Engl J Med 315:509, 1988

19. Hofstetter A, Schutz Y, Jéquier E et al: Increased 24-hour energy expenditure in cigarette smokers. N Engl J Med 314:79, 1986

20. Jéquier E, Gygax P-H, Pittet PH et al: Increased thermal body insulation: Relationship to the development of obesity. J Appl Physiol 36:674, 1974

21. Jéquier E: Energy expenditure in obesity. In James WPT (ed): Clinics in Endocrinology and Metabolism, pp 563–580. Philadelphia, WB Saunders, 1984

22. Nair KS, Halliday D, Garrow JS: Thermic response to isoenergetic protein, carbohydrate or fat meals in lean and obese subjects. Clin Sci 65:307, 1983

23. Ravussin E, Acheson KJ, Vernet O et al: Evidence that insulin resistance is responsible for the decreased thermic effect of glucose in human obesity. J Clin Invest 76:1268, 1985

24. Ravussin E, Bogardus C, Schwartz RS et al: Thermic effect of infused glucose and insulin in man: Decreased response with increased insulin resistance in obesity and non insulin-dependent diabetes mellitus. J Clin Invest 72:983, 1983

25. Ravussin E, Burnand B, Schutz Y et al: Twenty-four-hour energy expenditure and resting metabolic rate in obese, moderately obese, and control subjects. Am Clin Nutr 35:566, 1982

26. Ravussin E, Lillioja MB, Knowler WC et al: Reduced rate of energy expenditure as a risk factor for body-weight gain. N Engl J Med 318:467, 1988

27. Row JW, Young JB, Minaker KL et al: Effect of insulin and glucose infusions on sympathetic nervous system activity in normal man. Diabetes 30:219, 1981

28. Schutz Y, Thiébaud D, Acheson KJ et al: Thermogenesis induced by five different intravenous glucose/insulin infusions in healthy young men. Am J Clin Nutr 2:93, 1983

29. Thiébaud D, Acheson K, Schutz Y et al: Stimulation of thermogenesis in man following combined glucose-long chain triglyceride infusion. Am J Clin Nutr 37:603, 1983

30. Thiébaud D, Schutz Y, Acheson K et al: Energy cost of glucose storage in man during glucose/insulin infusion. Am J Physiol 244:E216, 1983

31. Thorin D, Golay A, Simonson DC et al: The effect of selective beta adrenergic blockade on glucose-induced thermogenesis in man. Metabolism 35:524, 1986

32. Welle S, Lilavivathana U, Campbell RG: Increased plasma norepinephrine concentrations and metabolic rates following glucose ingestion in man. Metabolism 7:806, 1980

33. Welle S, Lilavivathana U, Campbell RG: Thermic effect of feeding in man: Increased norepinephrine levels following glucose but not protein or fat consumption. Metabolism 30:953, 1981

34. Welle SL, Campbell RG: Normal thermic effect of glucose in obese women. Am J Clin Nutr 37:87, 1983

CHAPTER 11

Energy Expenditure During Exercise

BJÖRN EKBLOM

In general medicine and medical practice, the interest in energy expenditure is often focused on the basal metabolism rate (BMR). This is easy to understand, because variations in BMR in the range of 30% to 40%, which are found in patients with some diseases, may account for large increases or decreases in body weight if they persist for a long time.

However, the changes in metabolism during physical exercise, which may also influence postexercise BMR,[5] must be taken into account when analyzing an individual's energy balance. During short-term (a few minutes) hard dynamic muscular exercise carried out with large muscle groups, the metabolism may increase 10 to 15 times the BMR in untrained persons and up to 25 to 30 times the BMR in well-trained athletes in endurance events. Low-intensity exercise, which may require an energy expenditure corresponding to five to eight times the BMR, can be performed for hours even by untrained subjects. A game of soccer, which from a physiological point of view is high-intensity, noncontinuous exercise lasting about 90 minutes, requires an energy yield of between 6 and 8 MJ.[6] The energy cost of a marathon race (42 km) for an average 30- to 40-year-old man who is running the race in about 4 hours is about 12 MJ, or up to 20 to 22 MJ for 24 hours including and following the race. However, the training during the preceding 6 months before the race, needed for being capable of carrying out the race in 4 hours, can be calculated to be some 400 MJ,[7] equivalent to the energy content in approximately 15 kg of fatty tissue.

One cannot apply strict mathematical princi-

ples to biologic systems, but when analyzing energy balance for a longer period of time, energy metabolism during exercise must be taken into consideration. It is obvious that both the intensity and the duration are the main determinants of energy expenditure during exercise. However, many factors may modify the energy expenditure for a given rate of physical work and the total energy cost for certain activities. Thus it is difficult to give exact figures for the energy cost of exercise. Therefore, the discussion of energy expenditure should be based on individual conditions, and values given for certain activities or for groups of subjects are subject to large uncertainties.

The immediate source of energy for muscle contraction is derived from splitting of adenosine triphosphate (ATP) to adenosine diphosphate (ADP) and adenosine monophosphate (AMP). ATP must be restored, and the energy required can be obtained either by alactacid and lactacid anaerobic metabolism, the latter with glucose/glucogen as substrates and lactic acid as metabolite or by aerobic metabolism with fatty acids and glycogen/glucose as substrates and carbon dioxide and water as metabolites. The role of these energy-yielding systems during exercise is discussed next. It should be noted that in individuals in a good nutritional state, from a quantitative viewpoint, protein has a very limited role as a substrate for muscle contractions.

AEROBIC METABOLISM

For practical reasons, the determination of the energy release, used for the muscle metabolism during physical exercise, can mainly only be done by indirect calorimetry. For each liter of oxygen, between 19.7 and 21.2 kJ (4.70 to 5.05 kcal) is yielded during the aerobic metabolism. The variation in these figures depends on the type of substrate used. However, for most calculations of energy expenditure during exercise, a figure of 21 kJ (5 kcal) for each liter of oxygen can be used.

Oxygen Uptake Determination

For the determination of oxygen uptake at rest and during exercise, the Douglas bag system or automatic analysis systems, in which the oxygen and the carbon dioxide fractions along with the volume of expired air are measured, are most frequently used. The error of these methods for measuring oxygen uptake during submaximal exercise is now often less than 1% to 2%.

However, direct measurement of oxygen uptake can only be done with specific laboratory or field test equipment. Furthermore, in some activities, such as prolonged work, direct measurement of oxygen uptake is more or less impossible. Energy expenditure, based on calculations from oxygen uptake, must therefore most often be evaluated by other methods.

Estimation of Oxygen Uptake

Heart Rate

Measurement of heart rate during physical activity is one possible way to estimate oxygen consumption and energy expenditure. The background for this is that there is roughly a linear relationship between oxygen uptake and heart rate for most types of physical exercise under standardized conditions (Fig. 11-1).

However, it must be emphasized that the heart rate for a given absolute and even relative (percent of maximum) oxygen uptake can vary extensively, such as with age (see Fig. 11-1), different peak heart rates,[1] training status, diseases, psychological status and stress, medication (β-blockers), and many other factors. Therefore, each estimation of energy expenditure from heart rate recordings should be done individually, taking all these mentioned variations into consideration.

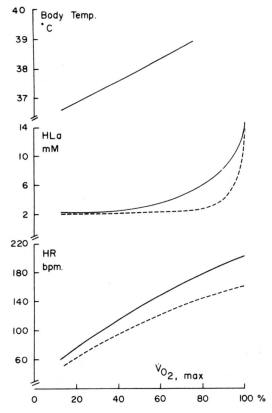

FIGURE 11-1

Schematic illustration of body temperature, blood lactate concentration (well-trained subjects, *broken line*), and heart rate (20-year-olds, *solid line*; 60-year-olds, *broken line*) in relation to relative maximal aerobic power.

This is done by first establishing the relationship between oxygen uptake and heart rate during increasing rates of exercise on a cycle ergometer or a treadmill, considering even the type of exercise that the subject is performing. The energy expenditure can thereafter be estimated by interpolation from heart rate recordings during the actual activity.

If all these measurements are done properly, the error of the method for estimation of energy expenditure from heart rate recordings during the actual work is in the range of ±15%.[4] However, this method is less accurate than direct measurement of oxygen uptake as a result of all the temporary variations in heart rate that may occur (e.g., during static exercise, during exercise with small muscle groups, during exercise at high altitude, in a hot environment, at hypohydration, and so on). Therefore, it must be emphasized that estimations of energy expenditure using this method must be done with great caution. On the other hand, in many situations, this method may be the only one available.

Core Temperature

Determination of core temperature during or after exercise may also be used for estimation of energy expenditure during dynamic exercise, because there is a close relationship between core temperature and relative oxygen uptake[12] (see Fig. 11-1). Thus, if the physical exercise has persisted for more than 25 to 30 minutes and is performed in normal conditions (e.g., within the air temperature range of approximately from 5°C to 35°C), a core temperature of 38°C indicates that the relative energy expenditure during the exercise is about 50% of maximal aerobic power.

It is obvious that even this method has its limitations, such as the inertia of the core temperature with time and changes in energy expenditure. However, this method may be very useful in some situations, such as intermittent work, in which rate of work may change rapidly, or during physical exercise with high levels of psychological stress. In these cases, core temperature determination may be one of the best estimations of energy expenditure.

ANAEROBIC METABOLISM

Anaerobic metabolism consists of the alactacid and lactacid energy turnover. In the former, ATP and creatine phosphate (CP) are split to metabolites with lower energy density. The alactacid energy yield is the immediate source of energy for muscle contraction and therefore is restored later by other energy-yielding systems. In the lactacid metabolism, glucose/glycogen are split to lactate. The lactacid energy yield is mainly used during static or heavy muscular exercise (see Fig. 11-1).

The performance capacity during heavy continuous muscular exercise, such as in sports, is heavily dependent on anaerobic metabolism.[4] However, it has been clearly shown that heavy manual occupational work can be carried out with very little or no increase in blood lactate concentration, if it is carried out as intermittent exercise and if the relationship between exercise and rest periods is appropriate.[2] Thus, if a rate of dynamic work that during continuous exercise would demand maximal oxygen uptake and result in high values of muscle and blood lactate concentrations and exhaustion within minutes is carried out as intermittent work with up to 10 to 30 seconds of alternating work and rest periods, the blood lactate concentration would be only insignificantly increased over resting values. The person would also subjectively perceive the rate of work to be much easier than during the continuous work, although the oxygen uptake would still be at maximum.

This phenomenon is explained by the fact that the energy needed for the exercise is derived from both the alactacid energy store and the stores of oxygen present in myoglobin and hemoglobin, which both would yield enough energy for even heavy muscular exercise during short periods of time. These energy-yielding stores can be restored during fairly short rest periods.

Determination of Anaerobic Metabolism

Blood Lactate Concentration

The appearance of lactate in the blood is a qualitative indicator for lactacid muscle metabolism, but the level of blood lactate concentration cannot be used for quantitative estimations because of the unknown volumes of body water, in which lactate is diluted, as well as other factors that modify the appearance and disappearance rates of lactate. Therefore, for more exact measurements of anaerobic energy yield during physical exercise, oxygen energy deficit or oxygen energy debt or both must be measured.

Oxygen Deficit

Oxygen energy deficit is the difference between the oxygen demand and the actual measured oxygen uptake for a given work task. This type of measurement can be used only when the energy requirement is known, which mainly is in strict laboratory conditions such as during exercise on a cycle ergometer.

Oxygen Debt

The oxygen energy debt is the "extra" oxygen uptake—the oxygen uptake more than the BMR—that can be measured after physical exercise mainly as a consequence of the anaerobic metabolism occurring during the exercise. The disadvantage of this method is that the oxygen debt is not only dependent on the oxygen used for "straightening up" or clearing away the alactacid and lactacid metabolism used during the exercise but also is influenced by many factors that are consequences of the exercise, such as increased core temperature, increased heart and ventilatory rate, increased epinephrine levels in the blood, and so on. Furthermore, it is still not known how much of the lactic acid produced during the exercise is oxidized and how much is used in glycogenesis.[4] Despite all these disadvantages, it can be calculated that the oxygen debt is about twice the oxygen deficit for many types of physical exercise and rates of work.

As mentioned earlier, anaerobic metabolism is of fairly moderate importance during occupational work and in most spare-time activities. On the other hand, during heavy muscular work, as in endurance sports, it can induce an increased oxygen uptake and oxygen debt for a long time after the termination of the exercise. However, the oxygen energy debt is seldom greater than 200 kJ.[5]

CALCULATIONS OF ENERGY EXPENDITURE DURING EXERCISE

For calculations of total energy expenditure for a given work task over a fairly short period (up to some hours), the power multiplied by time can simply be used with corrections for variations in power during the exercise. Theoretically, oxygen energy debt or oxygen energy deficit should also be added to these figures, but as mentioned earlier, lactacid anaerobic metabolism during occupational or normal spare-time activities is of little quantitative importance.

For calculation of energy expenditure for a longer period (days and weeks), energy balance studies can be used. Under the assumption that the body weight and body composition are not changed, the energy intake, measured by some acceptable method, equals the energy expenditure. It should be emphasized that there are normal variations in body weight of ± 2 kg between days, mainly as a result of variations in body water content, which may make energy balance studies with this method harder. Nevertheless, this method can be used in many situations, giving reliable results.

For instance, we studied a long-distance runner who ran 3520 km, from Helsinki, over the northern part of Norway, and down to Stockholm in 50 days.[13] His body weight did not change after 50 days. We calculated energy expenditure first from the heart rate, body temperature, and speed, "calibrated" to oxygen uptake during running on a treadmill, and second from the energy intake from dietary recordings. Using the two methods, we calculated the energy expenditure to be between 22 and 24 MJ/day, or a total of between 1100 and 1200 MJ for the whole run. However, it must be emphasized that measurements of energy intake are very time-consuming, particularly if many subjects are included in the study.

Power

During all types of dynamic physical exercise, such as walking, running, and bicycling, the energy expenditure increases linearly or curvilinearly with increasing rate of work (Fig. 11-2). During the lower submaximal rates of work, aerobic metabolism covers the energy expenditure, whereas during higher rates of work, the contribution from anaerobic metabolism, as indicated by blood lactate concentration, increases. During very heavy exercise, neither cardiac output nor oxygen extraction from arterial blood (arteriovenous oxygen difference) can increase any more, and the subject has reached maximal aerobic power.

Variations in Power

Variations in maximal aerobic power are due to age, genetic endowment, body size, and physical endurance fitness, among other factors. A high maximal aerobic power has several advantages, such as increased potential for high-level aerobic exercise, less fatigue during exercise, and, due to

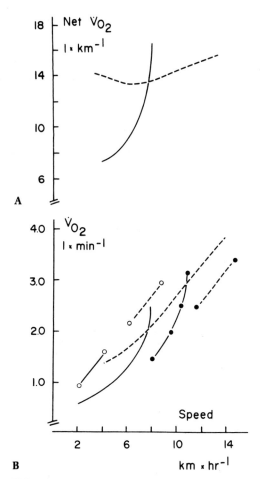

FIGURE 11-2

A: Net oxygen uptake (BMR subtracted) for walking and running, respectively. Body weight 75 kg. **B:** Oxygen uptake in relation to speed. *Solid line,* walking; *broken line,* running. *Open circles,* overweight subjects; *filled circles,* race walkers and long-distance runners, respectively.

increased energy needs when physically active, increased intake of essential nutrients.

Variations in power for a given submaximal rate of work are due to both individual variations in economy of locomotion, such as different technique, body composition, and temporary interindividual factors such as changes in core temperature, choice of energy substrate, and so on.

Figure 11-2 illustrates the energy expenditure during walking and running. At low speeds,

walking has a better energy economy—that is, lower oxygen uptake—than running with regard to both power (lower panel) and net energy cost per kilometer. However, at speeds faster than 6 to 8 km/hour, running is more effective. It should be emphasized that the net energy cost per kilometer in running is about the same for both low and high speeds—about 280 to 300 kJ/km for the average 70- to 75-kg man—whereas in walking the net energy cost increases with speed (see Fig. 11-2).

Women and children have lower energy cost than men for a given speed in walking and running because of their lower body weight. However, energy cost calculated per kilogram of body weight in men and women for both young and old adults has about the same values, whereas children have higher values.[3]

The variation in energy cost at a given speed is also illustrated in Figure 11-2. The energy cost is increased with increasing body weight[10] yet decreased at a given speed with increased energy economy, as for race walkers or long-distance runners. Thus, for a given low walking speed, the variation in energy cost can be up to 100% in a normal population.

Furthermore, the energy cost at a given speed varies with conditions such as surface, uphill or downhill walking, with or without wind resistance, and so on.[4] People with joint disease, an amputation, or other physical handicaps have decreased energy economy in running and walking.

In some types of exercise, in which technique is very important, such as in swimming, the energy cost at a given speed can vary up to more than 100% between good and poor swimmers for the same style of swimming or between the different swimming styles.[8] On the other hand, in bicycling, energy cost at lower speeds is about the same for well-trained cyclists and for runners, for example.

In high-speed activities, in which wind resistance increases energy cost curvilinearly, the style, position, or equipment can influence the energy cost of a given exercise. This is specifically true in cycling but is also true in other sports. For example, running behind another runner may save up to 6% in energy cost because of the wind protection.[11]

Different proportions of free fatty acids and

carbohydrate used as substrates for the energy-yielding processes influence the energy cost at a given rate of work. Because maximal oxygen flux through ventilation and circulation limits maximal aerobic performance during work with large muscle groups (e.g., running, bicycling, swimming, cross-country skiing), it is essential that carbohydrate is used as substrate because the energy yield is about 21.2 kJ per liter of oxygen compared with about 19.7 kJ when only free fatty acids are used. The disadvantage, however, is that the glycogen stores are limited and can be reduced or depleted during exercise, which may occur if the pre-exercise diet is inadequate or the exercise time is longer than 45 to 60 minutes. For a more accurate calculation of energy cost for a given work task of high intensity, it may be of importance to take the variation in R value into account as well as oxygen debt or deficit. The problem is that it is methodologically difficult to establish a true R value.

There are many other situations in which the energy cost for a given submaximal rate of work is changed, such as in hypothermia with shivering (increased oxygen cost), but in most such cases the magnitude of these increased costs is of quantitatively little importance. On the other hand, in many situations the oxygen cost for a given submaximal rate of work is not changed. There are no major changes in oxygen uptake for a given rate of submaximal work with variation in hot or cold climate (except if shivering), in acute hypoxia, with most types of medications, and in different diseases, although the physical performance capacity can be severely impaired. In these cases, although the power is not changed, the total energy expenditure for a longer period of physical exercise may be reduced because the individual fatigues earlier.

In Table 11-1, the maximal aerobic power and the energy expenditure during 1 hour of exercise at a rate of work corresponding to 50% of maximal aerobic power are presented. The latter values are presented because this rate of work is easily performed even by an untrained person during 1 hour. Furthermore, it also illustrates the energy expenditure during exercise in comparison with the BMR during 24 hours, which is around 7 MJ for an average 70- to 75-kg man.

The energy expenditure of endurance athletes during competition is based on data obtained in

our laboratory on well-trained endurance athletes during cross-country skiing, running, orienteering, and other endurance events. It indicates that these athletes on average tax their oxygen transport system to some 80% to 85% of their maximal aerobic power during competition, and in many cases higher than that.

Figure 11-3 illustrates maximal aerobic power in well-trained men and women who were 20 to 25 years of age and participated in different sports, indicating the energy demand when performing these sports. For increasing ages, the average energy cost decreases in parallel with the changes with age, as shown in Table 11-1.

The approximate energy cost for some activities, performed for more than 5 to 10 minutes, is shown in Table 11-2. The spread is the variation that can be expected in the age-group from 20 to 25 years.

SUMMARY AND DISCUSSION

Determination of oxygen consumption during and after exercise gives a reliable measure of energy yield during exercise, because 1 liter of oxygen used yields about 21 kJ (5 kcal). The power is mainly dependent on the intensity of the physical activity. However, it is not possible to give exact figures on the energy cost for different types of physical exercise because of all the fac-

TABLE 11-1

Maximal Aerobic Power and Energy Expenditure during 1 Hour of Exercise

	VO_{2max} (liters/min)	kJ/hour
Untrained women		
25 years	2.3	1400
50 years	1.9	1200
75 years	1.4	900
Untrained men		
25 years	3.3	2100
50 years	2.7	1700
75 years	2	1300
Endurance athletes		
Women	4–4.5	4200–4800
Men	5–7.4	5400–7800

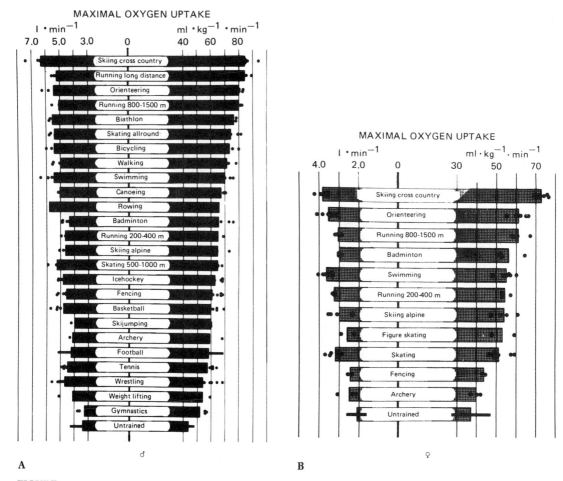

FIGURE 11-3

A, B: Maximal aerobic power in liters per minute and per kilogram of body weight, respectively, in well-trained male and female athletes participating in various sports. *Bars* represent means, and *filled circles* highest individual values. (Courtesy of Ulf Bergh)

tors that modify the power for a given rate of physical work.

This variation in oxygen cost for a given rate of work is of less importance from the weight-reduction point of view, because the total cost of an activity is mainly dependent on its duration. The total energy turnover during low-intensity exercise, in which the power is low but the work time can be very long without physical fatigue, can be much higher than in high-intensity exercise, in which fatigue may limit work time.

It has also been argued that low-intensity exer-

cise should be advantageous because of a higher proportion of free fatty acid oxidation (lower R value), mainly as a result of the preferential oxidation of free fatty acids in the slow-twitch (type 1) muscle fibers.

It is true that slow-twitch muscle fibers have a higher capacity to oxidize free fatty acids than untrained fast-twitch (type 2) muscle fibers. The capacity for fat oxidation in both fiber types increases as a consequence of endurance training, however, as indicated by reduced R values for a given rate of work. More important is the fact that although the R value increases with increasing rate of work, indicating a lower proportion of fat oxidation during high-intensity exercise, the energy turnover increases more than the change in R value. Therefore, the fat oxidation in absolute figures increases with increasing rate of work, up to some 75% of maximal aerobic power.

This observation can be illustrated in the following example comparing a low-intensity exercise (walking at a speed of 4 km/hour) and a high-intensity exercise (running at 8 km/hour). In the former, an untrained 30-year-old man with a body weight of 75 kg has an oxygen consumption of 0.8 liters/min and an R value of about 0.85, indicating an equal oxidation of glucose units and free fatty acids. During running, he may have an oxygen uptake of 2.1 liters/min and an R value of 0.90, indicating a relative proportion of fat oxidation of 33%. Taking these oxygen uptake and R values into account, the fat oxidation would account for the energy turnover of about 8 kJ/min during walking but about 15 kJ during running.

Furthermore, during 60 minutes of walking, the man yields about 1000 kJ, and he probably experiences fairly little physical fatigue. He would have to run for 25 minutes in order to use the same amount of energy. During 60 minutes of running, his energy expenditure would be about 2600 kJ. However, it is not very probable that an untrained man can run for 60 minutes at this speed—perhaps not even 25 minutes—and especially not perform this training program five to seven times per week without injury (overuse) problems. Therefore, the low-intensity program is advantageous from the weight-reduction point of view because of its potential for high total energy cost during a longer period and not because of the fat oxidation argument.

Finally, during rates of work yielding an energy turnover corresponding to more than 75% of maximal aerobic power, the fat oxidation contribution to the energy metabolism decreases and the carbohydrate stores are more stressed. However, after exercise, the energy taken in through the diet will, in the case of high-intensity exercise, first restore the glycogen stores and thereafter refill the reduced fat stores. If the exercise had taxed the carbohydrates to a lesser extent, then

TABLE 11-2

Average Energy Cost for Different Activities

	kJ × min^{-1}
Complete rest	4–7
Sitting	6–8
Standing	7–9
Standing, light activity	9–13
Light housework	13–30
Gardening activities	15–45
Walking	
3 km/hour	15–30
5 km/hour	20–40
7 km/hour	30–60
Running	
7 km/hour	30–50
9 km/hour	40–70
11 km/hour	50–90

the extra energy ingested after the exercise would have been stored in the fat cells directly. Thus, from the weight-reduction point of view, it is of little or no importance which type of substrate was used during the exercise.

However, there may be other reasons for choosing a high-intensity exercise, such as effects of physical training on health, on regulation of energy metabolism, and so on. It should be mentioned that it has been shown that an extra energy expenditure of about 8000 kJ (2000 kcal) per week or more through increased physical exercise above weekly energy output of sedentary controls is of importance for cardiovascular health.[9] Whether this should be carried out with high- or low-intensity exercise is unknown.

Figure 11-2 also illustrates the importance of low body weight and high maximal aerobic power for adults—especially the elderly—for maintaining good functional status. With increasing age, the maximal aerobic power decreases but the cost for moving a given body weight is in essence unchanged or somewhat increased. If the body weight increases, the energy cost for walking increases. For example, an overweight older woman, who according to Table 11-1 has a maximal aerobic power of 1.4 to 1.7 liters/min, may have difficulties in walking at a speed faster than 2 to 3 km/hour on level ground. If she encounters stairs, an uphill, or soft ground, she may become exhausted within minutes, and in such cases exercise is not a meaningful way of treating her obesity.

In our laboratory, we have even seen younger persons with these problems. A young former woman athlete, now weighing 120 kg, had been inactive for many years and had a maximal aerobic power of 1.2 liters/min. After 6 minutes of walking on the treadmill at a speed of 2.5 km/hour, she was exhausted. Her blood lactate concentration was 6 mg/dl, and her heart rate just above 190 beats per minute.

It is thus obvious that in extremely overweight untrained subjects, exercise intensity and duration will be so low and short, respectively, that the total energy expenditure for a given training session will be fairly low. In this context, it should be pointed out that in an obese person, the BMR for 24 hours corresponds to some 30 km of walking for the average adult. Thus, exercise should not be primary treatment for severe obesity. However, regular physical activity must be regarded as one of the most important factors for the prevention of obesity, but also, preferably, used in a latter part of a treatment program for obesity. It takes a long time to become obese; patients must accept that it takes time to lose the extra weight.

Reference

1. Åstrand I: Aerobic work capacity in men and women with special reference to age. Acta Physiol Scand (Suppl) 169, 1960

2. Åstrand I, Åstrand P-O, Christensen EH et al: Myohemoglobin as an oxygen store in man. Acta Physiol Scand 48:454, 1960

3. Åstrand P-O: Experimental Studies of Physical Working Capacity in Relation to Sex and Age. Copenhagen, Munksgaard, 1952

4. Åstrand P-O, Rodahl K: Textbook of Work Physiology, 3rd ed. New York, McGraw-Hill, 1986

5. Brehm BA: Elevation of metabolic rate following exercise: Implications for weight loss. Sports Med 6:72, 1988

6. Ekblom B: Applied physiology of soccer. Sports Med 3:50, 1986

7. Engström L-M, Ekblom B: Stockholm Marathon 1982. Participants, Motives and Training Preparations. Research Report 4. Stockholm, Department of Education, 1983

8. Holmer I: Physiology of swimming man. Acta Physiol Scand (Suppl) 407, 1974

9. Paffenbarger RF Jr, Hyde RT, Hsieh C-C et al: Physical activity, other life-style patterns, cardiovascular disease and longevity in physical activity in health and disease. Acta Med Scand (Suppl) 711:85, 1988

10. Passmore R, Durnin JVGA: Human energy expenditure. Physiol Rev 35:801, 1955

11. Pugh LGCE: The influence of wind resistance in running and walking and the mechanical efficiency of work against horizontal or vertical forces. J Physiol 213:255, 1971

12. Saltin B, Hermansen L: Esophageal, rectal and muscle temperature during exercise. J Appl Physiol 21:1757, 1966

13. Sjöström M, Friden J, Ekblom B: Endurance, what is it? Muscle morphology after an extremely long distance run. Acta Physiol Scand 130:513, 1987

Metabolic-Control-Logic: Its Application to Thermogenesis, Insulin Sensitivity, and Obesity

E. A. NEWSHOLME and R. A. J. CHALLISS

Energy expenditure is increased under various conditions when the body carries out either physical or chemical work; but not all the energy is converted into useful work, and the implicit assumption is that all of the energy not transformed into work can be classified as wasted. However, this view of energy consumption is myopic because it does not take into account the energy that is expended to provide for control and regulation of *all* the processes involved in the expenditure of energy. Regulation occurs at many different levels, and the preoccupation of biologists and physiologists with neural and endocrine control may explain a prevalent viewpoint—that the amount of energy expended in regulation is quantitatively trivial. This clearly is not the case. For example, it is well established that in most if not all cells, the large differences between extracellular and intracellular ionic concentrations (e.g., $[Ca^{2+}]_e/[Ca^{2+}]_i \simeq 10^4$) are maintained by two separate processes: a non–energy-requiring process sometimes known as a "leak," which transports the ion down its concentration gradient, and an active transport process requiring the expenditure of a considerable amount of energy. These two processes operate simultaneously and constitute a "translocation" cycle.[32] The translocation cycle is equivalent to a substrate cycle, which forms the basis of some of the discussion in this chapter. The differences in ionic concentrations are used to permit tran-

sient changes in the intracellular ionic concentrations, which can then be used in regulation of many different processes.

Of importance for discussion in this chapter, it is considered that *small* deficits in the precision of a regulatory mechanism can lead to pathology, such as obesity and type II diabetes mellitus. The importance of precision in regulation is illustrated by referring to one simple metabolic process in humans—the everyday occurrence of synthesizing glycogen from blood glucose. The pathway of conversion of glucose to glycogen involves four to five enzymes, but control of the pathway may require ten or more separate enzymes, illustrating the importance of *precise* regulation of this pathway. Why is this precision so important? The capacity to synthesize glycogen is sufficiently high that if fully activated under the wrong conditions it could lead to severe hypoglycemia; if the pathway were not activated sufficiently, it could lead to hyperglycemia.

Knowledge of the principles of what we call *metabolic-control-logic* is necessary to understand the significance of different metabolic control mechanisms. Such knowledge can then provide a basis from which to calculate how much energy may be involved in control and what may arise if these control mechanisms are impaired.

The application of logic to endocrinology allows a novel interpretation of, for example, the physiological significance of changes in insulin sensitivity and hence the phenomenon of insulin resistance. It may also help to explain at least one mechanism for thermogenesis. We consider that impairment of a common mechanism of control of both thermogenesis and insulin sensitivity may explain defective thermogenesis and some aspects of insulin resistance in obesity and type II diabetes. However, in order to explain this possible common defect it is necessary to understand the subject of sensitivity in metabolic control.

SENSITIVITY IN METABOLIC REGULATION

To understand one aspect of energy consumption, which is necessary in providing precision in regulation, it is important to appreciate the meaning of sensitivity in control.

Sensitivity in metabolic regulation can be defined as the quantitative relationship between the relative change in enzyme activity and the relative change in concentration of the regulator. If the concentration of a regulator (x) changes by Δx, the relative change is $\Delta x/x$; similarly, if the flux (J) changes by ΔJ, the relative change is $\Delta J/J$. The sensitivity of J to the change in concentration of (x) is given by the ratio $(\Delta J/J) : (\Delta x/x)$, and this sensitivity is indicated by the symbol s.[32] For example, if the concentration of a regulator increases twofold, the question arises, How large an increase in enzyme activity will this produce? The greater the response of enzyme activity to a given increase in regulator concentration, the greater is the sensitivity. To understand more clearly this principle, it is necessary to appreciate the process of equilibrium binding.

EQUILIBRIUM BINDING OF A REGULATOR TO AN ENZYME

It is likely that all regulators modify the activity of an enzyme by binding in a reversible manner to a protein. This protein may not be the immediate target enzyme but may be a regulatory protein of the target enzyme (e.g., in an interconversion cycle[34]). Such binding, which is described as equilibrium binding, controls the activity of the enzyme as follows:

$$E + R \rightleftarrows E^*R$$

where E is the inactive form of the enzyme and E^* is the active form. The asterisk indicates that the binding of R has changed the conformation of the catalytic site of the enzyme to the active form. The normal response of enzyme activity to the binding of the regulator is hyperbolic. Unfortunately, this response is relatively "inefficient" for metabolic regulation—for example, a twofold change in regulator concentration changes the enzyme activity by no more than twofold (i.e., the maximum sensitivity is unity). This concept may be difficult to accept when simply observing the steepness of the initial part of a hyperbolic curve. However, it must be appreciated that sensitivity is not the slope of the plot of activity versus concentration of substrate or regulator; it is the slope of the plot of the logarithm of activity versus the logarithm of regulator concentration. Because the hyperbolic response is the simplest relationship between protein and regulator, it can be considered as the basic response with which any mechanism for improving sensitivity can be compared. The basic limitation of this mechanism is given in Table 12-1. Four mechanisms for improving sensitivity are described.

MECHANISMS FOR IMPROVING SENSITIVITY AT NONEQUILIBRIUM REACTIONS

Multiplicity of Regulators

In the previous section, it was assumed that there is only one regulator for the enzyme. However, it is possible for an enzyme to be regulated by several different regulators that bind at different sites on the enzyme. In this case, if the concentrations of all the regulators change in the same direction (or in directions to change the activity of the enzyme in the same way), the effect of all the regulators is additive.

Cooperativity

For many enzymes that have a key role in metabolic regulation, the response of their activity to the substrate or regulator concentration is sigmoid. This phenomenon is known as positive cooperativity. For part of the concentration range of the regulator, the sensitivity is greater than that provided by the hyperbolic response (i.e.,

TABLE 12-1

The Change in Concentration of Regulator that Is Necessary to Increase the Activity of an Enzyme from 10% to 90% of Its V_{max}

Fractional saturation is calculated according to the simplest model of Monod et al[31]:

$$Y = \frac{\alpha (1 + \alpha)^{\eta-1}}{L + (1 + \alpha)^{\eta}}$$

It is assumed that n has a value of 4.

Allosteric Constant (L)	Concentration of Regulator Providing Fractional Saturation of		Increase in Concentration of Regulator Necessary to Increase Enzyme Activity from 10% to 90% of Maximum
	0.1	0.9	
0 (hyperbolic)	0.11	9.0	81.0
1	0.18	8.0	44.4
100	1.20	9.8	9.2
500	2.00	11.5	5.7
1000	2.60	12.6	4.8
10000	5.00	19.6	3.9
100000	9.60	32.6	3.4

greater than unity), and the quantitative significance of this can be estimated (see Table 12-1).[34]

Interconversion Cycles

A number of enzymes (e.g., glycogen phosphorylase, pyruvate dehydrogenase) are known to exist in two forms, conventionally designated a and b, one being a covalent modification of the other. The conversion of one form to the other is generally brought about by reaction with adenosine triphosphate (ATP), so that one form is a phosphorylated modification of the other. In general, only one of the two forms (a) has significant catalytic activity; therefore, the flux can be regulated by altering the amount of enzyme in this form. The interconversions between the forms are carried out by enzymes, one for each direction, that catalyze nonequilibrium reactions. The activity of one or both of these enzymes can be altered by regulators. Although the improvement in sensitivity provided by such cycles is likely to be large, it is dependent on the kinetic properties of both interconverting enzymes, and none of these

enzymes have been studied kinetically in detail. Highest sensitivity is achieved when the Km values of both interconverting enzymes for their substrates are much lower than the concentration of the substrates (i.e., the enzymes that are to be covalently modified). This has been termed zero-order ultrasensitivity. In other words, both interconverting enzymes catalyze processes that approach zero order—that is, they approach saturation with substrate.[25]

Substrate Cycle

A totally different mechanism for improving sensitivity is known as the substrate cycle. It is discussed at some length because it is considered to be important in the dissipation of chemical energy (see below).

It is possible for a reaction that is nonequilibrium in the forward direction of a pathway (i.e., A → B) to be opposed by a reaction that is nonequilibrium in the reverse direction of the pathway (i.e., B → A). Both reactions must be chemically distinct (different reactions) so that they

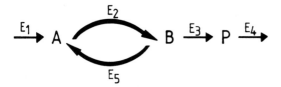

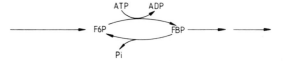

FIGURE 12-1

A substrate cycle in a hypothetical metabolic pathway. The enzymes E_1, E_2, E_3, and E_4 catalyze reactions in a metabolic pathway, but the nonequilibrium reaction is opposed by the reaction catalyzed by E_5. If enzymes E_2 and E_5 are simultaneously catalytically active, a substrate cycle results.

FIGURE 12-2

The fructose-6-phosphate/fructose/1,6-bisphosphate cycle.

will be catalyzed by separate enzymes. Then, a substrate cycle between A and B occurs if the two enzymes are simultaneously catalytically active. For every molecule of A converted to B and back again to A, chemical energy must be converted to heat, which is lost to the environment (Fig. 12-1). The role of substrate cycles in improving sensitivity should be appreciated by reference to Table 12-2.

An example of a substrate cycle is the fructose-6-phosphate/fructose-1,6-bisphosphate cycle (Fig. 12-2). This cycle is considered important in the control of the rate of degradation of glycogen to lactate, which provides energy for muscle under anaerobic or hypoxic conditions (e.g., at the beginning of exercise, climbing stairs, or sprinting). The operation of this cycle results in the hydrolysis of ATP to adenosine diphosphate (ADP) and phosphate (P_i), as fructose-6-phosphate is converted to fructose-1,6-bisphosphate and back again, so that the chemical energy available in the ATP molecule is converted into heat. Consequently, the greater the rate of cycling, the greater the rate of conversion of chemical energy into heat, which is then lost to the environment.

TABLE 12-2

Effect of Increase in Regulator Concentration on Net Flux Through a Reaction by a Substrate Cycle

Concentration of Regulator	Enzyme Activities* (units·min^{-1})		Net Flux A to B	Relative Fold Increase in Flux
	E_2	E_5		
Situation 1†				
Basal	10	9.8	0.2	
Fourfold above basal	90	9.8	81.2	406
Situation 2‡				
Basal	10	9.8	0.2	
Fourfold above basal	90	1.0	89.0	445

*The activities are hypothetical. See Fig 12-1 for reference to enzymes and the concept of cycling.

†In situation 1, the regulator has no effect on the reverse reaction catalyzed by E_5. The ratio of cycling rate:flux is 49.

‡In situation 2, the regulator not only increases the activity of E_2 but decreases that of E_5. The improvement in the relative change of the net flux is, however, not much greater than that in situation 1.

The role of substrate cycling in the provision of sensitivity and flexibility in metabolic regulation has been discussed in detail in several reviews.[32,34] The role of a cycle can best be understood when it is appreciated that in some conditions, an enzyme activity may have to be reduced to values closely approaching zero. Even with a sigmoid response, this would require that the concentration of an activator be reduced to almost zero or that of an inhibitor to an almost infinite level. Such enormous changes in concentration probably never occur in living organisms, because they would cause catastrophic osmotic and ionic problems and unwanted side-reactions. However, the net flux through a reaction can be reduced to very low values (approaching zero) by way of a substrate cycle. Thus, as the concentration of the product of the forward enzyme (E_2) (i.e., B in Fig. 12-1) increases, it is converted back to substrate A by the reverse enzyme (E_5), which maintains a low concentration of the product (B). This step ensures that the net flux (i.e., A to B) is very low despite a finite activity of the forward enzyme and a moderate concentration of the activator of the enzyme. If the concentration of this activator is increased by only a small amount above that at which the activities of the two enzymes are almost identical (and the flux is almost zero), the activity of E_2 increases so that the net flux through the reaction increases from almost zero to a moderate rate. Such a cycle, therefore, provides a large improvement in sensitivity; indeed, it can be seen as a means of producing a threshold (or almost threshold) response for a simple metabolic system.

Indeed the cycle provides an improvement in sensitivity without changing the properties or characteristics of the enzyme catalyzing the forward reaction in the pathway and for this reason can be seen to be different from the other mechanisms for improving sensitivity. This has also been shown to be the case when the precise quantitative role of substrate cycles in metabolic control is considered.[12]

One advantage of the substrate-cycling mechanism for increasing sensitivity is that the extent of this increase varies according to the rate of cycling; in other words, sensitivity is proportional to the ratio of cycling rate:flux.[32] In contrast, the increase in sensitivity provided by co-operativity, for example (see Table 12-1), is constant because it is dependent on the properties of the enzyme. It is considered that the variability of sensitivity in regulation provided by cycling is a major advantage of cycling. Such variations can be controlled by hormones or neural action, and although they can markedly change the sensitivity in control, such variations do not interfere in the basic cellular control mechanism.

The previous discussion has focused attention on the role of substrate cycles in regulation of metabolic flux. However, control of metabolic flux is only one aspect of the phenomenon of homeostasis. Control of the concentration of certain ions (e.g., intracellular Na^+ and Ca^{2+}), control of the concentration of key proteins (e.g., many regulatory enzymes), and control of the concentration of key metabolites (e.g., plasma glucose, intracellular cholesterol) must also occur. These concentrations may be maintained by what can be described as substrate cycles. The Na^+ concentration in many, if not all, cells may be precisely regulated by the balance between the Na^+-leak process and the Na^+-pump process, which has been described as a translocation cycle.[32] Indeed it is difficult to conceive of a process as effective as this translocation cycle for the regulation of the intracellular Na^+ concentration; furthermore, it provides a specific physiological function for the Na^+-leak process. Similarly, the Ca^{2+} concentration in the cytosol and especially in the mitochondrial matrix may be regulated by a similar translocation cycle.[36] Furthermore, in some cells, the intracellular cholesterol concentration may be regulated by the balance between esterification and hydrolysis of cholesterol ester.[34] Finally, the balance between protein synthesis and protein degradation may provide a precise mechanism for the regulation of concentration of many key proteins. It is well established that the rate of turnover of key regulatory enzymes is considerably faster than that of other enzymes that are less important in regulation.[34] As indicated earlier, a faster rate of cycling provides more precision in regulating the concentration of such key proteins. The obvious importance of maintaining the precise concentration of many proteins by such cycles may explain

TABLE 12-3

**List of Possible Substrate Cycles that Might Be
Involved in Thermogenesis and Control of
Metabolism**

Cycle	Tissues
Glucose/glucose-6-phosphate	Liver, kidney, intestine, brain
Glycogen/glucose-1-phosphate	Liver, muscle
Fructose-6-phosphate/fructose bisphosphate	Liver, kidney, muscle
Pyruvate/phosphoenolpyruvate	Liver, kidney, adipose
Triacylglycerol/fatty acid	Adipose, muscle, liver
Protein/amino acid	Many tissues
Cholesterol/cholesterol ester	Various tissues
AMP/adenosine	Liver
Acetyl CoA/acetate	Liver
Fatty acyl CoA/fatty acid	Liver, muscle, brain
Glutamine/glutamate	Kidney, liver, muscle
Na^+ leak/Na^+ pump (cell membrane)	Many tissues
Ca^{2+} leak/Ca^{2+} pump (cell membrane)	Many tissues
Ca^{2+} transport/Na^+-Ca^{2+} exchange (mitochondrial membrane)	Many tissues

why as much as 20% of the basal metabolic rate may be expended in protein turnover, which is, of course, the protein/amino acid substrate cycle.[34]

The potential quantitative importance of such cycles can perhaps be gleaned from reflection on the magnitude of the list of possible cycles given in Table 12-3.

In this way, hormones, for example, can markedly modify the response of a tissue to a given physiological stimulus. Control of the rate of substrate cycling may represent a *major* action of *some* hormones. This effect of hormones has largely been ignored by endocrinologists and nutritionalists, a lapse that may explain some myopic views on efficiency of metabolism.

SUBSTRATE CYCLES: THEIR RANGE AND QUANTITATIVE IMPORTANCE IN THERMOGENESIS

A substrate cycle requires the presence of enzymes in a cell that catalyze the forward and back reactions (different reactions and different enzymes). Thus the enzymic potential exists for a large number of cycles. However, the potential for substrate cycling does not prove that they exist. This must be demonstrated experimentally. Proof was first evidenced for the triacylglycerol/fatty acid substrate cycle *in vivo* in 1959[26] and *in vitro* in 1963.[42] In 1973, the use of dual isotopic labeling was developed for the measurement of the glucose/glucose-6-phosphate and the fructose-6-phosphate/fructose-1,6-bisphosphate cycle.[35] Since that time, the rates of several other cycles have been measured.

A very important question is the rate of substrate cycling in humans. A survey of some cycles in humans and their rates in some conditions is presented in Table 12-4. These results demonstrate the existence of some such cycles in humans, and the results have only been obtained in the past few years. Eventually, when a larger number of cycles has been investigated, it should be possible to elucidate the quantitative importance of substrate cycles in thermogenesis in humans. The currently available results indicate not only that they can account for considerable rates of thermogenesis, but that the rate of such cycles changes under conditions in which thermogenesis is known to change in humans.

TABLE 12-4

The Rates of Some Substrate Cycles in Humans

Substrate Cycle	Condition	Rate (Study)
Glucose/glucose-6-phosphate plus fructose-6-phosphate/ fructose bisphosphate	Euthyroid	6.8 μmol/kg/min (Shulman et al[41])
	Hyperthyroid	7.7 μmol/kg/min (Shulman et al[41])
	Hypothyroid	1.1 μmol/kg/min (Shulman et al[41])
Glucose/glucose-6-phosphate Fructose 6-phosphate/ fructose bisphosphate	Basal	1.8 μmol/kg/min (Karlander et al[21])
	Basal	0.7 μmol/kg/min (Karlander et al[21])
Glucose recycling (Cori cycle)	Euthyroid	1.3 μmol/kg/min (McCulloch et al[28])
	Hyperthyroid	4.7 μmol/kg/min ((McCulloch et al[28])
Triacylglycerol/fatty acid	Injured	3.3 μmol/kg/min (Carpentier et al[9])
	Basal	1.1 μmol/kg/min (Wolfe and Peters[46])
	Glucose infusion	2.5 μmol/kg/min (Wolfe and Peters[46])
	Normal	0.6 μmol/kg/min (Wolfe et al[44])
	Burn injury	10.1 μmol/kg/min (Wolfe et al[44])

SOME CONDITIONS CHARACTERIZED BY INCREASED RATES OF THERMOGENESIS THAT MAY INVOLVE SUBSTRATE CYCLES

At least two groups of hormones are known to be involved in thermogenesis: the catecholamines and thyroid hormones. These hormones are known to increase the rate of some substrate cycles. The possible importance of these hormones in thermogenesis is considered in two specific situations: after exercise and in digestion and absorption of food.

Postexercise Oxygen Consumption

When mechanical activity is undertaken by muscle tissue, more oxygen is used by the working muscle. The transition from rest to severe muscular effort can be immediate, but the increase in oxygen uptake on exercise is not immediate. It suffers a time lag. The adaptive processes in the heart, lungs, and blood vessels, which result in increased blood flow through the lungs and the muscle and hence in increased oxygen and fuel supply for the muscle, take a finite amount of time. During this lag period, energy is supplied within the muscle by processes that do not require molecular oxygen (i.e., creatine phosphate degradation and glycogen degradation to lactate).

During a relatively short period (from 30 seconds to 5 minutes), the rate of oxygen consumption in an exercising subject increases until it reaches a new steady-state value (Fig. 12-3). This new rate of oxygen consumption is sufficient to allow provision of energy at the required rate for the mechanically active muscles (unless the exercise rate is so high that it exceeds the maximum possible rate of oxygen consumption, when exhaustion soon ensues). The oxygen "missed" during the initial period of adjustment is defined as the oxygen deficit (see Fig. 12-3).

Termination of exercise can occur almost instantaneously and is accompanied by a time lag in the change in oxygen consumption. During this recovery period, oxygen is consumed in excess of that required to support the metabolism of the resting muscle. This extra oxygen consumption in recovery was noted in the early 1920s and for many years has been ascribed to the payment of an oxygen debt: Indeed, it was known as *oxygen debt*. Newer terms, *postexercise recovery oxygen* or *extra postexercise oxygen consumption* (EPOC), have replaced the word *debt*, which implied that it involved some form of reversal of the anaerobic processes that "saved" oxygen at the beginning of activity. Only part of EPOC can be explained by this mechanism, however (Table 12-5). The biochemical

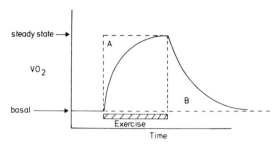

FIGURE 12-3

Stylized plot of oxygen consumption against time during and after exercise to show the relationship between oxygen deficit and oxygen debt. Portion A is the deficit, and portion B is the debt. The magnitude of B depends on how long the $\dot{V}O_2$ remains above the baseline. In some studies this is as long as 24 hours.[27]

mechanisms involved in the deficit and the debt have puzzled physiologists for more than 50 years.

Early Biochemical Explanations for Oxygen Debt

Lactate Theory. It is well established that lactate accumulates in the muscle and the blood during exercise. In the early 1920s, Hill and his collaborators[17] proposed that the extra oxygen used during recovery from exercise was utilized for the removal of this lactate. Because the formation of the lactate from the carbohydrate store in the muscle (i.e., glycogen) yields energy without using oxygen (i.e., an anaerobic process), Hill proposed that this was the mechanism by which oxygen was saved at the beginning of exercise. This theory predicts a simple relationship between the volume of the deficit and that of the debt. A simple relationship has not always been observed, however.

"Alactate" Theory. Some years after the pioneering work by Hill, Margaria and his group disputed the simple lactate explanation of the oxygen debt. Among the reasons for their doubts was the observation that in relatively mild exercise, an oxygen debt arose without any accumulation of lactate in the blood. Furthermore, during strenuous exercise, lactate accumulated, but its removal, and hence the decrease in concentration, did not coincide with the decline in oxygen consumption during recovery. Complete removal of lactate from the blood required about 1 hour, which was defined by Margaria as the "lactacid debt." However, an early component could not be related to lactate removal and this was termed the "alactacid debt." Several other explanations were put forward to explain its occurrence. During the initial deficit period, oxygen bound to hemoglobin in the blood and to myoglobin in the muscle and oxygen dissolved in the tissue water could provide the muscle with extra oxygen required for activity. During recovery, these stores of oxygen would be refilled, and because this could occur rapidly, it could provide an explanation for the fast component in oxygen debt. In addition, high-energy phosphate compounds (e.g., creatine phosphate) are known to provide energy for muscle contraction during the initial (i.e., deficit) period, and because these compounds are resynthesized rapidly during recovery, rapid extra oxygen consumption would result. Consequently, the resynthesis of creatine phosphate and refilling the oxygen stores could explain, at least in part, the fast component of the debt. Nonetheless, there remained the problem of the explanation for the slow component, which could not be accounted for by lactate removal.

Observations in Conflict with the Theories of Oxygen Debt

The total volume of recovery oxygen is not consistent with any of the theories that have been proposed to account for oxygen debt. Thus it is frequently greater than the deficit incurred at the onset of exercise. Theoretical considerations establish that the debt:deficit ratio should be 2 if all the lactate produced at the beginning of exercise were reconverted into glycogen during recovery. (Glycogen synthesis requires twice as much energy as is released during its breakdown to lactic acid.) However, the observed ratios (debt:deficit) are usually much greater than 2 whether or not lactate accumulates.

The utilization of each atom of oxygen should theoretically provide sufficient energy for the formation of three molecules of ATP in the muscle. However, it is observed that in experiments with isolated muscle preparations during recovery from exercise, the ratio obtained is considerably

TABLE 12-5

Calculations on Oxygen Consumption Required to Restore Metabolism to Normal for a 60-min Period After Extensive Intermittent Exercise

Recovery Process Requiring O_2 Consumption	Calculated O_2 Required	
	mmol/person	Percentage of EPOC
ATP and phosphocreatine resynthesis*	56	4.1
Lactate conversion to glycogen†	392	29
Repletion of oxymyoglobin plus oxyhaemoglobin‡	7.5	0.6
Increased work of heart§	43	3.2
Increased work of respiratory muscles‖	17.5	1.3
Total	516	38.2

The total measured EPOC during a 60-min period after exhaustive exercise was 1350 mmol O_2. The changes are taken from a study by Karlsson and Saltin.[22] The calculations provide similar results if data are taken from studies by Hermansen and Vaage[16] and by Hultman et al.[18] In all the calculations, a P:O ratio of 3 is assumed. Hence 1 mmol of O_2 consumed is assumed to be equivalent to 6 mmol of ATP synthesized.

*12 mmol of $\sim$ P per kg wet weight of muscle required to restore ATP and phosphocreatine levels to pre-exercise values: Therefore, assuming all muscles affected by the exercise equally, which is very unlikely, this is equal to $12 \times 40/100 \times 70/6 = 56$ mmol O_2, assuming 40% of body weight is muscle.

†21 mmol of lactate was removed from 1 kg muscle during 60 min: Formation of glycogen from 2 mmol of lactate requires 8 mmol ATP.

$$\text{Therefore, 21 mmol lactate requires } \frac{8}{6} \times 0.5 \times 21 = 14 \text{ mmol } O_2/\text{kg muscle}$$

$$= 392 \text{ mmol } O_2/\text{person}$$

‡Calculations were based on studies in dogs[36]: 1.5 ml/kg body weight estimated to have been released from venous blood; 0.9 ml/kg estimated to be released from stores of oxymyoglobin. Assuming this would be the same for a 70-kg person, oxygen required would be 168 ml or 7.5 mmol/person.

§Assuming that the increased work of the heart is due to carrying increased O_2 needed as recovery O_2, this is 30.2 liters. Assuming a utilization coefficient of O_2 in blood as 60% and an O_2 capacity of blood of 18.5 vol %, the amount of blood required to transport the extra O_2 is about 300 liters. The heart has to work against a mean pressure of 100 mg Hg, which is 0.132 atm. Work done by the heart $= 300 \times 0.132 = 39.6$ liter atm $= 965$ kcal. Assuming an efficiency of the heart of 25%, the amount of energy required is 3860 kcal or 772 ml of O_2. If further 25% is required for pulmonary circulation, that is 0.96 liter or 43 mmol O_2. ‖It is assumed that for the utilization of 1 liter of O_2, 35 liters of air are inspired.[17] Assuming the mean pressure in the pleural cavity is 15 mm Hg, the work done by the respiratory muscles in inspiring 35 liters is $35 \times 15/760 = 0.69$ liter atm. $= 16$ kcal. Therefore, for 30.2 liters of O_2 $= 16 \times 30.2 = 483$ kcal. Assuming 25% efficiency of the respiratory muscle $= 1852$ kcal $= 370$ ml O_2 or 17.5 mmol.

less than 3. Consequently, it is concluded that some of the energy obtained from the extra oxygen consumption is not used for the replenishment of creatine phosphate in the muscle.[38] Furthermore, during the deficit phase, a greater quantity of creatine phosphate is hydrolyzed than would be expected on the basis of the amount of oxygen saved (i.e., the phosphate:oxygen ratio is less than 3).[39] Both these observations indicate that some energy expended both at the beginning of activity and during recovery could not, at that time, be accounted for by any of the current theories.

Groups of animals that had undergone various surgical manipulations (e.g., removal of the viscera; removal of the liver) were exercised, and the quantity of oxygen consumed and the rate of removal of lactate were measured.[20] The volumes of oxygen required for the exercise and the oxygen debt were the same for all groups of animals, but the rate of disappearance of lactate from the blood varied greatly, depending on the surgical treatment. Furthermore, in certain groups, the lactate concentrations in the blood remained elevated even after the rate of extra oxygen consumption had declined to zero.

A number of experiments that result in the development of an oxygen deficit or the payment of an oxygen debt but that do not involve exercise have been carried out. These experiments have yielded interesting results in relation to the theories of oxygen debt.

The infusion of sodium lactate into the bloodstream has been used to simulate lactate accumulation in the blood during exercise. Infusion of lactate causes an elevation in oxygen consumption. However, the volume of extra oxygen consumed does not bear any simple relationship to the amount of lactate infused or the increased concentration of lactate in the blood.[2] Thus the volume of oxygen consumed is too large to be accounted for by any of the known biochemical processes for the utilization of lactate, especially its reconversion to glycogen.

Several methods that have been applied impose a relative oxygen lack on the tissues. (This is, of course, the situation that occurs in muscle at the beginning of exercise.) Such methods include the artificial decrease in blood flow from the heart,[1] breathing gas mixtures low in oxygen, and occlusion of major blood vessels by a pneumatic cuff. In all cases, the consumption of oxygen is decreased during the experimental period. However, in no case does the volume of the oxygen debt, which occurs during recovery from the hypoxia, bear any relationship to the oxygen deficit or the amount of lactic acid produced during hypoxia and subsequently removed during recovery.

When all the known factors that could be involved in recovery oxygen have been taken into account, there is still a large difference between that calculated and that observed (see Table 12-5). Despite the inaccuracies inherent in calculation of the energy requirement of these various processes, we do not consider them sufficient to explain the discrepancy shown in Table 12-5.

We consider that the oxygen not accounted for by these classic processes (see Table 12-5) may be due to stimulation of the rates of substrate cycles. The significance of increased rates of cycling would be to increase the sensitivity of metabolic control so that the increased rates of metabolism during exercise can return gradually and smoothly to the normal resting level during the recovery period. Stimulation of cycles after exercise could be caused by an elevation in the level of catecholamines. There is evidence that the plasma level of adrenaline is elevated after endurance exercise.[29] It has been shown that the rate of the triacylglycerol/fatty acid cycle is elevated after exercise in rats, guinea pigs, and humans.[4,30,43]

Important questions arose from this study of the literature on recovery oxygen. What is its magnitude, and how does it relate to endurance and intensity of the exercise? Although early studies indicated its existence and provided information about mechanisms to explain the phenomenon of EPOC, the variability in its magnitude and duration casts doubt on its significance. Hence in the 1980s, very carefully controlled systematic studies were carried out by a research group in Oslo. They have shown that after 60 to 90 minutes of exercise (at about 70% of $\dot{V}O_{2\,max}$) in human volunteers, oxygen consumption was elevated for at least 24 hours after cessation of exercise.[27] Similar findings were observed for this same level of exercise but lasting for shorter periods of time (20 and 40 minutes). There is in fact a linear relationship between the extent of EPOC and the time of exercise.[5] Of considerable importance is the fact that the respiratory exchange ratio was found to be lowered for the whole of the EPOC period, indicating a greater rate of fat oxidation after exercise.[27] Because these subjects were allowed to eat only simple carbohydrate meals after exercise and because the plasma glycerol and fatty acid levels were elevated, these findings suggest that triacylglycerol is being mobilized from the adipose tissue depots and the fatty acids are being utilized by muscle and perhaps other tissues. The carbohydrate in the diet thus could be converted to glycogen in muscle and liver rather than being oxidized. It also suggests that the rate of the triacylglycerol/fatty acid cycle should be enhanced. This is now known to be the case. Bahr and Hansson[4] have now measured the rate of the triacylglycerol/fatty acid cycle and have shown that for the extra oxygen consumption at 3 hours after cessation of exercise, at least 50% can be explained from the increased rate of this cycle. This observation is in general agreement with the discrepancy shown in Table 12-5.

Finally, a number of studies have shown that the thyroid status can affect the cycling rates of the glucose/glucose-6-phosphate and fructose-6-phosphate and fructose-1,6-bisphosphate cycles in both the rats and humans. In general, hypothyroidism decreases the rates of these cycles and hyperthyroidism decreases the rates *in vivo* in both humans and rats (Fig. 12-4).

Thermic Response to Food

The increase in heat production that occurs after a meal (the thermic response to food) has been divided into two parts: obligatory and facultative. Obligatory thermogenesis is released in the processes of transport, metabolism, and assimilation of the metabolites absorbed after digestion—for example, conversion of one molecule of glucose to glycogen requires the hydrolysis of three molecules of ATP to ADP. The remainder of the thermogenesis is facultative, although we suggest that it is due to control and cannot really be described in meaningful terms as facultative. Such control may include substrate cycles, which have many properties that are consistent

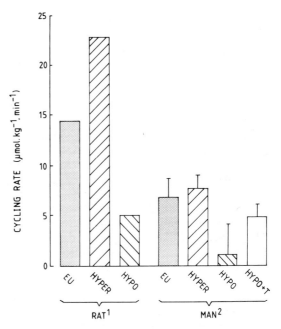

FIGURE 12-4

The effect of thyroid status on the rates of glucose/glucose-6-phosphate and fructose-6-phosphate/fructose bisphosphate cycles in rats[37] and humans.[41] (EU, euthyroid; HYPER, hyperthyroid; HYPO, hypothyroid; HYPO + T, hypothyroid patient treated with thyroxine for 6 months)

with their having a role in the thermic response to food.[32] (1) The increase in heat production varies with the type of food assimilated. (2) The extent and duration of the heat production is proportional to the amount of food ingested. (3) The increase can be observed after injection of monosaccharides or amino acids, so that it is not solely due to the digestive processes. (4) The increase is not dependent on oxidation of the food. Administration of glucose to dogs that had been starved for 3 weeks produced a pronounced thermic response, although most of the glucose was excreted in the urine.[13] (5) Removal of the liver from dogs abolishes the specific thermic response to protein but not that to carbohydrate or fat. (6) The thermic response is either zero or positive; it is never negative. Thus, changing from one food to another does not decrease the response.

These properties provide *indirect* support for

the hypothesis that increased rate of substrate cycling can explain in part the thermic response to food. It is, in fact, the only mechanism that can provide a satisfactory answer to the thermic response to glucose in dogs that had been starved for 3 weeks and in which there was little oxidation of glucose. An increase in the blood glucose concentration could increase the synthesis of glycogen in the liver; the elevated amounts of glycogen could increase the rate of degradation of glycogen, thus stimulating the rate of the glucose-1-phosphate/glycogen cycle. Similarly, there might be an increase in the rate of the glucose/glucose-6-phosphate cycle. However, if glycolysis were inhibited at the phosphofructokinase reaction and pyruvate oxidation were severely inhibited at pyruvate dehydrogenase, glucose and glycolytic residues would not be oxidized, glycolytic residues would be reconverted into glucose by gluconeogenesis, and the glucose would eventually be excreted by the kidneys.

More direct evidence is now available. It has been shown that the rate of the fructose-6-phosphate/fructose bisphosphate cycle in isolated muscle is decreased by starvation for 24 hours,[10] and it has been shown in rats and mice that the rate of the triacylglycerol/fatty acid cycle in white and brown adipose tissue in vivo is increased by feeding.[6] Furthermore, these effects are removed by administration of a β-adrenoreceptor blocker. This observation suggests that the stimulation of cycling rates during feeding is due to increased levels of catecholamines. In humans, it has been shown that infusion of glucose increases the rate of the triacylglycerol/fatty acid cycle.[46]

We suggest that one role of the increased sympathetic activity after a meal is to provide higher rates of substrate cycling for improved sensitivity of processes that control the rates of synthetic and degradative processes. This action would result in thermogenesis, but such thermogenesis cannot be considered as the primary role of the thermic response to food. The primary role, we argue, is to provide for sensitivity in control. That is, a significant proportion of the energy ingested in the meal must be lost as heat during assimilation to provide for sensitivity in metabolic control. It should be noted that these rates of cycling vary from condition to condition, from time to time, and from individual to individual. It is a known fact that facultative thermogenesis shows such variability.

An important factor that cannot be fully understood at the present time is the quantitative significance of cycles in relation to heat production in humans. The inability to provide precise quantitative information stems from two important points. First, our knowledge of metabolism is still very incomplete. For example, although

TABLE 12-6

Effects of Insulin on Rates of Lactate by the Stripped-Soleus-Muscle Preparation* Isolated from Rats that had Received Adrenaline Retard Tablets Implanted 0 to 120 hours Before Study

Insulin (μunits/mol)	Time After Retard Tablet Implantation (hours)	Rate (μmol/hour/g of tissue)				
		0 (control)	6	48	72	120
1		6.91	6.58	7.95	8.99†	8.30
10		8.62	6.58	8.05	9.90	11.88†
100		12.10	5.66†	8.15†	11.77	14.07†
1000		15.39	11.91†	13.30†	13.65	14.61
10000		15.24	15.33	15.85	15.98	13.99

(Data from Budohoski L, Challiss RAJ, Dubaniewicz A et al: Biochem J 244:655, 1987)

*Soleus muscles were incubated for 60 min in medium containing 5-mM glucose at the insulin concentrations listed above.

†Statistical significance of difference from control. (Minimum number of observations is 7.)

the stoichiometry of gluconeogenesis indicates that six ATP molecules need to be hydrolyzed to produce one glucose molecule, this equation fails to take into account any substrate cycling within the hepatocyte or any expenditure of energy for transportation of molecules across the cell and mitochondrial membranes. Second, the cycles given in Table 12-4 probably represent a minimum of cycles that are operative in humans and that can change in rate under different conditions. Finally, it should be noted that not all heat production in brown adipose tissue need be due to the activity of the uncoupling protein (thermogenin). It seems to be tacitly assumed that if heat is produced by this tissue, it must be due to thermogenin; some heat could be produced by the operation of the triacylglycerol/fatty acid cycle.

INSULIN SENSITIVITY

Several physiological conditions increase the sensitivity of glucose metabolism to insulin, including cold exposure, starvation, and exercise training. It has been shown that the soleus muscles removed from animals subjected to these conditions and incubated in vitro exhibit increased sensitivity of glucose utilization to insulin (Table 12-6). This appears to be a postreceptor effect. The evidence that catecholamines are involved in such changes is as follows.

The findings (summarized in reviews by Challiss and colleagues[11] and by Newsholme and associates[33]) indicate that chronic treatment in vivo with adrenaline or β-adrenoceptor agonists increases the sensitivity of glucose utilization by muscle incubated in vitro to insulin (Fig. 12-5). This effect may explain, at least in part, the improved sensitivity to insulin in vivo. What is the nature of this chronic effect of catecholamines?

The local hormones, adenosine and prostaglandins, are factors known to influence the sensitivity of glucose utilization in muscle to insulin. Adenosine and prostaglandins are produced continuously by most tissues (Figs. 12-6 and 12-7). It has been shown that lowering the adenosine concentration in the incubated isolated soleus muscle of the rat, by addition of adenosine deaminase to the incubation medium, dramatically increases the sensitivity of glucose utiliza-

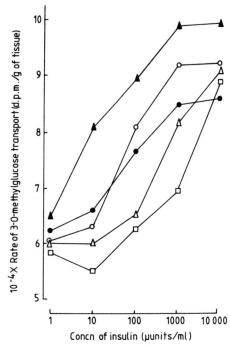

FIGURE 12-5

Effects of insulin on rates of 3-0-methyl-D[14C]-glucose uptake by the incubated soleus-muscle preparation isolated from rats receiving adrenaline retard-tablets for 0 to 120 hours before investigation in vitro. Each data point represents the mean of at least six separate muscle incubations for control (○) or 6 hours (△), 48 hours (□), 72 hours (●), and 120 hours (▲) after retard-tablet implantation. Error bars have been omitted for clarity, but the standard error of the mean was never greater than 8% of the mean.

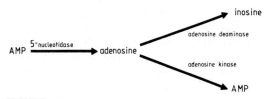

FIGURE 12-6

The formation and utilization of adenosine. Adenosine is produced from AMP by the action of 5'-nucleotidase and can then be converted either back to AMP by adenosine kinase or to inosine by adenosine deaminase. These three enzymes may have an important role in the precise regulation of the adenosine concentration.[3]

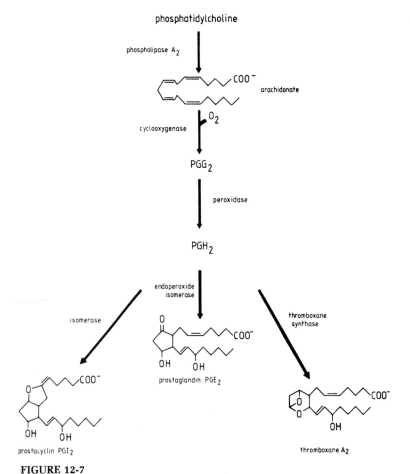

FIGURE 12-7

Pathway for the synthesis of prostaglandin PGE_2 and related compounds.

tion to insulin (Fig. 12-8). Similarly, increasing the concentration of prostaglandins E_1 or E_2 in the incubation medium increases the sensitivity of glucose utilization to insulin. It is likely that specific receptors are involved in these effects. Thus, adding adenosine receptor antagonists to the incubation medium increases the sensitivity to insulin; adding adenosine receptor agonists decreases the sensitivity of the isolated soleus muscle. These findings suggest that variations in the concentration of such local hormones or changes in the number or affinity of receptors to these local hormones in muscle could be a physiological mechanism for changing the sensitivity of glucose utilization to insulin. Hence, the

chronic effect of catecholamines or, more specifically, β-adrenoceptor agonists, in improving the sensitivity of glucose utilization in muscle, may be due to a change in the effectiveness of locally produced adenosine or prostaglandins or both.

How is it possible for such local hormones to cause a change in sensitivity of glucose transport to insulin? One possibility is the existence of a translocation cycle between an intracellular store of glucose transporters and those present in the cell membrane.[8] Thus the number of transporters present in the membrane at any one time may represent a balance between the flux of transporters into the membrane and out of the membrane.

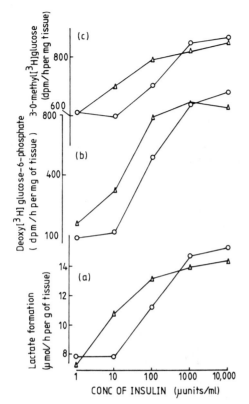

FIGURE 12-8

The effect of lowering the concentration of adenosine on the sensitivities of glucose conversion to lactate (a) phosphorylation of 2-deoxyglucose (b) and glucose transport (c) in response to insulin in the isolated incubated soleus muscle. For all three processes, lowering the adenosine concentration by addition of adenosine deaminase to the incubation medium increased the sensitivity to insulin (i.e., in each case the plot was moved to the left by the addition of deaminase). (O—O control incubation; △—△ addition of adenosine deaminase)

Insulin is known to increase the number of transporters in the cell membrane of skeletal muscle.[24] It could do this by an increase in the rate of efflux of transporters to the cell membrane, a decrease in their inward rate of transport, or both (Fig. 12-9). A decrease in the concentration of adenosine may lead to an increase in the rate of cycling of such transporters—that is, an increase in the rate of influx and an equal increase in the rate of efflux. In this way, changes in the local

hormone concentration would not change the rate of glucose transport in the basal state, but they would change the effectiveness of insulin. If the rate of cycling (i.e., influx and efflux) were increased, any change in insulin concentration below maximal would then have a greater effect on the number of transporters in the membrane—that is, the increase in the cycling of transporters would increase the sensitivity to insulin (see Fig. 12-9).

Whatever the mechanism for this chronic effect of catecholamines, the finding leads to a hypothesis for a *common mechanism* to explain both decreased rates of thermogenesis (not in the basal state, but in response to thermogenic stimuli) plus insulin resistance. Decreased rates of thermogenesis in response to thermogenic stimuli are common characteristics in some cases of obesity and type II diabetes mellitus.

A COMMON MECHANISM TO EXPLAIN CHANGES IN SENSITIVITY OF MUSCLE TO INSULIN AND TO CATECHOLAMINES

Evidence provided earlier supports the view that catecholamines can stimulate the rate of substrate cycles: Increased rates of cycling not only increase sensitivity in metabolic control but also increase the rate of thermogenesis. It is suggested that the increased rate of thermogenesis under conditions when catecholamines are elevated is due, in part, to increased rates of substrate cycling. It is also suggested that catecholamines have an additional, but totally different, role— that is, they chronically increase the sensitivity of glucose utilization in muscle to insulin. This latter effect of catecholamines is not, as far as we are aware, the result of an effect on substrate cycling, but it may be achieved by changing the effectiveness of locally produced modulators. If these two quite separate effects of catecholamines are considered together, they could explain that at least in some cases of obesity in experimental animals and in humans, insulin resistance coexists with decreased rates of thermogenesis in response to thermogenic stimuli (e.g., the rate of thermogenesis is decreased in response to glucose or in response to exercise).[23,40,47] Hence, if the muscle of these subjects

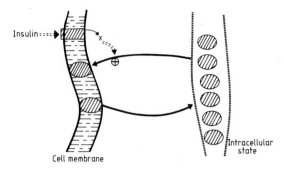

FIGURE 12-9

A control mechanism for the number of glucose transporters in the cell membrane. Insulin binds at its receptor in the cell membrane and increases the intracellular concentration of the second messenger (X). This action increases the rate of translocation of glucose transporter to the cell membrane. It is predicted that an increase in the level of prostaglandin E_2 or a decrease in that of adenosine will lead to equal increases in the rates of translocation to *and* from the cell membrane. This would increase the rate of translocation cycling and in an analogous manner to the substrate cycle will increase the sensitivity of the effect of X on the increase in the number of glucose transporters in the membrane.

were insensitive to catecholamines, the rates of cycling would be lower, resulting in decreased rates of thermogenesis together with decreased insulin sensitivity of muscle, which would result in insulin resistance *in vivo*. A similar condition would result from a lower activity of the sympathetic nervous system, which has been reported in some obese subjects,[19] or by pharmacologic blockade of β-adrenoceptor stimuli.[14]

In our view, the previous discussion provides *prima facie* evidence to support the hypothesis of a common mechanism for the control of thermogenesis, in response to specific stimuli, and the control of the sensitivity of glucose utilization in muscle to insulin. Because catecholamines are known to stimulate the rates of substrate cycling, thus increasing the rate of conversion of chemical energy into heat, an elevation in the plasma and tissue catecholamine concentration, either acutely or chronically, increases the rate of thermogenesis. However, chronic elevation in the catecholamine levels increases the sensitivity of glucose utilization by

muscle to insulin. Consequently, lowering the concentration of catecholamines in the plasma or within the muscle results in both decreased thermogenesis and decreased sensitivity to insulin.

References

1. Alpert NR: Am J Physiol 168:565, 1952
2. Alpert NR, Root WS: Am J Physiol 177:455, 1954
3. Arch JRS, Newsholme EA: Essays Biochem 14:82, 1978
4. Bahr R, Hansson P: Acta Physiol Scand (in press)
5. Bahr R, Ignes I, Vaage O et al: J Appl Physiol 62:485, 1987
6. Brooks BJ, Arch JRS, Newsholme EA: Biosci Rep 3:263, 1983
7. Budohoski L, Challiss RAJ, Dubaniewicz A et al: Biochem J 244:655, 1987
8. Burdett HE, Beeler T, Klip A: Arch Biochem Biophys 253:279, 1987
9. Carpentier YA, Asanazi J, Elwyn DH: J Trauma 19:649, 1979
10. Challiss RAJ, Arch JRS, Newsholme EA: Biochem J 231:217, 1985
11. Challiss RAJ, Leighton B, Lozeman FJ et al: In Gerlach E, Becker BF (eds): Topics and Perspectives in Adenosine Research, pp 275–285. New York, Springer-Verlag, 1987
12. Crabtree B, Newsholme EA: Curr Top Cell Regul 25:21, 1985
13. Dann M, Chambers WH: J Biol Chem 89:675, 1930
14. Dulloo AG, Miller DS: Metabolism 34:1061, 1985
15. Herndon DN, Jahoor R, Miyoshi H et al: N Engl J Med 371:403, 1987
16. Hermansen L, Vaage O: Am J Physiol 233:E422, 1977
17. Hill AV, Long CNH, Lupton H: Proc R Soc Lond [Biol] 97:846, 1925
18. Hultman E, Bergstrom J, McLennan-Anderson N: Scand J Clin Lab Invest 19:56, 1987
19. Jung RT, James WPT: Br J Hosp Med December, p 503, 1980
20. Kayne HL, Alpert NR: Am J Physiol 206:51, 1964
21. Karlander S, Roovete A, Vranic M et al: Am J Physiol 251:E530, 1986
22. Karlsson J, Saltin B: Acta Physiol Scand 82:115, 1971
23. Katzeff HL, O'Connell M, Horton ES et al: Metabolism 35:166, 1986
24. Klip A, Ramlal T, Young DA et al: FEBS Lett 224:224, 1987
25. Koshland DE, Goldbeter A, Stock JB: Science, 217:220, 1982

26. Le Beouf B, Flinn RB, Cahill GF: Proc Soc Exp Biol Med 102:527, 1959

27. Maehlum S, Grandmontagne M, Sejersted O et al: Metabolism 35:425, 1986

28. McCulloch AJ, Nosadini R, Pernet A et al: Clin Sci 64:41, 1983

29. Maron MB, Horvath SM, Wilkerson JE: Eur J Appl Physiol 36:231, 1977

30. Mattacks CA, Pond CM: Int J Obes 12:585

31. Monod J, Wyman J, Changen JP: J Mol Biol 12:88, 1965

32. Newsholme EA, Crabtree B: Biochem Soc Symp 41:61, 1976

33. Newsholme EA, Challiss RAJ, Leighton B et al: Nutrition 3:195, 1987

34. Newsholme EA, Leech AR: Biochemistry for the Medical Sciences. New York, John Wiley & Sons, 1983

35. Newsholme EA, Stanley JC: Diabetes Metab Rev 3:295, 1987

36. Nicholls DG, Crompton M: FEBS Lett 111:261, 1980

37. Okajima F, Ui M: Biochem J 182:565, 1979

38. Piiper J, Spiller PJ: J Appl Physiol 28:657, 1970

39. Piiper J, di Prampero PE, Cerretellii P: Am J Physiol 215:523, 1968

40. Ravussin E, Acheson KJ, Vernet O et al: J Clin Invest 76:1268, 1985

41. Shulman GI, Ladenson PW, Wolfe MH et al: J Clin Invest 76:757, 1985

42. Steinberg D: Biochem Soc Symp 24:111, 1963

43. Tagliaferro A, Dobbin S, Newsholme EA: Int J Obes (in press)

44. Wolfe RR, Margaria R, Edwards HT et al: Am J Physiol 106:689, 1933

45. Wolfe RR: Am J Physiol 252:E189, 1987

46. Wolfe RR, Peters EJ: Am J Physiol 252:E218, 1987

47. Zahorska-Markiewicz B: Eur J Appl Physiol 44:231, 1980

CHAPTER 13

Calorie Restriction and Longevity

EDWARD J. MASORO

In 1934, McCay and Crowell[30] reported the results of their seminal studies on the life-extending effects of restricting the food intake of rats. These findings have been confirmed by many laboratories using rats, mice, and hamsters[39] on several dietary regimens varying in composition. Survival curves typical of the effects of food restriction on longevity are presented in Figure 13-1.[42] Because of long life spans, it has not been feasible to carry out similar studies with other mammalian species.[23] In addition to extending the life span, food restriction also retards the age-associated deterioration of many physiologic systems and delays the occurrence or slows the progression (often preventing the clinical expression) of most age-associated disease processes.[22] On the basis of these diverse findings, it has been concluded that food restriction acts on the primary aging processes rather than on specific physiologic processes or the specific pathogenesis of a particular disease.[24]

Berg and Simms[3] proposed that food restriction increases longevity in rodents by reducing body fat content. This hypothesis probably stems from the widely held belief that even mild obesity in humans decreases longevity, a concept currently being debated.[1] Indeed, our initial interest in the food restriction phenomenon was that of determining what role, if any, adipose tissue has in its antiaging actions.

FOOD RESTRICTIONS AND ADIPOSE TISSUE

Bertrand and her associates[5] carried out a longitudinal life span investigation of body fat content of ad libitum fed and food-restricted (60% of the ad libitum intake) male Fischer 344 rats. Food-restricted rats were found to be leaner than ad libitum fed animals (Fig. 13-2). Cross-sectional studies were also carried out by Bertrand and colleagues[5,7] on the epididymal and perirenal fat depots of the ad libitum fed and food-restricted rats. The mass for both depots was greater for the ad libitum fed than for the food-restricted rats (Fig. 13-3); the mass of these depots peaked at 18 months of age in ad libitum fed rats and at 30 months of age in food-restricted rats, findings that are similar to what was observed in the longitudinal study of total fat mass. Mean fat cell volume was studied (Fig. 13-4). Food-restricted rats had smaller fat cells than ad libitum fed rats. Fat cell number was also studied (Fig. 13-5). Ad libitum fed rats had a greater number of fat cells per depot than did food-restricted rats.

The functioning of fat cells changes markedly with increasing age, and food restriction retards these changes. For example, the lipolytic response to glucagon precipitously falls during the first 6 months of life of male Fischer 344 rats (Fig. 13-6), and food restriction (60% of the mean ad libitum food intake) delays and partially prevents the loss of function.[6,27,36] Decreases in lipolytic responsiveness to glucagon with advancing age thus appear to be due to the loss of glucagon receptors.[4] Food restriction also retards the age-associated loss in the lipolytic response of rat adipocytes to epinephrine (Figs. 13-6 and 13-7).[40] These age changes in the response to epinephrine are not due to changes in β-adrenergic receptors, nor does the protective effect of food restriction act by way of these

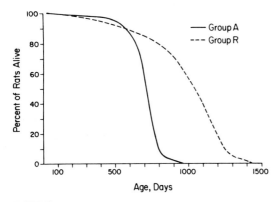

FIGURE 13-1

Survival curves for *ad libitum* fed male Fischer 344 rats (Group A, n = 115) and rats restricted to 60% of the mean *ad libitum* food intake (Group R, n = 115). (Yu BP, Masoro EJ, Murata I et al: Life span study of SPF Fischer 344 male rats fed *ad libitum* or restricted diets. J Gerontol 37:130, 1982)

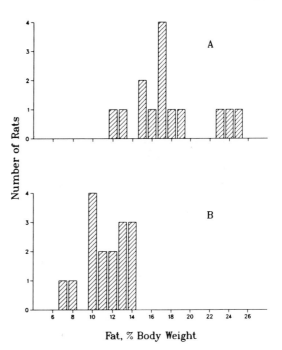

FIGURE 13-2

Body fat content of *ad libitum* fed and food-restricted male Fischer 344 rats. Panel **A** refers to the maximum fat content per unit body mass measured during the life span of *ad libitum* fed rats; Panel **B** refers to the maximum fat content per unit of body mass measured during the life span of rats restricted to 60% of the mean food intake of the *ad libitum* fed rats. (Data from Bertrand HA, Lynd FT, Masoro EJ et al: Changes in adipose mass and cellularity through the adult life of rats fed *ad libitum* or a life-prolonging restricted diet. J Gerontol 35:827, 1980)

receptors, but rather both relate to postreceptor events.[4]

Although age changes occur in adipose tissue function and food restriction retards these changes and also reduces fat mass, it does not appear that the effects of food restriction on adipose tissue have a causal role in its antiaging action. This conclusion is based on the following: First, Bertrand and colleagues[5] found that *ad libitum* fed male Fischer 344 rats had no correlation between body fat content and the length of life, and in the food-restricted rats, there was a significant positive correlation between the length of life and the body fat content. Similarly, Harrison and associates[15] have reported that food-restricted obese (ob/ob) mice are fatter and live longer than the *ad libitum* fed lean litter mates. Therefore, it seems reasonable to conclude that body fat content does not have a major role in the action of food restriction in extending longevity.

OTHER POTENTIAL MECHANISMS BY WHICH FOOD RESTRICTION RETARDS THE AGING PROCESSES

With the conclusion that adipose tissue mechanisms are not likely to play a major part in the antiaging actions of food restriction, our attention has focused on possible mechanisms not directly involving adipose tissue. The reason for our intense study of mechanisms is our belief that such knowledge will yield insights in regard to the nature of the primary aging processes and that it will provide a data base for the development of effective interventions of human aging.

The question arises about whether food restriction influences aging by reducing caloric intake or by restricting a specific dietary component. Evidence indicates calories to be the factor.[23] Restricting protein without restricting calories does increase longevity, but not nearly as markedly as

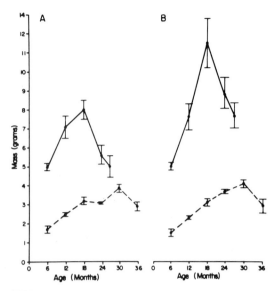

FIGURE 13-3

Changes with age in the mass of the epididymal depots (**A**) and the perirenal depots (**B**). The *solid lines* refer to the *ad libitum* fed rats and the *broken lines* to food-restricted rats. Values are means ± SEM for an n = 10 except for 27-month-old *ad libitum* fed rats, where n = 9. (Bertrand HA, Lynd FT, Masoro EJ et al: Changes in adipose mass and cellularity through the adult life of rats fed *ad libitum* or a life-prolonging restricted diet. J Gerontol 35:827, 1980)

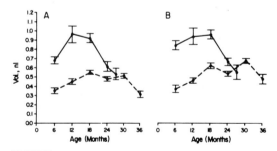

FIGURE 13-4

Changes with age in the mean volume of the adipocytes in the epididymal depot (**A**) and the perirenal depot (**B**). The *solid lines* refer to the *ad libitum* fed rats and the *broken lines* to food-restricted rats. Values are means ± SEM for an n = 10, except for the 27-month-old *ad libitum* fed rats, where n = 9. (Bertrand HA, Lynd FT, Masoro EJ et al: Changes in adipose mass and cellularity through the adult life of rats fed *ad libitum* or a life-prolonging restricted diet. J Gerontol 35:827, 1980)

when calories are restricted as well[41]; moreover, this manipulation appears to act solely by its ability to retard nephropathy and related problems[21] without having the many other antiaging actions of food restriction described earlier. Restricting fat or minerals to the same extent as in the food restriction studies without restricting calories did not influence longevity.[16,17] Our findings also provide indirect evidence that food restriction does not influence aging by specifically restricting carbohydrate or vitamins. Concern has been voiced that food restriction increases longevity by reducing the intake of toxic contaminants. Our findings do not support this view.[23]

McCay and Crowell[30] hypothesized that food restriction retards the aging processes and extends the length of life by decreasing the rate of growth and delaying maturation. This hypothesis was directly tested by Yu and colleagues.[41] The design of that study and the results are summarized in Figure 13-8. Rats in which food restriction was started at 6 months of age (i.e., well after sexual maturation and when almost full skeletal growth has taken place) were similar to rats restricted from 6 weeks of age on (i.e., 2 weeks after weaning) in regard to the age of tenth percentile survivors, the maximum length of life, and the retardation of age changes in physiological processes and age-associated diseases. In contrast, food restriction limited to from 6 weeks to 6 months of age (during rapid growth and development) was much less effective in these respects. These findings, which clearly do not support the hypothesis of McCay and Crowell, have turned attention away from growth and development to the influence of food restriction on postmaturational events.

In 1977, Sacher[34] postulated that food restriction retards the aging processes by decreasing the metabolic rate. This view is based on the long-held belief that the rate of aging is inversely related to the metabolic rate[33] and the evidence that the metabolic rate per unit of body mass decreases when food intake is reduced.[2] McCarter and associates[28] directly measured the metabolic rate of rats on life-prolonging food restriction regimens under the usual living conditions and found that food restriction did not decrease the metabolic rate per unit of lean body mass or per unit of "metabolic mass" over most of the life

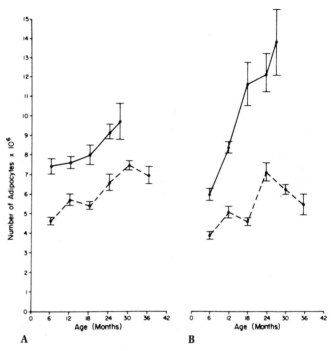

A   B

FIGURE 13-5

Changes with age in the number of adipocytes in the epididymal depot (**A**) and perirenal depot (**B**) the *solid lines* refer to the *ad libitum* fed rats and the *broken lines* to the food-restricted rats. Values are means ± SEM for n = 10, except for the 27-month-old *ad libitum* fed rats where n = 9. (Bertrand HA, Lynd FT, Masoro EJ et al: Changes in adipose mass and cellularity through the adult life of rats fed *ad libitum* or a life-prolonging restricted diet. J Gerontol 35:827, 1980)

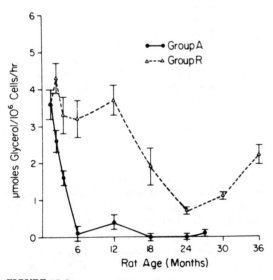

FIGURE 13-6

Glucagon-promoted lipolysis in adipocytes from *ad libitum* fed (Group A) and food-restricted (Group R) male Fischer 344 rats. Data are expressed as μmoles of glycerol released in the presence of 1 ng/ml glucagon per 10^6 cells per hour above the basal rate of glycerol release. Each point is a mean for nine or more rats. (Apfelbaum M: Adaptation to changes in caloric intake. Proc Nutr Soc 2:543, 1978)

span. The apparent discrepancy between this finding and the commonly held view was addressed by McCarter and McGee,[29] who found that metabolic rate did fall immediately after the initiation of food restriction but it returned to that of *ad libitum* fed rats within a few weeks. Since Yu and colleagues[41] showed that it is long-term food restriction that retards the aging processes, the currently available data do not support the metabolic rate hypothesis of Sacher (Figure 13-9).

Moreover, during our exploration of the metabolic rate hypothesis, it was discovered that for most of the life span, the intake of calories and other nutrients per unit of lean body mass was not reduced in the food-restricted rats.[26] Rather, on initiation of food restriction there is a rapid readjustment of lean body mass so that the intake of calories per unit of lean body mass is soon the same as in *ad libitum* fed rats. The question that must be addressed is how the decreased intake in calories per rat but not per unit of lean body mass is linked to the aging processes. Our working hypothesis, diagrammed in Figure 13-10,[24] is that food intake per rat is coupled to the aging processes by means of the endocrine or neural regulatory systems.

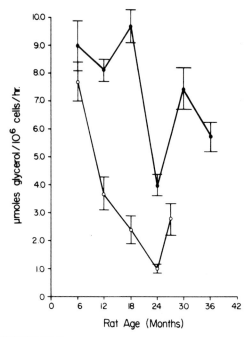

FIGURE 13-7

Effects of age and food restriction on the lipolytic response of rat fat cells to 10^{-3} M epinephrine. *Open circles* refer to *ad libitum* fed rats and *filled circles* to rats restricted to 60% of the food intake of *ad libitum* fed rats. Data are expressed as μmoles of glycerol released in response to epinephrine per 10^6 cells above that of the basal rate. Each point is a mean from seven or more rats. (Yu BP, Bertrand HA, Masoro EJ: Nutrition-aging influences on catecholamine-promoted lipolysis. Metabolism 29:438, 1980)

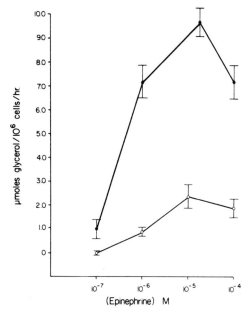

FIGURE 13-8

Dose-response curve for the lipolytic response to epinephrine of fat cells from 18-month-old *ad libitum* fed and food-restricted rats. *Open circles* refer to *ad libitum* fed rats and *filled circles* to rats restricted to 60% of the food intake of the *ad libitum* fed rats. Data are expressed as μmoles of glycerol released in response to epinephrine per 10^6 cells above that of the basal rate. Each point is a mean for 10 rats. (Yu BP, Bertrand HA, Masoro EJ: Nutrition-aging influences on catecholamine-promoted lipolysis. Metabolism 29:438, 1980)

Of the many afferent pathways (arrow 1 in Fig. 13-10) and neural or endocrine systems (box 2 in Fig. 13-10) that could be involved, is there a guide to which would be the most profitable to study? Our guide has been the following: the evidence that a particular endocrine or neural system is involved in aging and the likelihood that a particular system is influenced by food restriction.

On the basis of these criteria, the glucocorticoid system was chosen for study. Sapolsky and colleagues[35] proposed the glucocorticoid cascade theory of aging based on evidence that with age there is a loss of the regulatory control of glucocorticoid secretion in rats. They envision that the resulting hyperadrenocorticism causes further deterioration of the glucocorticoid regulatory system and promotes the aging processes in tissues throughout the body. In addition, Dallman[13] has summarized the large body of evidence showing a strong interaction between food intake and plasma glucocorticoid levels. Although unpublished data obtained in our laboratory are in accord with Dallman's view, our findings indicate that food restriction does not retard aging processes by preventing hyperadrenocorticism.

The insulin-glucose system has also become a focus of our research because of the concept of Cerami[9] that glucose may be a mediator of aging. Moreover, it is likely that food restriction influ-

			Length of Life, Days		
			Median	10th Percentile	Maximum
GROUP 1					
NNNNAAAAAAAAAAAAAAAAAAAAAAAAAAAAAAAAAAAAA			701	822	941
GROUP 2					
NNNNAARRRRRRRRRRRRRRRRRRRRRRRRRRRRRRRRRRR			1057	1226	1296
GROUP 3					
NNNNAARRRRRRRRRRRRRRRRRRRRAAAAAAAAAAAAAAA			808	918	1040
GROUP 4					
NNNNAAAAAAAAAAAAAAAAAAAAAAARRRRRRRRRRRRRR			941	1177	1299

1 month of age
1¼ months of age
6 months of age

N, Nursing
A, Ad libitum Fed
R, FFood Restricted

FIGURE 13-9

The effect of food restriction of various durations and times of initiation on longevity. (Data from Yu BP, Masoro EJ, McMahan CA: Nutritional influences on aging of Fischer 344 rats. I. Physical, metabolic and longevity characteristics. J Gerontol 40:657, 1985)

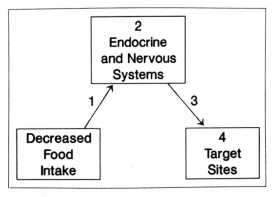

FIGURE 13-10

Schematic presentation of working hypothesis for the coupling of food restriction to the aging processes. (Masoro EJ: Retardation of the aging processes by food restriction: A search for mechanisms. ISI Atlas Sci Biochem 1:329, 1988)

ences glucose metabolism. Cerami proposed what might be called the glycation theory of aging. This theory is based on the fact that glucose reacts nonenzymatically with the amino groups of proteins to form Schiff bases, which rearrange to yield Amadori products. Because the Schiff bases and Amadori products are in equilibrium with each other as well as with glucose, the extent of their formation is directly influenced by the sustained plasma glucose concentration and the time of exposure to that concentration. Moreover, the Amadori products slowly and irreversibly form what Cerami calls "advanced glycation end-products," which cause cross-linking as well as other reactions within and between protein macromolecules. Such alterations change the functional characteristics of proteins such as their enzymatic activity, the binding of regulatory molecules, as well as the physical properties of the tissues in which they reside (e.g., compliance characteristics). Cerami views the alterations caused by glycation as fundamental aspects of aging. Data in one re-

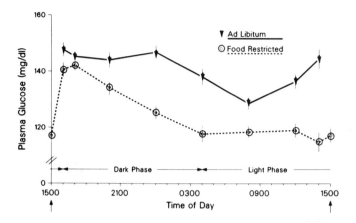

FIGURE 13-11

Diurnal pattern of plasma glucose concentrations in *ad libitum* fed and food-restricted rats in the age range of 4 to 6 months. (Masoro EJ, Katz MS, McMahan CA: Evidence for the glycation hypothesis of aging from the food-restricted rodent model. J Gerontol Biol Sci 44:B20, 1989)

port[25] from our laboratory clearly show that food-restricted rats have sustained plasma glucose concentrations below those of *ad libitum* fed rats (Fig. 13-11). Our findings also show the level of Amadori products in the hemoglobin to be less for food-restricted than for *ad libitum* fed rats. Further work is needed to determine if this difference in plasma glucose level will result in a difference in the extent to which advanced glycosylation end products accumulate and whether these effects have a causal role in the aging processes.

Research carried out in our laboratories and others has focused on the influence of food restriction on biochemical processes in target tissue (box 4 in Fig. 13-10). One aspect of this research is the influence of food restriction on free radical reactions and damage, events that have been proposed as being causally involved in the aging processes.[14] Cellular lipid peroxidation has been found to be decreased by food restriction.[12,19,20] Koizumi and colleagues[19] believe that this lipid peroxidation is caused by free radicals and that food restriction retards the occurrence of the lipid peroxidation by increasing catalase activity. Laganiere and Yu[20] suggest that in addition to its effects on catalase activity, food restriction decreases lipid peroxidation by maintaining a fatty acid composition of cellular membranes that is less susceptible to free radical-promoted peroxidation.

Another aspect of target tissue function under study is the influence of food restriction on protein turnover and gene expression. Cheung and

Richardson[11] hypothesized that a high level of protein turnover is needed for appropriate cellular function and that aging involves a reduction in the rate of protein turnover. Recent evidence indicates that food restriction maintains protein turnover at higher levels than in *ad libitum* fed rodents of the same age during most of the life span.[8,32,37,38] Moreover, food restriction maintains gene expression at youthful levels by retarding both age-associated decreases and increases in gene expression.[10,18,31]

CONCLUSIONS

Although caloric restriction influences fat mass, fat depot cellularity, and adipocyte function, its antiaging actions do not seem to be causally related to these effects on adipose tissue. Currently available evidence indicates that the neural and endocrine systems are involved in the coupling of caloric restriction to the aging processes. Findings indicate that influencing glycation reactions may at least in part be a mode by which caloric restriction retards the aging processes. Other provocative findings suggest that caloric restriction protects against free radical damage and retards age changes in gene expression; both of these actions may play an important role in the antiaging effects.

References

1. Andres R: Influence of obesity on longevity in the aged. In Borek C, Fenoglia CM, King DW (eds):

Aging, Cancer and Cell Membranes. Stuttgart, Thieme, 1980

2. Apfelbaum M: Adaptation to changes in caloric intake. Proc Nutr Sci 2:543, 1978

3. Berg BN, Simms HS: Nutrition and longevity in the rat. II. Longevity and onset of disease with different levels of intake. J Nutr 71:255, 1960

4. Bertrand HA, Anderson WR, Masoro EJ et al: Action of food restriction on age-changes in adipocyte lipolysis. J Gerontol 42:666, 1987

5. Bertrand HA, Lynd FT, Masoro EJ et al: Changes in adipose mass and cellularity through the adult life of rats fed ad libitum or a life-prolonging restricted diet. J Gerontol 35:827, 1980

6. Bertrand HA, Masoro EJ, Yu BP: Maintenance of glucagon-promoted lipolysis in adipocytes by food restriction. Endocrinology 107:591, 1980

7. Bertrand HA, Stacy C, Masoro EJ et al: Plasticity of fat cell number. J Nutr 114:129, 1984

8. Birchenall-Sparks M, Roberts MS, Staecker J et al: Effect of dietary restriction on liver protein synthesis in rats. J Nutr 115:944, 1985

9. Cerami A: Hypothesis: Glucose as a mediator of aging. J Am Geriatr Soc 33:626, 1985

10. Chatterjee B, Fernandes G, Yu BP et al: Calorie restriction delays age-dependent loss in androgen responsiveness of the rat liver. FASEB J 3:169, 1989

11. Cheung HT, Richardson A: The relationship between age-related changes in gene expression, protein turnover and the responsiveness of an organism to stimuli. Life Sci 31:605, 1982

12. Chipalkatti S, De AK, Aiyar AN: Effect of diet restriction on some biochemical parameters related to aging in mice. J Nutr 113:944, 1983

13. Dallman M: Viewing the ventromedial hypothalamus from the adrenal gland. Am J Physiol 246:R1, 1984

14. Harman D: The aging processes. Proc Natl Acad Sci USA 78:124, 1981

15. Harrison DE, Archer JR, Astole CM: Effects of food restriction on aging: Separation of food intake and adiposity. Proc Natl Acad Sci USA 81:1835, 1984

16. Iwasaki K, Gleiser CA, Masoro EJ et al: The influence of dietary protein source on longevity and age-related disease processes of Fischer rats. J Gerontol Biol Sci 43:B5, 1988

17. Iwasaki K, Gleiser CA, Masoro EJ et al: Influence of the restriction of individual dietary components on longevity and age-related disease of Fischer rats: The fat component and the mineral component. J Gerontol Biol Sci 43:B13, 1988

18. Kalu DN, Herbert DC, Hardin RR et al: Mechanisms of dietary modulation of calcitonin levels in Fischer 344 rats. J Gerontol Biol Sci 43:B121, 1988

19. Koizumi A, Weindruch R, Walford RL: Influences of dietary restriction and age on liver enzyme activities and lipid peroxidation in mice. J Nutr 117:361, 1987

20. Laganiere S, Yu BP: Anti-lipoperoxidation action of food restriction. Biochem Biophys Res Commun 145:1185, 1987

21. Maeda H, Gleiser CA, Masoro EJ et al: Nutritional influences on aging of Fischer 344 rats. II. Pathology. J Gerontol 40:671, 1985

22. Masoro EJ: Nutrition and aging: A current assessment. J Nutr 115:842, 1985

23. Masoro EJ: Food restriction in rodents: An evaluation of its role in the study of aging. J Gerontol Biol Sci 43:B59, 1988

24. Masoro EJ: Retardation of the aging processes by food restriction: A search for mechanisms. ISI Atlas Sci Biochem 1:329, 1988

25. Masoro EJ, Katz MS, McMahan CA: Evidence for the glycation hypothesis of aging from the food-restricted rodent model. J Gerontol Biol Sci 44:B20, 1989

26. Masoro EJ, Yu BP, Bertrand HA: Action of food restriction in delaying the aging processes. Proc Natl Acad Sci USA 79:4239, 1982

27. Masoro EJ, Yu BP, Bertrand HA et al: Nutritional probe of the aging process. Fed Proc 39:3178, 1980

28. McCarter R, Masoro EJ, Yu BP: Does food restriction retard aging by reducing the metabolic rate? Am J Physiol 248:E488, 1985

29. McCarter R, McGee J: Food restriction and metabolic rate: Different adaptive time course of BMR and 24-hour metabolic rate. FASEB J 2:A1208, 1988

30. McCay CM, Crowell MF: Prolonging the life span. Sci Monthly 39:405, 1934

31. Richardson A, Butler JA, Rutherford M et al: Effect of age and dietary restriction on the expression of $\alpha_2\mu$-globulin. J Biol Chem 262:12821, 1987

32. Ricketts WG, Birchenall-Sparks M, Hardwick JI et al: Effect of age and dietary restriction on protein synthesis by isolated kidney cells. J Cell Physiol 125:492, 1985

33. Rubner: Das Problem der Lebensdauer und seine Beziehungen zum Wachstum und Ernäbrung. Munich, Oldenbourg, 1908

34. Sacher GA: Life table modifications and life prolongation. In Finch C, Hayflick L (eds): The Biology of Aging. New York, Nostrand Reinhold, 1977

35. Sapolsky RM, Krey LC, McEwen BS: The neuroendocrinology of stress and aging: The glucocorticoid cascade hypothesis. Endocrinol Rev 7:284, 1986

36. Voss KH, Masoro EJ, Andersen W: Modulation of age-related loss of glucagon-promoted lipolysis by food restriction. Mech Ageing Dev 18:135, 1982

37. Ward WF: Enhancement by food restriction of liver

protein synthesis in the aging Fischer 344 rat. J Gerontol Biol Sci. 43:B50, 1988

38. Ward WF: Food restriction enhances the proteolytic capacity of aging rat liver. J Gerontol Biol Sci 43:B121, 1988

39. Weindruch R: Aging in rodents fed restricted diets. J Am Geriatr Soc 33:125, 1985

40. Yu BP, Bertrand HA, Masoro EJ: Nutrition-aging influences on catecholamine-promoted lipolysis. Metabolism 29:438, 1980

41. Yu BP, Masoro EJ, McMahan CA: Nutritional influences on aging of Fischer 344 rats. I. Physical, metabolic and longevity characteristics. J Gerontol 40:657, 1985

42. Yu BP, Masoro EJ, Murata I et al: Life span study of SPF Fischer 344 male rats fed *ad libitum* or restricted diets. J Gerontol 37:130, 1982

Electrophysiological and Neurochemical Approach to a Hierarchical Feeding Organization

LUIS HERNANDEZ, EURO MURZI, DAVID H. SCHWARTZ, and BARTLEY G. HOEBEL

To understand feeding behavior it is important to elucidate the neuronal circuitry that underlies it. Tracking this neuronal net requires identification of the cell groups in the circuit and the chemicals that they use to communicate. As with any other complex function, the neurons involved in feeding regulation are organized in clusters that are distributed in the central nervous system (CNS). This chapter discusses experiments in which stimulation of the lateral hypothalamus (LH) had both electrophysiologic effects on hindbrain taste cells and neurochemical effects in forebrain reward sites. All three levels interact in processing the reinforcing aspects of eating.

Neuronal groups that are located in the brainstem can integrate sensory inputs with feeding motor acts. The existence of such neuronal groups was first inferred from experiments with decerebrate animals. When the brainstem was cut at the collicular level in rats or cats, masticatory, salivary, and swallowing reflexes that were still present allowed them to eat when food was placed in their mouths.[6,76,102,120] A decerebrated rat can even regulate its food intake according to the degree of food deprivation.[27] However, a decerebrated animal is unable to search for food. If food is placed in front of the animal but not directly into its mouth, it is unable to eat. Searching and reaching for food require the integrity of neurons located above the colliculi.

Electrical stimulation of the LH region triggers locomotor activity, searching for food, reaching, and eating behavior in cats,[13,45] goats,[63] and rats,[48,56,73,77] and electrical stimulation of the ventromedial hypothalamus (VMH) inhibits feeding behavior in goats.[122] The exact location of the cell bodies of neurons underlying these effects has not been established. The early studies of lesions of the hypothalamus showed that lesions of the LH cause aphagia, adipsia, and body weight loss.[2] Animals with such lesions actively reject food placed in their mouths, although they eventually recover spontaneous feeding.[108,109] Lesions of the medial hypothalamus (MH) enhance feeding and cause adiposity.[46] These early experiments were the basis of the dual center theory proposed by Stellar.[105] According to this theory, feeding behavior is controlled by an LH feeding center and an MH satiety center. Electrophysiologic studies suggested a reciprocal relationship between the firing rate of some LH and VMH neurons.[3,32,34,85] The original Stellar proposal contained interactive pathways between the hypothalamus and the rest of the brain based on a hierarchical organization of the feeding neurons in the Jacksonian sense.[60] According to this view, the hypothalamus modulates the brainstem feeding centers by either magnifying or diminishing their activity, and the hypothalamus itself is under the control of higher centers.[84,95]

In the early 1970s, it was shown that dopa-

mine, norepinephrine, epinephrine, and serotonin cell bodies are located in the midbrain and
hindbrain. Their axons project up and down the
neuraxis, sending branches to many parts of
the CNS. Some of them project to the hypothalamus. Others project through the hypothalamus
to higher forebrain regions.[57,70,111] Depletion of
some of these pathways produced weight gain.
Lesions of the ventral noradrenergic bundle
caused hyperphagia and obesity.[36,49,50,67] Various techniques were used to disrupt the ascending serotonergic system, such as synthesis
inhibition,[10] electrolytic lesions, neurotoxic
lesions,[18,98,115] and pharmacologic activation of
inhibitory autoreceptors on the serotonin cell
bodies.[23] The consensus today is that disruption
of part of the serotonin system leads to obesity.[52,82] Depletion of other pathways can cause
weight loss. Neurotoxins used to kill dopamine inputs to the basal ganglia caused anorexia
or aphagia with akinesia and sensory neglect.[74,106,112]

Depletion of the noradrenergic input to the
paraventricular nucleus (PVN) causes modest
weight loss without the severe sensory or motor
deficits.[66] Microinjection of monoamines in various monoamine cell body and terminal areas can
affect feeding behavior. Depending on the injection site, the environment, and the state of the
animal, the same monoamine may either increase or decrease feeding. For example, when
injected into the LH, norepinephrine usually inhibits feeding,[66] although early studies reported
other effects with higher doses.[8,28,71,72,78] When
injected in the PVN, norepinephrine increases
feeding, particularly carbohydrate intake.[65] Dopamine decreases feeding when injected in the
LH.[64,86] In the prefrontal cortex, some components of feeding behavior, such as swallowing
reflexes, are affected by microinjections of dopamine.[4] Serotonin in the LH decreases some undetermined aspect of feeding,[86] although lower
doses are effective in the medial region and PVN,
suggesting these are more sensitive sites. At these
medial sites, serotonin blocks carbohydrate intake in the early dark period and blocks the feeding induced by norepinephrine.[68] The amygdala
is also intimately involved in feeding.[26,29,94,121]
Recording studies implicate the frontal cortex
and show cortical pathways to and from the hy-

pothalamus.[84] These experiments suggest that in
addition to the hindbrain, midbrain, and hypothalamus, much of the limbic system including
the prefrontal "limbic" cortex will eventually
have to be incorporated into our conception of
feeding circuitry.

In order to understand the neural basis of feeding, a temporal correspondence between feeding
behavior, neuronal activity, and neurotransmitter function has to be shown at the various levels
of organization and in the long pathways that
interconnect and modulate them. Then these cell
assemblies and pathways can be reliably placed
in a model of the feeding circuit.

In the past few years, we have used classic
electrophysiologic techniques and novel neurochemical techniques to explore this feeding circuit. A coherent picture is gradually emerging.[51]
Here we describe first the electrophysiologic followed by the neurochemical results.

ELECTROPHYSIOLOGIC STUDIES

As we mentioned before, both Stellar's model
and Jacksonian hierarchical organization predict
that the hypothalamus should be able to modulate the lower feeding centers of the brainstem.
We tested this prediction by using stimulation of
hypothalamic placements that elicited feeding to
drive gustatory neurons in the medullary taste
area, predominantly in the nucleus tractus solitarius (NTS) (Fig. 14-1).

Electrical stimulation was done with perma-
nently implanted bundles of small electrodes
in the perifornical region of the LH of 76 rats.
This region was chosen because electrical stimulation elicits feeding that resembles natural eating.[35,40,48] Electrical stimulation of each electrode
yielded different behaviors, but we focused our
study on feeding behavior. Screening these rats
gave us two groups of electrodes: those that elicited feeding and those that did not. Rats in both
groups were anesthetized, and with a glass-
insulated tungsten microelectrode, gustatory
unit activity was recorded in the medullary and
the pontine taste area. Gustatory neurons were
identified by sparging solutions of the basic tast-
ants on the tongue of the rat while recording the
electrophysiologic response in the NTS, which
is the first taste relay. About 22% of gustatory

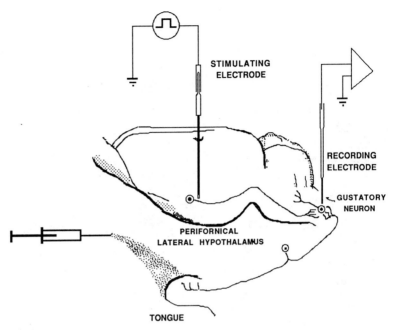

FIGURE 14-1

Schematic representation of an experiment in which a tastant dissolved in water was sparged on the tongue to localize gustatory neurons in the NTS. Electrical stimulation on the perifornical LH, which induced feeding when the rat was awake, drove gustatory neurons in the NTS and nucleus reticularis parvocellularis when the rat was anesthetized (see Fig. 14-2).

neurons responded to electrical stimulation of the perifornical LH. They responded predominantly to electrodes that had elicited feeding when the animal was awake (Fig. 14-2).

When we explored the gustatory neurons located in the parabrachial nucleus (PBN), which is the second taste relay, no effect was observed on firing rate during stimulation of the hypothalamus. This unexpected finding suggests that the PBN neurons did not receive direct inputs from the LH stimulation site, nor indirect inputs from stimulated NTS neurons. It is possible that the stimulated NTS neurons were involved in salivation or other local sensorimotor reflex circuits that did not involve the recorded PBN neurons.

A descending pathway has been discovered from the LH to the NTS and to the nucleus reticularis parvocellularis, which controls salivation.[17,58,99,107,114] Therefore, anatomical evidence supports the electrophysiologic finding that elec-

trical stimulation of the perifornical LH could modulate the afferent or the efferent portion of the feeding centers in medulla.

MICRODIALYSIS STUDIES

Electrical stimulation of the perifornical LH can trigger searching and hoarding as well as eating and self-stimulation behavior. Evidence strongly links the dopamine systems to locomotor activity,[61,88,91] self-stimulation reward,[11,19,25,51,119] and feeding behavior.[14,24,31,64,119] For this reason, we have explored some of the terminal fields of the dopaminergic systems with brain microdialysis.

In this technique, a double, concentric cannula with a porous cellulose tip for dialysis is inserted in the brain, and Ringer's solution flowing inside the cannula brings out extracellular brain chemicals as they diffuse in through the dialysis membrane[21,43,44,113,118] (Fig. 14-3). Femtomole amounts

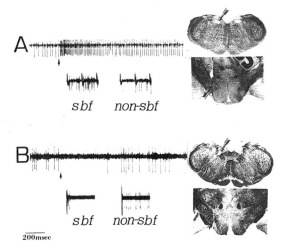

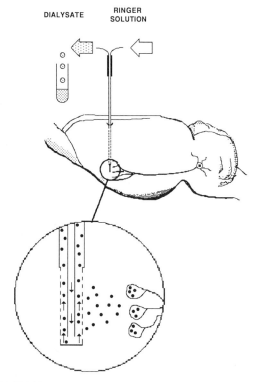

FIGURE 14-2

Excitatory (**A**) and inhibitory (**B**) responses of two NTS gustatory neurons: **A**: Upper record shows the excitatory response evoked by 0.03-M sucrose applied to the tongue at the time shown by the *arrow*. Lower records show superimposed traces of the stimulus artifact and spike discharges of the same cell during electrical stimulation of the LH through a stimulation-bound feeding electrode (sbf) and a non–stimulation-bound feeding electrode (non-sbf). Note that the sbf electrode had an effect similar to sucrose. **B**: Upper record shows the inhibitory response of a different NTS cell evoked by 0.03-M sucrose applied to the tongue. Lower record shows responses elicited by sbf and non-sbf electrodes. Again, the sbf electrodes mimicked the sucrose. The histologic sections at the right show the location (indicated by *arrows*) of the medullary recording sites and the perifornical LH stimulation sites.[81]

FIGURE 14-3

Schematic representation of brain microdialysis. A microdialysis probe is placed in a neuronal terminal field. The circle shows the tip of the probe and three synaptic terminals. The neurotransmitter released by the terminals diffuses into the microdialysis tip and is carried out to a collecting vial by the flow of Ringer's solution. The dialysate is injected into a high-pressure liquid chromatograph with electrochemical detection.

of monoamine neurotransmitters and their metabolites can be collected and identified by high-performance liquid chromatography with electrochemical detection. Microdialysis does not directly measure neuronal activity as electrophysiologic recording does, but it can show extracellular signals produced by a population of neurons. It is assumed that any chemical communication between cells will be expressed as a change in chemical concentration in the synapses and that many of these chemicals will reach the extracellular space near the microdialysis probe by diffusion.

First we used microdialysis to explore the neurochemical activity of dopamine terminals in the nucleus accumbens and in the striatum during feeding induced by electrical stimulation of the perifornical LH.[37,38,42] This is the same type of electrical stimulation that influenced cells in the NTS and mimicked good tastes, and it is the same stimulation that animals work to obtain in our self-stimulation experiment relating self-stimulation to eating.[40,47,51] Electrical stimulation with food available increased dopamine and its metabolites dihydroxyphenylacetic (DOPAC) and homovanillic acid (HVA) in the nucleus

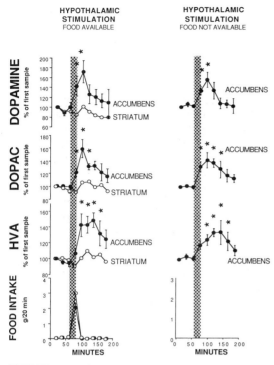

FIGURE 14-4

Left column shows the increase of extracellular dopamine, DOPAC, and HVA in the nucleus accumbens but not in the striatum during electrical stimulation of the perifornical LH with food available (*shaded area*). The right column shows stimulated release in the nucleus accumbens with no food available. The concentration of the chemicals is expressed as percent of the first sample. Samples were taken at 20-minute intervals.[38]

accumbens. The effect showed some anatomical specificity, because experimenter-delivered stimulation increased dopamine release and metabolism in the accumbens but an increase was not detectable in the striatum. The nucleus accumbens effect of experimenter-delivered stimulation occurred even without food available to eat.[38] This demonstrates stimulated release in the absence of operant requirements or eating (Fig. 14-4). In this respect, perifornical LH stimulation mimics eating, as suggested earlier on the basis of self-stimulation studies.[47,56] This experiment also suggests that the feeding area of the perifornical hypothalamus interacts with the dopamine

cells of the mesolimbic system, which project to the accumbens. It has been shown that dopamine in the accumbens can stimulate the second messenger, cyclic-adenosine monophosphate[52] and generate neural activity in postsynaptic cells there.[103] Animals presumably find this to be rewarding because they self-administer dopamine in the same region.[30]

Next, we explored the dopaminergic effect of natural feeding. Rats were food deprived until they reached 80% of their original body weight. Microdialysis probes were inserted into the nucleus accumbens, and dopamine release was measured before, during, and after eating. A significant increase in dopamine, DOPAC, and HVA was observed after the initiation of the meal (Fig. 14-5). Note that extracellular dopamine remained elevated for some time after eating stopped.

With a less drastic food deprivation schedule, rats at a normal body weight and after 20 hours of deprivation were trained to press a bar for food when a signal light was turned on. This time we explored three dopamine terminal regions: the nucleus accumbens, the striatum, and the prefrontal cortex.[39] An increase in extracellular dopamine and its metabolites was observed in the nucleus accumbens and the prefrontal cortex, but there was no measurable change in the striatum even during bar pressing for food (Fig. 14-6). Similar microdialysis or *in vivo* voltammetry findings in the accumbens have been reported by others.[20,90] As a control, turning the light on during an extinction schedule or simply leaving the animal in the experimental cage with the feeder disconnected did not increase dopamine release detectably in the nucleus accumbens (Fig. 14-7).

When the dopamine levels of the rats deprived to 80% body weight were compared with the dopamine levels of 20-hour deprived rats at a normal weight, we discovered that the underweight rats had less extracellular dopamine, DOPAC, and HVA than the control group. This finding was confirmed using rats as their own controls.[52,89] Food deprivation apparently lowers basal dopamine levels in the accumbens. Interestingly, a similar phenomenon has been observed for peripheral catecholamines. Fasting and weight loss decrease norepinephrine blood

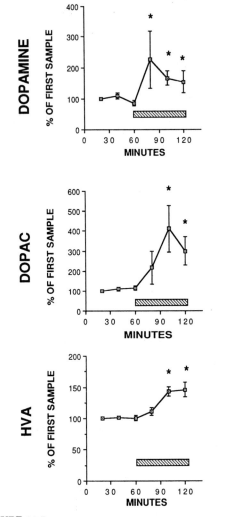

FIGURE 14-5

Increase of extracellular dopamine, DOPAC, and HVA in the nucleus accumbens during feeding (*horizontal hatched bar*) in chronically food-deprived rats. The concentration of the chemicals is expressed as percent of the first sample.[37]

levels and lower blood pressure.[9] The physiological significance of the accumbens dopamine depression by food deprivation is not known.

The problem now is to determine the role of the mesolimbic and mesocortical systems in feeding behavior. The mesolimbic system has been associated with arousal, stress, general lo-

comotion, reflex facilitation, appetitive behavior, and reward. Lesion and injection studies suggest that dopamine terminals in the nucleus accumbens can be capable of initiating central locomotor programs, facilitating swallowing reflexes,[4,116] and supporting different kinds of reinforced behaviors such as self-stimulation, conditioned place preference, drug self-administration,[30,55,119] and ingestive behaviors.[51,54] *In vivo* microdialysis and voltammetry show that dopamine is released not only during eating,[20,37-39,90] but also during cocaine self-administration,[87,117] drinking by water-deprived rats,[7,97] salt consumption by sodium-deficient rats,[15] self-stimulation of the hypothalamus,[59] self-stimulation of the ventral tegmental area,[25] and by intra-accumbens applications of drugs of abuse.[33,37,41,42] Dopamine in the prefrontal cortex is necessary for the successful learning, retention, and emission of delayed-alternation responses in rats and monkeys.[12,104] Therefore, activation of the mesocortical and mesolimbic system during bar pressing for food might be related to any or all of the higher CNS processes involved in foraging components of feeding behavior such as searching, choice behavior, and positive reinforcement.

Microdialysis can also be used to study serotonin function. We measured serotonin changes in both the MH and perifornical LH because feeding suppression effects have been associated with serotonin microinjections in the medial hypothalamus,[68,69] because serotonin is the most abundant monoamine in the lateral hypothalamus,[86,96] and because serotonergic drugs decrease food intake and self-stimulation.[53,82]

Food-deprived rats were trained to eat a mash of sweetened condensed milk and powdered Purina chow pellets. During 30 minutes, the animals could see and smell the food, then they were allowed to eat it. The extracellular concentration of serotonin increased detectably at both times. For some animals with low basal levels of serotonin, it was necessary to add fluoxetine to the perfusate in the microdialysis probe to boost basal levels by blocking serotonin reuptake into the nerve terminals (Fig. 14-8). This finding suggests that smelling food and eating food release serotonin in both the MH and LH.[100,101] Leibowitz and her colleagues have shown that a function

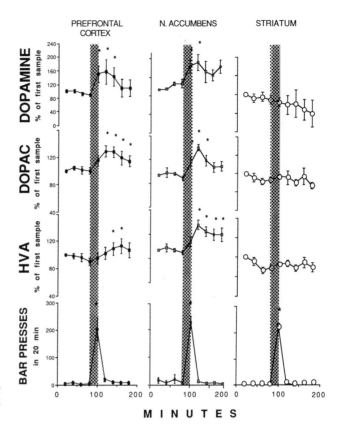

FIGURE 14-6

Increase of extracellular dopamine, DOPAC, and HVA in the prefrontal cortex and nucleus accumbens but not in the striatum during the emission of operant behavior for food (*shaded area*). The concentration of the chemicals is expressed as percent of the first sample (* = P < 0.001).[39]

of serotonin in the medial nuclei of the hypothalamus is to suppress carbohydrate intake in the first meal when rats awaken and become active.[69] The function of serotonin in the LH regions is not clear, but indirect evidence points to a role in suppressing a feeding reward system.[52,54,75]

In summary, the experiments reported here show that certain monoamines are released in the hypothalamus, the nucleus accumbens, and the prefrontal cortex during feeding. The hypothalamus seems to have a pivotal role. Stimulation of the perifornical LH activates the NTS and the nucleus accumbens, thus mimicking and inducing ingestive behavior. We noted that during feeding, dopamine was released in both the nucleus accumbens and the prefrontal cortex. Others have reported that the prefrontal cortex is connected with the nucleus accumbens, the hypothalamus, the NTS, the masticatory nucleus of the trigeminal nerve, and the medullary center

for swallowing.[5,58,62,79,83,92,110,114,116] This finding suggests that dopamine could modulate the various functions of both the accumbens and prefrontal cortex and thus serve as an overarching controller. To the extent that feeding is organized in a neural hierarchy, dopamine could modulate the whole hierarchy by its actions on the highest, most recently evolved regions, which in turn control the lower regions.

The brainstem feeding centers should represent the most fundamental and elementary organization level for feeding. These feeding centers contain the basic patterns of neural activity underlying consummatory behavior. For instance, swallowing is a sequence of an orderly contraction and relaxation of at least ten different muscles triggered by pharyngeal stimulation.[22] Apparently, once the sequence is triggered, no external feedback is required to keep the sequence going. Arousal level as well as different

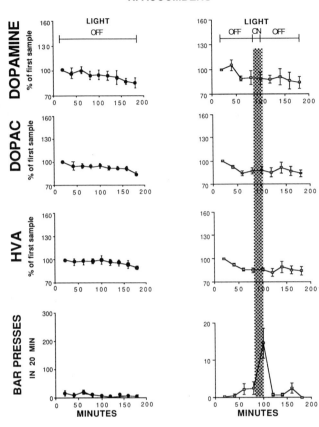

FIGURE 14-7

Control studies. Left graphs show no detectable changes in extracellular dopamine, DOPAC, and HVA in the nucleus accumbens when food was unavailable during the time the animals normally responded for food on prior days. Right graphs show no detectable changes during the extinction of the operant responding with the signal light turned on but with the feeder turned off.[38]

kinds of pharyngeal stimulation just modify the duration and the strength of deglutition.

Within the diencephalon, the hypothalamus triggers feeding action patterns that are more complex than the ones triggered by the brainstem. The motor acts triggered by hypothalamic stimulation are under external feedback control. For example, in an unpublished experiment, electrical stimulation of the perifornical hypothalamus triggered the searching and consummatory sequence characteristic of feeding; however, if animals found a piece of rubber instead of a food pellet, they held it in their forepaws and chewed it without any attempt to swallow it. This behavior continued for as long as the rat received electrical stimulation. This observation suggests that the next step in a central program for feeding (i.e., swallowing) could not proceed because the required sensory cue, pharyngeal stimulation by a wet and soft bolus, was absent.

The most complex level of feeding organization includes circuits that connect the cortex and the basal ganglia.[51] This level might be involved in cognitive aspects of feeding that are essential to foraging for food, including complex learning and memory functions.[16,84,93,94] Dopamine in the nucleus accumbens is positioned to play a prominent role in modulating the limbic inputs from the cortex, amygdala, and hippocampus,[80] which reinforce locomotion and operant behavior. Although the details of the wiring diagram are not well known yet, the emerging picture suggests a hierarchical organization of feeding systems with modulation by the monoamine systems.

This old idea is strengthened by new results showing that the lateral hypothalamus sends a descending signal that affects the NTS taste response; that during feeding, norepinephrine and serotonin are released in hypothalamic sites where these monoamines modulate feeding; and

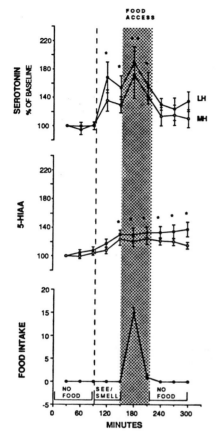

FIGURE 14-8

Increase of extracellular serotonin in the perifornical LH and MH during the sight and smell of food and subsequent eating of the food in mildly deprived rats.[100,101]

that dopamine is released in the highest levels of the hierarchy, where it modulates ongoing functions of those areas, including feeding functions.

Acknowledgment: This research was supported by USPHS grant DA03597, Campbell Soup Company and Servier Amerique.

References

1. Ahlskog JE, Hoebel BG: Overeating and obesity from damage to a noradrenergic system in the brain. Science 182:166, 1973
2. Anand BK, Brobeck JR: Hypothalamic control of food intake in rats and cats. Yale J Biol Med 24:123, 1951
3. Anand BK, Chhina GS, Sharma KN et al: Activity of single neurons in the hypothalamic feeding centers: Effect of glucose. Am J Physiol 207:1146, 1964
4. Bieger D, Giles SA, Hockman CH: Dopaminergic influences on swallowing. Neuropharmacology 16:245, 1977
5. Bieger D, Hockman CH: Suprabulbar modulation of reflex swallowing. Exp Neurol 52:311, 1976
6. Bignall KE, Schramm L: Behavior of chronically decerebrated kittens. Exp Neurol 42:519, 1974
7. Blander DS, Mark GP, Hernandez L et al: Angiotensin and drinking induce dopamine release in the nucleus accumbens. Soc Neurosci Abstr 14:527, 1988
8. Booth DA: Amphetamine anorexia by direct action on the adrenergic feeding system of the rat hypothalamus. Nature 217:869, 1968
9. Bray G: Factors leading to obesity: Physical (including metabolic) factors and disease states. In Bender AE, Brookes LJ (eds): Body Weight Control. New York, Churchill Livingstone, 1987
10. Breisch ST, Zemlan FP, Hoebel BG: Hyperphagia and obesity following serotonin depletion by intraventricular p-chlorophenylalanine. Science 192:382, 1976
11. Broekkamp CLE, Pijnenburg AJJ, Cools AR et al: The effect of microinjections of amphetamine into the neostriatum and the nucleus accumbens on self-stimulation behaviour. Psychopharmacologia 42:179, 1975
12. Brozoski TJ, Brown RM, Rosvold ME et al: Cognitive deficit caused by regional depletion of dopamine in prefrontal cortex of rhesus monkey. Science 205:929, 1979
13. Brugger M: Freestriab als hypothalamisches symptom. Helv Physiol Pharma Acta 1:183, 1943
14. Carr GD, White NM: Contributions of dopamine terminal areas to amphetamine-induced anorexia and adipsia. Pharmacol Biochem Behav 25:17, 1986
15. Chang VC, Mark GP, Hernandez L et al: Extracellular dopamine increase in the nucleus accumbens following rehydration or sodium repletion in rats. Soc Neurosci Abstr 14:527, 1988
16. Collier GH: Life in a closed economy: The ecology of learning and motivation. In Zeiler MD, Harzem P (eds): Advances in Analysis of Behavior. New York, John Wiley & Sons, 1983
17. Conrad LCA, Pfaff DW: Efferents from medial basal forebrain and hypothalamus in the rat. II. An autoradiographic study of the anterior hypothalamus. J Comp Neurol 169:221, 1976
18. Coscina DV: Effects of central 5,7-dihydroxytryptamine on the medial hypothalamic syndrome in

rats. In Jacoby JH, Lytle LD (eds): Serotonin Neurotoxins. Ann NY Acad Sci 305:627, 1978

19. Crow TJ: Specific monoamine systems as reward pathways: Evidence for the hypothesis that activation of the ventral mesencephalic dopaminergic neurones and noradrenergic neurones of the locus coeruleus complex will support self-stimulation responding. In Wauquier A, Rolls ET (eds): Brain-Stimulation Reward. New York, Elsevier, 1976

20. Damsma G, Yoshida M, Wenkstern D et al: Dopamine transmission in the rat striatum, nucleus accumbens and pre-frontal cortex is differently affected by feeding, tail pinch, and immobilization. J Neurosci Methods 29:272, 1989

21. Delgado JMR, Defeudis FV, Roth RH et al: Dialytrode for long term intracerebral perfusion in awake monkeys. Arch Int Pharmacodyn Ther 198:9, 1972

22. Doty RW, Bosma JF: An electromyographic analysis of reflex deglutition. J Neurophysiol 19:44, 1956

23. Dourish CT, Hutson PH, Curzon G: Characteristics of feeding induced by the serotonergic agonist 8-hydroxy-2-(di-n-propylamino) tetralin (8-OH-DPAT). Brain Res Bull 15:377, 1985

24. Evans KR, Vaccarino FJ: Intra-nucleus accumbens amphetamine: Dose-dependent affects on food intake. Pharmacol Biochem Behav 25:1149, 1986

25. Fibiger HC, Phillips AG: Reward, motivation, cognition: Psychobiology of mesotelencephalic dopamine systems. In Mountcastle VB (ed): Handbook of Physiology, Section 1, Vol IV, The Nervous System, 1986.

26. Fonberg E: The relation between alimentary and emotional amygdala regulation. In Novin D, Wyrwicka W, Bray G (eds): Hunger: Basic Mechanisms and Clinical Implications. New York, Raven Press, 1976

27. Grill HJ, Norgren R: Chronically decerebrate rats demonstrate satiation but not bait shyness. Science 201:267, 1978

28. Grossman SP: Direct adrenergic and cholinergic stimulation of hypothalamic mechanism. Am J Physiol 202:872, 1962

29. Grossman SP, Grossman L: Food and water intake following lesions or electrical stimulation of the amygdala. Am J Physiol 205:761, 1963

30. Guerin GF, Goeders NE, Dworkin SV et al: Intracranial self-administration of dopamine into the nucleus accumbens. Soc Neurosci Abstr 10:1072, 1984

31. Heffner TG, Hartman JA, Seiden LS: Feeding increases dopamine metabolism in the rat brain. Science 208:1168, 1980

32. Hernandez L: Glucostatic influence on self-stimulation and hypothalamic neurons. In Wauquier A, Rolls ET (eds): Brain-Stimulation Reward. New York, Elsevier, 1976

33. Hernandez L, Auerbach S, Hoebel BG: Phencyclidine (PCP) injected into the nucleus accumbens increases dopamine and serotonin as measured by microdialysis. Life Sci 42:1713, 1988

34. Hernandez L, Gottberg E: Systemic insulin decreases lateral hypothalamic unit activity. Physiol Behav 25:981, 1980

35. Hernandez L, Hoebel BG: Mutual supra-additive facilitation of contralateral self-stimulation and stimulation-induced feeding. Soc Neurosci Abstr 3:163, 1977

36. Hernandez L, Hoebel BG: Overeating after midbrain 6-hydroxydopamine: Prevention by central injection of selective reuptake blockers. Brain Res 245:333, 1982

37. Hernandez L, Hoebel BG: Food reward and cocaine increase extracellular dopamine in the nucleus accumbens as measured by microdialysis. Life Sci 42:1705, 1988

38. Hernandez L, Hoebel BG: Feeding and hypothalamic stimulation increase dopamine turnover in the accumbens. Physiol Behav 44:599, 1988

39. Hernandez L, Hoebel BG: Mesolimbic and mesocortical dopamine systems become active during feeding behavior. Appetite 12:215, 1989

40. Hernandez L, Hoebel BG: Food intake and lateral hypothalamic self-stimulation covary after medial hypothalamic lesions or ventral midbrain 6-hydroxydopamine injections that cause obesity. Behav Neurosci 103:412, 1989

41. Hernandez L, Lee F, Hoebel BG: Simultaneous microdialysis and amphetamine infusion in the nucleus accumbens. Pharmacol Biochem Behav 19:623, 1987

42. Hernandez L, Lee F, Hoebel BG: Microdialysis in the mesolimbic system during feeding or treatment with amphetamine, cocaine, or phencyclidine. In Kalivas PW, Nemeroff CB (eds): The Mesocorticolimbic Dopamine System. Ann NY Acad Sci 537:508, 1988

43. Hernandez L, Paez X, Hamlin C: Neurotransmitter extraction by local intracerebral dialysis in anesthetized rats. Pharmacol Biochem Behav 18:159, 1983

44. Hernandez L, Stanley BG, Hoebel BG: A small, removable microdialysis probe. Life Sci 39:2629, 1986

45. Hess WR: The Functional Organization of the Diencephalon. New York, Grune & Stratton, 1957

46. Hetherington AW, Ranson SW: The relation of various hypothalamic lesions to adiposity in the rat. J Comp Neurol 76:475, 1942

47. Hoebel BG: Feeding and self-stimulation. Ann NY Acad Sci 157-R2:758, 1969

48. Hoebel BG: Brain-stimulation reward and aversion in relation to behavior. In Brain-Stimulation Reward. Amsterdam, North Holland, 1976

49. Hoebel BG: Hyperphagia: A neurochemical analysis. In Iversen LL, Iversen SD, Snyder SH (eds): Handbook of Psychopharmacology, Vol 8. New York, Plenum, 1977

50. Hoebel BG: Neurotransmitters in the control of feeding and its rewards: Monoamines, opiates, and brain-gut peptides. In Stunkard AJ, Stellar E (eds): Eating and Its Disorders. New York, Raven Press, 1984

51. Hoebel BG: Neuroscience and motivation: Pathways and peptides that define motivational systems. In Atkinson RC, Herrnstein RJ, Lindzey G et al (eds): Stevens' Handbook of Experimental Psychology, 2nd ed, Vol 1, Perception and Motivation. New York, John Wiley & Sons, 1988

52. Hoebel BG, Hernandez L, Mark GP et al: Brain microdialysis as a molecular approach to obesity: Serotonin, dopamine and cyclic-AMP. In Obesity: Towards a Molecular Approach. New York, Alan Liss, 1990

53. Hoebel BG, Hernandez L, McClelland RC: Dexfenfluramine and feeding reward. Clin Neuropharmacol (Suppl 1) 11:S72, 1988

54. Hoebel BG, Hernandez L, Schwartz DH et al: Microdialysis studies of brain norepinephrine, serotonin and dopamine release during ingestive behavior. Ann NY Acad Sci 575:171, 1989

55. Hoebel BG, Monaco AP, Hernandez L: Self-injection of amphetamine directly into the brain. Psychopharmacology 81:158, 1983

56. Hoebel BG, Teitelbaum P: Hypothalamic control of feeding and self-stimulation. Science 135:375, 1962

57. Hokfelt T, Fuxe K, Goldstein M et al: Immunohistochemical evidence for the existence of adrenaline neurons in the rat brain. Brain Res 66:235, 1974

58. Hosoya Y, Matsushita M: Descending projections from the lateral hypothalamic area to the brain stem and spinal cord in the rat: A study by HRP and autoradiographic methods. In Sano Y, Ibata Y, Zimmerman EA (eds): Structure and Function of Aminergic and Peptidergic Neurons. Tokyo, Japan Scientific Society Press: Utrecht: VNU Science Press BV, 1983

59. Hunter GA, Hernandez L, Hoebel BG: Microdialysis shows increased dopamine turnover in the nucleus accumbens during lateral hypothalamic self-stimulation. Soc Neurosci Abstr 14:1100, 1988

60. Jackson JH: Selected Writings of John Hughlings Jackson. Taylor E (ed): New York, Basic Books, 1958

61. Kelly PH, Iversen SD: Selective 6-OHDA-induced destruction of mesolimbic dopamine neurones: Abolition of psychostimulant-induced locomotor activity in rats. Eur J Pharmacol 40:45, 1976

62. Kita H, Oomura Y: Reciprocal connections between the lateral hypothalamus and the frontal cortex in the rat: Electrophysiological and anatomical observations. Brain Res 213:1, 1981

63. Larsson S: On the hypothalamic organization of the nervous mechanisms regulating food intake. Acta Physiol Scand (Suppl) 32:115, 1954

64. Leibowitz SF: Identification of catecholamine receptor mechanisms in the perifornical lateral hypothalamus and their role in mediating amphetamine and L-DOPA anorexia. In Garattini S, Samanin R (eds): Central Mechanisms of Anorectic Drugs. New York, Raven Press, 1978

65. Leibowitz SF: Paraventricular nucleus: A primary site mediating adrenergic stimulation of feeding and drinking. Pharmacol Biochem Behav 8:163, 1978

66. Leibowitz SF: Neurochemical systems of the hypothalamus. Control of feeding and drinking behavior and water-electrolyte excretion. In Morgane PJ, Panskepp J (eds): Handbook of the Hypothalamus, Vol 3, Part A, Behavioral Studies of the Hypothalamus. New York, Marcel Dekker, 1980

67. Leibowitz SF, Brown LL: Histochemical and pharmacological analysis of catecholaminergic projections to the perifornical hypothalamus in relation to feeding inhibition. Brain Res 172:101, 1980

68. Leibowitz SF, Weiss GF, Shor-Posner G: Medial hypothalamic serotonin in the control of eating behavior. Int J Obes (Suppl 3) 11:109, 1987

69. Leibowitz SF, Weiss GF, Shor-Posner G: Hypothalamic serotonin: Pharmacological, biochemical, and behavioral analyses of its feeding-suppressive action. Clin Neuropharmacol (Suppl 1) 11:S51, 1988

70. Lindvall O, Bjorklund A: The organization of the ascending catecholamine neuron systems in the rat brain, as revealed by the glyoxylic acid fluorescence method. Acta Physiol Scand (Suppl) 412:1, 1974

71. Margules DL, Dragovich J: Studies on phentolamine-induced overeating and finickiness. J Comp Physiol Psych 84:644, 1973

72. Margules DL, Lewis MJ, Dragovich JA et al: Hypothalamic norepinephrine: Circadian rhythm and the control of feeding behavior. Science 178:640, 1972

73. Margules DL, Olds J: Identical "feeding" and "re-

ward" systems in the lateral hypothalamus. Science 174:523, 1962

74. Marshall JP, Richardson JS, Teitelbaum P: Nigrostriatal bundle damage and the lateral hypothalamic syndrome. J Comp Physiol Psych 87:808, 1974

75. McClelland RC, Sarfaty T, Hernandez L et al: The appetite suppressant, D-fenfluramine, decreases self-stimulation at a feeding site in the lateral hypothalamus. Pharmacol Biochem Behav 32:411, 1989

76. Miller FR, Sherrington CS: Some observations on the buccopharyngeal stage of reflex deglutition in the cat. Q J Exp Physiol 9:147, 1915

77. Miller NE: Experiments on motivation: Studies combining psychological, physiological and pharmacological techniques. Science 126:1271, 1957

78. Miller NE: Chemical coding of behavior in the brain. Science 148:328, 1965

79. Mishima K, Sasamoto K, Saeki K et al: Monosynaptic cortical projection to trigeminal motoneurons in the rat. Neurosci Let (Suppl) 13:S86, 1983

80. Mogenson GJ, Yim CY: Electrophysiological and neuropharmacological-behavioral studies of the nucleus accumbens: Implications for its role as a limbic-motor interface. In Chronister RB, DeFrance JF (eds): The Neurobiology of the Nucleus Accumbens. Brunswick, ME, Haer Institute, 1981

81. Murzi E, Hernandez L, Baptista T: Lateral hypothalamic sites eliciting eating affect medullary taste neurons in rats. Physiol Behav 36:829, 1986

82. Nicolaidis S (ed): Serotonergic System, Feeding and Body Weight Regulation. New York, Academic Press, 1986

83. Ohta M: Amygdaloid and cortical facilitation or inhibition of trigeminal motoneurons in the rat. Brain Res 291:39, 1984

84. Oomura Y: Neurophysiology of control: Metabolic receptors. In Ritter RC, Ritter S, Barnes CD (eds): Feeding Behavior: Neural and Humoral Controls. New York, Academic Press, 1986

85. Oomura Y, Kimura K, Ooyama H et al: Reciprocal activity of the ventromedial and lateral hypothalamic areas of cats. Science 143:484, 1964

86. Parada M, Hernandez L: Correlacion significativa entre la anorexia por anfetamina, serotonina, y dopamine intrahipotalamicas. XXXII Convencion anual de ASOVAC, Caracas, Venezuela, 1982

87. Pettit HO, Nicolaysen LC, Justice JB: The dopaminergic threshold of cocaine reward measured by in vivo microdialysis. Soc Neurosci Abstr 14:659, 1988

88. Pijnenburg AJJ, Honig WMM, Van Der Heyden JAM et al: Effects of chemical stimulation of the mesolimbic dopamine system upon locomotor activity. Eur J Pharmacol 35:45, 1976

89. Pothos E, Mark GP, Hernandez L et al: In vivo dialysis measurements of dopamine and serotonin release in the nucleus accumbens as a function of body weight. Appetite 12:231, 1989

90. Radhakishun FS, Van Ree JM, Westerink BHC: Schedule eating increases dopamine release in the nucleus accumbens of food-deprived rats as assessed with on-line brain dialysis. Neurosci Lett 85:351, 1988

91. Roberts DCS, Zis AP, Fibiger HC: Ascending catecholamine pathways and amphetamine-induced locomotor activity: Importance of dopamine and apparent non-involvement of norepinephrine. Brain Res 93:441, 1975

92. Roberts WW: [14C]Deoxyglucose mapping of first-order projections activated by stimulation of lateral hypothalamic sites eliciting gnawing, eating, and drinking in rats. J Comp Neurol 194:617, 1980

93. Rolls ET: The Brain and Reward. New York, Pergamon Press, 1975

94. Rolls ET: Processing beyond the inferior temporal visual cortex related to feeding, memory, and striatal function. In Katsuki Y, Norgren R, Sato M (eds): Brain Mechanisms of Sensation. New York, John Wiley & Sons, 1981

95. Rolls ET: Neuronal activity related to the control of feeding. In Ritter RC, Ritter S, Barnes D (eds): Feeding Behavior: Neural and Humoral Controls. New York, Academic Press, 1986

96. Saavedra JM, Palkovits M, Brownstein MJ et al: Serotonin distribution in the nuclei of the rat hypothalamus and preoptic region. Brain Res 77:157, 1974

97. Sabol KE, Freed CR: Effects of drinking on dopamine, DOPAC and HVA levels in the rat as measured by in vivo dialysis. Soc Neurosci Abstr 14:527, 1988

98. Saller CF, Stricker EM: Hyperphagia and increased growth in rats after intraventricular injection of 5,7-dihydroxytryptamine. Science 192:385, 1976

99. Saper CB, Lowey AD, Swanson LW et al: Direct hypothalamo-autonomic connections. Brain Res 117:305, 1976

100. Schwartz DH, Hernandez L, Hoebel BG: Serotonin release in the medial and lateral hypothalamus during feeding and its anticipation. Soc Neurosci Abstr 15:225, 1989

101. Schwartz DH, McClane S, Hernandez L et al: Feeding increases extracellular serotonin in the lateral hypothalamus of the rat as measured by microdialysis. Brain Res 479:349, 1989

102. Sherrington CS: Reflex elicited in the cat from pinna, vibrissae and jaws. J Physiol 51:404, 1917

103. Shimizu N, West MO, Lee RS et al: Dopaminergic involvement in striatal neural activity during locomotor behavior and its enhancement by cocaine. Soc Neurosci Abstr 13:979, 1987

104. Simon H, Scatton B, Le Moal M: Dopaminergic A10 neurones are involved in cognitive functions. Nature 286:150, 1980

105. Stellar E: The physiology of motivation. Psychol Rev 61:5, 1954

106. Stricker EM, Zigmond MJ: Brain catecholamine and the lateral hypothalamic syndrome. In Novin D, Wyrwicka W, Bray G (eds): Hunger: Basic Mechanisms and Clinical Observations. New York, Raven Press, 1976

107. Swanson LW, Kuypers HGJM: The paraventricular nucleus of the hypothalamus: Cytoarchitectonic subdivisions and organization of projections to the pituitary, dorsal vagal complex, and spinal cord as demonstrated by retrograde fluorescence double labeling methods. J Comp Neurol 194:555, 1980

108. Teitelbaum P, Epstein AN: The lateral hypothalamic syndrome: Recovery of feeding and drinking after lateral hypothalamic lesions. Psychol Rev 69:74, 1962

109. Teitelbaum P, Stellar E: Recovery from the failure to eat produced by hypothalamic lesions. Science 120:894, 1954

110. Terreberry RR, Neafsey E: Rat medial frontal cortex: A visceral motor region with a direct projection to the solitary nucleus. Brain Res 278:245, 1983

111. Ungerstedt U: Stereotaxic mapping of the monoamine pathways in the rat brain. Acta Physiol Scand (Suppl) 367:1, 1971

112. Ungerstedt U: Adipsia and aphagia after 6-hydroxydopamine induced degeneration of the nigrostriatal dopamine system. Acta Physiol Scand (Suppl) 367:95, 1971

113. Ungerstedt U: Measurement of neurotransmitter release by intracranial dialysis. In Marsden CA (ed): Measurement of Neurotransmitter Release In Vivo. New York, John Wiley & Sons, 1984

114. Van der Koy D, Koda LY, McGinty JF et al: The organization of projections from the cortex, amygdala, and hypothalamus to the nucleus of the solitary tract in the rat. J Comp Neurol 224:1, 1984

115. Waldbillig RJ, Bartness TJ, Stanley BG: Increased food intake, body weight, and adiposity in rats after regional neurochemical depletion of serotonin. J Comp Physiol Psychol 95:391, 1981

116. Weerasuriya A, Bieger D, Hockman CH: Basal forebrain facilitation of reflex swallowing in the cat. Brain Res 174:119, 1979

117. Weiss F, Hurd YL, Koob GF et al: In vivo microdialysis study of DA function in the rat nucleus accumbens after acute and repeated cocaine self-administration. Soc Neurosci Abstr 14:658, 1988

118. Westerink BHC, Damsma G, Rollema H et al: Scope and limitations of in vivo microdialysis: A comparison of its applications to various neurotransmitter systems. Life Sci 41:1763, 1987

119. Wise RA: Brain neuronal systems mediating reward processes. In Smith JE, Lane JD (eds): The Neurobiology of Opiate Reward Processes. New York, Elsevier Biomedical Publishers, 1983

120. Woods JW: Behavior of chronic decerebrate rats. J Neurophysiol 27:635, 1964

121. Wyrwicka W: Brain and Feeding Behavior. Springfield, IL, Charles C Thomas, 1988

122. Wyrwicka W, Dobrzecka C: Relationship between feeding and satiation centers of the hypothalamus. Science 132:805, 1960

Brain Neurotransmitters and Hormones in Relation to Eating Behavior and Its Disorders

SARAH FRYER LEIBOWITZ

Studies on brain neurochemical mechanisms have provided extensive evidence in support of their active role in controlling food intake, appetite for macronutrients, meal patterns, energy and nutrient metabolism, and body weight gain. The myriad of behaviors associated with food ingestion are complex and are believed to involve multiple neurotransmitter systems within the brain. These systems may function both independently and through close interaction, and they are responsive to both neural and humoral signals regarding the organism's nutritional status. In this process, the hypothalamus, with its rich innervation of neurochemical projections and dense concentration of neuroendocrine cells, is believed to have a critical responsibility in balancing signals for hunger and satiety and then in generating appropriate qualitative and quantitative adjustments in the ingestion and metabolism of energy, as well as nutrients for body growth.

Extensive biochemical, pharmacologic, and endocrine research into brain systems regulating appetite has generated several hypotheses to explain the physiological functions of the monoamines, neuropeptides, and hormones, not only in regulating total energy intake but also in determining the amount and pattern of macronutrient selection and in controlling energy expenditure and body weight gain. Although in classic models experimental subjects were generally offered a single diet of fixed nutritional composition, other studies have now provided separate macronutrient choices and have revealed how animals can display a similar capacity to regulate their intake of protein, carbohydrate, and possibly fat, with remarkable consistency for proper growth and stable body weight.[12,63,92,152] Evidence obtained in animals, as well as in humans, suggests that brain neurotransmitters, nutrients, and steroid or peptide hormones may, in part, mediate the alterations or disturbances in these feeding patterns and energy balance, which emanate from physiological events, environmental conditions, or experimental manipulations.[13,29,66-72,150,152,153] The amines and neuropeptides are highly responsive to drug administration and to circulating nutrients and hormones; they are also responsive to psychological and emotional variables that may contribute to the development of disturbed eating habits and body weight control.

In terms of brain areas involved, the hypothalamus is generally found to be the structure most sensitive to neurohumoral manipulations that modulate eating. Tests in various species indicate that, after injection directly into the hypothalamus, specific neurotransmitters can cause fully satiated animals to eat and even binge on a particular diet, induce hungry animals to stop eating and even rest in the presence of food, and produce dramatic changes in energy metabolism and body weight gain.[66-68,70,72,78,128] Important biochemical studies have yielded evidence indicating that these behavioral changes do in fact reflect the action of endogenous neurotransmitter systems that control the expression of natural feeding patterns.

The relevance of these findings to our understanding of human eating disorders can be seen in biochemical studies of human cerebrospinal fluid (CSF). These investigations demonstrate specific neurotransmitter abnormalities, associated with disturbances in eating behavior and body weight, that may be predicted from the patterns of results obtained in animals.[8,49-54]

Any integrative hypothesis that explains eating behavior must consider the organism as a whole and take into account various neurotransmitters, including the monoamines (i.e., norepinephrine [NE], epinephrine [EPI], dopamine [DA], and serotonin [5-HT]); the amino acids (e.g., gamma-aminobutyric acid [GABA], tryptophan, and tyrosine); and several neuropeptides (e.g., the pancreatic polypeptides, opioid peptides, hormone-releasing factors, and various gut-brain peptides). In considering each of these neurotransmitters, as well as the nature of their interactions, critical issues that must be evaluated include the identification of specific brain site(s) where these neurotransmitters act to produce their behavioral effects and a precise characterization of the natural conditions under which they act. Conclusions concerning physiological significance will be greatly limited by the absence of such information.

MONOAMINES AND NEUROPEPTIDES

The monoamines and peptides have been found to be potent and varied in their effects on eating behavior, in rats as well as in various other species.[68-72,78,80,82,83] When administered directly into the brain, at least six classes of neurotransmitters have been found to influence eating in a stimulatory manner, whereas a considerably larger number of substances are shown to inhibit the ingestion of food. The feeding-stimulatory transmitters include the catecholamine NE; the amino acid GABA; the releasing factor for growth hormone; and three classes of neuropeptides—namely, the opioids (β-endorphin, enkephalin, and dynorphin), the pancreatic polypeptides

(neuropeptide Y [NPY] and peptide YY [PYY]), and the peptide galanin (GAL). Studies that have injected these substances directly into the rat hypothalamus, as well as into several other species, have demonstrated that these drugs potentiate eating under satiated conditions.[46,60,68,103,104,130,131,142]

The feeding-inhibitory neurotransmitters in the brain, in contrast, include the monoamines 5-HT, DA, and under certain conditions NE and EPI when acting by way of β-adrenergic receptors[13,65,66]; and a long list of gut-brain peptides, most notably neurotensin, corticotropin releasing factor, cholecystokinin, calcitonin, and glucagon.[37,65,82,103,127] Extensive mapping and lesion studies, with the catecholamines tested in hungry rats, indicate that they act within the lateral perifornical hypothalamus to inhibit the ingestion of food. In contrast, newer studies have indicated that 5-HT is most effective within the medial hypothalamus, at the exclusion of all other hypothalamic or extrahypothalamic sites.[80] Although few such mapping studies have been conducted with the peptides, limited evidence to date demonstrates that exogenously administered peptides are apparently effective in multiple brain sites, including medial as well as lateral hypothalamic nuclei and both forebrain and hindbrain sites.[82] The ubiquitous nature of this sensitivity clearly indicates the necessity for further examination, in order to determine its significance relative to physiological function.

The main focus of this review is on two putative hypothalamic monoaminergic systems—namely, the α_2-noradrenergic and serotonergic systems. These systems are examined in terms of their function in controlling total energy intake, their impact on the amount and pattern of macronutrient selection, and their relation to energy metabolism and body weight gain. The nature of the interaction between these monoamines and various neuropeptides, hormones, and nutrients is then described, followed by a discussion of how these interactive substances may impact on circadian patterns of feeding behavior in animals and specific appetites in humans. The possibility that disturbances in these neurochemical and neuroendocrine systems may underlie abnormal eating patterns and body weight gain in humans is then evaluated.

HYPOTHALAMIC α_2-NORADRENERGIC AND SEROTONERGIC SYSTEMS IN CONTROL OF MEAL PATTERNS AND APPETITE FOR SPECIFIC NUTRIENTS

Norepinephrine

Intracerebral injection studies in rats have shown that hypothalamic stimulation with NE, acting by way of α_2-noradrenergic receptors,[35] produces a feeding response that is characterized by a rapid onset (<1 minute) and a short duration (<30 minute) and that is anatomically localized predominantly to the hypothalamic paraventricular nucleus (PVN).[64] Destruction of this nucleus, as opposed to other brain sites, dramatically disturbs an animal's ability to respond to NE,[66,68] as well as its ability to normally regulate carbohydrate and protein consumption.[1,116]

Serotonin

In contrast to NE, hypothalamic administration of 5-HT has a suppressive effect on eating behavior under various conditions, such as in spontaneously feeding animals, food-deprived animals, and animals induced to eat by drug stimulation.[71,80,84-86,119,146-148] This effect occurs with both peripheral and central administration of serotonergic drugs, which are believed to act through the release of endogenous 5-HT. Cannula mapping studies,[85,147,148] with 5-HT itself and with drugs that release endogenous 5-HT (D-norfenfluramine [DNF]) or block 5-HT reuptake (fluoxetine [FLU]), indicate that this phenomenon is anatomically localized, specifically to the medial hypothalamic nuclei (the PVN, ventromedial, dorsomedial, and suprachiasmatic nuclei), as opposed to the lateral hypothalamus or extrahypothalamic structures. With microdialysis procedures, PVN injection of DNF has been shown to produce a dose-related rise in extracellular levels of PVN 5-HT,[109] providing further support for a role of this medial hypothalamic nucleus in mediating the actions of endogenous 5-HT. Moreover, the receptor sites through which 5-HT functions to suppress feeding are the postsynaptic 5-HT_{1B} receptors that are concentrated in the medial hypothalamic nuclei and are responsive to food deprivation.[24,76]

Diurnal Rhythms

The activity of both the α_2-noradrenergic and 5-HT_{1B} receptor systems is closely linked to the light/dark cycle. That is, these systems, at the start of the active period (nocturnal cycle for rats), exhibit a sharp, unimodal peak in activity.[44,68,76,80,86,132,133,139,147,148] This finding is reflected in microinjection studies showing the animals' sensitivity to exogenous NE and 5-HT and to drugs that stimulate endogenous monoamines. It is also detected in microdialysis studies of extracellular PVN NE and 5-hydroxyindoleacetic acid, a 5-HT metabolite, as well as in radioligand binding studies of PVN α_2-receptor and 5-HT_{1B}-receptor density. Moreover, this peak in monoaminergic activity occurs in association with a natural rise in circulating levels of corticosterone (CORT),[55] which in turn may be controlled in part by endogenous PVN monoamines.[74,81]

Physiologic Function

With regard to the precise function of PVN NE, studies have considerably strengthened our knowledge of this neurotransmitter in the control of natural eating behavior. Although experiments have shown that noradrenergic stimulation of this nucleus increases intake of total calories in rats maintained on a single mixed diet, the primary effect of NE in animals given a choice of macronutrients is to selectively potentiate the consumption of carbohydrate (Table 15-1), although in some cases suppressing intake of protein and maintaining normal total calorie intake.[87,95,154] This specificity is similarly exhibited by drugs such as the α_2-receptor agonist clonidine (see Table 15-1) or the tricyclic antidepressants, which enhance the release of endogenous NE.[73] In contrast, a deficit in carbohydrate consumption and sometimes an enhancement of protein ingestion occur in response to agents that selectively block α_2 receptors (see Table 15-1),[21] inhibit NE synthesis,[154] or destroy noradrenergic neurons.[117] These data argue for a physiological function of PVN NE and local α_2 receptors in the control of diet composition, in particular, carbohydrate intake possibly in relation to protein.[68,73,87]

Hypothalamic administration of 5-HT, as well

TABLE 15-1

Change in Macronutrient Intake (kcal) After Injection of
α_2-Noradrenergic Agonists and Antagonists at Dark Onset

	Carbohydrate	Protein	Fat	Carbohydrate/Protein
α_2 Agonists				
PVN Norepinephrine	+8.0*	0.0	0.0	↑
i.p. Clonidine	+5.2*	0.0	0.0	↑
α_2 Antagonists				
i.p. Idazoxan	−2.0*	0.0	0.0	↓
i.p. Rauwolscine	0.0	+5.0*	0.0	↓

*$P < 0.05$

as systemic injection of serotonergic agents, produces feeding patterns opposite to those observed after α_2-noradrenergic stimulation. By reducing the proportion of carbohydrate in the diet and sparing protein intake (Fig. 15-1), 5-HT specifically in the medial hypothalamus (PVN, ventromedial and suprachiasmatic nuclei) appears to alter the ratio of carbohydrate to protein in the diet,[78,84-86,119] consistent with the earlier peripheral injection studies by Wurtman and Wurtman[151-153] and Li and Anderson.[94] A similar pattern of diet selection can be seen with PVN injections of DNF, which acts through the release of endogenous 5-HT, and also with FLU, which blocks the reuptake of presynaptic 5-HT.[147,148] Furthermore, these effects are opposite to the changes observed when brain 5-HT is reduced, through intraventricular injection of the serotonergic neurotoxin 5,7-dihydroxytryptamine.[4]

In addition to affecting macronutrient selection, the hypothalamic neurotransmitters are also believed to influence the animals' temporal patterns of food ingestion. To date, only the monoamines have been examined after central administration, and the evidence indicates that NE or clonidine in the PVN stimulates eating, first, by increasing meal size and duration rather than altering meal frequency and, second, by enhancing the rate of eating.[68,120] This evidence has led us to propose a role for NE in delaying or inhibiting satiety for carbohydrate, rather than in stimulating hunger and meal initiation. The

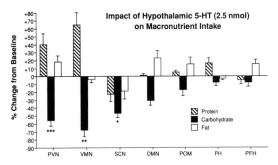

FIGURE 15-1

Responsiveness of seven hypothalamic sites to 5-HT injection, indicated by a percent change in feeding scores relative to vehicle control baseline. Measurements of protein, carbohydrate, and fat intake were taken 1 hour after 5-HT injection into the paraventricular nucleus (PVN), ventromedial nucleus (VMN), suprachiasmatic nucleus (SGN), dorsomedial nucleus (DMN), medial preoptic area (POM), posterior hypothalamus (PH), and lateral perifornical hypothalamus (PFH), just before the beginning of the nocturnal cycle. The three medial hypothalamic nuclei (PVN, VMN, and SCN) showed a significant response to 5-HT injection—namely, a strong suppression of carbohydrate ingestion, a tendency toward enhancement of protein intake, and no change in fat consumption. The DMN exhibited a smaller response, whereas no effect was observed in the POM, PH, and PFH. (*$P < 0.05$; **$P < 0.01$; ***$P < 0.001$) (Leibowitz SF, Weiss GF, Suh JS: Medial hypothalamic nuclei mediate serotonin's inhibitory effect on feeding behavior. Pharmacol Biochem Behav 37:735, 1990)

converse appears to occur with 5-HT and 5-HT-releasing drugs, which reduce meal size and duration as well as rate of eating while having little impact on the number of meals consumed.[13,119,153]

These findings suggest that NE and 5-HT act antagonistically through a medial hypothalamic satiety system to, respectively, inhibit or promote satiety for carbohydrate. This proposal is consistent with the evidence that electrolytic destruction of the PVN or ventromedial nuclei produces hyperphagia specifically for carbohydrate.[1,75,116]

This role of the medial hypothalamus, to produce satiety for carbohydrate, contrasts with that of the lateral hypothalamus, which has long been associated with the stimulation of feeding and processes relating to reinforcement. In this hypothalamic area, there is evidence to suggest that 5-HT may influence feeding by reducing the rewarding properties of food,[36] rather than by inhibiting satiety for a specific nutrient (see Fig. 15-1).[85] Moreover, the catecholamine DA may also act in this brain area through a different mechanism that controls the onset, rather than the termination, of feeding.

Specifically, when injected into the perifornical region of the lateral hypothalamus, both DA and the DA-releasing anorexic agent amphetamine have been shown to inhibit food intake and, in particular, to reduce appetite for protein and fat while having little impact on carbohydrate intake.[65,79] Blockade of the DA receptors in the lateral hypothalamus by injection of neuroleptics causes the opposite effect, a potentiation of protein and fat ingestion (Shor-Posner and Leibowitz, unpublished data). The function of the DA receptors in this brain area, in contrast to the medial hypothalamic 5-HT receptors, is to affect the process of eating initiation and, more specifically, to reduce food intake by delaying the onset of a meal rather than by altering the time of meal termination.[79]

As in animal studies, administration of drugs that increase the availability of 5-HT has been shown in humans to inhibit the ingestion of carbohydrate, as well as the craving for snacks rich in this macronutrient.[122,152,153] Moreover, injection of agents that antagonize serotonergic activity is found to cause an increase in calorie intake and hunger ratings in human subjects.[122]

Interaction Between Norepinephrine and Serotonin

The effects of medial hypothalamic 5-HT and NE stimulation on ingestive behavior suggest an important role for these neurotransmitters in modulating temporal patterns of feeding and appetite for particular macronutrients. The available evidence suggests that these monoamines may interact directly in the process of controlling appetite for carbohydrate and protein.[66,71,78,146] In addition to having opposite effects on nutrient intake and meal patterns, NE and 5-HT appear to act within the same brain area—namely, the medial hypothalamic nuclei—where they, respectively, inhibit or activate satiety mechanisms. They also appear to be activated at the same time of the diurnal cycle, at the onset of the active feeding period. Support for their direct interaction is obtained from the studies by Weiss and colleagues,[146] which reveal a potent inhibitory effect of PVN 5-HT injection on NE-induced eating. Moreover, biochemical studies provide further evidence for a specific antagonism between serotonergic and α_2-noradrenergic receptors in the hypothalamus.[32]

Using other experimental paradigms, such an interaction between noradrenergic and serotonergic systems in the control of feeding behavior may be further indicated. For example, the results of experiments on hyperphagia induced by 2-deoxy-D-glucose show that the serotonergic compounds DF and FLU inhibit this overeating effect.[18] Because it is believed that central noradrenergic transmission may have a role in mediating the feeding response to 2-deoxy-D-glucose administration,[65,99,105] one may interpret this phenomenon as reflecting an interaction between hypothalamic serotonergic and noradrenergic projections. A similar suggestion may be made in the case of the eating responses induced by the GABA agent muscimol and the opioid β-endorphin. These responses, which are believed to involve the noradrenergic circuit, are also potently inhibited by DF.[14,33,34,65,69,97]

ENDOCRINE PARAMETERS AND THEIR INTERACTION WITH HYPOTHALAMIC MONOAMINES

Two hormones, in particular—the adrenal glucocorticoid CORT and the pancreatic hormone insulin (INS)—are indicated by numerous studies to function synergistically with the central neurotransmitters to control behavior.[66-68] These hormones have long been known to be involved in the control of food ingestion, as well as glucose metabolism and availability. There is some evidence to suggest that they may exert their effects, in part, by acting directly on the hypothalamic monoaminergic systems. They may also function indirectly by altering circulating levels of glucose, which in turn influence brain neurotransmitter activity.

It is now believed that CORT and possibly INS interact directly with NE and its receptors in the hypothalamus, specifically to control carbohydrate (glucose) ingestion. When injected into the PVN, NE has been found to significantly enhance the release of CORT[74,81] and INS[26] into the circulation. Studies with CORT indicate that fluctuations in circulating levels of this steroid, in turn, cause changes in the release of brain NE,[43] in the availability of α_2-noradrenergic receptors to which NE binds,[41,44] and consequently in the animals' appetite for carbohydrate specifically at the onset of the active cycle.[56,57] Moreover, eating elicited by NE in the PVN is abolished by adrenalectomy, as well as by dissection of vagal fibers to the pancreas,[77,110,114] and this response is restored or potentiated by systemic injection of CORT or INS.[68]

Under normal conditions, a peak of both circulating CORT and hypothalamic NE activity occurs at the start of the active feeding cycle,[55,68] when carbohydrate meals naturally predominate.[141] Under abnormal conditions of adrenal insufficiency, this diurnal rhythm may be disturbed, particularly at the onset of the feeding period, and there may occur a specific deficit in the ingestion of high-energy foods.[9,56,57] The opposite pattern, overeating of carbohydrate-rich foods in particular, develops with high levels of circulating CORT, as demonstrated by systemic injection studies of CORT itself.[9]

Investigations with steroid implants in the brain suggest that the PVN is directly involved in the mediation of this neuroendocrine response.[137] This is demonstrated by the increase in carbohydrate ingestion produced by CORT administration into this nucleus of adrenalectomized rats, specifically at the start of the natural feeding period (Fig. 15-2). This effect of CORT

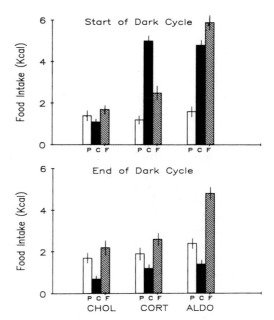

FIGURE 15-2

Effects of PVN implants of cholesterol (CHOL), corticosterone (CORT), and aldosterone (ALDO) on total (T), protein (P), carbohydrate (C), and fat (F) intake of adrenalectomized (ADX) rats. Implants of CORT, relative to CHOL, stimulated intake of carbohydrate only at the start of the dark period. PVN implants of ALDO, in contrast, potentiated ingestion of fat in both the beginning and end of the dark cycle but also increased consumption of carbohydrate at dark onset. No change in protein intake was observed with either steroid.

on carbohydrate feeding at this time may be distinguished from the proposed role of this glucocorticoid in maintaining normal 24-hour ingestion of fat.[19] It may also be contrasted with the feeding effect produced by the mineralocorticoid aldosterone. A PVN implant of this steroid[137] increases predominantly fat ingestion at both the start and end of the dark cycle (see Fig. 15-2), and a similar effect has been observed with peripheral injection of aldosterone.[27]

IMPACT OF CIRCULATING NUTRIENTS ON HYPOTHALAMIC NEUROTRANSMITTERS

The macronutrients selected by a normal animal to satisfy its internal needs may themselves influence the brain mechanisms that regulate food intake. Ingestion of food has been shown to alter plasma amino acid patterns, which in turn influence the entry of tryptophan and tyrosine into the brain and thus the synthesis of 5-HT and catecholamines, respectively.[29,30,93,150,152] Consumption of a large carbohydrate meal at the beginning of the active cycle causes a substantial release in INS, which results in an increase in the concentration of plasma tryptophan relative to the other neutral amino acids and consequently a rise in brain tryptophan and 5-HT synthesis. Protein ingestion, in contrast, decreases brain tryptophan uptake and thus reduces 5-HT synthesis. These effects, suggested to occur in humans[5,102] as well as in animals, have led to the proposal that brain 5-HT may function as a sensor of circulating amino acids, translating their blood levels and their ratio into neurotransmitter function.[150,152]

Additional evidence shows that precursor events may also influence the synthesis of hypothalamic catecholamines NE, DA, and EPI.[30] There is some suggestion that a protein meal may enhance their production owing to a relative increase in tyrosine levels, whereas a carbohydrate meal may reduce their production. This proposal is strengthened by the evidence that a carbohydrate-rich nutrient loaded into the stomach of rats inhibits endogenous NE release in the medial hypothalamus, specifically in the PVN.[106] Furthermore, in humans, a similar relationship, between the ingestion of pure protein and an increase in tyrosine levels, has been demonstrated.[102]

Small changes in glucose are found to occur immediately before the beginning of meals in animals,[16,17,88] and these changes may themselves have direct and rapid impact on central neurotransmitter systems controlling food ingestion. The α_2-noradrenergic system of the PVN appears to be particularly responsive to alterations in circulating glucose. A rapid decline in glucose levels, after tolbutamide injection or food deprivation, causes an increase in the turnover of medial hypothalamic NE, in association with a compensatory decline in PVN α_2-noradrenergic receptor density.[20,40,42] These studies have also shown that the restoration of circulating glucose levels, either through brief periods (15 minutes) of glucose ingestion or through metabolic processes, provides an adequate signal for reversing

these changes in noradrenergic activity. In addition, blood levels of glucose are significantly enhanced by medial hypothalamic administration of NE.[20]

IMPACT OF PEPTIDES ON NUTRIENT CHOICE AND THEIR INTERACTION WITH HYPOTHALAMIC MONOAMINES

Neuropeptide Y

NPY, a 36-amino-acid peptide, is among the most abundant peptides in neurons of the peripheral and central nervous systems.[107] Several studies have shown this peptide to mimic the action of NE, EPI, and the α_2-receptor agonist clonidine,[31,108] in stimulating food intake in rats as well as other species.[23,91,130] This response, which has a longer latency and duration than that induced by the amines, is similar to NE in being associated with a preferential enhancement of carbohydrate ingestion[126] and in being dependent on the adrenal steroid CORT.[129] In endocrine studies,[74,81] we have also observed similar effects of these neurotransmitters in the PVN on circulating hormone levels—namely, an increase in the release of CORT and vasopressin.

This evidence, revealing several similarities between the behavioral and endocrine effects of hypothalamic NE (or EPI) and NPY, has encouraged us to propose some degree of association between NPY and NE in their control of physiological processes.[70] This association is further strengthened by evidence that demonstrates the coexistence of NPY and NE (or EPI) within projections innervating the medial hypothalamus.[31,107] This coexistence may determine each other's pattern of release and receptor activity and thus allow for close interaction in their control of appetite for macronutrients.[70]

Other results, however, suggest that these coexisting neurotransmitters, although acting in a cooperative fashion, may actually function independently of each other. For example, pharmacologic studies have shown that the eating response induced by NPY is unaffected by local administration of general α-noradrenergic or selective α_2-noradrenergic receptor blockers,[46,59,91,131] and it remains intact after knife-cut damage to descending periventricular fiber projections that are critical to NE's feeding effect (Stanley and Leibowitz, unpublished data).[145] Moreover, NPY's actions are unaffected or even potentiated by local PVN administration of catecholamine synthesis inhibitors,[59,70] as well as after brainstem knife cuts that reduce hypothalamic NE and EPI levels.[48] These manipulations, which damage adrenergic afferents to the PVN, are both effective in antagonizing the behavioral effects of catecholamine-releasing drugs in this nucleus.[64,65,68] Based on this evidence and the finding that NPY acts in a broader range of hypothalamic sites than NE,[125] it may be concluded that although NE and NPY may act similarly and cooperatively in producing their behavioral and endocrine effects, NPY is not dependent on endogenous stores of NE for its stimulatory actions on feeding.

Galanin

Galanin, a 29-amino-acid peptide,[136] is another neuropeptide known to coexist with NE in neurons of the hypothalamus.[100] Research conducted by Kyrkouli and colleagues,[59-62] suggests that GAL, in contrast to NPY, may in some conditions require endogenous NE to produce its effects on feeding; however, in other conditions, GAL appears to act through separate neural mechanisms to induce behavioral and endocrine effects very different from NE.[70,72]

As with NE and NPY, direct injection of GAL into the PVN has been shown to have a stimulatory effect on food intake in satiated rats.[60,140] The GAL-induced feeding response, similar to that of NE but unlike NPY, is antagonized by local administration of α_2-noradrenergic blockers and unaffected by α_1-noradrenergic blockers.[59] Moreover, the response to GAL, unlike NPY, is attenuated by prior administration of catecholamine synthesis inhibitors, indicating that this peptide's action involves, in part, the release of endogenous NE. In fact, microdialysis studies have revealed an increase in extracellular NE levels after GAL, but not NPY, injection into the PVN.[61]

The most recent studies, testing the sensitivity of several hypothalamic and extrahypothalamic sites to the effects of GAL, show the PVN to be a primary site of action.[62] In particular, it appears to be the medial, as opposed to the lateral, portion of the PVN where the effects of this peptide

are strongest. In fact, preliminary evidence, with electrolytic lesions that destroy only the medial region of the PVN, shows that the feeding response to GAL, as well as to NE, is abolished by this lesion.[58] This finding suggests that the medial PVN is most critical in mediating the actions of these coexisting neurotransmitters and possibly in providing the mechanism for their interaction.

Evidence arguing for a dissociation between GAL and NE within the PVN is the additional finding that GAL, in contrast to NE, preferentially stimulates the ingestion of fat, an effect that occurs in conjunction with a smaller increase in carbohydrate ingestion.[140] This finding raises the possibility that although a component of GAL's effect on feeding (i.e., its potentiation of carbohydrate intake) may be mediated through the release of PVN NE, its stimulatory action on fat ingestion may involve a different neurochemical system.[70,72]

Further dissociation between these coexisting peptide and catecholamine neurotransmitters becomes apparent in studies of circulating hormones.[138] Administration of GAL into the PVN causes a dramatic decrease in blood levels of CORT and INS, with no change in glucose. This effect is diametrically opposite to the impact of NE in the PVN, which increases levels of CORT, INS, and also glucose.[20,26,74]

NEUROTRANSMITTER ACTIVITY IN RELATION TO DIURNAL PATTERNS OF FEEDING

Natural Feeding Patterns

The ability of animals to alter patterns of protein and energy intake in relation to need becomes especially apparent during the active period of the diurnal cycle, when feeding behavior is most pronounced.[2] The nocturnal feeding activity in rats is characterized by bursts of eating at the beginning and toward the end of the night, with a relatively stable trough in the middle of the cycle.[141] The burst of food intake at the start of the feeding period is characterized by a strong preference for carbohydrate; this pattern contrasts with the feeding in the later hours of the active cycle, when carbohydrate intake dramatically declines and protein and fat are preferred.

It is proposed that in animals as well as in humans,[2,3,5,25,88,134,141] food ingested during the first half of the night is used to fulfill immediate energy requirements and then to promote lipogenesis. In contrast, later in the night, nutrient and energy stores are to a large extent replenished and feeding is anticipatory in nature, geared toward ingestion of nutrients (fat and protein) that can be readily stored and subsequently utilized during the light cycle. This circadian pattern of nutrient intake and metabolism places particular demands on body energy stores, such that at the end of the inactive (light) cycle, when little food is ingested, hepatic glycogen stores are low and blood glucose levels may actually decline.

Norepinephrine

These findings obtained in normal animals, along with the previous pharmacologic results, lead us to propose that certain neurotransmitters of the hypothalamus, such as NE and 5-HT, participate and interact in coordinating the patterns of carbohydrate and protein meals that occur during the normal feeding cycle and, in particular, at the onset of this period.[66-68,84,85] A range of evidence suggests that when the organism is most hungry, such as at the start of the active feeding period, PVN NE is called on to initiate the eating process and thereby help to restore energy reserves.

In support of this hypothesis, several events are found to take place at the beginning of the nocturnal cycle, when spontaneous feeding naturally occurs in rats. They include an increase in α_2-receptor responsiveness to PVN NE (Fig. 15-3) and clonidine infusion[10,139]; an increase in α_2-receptor density exclusively within the PVN[44]; a sharp unimodal peak in circulating CORT[55]; a release of medial hypothalamic NE in association with eating[98,132,143]; a natural increase in meal size, rate of eating, and preference for a specific nutrient, namely, carbohydrate.[12,63,141]

Serotonin

After the consumption of the initial carbohydrate meal, there possibly occurs a rise in circulating levels of the amino acid tryptophan, an essential precursor for the synthesis of 5-HT.[29,152] With in-creased 5-HT synthesis in the hypothalamus, NE activity in the PVN should be inhibited, followed by the development of normal satiety for carbohydrate. In support of this idea is evidence described earlier that 5-HT, similar to NE, is most active at the start of the nocturnal cycle in controlling the ingestion of carbohydrate. Studies have shown that the first carbohydrate meal of the active period[141] is strongly inhibited by direct injection of 5-HT into the PVN (see Fig. 15-1), as well as by the serotonergic drugs DF or its active metabolite DNF.[80,86,119,147,148] In contrast, carbohydrate-rich meals later in the cycle, as well as protein- or fat-rich meals at any time, are minimally affected by serotonergic stimulation. Microdialysis studies support the proposal that endogenous serotonergic activity within the PVN peaks during the initial phase of the natural feeding cycle.[133]

In addition to reducing appetite for carbohydrate, 5-HT may play a role in switching the animals' preference toward protein. Protein is frequently the nutrient of choice during the second meal of the natural feeding cycle.[141] Moreover, some studies have actually demonstrated an increase in appetite for protein after central[86,147,148] and peripheral[94,151,152] administration of serotonergic stimulants. The opposite effect, a decrease in appetite for protein, also occurs after endogenous 5-HT has been depleted.[4] Thus, during the early stages of the natural feeding cycle, hypothalamic 5-HT appears to be physiologically active in balancing the ratio of carbohydrate to protein, perhaps in relation to the body's immediate energy requirements and need to replenish nutrient stores.

Neuropeptide Y

With regard to the role of NPY in modulating natural feeding patterns, it is proposed that this peptide, as a cotransmitter with NE in the PVN, becomes activated to stimulate carbohydrate intake specifically under conditions when energy stores are most depleted by an extended period of little eating. This may occur either after a period of food deprivation or, more naturally, at the end of the inactive, light period. The strongest evidence in support of this idea is the finding (Fig. 15-4) that NPY levels, in the parvocellular

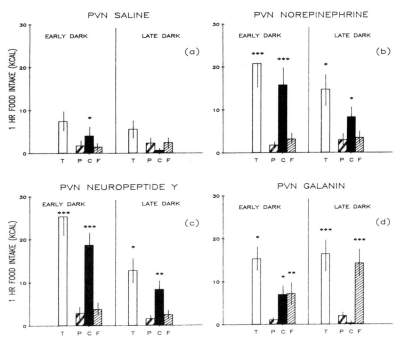

FIGURE 15-3

Macronutrient selection patterns after PVN injection of saline, NE, NPY, or GAL during the early and late dark periods of the nocturnal cycle. Relative to saline baseline scores, PVN NE and NPY produce a greater increase in total food intake and carbohydrate intake in the early dark period relative to the late dark period. PVN GAL enhances both carbohydrate and fat intake at the onset of dark, whereas at the end of the dark only fat ingestion is increased. (*$P < 0.05$; **$P < 0.01$; ***$P < 0.001$) (Temple DL, Leibowitz SF: Diurnal variations in the feeding responses to norepinephrine, neuropeptide Y and galanin in the PVN. Brain Res Bull 25:821, 1990)

region of the PVN as well as the arcuate and suprachiasmatic nuclei, peak just before the start of the active feeding cycle.[38] Moreover, PVN injection of NPY, like NE, is most effective in producing the carbohydrate feeding response at the start of the dark cycle (see Fig. 15-3), when the density of PVN α_2 receptors and the rats' natural carbohydrate preference also peak; in contrast, it is least effective later in the nocturnal period, when there is a sharp decline in both the α_2 receptors and carbohydrate consumption.[68,70,139] It is also relevant that NPY injected into the PVN stimulates the release of CORT,[81,144] which as mentioned earlier normally rises toward the onset of the dark cycle.[55] In fact, the action of NPY in stimulating feeding is dependent on high levels of circulating CORT.[48,129]

In addition to the nocturnal peak of hypothalamic NPY in relation to the onset of natural feeding, this peptide also appears to respond to the state of energy depletion that develops after environmentally imposed periods of food deprivation. Several studies have demonstrated that deprivation causes an increase in hypothalamic NPY content[7,112] and mRNA for NPY.[22,113] This increase in NPY occurs specifically in the PVN and arcuate nucleus, where NPY levels are found to rise just before the onset of the natural feeding cycle and then sharply decline after a brief episode of food ingestion.[38] This evidence suggests

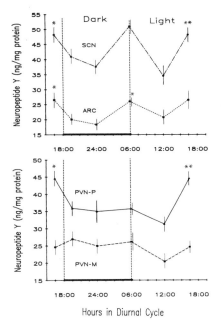

FIGURE 15-4

Diurnal rhythms of neuropeptide Y (NPY) concentration in the suprachiasmatic nucleus (SCN), arcuate nucleus (ARC), and parvocellular (PVN-P) and magnocellular (PVN-M) subdivisions of the paraventricular nucleus of the rat hypothalamus. (*$P < 0.05$; **$P < 0.01$; ***$P < 0.001$, as compared with values at preceding and succeeding time points) (Jhanwar-Uniyal M, Beck B, Burlet C et al: Diurnal rhythm of neuropeptide Y-like immunoreactivity in the suprachiasmatic, arcuate and paraventricular nuclei and other hypothalamic sites. Brain Res 536:331, 1990)

that NPY may mediate the preferential increase in carbohydrate and fat ingestion that occurs in response to food deprivation.[116,141]

Galanin

Studies with the peptide GAL implicate this potential neurotransmitter in the regulation of fat intake during the nocturnal cycle, perhaps in addition to carbohydrate intake specifically at the beginning of the feeding cycle.[72,139] As described earlier, studies with GAL injection into the PVN demonstrate that this peptide acts similarly to NE early in the active cycle, when both neurotransmitters stimulate the ingestion of carbohydrate (see Fig. 15-3) and act in cooperation to

control natural preference for this nutrient, as well as metabolic processes for replenishing circulating glucose levels.[70,72] In addition, however, GAL appears to act differently later in the active cycle, when it loses its capacity to potentiate carbohydrate ingestion and instead strongly stimulates the ingestion of fat (see Fig. 15-3). This effect on fat preference, which occurs independently of NE, can be observed throughout the dark cycle, although it is most potent and selective during the later portion of the dark period, when fat is naturally preferred.[141]

Thus, it is clear that appetite for the different nutrients changes across the natural feeding cycle and that various brain neurochemicals exhibit simultaneous temporal shifts in activity, possibly reflecting their role in the control of these natural appetites. It is very likely that other neurotransmitters, besides the monoamines, NPY, and GAL, are involved in this process. For example, one set of neurotransmitters that may influence the increase in protein and fat intake toward the end of the active cycle may be the opiate peptides, which act through different types of receptors (μ, δ, and κ) to stimulate food intake.[69,83,104] Microinjections of these peptides into the hypothalamus potentiate the rats' preference specifically for fat and protein. Similar effects are observed with systemic injections of the opiate agonists, whereas the opposite may occur with administration of the opiate antagonists naloxone and naltrexone. As described earlier, the catecholamine DA may also be involved in controlling fat and protein ingestion, which is inhibited by lateral hypothalamic injection of this amine.[79]

RELATIONSHIP BETWEEN BRAIN NEUROTRANSMITTERS AND BODY WEIGHT GAIN

In addition to modulating eating patterns and appetite for specific macronutrients, brain neurotransmitters, perhaps in conjunction with circulating peptide and steroid hormones, also appear to affect energy metabolism and body weight gain, in some cases leading to the development of obesity. Central infusion studies have revealed an increase in body weight with chronic administration of NE and clonidine into the PVN.[95,154]

This effect is strongest under conditions when the animals are given a single, mixed diet. With pure macronutrients, a smaller change in body weight occurs, as the subjects are allowed to overeat selectively their preferred diet (*i.e.,* carbohydrate) while maintaining a relatively stable total calorie intake by consuming less of the other nutrients, in particular, protein. In a separate study,[115] NE was chronically infused into the ventromedial hypothalamus and found to produce a stronger increase in body weight than it did in the PVN. This finding suggests that the ventromedial hypothalamic area may be more involved in controlling body weight gain, whereas the PVN acts to coordinate patterns of nutrient ingestion.[68]

Infusions of NPY into the PVN, however, have been shown to have the most potent stimulatory effect on body weight (Fig. 15-5).[124,128] In fact, the magnitude of this effect on weight gain exceeded what would be expected on the basis of the hyperphagia produced by NPY. This result suggests

that chronic NPY stimulation may, in fact, enhance the deposition of fat, in addition to potentiating consumption of energy-rich foods.

Studies examining the effect of NPY on energy metabolism have provided data that support this suggestion and also that further differentiate the actions of this peptide from those of the coexisting NE. When injected into the PVN, NE has been shown to reduce energy expenditure, independently of its effect on activity level.[123] Experiments demonstrate that PVN injection of NPY, in contrast to NE, has no effect on energy expenditure or activity level.[101] However, it has a potent stimulatory effect on respiratory quotient (Fig. 15-6), which increases in latency with increase in dose. This increase in respiratory quotient suggests that NPY potentiates fat synthesis preferentially from carbohydrate. This diversion of metabolism toward carbohydrate utilization and lipogenesis may be related to the preferential stimulatory effect of NPY on carbohydrate ingestion,[126] as well as to the finding that chronic NPY

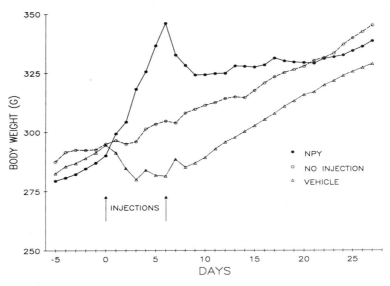

FIGURE 15-5

Body weights of three groups of female rats before, during, and after PVN injections of either NPY, vehicle, or no injection. (Stanley BG, Anderson KC, Grayson MH et al: Repeated hypothalamic stimulation with neuropeptide Y increases daily carbohydrate and fat intake and body weight gain in female rats. Physiol Behav 46:173, 1989)

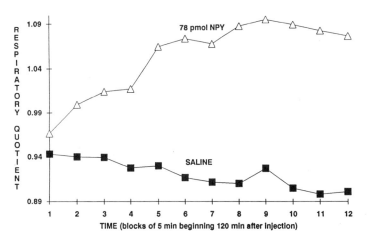

FIGURE 15-6

Mean respiratory quotient (5-minute blocks) over a 60-minute test period beginning 2 hours after PVN injection of either saline or NPY. (Menendez JA, McGregor IS, Healey PA et al: Metabolic effects of neuropeptide Y injections into the paraventricular nucleus of the hypothalamus. Brain Res 516:8, 1990)

injection has a potent effect on fat deposition and body weight, greater than would be predicted from its hyperphagic effect.[128,129] These findings agree with evidence showing ventricular NPY administration to promote white fat lipid storage while decreasing brown fat thermogenesis[11] and to reduce energy expenditure by controlling sympathetic activity to interscapular brown adipose tissue.[28]

In addition to these studies with NPY, other investigations have linked α_2-noradrenergic receptor sites in discrete hypothalamic nuclei to patterns of daily food intake and body weight gain.[39] This link has been demonstrated in rats exposed for 6 weeks to a high-fat diet, which caused variable changes in body weight in individual rats, ranging from low to severe levels of obesity. Analyses of hypothalamic α_2 receptors in these subjects indicated a significant increase in receptor number in the PVN of moderately and severely obese rats (Fig. 15-7) and also in the dorsomedial nucleus of severely obese rats, compared with dietary-resistant and chow-fed rats. No change in the density of α_2 receptors in other hypothalamic areas was detected.

A similar study was performed in genetically obese Zucker rats, which, in addition to enhanced lipogenesis and body weight gain, exhibit impaired thermogenesis, altered circadian rhythms of CORT release, and aggravated hyperphagia with a preference for carbohydrate- and fat-rich foods.[15] These obese animals, relative to their lean littermates, are found to have a greater number of available α_2-receptor sites (see Fig. 15-7), specifically in the PVN.[39] They also exhibit higher levels of NPY content, in the PVN as well as the arcuate and suprachiasmatic nuclei,[6] in addition to raised levels of hypothalamic NPY mRNA, suggesting enhanced peptide synthesis.[113] This evidence, together with additional findings showing a positive relationship between circulating CORT and hypothalamic α_2 receptors (see Fig. 15-7) or NPY synthesis,[149] suggests that both of these neurochemical systems may contribute significantly to the development of the abnormal metabolic, endocrine, and behavioral patterns characteristic of these obese animals.

In rats maintained on a high-fat diet that can potentiate body weight without producing hyperphagia,[90] a similar increase in α_2 sites was detected in animals that developed obesity, compared with rats that were resistant to the diet and exhibited normal body weight gain. This effect was detected in the PVN, as well as in a number of other hypothalamic sites. Further studies by Levin[89] suggest that these changes may be a consequence rather than a cause of body weight gain, because they were not detected in younger animals that were believed to be prone to gain weight but had not yet exhibited the weight gain.

In our laboratory, two studies have been performed in young animals in an attempt to characterize developmental patterns of nutrient intake and to understand the relationship between eating behavior early in life and behavioral patterns that develop in adulthood.[96,118] Our knowl-

FIGURE 15-7

[³H] p-aminoclonidine binding to α₂-noradrenergic receptors in the paraventricular nucleus of rats that became moderate to severely obese when kept on a high-fat diet (*left panel*); of lean and genetically controlled obese Zucker rats (*middle panel*); and of rats receiving either sham adrenalectomy (ADX) + cholesterol implants, ADX + cholesterol, or ADX + CORT (*right panel*). (*$P < 0.05$; **$P < 0.01$; ***$P < 0.001$ for direct comparisons between experimental and control groups) (Jhanwar-Uniyal M, Grinker JA, Finkelstein JA et al: Hypothalamic α₂-noradrenergic receptor system relation to dietary, genetic, and hormonally induced obesity. Ann NY Acad Sci 575:613, 1989)

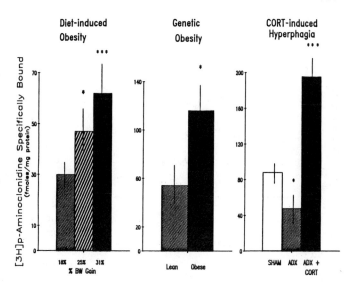

edge of this relationship is important, because several variables, including birth weight, rate of growth and development, and sex, may be predisposing factors in the development of certain eating and body weight disorders.

In these investigations, male and female Sprague-Dawley rats were maintained on pure macronutrient diets (protein, carbohydrate, and fat) since birth and were sacrificed at 77 days of age. The main findings of these studies were as follows: Body weight as early as 3 days of age, in male and female rats, is positively related specifically to preference for carbohydrate and sucrose after weaning and puberty (Table 15-2). Nutrient intake patterns at weaning closely reflect nutrient intake patterns at maturity (day 77). At puberty, females exhibit a strong preference for carbohydrate, whereas males prefer protein (Fig. 15-8). At maturity, body weight is strongly related to fat intake, appetite for sucrose, and blood levels of insulin. The density of α₂-noradrenergic receptor sites, in the PVN of female rats and dorsomedial nucleus of males rats, is positively related to total caloric intake, circulating levels of glucose, and body weight gain (see Table 15-2). Female rats, relative to male rats, demonstrate a higher density of 5-HT$_{1B}$ receptor sites in the PVN and greater responsiveness to the feeding-suppressive effect of serotonergic stimulants.[76]

These results reveal a close relationship between nutrient intake and appetite, body weight, circulating hormones, and neurotransmitter receptors in the hypothalamus. Taken together, the previous findings demonstrate that the α₂-noradrenergic and perhaps NPY receptors in the medial hypothalamus, known to have a role in the

TABLE 15-2

Correlations Between Body Weight, Nutrient Intake, and PVN α₂-Noradrenergic Receptors of Female Rats

Correlations Between Body Weight at Birth (Day 3) and Nutrient Intake After Puberty (Day 50)

Carbohydrate intake	r = + 0.65*
Sucrose intake	r = + 0.52*
Protein intake	r = + 0.37
Fat intake	r = + 0.24
Total kcal intake	r = + 0.08

Correlations Between PVN α₂-Noradrenergic Receptor Number and Physiological Measures at Maturity (Day 77)

Total kcal intake	r = + 0.78*
Blood glucose	r = + 0.74*
Body weight	r = + 0.67*

*$P < .05$

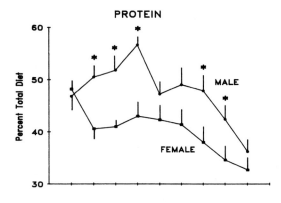

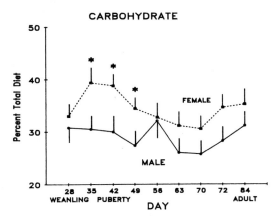

FIGURE 15-8

Preference for protein or carbohydrate (intake of either diet relative to total food intake) in freely feeding rats from weaning (day 21) to maturity (day 84). (*$P < 0.05$ for direct comparisons between scores of male and female rats)

control of energy intake as well as energy metabolism, exhibit dramatic changes in relation to dietary and genetic factors that are known to contribute to the onset and maintenance of obesity.

IMPLICATIONS FOR BRAIN NEUROTRANSMITTER CONTROL OF APPETITE IN HUMANS

In light of pharmacologic studies in animals and in humans[45,65,67,153] showing similar effects of antidepressants, antipsychotic agents, stimulants, and peptides on eating behavior, it is believed that the neurotransmitter systems just described

may to some extent act similarly in these different species to control food intake, appetite for specific nutrients, and body weight gain. It is clear from the available evidence that hypothalamic amines and peptides, in addition to circulating amino acids, glucose, and hormones, jointly participate in a complex network of systems that have distinct effects on patterns of eating behavior and metabolism of specific nutrients. Together with reports showing that medial and lateral hypothalamic damage in humans produces extremes of overeating and undereating similar to effects in animals, it is possible to consider that the pathogenesis of clinical eating disorders may, in part, involve specific disturbances in brain or hypothalamic neurochemical function.

This suggestion is consistent with studies that have detected abnormal concentrations of these neurotransmitters in the CSF of patients with anorexia nervosa or bulimia. For example, anorexic patients who have partially recovered their body weight exhibit a significantly reduced concentration of NE in CSF, in association with sustained behavioral abnormalities including disturbed appetite for calorically dense foods and abnormal recovery from episodes of food deprivation.[53,54] Furthermore, bulimia, a disorder characterized by compulsive eating but not necessarily obesity (because of self-indulged purging), has been associated with a disturbed release of brain 5-HT.[50-52] With reduced levels of 5-HT in the CSF, bulimic patients would be expected to exhibit the behaviors that they do, such as increasing meal size, particularly of energy-rich nutrients, and increasing the rate at which they consume these meals. Such a behavioral pattern may result from an overabundance of noradrenergic activation as a result of reduced activity of the central serotonergic system.

Studies of the pathophysiology of eating disorders have also detected in bulimic patients disturbances in CSF content of peptide YY (PYY), a pancreatic polypeptide closely related to NPY.[8,49] In particular, a dramatic increase in CSF PYY was detected in bulimic patients who had abstained from bingeing. This finding led to the proposal that bulimic patients, when they initiate a binge, may be responding to heightened levels of PYY.

Further evidence suggests a relationship between hypothalamic NPY, the onset of puberty, and the transition toward development of adult eating patterns in young females. It has been demonstrated that immunoreactive NPY content in the rat hypothalamus rises steadily from birth to the onset of puberty.[135] Moreover, a sharp rise in hypophysial-portal levels of NPY occurs only in female rats on the day of puberty onset, immediately before the prepubertal surge in luteinizing hormone secretion. Studies of feeding behavior in pubescent rats[118] indicate that female rats exhibit a natural rise in preference for carbohydrate at this time, in contrast to the preference for protein exhibited by male rats (see Fig. 15-8). It is possible that these simultaneous behavioral and endocrine events are related, because central injection of NPY induces luteinizing hormone secretion[47] and preferentially stimulates carbohydrate ingestion.[126] Furthermore, food deprivation increases NPY content within the PVN[7,112] while producing a strong increase in preference for carbohydrate and fat.

It is of interest that anorexia nervosa, a disturbance in appetite for energy-rich foods, occurs predominantly in females, most often around the time of puberty and as a consequence of dieting and malnutrition.[121] Moreover, CSF levels of NPY are altered in anorexic patients before and after weight restoration.[49] It is possible that abnormal peptide activity in anorexia nervosa may provide the link between disturbed appetite and menstrual function, as well as contribute to the vicious cycle characteristic of this eating disorder. In view of the link established between hypothalamic NPY and circulating CORT[81,129,144] or glucose,[111] any disturbances in such hormones or nutrients in the blood may be expected to alter the activity of the peptides, as well as the monoamines, in the brain and consequently produce changes in eating patterns and appetite for the different nutrients.

In light of the experimental evidence obtained in animals, the mentioned human studies of brain neurotransmitter systems suggest that disturbances in the monoamines, peptides, and their receptors may to some extent underlie these clinical disorders of eating behavior, energy metabolism, and body weight regulation. Further investigation is needed to determine to what extent these neurochemical abnormalities are a cause rather than a product of these disorders, and also

to evaluate the relationship between these changes in appetite and body weight and an array of emotional symptoms characteristic of eating disorders.

Acknowledgment: This research was supported by a grant from the National Institute of Mental Health, MH 43422.

References

1. Aravich PF, Saclfani A: Paraventricular hypothalamic lesions and medial hypothalamic knife cuts produce similar hyperphagia syndromes. Behav Neurosci 97:970, 1983
2. Armstrong S: A chronometric approach to the study of feeding behavior. Neurosci Biobehav Rev 4:27, 1980
3. Ashley DV, Barclay DV, Chauffard F et al: Plasma amino acid responses in humans to evening meals of differing nutritional composition. Am J Clin Nutr 36:143, 1982
4. Ashley DVM, Coscina DV, Anderson GH: Selective decrease in protein intake following brain serotonin depletion. Life Sci 24:973, 1977
5. Ashley DVM, Liardon R, Leathwood PD: Breakfast meal composition influences plasma typtophan to large neural amino acid ratios of healthy lean young men. J Neural Transm 63:271, 1985
6. Beck B, Burlet A, Nicolas JP et al: Hypothalamic neuropeptide Y (NPY) in obese Zucker rats: Implications in feeding and sexual behaviors. Physiol Behav 47:449, 1990
7. Beck B, Jhanwar-Uniyal M, Burlet A et al: Rapid and localized alterations of neuropeptide Y (NPY) in discrete hypothalamic nuclei with feeding status. Brain Res 528:245, 1990
8. Berrettini WH, Kaye WH, Gwirtsman H et al: Cerebrospinal fluid peptide YY immunoreactivity in eating disorders. Neuropsychobiology 19:121, 1988
9. Bhakthavatsalam P, Leibowitz SF: Morphine-elicited feeding: Diurnal rhythm, circulating corticosterone and macronutrient selection. Pharmacol Biochem Behav 24:911, 1986
10. Bhakthavatsalam P, Leibowitz SF: α_2-Noradrenergic feeding rhythm in paraventricular nucleus: Relation to corticosterone. Am J Physiol 250:1283, 1986
11. Billington CJ, Briggs JE, Levine AS: Effects of intracerebroventricular injection of neuropeptide Y on energy metabolism. Am J Physiol 260:R321-R327, 1991

12. Blundell JE: Problems and processes underlying the control of food selection and nutrient intake. In Wurtman RJ, Wurtman JJ (eds): Nutrition and the Brain, pp. 163–222. New York, Raven Press, 1983

13. Blundell JE: Serotonin and appetite. Neuropharmacology 23:1537, 1984

14. Borsini F, Bendotti C, Przewlocka B et al: Monoamine involvement in overeating caused by muscimol injection in the rat nucleus raphe dorsalis and the effects of D-fenfluramine and D-amphetamine. Eur J Pharmacol 94:109, 1983

15. Bray GA: Genetic and hypothalamic mechanisms for obesity: Finding the needle in the haystack. Am J Clin Nutr 50:891, 1989

16. Campfield LA, Brandon P, Smith FJ: On-line continuous measurement of blood glucose and meal pattern in free-feeding rats: The role of glucose in meal initiation. Brain Res Bull 14:605, 1985

17. Campfield LA, Smith FJ: Functional coupling between transient declines in blood glucose and feeding behavior: Temporal relationships. Brain Res Bull 17:427, 1986

18. Carruba MO, Mantegazza P, Memo M et al: Peripheral and central mechanisms of action of serotonergic anorectic drugs. Appetite 7:105, 1986

19. Castonguay TW, Dallman MF, Stern JS: Some metabolic and behavioral effects of adrenalectomy on obese Zucker rats. Am J Physiol 251:R923, 1986

20. Chafetz MD, Parko K, Diaz S et al: Relationship between medial hypothalamic α_2 receptor binding, norepinephrine, and circulating glucose. Brain Res 384:404, 1986

21. Cheung WK, Dietz CB, Alexander J et al: α_2-Noradrenergic receptor agonists and antagonists have opposite effects on carbohydrate and protein ingestion in the rat. Soc Neurosci Abstr 16:910, 1990

22. Chua SC, Leibel RL, Hirsch J: Food deprivation and age modulate neuropeptide gene expression in the murine hypothalamus and adrenal gland. Mol Brain Res 9:95, 1991

23. Clark JT, Kalra PS, Crowley WR et al: Neuropeptide Y and human pancreatic polypeptide stimulate feeding behavior in rats. Endocrinology 115:427, 1984

24. Curzon G: Serotonin and appetite. Ann NY Acad Sci 600:521, 1990

25. DeCastro JM: Circadian rhythms of the spontaneous meal pattern, macronutrient intake, and mood of humans. Physiol Behav 40:437, 1987

26. De Jong A, Strubbe JH, Steffens AB: Hypothalamic influence on insulin and glucagon release in the rat. Am J Physiol 233:E380, 1977

27. Devenport L, Knehans A, Thomas T et al: Macronutrient intake and utilization by rats: Interactions with type I adrenocorticoid receptor stimulation. Am J Physiol 260:R73-R81, 1991

28. Egawa M, Yoshimatsu H, Bray GA: Neuropeptide Y (NPY) suppresses sympathetic activity to interscapular brown adipose tissue in rats. Am J Physiol 260:R328-R334, 1991

29. Fernstrom JD: Dietary effects on brain serotonin synthesis: Relationship to appetite regulation. Am J Clin Nutr 42:1072, 1985

30. Fernstrom JD, Faller DV: Neutral amino acids in the brain: Changes in response to food ingestion. J Neurochem 30:1531, 1978

31. Fuxe K, Agnati LF, Harfstrand A et al: Morphofunctional studies on the neuropeptide Y/adrenaline costoring terminal systems in the dorsal cardiovascular region of the medulla oblongata. Focus on receptor-receptor interactions in cotransmission. Prog Brain Res 68:303, 1986

32. Galzin AM, Moret C, Langer SZ: Evidence that exogenous but not endogenous norepinephrine activates the presynaptic alpha-2 adrenal receptors on serotonergic nerve endings in the rat hypothalamus. J Pharmacol Exp Ther 228:725, 1984

33. Garattini S: Effects of D-fenfluramine on eating disorders. In Ferrari E, Brambilla F (eds): Advances in the Biosciences, Vol 60, pp 327–341. London, Pergamon Press, 1986

34. Garattini S, Mennini T, Bendotti C et al: Neurochemical mechanism of action of drugs which modify feeding via the serotonergic system. Appetite (Suppl) 7:15, 1986

35. Goldman CK, Marino L, Leibowitz SF: Postsynaptic α_2-noradrenergic receptors mediate feeding induced by paraventricular nucleus injection of norepinephrine and clonidine. Eur J Pharmacol 115:11, 1985

36. Hoebel BG, Hernandez L, Mark GP et al: Brain microdialysis as a molecular approach to obesity: Serotonin, dopamine, cyclic-AMP. In Bray G, Ricquier D, Spiegleman B (eds): Obesity: Toward a Molecular Approach. UCLA Symposia on Molecular and Cellular Biology New Series, Vol 132, Wiley-Liss Inc, New York, pp 45–61, 1990

37. Inokuchi A, Oomura Y, Nishimura H: Effect of intracerebroventricularly infused glucagon on feeding behavior. Physiol Behav 33:397, 1984

38. Jhanwar-Uniyal M, Beck B, Burlet C et al: Diurnal rhythm of neuropeptide Y-like immunoreactivity in the suprachiasmatic, arcuate and paraventricular nuclei and other hypothalamic sites. Brain Res 536:331, 1990

39. Jhanwar-Uniyal M, Grinker JA, Finkelstein JA et al: Hypothalamic α_2-noradrenergic receptor sys-

tem relation to dietary, genetic, and hormonally induced obesity. Ann NY Acad Sci 575:613, 1989

40. Jhanwar-Uniyal M, Leibowitz SF: Impact of food deprivation on α_1- and α_2-noradrenergic receptors in the paraventricular nucleus and other hypothalamic areas. Brain Res Bull 17:889, 1986

41. Jhanwar-Uniyal M, Leibowitz SF: Impact of circulating corticosterone on α_1- and α_2-noradrenergic receptors in discrete brain areas. Brain Res 368:404, 1986

42. Jhanwar-Uniyal M, Papamichael MJ, Leibowitz SF: Glucose-dependent changes in α_2-noradrenergic receptors in hypothalamic nuclei. Physiol Behav 44:611, 1988

43. Jhanwar-Uniyal M, Renner KJ, Bailo MT et al: Corticosterone-dependent alterations in utilization of catecholamines in discrete areas of rat brain. Brain Res 500:247, 1989

44. Jhanwar-Uniyal M, Roland CR, Leibowitz SF: Diurnal rhythm of α_2-noradrenergic receptors in the paraventricular nucleus and other brain areas: Relation to circulating corticosterone and feeding behavior. Life Sci 38:473, 1986

45. Johnson C, Stuckey M, Mitchell J: Psychopharmacological treatment of anorexia nervosa and bulimia. J Nerv Ment Dis 171:524, 1983

46. Kalra SP, Clark JT, Sahu A et al: Control of feeding and sexual behaviors by neuropeptide Y: Physiological implications. Synapse 2:254, 1988

47. Kalra SP, Crowley WR: Norepinephrine-like effects of neuropeptide Y on LH release in the rat. Life Sci 35:1173, 1984

48. Kalra SP, Dube MG, Kalra PS: Continuous intraventricular infusion of neuropeptide Y evokes episodic food intake in satiated female rats: Effects of adrenalectomy and cholecystokinin. Peptides 9:723, 1988

49. Kaye WH, Berrettini W, Gwirtsman H et al: Altered cerebrospinal fluid neuropeptide Y and peptide YY immunoreactivity in anorexia and bulimia nervosa. Arch Gen Psychiatry 47:548, 1990

50. Kaye WH, Ebert MH, Gwirtsman HE et al: Differences in brain serotonergic metabolism between nonbulimic and bulimic patients with anorexia nervosa. Am J Psychiatry 141:1598, 1984

51. Kaye WH, Gwirtsman HE, Brewerton TD et al: Bingeing behavior and plasma amino acids: A possible involvement of brain serotonin in bulimia nervosa. Psychiatry Res 23:31, 1988

52. Kaye WH, Gwirtsman HE, George DT et al: Altered feeding behavior in bulimia: Is it related to mood and serotonin? In Walsh BT (ed): Eating Behavior in Eating Disorders, Vol 13, pp 201–216. Washington, DC, American Psychiatric Press, 1988

53. Kaye WH, Gwirtsman HE, Jimerson DC et al: Catecholamine function in anorexia nervosa at low weight and after weight restoration. In Progress in Catecholamine Research, Part C: Clinical Aspects, pp 355–361. New York, Alan R Liss, 1988

54. Kaye WH, Jimerson DC, Lake CR et al: Altered norepinephrine metabolism following long-term weight recovery in patients with anorexia nervosa. Psychiatry Res 14:333, 1985

55. Krieger DT, Hauser H: Comparison of synchronization of circadian corticosteroid rhythms by photoperiod and food. Proc Natl Acad Sci 75:1577, 1978

56. Kumar BA, Leibowitz SF: Impact of acute corticosterone administration on feeding and macronutrient self-selection patterns. Am J Physiol 254:R222, 1988

57. Kumar BA, Papamichael M, Leibowitz SF: Feeding and macronutrient selection patterns in rats: Adrenalectomy and chronic corticosterone replacement. Pharmacol Biochem Behav 42:581, 1988

58. Kyrkouli SE, Seirafi RD, Stanley BG et al: Paraventricular hypothalamic lesions attenuate galanin-induced feeding. Proc Eastern Psychol Assoc 60:24, 1989

59. Kyrkouli SE, Stanley BG, Hutchinson R et al: Peptide-amine interactions in the hypothalamic paraventricular nucleus: Analysis of galanin and neuropeptide Y in relation to feeding. Brain Res 521:185, 1990

60. Kyrkouli SE, Stanley BG, Leibowitz SF: Galanin: Stimulation of feeding induced by medial hypothalamic injection of this novel peptide. Eur J Pharmacol 122:159, 1986

61. Kyrkouli SE, Stanley BG, Leibowitz SF: Galanin increases extracellular norepinephrine in the paraventricular hypothalamus as measured by microdialysis. Soc Neurosci Abstr 14:614, 1988

62. Kyrkouli SE, Stanley BG, Seirafi RD et al: Stimulation of feeding by galanin: Anatomical localization and behavioral specificity of this peptide's effects in the brain. Peptides 11:995, 1990

63. Leathwood PD, Arimanana R: Circadian rhythms of food intake and protein selection in young and old rats. Annu Rev Chronopharm 1:255, 1984

64. Leibowitz SF: Paraventricular nucleus: A primary site mediating adrenergic stimulation of feeding and drinking. Pharmacol Biochem Behav 8:163, 1978

65. Leibowitz SF: Neurochemical systems of the hypothalamus: Control of feeding and drinking behavior and water-electrolyte excretion. In Morgane PJ, Panksepp J (eds): Handbook of the

Hypothalamus, pp. 299–437. New York, Marcel Dekker, 1980

66. Leibowitz SF: Brain monoamines and peptides: Role in the control of eating behavior. Fed Proc 45:1396, 1986

67. Leibowitz SF: Hypothalamic neurotransmitters in relation to normal and disturbed eating patterns. Ann NY Acad Sci 499:137, 1987

68. Leibowitz SF: Hypothalamic paraventricular nucleus: Interaction between α_2-noradrenergic system and circulating hormones and nutrients in relation to energy balance. Neurosci Biobehav Rev 12:101, 1988

69. Leibowitz SF: Opioid, α_2-noradrenergic and adrenocorticotropin systems of hypothalamic paraventricular nucleus. In Weiner H, Baum A (eds): Perspectives in Behavioral Medicine, Eating Regulation and Discontrol, pp 113–135. Hillsdale, New Jersey, Lawrence Erlbaum, 1988

70. Leibowitz SF: Hypothalamic neuropeptide Y, galanin and amines: Concept of coexistence in relation to feeding behavior. Ann NY Acad Sci 575:221, 1989

71. Leibowitz SF: The role of serotonin in eating disorders. Drugs (Suppl 3) 39:33, 1990

72. Leibowitz SF: Hypothalamic galanin in relation to feeding behavior and endocrine systems. In Hokfelt T, Bartfai T (eds): Galanin: A New Multifunctional Peptide in the Neuro-Endocrine System. New York, Macmillan, 1991

73. Leibowitz SF, Brown O, Tretter JR et al: Norepinephrine, clonidine, and tricyclic antidepressants selectively stimulate carbohydrate ingestion through noradrenergic system of the paraventricular nucleus. Pharmacol Biochem Behav 23:541, 1985

74. Leibowitz SF, Diaz S, Tempel D: Norepinephrine in the paraventricular nucleus stimulates corticosterone release. Brain Res 496:219, 1989

75. Leibowitz SF, Hammer NJ, Chang K: Hypothalamic paraventricular nucleus lesions produce overeating and obesity in the rat. Physiol Behav 27:1031, 1981

76. Leibowitz SF, Jhanwar-Uniyal M: 5-HT$_{1A}$ and 5-HT$_{1B}$ receptor binding sites in discrete hypothalamic nuclei: Relation to circadian rhythm and gender. Soc Neurosci Abstr 16:294, 1990

77. Leibowitz SF, Roland CR, Hor L et al: Noradrenergic feeding elicited by the paraventricular nucleus is dependent upon circulating corticosterone. Physiol Behav 32:857, 1984

78. Leibowitz SF, Shor-Posner G: Hypothalamic monoamine systems for control of food intake: Analysis of meal patterns and macronutrient selection. In Carruba MO, Blundell J (eds): Pharmacology of Eating Disorders: Theoretical and Clinical Developments, pp. 29–49. New York, Raven Press, 1986

79. Leibowitz SF, Shor-Posner G, MacLow C et al: Amphetamine: Effects on meal patterns and macronutrient selection. Brain Res Bull 17:681, 1986

80. Leibowitz SF, Shor-Posner G, Weiss GF: Serotonin in medial hypothalamic nuclei controls circadian patterns of macronutrient intake. In Paoletti R, Vanhoutte PM (eds): Serotonin: From Cell Biology to Pharmacology and Therapeutics, pp 203–211. Netherlands, Kluwer Academic Publishers, 1990

81. Leibowitz SF, Sladek C, Spencer L et al: Neuropeptide Y, epinephrine and norepinephrine in the paraventricular nucleus: Stimulation of feeding and the release of corticosterone, vasopressin and glucose. Brain Res Bull 21:905, 1988

82. Leibowitz SF, Stanley BG: Brain peptides and the control of eating behavior. In Moody TW (ed): Neural and Endocrine Peptides and Receptors, pp 333–352. New York, Plenum, 1986

83. Leibowitz SF, Stanley BG: Neurochemical controls of appetite. In Ritter R, Ritter S (eds): Feeding Behavior: Neural and Humoral Controls, pp 191–234. New York, Academic Press, 1986

84. Leibowitz SF, Weiss GF, Shor-Posner G: Hypothalamic serotonin: Pharmacological, biochemical, and behavioral analyses of its feeding-suppressive action. Clin Neuropharmacol (Suppl) 11:s51, 1988

85. Leibowitz SF, Weiss GF, Suh JS: Medial hypothalamic nuclei mediate serotonin's inhibitory effect on feeding behavior. Pharmacol Biochem Behav 37:735, 1990

86. Leibowitz SF, Weiss GF, Walsh UA et al: Medial hypothalamic serotonin: Role in circadian patterns of feeding and macronutrient selection. Brain Res 503:132, 1989

87. Leibowitz SF, Weiss GF, Yee F et al: Noradrenergic innervation of the paraventricular nucleus: Specific role in the control of carbohydrate ingestion. Brain Res Bull 14:561, 1985

88. LeMagnen J: The metabolic basis of dual periodicity feeding in rats. Behav Brain Sci 4:561, 1981

89. Levin BE: Obesity-prone and -resistant rats differ in their brain 3H-paraminoclonidine binding. Brain Res 512:54, 1990

90. Levin BE: Increased brain 3H-paraminoclonidine (α_2-adrenoceptor) binding associated with perpetuation of diet-induced obesity in rats. Int J Obes 14:689, 1990

91. Levine AJ, Morley JE: Neuropeptide Y: A potent inducer of consummatory behavior in rats. Peptides 5:1025, 1984

92. Li ETS, Anderson GH: Meal composition influences subsequent food selection in the young rat. Physiol Behav 29:779, 1982

93. Li ETS, Anderson GH: Amino acids in the regulation of food intake. Nutr Abstr Rev Clin Nutr 53:169, 1983

94. Li ETS, Anderson GH: 5-Hydroxytryptamine: A modulator of food composition but not quantity? Life Sci 34:2453, 1984

95. Lichtenstein SS, Marinescu C, Leibowitz SF: Chronic infusion of norepinephrine and clonidine into the hypothalamic paraventricular nucleus. Pharmacol Biochem Behav 13:591, 1984

96. Lucas DJ, Jhanwar-Uniyal M, Leibowitz K et al: Developmental patterns of nutrient intake, specific appetites and body weight: Relation to hypothalamic α_2-noradrenergic receptor sites and circulating levels of glucose and insulin. Neuroscience Abstr 16:910, 1990

97. Majeed NH, Lason W, Przewlocka B et al: Differential modulation of the beta-endorphin and dynorphin systems by serotonergic stimulation in the rat. Neuropeptides 5:563, 1984

98. Martin GE, Myers RD: Evoked release of [^{14}C]norepinephrine from the rat hypothalamus during feeding. Am J Physiol 229:1547, 1975

99. McCaleb ML, Myers RD, Singer G et al: Hypothalamic norepinephrine in the rat during feeding and push-pull perfusion with glucose, 2-DG, or insulin. Am J Physiol 236:312, 1978

100. Melander T, Fuxe K, Harfstrand A et al: Effects of intraventricular injections of galanin on neuroendocrine functions in the male rat: Possible involvement of hypothalamic catecholamine neuronal systems. Acta Physiol Scand 131:25, 1987

101. Menendez JA, McGregor IS, Healey PA et al: Metabolic effects of neuropeptide Y injections into the paraventricular nucleus of the hypothalamus. Brain Res 516:8, 1990

102. Moller SE: Effects of various oral protein doses on plasma neutral amino acid levels. J Neural Transm 61:183, 1985

103. Morley JE, Levine AS, Gosnell BA et al: Peptides as central regulators of feeding. Brain Res Bull 14:511, 1985

104. Morley JE, Levine AS, Yim GK et al: Opioid modulation of appetite. Neurosci Biobehav Rev 7:281, 1983

105. Muller EE, Cocchi D, Mantegazza P: Brain adrenergic system in the response induced by 2-deoxy-D-glucose. Am J Physiol 223:945, 1972

106. Myers RD, McCaleb ML: Feeding: Satiety signals from intestine trigger brain's noradrenergic mechanism. Science 209:1035, 1980

107. O'Donohue TL, Chronwall BM, Pruss RM et al: Neuropeptide Y and peptide YY neuronal and endocrine systems. Peptides 6:755, 1985

108. Pernow J: Co-release and functional interactions of neuropeptide Y and noradrenaline in peripheral sympathetic vascular control. Acta Physiol Scand (Suppl) 568:1, 1988

109. Rogacki N, Weiss GR, Fueg A et al: Impact of hypothalamic serotonin on macronutrient intake. Ann NY Acad Sci 575:619, 1989

110. Roland RC, Bhakthavatsalam P, Leibowitz SF: Interaction between corticosterone and α_2-noradrenergic system of the paraventricular nucleus in relation to feeding behavior. Neuroendocrinology 42:296, 1986

111. Rowland NE: Peripheral and central satiety factors in neuropeptide Y-induced feeding in rats. Peptides 9:989, 1988

112. Sahu A, Kalra PS, Kalra SP: Food deprivation and ingestion induce reciprocal changes in neuropeptide Y concentrations in the paraventricular nucleus. Peptides 9:83, 1988

113. Sanacora G, Kershaw M, Finkelstein JA et al: Increased hypothalamic content of preproneuropeptide Y messenger ribonucleic acid in genetically obese Zucker rats and its regulation by food deprivation. Endocrinology 127:730, 1990

114. Sawchenko PE, Gold RM, Leibowitz SF: Evidence for vagal involvement in the eating elicited by adrenergic stimulation of the paraventricular nucleus. Brain Res 225:249, 1981

115. Shimazu T, Noma M, Saito M: Chronic infusion of norepinephrine into the ventromedial hypothalamus induces obesity in rats. Brain Res 369:215, 1986

116. Shor-Posner G, Azar AP, Insinga S et al: Deficits in the control of food intake after hypothalamic paraventricular nucleus lesions. Physiol Behav 35:883, 1985

117. Shor-Posner G, Azar AP, Jhanwar-Uniyal M et al: Destruction of noradrenergic innervation to the paraventricular nucleus: Deficits in food intake, macronutrient selection, and compensatory eating after food deprivation. Pharmacol Biochem Behav 25:381, 1986

118. Shor-Posner G, Brennan G, Jasaitis R et al: Developmental patterns of eating behavior. Ann NY Acad Sci 575:622, 1989

119. Shor-Posner G, Grinker JA, Marinescu C et al: Hypothalamic serotonin in the control of meal patterns and macronutrient selection. Brain Res Bull 17:663, 1986

120. Shor-Posner G, Grinker JA, Marinescu C et al: Role of hypothalamic norepinephrine in control of meal patterns. Physiol Behav 35:209, 1985

121. Silverman JA: Anorexia nervosa: clinical and

metabolic observations. Int J Eating Disorders 2:159, 1983

122. Silverstone T, Goodall E: Serotonergic mechanisms in human feeding: The pharmacological evidence. Appetite (Suppl)7:85, 1986

123. Siviy SM, Kritikos A, Atrens DM et al: Effects of norepinephrine infused in the paraventricular hypothalamus on energy expenditure in the rat. Brain Res 487:79, 1989

124. Stanley BG, Anderson KC, Grayson MH et al: Repeated hypothalamic stimulation with neuropeptide Y increases daily carbohydrate and fat intake and body weight gain in female rats. Physiol Behav 46:173, 1989

125. Stanley BG, Chin AS, Leibowitz SF: Feeding and drinking elicited by central injection of neuropeptide Y: Evidence for a hypothalamic site(s) of action. Brain Res Bull 14:521, 1985

126. Stanley BG, Daniel DR, Chin AS et al: Paraventricular nucleus injections of peptide YY and neuropeptide Y preferentially enhance carbohydrate ingestion. Peptides 6:1205, 1985

127. Stanley BG, Hoebel BG, Leibowitz SF: Neurotensin: Effects of hypothalamic and intravenous injections on eating and drinking in rats. Peptides 4:493, 1983

128. Stanley BG, Kyrkouli SE, Lampert S et al: Neuropeptide Y chronically injected into the hypothalamus: A powerful neurochemical inducer of hyperphagia and obesity. Peptides 7:1189, 1986

129. Stanley BG, Lanthier D, Chin AS et al: Suppression of neuropeptide Y-elicited eating by adrenalectomy or hypophysectomy: Reversal with corticosterone. Brain Res 501:32, 1989

130. Stanley BG, Leibowitz SF: Neuropeptide Y: Stimulation of feeding and drinking by injection into the paraventricular nucleus. Life Sci 35:2635, 1984

131. Stanley BG, Leibowitz SF: Neuropeptide Y injected in the paraventricular hypothalamus: A powerful stimulant of feeding behavior. Proc Natl Acad Sci USA 82:3940, 1985

132. Stanley BG, Schwartz DH, Hernandez L et al: Patterns of extracellular norepinephrine in the paraventricular hypothalamus: Relationship to circadian rhythm and deprivation-induced eating behavior. Life Sci 45:275, 1989

133. Stanley BG, Schwartz DH, Hernandez L et al: Patterns of extracellular 5-hydroxyindoleacetic acid (5-HIAA) in the paraventricular hypothalamus (PVN): Relation to circadian rhythm and deprivation-induced eating behavior. Pharmacol Biochem Behav 33:257, 1989

134. Strubbe JH, Keyser J, Dijkstra T et al: Interaction

135. Sutton SW, Mitsugi N, Plotsky PM et al: Neuropeptide Y (NPY): A possible role in the initiation of puberty. Endocrinology 123:2152, 1988

136. Tatemoto K, Rokaeus A, Jornvall H et al: Galanin: A novel biologically active peptide from porcine intestine. FEBS Lett 164:124, 1983

137. Tempel DL, Leibowitz SF: PVN steroid implants: Effect on feeding patterns and macronutrient selection. Brain Res Bull 23:553, 1989

138. Tempel DL, Leibowitz SF: Galanin inhibits insulin and corticosterone release after injection into the PVN. Brain Res 536:353, 1990

139. Tempel DL, Leibowitz SF: Diurnal variations in the feeding responses to norepinephrine, neuropeptide Y and galanin in the PVN. Brain Res Bull 25:821, 1990

140. Tempel DL, Leibowitz KJ, Leibowitz SF: Effects of PVN galanin on macronutrient selection. Peptides 9:309, 1988

141. Tempel D, Shor-Posner G, Dwyer D et al: Nocturnal patterns of macronutrient intake in freely feeding and food-deprived rats. Am J Physiol 256:R541, 1989

142. Vaccarino FJ, Bloom FE, Rivier J et al: Stimulation of food intake in rats by centrally administered hypothalamic growth hormone-releasing factor. Nature 314:167, 1985

143. Van der Gugten J, Slangen JL: Release of endogenous catecholamines from rat hypothalamus in vivo related to feeding and other behaviors. Pharmacol Biochem Behav 7:211, 1977

144. Wahlestedt C, Skagerberg G, Ekman R et al: Neuropeptide Y (NPY) in the area of the hypothalamic paraventricular nucleus activates the pituitary-adrenocortical axis in the rat. Brain Res 417:33, 1987

145. Weiss GF, Leibowitz SF: Efferent projections from the paraventricular nucleus mediating α_2-noradrenergic feeding. Brain Res 347:225, 1985

146. Weiss GF, Papadakos P, Knudson K et al: Medial hypothalamic serotonin: Effects on deprivation- and norepinephrine-induced eating. Pharmacol Biochem Behav 25:1223, 1986

147. Weiss GF, Rogacki N, Fueg A et al: Impact of hypothalamic D-norfenfluramine and peripheral D-fenfluramine injection on macronutrient intake in the rat. Brain Res Bull 25:849, 1990

148. Weiss GF, Rogacki N, Fueg A et al: Effect of hypothalamic and peripheral fluoxetine injection on natural patterns of macronutrient intake in the rat. Psychopharmacology (in press)

149. White BD, Dean RG, Martin RJ: Adrenalectomy

decreases neuropeptide Y mRNA levels in the arcuate nucleus. Brain Res Bull 25:711, 1990

150. Wurtman RJ, Heftl F, Melamed E: Precursor control of neurotransmitter synthesis. Pharmacol Rev 32:315, 1981

151. Wurtman JJ, Wurtman RJ: Drugs that enhance central serotoninergic transmission diminish elective carbohydrate consumption by rats. Life Sci 24:895, 1979

152. Wurtman RJ, Wurtman JJ: Nutrients, neurotransmitter synthesis and the control of food intake. In Stunkard A, Stellar E (eds): Eating and Its Disorders: Association for Research in Nervous and Mental Disease, pp 77–96. New York, Raven Press, 1984

153. Wurtman RJ, Wurtman JJ: Carbohydrate craving, obesity and brain serotonin. Appetite (Suppl)7: 99, 1986

154. Yee F, MacLow C, Chan IN et al: Effects of chronic paraventricular nucleus infusion of clonidine and α-methyl-para-tyrosine on macronutrient intake. Appetite 9:127, 1987

Hibernation: A Model of Adaptive Hyperlipogenesis and Associated Metabolic Features

WILLIAM A. BAUMAN

A hibernator fattens from spring to fall and then appears to survive winter by subsisting on body fat stores, shrinking to skin and bone by spring. Our present knowledge of hibernation does not extend beyond this fundamental insight. Careful observation and recent biochemical advances have significantly enriched our appreciation and understanding of this adaptive survival tactic.

The verb *hibernate* in Webster's dictionary is defined, "to pass the winter in a torpid or resting state, to become inactive, dormant." Thus reptiles, amphibians, fish, birds, and mammals, as well as some invertebrates and various plants, would be included in this broad definition. In the restricted scientific sense, *to hibernate* means to depress body temperature (T_b). Because T_b in mammals is usually maintained at a steady, high level, any downward deviation must be either pathologic or a species-specific adaptation.

Specific groups of mammalian hibernators profoundly lower their T_b, approaching 0°C for a period of days or weeks, and are capable of intermittently rewarming using only self-generated heat. These animals are designated *deep hibernators*. Although bears, as well as other similarly adaptive mammals, may undergo an annual weight cycle in association with some fluctuation in T_b, these animals depress T_b more modestly. The lowest recorded rectal temperature of black bears is 31.2°C.[1] In bears and other adaptive animals, this condition has been referred to as *torpor*. Surprisingly little is known about mammals that undergo periods of torpor during the winter, because it is a condition that is exceedingly difficult to produce and study in the laboratory. Thus this chapter is restricted to studies of deep hibernators, those that undergo a cycle of weight gain and weight loss and can be used as models to study body weight regulation.

The question may be posed: What is the physiological need that forces relatively small mammals in northern climates to gain body weight and hibernate? The relationship between body size and metabolic rate is of importance in the maintenance of euthermia. Generally, basal metabolic rate of euthermic animals varies more in proportion to body surface area than it does in relation to body weight. The rate of heat flow from an object to its surroundings is proportional to its surface area. A small animal has a larger ratio of body surface area to body weight than does a large animal. The rate at which energy is used in warm environments to maintain euthermia is approximately proportional to body weight $(W_b)^{3/4}$.[2] Smaller animals must gather enough food to sustain their relatively high metabolic demands. This demand is accentuated in small animals living in cold climates, where the rate at which energy is used to maintain euthermia is approximately proportional to $(W_b)^{1/2}$ (Fig. 16-1).[3]

Body insulation in the form of fat and fur are

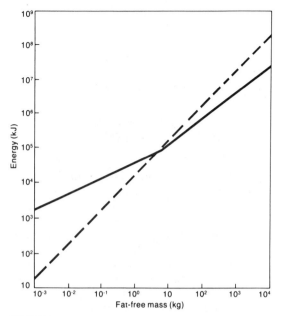

FIGURE 16-1

The energy available to mammals when fat is 50% of body weight (*broken line*) and the energy necessary to maintain high body temperatures (*solid line*) are related differently to body size. Energy requirements were calculated for mammals resting for a period of 6 months at a temperature of 5°C; the slope of the line changes because large mammals metabolize at basal levels at this temperature but small mammals do not. These relationships indicate that although large mammals consume more food each day, they can also go without eating for much longer periods than can small mammals. As lean body weight falls below about 5 kg, the energy available from body fat becomes increasingly inadequate for the continuous maintenance of high body temperatures, and the selection pressures for the use of hibernation increase commensurately. (French AR: The patterns of mammalian hibernation. Am Sci 76:569, 1988)

of vital importance to survival. A large animal can successfully insulate itself from heat dissipation in a cold environment, whereas the amount of insulation needed to perform a comparable task in a small animal would limit movement. Small mammals rely on insulation provided by shelters found or constructed in the wild to compensate for their lack of insulation. Because these small animals can store only a limited number of calories in the form of fat, they require a sufficient supply of food at frequent intervals. A reduction in T_b and basal metabolic rate would reduce or eliminate the need for a constant food supply. Although many mammals have adopted the strategy of hibernation, most have not. One could empirically reason that hibernation was an obligate adaptation to ensure survival in those species that do.

HIBERNATORS: A DIVERSE GROUP

Deep hibernators do not have identical or necessarily even similar characteristics. Absolute body weight, body weight gain or loss, hibernating patterns, and relationships between body weight and hibernation may differ among various species. Therefore, one cannot generalize from a single species that may have been arbitrarily chosen for study because it is convenient or because it adjusts to and is capable of hibernation in the laboratory. There are some characteristics that many hibernators share, however, and generalizations can be drawn. It is instructive to review and categorize the hibernators commonly used in research endeavors.

Most research in hibernation has been performed on the order Rodentia. Rodents are generally small, readily trapped in the wild, and can be made to hibernate without difficulty under the appropriate laboratory conditions. Subgroups of rodents that hibernate include Sciuromorpha, or squirrellike rodents, and Myomorpha, or mouselike rodents. The most studied hibernators are the Sciuromorpha. Generally, ground squirrels are hibernators, but there are several exceptions. "Seasonal" hibernators, such as the hibernating ground squirrel, are hyperphagic before hibernation, and certain species can double their body weight as a result of fat storage. These animals exhibit little or no food storage during the winter and, if food is present during periodic arousal between bouts of hibernation, eat a negligible amount.[4,5] In North America, the 13-lined ground squirrel (*Citellus tridecemlineatus*) has been widely studied. Other ground squirrels of investigative interest include the golden-mantled (*Citellus lateralis*), the Richardson's (*Citellus richardsonii*), the artic (*Citellus parryi*), and the California (*Citellus* beecheyi). The woodchuck (Marmota monax) and the yellow-bellied marmot (Marmota flaviventris) are the largest hibernators and have been less frequently investigated. The marmot and woodchuck may serve as models in the study of carbohydrate metabolism because they are large enough to permit intermittent blood sampling and placement of central arterial thermocouple devices. In Europe, the European ground squirrel (Citellus citellus) has been studied.

Many species of hamsters and the edible dormouse are "permissive" hibernators, and they store large amounts of food. The Syrian hamster (Mesocricetus auratus) has been investigated in North America and Europe because of its wide availability as a domestic rodent. It is a fickle hibernator in that it may not hibernate when exposed to the cold, and if it does, it may do so for unpredictably short bouts and may eat a substantial amount during periods of arousal. Turkish hamsters (Mesocricetus brandti) are about the same size as Syrian hamsters and hibernate more readily. Although the European hamster (Cricetus cricetus) is larger, it has not been the focus of much research interest. Various species of Myomorpha hibernate. The edible dormouse, Glis glis, is a frequently reported hibernator in the European literature. It is compared with squirrellike hibernators with regard to body weight cycles and carbohydrate metabolism later in this chapter.

Insectivora, the most primitive of eutherian mammals, include many species that may be hypothesized to be ideal candidates for hibernation, but few actually hibernate. Erinacidae is a family in which the European hedgehog (Erinaceus eurpaeus), a typical hibernator, is a member. This family contains other genera that may hibernate, but remarkably little is known about their habits. Therefore, much of the European research on hibernation has been performed on hedgehogs.

Chiroptera, insect-eating bats, of which several species hibernate, are the smallest and most energetically constrained of hibernators. These bats cannot store their food and compensate by becoming suitably fat by fall. Bats reportedly are not hyperphagic. To conserve energy, bats only intermittently arouse from hibernation. Thus, an investigator can be fairly confident that animals undisturbed during winter are in a state of deep hibernation, rather than recently having entered or been aroused from this state. Bats readily hibernate in the laboratory under the appropriate conditions, and certain species, such as Myotis lucifugus, are available in large numbers.

BODY WEIGHT SET-POINT AND PATTERNS OF HIBERNATION

A cycle in body weight and food intake is well appreciated in hibernators. In seasonal hibernators, body weight gradually increases from spring to fall, when there may be a period of hyperphagia and accelerated weight gain associated with reduced activity. Hypophagia predictably occurs before these animals enter hibernation.

Various manipulations have been used to study the relationships between regulation of body weight and hibernation. Barnes and Mrosovsky[6] observed golden-mantled ground squirrels that were experimentally deviated from their annual cycle of either weight gain or weight loss. During the weight-gain portion of their yearly cycle (Fig. 16-2A), food was withheld, with a resultant decrease in body weight. When food was reintroduced, the squirrels rapidly gained the amount of weight necessary to place them at the appropriate level for that time of year on an ascending curve of prehibernation weight gain. Conversely, during the weight-loss portion of their cycle (Fig. 16-2B), if extra palatable foodstuff was offered in addition to their usual food pellets during arousal, the animals were successfully tempted to eat more than the usual nominal amount and maintained body weight. Once this food was removed from the hibernaculum, the squirrels rapidly lost weight to a level appropriate for that time of year in their hibernation cycle. A sliding set-point for body weight appears to be operative in these animals.

What is the relationship, if any, that exists between food consumption and bouts of hibernation? Mrosovsky and Barnes[5] studied squirrels fasted at times when the hibernation bout length naturally changes (i.e., at the start or at the end of the hibernation season, when food consumption is decreasing or increasing, respectively). When food was totally withheld from these squirrels at the start of hibernation (Fig. 16-3A),

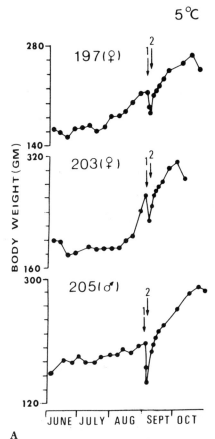

A

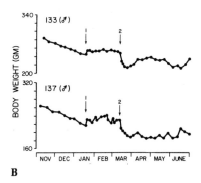

B

FIGURE 16-2

A: Body weight of ground squirrels during their weight-gain phase. For the animals, *arrow 1* shows when food was removed, and *arrow 2* shows when food was returned. The highest weights shown for each animal are their peak weights for that year. **B**: Body weights of ground squirrels during their weight-loss phase. For the animals, *arrow 1* shows when extra palatable food (wet mash) was offered, and *arrow 2* when it was removed. (Barnes DS, Mrosovsky N: Body weight regulation in ground squirrels and hypothalamically lesioned rats: Slow and sudden set point changes. Physiol Behav 12:251, 1974)

compared with a control group with unrestricted access to food, their body weight fell more precipitously and hibernation bout length increased more rapidly. Restricting food near the end of the hibernating season (Fig. 16-3B), when bout length normally begins to shorten, resulted in weight loss and an appropriate decrease in bout length from 7 to 4 days in both experimental and control squirrels. However, animals fasted near terminal hibernation failed to decrease hibernation bout length any more than 4 days or terminate hibernation unless given access to food. Thus, hibernators can reduce or accelerate weight loss by modulating the duration of the act of hibernation itself. Hibernation bout length increased when animals fasted in the fall, and it failed to be shortened beyond a certain number of days when animals fasted in the spring. These behaviors in fall and spring were designed to result in a conservation of body mass.

Food availability and body size appear to influence patterns of arousal during hibernation (Fig. 16-4). The marmot, the largest hibernator (>4 kg), by fall may have accumulated almost 2 kg of fat and, during the hibernation season, arouses every 7 to 10 days for 10 to 20 hours. The little brown bat, weighing only 6 to 8 g and surviving the entire winter on 2 to 3 g of fat, arouses no more than once a month, for periods as short as 1 hour. The act of hibernation appears to be species specific and is modified according to a mass-energy relationship depending on body size.

CARBOHYDRATE HOMEOSTASIS

There appear to be several biochemical similarities between the fasting state in humans and the hibernating state in several species of ground squirrels. In humans, after commencing a fast, the liver[7] and kidneys[8] become major sites for glucose production. Alanine is preferentially re-

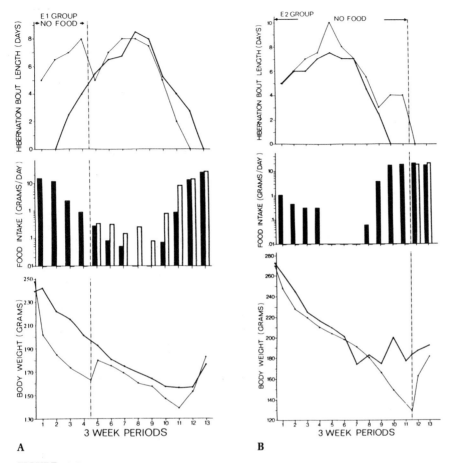

FIGURE 16-3

A and B: Median hibernation bout lengths (*top panel*), food intakes (*middle panel*), and body weights (*lower panel*) for control animals (*heavy lines and darker histogram*) and experimental animals (*lighter lines and lighter histogram*). Food intakes (*middle panel*) are plotted on a log scale. Data are expressed for 3-week periods. In the case of body weights (*lower panel*), data of the day on which food was removed (*first point on graph*) and the day when it was returned are also shown. (Mrosovsky N, Barnes DS: Anorexia, food deprivation and hibernation. Physiol Behav 12:265, 1974)

leased from muscle, probably by transamination of pyruvate[9] derived from glucose and amino acid metabolism.[10] The liver then takes up alanine by a virtually unsaturable transport mechanism[11] and converts it to glucose. In liver slices taken from hibernating 13-lined ground squirrels and incubated at 37°C, Whitten and Klain[12] noted a 20-fold increase in ^{14}C incorporation into glycogen from alanine in contrast to active, nor-

mothermic animals. Burlington and Klain[13] reported that the capacity of squirrel kidney slices to synthesize glucose at 6°C from all substrate precursors (α-ketoglutarate, L-glutamate, L-aspartate, glycerol, oxaloacetate, L-lactate, and pyruvate) was twice as great in animals during hibernation as in kidney slices taken from active animals in the spring. Glycerol released from triglycerides probably is the major precursor for

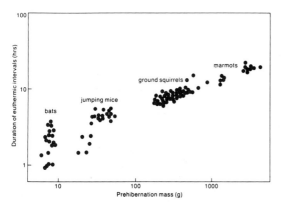

FIGURE 16-4

Large hibernators kept at 5°C spend more time at high body temperatures during each arousal episode in midwinter than do small hibernators. The duration of the arousal increases or decreases with mass$^{0.38}$, whereas the basal metabolic rate is proportional to mass$^{-0.38}$.[61] (French AR: The patterns of mammalian hibernation. Am Sci 76:569, 1988)

kidney gluconeogenesis. Galster and Morrison[14] estimated that in the arctic ground squirrel, about two thirds, or 430 mg of the 650 mg, of the carbohydrate reserve depleted during a single bout of hibernation and arousal could be replaced by glycerol serving as gluconeogenic substrate, assuming that oxygen consumption during the bout was totally due to fatty acid oxidation. This is a reasonable assumption, because in several studies the respiratory quotient during hibernation is near 0.7, a value consistent with lipid metabolism. Although the predominant source of energy during hibernation is derived from fat stores, cellular proteins must remain a vital source of gluconeogenic substrate. Tashima and colleagues[15] reported that the protein content of skeletal muscle of ground squirrels during hibernation or after arousal from hibernation was reduced by about 40% when compared with that of active, nonfasting animals.

Considerable attention has been focused on other endocrine organs, but the endocrine pancreas appears to have escaped notice until recently. It is thus a potential source of new information about endocrine physiology. Several animal models have been used to address body

weight and carbohydrate metabolism in hibernators. Castex and associates[16] studied pancreatic B-cell secretion by an *in situ* pancreatic perfusion technique in the edible dormouse. The researchers reported that mice maintained throughout the winter at an environmental temperature of 5°C lost weight by spring and had increased insulin secretion when compared with animals exposed during the winter to a more moderate environmental temperature, when body weight in these latter mice increased. Increased peripheral glucose utilization in the mice that lost weight was noted by calculating glucose disposal after administration of a central arterial glucose bolus.[16] This study did not explore the question of insulin resistance in the fall when the animals placed at 5°C are fat.[16] Mrosovsky[17] and Melnyk and colleagues[18-19] reported that in the dormouse, insulin resistance (as determined by reduced insulin-stimulated glucose utilization and impaired insulin binding and postreceptor events in isolated adiposites, as well as by decreased oral glucose tolerance) occurs after body weight begins to decline during the low food intake portion of their infradian cycle. This insulin resistance occurs in the absence of hyperinsulinemia despite normal pancreatic insulin content, and it is not corrected with weight loss.[17,19] Laurila and Suomalainen[20] evaluated carbohydrate metabolism in European hedgehogs and suggested that these animals had an annual rhythm in serum insulin concentration, with lower levels in the fall and winter when hibernating and higher values in spring and summer when the animals were more active and eating.

Florant and colleagues[21,22] have studied carbohydrate metabolism in yellow-bellied marmots. Marmots display clear circannual rhythms of body weight that result from increased food intake and enhanced lipogenesis during the summer and early fall. By fall, marmots have usually doubled their spring weight. They then cease to feed and enter a lipolytic metabolic state. Most animals have lost as much as 50% of their fall weight when, by midspring, they arise from hibernation and begin to feed, commencing the weight cycle once again. During intra-arterial glucose tolerance testing in euthermic animals, glucose values fell more slowly in summer and

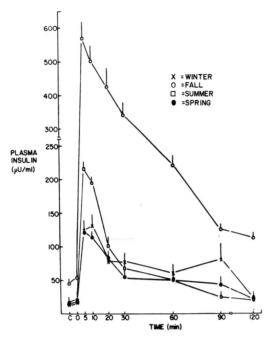

X = WINTER
O = FALL
□ = SUMMER
● = SPRING

PLASMA
INSULIN
(μU/ml)

TIME (min)

FIGURE 16-5

Plasma insulin concentrations in fasting marmots after dextrose administration (500 mg/kg) by season. Each point represents mean ± SEM. (Florant GL, Lawrence AK, Williams K et al: Seasonal changes in pancreatic B cell function in the euthermic yellow-bellied marmot [*Marmota flaviventris*]. Am J Physiol 249:R159, 1985)

fall than during winter months. Stimulated plasma insulin concentrations were increased during the summer and even more so in the fall, when the animals displayed markedly increased peripheral insulin resistance (Fig. 16-5).[21] This resistance was determined by several findings, including elevated fasting levels of insulin, an augmented insulin response to intra-aortic glucose, and no decline in basal serum glucose concentration during an insulin tolerance test. Maximal insulin resistance appeared to be highly correlated with peak body weight. After weight loss during the early winter, hyperinsulinemia and insulin resistance appeared to diminish.

The possibility that hibernating mammals regulate their circulating glucose concentration by means of pancreatic hormonal mechanisms was also addressed by Florant and colleagues.[22]

Three prior studies[23-25] reported that hibernators were not capable of pancreatic hormone responses to intra-arterial injection of glucose or arginine, suggesting that plasma glucose concentrations during hibernation may not be regulated by insulin or glucagon secretion. However, Florant and associates[22] reported that pancreatic A and B cells of marmots are sensitive to changes in circulating glucose and arginine levels, not only during euthermia but also during deep hibernation (T_b <10°C) (Fig. 16-6). These findings suggest that regulation of plasma glucose by pancreatic hormones occurs during euthermia and continues throughout the hibernation cycle.

It is not surprising that the pancreatic A and B cells of a hibernator are still functional during hibernation, because the permissive hibernators feed during arousal between bouts of hibernation, as do the seasonal hibernators but to a lesser degree.[4,5] The latter frequently have partially digested food in their gut during deep hibernation.[26] Whether the absorption of nutrients continues at low T_b is unclear. By use of the everted sac technique, increase of active absorption of glucose across isolated small-intestinal segments has been demonstrated in the 13-lined ground squirrel.[27] This phenomenon also occurs in many fasting mammals. It may be assumed, however, that if absorption does occur, even at a low rate, the pancreatic islets might be stimulated by the metabolic fuels absorbed into the circulation. Because many physiological processes such as T_b regulation have been shown to continue to function during hibernation, it was not surprising to discover, as has been shown by Florant and colleagues,[22] that pancreatic hormone secretory mechanisms also continue to function.

Earlier investigations concentrating on histologic observations of islet A and B cells failed to demonstrate a clear pattern, possibly partly because of the difficulty in obtaining quantitative information with this methodology, as well as the fact that species differences exist. The histology and relative ratios of pancreatic A to B cells in hibernators has been taken as a crude indicator of hormonal activity. The ratio of A to B cells has been reported to undergo no change during hibernation in golden hamsters and European ground squirrels but to increase in hedgehogs and European hamsters.[28] In a hibernating bat,

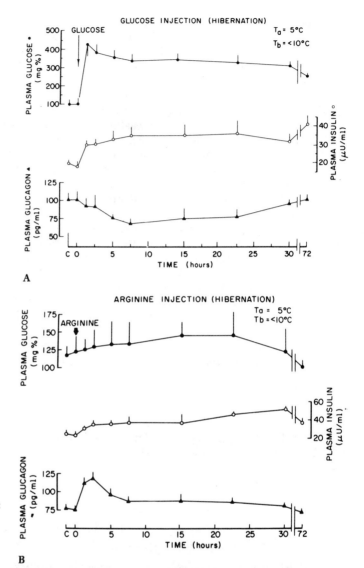

FIGURE 16-6

Studies performed in hibernating marmots. **A**: Changes in plasma glucose, insulin, and glucagon after administration (*arrow*) of glucose (500 mg/kg). **B**: Changes in plasma glucose, insulin, and glucagon after administration (*arrow*) of L-arginine (50 mg/kg). (Florant GL, Hoo-Paris R, Castex C et al: Pancreatic A and B cell stimulation in euthermic and hibernating marmots [*Marmota flaviventis*]: Effects of glucose and arginine administration. J Comp Physiol [B] 156:309, 1986)

Eptesicus fuscus, the ratio of A to B cells was reported to remain unchanged during hibernation.[29] In another hibernating bat, *Rhynolophs ferrum,* Mosca[30] noted a general decrease in B cell granulation while A cell granulation remained fairly constant, suggesting a reduction in pancreatic insulin with preservation of pancreatic glucagon. In support of reduced B-cell activity, Hinkley and Burton[29] reported that the blood glucose level in hibernating bats, *E. fuscus,* are

3.5 times higher than in active bats. In the fall, before hibernation, B-cell activity appeared histologically to be increased.[31] Raths and Kulzer[31] explained their findings on the basis of increased adiposity and probable insulin resistance in the fall.

Johansson and Senturia[32] have reported that the concentration of pancreatic insulin was reduced from 30 μg/g in nonhibernating European hedgehogs in July to 7 μg/g in January during hibernation. The weight of the pancreas was reduced by 65% during this period. Other pancreatic hormones were not measured.

Bauman and associates[33] have determined the effect of hibernation on the content and concentration of the pancreatic islet hormones in golden-mantled ground squirrels. The contents and concentrations of insulin, somatostatin, and pancreatic polypeptide were significantly reduced during hibernation in January compared with levels during euthermia in July. However, the content but not the concentration of glucagon was significantly lowered during hibernation (Fig. 16-7).

Bauman and DeSalvo[34] studied the pancreatic hormones in the little brown bat. In late spring, 2 months after arousal, pancreatic insulin and glucagon concentrations and contents were low. In the fall, when the animals were prepared for hibernation or in early hibernation (before pancreatic weight decreased), both insulin and glu-

cagon contents and concentrations are significantly increased (Fig. 16-8). Throughout the hibernation period, there was a further increase in concentration and content of these pancreatic hormones that reaches significance toward terminal hibernation. Pancreatic weight decreased 30% to 40% during the period of hibernation. The investigators hypothesized that pancreatic insulin increases in the fall are due to an increased absolute amount and percentage of body fat, with resultant insulin resistance.

Bauman and co-workers[33,34] found a fairly constant pancreatic glucagon concentration in the squirrel or elevated glucagon concentration in the bat during hibernation, raising the possibility that the glucagon concentration may be maintained during hibernation to ensure carbohydrate homeostasis during prolonged fasting. Glucagon is capable of rapidly inducing hepatic enzymes required for gluconeogenesis.[35,36] In addition, when the insulin concentration is suppressed,

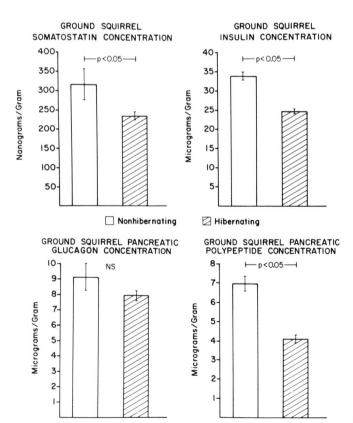

FIGURE 16-7

Ground squirrel pancreatic hormone concentration. Mean ± SEM. (Bauman WA, Meryn S, Florant GL: Pancreatic hormones in the nonhibernating and hibernating golden mantled squirrel. Comp Biochem Physiol [A] 86:241, 1987)

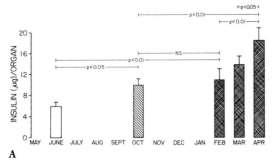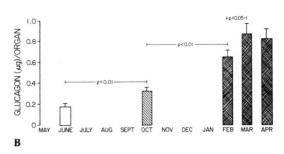

FIGURE 16-8

A: Pancreatic organ insulin content, mean ± SEM. The *open bar* represents active animals; *striped bar*, early or prehibernating animals; and *cross-hatched bars*, hibernating animals. **B**: Pancreatic organ glucagon content, mean ± SEM. (Bauman WA, DeSalvo CA: Pancreatic hormones in the nonhibernating and hibernating little brown bat (*Myotis lucifugus*). Pancreas [in press])

glucagon can induce ketogenesis in the liver.[37,38] Mild hypothermia (28°C) in a perfused rat pancreatic islet cell system reduces insulin release but has little effect on glucagon release.[39] Preservation of A-cell function may be an adaptive response in the rat, a nonhibernator, to ensure carbohydrate homeostasis at low T_b.

The apparent species differences in pancreatic insulin concentrations during hibernation noted in squirrels and bats do not necessarily imply a difference in basic physiology of carbohydrate homeostasis. Squirrels arise from hibernation in a rhythmic pattern. Hibernation bout length varies between 2 and 12 days, with shorter bout lengths at the beginning or at the end of the hibernation season, when feeding patterns are also changing. When aroused, squirrels do eat, albeit not sufficient calories to maintain body weight except near the end of the hibernation season. Bats, on the other hand, arouse much less frequently during hibernation and do not eat. Pancreatic insulin may vary in squirrels, depending on food consumption, absorption, and the precise time in the hibernation-arousal cycle. Furthermore, the concentration of insulin in the squirrel pancreas was not examined in the fall, when the animal was maximally obese and when pancreatic or plasma insulin may have been reasonably expected to be elevated. These matters remain to be addressed.

FAT METABOLISM

Hibernators become fat by fall and utilize fat reserves in the winter. Therefore, any discussion of fat metabolism should be divided into lipogenesis and lipolysis. Studies of these areas are incomplete and anecdotal, however. Fat metabolism may also influence carbohydrate metabolism, and vice versa, although this relationship has not been addressed in seasonal hibernators.

In 13-lined ground squirrels, Whitten and Klain[40] noted that the activity of three liver dehydrogenase enzymes involved in fat biosynthesis were twice as active in June as in September. Liver slices collected in June were more active in incorporating ^{14}C from glucose into fatty acids than were comparable slices in September. During hibernation, squirrels appear to turn off the hepatic enzymes necessary for fatty acid synthesis, with the activities of several enzymes falling to 5% or less of June levels. However, in the Syrian hamster, a permissive hibernator, the lipogenic activity of white adipose tissue has been found to differ from that of liver.[41-43] When animals were exposed to cold or when they entered hibernation, the capacity of white adipose tissue to synthesize lipid *in vitro* from acetate increased four- to sixfold.[41] However, after exposure to cold or with the eventual onset of hibernation, *in vitro* fatty acid synthesis markedly decreased in liver slices.[42,43]

Entenman and colleagues[44] addressed fatty acid oxidation by measuring the hepatic production of $^{14}CO_2$ from ^{14}C-labeled palmitate, a long-chain free fatty acid. Production of $^{14}CO_2$ at various incubation temperatures by liver slices collected from hibernating 13-lined ground squirrels was depressed compared with preparations taken from active euthermic animals at the same time of year. This result is unexpected, but perhaps a hibernator is capable of preserving its fat stores by the additional mechanism of lowering its lipid oxidation rate. Lipid utilization is an oxidative process that takes place intramitochondrially. In 13-lined ground squirrels, the number of mitochondria in myocytes has been reported to increase by about one third during hibernation[45] and the size to increase by about 30% during arousal.[46] Fat droplets near mitochondria in golden-mantled ground squirrels appear to double in number after 10 weeks of hibernating, suggestive of a switch to a lipid metabolism.[47] However, this finding has not been universally confirmed, and Olsson[48] reported the absence of seasonal changes in the absolute number of mitochondria in the myocardium of hedgehogs. Of interest, reserpine induced an increase in the size and number of lipid droplets and an increase in the number of glycogen granules in the myocardium of active but not in hibernating bats.[49] Reserpine-induced structural alterations in mitochondria occurred in both groups but were more pronounced during hibernation. The increase in lipid collection in nonhibernating animals may be merely the result of an absolutely higher fat utilization at euthermia, rather than indicative of a more predominant lipid metabolism. Direct measure of the oxidative capacity of additional tissues in permissive and seasonal hibernators is required to yield a clearer picture.

CENTRAL NERVOUS SYSTEM

This chapter has addressed questions related to appetite and body weight regulation and the endocrine-metabolic changes or their sequelae in hibernators. However, neurochemical studies of pertinent investigative interest have yet to be reported—that is, those related to the postulated appetite and satiety regions of the brain. Two reviews[50,51] have outlined the bioamine and pep-

tide neurotransmitters of investigative interest and the specific brain regions responsible for feeding behavior in nonhibernators. Some of these findings may be relevant to research opportunities in hibernators.

Grossman[52] reported that injection of norepinephrine into the hypothalamus of rats leads to hyperphagia, a prominent behavior of seasonal hibernators in the fall. Using microdialysis and high-pressure liquid chromatography with electrochemical detection, a daily cycle of release of norepinephrine in the rat paraventricular hypothalamus (PVN) was found[53] to peak at the beginning of the dark cycle, when a burst of natural feeding normally occurs. One may speculate that in the early fall, when a seasonal hibernator is hyperphagic, norepinephrine release by the PVN may be tonically elevated, whereas in the late fall, during the onset of hypophagia and eventual hibernation, norepinephrine release may be postulated to be suppressed. Two peptides, cholecystokinin[54,55] and neurotensin,[56,57] appear to inhibit feeding when infused into the PVN of rats. Stanley and associates[56] reported that neurotensin, when infused into the PVN, inhibited in a dose-dependent fashion eating induced by norepinephrine injected into the same region. Modulation of hypothalamic bioamine or peptide neurotransmission with receptor agonists or antagonists may alter seasonal weight gain or loss, as well as an animal's ability to hibernate. Recording regional brain bioamine fluctuations on a seasonal basis, possibly in association with α_2-noradrenergic receptor status in the PVN or D_2 receptors in the hypothalamus and posterior nucleus accumbens regions,[58,59] may yield fascinating insights into this adaptive behavior.

FUTURE DIRECTIONS AND CONCLUSIONS

Hibernation provides an endocrine-metabolic-neurophysiological model of body weight regulation on an infradian or annual body weight cycle. Because the same basic regulatory systems and neuroanatomical structures appear to exist in mammalian hibernators and in humans, it may be speculated that hibernation is an extension of regulatory systems found in nonhibernators. Indeed, the act of hibernation itself, as inferred from cortical electroencephalographic studies, is homologous with sleep, predominantly slow-wave sleep.[60] Thus it could be hypothesized that the hypothalamic set-point for T_b could have been lowered as an adaptive extension of the mild fall in T_b that occurs in nonhibernators during sleep. Elucidation of the control mechanisms in a hibernator may permit better understanding of those mechanisms that regulate body weight, T_b, and sleep cycles, among other functions, in humans. Several reports have addressed neurochemical changes in hibernators, but none to my knowledge have focused on appetite regulation. It would appear that studies directed at appropriate hypothalamic areas for specific bioamines and peptides related to satiation in seasonal hibernators may be a useful and productive avenue of future investigative interest. Studies involving integration of our knowledge of the endocrine and nervous systems will permit a more complete understanding of the fascinating adaptive behavior of hibernators, with potential application to nonhibernators, including humans.

Acknowledgment: I thank Arline Vargas for providing excellent secretarial assistance.

References

1. Hock RJ: Seasonal variations in physiologic functions of artic ground squirrels and black bears. Bull Mus Comp Zool 124:155, 1960

2. Kleiber M: Body size and metabolic rate. Physiol Rev 27:511, 1947

3. Herreid CF II, Kessel B: Thermal conductance in birds and mammals. Comp Biochem Physiol 21:405, 1967

4. Jameson EW: Food consumption of hibernating and nonhibernating *Citellus lateralis*. J Mammals 46:634, 1965

5. Mrosovsky N, Barnes DS: Anorexia, food deprivation and hibernation. Physiol Behav 12:265, 1974

6. Barnes DS, Mrosovsky N: Body weight regulation in ground squirrels and hypothalamically lesioned rats: Slow and sudden set point changes. Physiol Behav 12:251, 1974

7. Garber AJ, Menzel PH, Boden G et al: Hepatic ketogenesis and gluconeogenesis in humans. J Clin Invest 54:981, 1974

8. Owen OE, Felig P, Morgan AP et al: Liver and kidney metabolism during prolonged starvation. J Clin Invest 48:574, 1969

9. Felig P, Pozefsky T, Marliss E et al: Alanine: Key role in gluconeogenesis. Science 167:1003, 1970

10. Felig P: The glucose-alanine cycle. Metabolism 22:179, 1973

11. Mallette LE, Exton JH, Park CR: Control of gluconeogenesis from amino acids in the perfused rat liver. J Biol Chem 244:5713, 1969

12. Whitten BK, Klain GJ: Proteins metabolism in hepatic tissues of hibernating and arousing ground squirrels. Am J Physiol 214:1360, 1968

13. Burlington RF, Klain GJ: Gluconeogenesis during hibernation and arousal from hibernation. Comp Biochem Physiol 22:701, 1967

14. Galster W, Morrison PR: Gluconeogenesis in artic ground squirrels between periods of hibernation. Am J Physiol 228:325, 1975

15. Tashima LS, Adelstein SJ, Lyman CP: Radioglucose utilization by active, hibernating and arousing ground squirrels. Am J Physiol 218:303, 1970

16. Castex CH, Tahri A, Hoo-Paris R et al: Hibernation depth influences the edible dormouse pancreatic B cell during the spring arousal. Gen Comp Endocrinol 54:123, 1984

17. Melnyk R, Mrosovsky N, Martin J: Spontaneous obesity and weight loss: Insulin action in the dormouse. Am J Physiol 245: (Regul Integrative Comp Physiol) R396, 1983

18. Melnyk R, Mrosovsky N, Martin J: Spontaneous obesity and weight loss: Insulin binding and lipogenesis in the dormouse. Am J Physiol 245: (Regul Integrative Comp Physiol) R403, 1983

19. Mrosovsky N: Cyclical obesity in hibernators: The search for the adjustable regulator. In Van Itallie TB, Hirsch J (eds): Advances in Obesity Research, Vol 4. London, John Libbey & Co (in press)

20. Laurila M, Suomalainen P: Studies in the physiology of the hibernating hedgehog. Ann Acad Sci Fenn [A] 201:1, 1974

21. Florant GL, Lawrence AK, Williams K et al: Seasonal changes in pancreatic B cell function in the euthermic yellow-bellied marmot (*Marmota flaviventris*). Am J Physiol 249:R159, 1985

22. Florant GL, Hoo-Paris R, Castex C et al: Pancreatic A and B cell stimulation in euthermic and hibernating marmots (*Marmota flaviventis*): Effects of glucose and arginine administration. J Comp Physiol [B] 156:309, 1986

23. Castex C, Tahri A, Hoo-Paris R et al: Insulin secretion in the hibernating edible dormouse (*Glis glis*): *In vivo* and *vitro* studies. Comp Biochem Physiol [A] 79:179, 1984

24. Hoo-Paris R, Hamsany M, Sutter B et al: Plasma glucose and glucagon concentrations in the hibernating hedgehog. Gen Comp Endocrinol 46:246, 1982

25. Hoo-Paris R, Hamsany M, Castex CH et al: Pancreatic A cell response to arginine in the hibernating hedgehog (Erinaceus europaeus). Gen Comp Endocrinol 52:157, 1983

26. Musacchia XJ, Deavers D: The regulation of carbohydrate metabolism in hibernators. In Musacchia XJ, Jansky L (eds): Survival in the Cold: Hibernation and Other Adaptions, pp. 55–75. New York, Elsevier, 1981

27. Musacchia XJ, Westhoff DD: Absorption of D-glucose by segments of intestine from active and hibernating, irradiated and non-irradiated ground squirrels, Citellus tridecemlineatus. Ann Acad Sci Fenn [A] 71/25:347, 1964

28. Kayser C: The Physiology of Natural Hibernation. New York, Pergamon Press, 1961

29. Hinkley RE, Burton PA: Fine structure of the pancreatic islet cells of normal and alloxan treated bats (Eptesicus fuscus). Anat Rec 166:67, 1970

30. Mosca L: Changes in the islets of Langerhans associated with age and hibernation. Q J Exp Physiol 41:433, 1956

31. Raths P, Kulzer E: Physiology of hibernation and related lethargic states in mammals and birds. Bonn Zool Monogr 9:1, 1976

32. Johansson BW, Senturia JB: Seasonal variations in the physiology and biochemistry of the European hedgehog (Erinaceaus europaeus) including comparisons with nonhibernators, guinea pig and man. Acta Physiol Scand (Suppl)380:43, 1979

33. Bauman WA, Meryn S, Florant GL: Pancreatic hormones in the nonhibernating and hibernating golden mantled squirrel. Comp Biochem Physiol [A] 86:241, 1987

34. Bauman WA: Seasonal changes in pancreatic insulin and glucagon in the little brown bat (Myotis lucifugus). Pancreas 5:342, 1990

35. Taunton OD, Stifel FB, Greene HL et al: Rapid reciprocal changes of rat hepatic glycolytic enzymes and fructose-1,6-diphosphatase following glucagon and insulin injection in vivo. Biochem Biophys Res Commun 48:1663, 1972

36. Greene HL, Taunton OD, Stifel FB et al: The rapid changes of hepatic glycolytic enzymes and fructose-1,6-diphosphatase activities. J Clin Invest 53:44, 1974

37. Williamson RJ: Effects of fatty acids, glucagon, and anti-insulin serum on the control of gluconeogenesis and ketogenesis in rat liver. Adv Enzyme Regul 5:229, 1967

38. Liljenquist JE, Bomboy JD, Lewis SB et al: Effects of glucagon on lipolysis and ketogenesis in normal and diabetic men. J Clin Invest 53:190, 1974

39. Loubatieres-Mariani M, Chapal J, Puech R et al: Different effects of hypothermia on insulin and glucagon secretion from the isolated perfused rat pancreas. Diabetologia 18:329, 1980

40. Whitten BK, Klain GJ: NADP-specific dehydrogenases and hepatic lipogenesis in the hibernator. Comp Biochem Physiol 29:1099, 1969

41. Baumber J, Denyes A: Acetate-1-C[14] metabolism of white fat from hamsters in cold exposure and hibernation. Am J Physiol 205:905, 1963

42. Denyes A, Carter JD: Utilization of acetate-1-C[14] by hepatic tissue from cold exposed and hibernating hamsters. Am J Physiol 200:1043, 1961

43. Denyes A, Baumber J: Lipogenesis of cold-exposed and hibernating golden hamsters. Ann Acad Sci Fenn [A] 71:129, 1964

44. Entenman C, Ackerman PD, Walsh J et al: Effect of incubation temperature on hepatic palmitate metabolism in rats, hamsters and ground squirrels. Comp Biochem Physiol [B] 501:51, 1975

45. Moreland JE: Electron microscopic studies of mitochondria in cardiac and skeletal muscle from hibernated ground squirrels. Anat Rec 142:155, 1962

46. Zimny ML, Moreland JE: Mitochondrial populations and succinic dehydrogenase in the heart of a hibernator. Can J Physiol Pharmacol 46:911, 1968

47. Burlington RF, Bowers WD Jr, Damm RC et al: Ultrastructural changes in heart tissue during hibernation. Cryobiology 9:224, 1972

48. Olsson SOR: Ultrastructure of brown adipose tissue and myocardium. Acta Physiol Scand (Suppl) 380:117, 1972

49. Hagopian M, Gershon MD, Nunez EA: An ultrastructural study of the effect of reserpine on ventricular cardiac muscle of active and hibernating bats (Myotis lucifugus). Lab Invest 27:99, 1972

50. Hoebel BG: Neuroscience and motivation pathways and peptides that define motivational systems. In Atkinson RC, Herrnstein RJ, Lindzey G et al (eds): Stevens' Handbook of Experimental Psychology, Vol 1, 2nd ed, pp 547–625. New York, John Wiley & Sons, 1988

51. Leibowitz SF: Neurochemical systems of the hypothalamus: Control of feeding and drinking behavior and water-electrolyte excretion. In Morgane PJ, Panksepp J (eds): Handbook of the Hypothalamus, Vol 3, Part A, pp 299–437. New York, Marcel Dekker, 1980

52. Grossman SP: Direct adrenergic and cholinergic stimulation of hypothalamic mechanism. Am J Physiol 202:872, 1962

53. Stanley BG, Schwartz DH, Hernandez L et al: Patterns of extracellular norepinephrine in the paraventricular hypothalamus: Relationship to circadian rhythm and deprivation-induced eating behavior. (in press)

54. Morley JE: The ascent of cholecystokinin (CCK): From gut to brain. Life Sci 30:479, 1982
55. McCaleb ML, Myers RD: Cholecystokinin acts on the hypothalamic "noradrenergic system" involved in feeding. Peptides 1:47, 1980
56. Stanley BG, Hoebel BG, Leibowitz SF: Neurotensin: Effects of hypothalamic and intravenous injections on eating and drinking in rats. Peptides 4:493, 1983
57. Stanley BG, Leibowitz SF, Eppel N et al: Suppression of norepinephrine-elicited feeding by neurotensin: Evidence for behavioral, anatomical and pharmacological specificity. Brain Res 343:297, 1985
58. Hernandez L, Hoebel BG: Feeding and hypothalamic stimulation increase dopamine turnover in the accumbens. Physiol Behav 44:599, 1988
59. Parada MA, Hernandez L, Hoebel BG: Sulpiride injections in the lateral hypothalamus induce feeding and drinking in rats. Pharmacol Biochem Behav 30:917, 1988
60. Heller HC: Hibernation: Neural aspects. Ann Rev Physiol 41:305, 1979
61. French AR: Allometries of the durations of torpid and euthermic intervals during mammalian hibernation: A test of the theory of metabolic control of the timing of changes in body temperature. J Comp Physiol [B] 156:13, 1985
62. French AR: The patterns of mammalian hibernation. Am Sci 76:569, 1988

CHAPTER 17

Determinants of Food Intake Regulation in Obesity

JUDITH RODIN

Most investigators agree that fat storage in obesity is affected by three major factors: caloric intake, energy expenditure, and familial predisposition. A potentially sizable role in each domain is played by behavioral variables. In the discussion of caloric intake, there is continuing controversy regarding which aspects of eating behavior distinguish overweight from normal weight people.[1] However, most investigators assume that some feature of food intake or its determinants must be different. The most widely debated factor is the amount of food eaten. Although many studies have shown that obese persons do not consume more calories than nonobese subjects,[1-4] these studies often did not distinguish overweight people in the static (weight maintaining) phase from those in the dynamic (weight gaining) phase of obesity. Furthermore, overweight people may not overeat continuously, especially under scrutiny, but rather binge and restrict, thus appearing to eat little under testing conditions but eating a great deal at another time. Alternatively, overweight people may actually have a relatively low caloric intake and maintain their higher weight through metabolic adaptations resulting from earlier patterns of overeating and dieting.[5]

Activity accounts for only about a third of total energy expenditure and may not be the component of expenditure that most distinguishes obese from nonobese people. Most studies have focused on children, in a search for an etiologically significant role for exercise in the onset of obesity, but the data are contradictory. Stunkard and colleagues[6,7] have found no activity differences as a function of weight, while other studies find that obese children appear to be less active than their leaner counterparts.[8,9] Differences in metabolism, accounting for the larger component of thermogenesis, may be the more significant feature that distinguishes lean from overweight people and may have a strong genetic component. Again, it is possible that some of these metabolic differences result from behavioral factors such as the patterns of dieting and weight regain that are prevalent among overweight people.[10,11]

There are significant family influences in the predisposition to obesity.[12-14] In addition to shared genes, families share models for food-relevant behavior,[15] and there appear to be commonalities within families in dietary habits and activity patterns.[16,17]

Thus, in all the major determinants of obesity—caloric intake, energy expenditure, and familial determinants—a major role for behavioral factors exists. Behavioral factors may play both direct and indirect roles, for example, by influencing amount eaten or activity patterns (the direct effect) or by influencing resting metabolism in response to exercise or repeated cycles of gaining and losing weight (the indirect effect). Different behavioral factors may be important at different phases in the course of weight gain and weight maintenance. Overeating, eating too quickly or too much in a single meal, may contribute to weight gain but may play a less signifi-

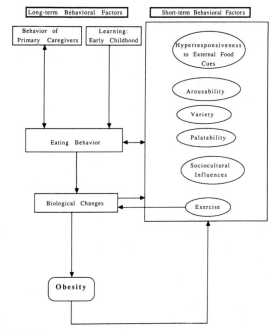

FIGURE 17-1

Behavioral factors relevant to the development of obesity.

cant role in weight maintenance. Inactivity may be important to maintain overweight but may account for less variance in weight gain.

A model of behavioral factors relevant to the development of obesity is presented in Figure 17-1. Note that behavioral factors are hypothesized to act largely through their effects on eating behavior and thus to influence obesity indirectly for the most part, through their effects on physiologic and biochemical processes. This figure does not specify the relevant biologic changes, an elaboration beyond the scope of the present discussion, but suggests a possible set of pathways through which behavior influences both the etiology and maintenance of obesity. The following discussion focuses on behavioral factors relevant to regulation of the food intake portion of the diagram.

BEHAVIORAL REGULATION OF FOOD INTAKE

Human eating behavior is an extremely complex process that involves multiple factors. Some of the earliest work on the determinants of food intake in humans[18-20] was undertaken because of the growing appreciation that interspecies differences in feeding behavior prevented a simple extrapolation from animal studies to people. The studies in humans showed that internal physiologic signals for repletion and depletion were insufficient to guide accurate control of food intake. It was suggested that oral, cognitive, and environmental variables might play a more important role in eating behavior in humans. An acknowledgment of the importance of such signals and an understanding of how they operate has led to a richer and more complex picture of the events involved in the initiation and maintenance of human eating behavior, and in the regulation of body weight.

Eating behavior, like other learned habitual behavior, arises from the complex interaction of biologic predisposition, learning history, and current context. This fact is true for all people, regardless of weight. As a result, individual differences rather than systematic between-group differences may account for the greater variance in studies of obese and nonobese subjects. Such variability among individuals does not render attempts to find general principles useless; it merely highlights the necessity of examining the underlying causes of different eating patterns rather than simply describing them and trying to link them to a particular sex or age or weight group.

Herman and Polivy[21] have proposed a boundary model of food intake regulation according to which consumption is regulated within boundaries rather than at a single point. The separation of boundaries, with hunger defining one boundary limit and satiety the other, suggests that outside the boundary—that is, under conditions of deficit or excess—physiologic controls may play a primary role in regulating consummatory behavior. Between the boundaries, on the other hand, appetitive factors based on social context and palatability, for example, tend to be more influential in regulating intake. Herman and Polivy argue that individual differences in boundary placement occur between dieters and nondieters. Dieters appear to have a lower hunger boundary and a higher satiety boundary.

OBESITY AND FOOD INTAKE REGULATION

Overall, major differences between obese and lean persons in food intake have been difficult to establish, although some differences have been found.

Palatability

Our review of the literature[1] suggests that palatability may be a potent determinant of food intake in the obese. In general, findings that overweight people eat more than normal weight people in response to highly palatable stimuli are stronger than findings of lowered intake in obese subjects under conditions of low palatability. Palatability may influence both the amount consumed at a given meal and the rate of consumption.[22-28] Palatability and hunger have similar effects on several aspects of eating behavior, including amount ingested, frequency of chewing movements, length of a meal, number of bites, total chewing time, and chewing speed.[23] Some studies suggest that obese subjects may be slower to terminate eating because the perceived pleasantness of taste sensations fails to decrease.[27,29-32] Some studies also suggest that obese children and adults may perceive foods differently, especially along the dimensions of tastiness–preference.[33,34]

The attractiveness of certain foods may be innately determined. Various species-specific preferences and aversions have been documented,[35] including a strong preference for sweet tastes in many human cultures.[36] In general, newborn infants show an aversion to bitter tastes[37-40] and a preference for sweet tastes.[41-46] However, infants born to overweight parents may actually show a preference for sweeter tastes, suggesting a possible innate risk factor for obesity.

Since certain taste preferences are innate, it is reasonable to hypothesize that individual differences in responsiveness to these stimuli may also be inborn. Individuals highly responsive to such stimuli as sweet tastes may be prone to overeat and gain weight. Support for hypothesized differences in baseline responsiveness comes from studies reporting individual differences in infants' responsiveness to taste stimuli, often only hours after birth.[37-40]

Both animals[41-46] and humans[32,47-49] can learn to modify food intake on the basis of orosensory cues in accordance with caloric density or nutritional value. The conditioned nature of these responses and the speed with which conditioning occurs have been shown to influence the development of specific hungers[45,50] and conditioned taste aversions in animals.[46,51] Thus, palatability is influenced by learning and conditioning.

There is evidence that children's food preferences can be altered by reinforcement of food selection,[52-54] which further supports the contention that certain food preferences are due to learning experiences. Madsen et al[53] found increased consumption of typical middle class breakfast foods when presentation of sweet treats and praise were made contingent on intake. Although only increased consumption was explicitly rewarded, this probably resulted in the tasting of unfamiliar foods and increased intake of nourishing foods.

The process whereby taste cues and eating become conditioned to a food's postingestive effects is not always infallible. Since a number of similar-tasting foods may differ in caloric density, taste does not always accurately guide amount consumed. Moreover, orosensory cues could become conditioned to other sensations besides those caused by a food's physiologic action. For instance, if a certain food is typically eaten under pleasurable circumstances, such as on holidays, the taste of that food may elicit a positive effect by virtue of this association, and may be more palatable on subsequent occasions. The opposite can occur if a food is eaten in an unpleasant context.

Although in a natural environment it may be adaptive to rely heavily on conditioned taste cues and innate preferences, since they often correlate with nutritional value, this may not be the case in a technologically advanced society. In the wild, if an organism encounters a sweet substance, that substance is likely to be nutritional and highly caloric, as well as safe to eat, whereas many bitter substances such as those in plants are poisonous and should be avoided.[54] Therefore, the use of taste preferences to guide behavior would be adaptive in a natural setting. However, modern science has developed many artificial substances and food substitutes that have approximately the same taste as their natural counterparts but different caloric densities and nutritional consequences. Most humans, therefore, may exhibit maladaptive eating behavior if they depend too strongly on taste cues.

Also, since highly palatable foods are consumed in greater amounts than less palatable foods[22-25,28,55-58] hyperresponsiveness to even informative taste cues can result in overeating. Maladaptive responses to taste cues are probably more likely to be elicited by novel than by familiar foods, as the association of taste with the metabolic consequences of ingesting the novel food has not yet been learned. If appropriate learning conditions prevail, theoretically the individual should develop the ability to regulate intake of a food based on this association.

At present, studies tell us relatively little about why overweight people tend to eat more of foods they find palatable. Again, issues of weight history and chronic energy deficit are major and are often overlooked. Humans and animals increase their preference for palatable foods after long periods of deprivation[31,59,60] and after losing weight.[61] If overweight subjects in these studies were currently dieting or had recently done so, differential consumption in response to good-tasting food would in fact be expected. Few of the cited studies measured and controlled for this factor. Furthermore, in most of these studies, it is unclear whether overweight subjects ate more because they perceived the foods as more palatable than the normal weight subjects, or whether they consumed more of food perceived to be equally palatable by both groups.

Studies that address these issues might provide data on the relation of increased taste responsiveness to the development and maintenance of obesity. If differences between overweight and normal weight persons prove relatively stable when diet history and level of chronic energy deficit are controlled for, and if increased responsiveness to palatability can be shown to precede obesity in some individuals, it might suggest a role for this variable in the etiology of at least some types of obesity. On the other hand, responsiveness to palatability may prove to be affected by factors such as dieting and energy deficit. If this is the case, increased responsiveness might be presumed to play a role in the

maintenance of obesity by providing a mechanism that guards against weight loss. Of note, these two possibilities are not mutually exclusive. It may be that there are individual differences in responsiveness to palatability; however, given these differences in baseline responsiveness, other factors such as deprivation may also produce transient changes.

Variety

Just as palatable foods may stimulate eating, presentation of a variety of palatable foods augments this response. Le Magnen[62] suggested that an oral satiety mechanism that is sensory specific operates through sensory stimulation of food passing through the mouth. Rats presented with distinctively flavored versions of their diet in succession ingested 72% more than those given only one flavor.[63] Le Magnen later concluded that oral satiety is effective only for the food eaten as a discriminated and specific sensory stimulus.[62]

Further evidence for specific satiety comes from an experiment by Rolls et al[64] which found that neuronal firing in the lateral hypothalamus (LH) of monkeys became attenuated on ingestion of food with which the animal was satiated, but continued to respond to other foods with which the animal was not satiated. It has also been shown that humans eating one food until satiated will begin eating again as if they were hungry when a new food is presented.[64] Satiety did not even generalize to other members of the same nutritional class as the ingested food (e.g., protein, carbohydrate, fat). A strong craving for foods can also be aroused in highly satiated subjects by the presentation of highly palatable novel foods.[65] The craving is primed by seeing and smelling the new food and leads subjects to consume more of that food and less of one that is equally palatable, when given a choice. In this case, sensory- or stimulus-specific craving (and consequent overeating) could be induced even in people who have just eaten a large and satisfying meal. This is true even when the new food is not a typical dessert food, for example, pizza rather than ice cream.

Variety may influence metabolic and digestive processes.[65-68] Since satiation is sensory specific, a cumulative insulin secretion induced by each successive or simultaneous flavor could delay satiation and meal termination.[69]

In light of the influence of palatability and variety on physiologic states and experience of satiation, it is not surprising that both contribute to hyperphagia and weight gain in animals.[55,70-73] This dietary obesity is the closest animal model to many forms of human obesity[74] and may be due in part to hyperinsulinemia.[75] Conversely, bland, monotonous diets resulted in decreased consumption and increased weight loss over three weeks in human subjects.[76] Pliner et al[56] suggest that both variety–monotony and palatability effects may account for these findings. Certainly some of the effects of very low calorie diets on weight loss may be due to their highly monotonous nature. Thus, there is weak and inferential data to support the assumption that variety may influence food intake regulation to a greater extent in obese than in lean individuals.

Social and Cultural Factors

Apart from innate preferences and personal experience with various foods and their metabolic consequences, humans base most of their food choices on culturally transmitted information. Religion, social class, ethnic group, and ecological factors all interact and exert much influence on human food preference and avoidance.[77] These same factors are clearly related to prevalence of obesity as well.[78] For example, in the United States obesity is most common among the lower classes, where sanctions against being overweight appear less strong than among the upper classes. Further, lower class persons who are upwardly mobile are thinner than those who are not.[79] Likelihood of obesity also correlates with ethnic group, perhaps in part because of differences among ethnic groups in their attitudes toward obesity.[80] The inverse relationship between socioeconomic status and prevalence of obesity seems unique to Western urban societies. In developing countries such as India and China, there appears to be a direct relationship between body weight or skin-fold thickness and rising standard of living.

Social and cultural rules and norms of weight, appearance, and behavior may disrupt the regulation of feeding and weight. If peopledo not meet the standards for appearance set by social rules, fashions, or family and peer pressures, they may be induced to diet in order to bring their weight within the range set by social norms. Dieting attempts induced by social pressures may then upset biologic processes and result in long-term weight gain.[81,82] These pressures appear greater for females than males.[83] A recent study of American 10- to 16-year-olds found that 68% of the girls, but only 16% of the boys, had dieted at least once. Furthermore, degree of dieting concern among the girls correlated with how feminine they believed themselves to be.[84] Rodin and colleagues have argued that pressures to be thin are increasing in all segments of society, leading to an escalation of disordered eating behavior.[85]

In addition to sociocultural attitudes regarding weight, the rules and norms imposed by society regarding meals and eating behavior may influence the normal regulation of feeding. The presentation of many courses in the typical meal makes it difficult to separate the metabolic consequences of each food and to learn to associate the appropriate orosensory characteristics with the corresponding physiologic effects. Also, the variety of foods and deliberate ordering of dishes according to increasing palatability facilitate consumption, even in the absence of an internal state of depletion (or in opposition to increasing repletion). Booth[86] has shown that the palatability of sweets declines less than the palatability of other foods in response to increasing satiation, and thus, sweets may still be eaten by replete subjects.

The social requirement that individuals eat at relatively fixed times, regardless of hunger, may contribute to overeating through conditioned responses or cognitions (eating in anticipation of future energy requirements and time until the next meal). This suggests that humans would regulate themselves differently in the absence of cues regarding appropriate meal time.

Bernstein and Sigmund[87] studied the meal patterns of three men who had been living for an extended period of time in an environment devoid of all time cues. Meal size was found to correlate with postprandial but not preprandial intervals: the larger a meal, the longer subjects waited to initiate the next meal. The authors suggested that the influence of social or time considerations on meal scheduling may prevent the use of this presumably short-term mechanism for regulation of food intake. The evidence seems to favor the interpretation that this mechanism is physiologic, although cognitive factors may be involved as well.

Overeating may also occur on specific occasions, such as holidays, when it is socially acceptable to do so and when external controls are relaxed. Here especially, different cultural norms regarding the type and quantity of foods to be eaten may prevail over physiologically determined signals.

Nutrient and Caloric Density

Hill and Blundell[88] have found that a high protein load reduces hunger and enhances satiety in the same way in obese and in lean people. In our own work, comparing regulation of food intake in response to different types of sugar, we found no differences as a function of weight.[1,89]

The majority of studies do not support the notion that the obese fail to respond to short-term manipulations of caloric preloading as accurately as normal weight subjects do (see Spitzer and Rodin[1] for review). However, experimentally induced increases in energy expenditure by fixed amounts (e.g., by cycling on a bicycle ergometer) do appear to be more accurately compensated for by energy intake in lean than obese subjects.[90] More extended manipulations of caloric density that controlled for cognitive and palatability factors showed no differences in regulation between obese and normal weight subjects.[49,91]

Longer-Term Factors

In recent years, many investigators have suggested that hunger has a large learned component.[92-94] These assertions challenge earlier views that hunger is simply the psychological experience of an innate biologic drive. Therefore, it is entirely plausible that mislearning or failure to learn about hunger can occur, probably quite early in the mother–child feeding interaction.

A second kind of learning that takes place during development is the learning of specific food preferences and aversions. Ever since the semi-nal studies of Garcia et al,[51] Revusky and Bedarf,[95] and Rozin and Kalat,[46] psychologists have been interested in these processes. Although some innate human preference for sugar or sweet is apparent, most other preferences and aversions are learned. Recently, Contreras and Kosten[96] found that neonatal consumption of high salt diets in animals led to a clear postweaning salt preference. Although Wurtman and Wurtman[97] failed to obtain the same result for sweet preference, Contreras suggests that their results are due to too delayed an introduction of the learning experiences.

It has also been shown that aversions can develop even after one learning trial, if that learning experience caused physical distress to the organism in association with a novel food taste.[95] There are as yet no comparable data in humans showing single-trial learning of food preferences except under extreme circumstances such as chemotherapy-related aversions.[87]

As it became clear that the preference for certain tastes and odors was learned, questions were raised about the possible function of such learning, other than simply to give pleasure. Le Magnen[98] suggested that the body possesses some mechanism for anticipating the metabolic consequences of food that is eaten, and that anticipation occurs on the basis of the food's flavor and odor. Following Le Magnen's suggestion, Booth and co-workers[47,99] showed persuasively that rather rapid learning occurs in which both odors and tastes of food come to predict the metabolic consequences of ingesting that particular food. The diagrammatic representation of these relationships is shown in Figure 17-2. This learning process leads the organism to take anticipatory action, prior to reliance on postabsorptive signals, to adjust the amount consumed.

There are good biologic reasons why all organisms, human and infrahuman alike, should be especially prepared to learn associations between the perceptual qualities of their food and the effect of that food on the body. This form of learning is an adaptive strategy. But certainly, this learning will not be the same in all individuals, and insufficient research addresses the consequences for body weight of differences that do arise.

Booth and co-workers[93,100] recently speculated

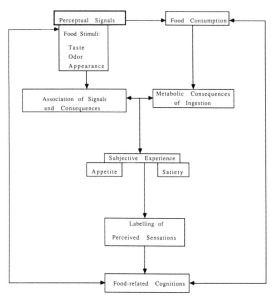

FIGURE 17-2

Postulated route by which anticipation of the metabolic consequences of food may be learned.

that individual differences in reactivity to salient environmental cues may affect the way individuals learn about the metabolic consequences of food. They found that overreactivity to the most obvious sensory characteristics of a food could distract from attention to that food's less obvious postingestional effects, and therefore could interfere with or block learning of an association between the predictive taste and texture of food cues and the postingestional effects of the food. Perhaps eating and weight problems would be more likely in these individuals.

A third significant childhood learning experience is learning self-control or self-regulation skills. Children receive early training in self-regulation, since part of childhood socialization involves instruction for, and enforcement of, self-controlling responses, especially learning to resist temptation.[101,102] The skills of self-regulation have been shown to depend on the ability to identify and maintain cues that can operate in the service of controlling one's own behavior.[103,104] Those cues may be environmental or internal to the organism (i.e., thoughts, feelings, or internal states).[58] Successful learning of self-regulation skills requires the combination of explicit instruction and a gradual weakening of external controls.

To take an example that might be important for the development of obesity, if parents control their child's eating behavior too extensively, the child may fail to experience and develop intrinsic, self-mediated control over the eating process. In the absence of external obstacles to eating, the typically constrained child may then overeat whenever food is attractive, salient, and available. This speculation is consistent with psychological theory,[105] which proposes that strong external rewards or punishments undermine a child's utilization of self-control strategies.

Finally, several childhood studies have also suggested behavioral factors that do not seem especially important to the development of obesity. Bottle feeding and the early introduction of solid foods have been studied[106-110]; however, there appears to be a relatively weak relationship between infant feeding methods and subsequent obesity in preschoolers.[27,38,40,95,102,105,111] Studies focusing on maternal nutritional knowledge or attitudes also do not find a direct correlation with fatness in children.[38,112]

CONCLUSION

How can we understand the relative paucity of differences in food intake regulation between obese and lean individuals? Although the factors reviewed in the foregoing discussion may play a role, they can hardly be of primary etiologic significance. People destined to become obese may expend energy differently because of their genetic destiny[113,114] or changes in metabolism, insulinemia, and LPL activity resulting from prior eating practices and dieting behavior.[115] Rolland-Cachera and Bellisle[4] present a further intriguing hypothesis, based on their findings that the lower a group's social status, the higher is the average caloric intake of that group, that the incidence of obesity is greatest in the groups of lowest status.

Rolland-Cachera and Bellisle[4] argue that social and cultural norms within a particular social class prescribe a certain level of caloric intake. At that level, obesity will develop in predisposed individuals—those at risk because of genetic characteristics, metabolic needs, or physical activity levels—even if these individuals do not eat differently than normal weight people of the same social group. They conclude "the daily diet that is typical of a social group challenges the regulating capacities of all individuals in the group; the higher the caloric value of the current diet, the larger the number of individuals who fail to regulate because of their constitutional features or particular lifestyle." This fascinating idea merits further empirical analysis, but it is consistent with the conclusion of many investigators that obesity is multiply determined. Except in extreme and unusual circumstances, aspects of food intake regulation alone do not play a role in isolation (i.e., as main effects). More complex models of interactions among genetic, metabolic, and lifestyle variables are needed.

References

1. Spitzer L, Rodin J: Human eating behavior: A critical review of studies in normal weight and overweight individuals. Appetite 2:293, 1981
2. Braitman LE, Aldin U, Stanton JL: Obesity and caloric intake: The National Health and Nutrition Examination Survey of 1971–1975 (HANES I). J Chronic Dis 38:727, 1985
3. Garrow JS: Energy Balance and Obesity in Man, 2nd ed. Amsterdam, Elsevier, 1978
4. Rolland-Cachera MF, Bellisle F: No correlation between adiposity and food intake: Why are working class children fatter? Am J Clin Nutr 44:797, 1986
5. Baeke JAH, Burema J, Frijter JER: Obesity in young Dutch adults: I. Sociodemographic variables and body-mass index. Int J Obes 7:1, 1983
6. Stunkard AJ, Pestka J: The physical activity of obese girls. Am J Dis Child 103:812, 1962
7. Waxman M, Stunkard A: Caloric intake and expenditure of obese boys. J Pediatr 96:198, 1980
8. Bullen BA, Reed RB, Mayer J: Physical activity of obese and nonobese adolescent girls appraised by motion picture sampling. Am J Clin Nutr 14:211, 1964
9. Klesges RC, Coates TJ, Moldenhauer-Klesges LM et al: The FATS: An observational system for assessing physical activity in children and associated parent behavior. Behav Assess 6:333, 1984
10. Brownell KD, Stunkard AJ: Behavioral treatment for obese children and adolescents. In Stunkard AJ (ed): Obesity. Philadelphia, 1980
11. Reed DR, Contreras RJ, Maggio C et al: Weight cycling in female rats increases dietary fat selection and adiposity. Physiol Behav 42:389, 1989
12. Garn SM, Bailey SM, Cole PE: Synchronous fatness changes in husbands and wives. Am J Clin Nutr 32:2375, 1979
13. Garn SM, Bailey SM, Solomon MA et al: Effect of remaining family members on fatness prediction. Am J Clin Nutr 34:148, 1981
14. Garn SM, Clark DC: Trends in fatness and the origins of obesity. Am Acad Pediatr 15:443, 1976
15. Harper L, Sanders K: The effects of adults' eating on young children's acceptance of unfamiliar foods. J Exp Child Psychol 20:206, 1975
16. Patterson TL, Kaplan RM, Sallis JF et al: Aggregation of blood pressure in Anglo-American and Mexican-American families. Prev Med (in press)
17. Sallis JF, Patterson TL, Buono MJ et al: Aggregation of physical activity habits in Mexican-American and Anglo families. J Behav Med 78:459, 1971
18. Hashim S, Van Itallie T: Studies in normal and obese subjects with a monitored food-dispensing device. Ann NY Acad Sci 131:654, 1965
19. Jordan HA, Weiland WF, Zebley SP et al: The direct measurement of food intake in man: A method for the objective study of eating behavior. Psychosom Med 28:836, 1966
20. Pierson A, Le Magnen J: Étude quantitative du processus de regulation des reponses alimentaires chez l'homme. Physiol Behav 4:61, 1969
21. Herman P, Polivy J: A Boundary Model for the Regulation of Eating. New York, Raven Press, 1984
22. Grinker JA: Obesity and taste: Sensory and cognitive factors in food intake. In Bray GA et al (eds): Obesity in Perspective. Washington, DC, US Government Printing Office, 1975
23. Hill SW: Eating responses of humans during dinner meals. J Comp Physiol Psychol 86:652, 1974
24. Hill SW, McCutcheon N: Eating responses of obese and nonobese humans during dinner meals. Psychol Med 37:395, 1975
25. McKenna RJ: Some effects of anxiety level and food cues in the behavior of obese and normal subjects. J Pers Soc Psychol 221:311, 1972
26. Nisbett RE: Taste, deprivation and weight determinants of food intake in obesity. J Pers Soc Psychol 10:107, 1968
27. Price JM, Grinker J: The effects of degree of obesity, food deprivation, and palatability on eating behavior of humans. J Comp Physiol Psychol 85:265, 1973
28. Rodin J: The effects of obesity and set point on taste responsiveness and intake in humans. J Comp Physiol Psychol 89:1001, 1975

29. Blundell JE, Hill AJ: On the mechanisms of action of dexfenfluramine: Effect on alliesthesia and appetite motivation in lean and obese subjects. Clin Neuropharmacol 11(1):121, 1988

30. Cabanac M, Duclaux R: Obesity: Absence of satiety aversion to sucrose. Science 168:496, 1970

31. Keys A, Brozek J, Henschek A et al: The Biology of Human Starvation, Vol. 1. Minneapolis, University of Minnesota Press, 1950

32. Wooley OW, Wooley SC: The experimental psychology of obesity. In Silverstone T, Finchman J (eds): Obesity: Its Pathogenesis and Management. Lancaster, England, Medical and Technical Publishing, 1975

33. Drewnowski A: Food perceptions and preferences of obese adults: A multidimensional approach. Int J Obes 9:201, 1985

34. Worsley A, Peters M, Worsley AJ et al: Australian 10-year-olds' perceptions of food: III. The influence of obesity status. Int J Obes 8:327, 1984

35. Kare MR, Ficken MS: Comparative studies on the sense of taste, p 285. In Zotterman Y (ed): Olfaction and Taste. Oxford, England, Pergamon Press, 1963

36. Jerome NW: Taste experience and the development of a dietary preference for sweet in humans: Ethnic and cultural variations in early taste experience. In Weiffenbach JM (ed): Taste and Development, p 235. Bethesda, Md, US Department of Health, Education, and Welfare, 1977

37. Desor JA, Maller O, Turner RE: Taste in acceptance of sugars by human infants. J Comp Physiol Psychol 58:63, 1973

38. Grinker JA: Infant taste responses are correlated with birthweight and unrelated to indices of obesity. Pediatr Res 12:371, 1978

39. Milstein RM: Responsiveness in newborn infants of overweight and normal weight parents. Appetite 1:65, 1980

40. Nisbett RE, Gurwitz S: Weight, sex, and the eating behavior of human newborns. J Comp Physiol Psychol 73:245, 1970

41. Le Magnen J: Quelques aspects des liens entre sensibilite chimique it appetit. Colloque CNRN: Le Comportement Alimentaire et l'Appetit, p 11. Paris, 1951

42. Le Magnen J: Role de la densite calorique dans le mecanisme d'etablissement des appetits. J Physiol (Paris) 49:274, 1957

43. Le Magnen J: Sur le mecanisme d'etablissement des appetits caloriques. Comp Rend Hebdom Seances Acad Sci 240:2346, 1955

44. Richter CP, Holt LE Jr, Burelare B Jr: Nutritional requirements for normal growth and reproduction in rats studied by the self-selection method. Am J Physiol 122:734, 1938

45. Rozin P: Specific hunger for thiamine: Recovery from deficiency and thiamine preference. J Comp Physiol Psychol 59:98, 1965

46. Rozin P, Kalat J: Specific hungers and poison avoidance as adaptive specializations of learning. Psychol Rev

47. Booth DA, Lee M, McAleavey C: Acquired sensory control of satiation in man. Br J Psychol 67:137, 1976

48. Jordan HA: Voluntary intragastric feeding: Oral and gastric contributions to food intake and hunger in man. J Comp Physiol Psychol 68:498, 1969

49. Spiegal TA: Caloric regulation of food intake in man. J Comp Physiol Psychol 84:24, 1973

50. Rozin P: Specific aversions as a component of specific hungers. J Comp Physiol Psychol 64:237, 1967

51. Garcia J, Hankins W, Rusiniak K: Behavioral regulation of the milieu interne in man and rat. Science 185:824, 1974

52. Epstein LH, Masek BJ, Marshall WR: A nutritionally based school program for control of eating in obese children. Behav Ther 9:766, 1978

53. Madsen CH Jr, Madsen CK, Thompson F: Increasing rural Head Start children's consumption of middle-class meals. J Appl Behav Anal 7:257, 1974

54. Rozin P, Fallon A: The psychological categorization of foods and non-foods: A preliminary taxonomy of food rejections. Appetite 1:193, 1980

55. Le Magnen J: Étude d'un phenomene de stimuli alimentaires sur le determinisme quantitatif de l'ingestion. Arch Sci Physiol 14:411, 1960

56. Pliner P, Polivy J, Herman CP et al: Short-term intake of overweight individuals and normal weight dieters and nondieters with and without choice among a variety of foods. Appetite 1:203, 1980

57. Rodin J: Research on eating behavior and obesity: Where does it fit in personality and social psychology. Pers Soc Psychol Bull 3:333, 1977

58. Rodin J, Maloff D, Becker H: Self-control: The role of environmental and self-generated stimuli. In Levison P (ed): Substance Abuse: Habitual Behavior and Self-Control. Boulder, Colo, Westview/Prager, 1986

59. Jacobs HL, Sharma KN: Taste versus calories: Sensory and metabolic signals in the control of food intake. Ann NY Acad Sci 157:1084, 1969

60. Nisbett RE: Hunger, obesity and the ventromedial hypothalamus. Psychol Rev 79:433, 1972

61. Rodin J, Slochower J, Fleming B: Effects of degree

of obesity, age of onset, and weight loss on responsiveness to sensory and external stimuli. J Comp Physiol Psychol 91:586, 1977

62. Le Magnen J: Advances in studies on the physiological control and regulation of food intake. In Stellar E, Sprague JM (eds): Progress in Physiological Psychology, p 203. New York, Academic Press, 1971

63. Le Magnen J: Hyperphagie provoquee chez le rat blanc par alteration du mecanisme de satiet peripherique. Comp Rend Sances Soc Biol 150:32, 1956

64. Rolls BJ, Rolls ET, Rowe EA: Specific satiety and its influence on feeding (abstr). Appetite 1:85–86, 1980

65. Cornell C, Rodin J, Weingarten H: Stimulus-induced eating when satiate. Physiol Behav 45:852, 1989

66. Rolls B: Sweetness and satiety. In Dobbing J (ed): Sweetness. London, Springer, 1987

67. Wooley OW, Wooley SC, Dunham RB: Deprivation, expectation and threat: Effects on salivation in the obese and nonobese. Physiol Behav 17:187, 1976

68. Wooley SC, Wooley OW: Salivation to the sight and thought of food: A new measure of appetite. Psychol Med 35:136, 1973

69. Le Magnen J: Efficacite des divers stimuli alimentaires dans l'etablissement et la commande d'un appetit chez le rat blanc. J Physiol (Paris) 51:987, 1959

70. Bellisle F: Human feeding behavior. Neurosci Biobehav Rev 3:163, 1979

71. Panksepp J: Hypothalamic regulation of energy balance and feeding behavior. Fed Proc 33:1150, 1974

72. Rogers PJ, Blundell JE: Investigation of food selection and meal parameters during the development of dietary induced obesity (abstr). Appetite 1:85, 1980

73. Rowe EA, Rolls BJ: Persistent dietary obesity and regulatory challenges (abstr). Appetite 1:86–87, 1980

74. Rothwell NJ: Reversible obesity induced by "cafeteria" diets (abstr). Appetite 1:87, 1980

75. Sclafani A, Springer D: Dietary obesity in adults rats: Similarities to hypothalamic and human obesity syndromes. Physiol Behav 17:461, 1971

76. Cabanac M, Rabe EF: Influence of a monotonous food on body weight regulation in humans. Physiol Behav 17:675, 1976

77. Wooley SC, Wooley OW, Bartoshuk LM et al: Psychological aspects of feeding: Group report. In Silverstone T (ed): Appetite and Food Intake. Berlin, Abakon Verlagsgesellschaft, 1976

78. Stunkard AJ: Obesity and the social environment. In Howard A (ed): Recent Advances in Obesity Research, Vol I. London, Newman Publishing Ltd, 1975

79. Goldblatt PB, Moore ME, Stunkard AJ: Social factors in obesity. JAMA 192:1039, 1965

80. Stunkard AJ: Environment and obesity: Recent advances in our understanding of the regulation of food intake in man. Fed Proc 27:1367, 1968

81. Rodin J: The current status of the internal-external obesity hypothesis: What went wrong. Am Psychol 36:3, 1981

82. Wooley SC, Wooley OW, Dyrenforth S: Theoretical, practical, and social issues in behavioral treatment of obesity. J Appl Behav Anal 12:3, 1979

83. Rodin J, Silberstein L, Striegel-Moore R: Women and weight: A normative discontent. In: Nebraska Symposium on Motivation. Lincoln, Neb, University of Nebraska Press, 1985

84. Davis S, Woodruff J, Hawkins R: Dieting concern and masculinity-femininity traits during childhood and adolescence. Presented at the annual convention of the Southwestern Society for Research in Human Development, Lawrence, Kansas, 1980

85. Spitzer L, Rodin J: Effects of fructose and glucose preloads on subsequent food intake. Appetite 36:284, 1987

86. Booth DA: Appetitive and satiety as metabolic expectancies. In Katsuki Y, Sato M, Takagi SF et al (eds): Food Intake and Chemical Senses, p 317. Tokyo, University of Tokyo Press, 1977

87. Bernstein I, Sigmundi R: Tumor anorexia: A learned food aversion? Science 209:416, 1980

88. Hill AJ, Blundell JE: Sensitivity of the appetite control system in obese subjects to nutritional and serotoninergic challenges. (unpublished manuscript)

89. Rodin J, Reed D, Jamner L: Metabolic effects of fructose and glucose: Implications for food intake. Am J Clin Nutr 47:683, 1988

90. Durrant M, Rayston JP, Wloch RT: Effect of exercise on energy intake and eating patterns in lean and obese humans. Physiol Behav 29:449, 1982

91. Porikos KP, Booth G, Van Itallie TB: Effort of covert nutritive dilution on the spontaneous intake of obese individuals: A pilot study. Am J Clin Nutr 30:1638, 1977

92. Blundell J: Hunger, appetite and satiety: Constructs in search of identities. In Turner M (ed):

Nutrition and Lifestyles, p 21. London, Applied Science Publishing, 1979

93. Booth DA: Hunger and satiety and conditioned reflexes. In Weiner H, Hofer M, Stunkard AJ (eds): Brain, Behavior and Bodily Disease. New York, Raven Press (in press)

94. Robbins T, Fray P: Stress-inducing eating: Fact, fiction or misunderstanding. Appetite 1:103, 1980

95. Revusky S, Bedarf E: Association of illness with prior ingestion of novel foods. Science 155:219, 1967

96. Contreras R, Kosten T: Salt preference in neonatal rats. J Nutr 113:1051, 1982

97. Wurtman J, Wurtman R: Sucrose consumption early in life fails to modify the appetite of adult rats for sweet food. Science 205:321, 1979

98. Le Magnen J: Metabolically driven and learned feeding responses in man. In Bray GA (ed): Recent Advances in Obesity Research, II, p 45. London, Newman, 1978

99. Booth DA: Satiety and appetite are conditioned reactions. Psychosom Med 39:76, 1977

100. Fuller J: Caloric Learning in Human Appetite. Thesis, University of Birmingham, England, 1980

101. Aronfreed J: Conduct and conscience: The socialization of internalized control over behavior. New York, Academic Press, 1968

102. Mischel W: Processes in delay of gratification. In Berkowitz L (ed): Advances in Experimental Social Psychology, Vol 7. New York, Academic Press, 1974

103. Kanfer FH: Self-regulation: Research issues and speculation. In Neuringer C, Michael J (eds): Behavior Modification in Clinical Psychology. New York, Appleton-Century-Crofts, 1970

104. Kaplan HI, Kaplan HS: The psychosomatic concept of obesity. J Nerv Ment Dis 125:181, 1957

105. Lepper MR, Greene D: Turning play into work: Effects of adult surveillance and extrinsic rewards on children's intrinsic motivation. J Pers Soc Psychol 31:479, 1975

106. Nisbett RE, Storms MD: Cognitive, social, and physiological determinants of food intake. In London H, Nisbett RE (eds): Cognitive Modification of Emotional Behavior. Chicago, Aldine, 1975

107. Nisbett RE, Temoshok L: Is there an external cognitive style? J Pers Soc Psychol 33:36, 1976

108. Penick S, Prince H, Hinkle L: Fall in plasma content of free fatty acids associated with sight of food. N Engl J Med 175:416, 1971

109. Piaget J: The Construction of Reality in the Child. London, Routledge and Kegan Paul, 1955

110. Poskitt E: Overfeeding and overweight in infancy and their relation to body size in early childhood. Nutr Metab 21:54, 1977

111. Price JM, Sheposh JP, Tiano FE: A direct test of Schachter's internal-external theory of obesity in a naturalistic setting. In Howard A (ed): Recent Advances in Obesity Research, Vol I, p. 204. London, Newman, 1975

112. Grinker JA: Development of the sensory system. Presented at the Satellite Symposium to the 3rd International Congress on Obesity, Anacapri, Italy, 1980

113. Ravussin E, Lillioja S, Knowler WC et al: Reduced rate of energy expenditure as a risk factor for body-weight gain. N Engl J Med 18:467, 1988

114. Roberts SB, Savage J, Coward WA et al: Energy expenditure and intake in infants born to lean and overweight mothers. N Engl J Med 318:000, 19xx

115. Brownell KD, Greenwood MRC, Stellar E et al: The effects of repeated cycles of weight loss and regain in rats. Physiol Behav 38:459, 1987

PART FOUR

ANIMAL MODELS OF OBESITY

CHAPTER 18

Genetic Models of Animal Obesity

DAVID A. YORK

In the past 20 years our understanding of the factors contributing to the development of obesity, and of the endocrine and metabolic consequences of obesity, has developed rapidly. Much of this understanding has come from studies of animal models of obesity. This chapter reviews the genetic models of obesity that are available for the research worker and considers their relevance to the study of human obesity. Further details are available in a number of more comprehensive reviews.[3-5,7,30]

GENETIC MODELS

A large number of genetically inherited forms of obesity have been described in the literature (Table 18-1), but not all are readily available to the researcher. Some, notably the commonly used ob/ob mouse, db/db mouse, and fa/fa rat, are available commercially; others can only be supplied by individual research laboratories.

The obesity may be inherited either through a single gene defect or as a result of the coincidence of multiple genes, i.e., polygenic inheritance. The single gene defects have been of particular interest as they promise to be useful in identifying single protein defects that cause obesity. To date, this goal has not been achieved for any of the models, but the availability of molecular biology techniques may hasten a breakthrough, particularly as the chromosome location of the defect is known for some of the mouse obesities. The single gene obesities may reflect either a defect in expression of a dominant gene,

in which the heterozygote becomes obese and the homozygous dominant allele is sometimes fatal (e.g., A^Y/A^Y), or the presence of a recessive gene. In the latter case, only the homozygous recessive animal becomes phenotypically obese and the heterozygote remains lean, although some moderate effects of the single gene have been reported. The maintenance of these single genes on inbred backgrounds has provided a readily available nonobese control animal. In practice, the majority of studies have utilized a mixture of lean animals—homozygous dominant and heterozygotes—as the lean controls, since the infertility of the obese genotypes when fed ad libitum has necessitated breeding from lean heterozygotes.

The comparison of heterozygotes and homozygous recessives may mask some differences associated with the defective gene. A change in background genome may significantly alter the phenotype expression of these obesity genes; comparison of the degree of obesity and severity of diabetes in the Aston strain ob/ob, C57BL/6J ob/ob, and C57BL/Ks ob/ob mice illustrates this point, as does comparison of the db, db^{2J}, and db^{ad} alleles. When the ob/ob gene is on the C57BL/6J background strain, the mice become very obese and mildly diabetic, with very high levels of circulating insulin maintained throughout life (Fig. 18-1). When the ob/ob gene is placed on the C57BL/Ks background, early development of the obese syndrome is similar, but by three to four months of age pancreatic insufficiency develops and the diabetes becomes more

TABLE 18-1

Genetic Models of Animal Obesity

Animal Models	Obese Genotype	Chromosome No.	Alleles	Comment
Autosomal Dominant				
Yellow mouse	A^y/a	2	A^{iy} intermediate	
			A^{vy} viable	
Autosomal Recessive				
Obese mouse	ob/ob	6	db^{ad} (adipose)	Expression varies with background genome
Diabetes mouse	db/db	4	db^{2J}, db^3	
Fatty rat	fa/fa	?	$fa^{k'}$ (Kolesky)	
Corpulent rat	SHR/LNcp	8		
Fat mouse		?		Slow-developing obesity, nondiabetic
Tubby	tub	7		
Polygenic				
New Zealand mouse	NZO			
Japanese mouse	KK			
Paul Bailey	PBB/Ld			
black mouse				
Psamonomys obesus				⎧ Expressed when animal
(sand rat)				⎪ transferred
Acomys cahirinus				⎨ to high carbohydrate
(spiny mouse)				⎪ laboratory diet
Genomys tolarum				⎩
(tuco tuco)				
Osborne-Mendel rat				When fed a high fat diet
Sprague-Dawley rat				When fed a cafeteria diet
Obese chickens				
Obese swine				

severe as β-cell atrophy leads to a reduction in insulin secretion and early death. A reverse picture is observed when the db/db genotype is moved from its normal C57BL/Ks background to a C57BL/6J background.[9,21]

Transfer of obese genes to other background strains may enhance and expand the suitability of the animal model. An example is provided by the fa/fa Zucker obese genotype, which is not hypertensive normally and thus not suitable for studies of the interrelationship between obesity and hypertension. However, when the fa gene is transferred to differing background strains, as in the Koletsky (fa[k]) or the SHR-fafa rat,[6,29] strains that are obese and hypertensive are created.

The polygenic forms of obesity are more diverse and more difficult to use as no congenic lean control groups are available as controls. A number of these obesities illustrate the impact of diet on the genome; they require an environmen-

tal, normally dietary, change to initiate the deposition of excess fat. The desert rodents *Acomys cahirinus* (spiny mouse), *Psammomys obesus* (sand rat), and *Genomys tolarum* (tuco tuco) are typical of this group and only develop obesity when they are transferred to the laboratory environment and its plentiful supply of high carbohydrate diet. It is also possible to include in this group those species of laboratory rodent that are particularly prone to a diet-induced form of obesity such as high fat feeding to the Osborne-Mendel rat[12] and cafeteria feeding to the Sprague-Dawley rat.[24] Indeed, this genetic predisposition to the development of obesity on diets of high energy density may be a particularly appropriate model for the majority of human obesities. A number of nonrodent obesities have also been reported in, for example, chickens and swine. These obesities are typically derived in cross-breeding experiments with selection over a

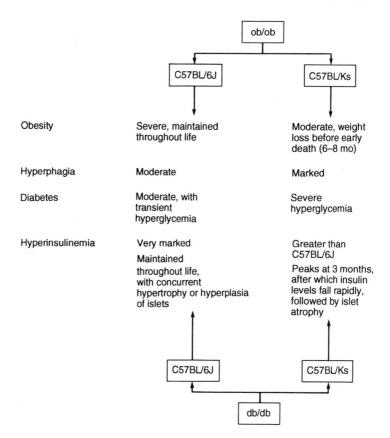

FIGURE 18-1

Effect of background genome (shown here for C57BL/6J and C57BL/Ks) on the phenotypic expression of the obese (ob/ob) and diabetes (db/db) genotypes.

number of generations for the fatter offspring. This type of obesity is assumed to be polygenic in nature.

CHARACTERISTICS OF THE GENETIC OBESITIES

The genetic obesities provide a range of obese models that vary not only in their modes of inheritance but also in the type of obesity and the severity of the associated metabolic changes. Some of these differences are listed in Table 18-2, which presents a general summary of the differing types of genetic obesity. The initial deposition of excess fat may begin at birth or shortly thereafter (ob/ob, db/db, fa/fa), as in the recessive obesities, or be evident shortly after weaning, as in the dominant yellow $A^Y a$ mouse. Obesity of polygenic origin may begin in the more mature animal (8–12 weeks in the New

Zealand obese [NZO] mouse), as it apparently can be triggered at any age by some environmental or diet change.[3,4] The location of the excess fat varies from predominantly subcutaneous (e.g., young fa/fa rats) to predominantly intra-abdominal (e.g., the NZO mouse). The severity of the obesity is variable; the greatest obesity is generally seen in the recessive obesities in apparent association with hyperplastic hypertrophic growth of adipose depots. In some species expressing more moderate obesity (e.g., the polygenic NZO mouse), hyperplasia of fat cells is not evident until fat deposition is further stimulated by a high fat diet. A number of species also exhibit a reduction in linear growth.

Hypersecretion of insulin is a common feature that initially becomes evident in the recessive obesities when preobese pups are weaned to high-carbohydrate diets, although a mild degree of insulin hypersecretion may be present even

TABLE 18-2

General Characteristics of Different Forms of Genetic Obesity

Characteristic	Mode of Inheritance/Derivation		
	Dominant	*Recessive*	*Polygenic*
Obesity	Moderate	Severe	Variable
Time of onset	After weaning	Birth or soon afterwards	2–3 mo, or when diet is changed
Linear growth	Increased	Decreased	Unchanged?
Hyperphagia	Moderate, not necessary for obesity	Marked, not necessary for obesity	Variable, diet change often necessary for obesity
Metabolic rate ($/wt^{0.75}$)	Decreased	Decreased	Increased or normal
Location of excess fat	SC or IA	SC > IA	(NZO)
Hyperinsulinemia	Moderate	Severe; early onset	Moderate; late onset or initiated by diet change
Diabetes	Mild	Variable: db/db—severe ob/ob—moderate fa/fa—mild or absent	

Abbreviations: SC, subcutaneous; IA, intra-abdominal; NZO, New Zealand obese.

during the suckling period.[10,11,18,23,32] The progressive hypersecretion of insulin leads to hyperinsulinization of certain tissues and metabolic pathways (e.g., hepatic lipogenesis) but a progressive development of insulin resistance elsewhere (e.g., muscle glucose metabolism and adipocyte lipogenesis).[11,17,28] In some species this insulin insensitivity may develop into overt diabetes that eventually leads to pancreatic failure, weight loss, and death (db/db); in others, such as the ob/ob mouse, it leads to mild diabetes. By contrast, in the fa/fa rat, blood glucose levels remain close to normal.[3-5,7,30] There is less information on insulin sensitivity and glucose homeostasis in the other forms of obesity, but, as with the recessive genotypes, there appears to be a spectrum of metabolic changes.

ENERGY BALANCE

An excessive food intake has been reported in all genetically obese strains fed *ad libitum*, although in no case has excessive food intake been shown to be an essential requirement for the development of obesity, and the degree of the hyperphagia is quite variable. Because physical activity, when measured, has been shown to be normal

until gross obesity is evident, a reduction in energy expenditure must provide the energy imbalance necessary for the deposition of excess fat when hyperphagia is prevented. Thus in some models the depression in metabolic rate (oxygen consumption) in suckling pups can be used to identify the preobese genotypes,[13,22] while an impairment in brown adipose tissue thermogenesis in response to dietary stimuli and sometimes also in response to cold stimuli has been reported in all those genotypes in which it has been investigated.[2,31] The coincidence of abnormalities in feeding behavior and in energy expenditure in the genetic obesities has focused attention on the hypothalamus as a possible site for the expression of the gene defects, since it is evident that the hypothalamic centers that control feeding also have important functions in controlling energy expenditure through their ability to modulate peripheral autonomic balance.[3]

POSSIBLE GENETIC DEFECTS

The identification of defects in the control of energy intake and energy expenditure, while focusing attention on the hypothalamus, does not nec-

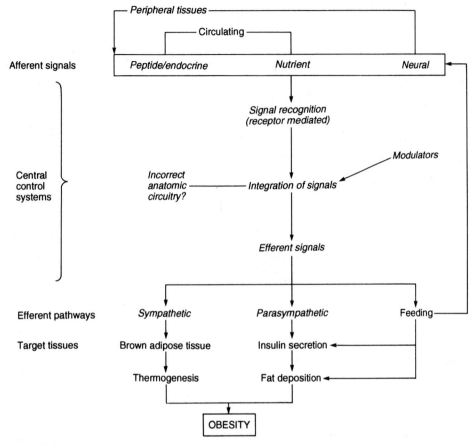

FIGURE 18-2

Possible sites for the expression of a genetic defect. Shown are some of the interrelationships involved in the control of energy balance in rodents. Sites or processes underlined represent possible locations for the expression of a genetic defect that could lead to the development of obesity and the characteristic changes in feeding and autonomic balance.

essarily imply that the gene defects are expressed in or solely in that tissue. Indeed, parabiotic studies suggest that either an absence of circulating factors or an inability to respond to circulating factors may be fundamental to the development of obesity.[8,19] Thus, the gene defects could be expressed in a variety of ways (Fig. 18-2). The gene defect could result in inappropriate afferent information reaching the hypothalamus either from the periphery or higher centers, or it could result from a defect in the coupling of afferent information to the efferent pathways controlling energy expenditure or feeding, which might itself result from a number of possible derangements, such as absence of receptor recognition, loss of neuromodulation, or an anatomic or chemical change in the efferent pathways themselves. Identification of the proteins coded by the defective genes in the genetic obesities may be a major development in our understanding of the hypothalamic regulation of energy balance. Possible defects in some of the genetic obesities are reviewed below.

1. *Autonomic defects.* There is evidence for

some degree of autonomic imbalance in all of the genetic obesities that have been studied; the attenuated sympathetic drive to brown adipose tissue at normal housing temperatures (mild cold acclimation for rats and mice) and in response to dietary stimuli reduces the proportion of energy intake dissipated as thermal energy.[5,20] In contrast, the hypersecretion of insulin, which may reflect an overactivity of the parasympathetic system,[23] stimulates energy deposition as fat. Hypothalamic centers control this autonomic balance in response to external and internal stimuli. Adrenalectomy, which prevents the development of all genetic obesities, is associated with a restoration of autonomic balance, suggesting that the adrenal-pituitary-hypothalamic systems controlling glucocorticoid secretion may have an important function in the development of obesity.[1,2,5,26,31] Early evidence suggests that the influence of glucocorticoid status on the development of obesity may reflect in part the reciprocal changes in corticotropin-releasing factor (CRF) secretion in the hypothalamus; CRF injection or infusion into the third ventricle prevents obesity, abolishes the hyperphagia, and stimulates sympathetic drive to brown adipose tissue.[31] Whether a defect in CRF action could cause obesity is, however, questionable. Adrenalectomy prevents all forms of obesity, not just the genetically inherited obesities, and therefore the weight-reducing responses to adrenalectomy may reflect excessive activity of CRF responsive systems that override the inborn errors in the control of energy balance. However, it should be recognized that adrenalectomy results in changes in the secretory patterns of multiple neuropeptides, not just CRF, and glucocorticoid control of these systems may be important in the development of obesity. It is difficult, though, to interpret some of the parabiotic studies[8,19] in the context of a primary gene-encoded defect in secretion of a neuropeptide unless these circulating factors normally enhance CRF secretion.

2. *Agouti coat color: abnormality in peptide acetylation?* The obesity of the yellow obese mouse is associated with the loss of normal coat color. A number of alleles of the dominant gene occur in which the severity of the obesity has been linked with the degree of yellow pigmentation of the coat. This association of obesity with the agouti coat color suggests that the genes controlling obesity and those controlling agouti coat color are closely linked or even identical. Geschwind et al[16] first reported that the yellow obese mouse responded normally to α-MSH (melanocyte-stimulating hormone), developing black pigmentation of the coat, which indicated the responsiveness of the hair follicle melanocytes to stimulation. More recently it has been shown that yellow obese mice secrete α-MSH but that the ratio of acetyl-MSH to desacetyl-MSH is reduced, possibly indicative of a defect in the acetylation process. Desacetyl-MSH is biologically inactive in inducing coat pigmentation but does stimulate food intake independently of its ACTH-like effects on glucocorticoid secretion. Because the activity of numerous other neuropeptides is also altered by N-terminal acetylation, Shimizu and colleagues have proposed the hypothesis that an abnormality in peptide acetylation may cause the obesity of the yellow obese mouse.[25]

3. *Absence of pancreatic polypeptide.* Islet transplantation studies performed by Gates and colleagues[14] showed absence of a pancreatic factor in the NZO mouse. This factor was subsequently identified as pancreatic polypeptide which, when injected into the NZO mouse, prevented the development of obesity.[15] The possible importance of pancreatic polypeptide as a circulating factor that is monitored centrally as a signal in the control of energy balance has not been thoroughly investigated.

RELEVANCE OF GENETIC MODELS TO HUMAN OBESITY

Clinicians and research funding bodies may question the relevance of the study of the genetic animal model to the human obese condition. The genetic obesities provide good models for investigating the physiologic control systems responsible for maintaining energy balance and for investigating the secondary effects of excess adiposity. Human and rodent obesities may differ in their relative distributions of body fat, but the metabolic status of the obese rodent and obese human has many similarities, including hyperinsulinemia, insulin resistance, and the development of diabetes. Indeed, prospective studies in the genetic model have been of value in clearly demonstrating that hyperinsulinemia precedes the development of insulin resistance in obesity.[11,18]

The single gene forms of animal obesity have been popular models, and their study will eventually lead to the identification of protein defects that can cause obesity. Whether such defects will also be observed in humans will not be known until definitive tests are available. A few clearly defined, genetically inherited obesities described in man have similarities to the homozygous recessive obesities of rodents. However, such inborn errors are rare and do not contribute significantly to the growing obese population. Nevertheless, recent research has emphasized the very strong genetic component in the determination of body fatness in man,[27] suggesting that genetic inheritance may be the most important determinant of obesity in individuals consuming a Western diet. Indeed, the animal studies might suggest that the apparent infinite varieties of obesities in humans may only reflect the variety of phenotypic expressions of a relatively few genetic components on the infinitely variable background genome of *Homo sapiens.*

Bray and colleagues have recently drawn attention to the essential afferent, central, and efferent components in the homeostatic system for control of body energy content (see Fig. 18-2).[5] They emphasized that there was evidence for some degree of efferent autonomic imbalance between the sympathetic control of brown adipose tissue thermogenesis and parasympathetic control of insulin secretion in all forms of animal obesity. Whether similar changes in the activity of these efferent pathways is also the ultimate cause of obesity in man awaits more detailed study of individual components of the autonomic system, although some supportive evidence has been reported. A better understanding of the interrelationships between food intake and autonomic activity will also be necessary since the majority of the investigations in human obesity are undertaken during a static phase, or when gross obesity is already apparent.

The advent of molecular biology and the possible resolution of some of the genetic defects underlying the animal obesities should make the next decade an exciting and stimulating period.

If new approaches to the treatment and prevention of obesity are the result, then clearly the study of animal models will have been justified.

References

1. Allars J, Holt S, York DA: Energetic efficiency and brown adipose tissue uncoupling protein of obese Zucker rats fed high carbohydrate and high fat diets: The effect of adrenalectomy. Int J Obes 11:591, 1987
2. Bray GA: Regulation of energy balance: Studies on genetic, hypothalamic and dietary obesity. Proc Nutr Soc 41:95, 1982
3. Bray GA, York DA: Genetically transmitted obesity in rodents. Physiol Rev 51:598, 1971
4. Bray GA, York DA: Hypothalamic and genetic obesity in experimental animals: An autonomic and endocrine hypothesis. Physiol Rev 59:719, 1979
5. Bray GA, York DA, Fisler J: Experimental obesity: A homeostatic failure due to defective nutrient stimulation of the sympathetic nervous system. Vitam Horm 45:1, 1989
6. Chanh PH, Kaiser R, Laserre B et al: Creation of a strain of genetically obese-hypertensive rats. Int J Obes 12:141, 1988
7. Coleman DL: Genetics of obesity in rodents. In Bray GH (ed): Recent Advances in Obesity Research, Vol 2, p 142. Newman, London
8. Coleman DL: Obese and diabetes: Two mutant genes causing diabetes-obesity syndrome in mice. Diabetologia 14:141, 1978
9. Coleman DL, Hummel KP: The influence of genetic background on the expression of the obese (ob) gene in the mouse. Diabetologia 9:287, 1973
10. Coleman DL, Hummel KP: Hyperinsulinemia in preweaning diabetes (db) mice. Diabetologia 10:607, 1974
11. Crettaz M, Jeanrenaud B: Progressive establishment of insulin resistance in skeletal muscles of obese rats. In Bjorntorp P, Cairella M, Howard A (eds): Recent Advances in Obesity Research, Vol 3, p 268. London, J. Libbey & Co Ltd, 19xx
12. Fisler J, Bray GA: Dietary obesity: Effects of drugs on food intake in S5B/Pl and Osborne-Mendel rats. Physiol Behav 34:225, 1988
13. Fred GH: Oxygen consumption rates of litters of thin and obese-hyperglycemic mice. Am J Physiol 225:209, 1973
14. Gates RJ, Hunt M, Lazarus N: Further studies in amelioration of characteristics of New Zealand obese (NZO) mice following implantation of islets of Langerhans. Diabetologia 10:401, 1974
15. Gates RJ, Lazarus NR: The ability of pancreatic

polypeptide (APP and BPP) to return to normal the hyperglycemia, hyperinsulinemia and weight gain of New Zealand obese mice. Horm Res 8:189, 1977

16. Geschwind II, Husbeby RA, Nishioka R: The effect of melanocyte stimulating hormone on coat colour in the mouse. Rec Prog Horm Res 28:91, 1972

17. Godbole V, York DA: Lipogenesis in situ in the genetically obese Zucker fafa rat: Role of hyperphagia and hyperinsulinemia. Diabetologia 14:191, 1978

18. Grundleger ML, Godbole VY, Thenen SW: Age-dependent development of insulin resistance of soleus muscles in genetically obese obob mice. Am J Physiol 239:R363, 1980

19. Harris RB, Hervey E, Hervey GR et al: Body composition of lean and obese Zucker rats in parabiosis. Int J Obes 11:274, 1987

20. Holt SJ, York DA: Studies on the sympathetic efferent nerves of brown adipose tissue of lean and obese Zucker rats. Brain Res 481:106, 1989

21. Hummel KP, Coleman DL, Lane PW: The influence of genetic background on the expression of mutations at the diabetes locus in the mouse: I. C57BL/KsJ and C57BL/6J strains. Biochem Genet 7:1, 1972

22. Planche E, Joliff M, DeGasquet P et al: Evidence of a defect in energy expenditure in 7 day old Zucker rat (fafa). Am J Physiol 245:E107, 1983

23. Rohner-Jeanrenaud F, Jeanrenaud B: Involvement of the cholinergic system in insulin and glucagon oversecretion in preobesity. Endocrinology 116:830, 1985

24. Rothwell NJ, Saville EM, Stock MJ: Effects of feeding a cafeteria diet on energy balance and diet-induced thermogenesis in four strains of rat. J Nutr 112:1515, 1982

25. Shimizu H, Bray GA, Retzios AD et al: Increased pituitary des-acetyl-MSH: An explanation for the genetically obese yellow mouse. In Bjorntorp P, Rossner S (eds): Obesity in Europe 88. London, J. Libbey & Co, 1988

26. Smith CK, Romsos DR: Effects of adrenalectomy on energy balance of obese mice are diet dependent. Am J Physiol 249:R13, 1985

27. Stunkard AJ, Thorkild IA, Sorensen M et al: An adoption study of human obesity. N Engl J Med 314:193, 1986

28. Terrataz J, Assimacopoulos-Jeannet F, Jeanrenaud B: Severe hepatic and peripheral insulin resistance as evidenced by euglycaemic clamps in genetically obese fafa rats. Endocrinology 118:674, 1986

29. Yen T, Shaw WN, Yu PL: Genetics of obesity in Zucker rats and Koletsky rats. Heredity 38:373, 1977

30. York DA: Animal models for the study of obesity. In Curtis-Prior PB (ed): Biochemical Pharmacology of Obesity, p 67. London, Elsevier Science Publishers, 1983

31. York DA, Holt SJ, Allars J et al: Glucocorticoids and the central control of sympathetic activity in the obese fafa rat. In Bjorntorp P, Rossner S (eds): Obesity in Europe 88. London, J. Libbey & Co, 1988

32. York DA, Shargill NS, Godbole V: Serum insulin and lipogenesis in the suckling fatty 'fafa' rat. Diabetologia 21:143, 1981

CHAPTER 19

Dietary Obesity Models

ANTHONY SCLAFANI

A number of different animal models have been developed to study the causes and consequences of obesity.[55] Among the most extensively studied models are the various forms of dietary obesity in rodents. Although the role of dietary factors in human obesity has not been precisely identified, laboratory research clearly establishes that certain diets promote overeating, overweight, and obesity in animals. This chapter briefly describes the dietary manipulations that lead to obesity in rodents. Most research has focused on the nutrient composition of the diet, in particular its fat and sugar content. However, as indicated in Table 19-1, many other features of the diet, including its physical form, flavor, and variety, influence its obesity-promoting effect. In addition, the degree of overeating and obesity obtained with a given diet is affected by subject variables such as the age, strain, and sex of the animal, and by environmental variables such as ambient temperature and housing conditions.

BASIC CONCEPTS

Dietary-induced overeating and obesity are typically evaluated in reference to a control group of animals fed a dry chow or semisynthetic diet that is high in starch and low in fat. It should be noted, however, that adult rats given free access to chow have up to 20% or more body fat, which some investigators consider excessive.[3] That is, compared to animals fed restricted amounts of food, rats fed chow *ad libitum* are not only fatter but have decreased longevity, reduced fertility,

and greater susceptibility to disease.[3,4] Thus, the control condition used to assess dietary obesity, the chow-fed animal, may arguably represent a form of mild obesity.

Dietary manipulations often produce the three O's—overeating, overweight, and obesity—but these effects can be dissociated. That is, relatively small increases in body fat can occur without body weight being affected, and increases in body weight or body fat can occur in the absence of increased food intake. Obesity without hyperphagia is possible because changes in the nutrient composition or form of the diet can alter the efficiency of food utilization and thereby increase the amount of body fat stored per calorie consumed. Increased feed efficiency can result from increased absorption of ingested food or enhanced storage of absorbed energy in body fat stores. It could be argued that any level of food intake that leads to excess fat disposition represents a form of hyperphagia,[66] but in the present discussion hyperphagia refers only to those cases in which caloric intake exceeds control levels.

When hyperphagia does occur it is frequently attributed to the *palatability* of the diet. The concept of palatability requires clarification since it is often used in circular fashion.[34,58] Diets are described as palatable if they promote overeating; overeating in turn is "explained" by the palatability of the diet. In order to assess the role of palatability in dietary-induced hyperphagia it is necessary to measure palatability and food intake independently; such measures are often not included in dietary obesity experiments. There are

TABLE 19-1

Variables Influencing Dietary-Induced Overeating and Obesity

Diet Variables	Subject Variables	Environmental Variables
Nutrient composition	Age	Ambient temperature
Physical form (hydration)	Strain	Housing conditions
Flavor	Sex	
Palatability	Individual differences	
Variety	Neural/endocrine disorders	
Availability		

many ways to evaluate food palatability in animals. One simple procedure is the two-choice preference test.[56,58] If an animal prefers food A to B, then it can be assumed that food A is more palatable than B. Recent studies indicate that increasing palatability (preference) can, in some cases, promote hyperphagia, but that preferred foods are not always overconsumed, and foods that are overconsumed are not necessarily preferred to other foods.[21,26,33] These and other findings demonstrate that while palatability is a contributing factor, it is not the only determinant of dietary-induced overeating.[34,58]

A second important issue concerns the origin of diet palatability. Palatability, which means "pleasing to the palate or taste," is often assumed to be a function solely of the orosensory properties—taste, odor, texture—of foods. It is now clear, however, that food preferences can change as the animal associates the flavor of a food with its postingestive effects. For example, recent studies demonstrate that rats learn to prefer flavors that are paired with intragastric starch or fat infusions.[22,63] Thus, the palatability of food is determined both by unlearned responses to flavor (e.g., innate preference for sweet taste) and by learned responses based on the food's postingestive actions (e.g., rise in plasma glucose).[58]

According to this analysis, dietary-induced obesity can result from a combination of factors. As illustrated in Figure 19-1, the orosensory (taste, smell, texture) and postingestive effects of food together determine palatability; palatability in turn can promote overeating. High palatability is not a necessary condition for overeating to occur, however; some postingestive actions of food

may stimulate food intake without enhancing palatability.[33] Also, the postingestive effects of some nutrients can enhance body fat deposition in the absence of overeating. Clearly, overeating and obesity will be greatest when all contributing factors are present.

OBESITY-PROMOTING DIETS

In one of the earliest reports of dietary obesity, Ingle[13] in 1949 observed excessive weight gain in rats fed a semiliquid, medium-carbohydrate diet and housed in small cages that severely limited their physical activity. A subsequent study confirmed these findings but also reported that rats would get just as fat when housed in standard-size cages and fed either Ingle's medium-carbohydrate diet or a high-fat ration.[24] Since this early work, many different diets have been formulated that promote overeating and/or obesity in laboratory rodents.

High-Carbohydrate Diets

The effects of dietary carbohydrate, particularly sucrose, on food intake and body weight have been extensively investigated.[32,56] Many studies have used the *composite diet method* in which animals are fed a single, nutritionally complete diet that varies in its carbohydrate type or amount. A number of studies demonstrate that, compared to starch-based diets, high-sucrose (30%–80%) composite diets increase body weight and/or body fat, but this is not always the case.[32,56] A number of factors influence the obesity-promoting effect of high-sugar diets.[32]

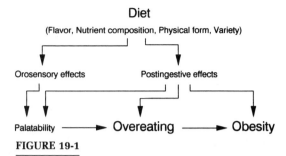

FIGURE 19-1

Conceptual model illustrating various ways that dietary factors can produce obesity.

Diet hydration is one important factor; recent work indicates that adding water to high-sucrose composite diets significantly increases food intake and weight gain.[31]

Overeating, overweight, and obesity are reliably produced by offering animals a sugar solution as an option to their chow diet (*diet option method*).[32,56] Adult rats given access to a 32% sucrose solution, plus chow and water, typically take 60% of their calories as sugar, increase their total caloric intake by about 20%, and gain more body weight and fat than animals fed only chow.[57] Similar effects have been obtained with glucose and fructose solutions.[16] If the sugar is offered as powdered sucrose rather than as a sucrose solution, however, there is little increase in food intake and body weight.[16,57]

Sugars are not the only carbohydrates to promote obesity. In particular, offering rats a solution of partially hydrolyzed starch (e.g., 32% Polycose) plus chow and water increases caloric intake, body weight, and body fat as much as do sucrose and glucose solutions.[57] Even unprocessed starch can produce overeating and obesity if it is presented in a hydrated form, although the effects are less than those obtained with sugar and hydrolyzed starch diets.[31,65] Taken together, these results indicate that both the type and the form of carbohydrate determine food intake, body weight and adiposity. Sugars and hydrolyzed starch increase food intake and body weight more than raw starch, and hydrated carbohydrate diets are more effective than dry diets. Why adding water to carbohydrate diets promotes overeating is not fully understood, but

hydration appears to improve the palatability of the food as well as to facilitate digestion.[58,65]

High-Fat Diets

High-fat composite diets have long been used to produce obesity in laboratory rodents. Compared to animals fed a low-fat control diet, rats fed a high-fat composite diet (30%–60% fat) gain more weight and deposit more body fat, sometimes to the point of extreme obesity.[14,24,27,52,53] High-fat composite diets, however, have variable effects on caloric intake. In many cases high-fat diets increase caloric intake by 10% to 20%,[52,53] whereas in other cases caloric intake remains unchanged even though the rats become obese.[14,27] The degree of overeating, overweight, and obesity is influenced by the concentration and type of fat included in the diet. Weight gains tend to be proportional to fat concentration, are enhanced when solid fats (vegetable shortening, lard) rather than vegetable oils are used, and are enhanced when the fat contains long-chain triglycerides rather than short-chain triglycerides.[2,5,8,51] Contrary to the results obtained with high-carbohydrate composite diets, adding water to high-fat composite rations has little impact on the diet's hyperphagia- and obesity-promoting effects.[31]

Obesity can also be produced by offering rats a pure fat source as an option to a chow diet. For example, in one study rats fed corn oil as an option consumed somewhat more calories (4%–10%) and gained significantly more body weight than did chow-fed controls.[21] Presenting the corn oil as a 35% oil-water emulsion rather than as pure oil reliably increased fat and total calorie intake and weight gain. Overeating and overweight were also enhanced when the fat source was vegetable shortening rather than corn oil.[21] Thus, the feeding response to a fat option is influenced by the type of fat used, and, with corn oil at least, by presenting the fat in an emulsified form.

High-Fat, High-Sugar Diets

Because overeating and obesity can be produced by either high-fat or high-sugar foods it might be expected that combining both fat and sugar in the same diet would result in an exaggerated hyperphagia and obesity response. Although obesity has been obtained in animals fed foods high in both fat and sugar,[19,27] few experiments have systematically manipulated dietary fat and sugar levels. In two studies, adding sucrose to a high-fat diet failed to potentiate the diet's obesity-promoting effect and in fact tended to reduce it.[26,35] However, in other experiments the addition of sucrose to a high-fat diet significantly increased caloric intake and body weight gain.[1,23] In the latter study rats that were fed chow plus a 35% corn oil emulsion containing 8% sucrose consumed more fat, more total calories, and gained more weight than did rats given a plain corn oil emulsion. The feeding enhancing effect of the sucrose was due in part to its sweet taste, since adding saccharin to the corn oil emulsion also increased fat and total caloric intake.[23]

Thus, there are some diet formulations in which combining sugar and fat potentiate the overeating and obesity response. The specific form or choice of foods available appears to be a critical factor.

Cafeteria Diets

With the cafeteria diet animals are fed, in addition to a standard chow diet, a variety of food items that differ in their taste, texture, and nutritional composition. Most commonly the diet includes foods marketed for human consumption such as cookies, cheese, chocolate candy, marshmallows, peanut butter, salami, and sweetened condensed milk; in some experiments the foods may actually be leftovers from a real cafeteria. This dietary regimen was originally developed to produce rapid weight gains in adult rats.[64] Although systematic comparisons are lacking, the hyperphagia and obesity produced with cafeteria diets are generally much greater than that obtained with standard high-fat or high-sugar diets. Furthermore, the cafeteria diet can produce obesity in strains of rats that do not become obese when fed the high-fat or high-sugar diets.[9] Because of the complexity of the cafeteria diet, it is difficult but not impossible to obtain accurate caloric intake measures, and nutrient selection can vary from animal to animal. This has been a source of controversy, particularly with regard to studies of diet-induced thermogenesis.[25,48]

The effectiveness of the cafeteria diet in producing overeating, overweight, and obesity is attributable to several factors. Most of the food items are high in fat or sugar, are moist, and have been formulated to be very tasty (at least to humans). Variety is another important aspect of the diet. Rats given simultaneous access to two or three cafeteria foods in addition to chow consume more total food and gain more weight than do rats fed only a single food.[39,43] Overeating and obesity have also been observed in rats fed a variety of lab chows that differ in flavor and nutrient composition, but not in rats fed rations that differ only in flavor.[20,26] Variety in the diet may promote overeating by counteracting the effect of "sensory-specific" satiety. Rats, like people, eat more food in a meal when offered different foods rather than a single food.[40] In addition, individual animals have specific food preferences, and providing a varied diet would ensure that all rats had preferred foods available.[30,39,64]

Rats made obese with a cafeteria diet typically undereat and lose weight to control levels when they are returned to a chow-only diet.[10,38,45,62,64] The undereating response has been attributed to a suppressive effect of obesity on chow intake and to a "negative contrast" effect related to the change from the tasty cafeteria diet to the monotonous chow diet.[38] Cafeteria diet–induced obesity is not always reversible, however; in some cases rats stop gaining weight when the cafeteria-type foods are removed but do not lose weight to control levels.[41,42] Several factors may influence the reversibility of dietary obesity, including age, sex, and length of time on the cafeteria diet. Prolonged overfeeding of a cafeteria diet can produce adipocyte hyperplasia, which may be responsible for the persistent obesity observed following the return to the chow diet.[68]

Macronutrient Self-Selection Diets

Another diet that involves multiple food choices is the macronutrient self-selection (MNSS) diet. In this case animals are given the choice between separate sources of pure fat, protein, and carbohydrate supplemented with vitamins and minerals. Female but not male rats fed a MNSS diet gain more weight and accumulate more body fat than do chow-fed controls.[1,37] This effect is attributable to the high fat intake self-selected by the rats; animals maintained on a composite diet that matched the nutrient composition chosen by self-selecting rats (50% fat, 28% protein, 22% carbohydrate) had nearly identical weight gains.[1]

In an interesting variation of the weight cycling or "yo-yo" dieting procedure,[6] rats were placed on a feeding regimen in which *ad libitum* access to an MNSS diet was alternated with *ad libitum* access to chow.[37] During MNSS refeeding periods, the cycled group selected more fat than did rats maintained on the MNSS diet throughout. Furthermore, the MNSS/chow cycled group gained more weight and significantly more fat than did the noncycled group. These results demonstrate that variations in diet availability can influence macronutrient self-selection and adiposity.

DETERMINANTS OF DIETARY OBESITY

Subject Variables

A number of factors influence the degree of overeating, overweight, and obesity produced by the diets described in the previous section. Among the most important are the age and genetic background of the animal. Dietary-induced hyperphagia and adiposity are most pronounced in older animals. Feeding young rats (20–60 days old) high-fat, high-sugar, or cafeteria diets typically does not produce overeating or accelerated weight gain until the animals are 60 to 90 days old; however, body fat stores may increase before this age.[15,28,46] Furthermore, during adulthood the obesity response to high-fat or cafeteria diets increases with age.[28,62] Some evidence suggests that feeding rats a high-fat diet from an early age increases the ultimate level of adiposity attained during adulthood.[28] On the other hand, early exposure to a cafeteria diet may reduce the diet's obesity-promoting effect when it is reintroduced later in life.[46]

Genetic background is another major determinant of dietary obesity. Substantial strain differences have been observed in the overeating and obesity response to high-fat, high-sucrose cafeteria diets.[9,36,44,53] For example, in one study rats of the Osborne-Mendel strain fed a high-fat ration gained 50% more weight than their chow-fed controls, whereas rats of the S 5B/P1 strain gained only slightly more than controls.[53] Other

strains of rats showed intermediate weight gains on the high-fat diet. The differential weight gain response of Osborne-Mendel and S 5B/P1 rats was reduced when the animals were fed a cafeteria diet rather than a high-fat ration.[9] Therefore, diet and heredity interact in the determination of body weight and adiposity.

Within a given strain of animals, marked individual differences exist in the overeating and obesity response to particular diets. For example, in one study all (n = 26) rats fed a cafeteria diet outgained the chow-fed controls, but there was considerable variability in their weight gains, with some animals gaining only 14% more than the heaviest control and others gaining as much as 188% more.[64] In another study only half the rats fed a high-fat, high-sugar composite diet outgained the chow-fed controls.[19] The differential predisposition to dietary obesity on this diet was found to be related to pre-existing differences in the rats' sympathetic response to glucose loads.[18]

The individual differences observed in dietary obesity may be specific to the particular foods used. This is suggested by preliminary results obtained with rats selected for high or low weight gain on a cafeteria diet; the rats were the offspring of Sprague-Dawley females who were rapid or slow gainers on the cafeteria diet.[60] As expected, when fed the cafeteria foods, the offspring of the obese-prone mothers outgained the offspring of the lean-prone mothers. However, when subsequently tested with a high-sucrose diet (sucrose solution plus chow), the supposedly lean-prone offspring actually gained more weight than the obese-prone offspring. The cafeteria and sucrose diets differed in their fat and sugar content. These results indicate that even within a single strain of animals there may be genetically determined, nutrient-specific differences in dietary obesity.

The sex of the animal is another variable that influences development of dietary obesity. Sex-related differences have been reported in the degree of obesity, body fat distribution, feed efficiency, relative weight gain, and obesity-inhibitory effect of activity.[12,14,17,41,54,62] Also, as previously noted, only female rats have been reported to develop obesity on macronutrient self-selection diets.

In addition to producing overeating and overweight in otherwise normal animals, high-fat, high-sugar, and cafeteria diets also increase food intake and body weight in rats with pre-existing obesity. In particular, rats with hypothalamic obesity display exaggerated responses to these diets compared to neurologically intact controls.[59,61] The weight gain and adiposity of ovariectomized rats and genetically obese animals is also potentiated by high-fat and cafeteria diets.[7,10,61]

Environmental Variables

Laboratory rodents are usually housed in small cages that limit their physical activity. When given access to an activity wheel, rats will engage in a considerable amount of running behavior. This voluntary activity can substantially reduce or even eliminate the obesity-promoting effect of cafeteria and high-sucrose diets.[12,41,64] Not surprisingly, forced exercise (e.g., swimming, treadmill running) also suppresses dietary-induced obesity.[11,29] In contrast, the physical activity associated with housing rats in social groups or in large, multilevel cages does not alter the weight-promoting effect of cafeteria diets.[50,64] Most likely the animals in these latter studies exercise less than animals given access to an activity wheel or forced exercise.

Dietary-induced overeating and obesity are also influenced by ambient temperature. Compared to a normal room temperature (25°C), a very cold (4°C) temperature can inhibit weight gain whereas a moderately cold (18°C) temperature can facilitate weight gain in rats fed a cafeteria diet.[49,67] Body fat deposition may also be enhanced by maintaining rats at warm temperatures (29°C).[47]

SUMMARY

Obesity can be produced in laboratory animals by a variety of dietary manipulations. These include increasing the fat, sugar, or hydrolyzed starch content of the diet, adding water to the diet, and increasing the palatability or variety (or both) of foods available. The adiposity may result from increased caloric intake or increased efficiency of food utilization (or both). Dietary obesity is usually associated with overweight, but in some cases adiposity may increase without body

weight being elevated. The age, sex, and genetic background of the animal as well as its housing conditions all influence the development of dietary obesity. Dietary manipulations can also exaggerate the adiposity of animals with pre-existing obesity, such as the hypothalamic or genetically obese rodent.

Much remains to be learned about the behavioral and physiologic mechanisms involved in dietary-induced overeating and obesity. A greater understanding of how changes in the nutrient composition, flavor, physical form, and variety of the diet stimulate overeating and increase feed efficiency in laboratory animals may enhance our ability to prevent and treat obesity in humans.

Acknowledgment: This study was supported by grants from the National Institute of Diabetes and Digestive and Kidney Diseases (DK-31135) and the Faculty Research Award Program of the City University of New York.

References

1. Ackroff K, Sclafani A: Sucrose-induced hyperphagia and obesity in rats fed a macronutrient self-selection diet. Physiol Behav 44:181, 1988
2. Barboriak JJ, Krehl WA, Cowgill GR et al: Influence of high-fat diets on growth and development of obesity in the albino rat. J Nutr 64:241, 1958
3. Berg BN: Nutrition and longevity in the rat. I. Food intake in relation to size, health and fertility. J Nutr 71:242, 1960
4. Berg BN, Simms HS: Nutrition and longevity in the rat. II. Longevity and onset of disease with different levels of food intake. J Nutr 71:255, 1960
5. Bray GA, Lee M, Bray TL: Weight gain of rats fed medium-chain triglycerides is less than rats fed long-chain triglycerides. Int J Obes 4:27, 1980
6. Brownell KD, Greenwood MRC, Stellar E et al: The effects of repeated cycles of weight loss and regain in rats. Physiol Behav 38:459, 1986
7. Faust IM, Johnson PR, Stern JS et al: Diet-induced adipocyte number increase in adult rats: A new model of obesity. Am J Physiol 235:E279, 1978
8. Fenton PF, Carr C: The nutrition of the mouse: Responses of four strains to diets differing in fat content. J Nutr 45:225, 1951
9. Fisler JS, Lupien JR, Wood RD et al: Brown fat thermogenesis in a rat model of dietary obesity. Am J Physiol 253:R756, 1987

10. Gale SK, Van Itallie TB, Faust IM: Effects of palatable diets on body weight and adipose tissue cellularity in the adult obese female Zucker rat (fa/fa). Metabolism 30:105, 1981

11. Hill JO, Davis JR, Tagliaferro AR et al: Dietary obesity and exercise in young rats. Physiol Behav 33:321, 1984

12. Hirsch E, Ball E, Godkin L: Sex differences in the effects of voluntary activity on sucrose-induced obesity. Physiol Behav 29:253, 1982

13. Ingle DJ: A simple means of producing obesity in the rat. Proc Soc Exp Biol Med 72:604, 1949

14. Jen K-LC, Greenwood MRC, Brasel JA: Sex differences in the effects on high-fat feeding on behavior and carcass composition. Physiol Behav 27:161, 1981

15. Kanarek RB, Marks-Kaufman R: Developmental aspects of sucrose-induced obesity in rats. Physiol Behav 23:881, 1979

16. Kanarek RB, Orthen-Gambill N: Differential effects of sucrose, fructose, and glucose on carbohydrate-induced obesity in rats. J Nutr 112:1546, 1982

17. Lemonnier D: Effect of age, sex, and site on the cellularity of the adipose tissue in mice and rats rendered obese by a high-fat diet. J Clin Invest 51:2907, 1972

18. Levin BE, Sullivan AC: Glucose-induced norepinephrine levels and obesity resistance. Am J Physiol 253:R475, 1987

19. Levin BE, Triscari J, Sullivan AC: Relationship between sympathetic activity and diet-induced obesity in two rat strains. Am J Physiol 245:R367, 1983

20. Louis-Sylvestre J, Giachetti I, Le Magnen J: Sensory versus dietary factors in cafeteria-induced overweight. Physiol Behav 32:901, 1984

21. Lucas F, Ackroff K, Sclafani A: Dietary fat induced hyperphagia in rats as a function of fat type and physical form. Physiol Behav 45:937, 1989

22. Lucas F, Sclafani A: Flavor preferences conditioned by intragastric fat infusions in rats. Physiol Behav 46:403, 1989

23. Lucas, F, Sclafani A: Hyperphagia in rats produced by a mixture of fat and sugar. Physiol Behav 47:51, 1990

24. Mickelsen O, Takahashi S, Craig C: Experimental obesity. I. Production of obesity in rats by feeding high-fat diets. J Nutr 57:541, 1955

25. Moore BJ: The cafeteria diet: An inappropriate tool for studies of thermogenesis. J Nutr 117:227, 1987

26. Naim M, Brand JC, Kare MR et al: Energy intake, weight gain and fat deposition in rats fed flavored, nutritionally controlled diets in a multichoice ("cafeteria") design. J Nutr 115:1447, 1985

27. Oscai LB, Brown MM, Miller WC: Effect of dietary fat on food intake, growth and body composition in rats. Growth 48:415, 1984

28. Peckham SC, Entenman C, Carrol HW: The influence of a hypercaloric diet on gross body and adipose tissue composition in the rat. J Nutr 77:187, 1962

29. Pitts GC, Bull LS: Exercise, dietary obesity, and growth in the rat. Am J Physiol 232:R38, 1977

30. Prats E, Monfar J, Castella R et al: Energy intake of rats fed a cafeteria diet. Physiol Behav 45:263, 1989

31. Ramirez I: Feeding a liquid diet increases energy intake, weight gain and body fat in rats. J Nutr 117:2127, 1987

32. Ramirez I: When does sucrose increase appetite and adiposity? Appetite 9:1, 1987

33. Ramirez I: Overeating, overweight and obesity induced by an unpreferred diet. Physiol Behav 43:501, 1988

34. Ramirez I, Tordoff MG, Friedman MI: Dietary hyperphagia and obesity: What causes them? Physiol Behav 45:163, 1989

35. Rattigan S, Clark MG: Effect of sucrose solution drinking option on the development of obesity in rats. J Nutr 114:1971, 1984

36. Rattigan S, Howe PRC, Clark MG: The effect of a high-fat diet and sucrose drinking option on the development of obesity in spontaneously hypertensive rats. Br J Nutr 56:73, 1986

37. Reed DR, Contreras RJ, Maggio C et al: Weight cycling in female rats increases dietary fat selection and adiposity. Physiol Behav 42:389, 1988

38. Rogers PJ: Returning "cafeteria-fed" rats to a chow diet: Negative contrast and effects of obesity on feeding behavior. Physiol Behav 35:493, 1988

39. Rogers PJ, Blundell JR: Meal patterns and food selection during the development of obesity in rats fed a cafeteria diet. Neurosci Biobehav Rev 8:441, 1984

40. Rolls BJ: How variety and palatability can stimulate appetite. Nutr Bull 5:78, 1979

41. Rolls BJ, Rowe EA: Exercise and the development and persistence of dietary obesity in male and female rats. Physiol Behav 23:241, 1979

42. Rolls BJ, Rowe EA, Turner RC: Persistent obesity in rats following a period of consumption of a mixed, high energy diet. J Physiol (Lond) 298:415, 1980

43. Rolls BJ, Van Duijvenvoorde PM, Rowe EA: Variety in the diet enhances intake in a meal and contributes to the development of obesity in the rat. Physiol Behav 31:21, 1983

44. Rothwell NJ, Saville ME, Stock MJ: Effects of feeding a "cafeteria" diet on energy balance and diet-induced thermogenesis in four strains of rat. J Nutr 112:1515, 1982

45. Rothwell NJ, Stock MJ: Regulation of energy balance in two models of reversible obesity in the rat. J Comp Physiol Psychol 93:1024, 1979

46. Rothwell NJ, Stock MJ: Effects of early overnutrition and undernutrition in rats on the metabolic responses to overnutrition in later life. J Nutr 112:426, 1982

47. Rothwell NJ, Stock MJ: Influence of environmental temperature on energy balance, diet-induced thermogenesis and brown fat activity in "cafeteria"-fed rats. Br J Nutr 56:123, 1986

48. Rothwell NJ, Stock MJ: The cafeteria diet as a tool for studies of thermogenesis. J Nutr 118:925, 1988

49. Rowe EA, Rolls BJ: Effects of environmental temperature on dietary obesity and growth in rats. Physiol Behav 28:219, 1982

50. Sahakian BJ, Burdess C, Luckhurst H et al: Hyperactivity and obesity: The interaction of social isolation and cafeteria feeding. Physiol Behav 28:117, 1982

51. Schemmel R: Physiological considerations of lipid storage and utilization. Am Zool 16:661, 1976

52. Schemmel R, Mickelsen O, Fisher L: Body composition and fat depot weights of rats as influenced by ration fed dams during lactation and that fed rats after weaning. J Nutr 103:477, 1973

53. Schemmel R, Mickelsen O, Gill JL: Dietary obesity in rats: Body weight and body fat accretion in seven strains of rats. J Nutr 100:1041, 1970

54. Schemmel R, Mickelsen O, Tolgay Z: Dietary obesity in rats: influence of diet, weight, age, and sex on body composition. Am J Physiol 216:373, 1969

55. Sclafani A: Animal models of obesity: Classification and characterization. Int J Obes 8:491, 1984

56. Sclafani A: Carbohydrate taste, appetite, and obesity: An overview. Neurosci Biobehav Rev 11:131, 1987

57. Sclafani A: Carbohydrate-induced hyperphagia and obesity in the rat: Effects of saccharide type, form, and taste. Neurosci Biobehav Rev 11:155, 1987

58. Sclafani A: Dietary-induced overeating. Ann NY Acad Sci 575:281, 1989

59. Sclafani A, Aravich PF, Landman M: Vagotomy blocks hypothalamic hyperphagia in rats on a chow diet and sucrose solution, but not on a palatable mixed diet. J Comp Physiol Psychol 95:720, 1981

60. Sclafani A, Assimon SA: Influence of diet type and maternal background on dietary-obesity in the rat: A preliminary study. Nutr Behav 2:139, 1985

61. Sclafani A, Gale SK: Comparison of ovarian and hypothalamic obesity syndromes in the female rat: Effect of diet palatability on food intake and body weight. J Comp Physiol Psychol 91:381, 1977

62. Sclafani A, Gorman AN: Effects of age, sex, and prior body weight on the development of dietary obesity in adult rats. Physiol Behav 18:1021, 1977

63. Sclafani A, Nissenbaum JW: Robust conditioned flavor preference produced by intragastric starch infusions in rats. Am J Physiol 255:R672, 1988

64. Sclafani A, Springer D: Dietary obesity in adult rats: Similarities to hypothalamic and human obesity syndromes. Physiol Behav 17:461, 1976

65. Sclafani A, Vigorito M, Pfeiffer CL: Starch-induced overeating and overweight in rats: Influence of starch type and form. Physiol Behav 42:409, 1988

66. Slattery JM, Potter RM: Hyperphagia: A necessary precondition to obesity? Appetite 6:113, 1985

67. Vallerand AL, Lupien J, Bukowiecki LJ: Cold exposure reverses the diabetogenic effects of high-fat feeding. Diabetes 35:329, 1986

68. Walks D, Lavau M, Presta E et al: Refeeding after fasting in the rat: Effects of dietary-induced obesity on energy balance regulation. Am J Clin Nutr 37:387, 1983

CHAPTER 20

Neuroendocrinology of Type II Diabetes in Animal Models

BERNARD JEANRENAUD, ISABELLE CUSIN, and FRANÇOISE ROHNER-JEANRENAUD

POSTULATION: CNS DYSREGULATIONS UNDERLIE THE AUTONOMIC NERVOUS SYSTEM DYSREGULATIONS PRODUCING OBESITY

Several years ago we found that glucose-induced insulin output increased rapidly (within minutes) following the acute creation of ventromedial hypothalamic (VMH) lesions in normal anesthetized rats. Moreover, subsequent bilateral vagotomy reversed the VMH lesion–induced insulin oversecretion but had no effect in control animals.[1-4] It was concluded that acute VMH lesions altered central nervous system (CNS) homeostasis, a perturbation that somehow favored an increase in the parasympathetic efferents reaching the endocrine pancreas. Analogous observations were made for glucagon secretion, which was increased after lesions of the VMH and was also a vagus nerve–mediated abnormality.[3]

The activity of the sympathetic pathways was then investigated by measuring the spontaneous activity of the efferent sympathetic nerve reaching the brown adipose tissue as recorded by electrophysiologic means. In normal anesthetized rats, 3.1 spikes per second were recorded. By contrast, spike frequency diminished to 0.67 per second 30 minutes after VMH lesions were created.[5]

Because the VMH lesion represented an experimental situation, we wondered whether similar alterations could occur in a spontaneous, genetically determined syndrome such as that of the fa/fa obese rat. To answer this question, we tested the insulinemic response to an arginine bolus in lean and preobese (i.e., those destined to become obese) pups. Lean and preobese pups were 17 days old and were indistinguishable from each other. Arginine-induced insulinemia was greater in preobese than in lean pups.[6] We then questioned whether the abnormally high levels of insulinemia of the preobese animals could be related to an overactive vagus nerve. That such was the case was shown by the observation that acute atropine administration just prior to the arginine administration normalized the hyperinsulinemia in preobese pups but did not alter insulinemia in lean pups. The same conclusion could be drawn for glucagon: increased secretion in genetically preobese pups was normalized with atropine.[6]

The activity of the sympathetic efferents was also assessed in genetically obese (fa/fa) rats. In these experiments, efferent sympathetic nerve activity was assessed via its in vivo stimulatory action on glucose uptake by brown adipose tissue, using the labeled 2-deoxy-D-glucose method.[7] At normal room temperature, basal glucose uptake in brown adipose tissue was similar in lean and obese animals. However, when the animals were chronically exposed to a cold environment (4°C), the resulting overall activation of the sympathetic efferents markedly stimulated glucose uptake by normal brown adipose tissue, whereas such stimulation was moderate in the obese rodents, indicative of a blunted sympathetic nerve response.[8,9] This was in keeping with the reported decrease in brown adipose tissue thermogenesis measured in 7-day-old pre-obese pups.[10] These and other data led us to propose that in the genetically obese fa/fa rats (as well as in rats with VMH lesions), CNS dysregulations probably occur spontaneously and are somehow responsible for abnormal regulations of the autonomic nervous system. These abnormal regulations result in increased parasympathetic tone reaching the endocrine pancreas, thereby producing hyperinsulinemia and hyperglucagonemia, and in decreased sympathetic tone reaching the periphery (the brown adipose tissue in particular), resulting in decreased energy dissipation as heat.[11]

ROLE OF HYPERINSULINEMIA

Hyperinsulinemia was a key factor in producing obesity.[12] This conclusion was based on the following observations. Livers of lean fasted (17 hours) rats were taken as the reference standard, as fasting markedly decreased the plasma insulin levels. With refeeding of the fasted lean rats, hepatic glycolysis increased, attributable to increases in portal insulinemia and glycemia, and the increased glycolysis was associated with stimulation of phosphofructokinase 1 (PFK_1) and pyruvate kinase activities. Indeed, there was a marked augmentation in the concentration of the substrates of PKF_1 (fructose-6-phosphate in equilibrium with glucose-6-phosphate) and in its product (fructose-1,6-bisphosphate, triosesphosphate).[12] These changes were consistent with stimulation of PFK_1 by the stimulator of glycolysis, fructose-2,6-bisphosphate, which increased on refeeding of such normal rats. In refed lean rats, an additional stimulatory effect of insulin at the level of pyruvate kinase was suggested by the accumulation of its product (pyruvate) and a decreased concentration of its substrate (phosphoenol pyruvate). Even when fasted, the obese rats remained markedly hyperinsulinemic. Hepatic glycolysis in obese rats was stimulated as much as in fed normal animals, owing to the hyperinsulinemia of the former, which remained

high (even after a 17-hour fast), at about 40 ng/ml portal blood. Refeeding the obese rats resulted in a small additional increase in glycolysis at the level of both PFK_1 and pyruvate kinase. Finally, whatever the feeding situations, the hepatic concentrations of fructose-2,6-bisphosphate (the glycolysis stimulator) were always much higher in obese rats than in controls.[12]

It was concluded at this point that livers of obese fa/fa rats exhibit abnormal regulation of hepatic glycolysis in the sense that glycolysis is continuously overstimulated by hyperinsulinemia (i.e., this process never becomes insulin resistant).[12] This produces an increase in hepatic lipid synthesis and very low-density lipoprotein (VLDL) secretion in obese animals.[11] Because adipose tissue lipoprotein lipase activity always remains higher than normal in obese rats, the increased VLDL secretion is accompanied by increased VLDL-TG accumulation within adipocytes, resulting in intractable obesity.[11] Other metabolic pathways do, however, become insulin resistant.

INSULIN RESISTANCE AND GLUCOSE TRANSPORT IN PERFUSED HEART MUSCLE FROM NORMAL AND GENETICALLY OBESE RATS

Insulin resistance has been shown to lie at the level of glucose utilization by peripheral tissues and at the level of glucose production,[13] the two abnormalities underlying the abnormal oral glucose tolerance (OGT) clearly observed in conscious, genetically obese fa/fa rats.[14] When glucose metabolism (representing mostly that of the muscle mass) was tested by euglycemic clamp, it was observed that, while insulin stimulated glucose utilization in normal rats as expected, it failed to do so in obese fa/fa rats.[13] This led to attempts to determine the abnormalities responsible for insulin resistance in muscles.

Because glucose transport is the rate-limiting step for glucose utilization, efforts were concentrated on the glucose transport process. The technically easy preparation of the perfused heart was chosen for study, as this organ, when perfused at low pressure, uses mainly glucose as an energy source and responds to insulin. Also, it was of importance to define the state of the glucose transporters, and the heart provides a single muscle type that is big enough to allow preparation of the plasma and microsomal membranes necessary for measuring the glucose transporters.[15] As expected, hearts of genetically obese fa/fa rats were insulin resistant.[16] Therefore the likely pathology of heart glucose transporters was investigated. This was performed by measuring the glucose transporter translocation process under the influence of insulin, as well as the changes in the functional properties of the glucose transporters brought about by the hormone. We used a modified labeled cytochalasin B assay, in which the D-glucose–displaceable cytochalasin B permits quantitative and qualitative analysis of the glucose transporters.[17]

In normal hearts, insulin favored the translocation of glucose transporters from an intracellular pool to the plasma membrane without altering total transporter number (plasma plus microsomal membrane transporters), in agreement with the data reported by others for fat cells.[15] Moreover, in normal hearts insulin activated the glucose transporters once inserted into the plasma membranes, as evidenced by insulin-induced increases in the Hill coefficient (an index of positive cooperativity among transporters) and by the affinity values of plasma membrane transporters for glucose.[15] The total number of glucose transporters was halved in the hearts of obese animals. The translocation process was operating, but, as total transporter number was decreased, fewer transporters were translocated into the plasma membrane. Moreover, insulin failed to activate the transporters already in the plasma membrane. It is tentatively proposed that these defects may be similar to those that occur in skeletal muscles.[18]

DYSREGULATIONS AFFECTING HEPATIC GLUCOSE PRODUCTION

The abnormal hepatic glucose production by obese insulin-resistant rodents could be due to several regulatory defects, currently under investigation: (1) dysregulation of insulin counterregulatory hormones, in particular glucagon and glucocorticoids, which appear to be oversecreted in obesity syndromes; (2) abnormal neural control of the hepatic parenchyma; or (3) abnormal

regulation of glycogenolytic or gluconeogenic liver enzymes. One example of such a series of dysregulations is provided. Lean, genetically obese fa/fa rats were tested during a meal after a 17-hour fast. Refeeding of normal rats produced increases in portal insulin and glycemia levels that suppressed hepatic phosphorylase activity (livers were subsequently isolated).[12] In contrast, the very high, meal-induced increases in portal insulin and glycemia levels in the obese rats did not result in inhibition of this glycogen-degrading enzyme. Thus, increased glycogenolysis could be partly responsible for the increased hepatic glucose production noted in obese rodents.[12]

In normal rats studied during a euglycemic clamp, the suppression of hepatic glucose production by insulin is partly due to an insulin-mediated increase in glycolysis, an effect that is accompanied by a decrease (due to its utilization in the glycolytic pathway) of hepatic glucose-6-phosphate (G-6-P) concentrations.[19] In contrast, G-6-P concentrations in livers of genetically obese fa/fa rats often are higher than in livers of normal animals.[11,12] This is a surprising observation in view of the fact that livers of obese rats, even after a prolonged fast, are continuously and spontaneously "clamped" by their own high basal insulinemia (see above). However, the observation is in keeping with the postulation that the high G-6-P concentrations in obese animals could be due to increased gluconeogenesis, favored by one or several insulin counterregulation hormones. This would be possible via the existence of metabolic zonation, by which increased gluconeogenesis (and hence increased hepatic glucose production) would occur at the same time as increased glycolysis.[11]

Using a double tracer technique that permitted measurement of glucose turnover under non-steady-state conditions, we studied normal and genetically obese animals in the conscious state and following the spontaneous ingestion of a glucose load. Despite the presence of glucose transport and transporter defects, the rate of glucose utilization was higher in obese rats than in lean rats.[20] When the metabolic clearance rates of glucose were calculated (MCR_G), it was found that pre- and postprandial glucose clearances were identical in lean and obese rats. However, achieving normal glucose clearance in the obese animals exacted a cost: the normal glucose clearance in these animals was accompanied by basal and postprandial hyperinsulinemia and hyperglycemia.[20] Thus, as glucose clearance was ultimately normal in the obese rodents (albeit at the expense of increased insulin secretion), it could not be held responsible for the observed abnormal results on the oral glucose tolerance test (OGTT) in the obese group. Abnormal OGTT results had to be due to metabolic defects of another organ, evidently the liver.[20] In keeping with previous observations,[13] hepatic production was not adequately suppressed in obese animals following the glucose meal, as it was in normal rats.[20]

The pathologic situation prevailing in genetic obesities may be summarized as follows. Central nervous system–autonomic nervous system disorders are of fundamental etiological importance and appear to result in insulin oversecretion and in dysregulations of insulin counterregulatory hormones. On the basis of recent data obtained in rodents, insulin may be an important driving force in bringing about insulin resistance of muscle metabolism.[21] However, as under conditions close to physiologic ones (meal ingestion) glucose clearance appears to be normal in obese rats, it cannot be the main defect that ultimately produces abnormal OGT. The abnormalities of the glucose transport and glucose transporter system probably have a positive feedback effect on the endocrine pancreas, thereby producing basal and postprandial hyperinsulinemia. Actual abnormal OGT is most likely due to unsuppressed hepatic glucose production, partly through dysregulations of the insulin counterregulatory hormones.[11] Together with the continuous stimulation, by the hyperinsulinemia, of hepatic glycolysis and lipid synthesis and secretion in obese animals, these findings suggest an explanation for the occurrence and maintenance of an obesity associated with non-insulin-dependent diabetes mellitus (NIDDM).[11]

MODIFICATION OF OBESITY BY CRF INFUSION: SUPPORT FOR AUTONOMIC NERVOUS SYSTEM DEFECTS

Given the disorders of the autonomic nervous system seen in obese animals, we were interested

in finding a compound that, when administered into the CNS of obese animals, would correct at least some of these disorders. Corticotropin-releasing factor (CRF) appeared to be a candidate. Apart from its main effect on the hypothalamic-pituitary-adrenal axis, CRF injected into the cerebral ventricles stimulates sympathetic outflow in normal rats.[22] In addition, CRF inhibits gastric emptying and acid production by interfering with the vagal activation needed to elicit these processes.[23,24] Finally, CRF decreases food intake.[25]

Another reason to select CRF was the observation that adrenalectomy reverses the obesity syndrome in the fa/fa rat,[26] this manipulation being accompanied by an increase in central CRF drive.[27] We therefore decided to determine whether the chronic intracerebroventricular (ICV) infusion of ovine CRF (oCRF) to adult obese fa/fa rats could modify the trend toward obesity and its accompanying defects.[28] For comparison, similar ICV oCRF treatment of lean rats was also evaluated.

Male lean (FA/?) and genetically obese (fa/fa) rats were anesthetized and guiding cannulas were placed into the right lateral cerebral ventricle. A mandrel was inserted into each cannula and the cannulas were cemented to the skull. The animals were allowed to recover for one week, during which time body weight and food intake were measured daily. Injection cannulas were then connected via a polyethylene catheter to osmotic minipumps containing either oCRF or vehicle. The minipumps were initialized, the mandrels removed from the guiding cannulas, and the injection cannulas placed via the guiding cannulas. The minipumps were placed subcutaneously in the backs of the animals under slight ether anesthesia.[28]

Because oCRF treatment transiently decreased food intake (for about two days), the oCRF-treated animals were always studied one day before the vehicle-treated animals. This allowed us to perform pair-feeding of the two groups by giving the vehicle-treated rats the amount of food consumed on the previous day by the oCRF-treated rats. On day 7 of the experiment the animals were killed by decapitation. Trunk blood was collected and was kept until assayed, and various organs were removed.[28]

To minimize the effects of ICV oCRF on

hypothalamic-pituitary-adrenal function (glucocorticoids aggravate obesity syndromes), initial experiments were directed toward finding a dose of oCRF which, when given ICV to obese fa/fa rats for seven days, had no effect on plasma adrenocorticotropin (ACTH) and corticosterone levels. This requirement was met with a dosage of 5 μg/day. Higher concentrations of the peptide produced significant increases in both plasma ACTH and corticosterone levels and therefore were not further tested.[28]

With the pair-feeding method the overall food consumption was identical in both experimental groups. Despite analogous food consumption, the evolution of body weight gain was quite different in vehicle- and oCRF-treated obese rats. The vehicle-treated obese rats gained weight, such that on day 6 the mean delta body weight gain was 29 ± 4 g more than the initial body weight ($P < .05$). By contrast, the oCRF-treated animals did not gain weight during the same period; their mean body weight on day 6 was not statistically different from the mean initial body weight.[28]

The high values of basal insulinemia in vehicle-treated obese animals were greatly reduced by oCRF treatment while the basal glycemia, plasma free fatty acid levels, and triglyceride levels were unaltered by such treatment. The total weight of the interscapular brown adipose tissue was increased by oCRF administration, as were the protein content, the NADPH-cytochrome c reductase, and the cytochrome c oxidase activities.[28] These changes occurred without any alterations in lipid or DNA content of the tissue. The increase in intrascapular brown adipose tissue weight induced by oCRF administration contrasted with the decrease in the weight of the epididymal fat pad and the weight of the liver, whose glycogen content was also reduced by the chronic oCRF infusion. Adrenal weight was unaltered by oCRF treatment.[28]

The food efficiency (i.e., body weight gain in relation to food intake from days 2 to 6) was about fourfold lower in oCRF-treated rats than in vehicle-treated obese animals.[28]

Lean heterozygote (FA/?) rats of the same age as the obese rats were also treated with oCRF (5 μg/day) or with vehicle. oCRF treatment had no effect on any of the parameters measured. In keeping with these data, the evolution of body weight gain in the lean rats was similar whether they received vehicle or oCRF. Moreover, oCRF treatment of lean rats did not change food efficiency.[28]

The effects of CRF observed in obese rats may be mediated by an influence of this peptide on the autonomic nervous system. Several findings indirectly support this concept. Basal hyperinsulinemia in obese rats was markedly decreased by oCRF administration, an inhibitory effect that could be due either to stimulation of the α-adrenergic system, inhibitory to insulin output,[29] or to inhibition of the vagus nerve–mediated increase in insulin secretion.[29] The decrease in basal hyperinsulinemia in obese rats given oCRF is further evidence of a lack of CRF effect on the pituitary-adrenal axis, since ACTH has been reported to stimulate insulin output in rodents.[30] Decreased basal insulinemia together with normal basal glycemia of the oCRF-treated obese rats is suggestive of an amelioration of insulin sensitivity in these insulin-resistant animals. Liver weight and liver glycogen content decreased with oCRF treatment in obese rats. These effects are compatible with restoration of an increased sympathetic tone that would favor glycogenolysis.[31] The weight of the epididymal fat pad was decreased and the weight of the interscapular brown adipose tissue was increased in oCRF-treated obese rats, consistent with increased sympathetic tone acting at the level of these two tissues.[32,33] Increased oCRF-induced brown adipose tissue activity was also suggested by the finding of an elevation in the activities of two enzymes that are respectively markers of microsomal and mitochondrial activity of this tissue. The protein, lipid, and DNA contents of the brown adipose tissue of oCRF-treated obese rats remained the same (measured as mg/g tissue), which suggested that CRF had induced a hyperplasia of the tissue without reactivating each single brown adipocyte. This observation is consistent with the report showing that β-agonist stimulation results in brown adipocyte proliferation.[33]

The final effect of chronic (seven days) ICV administration of oCRF was a marked diminution in food efficiency, thereby leading to a decrease in the excessive rate of weight gain of the fa/fa rats, probably resulting from an increased sympathetic tone.

The finding of an inhibitory effect of central oCRF administration on body weight gain and other peripheral metabolic or endocrine abnormalities of the obese fa/fa rats substantiates the concept that CNS defects may be important etiological determinants of the fa/fa syndrome. This postulation is also consistent with the many similarities existing between the genetically determined disorders in this animal model and the results obtained by experimentally destroying the VMH area.[11,34] The observation that oCRF treatment was ineffective in lean animals strengthens the hypothesis that such a treatment has beneficial effects only when defective autonomic nervous system mechanism(s) actually prevail.

Acknowledgment: This study was supported by grant No. 3,822,086 of the Swiss National Science Foundation (Berne) and by a grant-in-aid of Nestlé S.A. (Vevey, Switzerland).

References

1. Berthoud HR, Jeanrenaud B: Acute hyperinsulinemia and its reversal by vagotomy after lesions of the ventromedial hypothalamus in anesthetized rats. Endocrinology 105:146, 1979
2. Rohner-Jeanrenaud F, Jeanrenaud B: Consequences of ventromedial hypothalamic lesions upon insulin and glucagon secretion by subsequently isolated perfused pancreases in the rat. J Clin Invest 65:902, 1980
3. Rohner-Jeanrenaud F, Jeanrenaud B: Possible involvement of the cholinergic system in hormonal secretion by the perfused pancreas from ventromedial-hypothalamic lesioned rats. Diabetologia 20:217, 1981
4. Rohner-Jeanrenaud F, Bobbioni E, Ionescu E et al: Central nervous system regulation of insulin secretion. In Szabo AJ (ed): Advances in Metabolic Disorders, vol 10, pp 193–220. Orlando, Fla, Academic Press, 1983
5. Niijima A, Rohner-Jeanrenaud F, Jeanrenaud B: Electrophysiological studies on the role of the ventromedial hypothalamus on the sympathetic efferent nerve activity of brown adipose tissue in the rat. Am J Physiol 247:R650, 1984
6. Rohner-Jeanrenaud F, Jeanrenaud B: Involvement of the cholinergic system in insulin and glucagon oversecretion of genetic pre-obesity. Endocrinology 116:830, 1985
7. Ferré P, Leturque A, Burnol A-F et al: A method to quantify glucose utilization in vivo in skeletal muscle and white adipose tissue of the anaesthetized rat. Biochem J 228:103, 1985
8. Greco R, Zaninetti D, Assimacopoulos-Jeannet F et al: Stimulatory effect of cold adaptation on glucose utilization by brown adipose tissue: Relationship with changes of the glucose transporter system. J Biol Chem 262:7732, 1987
9. Greco-Perotto R, Bobbioni E, Assimacopoulos-Jeannet F et al: Properties of glucose transporters after cold-adaptation or insulin in brown adipose tissue of normal and obese rats. In: Lessons in Animal Diabetes, vol II, p 250, 1987
10. Planche E, Joliff M, De Gasquet P et al: Evidence of a defect in energy expenditure in 7-day-old Zucker rat (fa/fa). Am J Physiol 245:E107, 1983
11. Jeanrenaud B, Halimi S, van de Werve G: Neuroendocrine disorders seen as triggers of the triad: obesity–insulin resistance–abnormal glucose tolerance. Diabetes Metab Rev 1:261, 1985
12. Van de Werve G, Jeanrenaud B: The onset of liver glycogen synthesis in fasted-refed lean and genetically obese (fa/fa) rats. Diabetologia 30:169, 1987
13. Terrettaz J, Assimacopoulos-Jeannet F, Jeanrenaud B: Severe hepatic and peripheral insulin resistance as evidenced by euglycemic clamps in genetically obese fa/fa rats. Endocrinology 118:674, 1986
14. Ionescu E, Sauter JF, Jeanrenaud B: Abnormal oral glucose tolerance in genetically obese (fa/fa) rats. Am J Physiol 248:E500, 1985
15. Zaninetti D, Greco-Perotto R, Assimacopoulos-Jeannet F et al: Effect of insulin on glucose transport and glucose transporters in rat heart. Biochem J 250:277, 1988
16. Zaninetti D, Crettaz M, Jeanrenaud B: Dysregulation of glucose transport in hearts of genetically obese (fa/fa) rats. Diabetologia 25:525, 1983
17. Greco-Perotto R, Assimacopoulos-Jeannet F, Jeanrenaud B: Insulin modifies the properties of glucose transporters in rat brown adipose tissue. Biochem J 247:63, 1987
18. Zaninetti D, Greco-Perotto R, Assimacopoulos-Jeannet F et al: Dysregulation of glucose transport and transporters in perfused hearts of genetically obese (fa/fa) rats. Diabetologia 32:56, 1989
19. Terrettaz J, Assimacopoulos-Jeannet F, Jeanrenaud B: Inhibition of hepatic glucose production by insulin in vivo in the rat: Contribution of glycolysis. Am J Physiol 250:E346, 1986
20. Rohner-Jeanrenaud F, Proietto J, Ionescu E et al: Mechanism of abnormal oral glucose tolerance of genetically obese fa/fa rats. Diabetes 35:1350, 1986
21. Cusin I, Rohner-Jeanrenaud F, Terrettaz J et al: In-

sulin infusion in normal rats produces muscle insulin resistance while overstimulating white adipose tissue. In Björntorp P, Rössner S (eds): Obesity in Europe 88, pp 173–175. London, John Libbey, 1988

22. Brown MR, Fisher LA: Corticotropin-releasing factor: Effects on the autonomic nervous system and visceral systems. Fed Proc 44:243, 1985
23. Taché Y, Maeda-Hagiwara M, Turkelson CM: Central nervous system action of corticotropin-releasing factor to inhibit gastric emptying in rats. Am J Physiol 253:G241, 1985
24. Taché Y, Gunion M: Corticotropin-releasing factor: Central action to influence gastric secretion. Fed Proc 44:255, 1985
25. Morley YE, Levine AS, Gosnell BA et al: Peptides as central regulators of feeding. Brain Res Bull 14:511, 1985
26. Yukimura Y, Bray GA: Effects of adrenalectomy on body weight and the size and number of fat cells in the Zucker rat. Endocr Res Commun 5:189, 1978
27. Dallman MF, Makaro GB, Roberts JL et al: Corticotrope response to removal of releasing factors and corticosteroids in vivo. Endocrinology 117:2190, 1985
28. Rohner-Jeanrenaud F, Walker C-D, Greco-Perotto R et al: Central corticotropin releasing factor administration prevents the excessive body weight gain of genetically obese (fa/fa) rats. Endocrinology 124:733, 1989
29. Miller RE: Pancreatic neuroendocrinology: Peripheral neural mechanisms in the regulation of the islets of Langerhans. Endocr Rev 2:471, 1981
30. Lebovitz HE, Pooler K: ACTH-mediated insulin secretion: Effect of aminophylline. Endocrinology 81:558, 1967
31. Shimazu T, Fukuda A: Increased activities of glycogenolytic enzymes in liver after splanchnic-nerve stimulation. Science 150:1607, 1965
32. Weiss B, Maickel RP: Sympathetic nervous control of adipose tissue lipolysis. Int J Neuropharmacol 7:395, 1968
33. Géleon A, Collet AJ, Guay G et al: β-adrenergic stimulation of brown adipocyte proliferation. Am J Physiol 254:C175, 1988
34. Bray GA, Inoue S, Nishizawa Y: Hypothalamic obesity: The autonomic hypothesis and the lateral hypothalamus. Diabetologia 20(suppl):366, 1981

CHAPTER 21

Obesity and Diabetes in Monkeys

BARBARA C. HANSEN

Spontaneous obesity has been observed in free-ranging protected rhesus monkeys provided chow *ad libitum* on the island of Cayo Santiago,[65] as well as in laboratory-reared, similarly fed monkeys.[16,39,74] The obese animals of Cayo Santiago were older than the general population of the island by approximately two years; and approximately 7% of a total sample aged four years and older were identified as obese (defined as 2 SD above the sample mean, using body weight, abdominal skin fold, or a Quetelet index: weight/height^2).[65] Kemnitz[42] has reviewed a number of cases of spontaneous or induced obesity in various macaque species.

In general, however, there have been few studies of obesity in nonhuman primates, probably because obesity develops spontaneously only in middle age. Early attempts were made to develop a model of obesity in the young rhesus monkey through ventromedial hypothalamic lesions.[17] The lesions were frequently inconsistent in their effects, perhaps because of the imprecision with which lesions were created at that time. Nevertheless, this method has been rarely used in monkeys. Forced overfeeding has also been used to induce obesity in young rhesus monkeys.[21-23,37]

FORMS OF SPONTANEOUS OBESITY AND DIABETES IN WILD OR ZOO-HELD NONHUMAN PRIMATES

In the laboratory-reared rhesus monkey, obesity develops after age seven years, with the greatest increase in adiposity occurring between ages 10 and 15 years, which is "middle age" for a monkey. Obesity in rhesus monkeys is relatively truncal in its distribution with a correlation of r > .77 between abdominal circumference and total body fat as determined by the tritiated water dilution method.[29]

Some obese monkeys spontaneously develop overt type 2 diabetes mellitus, as reported from time to time by veterinarians observing zoo-held primates. For example, the 1970 Annual Report of the National Zoo, Washington, DC, described an aged male rhesus monkey who was generally debilitated and was found to have urine 4+ for glucose and a glucose serum level as high as 400 mg/dl. The veterinarian considered the condition "pseudodiabetes."[13] Occasionally, other single cases of diabetes have been identified.[8,20,45,59]

A high-sucrose diet that was used in a study of periodontal disease may have induced or exacerbated the development of diabetes in three monkeys (*Macaca fascicularis*) in a colony of 300 monkeys.[41] All three had lost weight and had blood glucose levels above 140 mg/dl. Jones noted the similarity between the human and simian diabetes and surmised that several years of ingestion of a high-sucrose diet may have added to the stress of captivity in producing the diabetes. Jones[41] also reported, in reviewing past cases, that Froehner had observed a case of diabetes in an unspecified primate in 1892, perhaps the earliest written description of diabetes in monkeys. Cromeens and Stephens[5] described a case of diabetes in *Macaca fascicularis*. The 14-year-old female had experienced significant weight loss and glucose levels of 473 mg/dl prior to treatment. The animal was treated for 60 days on insulin, then recopsied. The pancreatic islets were stained and all had partial or total replacement with amyloid. Intact islet cells were principally beta cells with reduced glucagon and somatostatin cells.

Prosimians and other Old World monkeys have been reported to develop diabetes, including two tree shrews (*Urogali everetti*) with bilateral cataracts,[55] one bush baby (*Galago crassicaudatus kikuyuensis*),[30,41] and two squirrel monkeys (*Saimiri sciureus*). Davidson et al[6] and Martin et al[50] observed clinical diabetes or glucose intolerance in newly captured monkeys and have suggested that the disease may be present in the wild.

In addition to several reports on rhesus monkeys, other Old World monkeys and apes have occasionally been observed to develop diabetes. Diabetes has been observed in several Gray Guenons (*Cercopithecus* spp), one of which had an "enlarged pancreas."[31] One sacred baboon (*Papio hamadryas*) with diabetes was described by Sokoloverova[67] in a report thought by Stokes to be the first detailed clinical report of diabetes mellitus in this species.[68]

A form of probable hereditary diabetes was reported in 1972 by R. Howard to develop in the Celebes ape (*Macaca nigra*), and C.F. Howard has published an extensive series of articles describing the nature of this special type of diabetes, which is associated with amyloid formation in the pancreas.[32,33] More than 70% of older *Macaca nigra* animals studied have diabetes-related abnormalities. The form of diabetes that develops in *Macaca nigra* is not associated with obesity. With varying degrees of diabetes, the animals show impaired insulin response to glucose, decreased glucose clearance, and slightly impaired or abnormal responses on glucose tolerance tests. Diabetic *Macaca nigra* have fasting glucose levels above 140 mg/dl and minimal insulin secretion, and less than 5% of the islet cells have been found to be beta cells. C.F. Howard has reported that amyloid infiltration of an islet appears in *Macaca nigra* prior to overt diabetes and is not secondary to the development of the disease.[34] Shirgi et al[66] have also suggested possible virus involvement in the *Macaca nigra* diabetes syndrome. Detailed immunohistochemical studies

of the islet amyloid of the *Macaca nigra* have been carried out and are continuing.[10]

Diabetes has been described in two chimpanzees (*Pan troglodytes*), one zoo animal identified by Reuther[58] in 1967 (the animal responded to tolbutamide) and one identified by Rosenblum et al in the early 1980s.[60-62]

The pigtailed macaque (*Macaca nemestrina*) has also been found to develop diabetes.[48] Leathers and Schedewie[48] described the full diabetic syndrome in an eight- to ten-year-old male pigtailed macaque, including hypertriglyceridemia and hyperinsulinemia. Cases of spontaneous diabetes mellitus have also been reported in the ringtailed lemur.[51,53]

Gestational diabetes has occasionally been reported in older *macaca mulatta* with impaired glucose tolerance.[44,46,64,69]

EXPERIMENTAL OBESITY AND DIABETES IN PRIMATES

Diabetes has been induced experimentally in primates, primarily by pancreatectomy or by administration of beta cell toxic agents; those experimental models were reviewed by C.F. Howard in 1983.[33] Streptozotocin has been used to induce diabetes in various nonhuman primates, including baboons and rhesus monkeys.[60,61]

Jones et al[40] have concluded that the diabetes-like state induced by the administration of streptozotocin to monkeys resembles juvenile-onset human diabetes both in the hormone levels induced and in the decreased beta cell percent volume and numerical percentage of islets. The specificity of the effects of streptozotocin on the pancreas of rhesus monkeys has been shown by Takimoto et al.[71] Streptozotocin produces a selective pancreatic beta cell destruction that results from the direct action of the agent.[70] Kemnitz et al[43] reported fetuses large for gestational age in the streptozotocin-induced hyperglycemic and hypoinsulinemic animals.

Tso and others,[72,73] Harano et al,[28] and Yasuda et al[76] have used streptozotocin or alloxan to produce hyperglycemia for the purpose of studying the complications of diabetes.

Various hypothalamic lesions have been found to produce diabetes-like syndromes.[19,47,56] One male rhesus monkey showed rapid weight gain

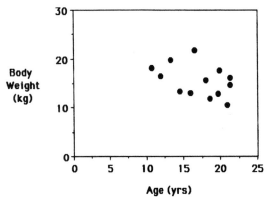

FIGURE 21-1

Age and body weight at diagnosis of non-insulin de-pendent diabetes mellitus (FPG > 140 mg/dl and glu-cose intolerance as defined by the National Diabetes Data Group, 1977, with $K_G < 1.5$).

following bilateral ventromedial hypothalamic lesions, and within seven months of the electro-lytic lesion, levels of urinary glucose were ele-vated.[15] Blood glucose was not determined until three years after the lesions and at that time was over 160 mg/dl. Insulin treatment was then initi-

ated. The animal remained diabetic and was fol-lowed in the laboratory for approximately ten years. Irradiation has also been reported to cause glucose intolerance and diabetes in nonhuman primates.[63]

FROM OBESITY TO DIABETES IN RHESUS MONKEYS: PERSONAL SERIES

In our laboratory we have extended the work of Hamilton and Ciaccia,[18] who first described the transition from obesity to diabetes in two rhesus monkeys. A portion of Hamilton's colony served as the original source of spontaneously obese monkeys in our longitudinal studies. We have focused on the factors involved in the develop-ment of insulin resistance and impaired glucose tolerance in these *ad libitum* fed animals with the aim of identifying the earliest markers of im-pending diabetes and the mechanisms underly-ing the earliest observable defects.[24,25] The youn-gest animal under study in our laboratory at the time of diagnosis of overt diabetes was 10 years old; the oldest was 21 years old (X ± SD, 17.1 ± 3.6 years). The average body weight at diagno-sis of diabetes was 15.6 ± 3.3 kg (range, 10–25

TABLE 21-1

Phases of Type 2 Diabetes

	Normal Lean (<10 yr)	Normal Obese and Lean (>10 yr)	Early Progression			Transition		Early Advanced NIDDM	
Phase	1	2	3	4	5	6	7	8	9
Fasting plasma glucose	—	—	—	—	—	—	↑	↑	↑↑
Fasting plasma insulin	—	—	↑	↑	↑	↑↑	↑↑	—	—
Acute insulin response	—	↑	↑	↑	↑↑	↑↑	↑↑	—	—
Adipose tissue response to insulin	—	↑			↑↑			↓	↓↓
Insulin induced peripheral glucose uptake	—	↓	↓	↓	↓	↓	↓	↓	↓
Hepatic glucose production	—	—	—	—	—	—	—	↑	↑↑

Note: Arrows show direction of change relative to values in normal young lean animals (phase 1).

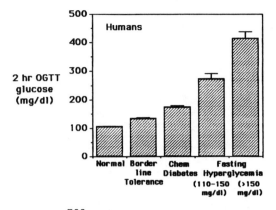

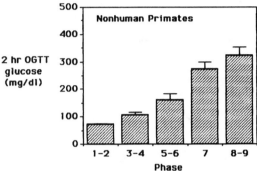

FIGURE 21-2

Comparison of data arrayed sequentially by phase from nonhuman primates with data obtained cross-sectionally from humans. Data shown represent plasma glucose levels at the two-hour point of an oral glucose tolerance test. (Adapted with permission from Reaven et al.[57])

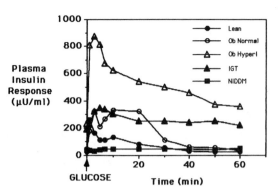

FIGURE 21-3

Insulin response to an intravenous glucose load (50% dextrose, 0.5 ml/kg) in five monkeys representing a range from normal to overtly diabetic: lean young adult; obese animal with normoinsulinemia and normoglycemia; obese animal with hyperinsulinemia; obese animal with impaired glucose tolerance; and obese diabetic (NIDDM) animal.

kg). As shown in Figure 21-1, both body weight and age varied widely at the time obese monkeys become overtly diabetic, with minimal thresholds of 10 years old and 10 kg body weight. Thus, while obesity may be permissive or facilitative, relative degree of obesity appears to play little or no role in the propensity to develop type 2 diabetes in rhesus monkeys.

Normal fasting plasma glucose values for a rhesus monkey generally range between 55 and 85 mg/dl. By convention, we have adopted the same threshold of fasting glucose for the diagnosis of non-insulin-dependent diabetes mellitus (NIDDM) in rhesus monkeys as has been agreed upon for humans—140 mg/dl,[54] although, because of the lower normal level in monkeys, a lower diagnostic threshold for diabetes may be

appropriate.[38,52] Fasting plasma glucose was not related to body weight, although no animals had elevated fasting plasma glucose levels before reaching a body weight of 10 kg or more. Fasting plasma glucose levels were sometimes in excess of 500 mg/dl prior to initiation of insulin therapy.

To describe the progressive process and sequence of events leading from lean to obese to diabetes in rhesus monkeys, we have identified a series of phases (Table 21-1). Cross-sectional data previously obtained from human subjects varying in glucose tolerance show remarkable similarities to data obtained longitudinally and prospectively in rhesus monkeys. For the purpose of this comparison, several phases have been combined in the monkeys in Figure 21-2. The upper panel shows the two-hour plasma glucose level following an oral glucose tolerance test in humans, with the humans classified by Reaven et al[57] into groups—a grouping then thought to reflect the heterogeneity of glucose tolerance. Data for monkeys are similarly arrayed in the lower panel. Note that each of the bars is the temporal predecessor of the next bar, i.e., part of a progressive process rather than simple heterogeneity. Thus, the classifications described by Reaven are similar to the phases identified longitudinally during the development of diabetes in nonhuman primates (rhesus monkeys).[25] The phase numbers 1 through 9 indicate sequential

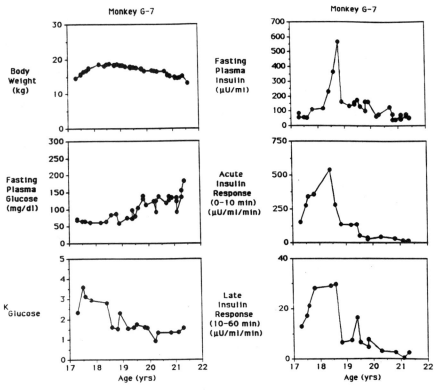

FIGURE 21-4

Longitudinal study of monkey G-7 progressing from normal glucose tolerance
and normal fasting glucose to overt diabetes at approximately age 20 years.
Fasting plasma insulin levels increased, then decreased. Note acute and late
insulin responses to intravenous glucose administration prior to hyperglycemia (FPG > 140 mg/dl) and overt diabetes.

steps in the progressive development of overt diabetes.

Plasma insulin responses following intravenous injection of glucose vary widely in monkeys (Fig. 21-3). Data are shown for representative monkeys, one from each of five groups: (1) a
lean, young, normal animal, (2) an obese animal
with normal fasting insulin levels and a slight
increase in insulin output during the first 20
minutes following bolus glucose administration,
(3) an obese animal with fasting hyperinsulinemia and an exceedingly exaggerated insulin
response, (4) the impaired—or relatively normal
—insulin response of a hyperinsulinemic animal
developing impaired glucose tolerance, and (5)
the low fasting plasma insulin level and absent

insulin response of an overtly diabetic animal.
The exaggerated early insulin response appears
to be part of the prodrome leading to type 2 diabetes in monkeys, and this is likely to be true of
humans as well, at least as can be judged from
cross-sectional data.[57] The beta cell subsequently
appears to show a decrease in the acute response
to glucose prior to the decrease in fasting plasma
insulin level. These five monkeys are also representative of the changes observed longitudinally
in single animals progressing to diabetes.

We followed the prospective development of
diabetes in individual obese animals from the
point of normal plasma glucose and insulin levels and normal glucose tolerance with normal
insulin response. The data for monkey G-7,

shown in Figure 21-4, are typical of the pattern observed within a single animal during this progressive process. The time course of changes in body weight, fasting plasma glucose, fasting plasma insulin, and $K_{glucose}$ is shown for an animal that became overtly diabetic at age 20. The absence of a change in body weight to parallel the change in fasting hyperinsulinemia is evident.

Not all monkeys develop diabetes, nor, under identical experimental conditions, including diet and food availability, do they necessarily develop obesity. Further, some obese monkeys appear to remain normal, never progressing to impairment in glucose tolerance, as shown in Figure 21-5 for monkey H-6.

The longitudinal study of the development of obesity and diabetes allowed us to look more critically at the relationship between fasting plasma glucose levels and changes in glucose tolerance (glucose disappearance rate during an intravenous glucose tolerance test, K_G). Figure 21-6 indicates the time sequence of events in this bivariate analysis. Monkeys in phase 1 were lean, young animals. Those in phases 2 through 6 were obese, with gradual deterioration in $K_{glucose}$ without significant change in fasting plasma glucose. Monkeys in phase 7 were in the transition to overt diabetes (phase 8). Those in phase 9 were severely diabetic and needed insulin to prevent weight loss and death.

The beta cell response to glucose in the first 10 minutes following the intravenous glucose tolerance tests (acute insulin release, AIR) is also shown in Figure 21-6 across the same sequence of phases. AIR shows progressive increases across phases 1 through 5, followed by decline toward normal in phases 6 and 7. With the initia-

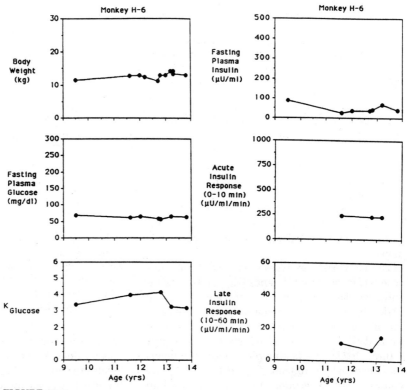

FIGURE 21-5

Monkey H-6, studied between ages 9 and 14 years, showing no changes in glucose tolerance or other variables with age.

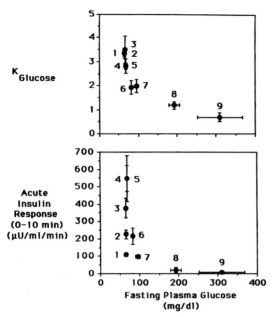

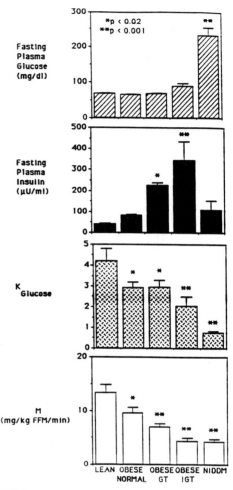

FIGURE 21-6

Relationships between changes in fasting plasma glucose levels and glucose disappearance rate and acute insulin response during an intravenous glucose tolerance test ($K_{glucose}$). The numbers represent a phase progression from normal lean adult animals (phase 1) to initial diagnosis of overt diabetes (phase 8) and severe diabetes (phase 9), as identified in Table 21-1.

tion of overt diabetes (phase 8), the acute insulin release in response to glucose is virtually absent. Since phases 2 through 6 may all occur in equally obese animals, it is understandable why previous reports indicated a wide range of insulin levels and insulin responses in obese humans.

These bivariate analyses of fasting plasma glucose levels, glucose tolerance (K_G), and acute insulin release in response to intravenous glucose (AIR) clearly show the wide range of values and the inadequacy of correlational approaches to these data. $K_{glucose}$ ranged widely during phases 1 through 7, while fasting plasma glucose levels remained below 100 mg/dl (see Fig. 21-6). By contrast, AIR in response to glucose showed an inverted U-shaped curve, with most of the change in AIR occurring before any elevation in fasting plasma glucose levels (see Fig. 21-6).

Data from monkeys studied cross-sectionally

FIGURE 21-7

Fasting plasma glucose (FPG), fasting plasma insulin (IRI), glucose tolerance (K_G), and insulin-stimulated glucose uptake (M) in a cross section of monkeys grouped according to progression to diabetes. *Left to right:* young, metabolically normal monkeys; older obese normals; obese hyperinsulinemic glucose-tolerant; obese hyperinsulinemic impaired–glucose tolerant; and NIDDM (overt type 2 diabetes).

and grouped on the basis of body weight, fasting plasma glucose levels, and fasting plasma insulin levels are shown in Figure 21-7. Peripheral insulin resistance, as indicated by glucose uptake/fat-free mass/min during a euglycemic hyperinsulinemic clamp (M), decreased very early and gradually as monkeys progressed toward impaired glucose tolerance.[1,3] No difference in peripheral glucose uptake was detected between monkeys with impaired glucose tolerance and overt diabetes. The greatest drop in glucose disappearance rate in response to an intravenous glucose tolerance test was observed in the transition from impaired glucose tolerance to diabetes.[1]

Adipocytes have been removed from the abdominal subcutaneous tissue of four groups of rhesus monkeys: lean, obese, obese with significant hyperinsulinemia, and diabetic. Neither obese animals nor obese hyperinsulinemic animals showed reduced lipid synthesis or glucose oxidation in response to increasing concentrations of insulin.[27] Insulin binding to adipocytes, however, was reduced in both obese and diabetic animals. Adipocytes from overtly diabetic animals or those about to become diabetic did show reduced sensitivity to insulin.

Lockwood et al[49] found decreased insulin binding to partially purified liver membranes in both obese nondiabetic and obese diabetic monkeys. They attributed the impaired insulin binding to decreased numbers of available receptor sites and not to a change in affinity.

In summary, peripheral insulin resistance, as assessed by the euglycemic clamp (thought principally, though not solely, to represent the resistance of muscle), appears to develop early, well before hyperglycemia develops, and is associated with obesity (but not severity of obesity). Insulin resistance of adipose tissue (as measured in isolated adipocytes) appears to develop at a later point in the progression to diabetes, close to the development of the overt clinical disease. Bodkin et al[1] found an even later hepatic manifestation of insulin resistance: insulin's ability to suppress basal hepatic glucose production was lost in parallel with the development of fasting hyperglycemia. These data from obese and diabetic primates suggest that "insulin resistance" is a term that should not be applied to the whole body but rather should be identified with respect to specific organs or cells and that further attention should be given to the antecedents of diabetes—obesity and changes in insulin and secretion.

Acknowledgment: Noni Bodkin, K.-L. Catherine Jen, and T. Russell, D. Harman, C. Sweeley, H. Ortmeyer, D. Doherty, T. Alexander, and S. Fluck contributed siginficantly to the work reviewed here. Scientific illustrations were drawn by H. Ortmeyer. This study was supported by National Institutes of Health grant DK 37717, and by the International Health Foundation.

References

1. Bodkin NL, Hansen BC: Discrete yet serial indications of the development of type 2 diabetes in the rhesus monkey: Marked similarity to human NIDDM. In Howard CF Jr (ed): Monographs in Primatology. Vol 12: Nonhuman Primate Studies on Diabetes, Carbohydrate Intolerance, and Obesity, p 7. New York, Alan R Liss, 1988
2. Bodkin NL, Hansen BC, Harman DM: Early changes in insulin resistance in monkeys progressing toward NIDDM. Diabetes 35:55A, 1986
3. Bodkin NL, Metzger BL, Hansen BC: Hepatic glucose production and insulin sensitivity preceding diabetes in monkeys. Am J Physiol 256:E676, 1989
4. Clarkson TB, Koritnik DR, Weingand KW et al: Nonhuman primate models of atherosclerosis: Potential for the study of diabetes mellitus and hyperinsulinemia. Metabolism 34:51, 1985
5. Cromeens DM, Stephens LC: Insular amyloidosis and diabetes mellitus in a crab-eating macaque (*Macaca fascicularis*). Lab Anim Sci 35:642, 1985
6. Davidson FWF, Lang CM, Blackwell WL: Impairment of carbohydrate metabolism of the squirrel monkey. Diabetes 16:395, 1967
7. DeSomery C, Walike BC: Effects of parenteral nutrition on voluntary food intake and gastric motility in monkeys. In Batey M (ed): Communicating Nursing Research, Vol 8. Boulder, Colo, Western Interstate Commission on Higher Education, 1976
8. DiGiacomo RF, Myers RE, Baez LR: Diabetes mellitus in a rhesus monkey (*Macaca mulatta*): A case report and literature review. Lab Anim Sci 21:572, 1971
9. Dubey AK, Hanukoglu A, Hansen BC et al: Metabolic clearance rates of synthetic human growth hormone in lean and obese male rhesus monkeys (*Macaca mulatta*). J Clin Endocrinol Metab 67:1064, 1988
10. Fang, T-Y, Howard CF Jr: Immunohistochemical study of islet amyloid in diabetes mellitus. Pancreas 1:293, 1986
11. Froehner E: Über Zuckerharnruhr beim Hunde. Monatsh Prakt Tierheilk 3:149, 1892
12. Goodner CJ, Walike BC, Koerker DJ et al: Insulin, glucagon, and glucose exhibit synchronous, sustained oscillations in fasting monkeys (*Macaca mulatta*). Science 195:177, 1977
13. Gray GW, Mikolajczyk EE, Scheider TG: Pseudodiabetes—rhesus monkey (*Macaca mulatta*). Ani-

mal Health Department 1970 Annual Report, National Zoological Park, Smithsonian Institution, p 59. Washington, DC, Smithsonian Institution Press, 1972

14. Hamerton AW, Rewell AE: Report of the pathologist for the year 1946. Proc Zool Soc (Lond) 117:663, 1947

15. Hamilton CL: An observation of long-term experimental obesity and diabetes mellitus in the monkey. J Med Primatol 1:247, 1972

16. Hamilton CL: Control of food intake in normal and obese monkeys. Ann NY Acad Sci 131:583, 1965

17. Hamilton CL, Brobeck JR: Hypothalamic hyperphagia in the monkey. J Comp Physiol Psychol 57:271, 1964

18. Hamilton CL, Ciaccia PJ: The course of development of glucose intolerance in the monkey (Macaca mulatta). J Med Primatol 7:165, 1978

19. Hamilton CL, Ciaccia PJ, Lewis DO: Feeding behavior in monkeys with and without lesions of the hypothalamus. Am J Physiol 230:818, 1976

20. Hamilton CL, Kuo PT, Feng LY: Experimental production of syndrome of obesity, hyperinsulinemia and hyperlipidemia in monkeys. Proc Soc Exp Biol Med 140:1005, 1972

21. Hansen BC: Does overfeeding produce sustained changes in physiology and behavior? In Hansen BC (ed): Controversies in Obesity, p 152. New York, Praeger, 1983

22. Hansen BC: Induction and remission of obesity in monkeys: Behavioral and physiological correlates. In Morrison AR, Strick PL (eds): Changing Concepts of the Nervous System, p 609. New York, Academic Press, 1982

23. Hansen BC: Induction of obesity in nonhuman primate models of human obesity. In Hayes KC (ed): Primates in Nutritional Research, p 291. New York, Academic Press, 1979

24. Hansen BC: Prospective study of the development of diabetes in spontaneously obese monkeys. In Berry EM, Blondheim SH, Eliahou HE et al (eds): Recent Advances in Obesity Research, vol V, p 33. London, John Libbey, 1987

25. Hansen BC, Bodkin NL: Heterogeneity of insulin responses: Phases in the continuum leading to non-insulin-dependent diabetes mellitus. Diabetologia 29:713, 1986

26. Hansen BC, Bodkin NL, Schwartz J et al: Beta cell responses, insulin resistance and the natural history of noninsulin diabetes in obese rhesus monkeys. In Shafrir E, Renold AE (eds): Frontiers in Diabetes Research: Lessons from Animal Diabetes II, p 279. London, John Libbey, 1988

27. Hansen BC, Jen K-LC, Schwartz J: Changes in insulin responses and binding in adipocytes from mon-

keys with obesity progressing in diabetes. Int J Obes 12:391, 1988

28. Harano Y, Yasuda H, Kosugi K et al: Study of microangiopathy in diabetic Macaca fuscata induced by streptozotocin. In Abe H, Hoshi M (eds): Proceedings of the International Symposium on Epidemiology of Diabetic Microangiopathy, March 18–20, 1982, Osaka, Japan, p 479. Tokyo, University of Tokyo Press, 1983

29. Harman DM, Hansen BC: Regional fat distribution and levels of obesity in male rhesus monkeys. Fed Proc 46:576, 1987

30. Hill WCO: Report of the Society's prosector for the year 1950. Proc Zool Soc Lond 121:641, 1951

31. Hill WCO: Report of the Society's prosector for the years 1955 and 1956. Proc Zool Soc Lond 129:431, 1956

32. Howard CF: Basement membrane thickness in muscle capillaries of normal and spontaneously diabetic Macaca nigra. Diabetes 24:201, 1975

33. Howard CF Jr: Diabetes and carbohydrate impairment in nonhuman primates. In Dukelow WR (ed): Nonhuman Primate Models for Human Diseases, p 1. Boca Raton, Fla, CRC Press, 1983

34. Howard CF Jr: Longitudinal studies on the development of diabetes in individual Macaca nigra. Diabetologia 29:301, 1986

35. Howard CF Jr, Kessler MJ, Schwartz S: Carbohydrate impairment and insulin secretory abnormalities among Macaca mulatta from Cayo Santiago. Am J Primatol 11:147, 1986

36. Howard R: Spontaneous diabetes in Macaca nigra. Diabetes 21:1077, 1972

37. Jen K-LC, Hansen BC: Feeding behavior during experimentally induced obesity in monkeys. Physiol Behav 33:863, 1984

38. Jen K-LC, Hansen BC: Glucose disappearance rate in rhesus monkeys: Some technical considerations. Am J Primatol 14:153, 1988

39. Jen K-LC, Hansen BC, Metzger BL: Adiposity, anthropometric measures, and plasma insulin levels of rhesus monkeys. Int J Obes 9:213, 1985

40. Jones CW, Reynolds WA, Hoganson GE: Streptozotocin diabetes in the monkey: Plasma levels of glucose, insulin glucagon, and somatostatin, with corresponding morphometric analysis of islet endocrine cells. Diabetes 29:536, 1980

41. Jones SM: Spontaneous diabetes in monkeys. Lab Anim 8:161, 1974

42. Kemnitz JW: Obesity in macaques: Spontaneous and induced. Adv Vet Sci Comp Med 28:81, 1984

43. Kemnitz JW, Eisele SG, Lindsay KA et al: Changes in food intake during menstrual cycles and pregnancy of normal and diabetic rhesus monkeys. Diabetologia 26:60, 1984

44. Kessler MJ, Howard CF, London WT: Gestational diabetes mellitus and impaired glucose tolerance in an aged *Macaca mulatta*. J Med Primatol 14:237, 1985

45. Kirk JH, Casey HW, Harwell JF Jr: Diabetes mellitus in two rhesus monkeys. Lab Anim Sci 22:245, 1972

46. Kohn LAP, Bennett KA: Fluctuating asymmetry in fetuses of diabetic rhesus macaques. Am J Phys Anthropol 71:477, 1986

47. Krey LC, Hess DL, Butler WR et al: Medial base hypothalamic disconnection and the onset of puberty in the female rhesus monkey. Endocrinology 108:1944, 1981

48. Leathers CW, Schedewie HK: Diabetes mellitus in a pigtailed macaque (*Macaca nemestrina*). J Med Primatol 9:95, 1980

49. Lockwood DH, Hamilton CL, Livingston JN: The influence of obesity and diabetes in the monkey on insulin and glucagon binding to liver membranes. Endocrinology 104:76, 1979

50. Martin JE, Kroe DJ, Bostrom RE et al: Rhino-orbital phycomycosis in a rhesus monkey. J Am Vet Med Assoc 155:1253, 1969

51. Meier J: Veterinary rounds: Diabetes mellitus in a ringtailed lemur. Zoonooz 65(1):17, 1981

52. Metzger BL, Hansen BC, Speegle LM et al: Characterization of glucose intolerance in obese monkeys. J Obes Weight Regul 4:153, 1985

53. Murata K: A case report on hyperglycemia in a ringtailed lemur. J Jpn Vet Med Assoc 39:59, 1986

54. National Diabetes Data Group: Classification and diagnosis of diabetes mellitus and other categories of glucose intolerance. Diabetes 28:1039, 1979

55. Rabb GB, Getty RE, Williamson WH et al: Spontaneous diabetes mellitus in tree shrews. Diabetes 15:327, 1966

56. Ranson SW, Fisher C, Ingram WR: Adiposity and diabetes mellitus in a monkey with hypothalamic lesions. Endocrinology 23:175, 1938

57. Reaven GM, Berstein R, Davis B et al: Nonketotic diabetes mellitus: Insulin deficiency or insulin resistance? Am J Med 60:80, 1976

58. Reuther RT: Primate notes from the San Francisco zoological gardens. Lab Primatol Newslett 6:19, 1967

59. Rosenberg DP, Gold EM, Prahalada S: Hyperosmolar non-ketotic diabetic coma in the nonhuman primate, a first report. Horm Metab Res 15:116, 1983

60. Rosenblum IY, Barbolt TA, Howard CF: Diabetes mellitus in the chimpanzee (Pan troglodytes). J Med Primatol 10:93, 1981

61. Rosenblum IY, Barbolt PA, Billhymer B et al: Biochemical and histological characterization of chemical-induced diabetes mellitus in the rhesus monkey (*Macaca mulatta*). Ecotoxicol Environ Safety 5:513, 1981

62. Rosenblum IY, Coulston F: Impaired renal function in diabetic chimpanzees (Pan troglodytes). Exp Mol Pathol 38(2):224, 1983

63. Salmon YL, Yochmowitz MG, Wilb BH: Delayed effects of proton irradiation in *Macaca mulatta*. III. Glucose intolerance. Interim Report No. UFAFFAM-TR-84-7. Brooks Air Force Base, Tex, US Air Force School of Aerospace Medicine, 1984

64. Schwartz R, Susa J: Fetal macrosomia: Animal models. Diabetes 430, 1980

65. Schwartz SM: Spontaneous obesity in the Cayo Santiago macaque. Am J Primatol 12(3):370, 1987

66. Shirgi SM, Wesson BJ, Marrey A et al: Virus-associated deficiencies in the mitogen reactivity in celebese black macaques (*Macaca nigra*). Critical immunology and immunopathology 35(2):200, 1985

67. Sokoloverova IM: Spontaneous diabetes mellitus in a monkey. In Utkin IA (ed): Theoretical and Practical Problems of Medicine and Biology in Experiments on Monkeys, p 171. New York, Pergamon, 1960

68. Stokes WS: Spontaneous diabetes mellitus in a baboon (*Papio cynocephalus anubis*). Lab Anim Sci 35(5):529, 1986

69. Susa JB, Widness JA, Hintz R et al: Somatomedins and insulin in diabetic pregnancies: Effects on fetal macrosomia in the human and rhesus monkey. J Clin Endocrinol Metab 58:1099, 1984

70. Takimoto G, Jones C, Lands W et al: Biochemical changes in rhesus monkeys during the first days after streptozotocin administration are indicative of selective β cell destruction. Metabolism 37:364, 1988

71. Takimoto GS, Jones CW, Bauman AF et al: Experimental insulin deficient diabetes in rhesus monkey. Am J Primatol 10:435, 1986

72. Tso NOM: Animal modeling of cystoid macular edema. Surv Ophthalmol 28:512, 1984

73. Tso NOM, Kurofawa A, Bauman A et al: Microangiopathic retinopathy in experimental diabetic monkeys. Invest Ophthalmol Vis Sci 27:145, 1986

74. Walike BC, Goodner CJ, Koerker DJ et al: Assessment of obesity in pigtail monkey (*Macaca nemestrina*). Med J Primatol 6:151, 1977

75. Widness JA, Schwartz R, Thompson D et al: Hemoglobin A_{Ic} in the glucose-intolerant, streptozotocin-treated or pancreatectomized macaque monkey. Diabetes 27:1182, 1978

76. Yasuda H, Harano Y, Kosugi K et al: Development of early lesions of microangiopathy in chronically diabetic monkeys. Diabetes 33:415, 1984

CHAPTER 22

Animal Models of Obesity: Hypothalamic Lesions

SHUJI INOUE

Hypothalamic lesions can produce obesity, a condition known as hypothalamic obesity. Until recently, hypothalamic obesity was defined as obesity produced by bilateral lesions of the ventromedial nuclei in the hypothalamus.

Ventromedial hypothalamic (VMH) obesity has been recognized for more than 150 years and was defined experimentally by Hetherington and Ranson in 1940.[1] In experimental studies lesions of the ventromedial nuclei are created in rats by passing an electrical current through an electrode,[1] in mice by the intraperitoneal (IP) injection of a chemical product, gold thioglucose.[2]

It is now known that obesity can be produced by destroying other regions of the hypothalamus. Bilateral electrolytic lesions of the paraventricular nuclei (PVH)[3] and dorsolateral tegmental regions (DLT)[4] can produce obesity, as can hypothalamic islands made with the Halasz knife.[5] Monosodium glutamate (MSG), which mainly damages the arcuate nuclei bilaterally, can also produce obesity.[6] Parasagittal knife cuts between the ventromedial and lateral nuclei produce a syndrome somewhat different from VMH lesion–induced obesity.[7]

Hypothalamic lesions are associated with number of derangements, including hyperphagia, hyperinsulinemia, impaired thermogenesis, disorders of autonomic nervous function, and so forth. The derangements and the pathogenesis of the obesity differ with different hypothalamic lesion sites.

This chapter describes the heterogeneity of de-rangements in relation to the pathogenesis of hypothalamic obesity and the different pathogenic states induced by different hypothalamic lesions.

HETEROGENEITY OF DERANGEMENTS OF HYPOTHALAMIC LESIONS

Food Intake

Hyperphagia and hyperinsulinemia are the characteristic features of obesity-producing hypothalamic lesions. Animals with VMH, PVH, and DLT lesions exhibit hyperphagia with hyperinsulinemia.[4,7,8] In VMH-lesioned rats, the diurnal pattern of food intake is disturbed,[8] whereas in PVH-lesioned rats it seems not to be disturbed.[9] Lesions created by knife cuts result in hyperphagia with or without hyperinsulinemia.[7,10] Animals with hypothalamic islands also have hyperphagia without hyperinsulinemia.[5] By contrast, MSG-treated animals with arcuate nucleus lesions do not show hyperphagia despite having hyperinsulinemia.[11]

The cause of hyperphagia in animals with different hypothalamic lesions seems to be different. In VMH-lesioned rats, in which hyperinsulinemia is associated with disorder of the autonomic nervous system, food intake increased by 70% after VMH lesions, whereas without hyperinsulinemia associated with disorder of autonomic nervous system, food intake increased by only 20%.[8] This suggests that hyperphagia in VMH-lesioned rats is mainly due to the hyperinsulinemia associated with disorder of the autonomic nervous system, but other mechanisms for the increase in food intake exist. The mechanism of hyperphagia produced by hyperinsulinemia in VMH-lesioned rats requires further investigation. Several possibilities can be postulated: (1) the increased peripheral glucose utilization resulting from hyperinsulinemia could serve as a signal for food-seeking behavior, although hyperphagia in response to real hypoglycemia caused by hyperinsulinemia has been denied[12]; (2) glucose deprivation by insulin in cerebral glucoreceptor cells could stimulate food intake[13]; (3) insulin receptors in the nuclei of the lateral hypothalamus could account for the hyperphagia associated with hyperinsulinemia[14]; and (4) hyperinsulinemia may be closely related to the activity of a neurotransmitter or neuromodulator that stimulates or inhibits food intake.

The cause of increased food intake in the absence of hyperinsulinemia is also unknown. Recently, a reciprocal relation between food intake and the activity of the sympathetic nervous system has been found.[15] Therefore, hypoactivity of the sympathetic nervous system after VMH lesions may contribute to increased food intake. Disturbance of histaminergic or γ-aminobutyric acid (GABA) receptors may be other candidates.[16,17]

On the other hand, in PVH- and DLT-lesioned rats, hyperphagia may occur independently of hyperinsulinemia.[18,19] Hyperphagia in rats with knife cut hypothalamic lesions and hypothalamic islands may also be independent of hyperinsulinemia or disorders of the autonomic nervous system.[5] A possible cause of this hyperphagia is damage to the parasagittal fibers that connect the ventromedial and lateral hypothalamus.[7]

It is an open question at present what mechanisms of neurotransmitter or neuromodulator systems do work in the hyperphagia seen in different hypothalamic lesions. It is possible that VMH lesions damage histaminergic or GABAnergic receptors in the hypothalamus.[16,17] On the other hand, Leibowitz et al[20] have suggested that PVH lesions damage feeding-related noradrenergic receptors in the PVH, producing hyperphagia.

Hormonal Factors

A variety of endocrine disturbances follow hypothalamic lesions. Of these, insulin and corticosterone release are the most relevant to the pathogenesis of obesity.

Insulin Release

Hyperinsulinemia with or without hyperphagia occurs after VMH lesions. Restricted food intake or pair-feeding to controls preserves hyperinsulinemia in VMH-lesioned rats.[21,22] Hyperinsulinemia occurs within minutes after the creation of VMH lesions.[23] These results suggest that hyperinsulinemia is the primary event and is not secondary to hyperphagia in VMH-lesioned rats. The cause of hyperinsulinemia in VMH-lesioned rats is related to a disorder of the autonomic nervous system, since (1) subdiaphragmatic vagotomy restored hyperinsulinemia[24,25] and (2) VMH lesions failed to produce hyperinsulinemia in rats with pancreatic transplants placed beneath renal capsule, which eliminated nerve connections between the pancreas and the hypothalamus.[8] Not only hyperactivity of vagal nerves but also hypoactivity of the sympathetic nervous system contribute to the hyperinsulinemia in VMH-lesioned rats.[26]

In PVH-lesioned rats, hyperinsulinemia appears in the fed condition when rats show hyperphagia, but it disappears when hyperphagia is inhibited by pair-feeding to controls.[7,9,27] Hyperinsulinemia is associated with hyperglycemia in PVH-lesioned rats, whereas hyperinsulinemia is not associated with hyperglycemia in VMH-lesioned rats.[9] These results suggest that hyperinsulinemia in PVH-lesioned rats is secondary to hyperphagia.

Rats with knife cut hypothalamic lesions become hyperinsulinemic or normoinsulinemic with hyperphagia.[10,28] The discrepancy may depend on the size and location of the knife cut. The cause of hyperinsulinemia in rats with knife cut lesions is suggested to be dependent on hyperphagia.[10]

MSG-treated rats exhibit hyperinsulinemia without hyperphagia.[11] The cause of hyperinsulinemia may be due in part to vagal nerve firing, since vagotomy restored hyperinsulinemia.[29]

In DLT-lesioned rats, hyperinsulinemia occurs

at night and during the day in the fed condition; however, moderate hyperphagia only occurs during the day.[4] The cause of this phenomenon is not known; however, Wellman et al[4] suggested that hyperphagia is not secondary to hyperinsulinemia.

Rats with hypothalamic islands also become hyperinsulinemic.[30] The cause of the hyperinsulinemia is not known; however, it may not depend on hyperphagia, since streptozotocin-treated rats with hypothalamic islands have hyperphagia without hyperinsulinemia.[30]

Corticosterone Release

The diurnal variation in plasma corticosterone levels is abolished or blunted in VMH-lesioned rats.[9,31] Elevated basal plasma corticosterone levels were also reported,[32] but there have been no reports of remarkable hypersecretion of corticosterone in rats with VMH lesions created with electrical current. GTG-induced VMH-lesioned rats were believed to have elevated corticosterone secretion.[33] The diurnal variation in plasma corticosterone levels is also blunted in PVH-lesioned rats.[9,18,27] Plasma corticosterone was reported to be increased or decreased in PVH-lesioned rats[18,34] and decreased in rats with knife cut hypothalamic lesions.[35]

The cause of the disturbance in diurnal rhythms in plasma corticosterone levels is not known for VMH- or PVH-lesioned rats; however, it may be secondary to hyperphagia or a disturbance of the diurnal rhythm of food intake, since pair-feeding restored normal diurnal rhythms in corticosterone levels.[9,36]

The role of corticosterone in the pathogenesis of hypothalamic obesity has recently attracted attention. Adrenalectomy reverses obesity associated with VMH and PVH lesions and knife cut lesions.[37-39] If corticosterone plays the primary role in the pathogenesis of hypothalamic obesity, a disturbance in corticosterone secretion should be the primary event in these hypothalamic-lesioned rats.

Autonomic Nervous System

The function of the autonomic nervous system is altered in VMH-lesioned rats. This involves hyperactivity of the vagus nerve and hypoactivity of the sympathetic nervous system.[26,40]

Evidence for vagal hyperactivity came first from measurement of gastric acid. Ridley and Brooks[41] demonstrated that VMH-lesioned rats had gastric hyperacidity, a phenomenon related to vagal overactivity. This result subsequently was confirmed by Powley and Opsahl[24] and by Inoue and Bray.[25]

Vagal nerve hyperactivity in VMH-lesioned rats appears to be involved in the pathogenesis of VMH-lesion–induced obesity since vagotomy[24,25] or scopolamine, which inhibit vagal function,[42] partly reduced body weight gain of VMH-lesioned rats. On the other hand, small or negligible changes in the function of the vagus nerve occur in PVH-lesioned rats and rats with knife cut hypothalamic lesions.[43,44]

The sympathetic nervous system becomes hypoactive after VMH lesions. This was first indicated by Inoue et al,[45] who observed enlarged salivary glands with reduced serum glucagon levels in VMH-lesioned rats. Inoue and Bray[40] also found impaired β-hydroxylase release into the circulation after treadmill stress. Subsequently this observation was supported by the finding that mobilization of free fatty acids was impaired by various stresses.[46] The results of electrophysiologic recordings of sympathetic nervous system activity to brown adipose tissue and pancreatic tissue also supported the proposed hypoactivity of sympathetic nervous activity, as the firing rate of the sympathetic nerves was reduced.[47,48]

The results of norepinephrine (NE) turnover, an indicator of sympathetic activity, are controversial. Romsos's group reported that NE turnover was reduced in weanling and adult VMH-lesioned rats.[49,50] In contradistinction to this report, Young and Landsberg[51] found that NE turnover was not suppressed in mice with VMH lesions created by injection of gold thioglucose. Finally, Yoshida and Bray[52] reported that NE turnover was increased in adult VMH-lesioned rats.

The discrepancy in findings regarding NE turnover in VMH-lesioned rats is difficult to explain. Two explanations are possible. First, the effects of VMH lesions on sympathetic activity may differ according to the size of the lesions or their location within or near the VMH. Second, the effects of VMH lesions on sympathetic nervous system activity may not be similar and may depend on the working situation or the site of sympathetic nervous system. It is reported that the activity of brown adipose tissue was reduced when animals were fed a cafeteria diet but was not reduced when animals were exposed to cold.[53] Yoshida and Bray[52] reported that NE turnover was increased in the brown adipose tissue but not in the pancreas. Yoshimatsu et al[54] reported that the sympathetic nervous system drive to brown adipose tissue was reduced but drive to the adrenal gland was increased.

The activity of the sympathetic nervous system in rats with knife cut hypothalamic lesions may also be slightly reduced since responsiveness of the activity of brown adipose tissue was impaired in animals fed a cafeteria diet or a high-fat diet[55]; however, it has not been reported that the activity of sympathetic nervous system is reduced in PVM-lesioned rats. NE turnover was reportedly reduced in obesity associated with MSG treatment.[56]

Thermogenesis

Brown adipose tissue is the major site for both cold-induced thermogenesis and diet-induced thermogenesis in rodents. Recently a defect in thermogenesis has been proposed as a pathogenic factor in the development of obesity.

Hogen et al[53] reported that diet-induced thermogenesis was reduced in VMH-lesioned rats but that cold-induced thermogenesis was not reduced. These observations were confirmed by other investigators.[57] The defective thermogenesis in brown adipose tissue is due to hypoactivity of the sympathetic nervous system in VMH-lesioned rats.

It is suggested that diet-induced thermogenesis is defective in rats with knife cut hypothalamic lesions and that the cause of this defect depends on adrenal function (probably corticosterone), since adrenalectomy restored GDP binding and cytochrome c oxydase activity to normal.[39,55]

HETEROGENEITY OF PATHOGENESIS OF HYPOTHALAMIC OBESITY

VMH Lesion–Induced Obesity

Brobeck[58] first reported hyperphagia in association with VMH lesion–induced obesity in 1946. Subsequently, the pathogenesis of VMH lesion–induced obesity was attributed to the destruction of a "satiety center" in the VMH. Ablation of this satiety center was believed to remove the inhibitory influences to a "hunger center" in the lateral hypothalamus and allow excess feeding. The excessive food intake made animals obese.[59]

Several investigations have suggested that this interpretation is incorrect. Han and Liu[60] demonstrated that VMH-lesioned rats became obese even if hyperphagia was prevented by force-feeding.

When increased concentrations of insulin were first reported in VMH lesion–induced obesity, the hyperinsulinemia was presumed to be secondary to hyperphagia, since the former disappeared after long fasting. However, restricted feeding or pair-feeding failed to eliminate the hyperinsulinemia.[21,22] The hyperinsulinemia occurs within minutes or in the first few days after VMH lesions even without hyperphagia.[22,23,61] York and Bray[62] and Goldman et al[63] demonstrated that when beta cells of the pancreas were destroyed beforehand with streptozotocin to prevent the increase in insulin after VMH lesions, obesity and hyperphagia were prevented or remarkably attenuated.

Since insulin treatment can produce hyperphagia and obesity, the focus of attention gradually shifted to the hyperinsulinemia. However, in the 1970s it was not known whether hyperphagia or hyperinsulinemia was the most important factor in the development of VMH lesion–induced obesity. The mechanism for the increase in insulin after VMH lesions also was not known. An increase in insulin is not secondary to hyperphagia or obesity, because hyperinsulinemia occurs even when food intake is limited and the increase in body weight is prevented.[21,22,61] Two hypotheses have been advanced. One hypothesis suggests humoral mediation, postulating that a hypothalamic factor that stimulates or suppresses pancreatic beta cells is released into the circulation from the hypothalamus and this increases release of insulin.[64] The second hypothesis proposes neural mediation, which implies that stimuli for increased release of insulin by the beta cells occurs via the autonomic nervous system.[65]

To clarify these questions, Inoue et al[8,66] performed the following experiment. In inbred Lewis rats, pancreatic beta cells were destroyed

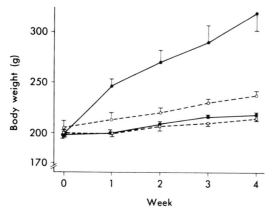

FIGURE 22-1

Body weight of VMH-lesioned and sham-lesioned rats. Data from each group are plotted as mean ± SE. N, intact pancreas; T, pancreatic transplants; ● N-VMH; ○ T-VMH; ■ N-sham-VMH; ○ T-sham-VMH. Modified with permission.[66]

by treatment with streptozotocin. Subsequently, several fetal pancreases were transplanted underneath the renal capsule. By this method rats with denervated pancreatic tissue were produced. After rats had recovered from the diabetes, VMH lesions were created and the rats were observed for four weeks.

VMH-lesioned rats with an intact pancreas gained weight rapidly after creation of the lesions, whereas VMH-lesioned rats with the pancreatic transplants gained weight slowly, in line with the weight gain in nonlesioned control rats (Fig. 22-1). Body fatness was compared by the methods of body density and the Lee Index (Table 22-1). VMH-lesioned rats with an intact pancreas were fatter than nonlesioned control rats on both comparisons, while VMH-lesioned rats with pancreatic transplants were not.

Insulin levels in VMH-lesioned rats with an intact pancreas were threefold higher than in nonlesioned control rats with an intact pancreas, whereas insulin levels in VMH-lesioned rats with pancreatic transplants were the same as in nonlesioned rats with pancreatic transplants (Fig. 22-2). The differences in serum insulin levels between control rats with an intact pancreas and those with pancreatic transplants may be explained by the fact that insulin is released into circulation and does not immediately traverse the liver in rats with pancreatic transplants.[67]

Food intake in VMH-lesioned rats with an intact pancreas increased by 70%, whereas in VMH-lesioned rats with pancreatic transplants food intake increased by 20% when hyperinsulinemia was prevented (see Table 22-2). If a humoral factor were the stimulus to pancreatic beta cells, this factor should stimulate insulin release from the pancreatic tissue beneath the renal capsule. The results supported the hypothesis that the hyperinsulinemia seen in VMH lesion–induced obesity is neurally mediated and is the most important factor in the development of VMH lesion–induced obesity.

Both the sympathetic and parasympathetic nervous systems appear to be involved in the hyperinsulinemia of VMH-lesioned rats.[26] In 1974 Powley and Opsahl[24] demonstrated that interruption of the vagus nerves below the dia-

TABLE 22-1

Effects of VMH Lesions on Body Fatness and Food Intake

Group	Body density*	Lee Index*	Food intake† (g/day)
VMH, intact pancreas	1.0253 ± 0.0167	0.327 ± 0.004	29.8 ± 0.8
Sham, intact pancreas	1.0770 ± 0.0030	0.288 ± 0.002	17.1 ± 0.4
VMH, pancreatic transplants	1.0654 ± 0.0116	0.296 ± 0.002	20.5 ± 0.5
Sham, pancreatic transplants	1.0794 ± 0.0046	0.292 ± 0.003	16.7 ± 0.4

Values are means ± SE. Lee Index = $\sqrt[3]{\text{body wt}}$ (g)/length (cm).

*Data were obtained four weeks after VMH lesions.

†Data were obtained during second week.

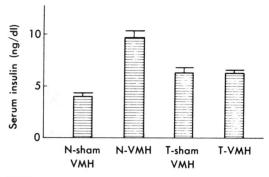

FIGURE 22-2

Serum insulin in VMH-lesioned and sham-lesioned rats. N, intact pancreas; T, pancreatic transplants. Modified with permission.[8]

phragm could reverse the obesity that follows VMH lesions. They suggested that hypersecretion of insulin was reduced after vagotomy and that reversal of obesity occurred because the hyperinsulinemia was removed. Inoue and Bray[25] repeated this study and found that the reversal of body weight after subdiaphragmatic vagotomy was due to restriction of food intake secondary to slowed gastric emptying. Nevertheless, in the same experiment they found a positive correlation between serum insulin levels and gastric acidity in VMH-lesioned rats. Berthoud and Jeanrenaud[23] reported that acute hyperinsulinemia,

which started within minutes after the creation of VMH lesions, could be reversed by acute vagotomy. These findings suggest that hyperactivity of the vagus nerve contributes to the hyperinsulinemia seen in VMH-lesioned rats.

To further investigate the role of vagus nerve activity in hyperinsulinemia after VMH lesions, Inoue et al[68] examined the effect of selective vagotomy of the pancreatic branch. During oral glucose tolerance tests, selective vagotomy decreased basal insulin levels by 42% and inhibited glucose-induced insulin secretion at peak value by 34% in VMH-lesioned rats. In contrast, no significant effect was observed in control rats. Of note, selective vagotomy did not completely restore insulin secretion to normal in VMH-lesioned rats.

The sympathetic nervous system appears to be hypoactive after VMH lesions. This factor may also contribute to the hyperinsulinemia seen after the creation of VMH lesions.

In order to explore the relative contribution of the autonomic nervous system to this hyperinsulinemia, Inoue et al[26] performed the following experiments. Four weeks after the creation of VMH lesions, overnight-fasted rats were infused with epinephrine (1.0 μg/min/kg) to remove the effects of the sympathetic nervous system. Firing of the vagus nerve was inhibited by administration of atropine (1 mg/kg IP and 1 mg/kg SC). When epinephrine was infused, basal insulin

TABLE 22-2

Effects of VMH Lesions on Body Fatness and Food Intake

Group	Body Density[a]	Lee Index[a]	Food Intake[b] (g/day)
VMH intact pancreas	1.0253±0.0167	0.327±0.004	29.8±0.8
Sham intact pancreas	1.0770±0.0030	0.288±0.002	17.1±0.4
VMH pancreatic transplants	1.0654±0.0116	0.296±0.002	20.5±0.5
Sham pancreatic transplants	1.0794±0.0046	0.292±0.003	16.7±0.4

Values are means ± SE. Lee Index = $\sqrt[3]{\text{body wt}}$ (g)/length (cm).

[a]Data were obtained four weeks after VMH lesions.

[b]Data were obtained during second week.

levels decreased and glucose-induced insulin secretion was inhibited by 83% in VMH-lesioned rats. When atropine was given, it also significantly decreased basal insulin levels and inhibited glucose-induced insulin secretion by 42% in VMH-lesioned rats. When the effects of epinephrine and atropine were combined, basal insulin levels decreased markedly and glucose-induced insulin secretion was completely inhibited in VMH-lesioned rats.

These results suggest that stimulation of the vagus nerve and suppression of sympathetic nerves both contribute to the hyperinsulinemia that follows VMH lesions.

Obesity is a consequence of excessive fat accumulation. Three factors can contribute to the process: increased lipogenesis in the liver and adipose tissue, increased fat deposition in the adipose tissue, and reduced lipolysis from the adipose tissue. Inoue and Bray[40] investigated the role of hyperinsulinemia in excessive fat accumulation in VMH-lesioned rats.

To investigate hepatic lipogenesis in the liver, the triglyceride secretion rate from the liver and serum insulin levels were examined.[69] Both triglyceride secretion rate and serum insulin levels increased significantly in VMH-lesioned rats, exhibiting a positive correlation. To assess lipogenic capacity in the adipose tissue, the activity of a key lipogenic enzyme, pyruvate dehydrogenase, and serum insulin levels were determined.[70] VMH-lesioned rats showed significantly increased pyruvate dehydrogenase activity and serum insulin levels in the fed state, which decreased significantly after 48 hours of fasting; there was a positive correlation between the two factors.

To investigate serum triglyceride deposition in adipose tissue, heparin-releasable lipoprotein lipase activity and insulin levels in the blood of fed rats were measured.[71] Both lipoprotein lipase activity and serum insulin levels increased significantly in VMH-lesioned rats, exhibiting a positive correlation.

To investigate lipolysis in adipose tissue, glycerol release and serum insulin levels were determined. Under basal conditions, there was no difference in glycerol release between VMH-lesioned rats and control rats (Fig. 22-3). VMH-lesioned rats showed significantly lower

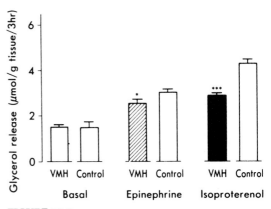

FIGURE 22-3

Plasma glycerol concentrations in basal state and after epinephrine and isoproterenol stimulation. $*P < .05$, $***P < .001$.

glycerol release in response to epinephrine and isoproterenol, with higher serum insulin levels. There was a weak but significantly negative correlation between serum insulin and epinephrine-induced glycerol release ($r = .76$, $P < .02$).

These results indicate that hyperinsulinemia after VMH lesions contributes to excessive fat accumulation.

Based on these results, Inoue and Bray[72] advanced an "autonomic hypothesis" for the pathogenesis of VMH lesion–induced obesity. This hypothesis could explain the pathogenesis of obesity in a framework like that shown in Figure 22-4. VMH lesions might produce derangement of the autonomic nervous system, suppressing the sympathetic nervous system and stimulating the vagus nerve. The combined effects would result in hyperinsulinemia. The hyperinsulinemia would increase lipogenesis in liver and adipose tissue; increase lipoprotein lipase activity, resulting in acceleration of deposition of exogenous (chylomicron) and endogenous (very low density lipoprotein triglyceride) lipids into adipose tissue; and reduce lipolysis in adipose tissue. Hyperphagia, which is enhanced mainly by hyperinsulinemia, would provide excessive foodstuffs for lipogenesis and chylomicrons for fat deposition. All of these effects might cooperate in the excessive fat accumulation and contribute to the development of VMH lesion–induced obesity.

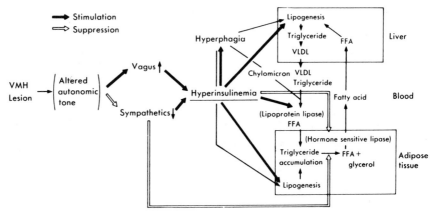

FIGURE 22-4

Schema for the pathogenesis of VMH obesity (see text).

This hypothesis has been criticized on three fronts. First, the primary role of hyperinsulinemia in the pathogenesis of obesity has been questioned. Sclafani[10] indicated that a 20% increase in food intake without hyperinsulinemia in VMH-lesioned rats with pancreatic transplants[8,66] could have led to obesity if the observation period had been extended to more than four weeks after the creation of VMH lesions. As mentioned earlier, hyperinsulinemia and hyperphagia are independent events in animals with hypothalamic lesions. Therefore, this criticism may be appropriate. However, it is also true that without hyperinsulinemia, VMH-lesioned rats that are not hyperinsulinemic fail to manifest the characteristic features of remarkable hyperphagia and rapid weight gain that lead to obesity. Thus, the hyperinsulinemia associated with a disorder of the autonomic nervous system may not be essential but may be substantially the most important factor in the development of VMH lesion–induced obesity.

A second criticism is that glucocorticoid may be the primary factor in the pathogenesis of VMH lesion–induced obesity, since adrenalectomy reverses this obesity[33,37] and replacement of glucocorticoid inhibits the effect of adrenalectomy.[73] However, King and Smith[37,74] noted that hypophysectomy or incomplete adrenalectomy failed to inhibit the development of obesity, and that only a small amount of corticosterone replacement is sufficient for the development of

obesity in completely adrenalectomized rats with VMH lesions. Based on these results, they regarded the role of corticosterone as permissive or indirect and not direct in the development of VMH lesion–induced obesity.

A third criticism is directed toward the thermogenic defect, which probably depends on dysfunction of brown adipose tissue. Dysfunction of brown adipose tissue is supposed to result from hypoactivity of the sympathetic nervous system after VMH lesions. However, Powley et al[75] demonstrated that guanethidine sympathectomy only potentiated the effects of VMH lesions on body weight gain.

The author does not deny that these three factors contribute in part to the pathogenesis of VMH lesion–induced obesity.

PVH Lesion–Induced Obesity

It is reported hyperphagia is the primary event in PVH-lesioned rats.[18,43] Therefore, hyperphagia may be the most important factor in the pathogenesis of this obesity. Hyperinsulinemia secondary to hyperphagia or hyperglycemia (or both) may exert an enhancing effect on fat accumulation.

It is also reported that adrenalectomy reverses this obesity.[38] The cause of this phenomenon cannot be explained at present, since (1) a disorder of the sympathetic nervous system that may produce a thermogenic defect in brown adipose tissue is not observed, and (2) serum corticosterone levels are rather low in PVH-lesioned rats.[18] However, one possible explanation is that adrenalectomy corrects the damage to feeding-related noradrenergic receptors that is produced by PVH lesions.[20,76]

Knife Cut Lesion–Induced Obesity

As in PVH-lesioned rats, it is reported that hyperphagia is the primary event in rats with knife cut hypothalamic lesions.[10] Therefore, hyperphagia may be the most important factor in the pathogenesis of knife cut–induced obesity. However, restriction of food intake did not prevent knife cut–induced obesity.[50]

Adrenalectomy could reverse this obesity, and a thermogenic defect in brown fat was suggested to be correctable with adrenalectomy.[39] A defect in energy expenditure may also contribute to the pathogenesis of this obesity.

Arcuate Nucleus Lesion–Induced Obesity

MSG treatment mainly damages the arcuate nuclei in the hypothalamus; it also damages some parts of the VMH.[77] MSG-treated animals showed hyperinsulinemia without hyperphagia.[11] Thus, hyperinsulinemia is probably the most important factor in the development of arcuate nucleus lesion–induced obesity. A defect in energy expenditure may contribute, in part, to the pathogenesis of this obesity.[56]

DLT Lesion–Induced Obesity

The pathogenesis of DLT lesion–induced obesity has not been unequivocally identified. Hyperphagia resulting from destruction of the ventral noradrenergic bundle is the most probable candidate.[78] Hyperinsulinemia with hyperphagia at night or without hyperphagia during the day may contribute to the pathogenesis of this obesity.[4] Wellman et al[4] suggested that reduced brown adipose tissue may also contribute to the pathogenesis of this obesity.

Obesity with Hypothalamic Islands

Onai et al[30] recently reported that streptozotocin-treated rats with hypothalamic islands increased food intake but failed to become obese, which suggests that hyperphagia and hyperinsulinemia cooperatively contribute to the pathogenesis of this obesity.

CONCLUSION

Obesity-inducing lesions in different regions of hypothalamus result in heterogeneous derangements and different pathogenesis; further, the pathogenesis of each obesity is multifactorial. Some investigators believe that glucocorticoid plays an essential role in all forms of obesity since adrenalectomy reverses or attenuates all forms of obesity. However, the effects of adrenalectomy have not yet been fully examined for any form of hypothalamic obesity and the available evidence is insufficient. We must be cautious in interpreting the results of adrenalectomy since adrenalectomized animals, especially mice, are extremely sensitive to any manipulations.

Further investigation of the interrelationship among hyperphagia, hyperinsulinemia, and corticosterone action may clarify the pathogenesis of hypothalamic obesity associated with different hypothalamic lesions. The role of corticotropin-releasing hormone in the pathogenesis of obesity also deserves investigation in the pathogenesis of hypothalamic obesity resulting from different hypothalamic lesions.

References

1. Hetherington A, Ranson SW: Hypothalamic lesions and adiposity in the rat. Anat Rec 78:149, 1940
2. Brecher G, Waxler SH: Obesity in albino mice due to single injection of gold thioglucose. Proc Soc Exp Biol Med 70:498, 1949
3. Leibowitz SF, Hammer NJ, Chang K: Hypothalamic paraventricular nucleus lesions produce overeating and obesity in the rat. Physiol Behav 27:1031, 1981
4. Wellman PJ, Elissalde M, Watkins PA et al: Hyperinsulinemia and obesity in the dorsolateral tegmental rat. Physiol Behav 32:1, 1984
5. Ohshima K, Okada S, Onai T et al: The characteristics of obese rats induced by medial basal hypothalamic deafferentation. Proceedings of the 5th Congress of the Japan Society for the Study of Obesity, p 114, 1985
6. Olney JW: Brain lesions, obesity, and other disturbances in mice treated with mono-sodium glutamate. Science 164:719, 1969
7. Sclafani A, Aravich PF: Macronutrient self-selection in three forms of hypothalamic obesity. Am J Physiol 244:R686, 1983

8. Inoue S, Bray GA, Mullen YS: Transplantation of pancreatic beta-cells prevents the development of hypothalamic obesity in rats. Am J Physiol 235: E266, 1978

9. Tokunaga K, Fukushima M, Kemnitz JW et al: Comparison of ventromedial and paraventricular lesions in rats that become obese. Am J Physiol 251:R1221, 1986

10. Sclafani A: The role of hyperinsulinemia and the vagus nerve in hypothalamic hyperphagia reexamined. Diabetologia 20:402, 1981

11. Scallett AC, Olney JW: Components of hypothalamic obesity: Bipieridyl-mustard lesions add hyperphagia to monosodium glutamate-induced hyperinsulinemia. Brain Res 374:380, 1986

12. Bray GA, Gallagher TF Jr: Manifestations of hypothalamic obesity in man: A comprehensive investigation of eight patients and a review of the literature. Medicine 54:301, 1975

13. Smith G, Epstein A: Increased feeding in response to decreased utilization in the rat and monkey. Am J Physiol 217:1083, 1969

14. Oomura Y, Kita H: Insulin acting as a modulator of feeding through the hypothalamus. Diabetologia 20(suppl):290, 1981

15. Sakaguchi T, Takahashi M, Bray GA: Diurnal changes in sympathetic activity: Relation to food intake and to insulin injected into the ventromedial or suprachiasmatic nucleus. J Clin Invest 82:282, 1988

16. Sakata T, Ookuma K, Fukagawa K et al: Blockade of the histamine H_1-receptor in the rat ventromedial hypothalamus and feeding elicitation. Brain Res 441:403, 1988

17. Orosco M, Jacquot C, Cohen Y: Brain catecholamine levels and turnover in various models of obese animals. Gen Pharmacol 12:267, 1981

18. Shor-Posner G, Azar P, Insinga S et al: Deficits in the control of food intake after hypothalamic paraventricular nucleus lesions. Physiol Behav 35:883, 1985

19. Aravich PF, Sclafani A: Paraventricular hypothalamic lesions and medial hypothalamic knife cuts produce similar hyperphagia syndromes. Behav Neurosci 97:970, 1983

20. Leibowitz SF, Hammer NJ, Chang K: Feeding behavior induced by central norepinephrine injection is attenuated by discrete lesions in the hypothalamic paraventricular nucleus. Pharmacol Biochem Behav 19:945, 1983

21. Han PW, Frohman LA: Hyperinsulinemia in tube-fed hypophysectomized rats bearing hypothalamic lesions. Am J Physiol 219:1632, 1970

22. Hustvedt BE, Løvø A: Correlation between hyperinsulinemia and hyperphagia in rats with ventromedial hypothalamic lesions. Acta Physiol Scand 84:29, 1972

23. Berthoud HR, Jeanrenaud B: Acute hyperinsulinemia and its reversal by vagotomy after lesions of the ventromedial hypothalamus unanesthetized rats. Endocrinology 105:146, 1979

24. Powley TL, Opsahl CA: Ventromedial hypothalamic obesity abolished by subdiaphragmatic vagotomy. Am J Physiol 226:25, 1974

25. Inoue S, Bray GA: The effect of subdiaphragmatic vagotomy in rats with ventromedial hypothalamic obesity. Endocrinology 100:108, 1977

26. Inoue S, Mullen YS, Bray GA: Hyperinsulinemia in rats with hypothalamic obesity: Effects of autonomic drugs and glucose. Am J Physiol 245:R372, 1983

27. Fukushima M, Tokunaga K, Lupien J et al: Dynamic and static phases of obesity following lesions in PVH and VMH. Am J Physiol 253:R523, 1987

28. Bray GA: Regulation of energy balance: Studies on genetic, hypothalamic and dietary obesity. Proc Nutr Soc 41:95, 1982

29. Hirose Y, Ishiharak, Utsumi M et al: Studies on hypersomatostatinemia in the development of MSG-induced hypothalamic obesity in rats. Proceedings of the 2nd Congress of the Japan Society for the Study of Obesity, p 45, JASSO, Tokyo, 1981

30. Onai T, Ohshima K, Okada S et al: The role of insulin in the development of obesity in hypothalamic deafferented rats: Studies of the effects of insulin in feeding behavior. J Jpn Diabetic Soc 164:719, 1990

31. Krieger DT: Ventromedial hypothalamic lesions abolish food-shifted circadian adrenal and temperature rhythmicity. Endocrinology 106:649, 1980

32. King BM, Calvert CB, Esquerre KR et al: Relationship between plasma corticosterone and insulin levels in rats with ventromedial hypothalamic lesions. Physiol Behav 32:991, 1984

33. Debons AF, Siclari E, Das KC et al: Gold thioglucose-induced hypothalamic damage, hyperphagia, and obesity: Dependence on the adrenal gland. Endocrinology 110:2024, 1982

34. Leibowitz SF, Roland CR, Hor L et al: Noradrenergic feeding elicited via the paraventricular nucleus is dependent upon circulating corticosterone. Physiol Behav 32:857, 1984

35. Sylvan A, Fecko J, Gold RM et al: Adrenal suppression following hypothalamic knife cuts that produce obesity (abstr). Neurosci 11:56, 1985

36. Krieger DT: Restoration of corticosteroid periodicity in obese rats by limited A.M. food access. Brain Res 171:67, 1979

37. King BM, Smith RL: Hypothalamic obesity after

hypophysectomy or adrenalectomy: Dependence on corticosterone. Am J Physiol 249:R522, 1985

38. Tokunaga K, Fukushima M, Lupien JR et al: Effects of food restriction and adrenalectomy in rats with VMH and PVH lesions. Physiol Behav 45:1131, 1989

39. Romsos DR, VanderTuig JG, Kerner J et al: Energy balance in rats with obesity-producing hypothalamic knife cuts: Effects of adrenalectomy. J Nutr 117:1121, 1987

40. Inoue S, Bray GA: Role of the autonomic nervous system in the development of ventromedial hypothalamic obesity. Brain Res Bull 5(suppl 4):119, 1980

41. Ridley PT, Brooks FP: Alterations in gastric secretion following hypothalamic lesions producing hyperphagia. Am J Physiol 209:319, 1965

42. Carpenter RG, Stamoutsos BA, Dalton LD et al: VMH obesity reduced but not reversed by scopolamine methylnitrate. Physiol Behav 23:955, 1979

43. Weingarten HP, Chang PK, McDonald TJ: Comparison of the metabolic and behavioral disturbances following paraventricular and ventromedial hypothalamic lesions. Brain Res Bull 14:551, 1985

44. Sawchenko PE, Gold RM: Effects of gastric vs. complete subdiaphragmatic vagotomy on hypothalamic hyperphagia and obesity. Physiol Behav 26:281, 1981

45. Inoue S, Campfield LA, Bray GA: Comparison of metabolic alterations in hypothalamic and high fat diet-induced obesity. Am J Physiol 223:R162, 1977

46. Nishizawa Y, Bray GA: Ventromedial hypothalamic lesions and the mobilization of fatty acids. J Clin Invest 61:714, 1978

47. Niijima A, Rohner-Jeanrenaud F, Jeanrenaud B: Role of ventromedial hypothalamus on sympathetic efferents of brown adipose tissue. Am J Physiol 247:R650, 1984

48. Yoshimatsu H, Niijima A, Oomura Y et al: Effects of hypothalamic lesion on pancreatic autonomic nerve activity in the rat. Brain Res 303:147, 1984

49. VanderTuig TG, Knehans AW, Romsos DR: Reduced sympathetic nervous activity in rats with ventromedial hypothalamic lesions. Life Sci 30:913, 1982

50. VanderTuig JG, Kerner J, Romsos DR: Hypothalamic obesity, brown adipose tissue, and sympathoadrenal activity in rats. Am J Physiol 248:E607, 1985

51. Young JB, Landsberg L: Impaired suppression of sympathetic activity during fasting in the gold thioglucose treated mouse. J Clin Invest 65:1086, 1980

52. Yoshida T, Bray GA: Catecholamine turnover in rats with ventromedial hypothalamic lesions. Am J Physiol 246:R558, 1984

53. Hogan S, Coscina DV, Himms-Hagen J: Brown adipose tissue of rats with obesity-inducing ventromedial hypothalamic lesions. Am J Physiol 243:E338, 1982

54. Yoshimatsu H, Oomura Y, Katafuchi T et al: Lesions of the ventromedial hypothalamic nucleus enhance sympatho-adrenal function. Brain Res 339:390, 1985

55. Coscina DV, Chambers JW, Park I et al: Impaired diet-induced thermogenesis in brown adipose tissue from rats made obese with parasagittal hypothalamic knife-cuts. Brain Res Bull 14:585, 1985

56. Yoshida T, Nishioka H, Nakamura Y et al: Reduced norepinephrine turnover in brown adipose tissue of pre-obese mice treated with monosodium-L-glutamate. Life Sci 36: 931, 1985

57. Ito M, Inokoshi Y, Shimazu T: Brown adipose tissue after ventromedial hypothalamic lesions in rats. Am J Physiol 248:E20, 1985

58. Brobeck JR: Mechanism of development of obesity in animals with hypothalamic lesions. Physiol Rev 26:541, 1946

59. Brobeck JR: Food and temperature. Recent Prog Horm Res 16:439, 1960

60. Han PW, Liu AC: Obesity and impaired growth of rats force-fed 40 days after hypothalamic lesions. Am J Physiol 211:229, 1966

61. Martin JM, Konijnendijk W, Bouman PR: Insulin and growth hormone secretion in rats with ventromedial hypothalamic lesions maintained on restricted food intake. Diabetes 23:203, 1974

62. York DA, Bray GA: Dependence of hypothalamic obesity on insulin, the pituitary and the adrenal gland. Endocrinology 90:885, 1972

63. Goldman JK, Schnatz JD, Bernardis LL et al: Effects of ventromedial hypothalamic destruction in rats with pre-existing streptozotocin induced diabetes. Metabolism 21:132, 1972

64. Idahl LA, Martin JM: Stimulation of insulin release by a ventrolateral hypothalamic factor. J Endocrinol 51:601, 1971

65. Bernardis LL, Frohman LA: Effect of lesion size in the ventromedial hypothalamus on growth hormone and insulin levels in the weanling rat. Neuroendocrinology 6:319, 1970

66. Inoue S, Bray GA, Mullen Y: Effect of transplantation of pancreas on development of hypothalamic obesity. Nature 226:742, 1977

67. Weber CJ, Hardy MA, Lerner RL et al: Hyperinsulinemia and hyperglucagonemia following pancreatic islet transplantation in diabetic rats. Diabetes 25:944, 1976

68. Inoue S: Mechanism of increase in insulin secretion in ventromedial hypothalamic lesioned rats. In Serrano-Rios M, LeFebvre PJ [eds]: Diabetes 1985, p 263. Excerpta Medica, Amsterdam, 1986

69. Satoh S, Inoue S, Egawa M et al: Increased triglyc-

eride secretion rate and hyperinsulinemia in ventromedial hypothalamic lesioned rats in vivo. Acta Endocrinol 110:6, 1985

70. Inoue S, Bray GA: Ventromedial hypothalamic obesity and autonomic nervous system: An autonomic hypothesis. In Cioffi LA et al (eds): The Body Weight Regulatory System: Normal and Disturbed Mechanisms, p 61. New York, Raven Press, 1981

71. Inoue S, Murase T: Increase of postheparin plasma-lipoprotein-lipase activity in ventromedial hypothalamic obesity in rats. Int J Obes 6:259, 1982

72. Inoue S, Bray GA: An autonomic hypothesis for hypothalamic obesity. Life Sci 25:561, 1979

73. Bruce BK, King BM, Phelps GR et al: Effects of adrenalectomy and corticosterone administration on hypothalamic obesity in rats. Am J Physiol 243:E152, 1982

74. King BM: Glucocorticoids and hypothalamic obesity. Neurosci Biobehav Rev 12:29, 1988

75. Powley TL, Walgren MD, Laughton WB: Effects of guanethidine sympathectomy on ventromedial hypothalamic obesity. Am J Physiol 245:R408, 1983

76. Leibowitz SF, Hor L: Endorphinergic and alpha-noradrenergic systems in the paraventricular nucleus: Effects on eating behavior. Peptides 3:421, 1982

77. Tanaka K, Shimada M, Nakao K et al: Hypothalamic lesion induced by injection of monosodium glutamate in suckling period and subsequent development of obesity. Exp Neurol 62:191, 1978

78. Peters RH, Blythe BL, Sensenig LD: Electrolytic current parameters in the dorsolateral tegmental obesity syndrome in rats. Physiol Behav 34:57, 1985

PART FIVE

HUMAN OBESITY: GENERAL ASPECTS

CHAPTER 23

Obesity: Historical Development of Scientific and Cultural Ideas

GEORGE A. BRAY

Massive obesity has been recognized for thousands of years, yet interpretation of this condition has varied from age to age, reflecting the cultural and scientific values of the observers. This chapter examines some earlier concepts about obesity from a historical perspective. In addition, it considers the relation of the moral stigma of obesity to the clinical concept of obesity as a pathology.

A number of synonyms have been used to describe obesity, including corpulence, excess adipose, *grand embonpoint*, pinguedinis, and polysarcia. In 1864 Down wrote, "The term polysarcia has been so long accepted as a designation of that condition of the body in which the purely adipose constituents are developed in excess, that I am induced to employ it, although its literal significance is not strictly in accordance with the pathological state." In less than 20 years, however, this term was almost completely abandoned. In the present discussion, we will use several of these terms, usually in the context in which they appeared historically.

OBESITY IN PREHISTORIC TIMES

The earliest artifacts indicating the presence of human obesity come from Stone Age statuettes showing excessive roundness of the human female form. The best known of these is the Venus

of Willendorf, a small statuette dating from approximately 25,000 years ago and currently housed in the Vienna Natural History Museum. This statue with large abdomen and pendulous breasts is one of a group of statues from this period. A major interpretation of these early Stone Age figures is that they represent maternal or fertility symbols.[45] A second statue in the same museum, a seated pregnant figure with fat on the lower abdomen and thighs, may be viewed as a mother goddess figure.[45]

OBESITY IN GRECO-ROMAN MEDICINE

According to Hippocrates there were two routes to knowledge about disease. The first was observation of the individual's symptoms. The second was the study of structure and function of the body at a time when human dissection was not possible. The Hippocratic works contain various theories of the body's functioning based largely on the elements and humors. There were four elements which had corresponding humors in the body. Health was associated with an appropriate balance among these humors; disease was a state of imbalance.[58,59]

The hazards of obesity to human health were clearly noted in medical writings of the Greco-Roman period. The Hippocratic texts state that "Sudden death is more common in those who are naturally fat than in the lean."[58] The hippocratic writings also note that obesity was a cause of infertility in women and that the frequency of menses was reduced. Infertility was thought to occur because of difficulty in copulation and be-

Reprinted with permission of Journal of Obesity, Volume 14, November 1990, Obesity: Historical development of scientific and cultural ideas. By George Bray.

cause accumulated fat closed the uterus to the admission of seminal fluids.

A moral tone is evident from Hippocrates' recommendations for treatment of obesity:

> Obese people with laxity of muscle and red complexion, because of their moist constitution, need dry food during the greatest part of the year. . . . Obese people and those desiring to lose weight should perform hard work before food. Meals should be taken after exertion and while still panting from fatigue and with no other refreshment before meals except only wine, diluted and slightly cold. Their meals should be prepared with sesame or seasoning and other similar substances and be of a fatty nature as people get thus satiated with little food. They should, moreover, eat only once a day and take no baths and sleep on a hard bed and walk naked as long as possible.[90]

Galen, following in the hippocratic tradition, adhered to the principles of the four elements and four humors (Table 23-1).[3] In addition, Galen postulated as a basic principle of life a spirit (pneuma) that was inhaled with the air and mixed with blood in the left ventricle where it was converted into "vital spirit." The blood left the ventricle for the brain, where the "vital spirit" was converted into "animal spirit," which traveled down the nerves, endowing them with sensation and the ability to cause movement. Another spirit, the "natural spirit," was thought to arise in the liver and separated food into "earthy" matter, which went to the spleen, "yellow bile," which went to the gallbladder, and "watery" matter, which went to the kidneys.[3]

Galen wrote more than 125 medical books concerning all aspects of anatomy, physiology, therapeutics, and hygiene. He identified two types of obesity, one moderate, the other immoderate.

The former was regarded as natural, the other as morbid. In De Sanite Tuenda, Galen wrote, "The hygienic art promises to maintain in good health those who obey it; but to those who are disobedient, it is just as if it did not exist at all."[49] This is the clearest indication that Galen viewed obesity as a reflection of personal inadequacy:

> Now, I have made any sufficiently stout patient moderately thin in a short time by compelling him to do rapid running, then wiping off his perspiration with very soft or very rough muslin, and then massaging him maximally with diaphoretic inunctions, which the younger doctors customarily call restoratives, and after such massage leading him to the bath, after which I did not give him nourishment immediately, but bade him rest for a while or do something to which he was accustomed, then led him to the second bath and then gave him abundant food of little nourishment, so as to fill him up but distribute little of it to the entire body.[49,p156]

The concept he articulated is that obesity resulted from disobedience to nature.

BYZANTINE AND ARABIC CONCEPTS OF OBESITY

With the decline in Roman influence, scholarly activity shifted from Rome to Byzantium[37,66] and then to the Arabic world. One of the leading figures of Arabic medicine was Avicenna, who like Galen was a highly influential author. The Cannon of Avicenna is the most important of his more than 100 books. It was translated into Latin in the 12th century and continued to be an important textbook of medicine through the 15th century. Obesity was well known to the Arabic physician. The first book of the Cannon describes how to reduce obesity.

TABLE 23-1

Relationship of the Four Elements to the Theory of Humors

Elements	Humors	Characteristics	Personality
Earth	Black bile	Dry and cold	Melancholy
Air	Yellow bile	Hot and dry	Choleric
Fire	Blood	Hot and wet	Sanguine
Water	Phlegm	Cold and wet	Phlegmatic

[For] The regimen which will reduce obesity. (1) Procure a rapid descent of the food from the stomach and intestines, in order to prevent completion of absorption by the mesentery. (2) Take food which is bulky but feebly nutritious. (3) Take the bath before food, often. (4) Hard exercise. . . .[50,p441]

17TH CENTURY MEDICINE

The first monographs in which obesity was the primary subject appeared in the late 16th century,[106] with several others appearing in the 17th century.[39,48,55,75,122] Written in Latin, all of these theses dealt primarily with the clinical aspects of obesity. The teachings of Hippocrates and Galen were quoted. These works also show the influence of the new physical and chemical thinking which was beginning to be used as a theoretical basis for understanding bodily function.[3] Physical interpretations of bodily function were strong in the work of Borelli, an Italian, who was in the center of the arena for new work in mechanics. The circulation of the blood described by William Harvey in 1628, the movement of the limbs, and breathing could all be explained in terms of mechanical principles. Using these concepts, Borelli and others developed what became known as the Iatromechanical School. Two theses took an iatromechanical approach in discussing obesity.[41,118] Since mechanics is not an area of personal responsibility, the iatromechanicists would be less moralistic toward the obese than Galen.

Another school of thought on the origin of disease was based on ideas about fermentations and putrefaction. These early chemical concepts of change preceded our knowledge of bacteria and biochemistry. Nonetheless, they served as the basis for a theory of disease called the Iatrochemical School. Two theses[55,75] cite the work of van Helmont,[57] thus putting their discussion of obesity into a iatrochemical framework.

Sydenham was the greatest clinician of the 17th century and is often acclaimed as the modern Hippocrates. He argued that bedside experience was the best teacher since the human mind is limited and theories are of little value.[116] It was his belief that diseases are clinically specific and can be identified much as flowers or animals can be identified. He initiated the movement for

grouping symptoms that culminated in the great clinical catalogues of disease in the 18th century

18TH CENTURY MEDICINE

The medical history of the 18th century can be divided into two parts. In the first half of the century, the medical world was dominated by the teachings of Boerhaave, who was successively professor of Chemistry, Botany, and Medicine at Leiden. Boerhaave was an eclectic. He included much of Galen and Hippocrates, as well as ideas from the iatrochemical and iatromechanical schools. Boerhaave believed that health resulted from the proper interaction of the vessels and the fluids. Disease was the improper action of either the vessels or the fluids. Treatment of disease was thus aimed at opening up the vessels, or restoring the fluids to proper balance. In the 18th century at least 34 doctoral theses dealing with obesity were published, indicating the rising awareness of this problem.* The first half of the 18th century also saw the first English-language monographs on obesity.[42,113] An understanding of these two monographs requires knowledge about the clinical setting in which health and disease were viewed in the 18th century. Although the details of Galen's system had been rejected by this time, fundamental assumptions about health and disease as representing states of balance or imbalance were common in medical thought. In the 17th and 18th centuries, the symptoms were regarded as the disease. The interaction between physician and patient consisted of a dialogue in which the doctor asked questions and the patient responded. Physical examination as we know it today did not exist, except for feeling the pulse and observing the urine, sputum, feces, and blood.

Eighteenth century medical education, epitomized by the teachings of Boerhaave in Leiden, consisted primarily of lectures. Subjects included Anatomy, Physiology, Materia Medica, the Institutes of Medicine, and the Practice of Physick, the course on clinical medicine. Disease

---

*9, 11, 13, 15, 30, 35, 41, 60, 62, 64, 65, 70, 73, 76, 77, 83, 85, 86, 88, 89, 92, 95, 96, 97, 99, 109, 110, 112, 114, 115, 117, 118, 119, 122, 123, and 127.

could be a disorder of the quality or quantity of either the solids or humors, or it could be a combination of both. Inflammation would be an example of a disease in which both solids and humors were involved.

Important factors in the cause of disease included the type of air one breathed; the types and quantity of food and fluid that were ingested; the type of evacuations; the amount of rest and exercise; the emotional state of mind; and the quantity and quality of sleep. These qualities of individual life were subsumed under the heading of "nonnaturals." They were believed to be largely under individual control. Thus, gluttony would be a condition with individual responsibility for overeating, i.e., a moral attribution to the patient.

A miasmatic model provided one of the principal bases for explaining disease in the 18th century. Thus, stagnation of air or the presence of excess moisture in the air were believed to be important features in the development of disease. The clinical encounter between physician and patient consisted of evaluating the various factors (nonnaturals) that might be out of order. Therapy was aimed at correcting this imbalance. If perspiration was reduced, then a therapeutic agent was needed to produce perspiration. If evacuations were infrequent, a laxative was needed; if gluttony was present, abstinence from excessive eating was the remedy.

Against this background we can examine the views of Thomas Short (1727) on the origin of corpulence.[113] He began by saying, "I believe no age did ever afford more instances of corpulency than our own." The corpulency of which Short spoke was "undeniably a morbid state," thus restating the aphorism of Hippocrates. The primary cause of corpulency, according to Short, was "a great plenty of blood stor'd with oily parts and not sufficiently attenuated and discharged by perspiration." Since defective perspiration was the cause, the treatment was to increase perspiration. Short thought that fat was separated from the blood and stored in "little bags" composing the whole of the membranae adiposae and filled with pinguiferous (fatty) globules. The concept of a fat cell did not then exist.

In addition to the proximate or immediate cause of corpulency, Short identified a number of remote or secondary causes. The first was the air one breathed. "A warm and soggy air prevents perspiration and relaxes the fibers of the body," leading to obesity. Corpulency was also common in countries like Holland, where there was a constant wet air. Marshy countries also predisposed to corpulency as did city air.

A second remote cause was "plenty of eatables and drinkables, of a soft, smooth, . . . nature." "Sweet, fat or oily things" and food that was easily assimilated also tended to produce corpulency. Although not stated by Short, implicit in this choice of foods was the responsibility of the individual for choosing the foods that were eaten.

A more clear-cut moral statement by Short regarding personal responsibility for corpulency occurred in his discussion of exercise:

[T]otal remission of usual and necessary exercise is a more effectual cause of a morbid corpulency; for by sloth and idleness the natural and necessary evacuations, especially by perspiration are diminished, the vessels are distended with fluids and this distension spoils or impairs the vigor of the solids.[113]

Short thus viewed the obese as idle and slothful, responsible for their own predicament.

The state of mind was also considered important in the development of corpulence. "A cheerful temper contributes much to fatten the body, hence the proverb 'laugh and be fat' is not without its reason and philosophy," Short said.[113] "Frequent tippling and drinking . . . probably explain the reason why ale-house keepers and pot-companions are generally of pretty bulky bodies." Too much sleep, too much "lying soft and warm," and moderate venery all were considered to promote corpulency. These remote or secondary causes were basically disturbances in the so-called nonnaturals. They also included several of the seven deadly sins (gluttony, venery, and sloth), for which the corpulent individual bore responsibility.

Treatment of corpulency entailed restoring the balance in the nonnaturals that made up the remote or secondary causes of obesity. A residence was ideally situated where the air was not too moist or too soggy, not in flat wet countries, the city, or in woodlands. These can be viewed as "moral imperatives." Exercise was important.

Diet was to be "moderate spare and of the more detergent kind." Meat was to be of the less nutritious kind, such as fish. Short sleep was best, and the "elevating passions ought not to be too much indulged." Again, the moral imperative. "Gentle evacuations are helpful to reduce the body." "Smoking of tobacco by stimulating the nerves of the mouth draws out phlegm from the salival glands and diminishes the fluids." Thus, Short viewed corpulence as both unhealthy and in some sense immoral, since it was a product of the failure of the individual to exert self-control over those factors in life over which he could have control.

MEDICINE IN EDINBURGH: 1750–1800

By the second half of the 18th century, the center of medical teaching had shifted from Leiden in The Netherlands to Edinburgh. Monro, a founder of the Edinburgh School, trained in Leiden under Boerhaave and returned to Edinburgh in 1726. During the remainder of the century, Edinburgh was the leading center for medical education. Monro lectured in English, as opposed to Latin, which had been the language used in Leiden and other early centers of medical education. The medical courses consisted of Anatomy and Surgery, Chemistry, the Institutes of Medicine, Materia Medica, and the Practice of Physick. The order in which these courses were taken was up to the student. Since Cambridge and Oxford were not open to "religious dissenters" such as Quakers, Puritans, or Unitarians, persons of these persuasions sought a medical education in Edinburgh. In the latter half of the 18th century, William Cullen, Professor of Chemistry and subsequently Professor of the Institutes of Medicine, became the leading clinical teacher in Edinburgh. In 1769 Cullen published his classification of disease,[25] which was based on the principles developed by Linnaeus for classifying plants. This system assumed that every disease had a constellation of symptoms which were the same. Each disease had a genus and species to describe it. Thus obesity, corpulency, or polysarcia (species) were classed among the cachexias (genus).[25,105]

An English-language monograph on corpulency was published in 1760, during the Edinburgh period, by Malcolm Flemyng, M.D.[42] Like Short, Flemyng viewed corpulency as a disease: "[C]orpulency, when in an extraordinary degree, may be reckoned a disease, as it in some measure obstructs the free exercise of the animal functions; and hath a tendency to shorten life, by paving the way to dangerous distempers."

Flemyng listed four causes for corpulency. The first cause was "the taking in of too large a quantity of food, especially of the rich and oily kind." This description of the first cause is close to a description of gluttony. However, he noted the differences between large and small eaters and obesity. "Not that all corpulent persons are great eaters; or all thin persons spare feeders. We daily see instances of the contrary. Tho' a voracious appetite be one cause of Corpulency, it is not the only cause; and very often not even the conditio sine qua non thereof."[42] The second cause of corpulency was "too lax a texture of the cellular or fatty membrane . . . whereby its cells or vesicles are liable to be too easily distended." He related this problem to a laxity of the solids. In the 18th century, solids and fluids were considered the major components of the body. Flemyng believed that "laxity of the solids" tended to run in families and thus suggested a familial basis for corpulency. Although this concept may have been proposed before[13] and was indeed suggested subsequently,[22,78] it did not advance significantly until the concept of genetics had been put on a firmer basis.[29]

The third cause of corpulence in Flemyng's view was an abnormal state of the blood that facilitated the storage of fat in vesicles. Finally, Flemyng included "defective evacuation" as a cause of corpulency. He believed that sweat, urine, and feces all contained oil, and that to keep from becoming corpulent, the dietary oil had to be evacuated by one of these routes.

In keeping with the concept that disease resulted from an imbalance between the humors and the solids, the appropriate treatment was to restore this balance. "Diseases, like other faults and imperfections, are, in a general way, to be attacked and conquered by remedies, opposite or contrary to the causes that brought them on; and that is exquisitely the case with regard to Corpulency."[42] First, the diet ought to be moderate in quantity. Individuals should get up from the table while still having an "appetite." This is a direct statement of individual responsibility. In some cases Flemyng advised "damping the stomach" by eating fruits or sweetmeats or drinking a glass of sweet wine before meals. He also advised limiting the variety of foods available at meal times. "Coarse brown bread" was recommended over white bread. Roots, greens and other succulent vegetables were also recommended, but with sparing use of butter.

The second problem, according to Flemyng, was the "flabby, relaxed state of the membranous texture." Diminution of the quantity of fat was the primary goal of treatment, along with a strengthening of the "solids" by exercise, proper diet, and cold bathing. Cold bathing tested one's resolve to adhere to a regimen for modifying the causes of corpulency. Since corpulency resulted from a "too easy separation of the oily particles of the blood," it was necessary to diminish the daily supply of fresh oily matter in the blood.

The final approach to treatment was to increase evacuations. Since Flemyng thought that oil must leave the body through sweat, urine, or feces, he believed these evacuations needed to be increased.[42] Flemyng considered purgatives dangerous, but he encouraged walking for its promotion of evacuation. The safest way of increasing the evacuation of oil in the sweat, according to Flemyng, was to increase muscular motion. Flemyng also recommended soap to increase evacuations. He viewed soap as a diuretic, noting that soap can remove greasy substances. He recorded the medical history of a man who lost 28 pounds (from 291 to 263 pounds) during a two-year period in which he consumed a mild castile soap in quantities varying from 2 to 4 drams daily.

One concept about the origin of obesity began as a rift in the faculty of the Edinburgh Medical School. John Browne, an Edinburgh physician at the height of its fame, was secretary to William Cullen, a leading teacher of the Edinburgh School. Browne and Cullen had a parting of the ways. Browne asserted that the classification of diseases by symptoms as proposed by Cullen was nonsense. Browne believed that there was only one principle of life, and that was excitability. Diseases according to Browne were of two types, those characterized by a lack of stimulation, which he labeled "asthenic diseases," and those

resulting from too much stimulation, which were called "sthenic diseases."

Thomas Beddoes, M.D., was the best-known disciple of Browne. He was educated at Oxford and received his medical degree from Edinburgh. Although he returned to Oxford, he was dismissed and thereafter settled in Bristol, where he established a Pneumatic Institute. Beddoes offered an interesting hypothesis about the origin of corpulence.[10] He believed that corpulence was the result of too little oxidation of fat. This, he claimed, was due to the reduced oxygen supplies available during exercise, which limited the ability to utilize fat. Treatment was therefore directed toward increasing the supply of oxygen.

Another explanation for obesity was offered by Rigby in 1785.[100] It is remarkably close to current concepts. "A quantity of nutriment, . . . admitted into the system, more than is sufficient for animal support, must, in all cases, be considered as the principal cause of preternatural fatness; and this may be produced either by intemperance [gluttony?] respecting the quantity of food eaten, by a more than usual disposition in the organs of digestion to convert the food into nutriment, or by circumstances which render the waste of nutriment unequal to the supply." Further, "retention of a matter of heat is a principal cause of animal fat." Regardless of the cause, Tweedie at the end of the 18th century could write, "Corpulency is in very different degrees in different persons; and may be often considerable without being considered a disease; but, however, there is a certain degree of it which will generally be allowed to be a disease."[120]

CLINICAL MEDICINE 1800–1850

From Edinburgh the focus of medical teaching shifted to Paris.[2] After the French Revolution a new vitality emerged in clinical medicine and lasted for more than 30 years. There were four major accomplishments of the Paris clinical school. First, surgery and internal medicine were joined in a single curriculum of medical education. Second, the center of clinical practice and research shifted to the hospital. Third, new methods for physical diagnosis appeared. And finally, pathological anatomy based on tissue theory made its appearance. "Paris medicine" was at its zenith during the first three decades of the 19th century. During this time, Laennec invented the stethoscope,[72] and Bichat founded a school that focused on tissue theory for disease localization.[12] Physical examination as we know it made its appearance with percussion and mediate auscultation through the stethoscope. Large Paris hospitals like the Hôtel Dieu et Pitie became the center of clinical teaching and pathological study. Of interest relative to the history of obesity is that Laennec in the introduction to his monograph describing the stethoscope indicated that the patient who prompted him to roll up a piece of paper to use as the first "stethoscope" in 1816 was an obese girl.[72]

At the time of Paris Medicine, a series of doctoral theses appeared in French dealing with obesity or polysarcie, Sauvages' term for obesity. The number of theses was fewer than in the 18th century, but the number of monographs increased sharply from two to nine.*

The fruits of the clinical approach known as Paris Medicine appeared in the identification of specific types of obesity.[1] The first case of pituitary obesity was probably described by Chapman in 1814,[23] although the credit is often given to Rayer (1823)[94] or Mohr (1840).[81] However, the syndrome of hypothalamic obesity as we know it only became clearly delineated at the beginning of the 20th century.[6,44] Subsequent case reports in English identify a syndrome with all of the characteristics of the modern-day Prader-Willi syndrome.[16,32] A case of obesity-hypoventilation syndrome,[104] also known as the pickwickian syndrome, was also described. Identification of glandular causes of obesity, however, had to wait until the 20th century.[26]

The state of knowledge about obesity at the end of the first half of the 19th century has been aptly summarized in Hufeland's *Textbook of Medicine* (1842), which still used the classification developed by Sauvages and Cullen. Hufeland used the term "polysarca" with a subtitle "adiposis."[63] He wrote,

> Diagnosis. Excessive accumulation of fat either in the whole system or in single parts; forming externally adipose tumors (steatoma); internally, accumulating around the heart, in the omentum, and about

the kidneys.—Its effects are: to impede the functions of the part concerned; and when it is universal, to embarrass motion, to overload the individual, to molest the whole economy, to oppress the circulation, to obstruct secretion and excretion; to dispose to external erysipelatous inflammations and abcesses; finally, transition into cachexy and dropsy.

> Pathogenesis. Immoderate use of nutritive, especially animal food, while exercise and elimination is wanting; a phlegmatic temperament, lax fibre and constitution, cessation of habitual hemorrhages, therefore occurring in women after the cessation of the menses. In general a congenital disposition has a great influence; hence some men continue lean though supplied with the richest food, and others grow fat though subject to restriction.

> Therapeutics. The leading idea of cure is to diminish the accession, and to increase the elimination of the aliments. The principal remedies, are consequently, scanty, unnutritive, vegetable, watery food; strong corporeal exercise; little sleep, excitement of mental affections, promotion of all the secretions, especially that of perspiration and the discharge from the bowels; fasting, mercurial treatment, in extreme cases iodine.

Use of "immoderate" and "phlegmatic" imputes individual responsibility for their plight.

GERMAN LABORATORY MEDICINE

After 1830, when Paris medicine passed its zenith,[2] the focus shifted to what became known as German Laboratory Medicine. There were important parallels with Scotland that led to the rise of German medicine. Germany in the first two thirds of the 19th century consisted of a number of independent states. Each had a strong university system with competition between the various states and universities. The predominant *Naturphilosophy* which claimed that there was a unity in nature and that nature had a temporal history provided important philosophical underpinnings for the growth of German Laboratory Medicine.

The cell theory announced in 1837 by Schwann and Schleiden was one of the singular outcomes of this new philosophical approach.[111] It proposed that the cell was the fundamental unit of living things, thus providing a basis for the science of biology. Shortly thereafter the first descriptions of the growth and development of the fat cell were published.[61] Analysis of fatty

---

*17, 27, 28, 33, 36, 40, 43, 46, 67, 68, 69, 71, 78, 79, 80, 96, 87, 97, 121, and 130.

acid composition appeared at about the same time.[71,91,101] Of more interest was the suggestion by Hassall[54] that certain types of obesity might result from an increased number of fat cells.

The compound microscope and the experimental approach of German Laboratory Medicine also provided the tools for the development of the germ theory of disease. This proved to be an effective replacement for the miasmatic theory of the previous century.

Other important contributions from the German Laboratory school included new methods for exploring disease, such as the various endoscopes (cystoscope, laryngoscope), the ophthalmoscope, the sphygmomanometer, and X-rays.

Another key development of the German school was the theory of the conservation of energy. The laboratory of Johannes Müller provided a training and nurturing ground for many of the outstanding physician scientists of the 19th century, as the institutionalization of scientific medicine in Germany began. From studies on the release of energy associated with muscular activity, Helmholtz concluded that during muscular activity, mass and energy were conserved. This provided the basis for the application of calorimetry[74,100] to pursue the question of whether corpulent individuals could deviate from this law.[5,103]

In addition, this emphasis on measurement stimulated the application of quantitative methods to the study of disease. To do so effectively, it was necessary to have a normal range of values against which to compare individual values. Thus there gradually arose the concept of statistical medicine, which was the basis for actuarial assessment for life insurance and for population studies of health. The publications of Quetelet are among the most important to the current definitions of obesity.[94] Quetelet studied the biologic values of human populations in Belgium and developed the concept that weight could be corrected for height by using the formula kg/m^2. Shortly afterward a manual for anthropometry was published.[102]

ENGLISH CLINICAL MEDICINE IN THE 19TH CENTURY

English medicine during most of the 19th century did not result in important contributions to the clinical understanding of disease and its localization, such as came from the Paris School, or to fundamental understanding of disease, which came from the growth of physiology and German Laboratory Medicine. However, several important figures advanced the concept of tissue pathology that had grown out of the work of Bichat and Laennec in Paris. These individuals included Graves, Stokes, and Corrigan from the Dublin School and Hodgkin, Bright, Addison, and Gull from the London School.

The English contributions to the study of obesity in the 19th century are reflected in books and clinical cases that are almost entirely descriptive.[7,21,22,52,53,125,126] Three of these deserve comment. The first is the 1829 book by Wadd entitled "Comments on Corpulency, Lineaments of Leanness."[22] In this book Wadd presented a series of clinical cases, many with illustrations of massively obese individuals. Most cases came to him through correspondence, a common way of "consulting patients," since the physical examination was not part of the usual examination. Of the 12 cases Wadd presented, all but one occurred in men. Weights were noted in five patients and ranged from 106 kg (16 stones 10 pounds, or 234 pounds) to 146 kg (23 stones 2 pounds, or 324 pounds). Two of the cases examined at post-mortem had enormous accumulations of fat. Although autopsy observations of obese individuals had been made previously,[14,34,51] this was the first instance in a monograph devoted to obesity.

Wadd noted that sudden death is not uncommon in the corpulent, thus restating Hippocrates: "A sudden palpitation excited in the heart of a fat man has often proved as fatal as a bullet through the thorax. . . ." In several cases, the corpulent patients had sought specific pills to treat their obesity. Wadd distinguished between the therapeutic activists and those favoring less aggressive therapy, with the homeopathists being at the far extreme with minimal dosage of medication: "Truly it has been said—some Doctors let the patient die, for fear they should kill him; while others kill the patient, for fear he should die." This is a succinct representation of the extremes of therapeutic intervention in the early 19th century. In Wadd's book there is little to suggest the opprobrium toward the obese that was evident in the works of Short and Flemyng.

Cases of massive obesity, like those described by Wadd, have been noted since antiquity.[20] In the 19th century, Dubourg[33] discussed 25 cases, Schindler[107] identified 17 cases, and Maccary 11.[78] Individual cases were also reported by many other authors. These individuals were frequently noted for their "odd" or "monstrous" appearance. The outlook for this group was particularly bleak, both from a clinical and a social perspective.

The most interesting English-language book on obesity during the 19th century was written by Chambers in 1850.[22] He indicated that "an increase in weight of a healthy adult may be safely considered to be due to fat deposited in some part." He also discussed the concept of "normality" in deciding who is overweight, and included a table with data produced by Hutchinson, based on normal values in 2560 healthy men. These data apparently precede those of Quetelet. Chambers said, "if a man considerably exceeds the average weight of others not taller than himself, we never find this large excess due to muscle or bone, but to adipose tissue."

In his discussion of the origin of fat, Chambers concluded that it arose from the oleaginous parts of the foods that were ingested, but that it might also arise from the conversion of nonoleaginous components of the diet into fat within the body. He discounted the idea that conversion of body tissues into fat plays a significant role in the origin of this disease. In his summary of pathophysiology, Chambers wrote, "For the formation of fat it is necessary that the materials be digested in a greater quantity than is sufficient to supply carbon to the respiration." This concept of excess of intake over expenditure for positive carbon balance followed from the calorimetry work of Lavoisier[74] and from the statement of the first law of thermodynamics by Helmholtz.[56]

Chambers' book is also noteworthy in providing data on 38 cases of obesity. In 13, obesity began before age 18; in the others either the age at onset was not indicated or onset occurred later in life. In seven of the ten individuals with obesity beginning before age 18, there was a hereditary tendency, which was also present in 19 of the 22 patients whose obesity began after age 18 (data on the other cases were inadequate to assign them).

The development of obesity in Chambers' monograph was described under four categories. (1) Infantile obesity: when massive in degree, it was usually lethal before puberty, but most instances of infantile obesity were considered reversible. (2) Childhood onset obesity: occurring between infancy and puberty, it was, Chambers believed, largely hereditary. In girls with this form of obesity, menstruation was thought to be usually precocious. (3) Adult onset: among adults the principal age at onset was between 18 and 30 years. This concept of obesity is singularly modern. In his discussion of treatment, Chambers encouraged a modest low-fat diet and walking, and also suggested that liquor potassae (potash) taken with milk might be helpful. He did not approve of the use of vinegar or iodine.

The final book from 19th century English medicine relating to obesity that deserves comment was by Banting, a layman,[7] and was based on advice he received from his physician, William Harvey.[53] In 1863 Banting wrote what is probably the first popular diet book,[7] a pamphlet entitled "A letter on corpulence addressed to the public." In this pamphlet Banting outlined the dietary method by which he had reduced his weight. It was translated into French, German, and Polish and was the basis for at least one conference.[82,84,121,124] Unlike the medical authorities cited above, Banting did not consider obesity an immoral state related to gluttony or sloth. In this regard his view was closer to that of Wadd with compassion for the afflicted.

20TH CENTURY AMERICAN MEDICINE

The 20th century has seen the continued growth in knowledge about obesity. The terms *corpulence* and *polysarca*, frequently used in the 19th century, have been almost entirely replaced by *obesity*. If the first part of the 19th century was dominated by Paris Medicine and the second part, up to World War I, by German Laboratory Medicine, clearly the 20th century would have to be considered the century of American medicine. Themes appearing in the 19th century have been expanded, and new themes, particularly the experimental study of obesity and the concept that obesity is a syndrome with many etiologies, have greatly expanded. In addition, metabolic studies have greatly increased as the physiologic and biochemical understanding of the basic biologic processes has increased. At least two areas of study have received their major advances during the 20th century. These are the studies of food intake and its control,[18,19] and the use of behavioral methods for the therapeutic approach to obesity. The stigmatization of obesity has become widely recognized and articulated, though its roots lie deep in medical history, dating at least to the time of Hippocrates and Galen.

Acknowledgment: The bibliography for this paper began with the thesis of Worthington and the monograph of Kisch. The papers in these bibliographies were individually verified through the historical collections of medical works at the Wellcome Library in London; The British Library, London; the Bibliotheque de l'Ecole de Medicine, Paris; the UCLA Medical Library, Los Angeles; the Countway Library of the Harvard Medical School, Boston; and the National Library of Medicine, Bethesda. Additional material was identified by cross-checking these sources and through the collection at the National Library of Medicine. Marilyn McClanahan was instrumental in obtaining the French theses.

References

1. Ackerknecht EH: The history of metabolic diseases. Ciba Symp 6:1834, 1944

2. Ackerknecht EH: Medicine at the Paris Hospital: 1794–1848. Baltimore, Johns Hopkins University Press, 1967

3. Ackerknecht EH: A Short History of Medicine. New York, Ronald Press, 1955

4. Anonymous: The life of that wonderful and extraordinarily heavy man, Daniel Lambert, from his birth to the moment of his dissolution; with an account of men noted for their corpulency, and other interesting matter. New York, Samuel Wood & Sons, 1818

5. Atwater WO, Benedict FG: A respiration calorimeter with appliances for the direct determination of oxygen. Washington, DC, Carnegie Institution of Washington, 1905

6. Babinski MJ: Tumeur du corps pituitaire sans acromegalie et avec de developpement des organes genitaux. Rev Neurol 8:531, 1900

7. Banting W: A letter on corpulence addressed to the public, 3rd ed, iv, p 5. London, Harrison and Sons, 1863

8. Barkhausen: Merkwurdige allgemeine Fettablagerung bei einem Knaben von 5 1/4 Jahren. Hannov Ann Ges Heilk 8(n.f. 3):200, 1843

9. Bass G: Dissertationem inauguralem medicam de obesitate nimia, 24 pp. Erfordiae, Preolo Heringii, 1740

10. Beddoes T: Observations on the nature and cure of calculus, sea scurvy, consumption, catarrh and fever: Together with conjectures upon several other subjects of physiology and pathology. London, John Murray, 1793

11. Bertram JW: Dissertatio inauguralis medica de pinguedine, quatro (2), 36 pp. Halae Magdeb, JC Hilligeri, [1739]

12. Bichat FX: Anatomie generale, appliquee a la physiologie et a la medicine. Paris, Chez Brosson, Gabon et Cie, 1801

13. Bon J: Dissertatio medica inauguralis: De mutatione pinguedinis. . . . Harderovici, Apud Johannem Moojen, [1742]

14. Bonetus Th: Sepulchretum, sive Anatomia practica, ex cadaveribus morbo denatis, proponens historias omnium humani corporis affectum . . . vol 1, p 552, L 3, sect xxi. Genevae, Sumptibus Cramer & Perachon, 1700

15. Bougourd O: An obesis somnus brevis salubrior? Paris, [1733], pp 1–4. In Heerkens, Quaes, Paris, [1754], pp 88–93

16. Bray GA: The Obese Patient. Philadelphia, WB Saunders, 1976

17. Caillaud L: De l'obesite (thesis No. 265). Paris, A Parent, 1865

18. Cannon WB, Washburn AL: An explanation of hunger. Am J Physiol 29:441, 1912

19. Carlson AJ: The Control of Hunger in Health and Disease. Chicago, University of Chicago Press, 1916

20. Celsus AAC: De Medicina. Spencer WG (trans): London, Heinemann, 1935–38

21. Chambers TL: On corpulence. Lancet 1:557, 1850

22. Chambers TL: Corpulence, or Excess of Fat in the Human Body. London, 1850

23. Chapman R: A remarkable case of obesity without any external appearance of corpulence, accompanied with hydrocephalus. Lond Med Repos 2:378, Aug 1814

24. Coe T: A letter from Dr. T. Coe, Physician at Chelmsford in Essex, to Dr. Cromwell Mortimer, Secretary R.S. concerning Mr. Bright, the Fat man at Malden in Essex. Philosoph Trans 47:188, 1751–1752

25. Cullen W: Synopsis and nosology, being an arrangement and definition of diseases, 2nd ed, p 48 (trans). Springfield, Edward Gray, 1793

26. Cushing H: The Pituitary Body and Its Disorders: Clinical States Produced by Disorders of the Hypophysis Cerebri. Philadelphia, JB Lippincott, 1912

27. Dancel JF: Traite theorique et pratique de l'obesite (trop grand embonpoint): Avec plusieurs observations de guerison de maladies occasionees ou entretienues par cet etat anormal. Paris, JB Bailliere et fils, 1863

28. Dardonville H: Dissertation sur l'obesite (thesis no. 22, v. 82). Paris, Didot Jeune, [1811]

29. Davenport CB: Body-Build and Its Inheritance. Washington, DC, Carnegie Institution of Washington, 1923

30. Dissertatio inauguralis medica de obesitate. Viennae, Typis Joan Thomae Nobil. de Trattnern, [1776]

31. Don WG: Remarkable case of obesity in a Hindoo boy aged twelve years. Lancet I:363, 1859

32. Down JLH: On polycarcia and its treatment. Clin Lect Rep London Hosp Rep 1:97, 1864

33. Dubourg L: Recherches sur les causes de la polysarcie (thesis No. 43). Paris, A Parent, [1864]

34. Dupytren: Observation sur un cas d'obesite, suivie de maladie du coeur et de la mort. J Med Chir Pharm 12:262, 1806

35. Ebart FCW: Dissertatio inauguralis medica de obesitate nimia et morbis inde orindus. Gottingen, Lit JH Schulzii, [1780]

36. Ebstein W: Die Fettleibigkeit (Korpulenz) und ihre Behandlung nach physiologischen Grundsatzen. Weisbaden, Bergmann, 1882

37. Eltychiades A: He pachusarkia kai he antimetopisis autes kata ten Byzantines iatriken. (Obesity and its treatment in Byzantine Medicine.) Nosokom Chron 43:290, 1981. (English abstract in Society of Ancient Medicine Newsletter, No. 9, p 20, 1982)

38. Eschenmeyer: Beschreibung eines monstrosen fett Mädchen, das in einem Alter von 10 Jahren starb, nach dem es eine Hohe von 5 Fuss 3 zoll und ein Gewicht von 219 Pfund erreicht hatte. Tubing Bl Naturw Arzn 1(3):261, 1815

39. Ettmueller M: Pratique de medicine speciale . . . sur les maladies propres des hommes, des femmes & des petits enfans, avec des Dissertations . . . sur l'epilepsie, l'yvresse, le mal hypochondriaque, la douleur hypochondriaque, la corpulence, & la morsure de la vipere (trad nouv). Lyon, Thomas Amaulry, 1691

40. Faurot A: Essai sur l'obesite (thesis No. 4, v. 65). Paris, Didot Jeune, [1807]

41. Fecht EH: Disputatio medica inauguralis de obesitate nimia. Rostochi, J Wepplingii, 1701

42. Flemyng M: A discourse on the nature, causes and cure of corpulency. Illustrated by a remarkable case, read before the Royal Society, November 1757, and now first published. London, L Davis and C Reymers, 1760

43. Foubert: Traitement de l'obesite par les eaux clorurees sodiques et par l'eau de mer en particulier. Paris, Germer Balliere, 1869

44. Frohlich A: Ein Fall von Tumor der Hypophysis Cerebri ohne Akromegalie. Wiener Klin Rdsch 15:883, 1901

45. Gimbutas M: The goddesses and gods of old Europe. 6500–3500 B.C. Myths and cult images. London: Thames and Hudson, 1974

46. Glais J: De la grossesse adipeuse (thesis No. 164). Paris, A Parent, [1875]

47. Gordon S: Art. XV. Reports of rare cases. IV. Case of extensive fatty degeneration in a boy 14 years of age. Death from obstructed arterial circulation. Dublin Q J Med Sci 33:340, 1862

48. Gosky AU: Disputatio solennis de marasmo, sive marcore: macilentia item & gracilitate sanorum; macilentia & gracilitate aegrotantium; crassitie & corpulentia sanorum naturali; crassitie & magnitudine corporis morbosa aegrorum. . . . Argentinae, Typis Eberhardii Welperi, [1658]

49. Green RM: A Translation of Galen's Hygiene (De Sanitate Tuenda). Springfield, Ill, Charles C Thomas, Publisher, 1951

50. Gruner OC: A treatise on the Canon of Medicine of Avicenna incorporating a translation of the first book. London, Luzac & Co, 1930

51. Haller A von: Corpulence ill cured; large cryptae of the stomach [etc]. In his Path Observ, 1756, p 44

52. Harvey J: Corpulence, Its Diminution and Cure Without Injury to Health, 3rd ed. London, Smith, 1864

53. Harvey W: On Corpulence in Relation to Disease: With Some Remarks on Diet. London, Henry Renshaw, 1872

54. Hassall A: Observations on the development of the fat vesicle. Lancet 1:63, 1849

55. Held JF: Disputationem medica de corpulentia nimia. Publicae . . . censurae . . . submittit. Jenae, Nisianis, [1670]

56. von Helmholtz HLF: Über die Erhaltung der Kraft, eine physikalische Abhandlung. Berlin, G Reimer, 1847

57. Helmont JB von: Ortus medicinae, id est initia physicae inavdita progressus medicinae mouusm, in morborum ultionem ad vitam longam, 4th ed. Lugduni, Joannis Baptiste Deuenet, 1655

58. Hippocrates: The Genuine Works of Hippocrates Translated from the Greek with a Preliminary Discourse and Annotations (Adams F, trans). London, Sydenham Society, 1849

59. Hippocrates: Oeuvres completes d'Hippocrate. Traduction nouvelle avec le texte gren en regard . . . par E. Littre. Paris, JB Balliere, 1839–61

60. Hoelder FB: Obesitatis corporis humani nosologia. Tubingae, Lit Schrammianis, [1775]

61. Hoggan G, Hogan FE: On the development and retrogression of the fat cell. J R Microscop Soc 2:353, 1879

62. Homeroch CF: De pinguidine ejusque sede tam secundum quam praeter naturam constitutis. . . . Lipsiae, Ex Offician Langenhemiana, [1738]

63. Hufeland CW: Enchiridion medicum: Or manual of the practice of medicine, the result of fifty years experience (Bruchhausen C, trans). Revised from the 6th German ed R. Nelson. New York, William Radde, 1852

64. Hulsebusch JF: Dissertatio inauguralis medica sistens pinguedinis corporis humani, sive panniculi adiposi veterum, hodie membranae cellulosae dictae fabricam, ejusque, & contenti olei historiam, usum, morbos. . . . Lugduni Batavorum, Joh. Arnold Langerak, [1728]

65. Jansen W-X: Pinguedinis animalis consideratio physiologica et pathologica, p 142, 1, IV. Lugduni Batavorum, J Hazebroek, A van Houte et Andream Koster, [1784]

66. Jeanselme ME: Comment on traitait les obese a Byzance. Bull Soc Fr Hist Med 20:388, 1926

67. Jeger G-F: Vergleichung einiger durch Fettigkeit oder colossale Bildung ausgezeichneter Kinder und einiger Zwerge. Stuttgart, JB Metzler, [1821]

68. Juette A: De adipis genesi. Berolini, B Schlesinger, [1850]

69. Kisch EH: Die Fettleibigkeit (lipomatosis universalis): Auf grundlage Zahlreicher beobachtungen klinisch Dargestellt. Stuttgart, Ferdinand Enke, 1888

70. Kroedler JS: Theses inauguralis medicae de eo quod citius moriantur obesi, quam graciles secundum Hippocratis aphorismum XLIV. Sect II. Erfordiae, Typis Groschianis, [1724]

71. Kuehn HE: De pinguedine imprimis humana. Lipsiae, Litteris Staritii, [1825]

72. Laennec RTH: De l'auscultation mediate, ou traite du diagnostic des maladies des poumons eet du couer. Paris, J-A Brosson et J-S Chaude, 1819

73. Lassone JMF: An in macilentis liberior quam in obesis circulatio. Paris, Quillau, [1740]

74. Lavoisier A-L: Traite elementaire de chemie, presente dans un order nouveau et d'apres les couvertes modernes. . . . Paris, chez Cuchet, 1789

75. Leisner KC: Dissertatio medica de obesitate exsuperante. Jenae, Typ Gollnerianis, [1683]

76. Locke SCJ: De celeri corporum incremento causa debilitatis in morbis. Lipsiae, Ex Officina Langenhemia, [1760]

77. Lohe AW: Exhibens de morbis adipis humani principia generalia. Duisburg, [1772]

78. Maccary A: Traite sur la polysarcie. Paris, Crochard, [1811]

79. Marcuse H: De obesitate nimia. Berolini, Typ AG Schadii, [1819]

80. Minel C-C: De l'obesite (thesis No. 472, 2.s, v. 26). Strasbourg, G. Silbermann, [1859]

81. Mohr B: Hypertrophie der Hypophysis cerebri und dadurch bedingter Druck auf die Hirngrundflache, insbesondere auf die Sehnerven, das Chiasma derselben und den linkseitigen Hirnschenkel. Wochenschr Ges Heilk 6:565, 1840

82. Mokricki T: Mleko jako srodek przeciwko otylosci. Pam tow Lek Warszaw 69:328, 1873

83. Muller PA: Dissertatio physiologica de pinguedine corporis. Hafniae, Typis Andreae Hartvigi Godiche, [1766]

84. Niemeyer F: Die Behandlung der Korpulenz nach dem sogenannten Bantingsystem: Ein popularwissenschaftliger Vortrag gehalten zu Stuttgart. Berlin, A Hirschwald, [1866]

85. Oswald JH: Obesitatis corporis humani therapia. Tubingae, Litteris Schrammianis, [1775]

86. Person C: Quaestio medica. An parcior obesis, quam macilentis sanguinis missio? Paris, Quillau, [1748]

87. Philbert: Du traitment de l'obesite et de la polysarcie. Paris, [1984]

88. Pohl JC: Dissertationem inauguralem de obesis et voracibus eorumque vitae incommodis ac morbis. Lipsiae, JC Langenhemii, [1734]

89. Polonus SI: Dissertatio medica inauguralis de pinguedine. Harderovici, Typis Everardi Tyhoff, [1797]

90. Precope J: Hippocrates on diet and hygiene. London, "Zeno," 1952

91. Putnam MC: De la graisse neutre et des acides gras, No. 33. Paris, A Parent, [1871]

92. Quabeck KJ: Dissertatio inauguralis medica de insolito corporis augmento frequenti morborum futurorum signo. Halae Magdeb, JC Hendelii, [1752]

93. Quetelet A: Sur l'homme et le developpement de ses facultes, ou essai de physique sociale. Bruxelles, L Hauman & Cie, 1836

94. Rayer PFO: Observations sur les maladies de l'appendice sus-sphenoidal (glande pituitaire) du cerveau. Arch Gen Med 3:350, 1823

95. Redhead J: Dissertatio physiologica-medica, inauguralis, de adipe, quam annuente summo numine. Edinburgh, Balfour et Smellie, [1789]

96. Reichel OF: De malis ex adipe nimio oriundis. Berolini, Typ JF Starchii, [1824]

97. Reussing HCT: Dissertatio inauguralis medica de pinguedine sana et morbosa. Jenae, Ex Officina Fiedleriana, [1791]

98. Riegels ND: De usu glandularum superrenalium

in animalibus nec non de origine adipis. Hafniae, [1790]

99. Riemer JA: De obesitatis causis praecipuis. Halae and Salem, Stanno Hendeliano, [1778]

100. Rigby E: An Essay on the Theory of the Production of Animal Heat, and on Its Application in the Treatment of Cutaneous Eruptions, Inflammations, and Some Other Diseases. London, Joseph Johnson, 1785

101. Robin C: Anatomie et physiologie cellulaires, ou des cellules animales et vegatales du protoplasma et des elements normaux et pathologiques qui en derivent. Paris, Bailliere, 1873

102. Roberts C: A manual of anthropometry or a guide to the physical examination and measurement of the body: Containing a systematic table of measurements, an anthropological chart or register, and instructions for making measurements on a uniform plan. London, J & A Churchill, 1878

103. Rubner M: The laws of energy consumption in nutrition. Markoff A, Sandri-White A (trans): New York, Academic Press, 1982

104. Russel J: A case of polysarka, in which death resulted from deficient arterialisation of the blood. Br Med J 1:220, 1866

105. Sauvages FB: De Nosologie methodique dans laquelle les maladies son rangees par classes suivant le systeme de Sydenham, et l'ordre des botanistes, Vol III, p 277. Paris, Herissant le fils, 1770

106. Schenkio MM (resp): De pinguedinis in animalibut generatione et concretione. In Erastus Th: Philosophi et medici celeberrimi disputationum et epistolarum medicinalium, volumen doctissimum, p 67. Tiguri, Johan Wolphium, 1595

107. Schindler CS: Monstrose Fettsucht. Wien Med Presse 12(16):410, 12(17):436, 1871

108. Schroeder CF: De adipis sani et morbosi causis. Berolini, formis Brueschckianis, [1832]

109. Schroeder PG: Dissertatio inauguralis medica de obesitate vitanda. Rintelii, JG Enax, [1756]

110. Schulz C: Disputatio medica inauguralis de obesitate quam, annuente summo numine. Lugduni Batavorum, Conradum Wishoff, [1752]

111. Schwann T: Mikroscopische Untersuchungen über die Uebereinstimmung in der Struktur un dem Wachsthum der Thiere und Pflanzen. Berlin, Sander, 1839

112. Seifert PDB: Dissertatio physiologico-pathologico de pinguedine. Gryphiswaldiae, IH Eckhardt, [1794]

113. Short T: Discourse on the causes and effects of corpulency together with the method for its prevention and cure, pp vi, 79. London, J Roberts, 1727

114. de la Sone JMF: An in macilentis liberiur quam in obesis circulatio. Paris, [1740]

115. Steube JS: Dissertatio medica de corpulentia nimia. Jenae, Litteris Mullerianus, [1716]

116. Sydenham T: The Works of Thomas Sydenham, M.D. Translated From the Latin Edition of Dr. Greenhill With a Life of the Author by R.G. Latham, 2 vols. London, Sydenham Society, 1848

117. Tralles BL: Dissertatio de obesorum ad morbos mortemque declivitte. Halae Magdeb, Litteris Hilligerianis, [1730]

118. Triller DW: De pinguedine seu succo nutritio superfluo. Halae, Typ C. Henklii, [1718]

119. Trouillart G: Dissertatio physiologico-practica inauguralis de pinguedine, et morbis ex nimia ejus quantitate. Harderovici, Apud Joannem Moojen, [1767]

120. Tweedie J: Hints on temperance and exercise; shewing their advantage in the cure of dyspepsia, rheumatism, polysarcia and certain stages of palsy. London, T Rickaby, 1799

121. Vacher L: De l'obesite et de son traitement. Paris, Savy, [1873]. With Niemeyer: Du Traitement de l'obesite part la methode Banting. Conference, pp 41–67

122. Vaulpre J-M: De obesitate, comodis et noxis. Montepellier, Joannem-Franciscum Picot, [1782]

123. Verdries JM: Dissertatio medica inauguralis de pinguedinis usibus et nocumentis in corpore humano. Giessae Hassorum, JR Vulpius, [1702]

124. Vogel J: Korpulenz ihre Ursachen, Verhutung und Heilung durch einfache diatetische mittel, mit Benutzung der Ernfahrungen von William Banting. Leipzig, L Denicke, 1864

125. Wadd W: Cursory Remarks on Corpulence; Or, Obesity Considered as a Disease, With a Critical Examination of Ancient and Modern Opinions, Relative to Its Causes and Cure, 3rd ed, Containing a Reference to the Most Remarkable Cases That Have Occurred in This Country. London, Callow, 1816

126. Wadd W: Comments on corpulency, lineaments of leanness mems on diet and dietetics. London, Johnn Ebers & Co, 1829

127. Widemann GM: Disputatio medica de corpulentia nimia. Lipsiae, Typ Krugerianus, [1681]

128. Wood T: The case of Mr. Thomas Wood, a miller of Billericay, in the County of Essex, communicated by the same. Med Trans (Coll Phys Lond) 2:259, 1772

129. Wood T: A sequel to the case of Mr. Thomas Wood, of Billericay, in the County of Essex, by the Same. Med Trans (Coll Phys Lond) 3:309, 1785

130. Worthington LS: De l'obesite: Etiologie, therapeutique et hygiene. Paris, E Martinet, 1875

CHAPTER 24

An Approach to the Classification and Evaluation of Obesity

GEORGE A. BRAY

CLINICAL CLASSIFICATION OF THE OBESITIES

The term "obesities" is used to indicate that excess fat deposition is multifactorial. "Obesity" is often used in place of the plural form, but unless a specific type of obesity is being referred to, "obesities" is more appropriate.

Obese individuals can be classified in several ways: according to the anatomical characteristics of the adipose tissue and its distribution, according to the age at onset of obesity, and according to etiological factors.

Anatomical Characteristics of Adipose Tissue

The anatomical classification is based on the number of adipocytes and the regional distribution of fat.

Number of Fat Cells

The number of fat cells can be estimated when there is a measure of total body fat and an estimate of average fat cell size. Because fat cells differ in size from one region to another, a reliable estimate of the total number of fat cells should be based on the average of fat cell sizes from more than one location. The upper limits of normal fat cell number in adults are 40 to 60 $\times$ 10^9 cells. The number of fat cells increases most rapidly during late childhood and puberty but may increase even in adult life. The number of fat cells can increase by three to five times normal when obesity occurs in childhood or adolescence. *Hypercellular obesity* shows varying degrees of enlargement of fat cells. This type of obesity usually begins in early or middle childhood, but may also occur in adult life. An increased total number of fat cells is usually present in individuals who are more than 75% above their desirable weight.[2,3] When the onset of obesity is during adult life or during pregnancy, it is called *hypertrophic obesity* and involves mainly enlargement of adipose tissue cells with lipids. Hypertrophic obesity tends to correlate with an android or truncal fat distribution and is often associated with metabolic disorders such as glucose intolerance, hyperlipidemia, hypertension and coronary artery disease.[4-7]

Fat Distribution

Fat distribution can be estimated by skin folds, by circumferences, or by sophisticated techniques employing ultrasound, computed tomography, or magnetic resonance imaging. One of the most widely used techniques estimates central fat from the ratio of the circumference of the waist or abdomen to the circumference of the hips. The subscapular skin-fold thickness has also been used to estimate central fat.[8,9] A more sophisticated technique uses principal components analysis of skin folds at several sites on the body.[10,11] The principal components analysis groups together those skin folds that are best correlated and gives an estimate of total fat, central fat, and peripheral fat.

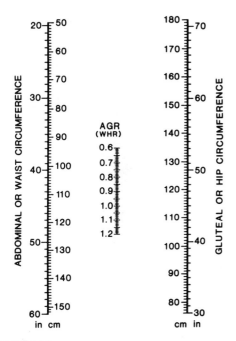

FIGURE 24-1

Nomogram for determining abdominal (waist) to gluteal (hips) ratio. Place a straight edge between the column for waist circumference and the column for hip circumference and read the ratio from the point where this straight edge crosses the AGR or WHR line. The waist or abdominal circumference is the smallest circumference below the rib cage and above the umbilicus, and the hips or gluteal circumference is taken as the largest circumference at the posterior extension of the buttocks. (© George A. Bray, 1987. Reproduced with permission.)

A nomogram for determining the abdominal to gluteal circumference ratios (AGR) or WHR is shown in Figure 24-1. The percentile distribution of these values for men and women in relation to age is shown in Figure 24-2, plotted from data published in the Canadian Fitness Survey.

Age at Onset of Obesity

Obesity can begin at any age. Birth weight of children who will become obese later in childhood has the same frequency distribution as for those who will maintain normal weight in later life.[1,12] The first appearance of obesity is in infancy, when body fat rises rapidly. During the first year of life the size of fat cells increases nearly two-fold, but there is no measurable increase in the number of fat cells.[13,14] Obesity in the first year of life is a relatively poor guide to the likelihood of becoming obese later, however. A second period of childhood obesity is between the ages of 4 to 11 years.[15] When obesity appears in this age group, there can be a progressive deviation of body weight from the upper limits of normal for height age. This may be called progressive obesity.[1] This type of obesity is usually lifelong and is associated with an increase in the number of fat cells. Obesity frequently appears during puberty in both black and white girls.[16] In this type of obesity the onset of menstruation usually occurs at an earlier age.[1]

Childhood-Onset Obesity

Childhood obesity does not necessarily predict obesity in adult life. A recent prospective follow-up over 36 years emphasized the variability in body weight with age.[17] At age 36, 3322 individuals from the cohort of 5362 individuals born in March 1946 were interviewed and subdivided into weight categories, using the body mass index (BMI). It was found that 5.3% of the men and 8.4% of the women were severely overweight (BMI > 30 kg/m^2) and 38.0% of the men and 24.2% of the women were overweight (BMI = 25–29.9 kg/m^2). The correlation between BMI at age 26 and 36 was $r = .64$ for men and $r = .66$ for women. From these studies, the authors draw several important conclusions. First, there is a subgroup of about 25% of individuals who were obese in both childhood and adult life. Second, the remaining 75% of obese 36-year-olds first became obese in adult life; obesity in these subjects could not be reliably predicted from weights before age 20. Those individuals who became obese between ages 11 and 36 often were not the most overweight subjects in childhood. However, only 50% to 60% of men and women in the top decile for weight at age 36 could be correctly predicted at age 26 using all the socio-economic, demographic, and weight data available.

Adult-Onset Obesity

Most obesity develops after the end of puberty. Estimates from several sources have suggested

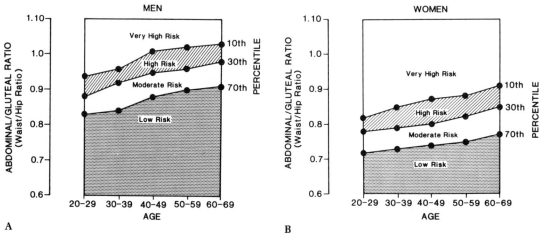

FIGURE 24-2

Percentiles for fat distribution. The percentiles for the ratio of abdominal circumference to gluteal circumference (ratio of waist to hips) are depicted for
men **(A)** and women **(B)** by age groups. The relative risk associated with these
percentiles is indicated, based on the available information. (Plotted from tab-
ular data in the Canadian Standardized Test of Fitness, 3rd ed, 1986. ©
George A. Bray, 1987.)

that less than one third of obese adults were
obese in childhood.[1] The early years of adult life
are important for the development of obesity in
both men and women. For women, the central
event is pregnancy. The woman who becomes
pregnant will be several kilograms heavier two
years after the pregnancy than the woman who
was not pregnant.[18] In addition, there are a few
women for whom pregnancy is a time of major
weight gain, with reports of weights increasing
by more than 50 kg. For fetal outcome, the optimal weight gain for normal weight women is 10
to 12 kg. As the body weight increases, the optimal weight gain to minimize fetal loss declines;
for women who are more than 50 kg above desirable weight, a weight gain of 6 to 8 kg is optimal
for fetal survival.[19] Weight loss during pregnancy
is never desirable.

For many men, the transition from the active
life-style associated with the teenage years to a
more sedentary style of the early adult years is
associated with weight gain. There is clear evidence provided by the National Center for Health
Statistics,[16] the Life Insurance Industry,[20] and
from the induction statistics from the military

that men and women have become progressively
heavier for height during this century.[1] A rise in
body weight continues through adult years until
the sixth decade. From age 54 to 62 years, relative weight remains stable, and then begins to
decline in both sexes. The development of obesity in older years is thus an unusual event suggesting some marked disturbance in energy
balance.

Etiological Factors in Obesity

There are a number of etiologic causes for obesity
(Table 24-1).[1,21] Genetic factors play a role in the
onset of obesity. Endocrine alterations are a second cause for obesity but are rare, even though
obesity influences the function of the endocrine
system.[23] The increase in body fat observed with
human endocrine diseases is usually small. Hyperinsulinism, produced by islet cell tumors or
by injection of excess quantities of insulin, results in increased food intake and increased fat
storage. The magnitude of this effect is small, but
the condition may be associated with larger
weight gains in some cases.

TABLE 24-1

An Etiological Classification of the Obesities

Neuroendocrine obesities

Hypothalamic syndrome
Cushing's syndrome
Hypothyroidism
Polycystic ovary (Stein-Leventhal) syndrome
Pseudohypoparathyroidism
Hypogonadism
Growth hormone deficiency
Insulinoma and hyperinsulinism

Iatrogenic obesities

Drugs (psychotropic; corticosteroids)
Hypothalamic surgery (neuroendocrine)

Obesities due to nutritional imbalance

High-fat, particularly saturated fat, diet
Cafeteria diets

Obesities due to physical inactivity

Enforced (postoperative)
Aging

Genetic (Dysmorphic) Obesities

Autosomal recessive
X-linked
Chromosomal

Genetic Causes of Obesity

Rare Genetic Syndromes. Evidence suggests that genetic factors are of major importance in causing obesity in a group of rare diseases with associated dysmorphic features. Several of these syndromes are compared in Table 24-2. For a more detailed discussion the reader is referred elsewhere.[24]

Genetic Diathesis. Family studies show that obesity runs in families, but they do not critically separate environmental from genetic factors.[1] This can be done through studies of adopted children or twins. Using the Danish adoption registry, Stunkard and his colleagues examined a sample of 800 adoptees.[25] There was no relationship between the BMI of the adoptive parents and their children. The BMI of the biological parents, on the other hand, increased with increasing weight status of the children. These data sug-

gest that inheritance plays an important role in the risk of developing obesity and are consistent with most, but not all, other studies of adopted children.[1,25]

The most definitive evidence for genetic versus environmental factors in obesity comes from the examination of body weight in twins.[1,27,28] Since monozygotic twins have identical genetic material, whereas dizygotic twins have the genetic diversity of brothers or sisters but the environmental closeness of monozygotic twins, evaluation of these groups of twins along with other siblings and more distant relatives should make it possible to identify genetic factors in obesity. Using BMI as the criterion for obesity, Stunkard et al[27] compared 1983 male monozygotic and 2104 male dizygotic twins from the Veterans Administration twin registry. Monozygotic twins had a higher correlation between their body weights than the dizygotic twins, and calculations of the heritability for obesity suggested that nearly two thirds of the variability in BMI was attributable to genetic factors.

Bouchard et al examined the skin-fold thickness and total body fat in various groups of individuals with differing degrees of genetic relationship, including monozygotic and dizygotic twins.[28] In adopted siblings, there is a very low order of correlation. Biological siblings, however, showed a higher correlation, which was highest among the monozygotic twins. Biological siblings had a lower order of correlation for all of the variables than did the dizygotic twins, although both groups have the same genetic variability, implying that there was an environmental influence operative in the dizygotic twins which was absent in their biological siblings. Based on a technique called path analysis these data on the genetic and nongenetic components for body fat and BMI can be partitioned into transmissible and nontransmissible components (Fig. 24-3). Approximately half of the distribution of body fat is transmissible and approximately 25% is genetic.

In summary, both single and polygenic inheritances are involved in the transmission of obesity in man. The best estimates suggest that genetic and environmental factors may be of equal importance in the overall determination of body fat and that genetic factors may be more important

TABLE 24-2

A Comparison of Syndromes of Obesity, Hypogonadism, and Mental Retardation

Feature	Syndrome				
	Prader-Willi	*Bardet-Biedl*	*Ahlstrom*	*Cohen*	*Carpenter*
Inheritance	Sporadic 2/3 have defective Chr 15(q:1,2)	Autosomal recessive	Autosomal recessive	Probably autosomal recessive	Autosomal recessive
Stature	Short	Normal, infrequently short	Normal, infrequently short	Short or tall	Normal
Obesity	Generalized, moderate to severe, onset at 1–3 yr	Generalized, early onset at 1–2 yr	Truncal, early onset at 2–5 yr	Truncal, mid-childhood onset at age 5	Truncal, gluteal
Cranofacies	Narrow bifrontal diameter, almond-shaped eyes, strabismus, V-shaped mouth, high arched palate	Not distinctive	Not distinctive	High nasal bridge, arched palate, open mouth, short philitrum	Acrocephaly, flat nasal bridge, high arched palate
Limbs	Small hands and feet, hypotonia	Polydactyly	No abnormalities	Hypotonia, narrow hands and feet	Polydactyly, syndactyly, genu valgum
Reproductive status	Primary hypogonadism	Primary hypogonadism	Hypogonadism in males but not in females	Normal gonadal function or hypogonadotrophic hypogonadism	Secondary hypogonadism
Other features	Enamel hypoplaria, hyperphagia, temper tantrums, nasal speech			Dysplastic ears, delayed puberty	
Mental retardation	Mild to moderate	Mild	Normal IQ	Mild	Slight

than environmental factors in determining fat distribution.

Neuroendocrine Causes

Hypothalamic Obesity

Hypothalamic obesity is a rare syndrome in humans[29] but can be regularly produced in animals by injury to the ventromedial region of the hypothalamus (VMH).[21] This region is responsible for integrating information about energy stores. When the VMH is damaged, hyperphagia develops and obesity follows. Disturbances in the function of the autonomic nervous system may play an important etiological role in this syndrome.

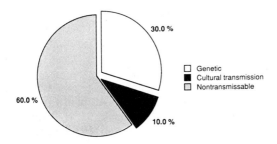

FIGURE 24-3

Genetic factors in obesity. The genetic and nongenetic transmission of fat-free mass and the ratio of subcutaneous fat to fat mass are presented from the analysis in Bouchard.[22] (Reprinted with permission.)

TABLE 24-3

Clinical Features Among 77 Patients with Hypothalamic Obesity Due to Tumors

Feature	No.*	(%)
Headache	50	(65)
Impaired vision	49	(64)
Impaired reproductive function	39	(51)
Diabetes insipidus polyuria or polydipsia	24	(31)
Somnolence	28	(36)
Behavioral changes	15	(19)
Impaired growth	7	(9)
Convulsions	5	(6)

*Number of patients with each symptom

Hypothalamic obesity is produced in human beings by malignancy, surgery, trauma, and inflammatory disease involving the VMH.[29] The clinical features that accompany this syndrome are listed in Table 24-3. These symptoms can be divided into three groups. The first group is related to changes in intracranial pressure and includes headache and diminished vision due to papilledema. Symptoms in the second group are manifestations of endocrine alterations and include impaired reproductive function with amenorrhea or impotence, diabetes insipidus, and thyroid or adrenal insufficiency. Symptoms in the third group are a variety of neurological and physiological derangements, including convulsions, coma, somnolence, and hypothermia or hyperthermia. Treatment of the syndrome requires treating the underlying disease and giving appropriate endocrine support.[74]

Ovarian Disease

The syndrome of polycystic ovaries described by Stein and Leventhal[30] may be a combination of hypothalamic and endocrine obesity. The complex consists of reduced or absent menses and of moderate hirsutism and weight gain, which usually develops in young women shortly after menarche. These women are often infertile. Menstruation and fertility can frequently be restored by wedge resection of the ovary. Studies on these women have failed to clarify the mechanism for the abnormalities in the ovary. Hypersecretion of the adrenal gland, which is often observed in

these patients, is also unexplained and may well be caused by several factors. However, the complex of hyperphagia, hypofunction of the gonads, and hyperfunctioning of the pituitary adrenal system is reminiscent of some of the defects observed in experimental animals with obesity, particularly the yellow obese mouse, in which obesity, mild hyperglycemia, and enlarged adrenal glands develop at or just after puberty.

Hyperinsulinism

Shortly after the discovery of insulin it was noted that its use could lead to increased body weight and body fat. The spontaneous hypersecretion of insulin that occurs in insulinoma can also increase body weight, but the effect is usually small.

Physical Inactivity and Obesity

Physical inactivity plays an important role in the development of obesity. Gross obesity in rats can be produced by severe restriction of activity. In a modern affluent society, energy-sparing devices also reduce energy expenditure and may enhance the tendency to become fat.[1] In one clinical study the onset of obesity was associated with inactivity in 67.5% of the patients. In epidemiological studies the highest frequency of overweight men was found in the groups with sedentary occupations. These observations suggest the importance of shifting patterns of physical activity in the regulatory systems controlling the storage, distribution, and utilization of calories.

Diet and Obesity

The composition of the diet is another etiological factor in obesity. This is particularly prominent in experimental animals but may also play a role in the development of human obesity. When rodents eat a high-fat diet,[31] drink sucrose-containing solutions,[32] or eat a cafeteria type of diet,[33] most strains are unable to regulate energy balance appropriately and ingest more energy than is needed for weight maintenance. The excess energy is accumulated as fat and the animals become obese to variable degrees.

Overfeeding may be of importance in the onset of childhood obesity. Infants fed an artificial formula were significantly heavier than expected from height and weight tables, whereas breast-fed infants showed a less dramatic weight gain.[34] Studies on the weight gain and milk intake of infants during the first 112 days of life showed that bottle-fed infants at the 10th percentile for birth weight were similar in weight to breast-fed infants at all ages up to 112 days. However, infants at the 90th percentile for birth weight who were fed by bottle were heavier and longer at 112 days of age than those who were breast-fed. When bottle-fed infants were divided into two groups, one fed formula that contained 67 kcal/100 ml and another fed formula that provided 133 kcal/100 ml, the infants receiving the more concentrated food drank less than the other group. Of particular interest was the gain in body weight. During the first six weeks the infants receiving the more concentrated formula ingested more calories each day and gained more weight. It is this same period of life that some authors think is predictive of obesity in children at age six. However, other researchers cannot find any relation between the rate of weight gain in children and whether as infants they received early nutrition from a bottle or from the breast.

The relationship of the frequency of eating to the development of human obesity remains an unsettled question. It has been observed clinically that obese individuals frequently eat fewer meals than normal-weight people, but this is a difficult point to document. Direct evidence on the relation of obesity to the frequency of food intake was obtained in a survey of 379 men ages 60 to 64 years.[34] The men who ate one or two meals per day were heavier, had thicker skin folds, had higher levels of cholesterol, and frequently had impaired glucose tolerance when compared with men who ate three or more meals per day. This finding was confirmed in a study of school children: those children who were fed only three meals per day tended to gain more weight than children who ate five to seven meals per day.

The frequency of eating also changes the metabolism of glucose and the concentration of cholesterol. When normal volunteers ate several small meals a day, they had lower concentrations of cholesterol than when the same total intake was consumed in a few large meals.[35] This reduction in cholesterol with frequent ingestion of small meals has been confirmed many times. Glucose tolerance curves are also improved when three or more meals are eaten as compared with one or two large meals. In one laboratory study,[36] six grossly obese patients were fed a 5000-calorie diet for eight weeks. During one four-week period the calories were divided into 20 small meals and during the other four weeks they were eaten as one large meal. The period with one large meal per day was associated with more rapid formation of fat as measured by incorporation of carbon from glucose into fatty acids in adipose tissue.[36] Of the enzymatic changes that were studied, the only one that showed a significant alteration during the rapid food ingestion was the cytoplasmic glycerol-3-phosphate dehydrogenase. This contrasts with the numerous enzymatic changes that have been observed in the adipose tissue of rats trained to eat large meals rather than to nibble. Recent epidemiologic evidence indicates that in middle-aged women there is a positive correlation between fat intake, particularly saturated fat, and rising BMI.[37]

Drugs and Obesity

Several drugs can lead to an increase in body weight (Table 24-4). Glucocorticoids are widely used in treating chronic immunologic disease, and one of the side-effects of the treatment is weight gain, similar to that seen in Cushing's syndrome. Amitriptylline (Elavil) is a tricyclic

TABLE 24-4

Drugs Associated with Weight Gain

Tricyclic antidepressants, particularly amitriptyline
Glucocorticoids
Phenothiazines
Cyproheptadine
Medroxyprogesterone
Lithium

antidepressant that is particularly likely to produce weight gain. Cyproheptadine (Periactin) has been shown to increase food intake in human subjects without an alteration in metabolism. This drug and the phenothiazines are among the major drugs that increase body fat. One study found that on admission to a mental institution, men averaged five pounds less than "desirable" for their height. They gained seven pounds during an average stay of 35 months,[1] and the use of phenothiazines probably played an important role in this weight gain. Although estrogens alone or in birth control pills have been reported to produce weight gain, this is largely the result of fluid retention and probably not the result of increased fat accumulation. Progestins, including medroxyprogesterone, are more likely to increase weight. There is a large body of data about weight gain, increased food intake, and hunger following cessation of cigarette smoking, suggesting that nicotine may reduce food intake.

Social, Economic, and Psychological Factors in the Development of Obesity

Obesity in the United States is more prevalent in the lower socioeconomic groups.[1,16] Using a scale of 12 to divide socioeconomic groups, Goldblatt et al[38] found that among the highest groups (i.e., the most educated and affluent) only 4% were overweight, whereas in the lowest socioeconomic groups 36% were overweight. These effects are most prominent in women. Similar conclusions have been drawn from data reported by the National Center for Health Statistics.[16,39] There was significantly more obesity as assessed by skin-fold thickness in the lower socioeconomic groups. Ethnic differences were also present.[39] Black males were generally less obese than white males. Black women, on the other hand, showed a consistently higher prevalence of obesity at all ages than white women. Both black and white males at lower income levels had a higher prevalence of obesity than black or white males at higher income levels. The effect of income level produced a more complex picture in women. Among older women both black and white, lower income was associated with a lower prevalence of obesity. For younger women, the relationship was not clear-cut. In some age groups obesity was more prevalent in women from lower income groups, but not in all. The importance of social factors can also be seen in children. Overweight children were detected among first graders from the lower socioeconomic groups but there were no overweight children from the highest socioeconomic groups at this age. When overweight did appear, it was less prevalent in children from the higher social classes than in those from the lower classes.

Psychological factors in the development of obesity are widely recognized, but attempts to define a specific personality type for obese individuals has been unsuccessful. Much of the early work on the psychological factors of obesity came from studies of single patients who had undergone intensive psychiatric analysis. Formulations based on these cases were tantalizing and tended to focus on the oral features of obese patients as important in the development of this syndrome. A review of psychological factors in obesity indicates several different approaches to the problem. One of these comes from the extensive studies of Bruch.[40] She identifies two types of obesity. The first is called reactive obesity and results from ingestion of excess food as an emotional reaction to situations in the environment. According to Bruch,[40] this type of abnormality is a reflection of inappropriate responses to the feeding situation during growth and development of the child. The second type of obesity she calls developmental. In these individuals, emotional problems are minimal. From an analysis of profiles on the Minnesota Multiphasic Personality Inventory (MMPI) and the Thematic Apperception Test (TAT), certain features stood out, forming what has been labeled the obese trait. Depression was common but not severe. Ingestion of food had frequently been used to reduce the feelings of emotional deprivation that had been present since early childhood and were historically associated with unstable marriages in the family of many of these patients. Such characteristics as stubbornness, defiance, the need for autonomy, and wariness of entangling relationships, as well as conflicts over exhibitionism, were prominent features in the personality structures of these patients. These characteristics contribute to the traditional reputation of the obese as "difficult" patients.

CLINICAL EVALUATION OF THE OBESE PATIENT

Assessment of the obese patient requires both clinical and laboratory techniques. The information collected can be used to characterize the type of obesity and to provide a basis for making recommendations about treatment. It can also aid in understanding the natural history and prognosis of obesity. This section provides methods for collecting the desired information and a rationale for its collection. The approach is predicated on the assumption that there are many types of obesity with differing degrees of associated risk. Some types of obesity can be isolated and the relative risks identified.

Overweight

Accurate measurement of body fat requires sophisticated techniques. These techniques include measurements of body density, determination of fat or water by isotopic or chemical dilution, and measurement of the naturally occurring isotope of potassium (^{40}K). Although these accurate techniques for measurement of body fat are not yet widely available, the technique of bioelectric impedance analysis (BIA) may remedy that deficiency in the near future and should be considered by anyone wanting accurate estimates of body fat.[41]

Accurate measurement of height and weight is the initial step in the clinical assessment of overweight. Overweight, as distinct from obesity, is defined in relation to tables of desirable weight

that have generally been prepared from insurance company information. Desirable weights are those which are associated with the most favorable mortality experience.

The degree of overweight can be expressed in several ways, but the most useful is the BMI. This index is the body weight (kg) divided by the height (m) squared (Wt/Ht^2) and can be obtained from the nomogram in Figure 24-4. Frankel has recently published another type of nomogram that can also be used for this purpose.[42] BMI correlates with body fat and is relatively unaffected by height. Overweight is defined as a BMI between 25 and 30, and obesity as a BMI above 30. Recommended ranges of BMI for given ages are shown in Table 24-5.

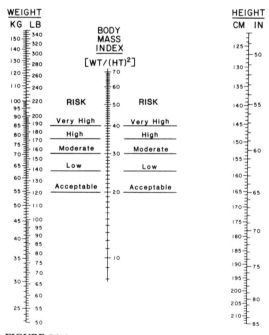

FIGURE 24-4

Nomogram for determing body mass index. To use this nomogram, place a straight edge between the body weight in kilograms or pounds (without clothes) on the left-hand line and the height in centimeters or in inches (without shoes) on the right-hand line. The body mass index is read from the middle of the scale and is in metric units. (© George A. Bray, 1978. Used by permission.)

TABLE 24-5

Desirable Body Mass Index Range in Relation to Age

Age Group (yr)	Body Mass Index* (kg/m²)
19–24	19–24
25–34	20–25
35–44	21–26
45–54	22–27
55–64	23–28
65 +	24–29

From Bray.[1] Reproduced by permission.

*Body mass index can be determined from the nomogram in Figure 24-3.

Regional Fat Distribution

The localized distribution of fat can be evaluated be measuring skin-fold thicknesses on the trunk and extremities or by measuring the circumference of the body in the abdominal region (waist) and the gluteal region (hips), producing the WHR ratio (also known as the android-gynoid ratio). The abdominal or waist circumference is measured with a flexible tape placed in a horizontal plane at the level of the natural waist line or narrowest part of the torso as seen from the anterior view. The gluteal (hip) circumference is measured in the horizontal plane at the level of maximal circumference, including the maximum extension of the buttocks posteriorly. A nomogram is shown in Figure 24-1.

It has long been noted that people differ with respect to the location of fat deposition.[6] In particular, men tend to have more abdominal fat, giving them the android or male pattern of fat distribution. Women tend to have greater amounts of gluteal fat and thus have larger hip circumferences, giving them the so-called gynoid or female pattern of fat distribution. The relative preponderance of one pattern or the other may be expressed by the WHR.

The major complications of obesity, including cardiovascular disease, diabetes mellitus, hypertension, and hyperlipidemia, are associated with increased abdominal fat.[43] Although the abdominal fat distribution pattern is more common in

men, both men and women show increased risk of heart disease with greater abdominal fat. Men may be considered at increased risk if the WHR is greater than 0.90,[44] and women if the WHR is greater than 0.80.[7,45]

Fat Cell Size and Number

The number and size of fat cells can be measured on a sample of adipose tissue obtained by needle biopsy, although this is not a common clinical procedure. A presumptive diagnosis of hypercellular obesity may be made on clinical grounds when the individual is grossly obese with a body weight more than 75% above the desirable weight (body mass approximately 35 kg/m²; see Table 24-2). On the other hand, when the onset of obesity is during adult years or during pregnancy, it often involves mainly enlargement of adipose tissue cells with lipid. This type of obesity is referred to as hypertrophic obesity and tends to correlate with an abdominal or android fat distribution. Obesity with enlarged fat cells is often associated with metabolic disorders such as glucose intolerance, hyperlipidemia, hypertension, and coronary artery disease.[46]

Etiological Factors

The presence of etiological factors should be noted. A family history of obesity and of abdominal fat distribution is an indication of potential genetic factors. Endocrine diseases, though rare, should be excluded. Diet history should be recorded with a focus on intake of fat and saturated fat intake. Levels of physical activity may play an etiological role. Since some drugs are associated with hyperphagia and weight gain (Table 24-5), they should be recorded. A smoking history is obviously relevant. Finally, any associated events need to be identified. All of the following factors have been associated with the occurrence of obesity: pregnancy, changes in physical activity associated with a new occupation, and surgical operations.

Developmental Factors

Obesity can develop at any age and in association with many factors, and these should be noted.

The onset of obesity in the childhood years is usually associated with hypercellularity of fat tissue. In contrast, obesity that occurs during adult life is usually hypertrophic in type. A patient's age is important in determining the risk for obesity. Age 40 is an arbitrary dividing line, as the risk for a given degree of obesity seems to be greater in people less than 40 years old than in those 40 years or older.[47] Duration of obesity and its progression are also important and may influence the associated risks. Longitudinal studies have shown that weight gain confers a greater risk of cardiovascular disease than an unchanging level of obesity.[48] Thus an attempt at determination of the age at onset of obesity is important in the evaluation of an obese patient.

Sex is another variable with great impact on the development of obesity. From puberty onward, women are fatter than men, and women tend to gain more fat during adult life than men. Yet women have a lower risk associated with any degree of extra body fat. This may be explained partly by differences in fat distribution. In one study an extra 20 kg of fat was needed by a woman to produce the same impairment in glucose tolerance as in a man.[7]

Functional Associations

Detection and description of the functional impairments associated with obesity is important both clinically and prognostically. It is well established that obese subjects have an increased frequency of high blood pressure, diabetes mellitus, and coronary artery disease.[48-52] This highlights the importance of delineating the presence of any cardiac risk factors such as hypertension, hyperlipidemia, glucose intolerance, and cigarette smoking. Menstrual disorders, including irregular bleeding and amenorrhea, are common in obese women.[53] Although some studies have shown that obesity is associated with osteoarthritis, others have not, and the role of excess body weight in the etiology of this condition remains controversial.[54,55] Morbid obesity can cause pulmonary compromise with possible sleep apnea. The Pickwickian syndrome of obesity and alveolar hypoventilation, often associated with sleep apnea, may be improved by weight loss.[56] Finally, obese people may experience psychologi-

cal and social problems, and these should be identified. Body image may be severely distorted in people with childhood-onset obesity, and obese people may experience discrimination in the school and workplace. A recent prospective study from Denmark found that obese military recruits attained much lower social class status than lean recruits after an average 12.5 years of follow-up.[57] Therefore it is important to find out about these functional impairments and to measure blood pressure, blood cholesterol and triglyceride levels, and blood glucose. If history warrants, evaluation of the gallbladder by ultrasonography or oral cholecystography and measurement of pulmonary function may be performed.

Algorithm

An algorithm has been developed to organize the appropriate evaluation of the obese patient (see Figure 24-5). It is a flow chart that incorporates most of the important information about obesity. Use of the algorithm is simple and straightforward. Questions begin in the upper left-hand corner and proceed via the appropriate arrows. At each point a positive answer to the question leads to suggestions for workup. For example, once the presence of overweight has been established, the possibility of hypertension is addressed. If hypertension is present, the physician is directed to search for clinical signs of Cushing's syndrome. If these are present, a dexamethasone suppression test is recommended; if they are not, a hypertension workup is suggested. In turn, the algorithm directs the physician to search for clinical clues of hypothyroidism, glucose intolerance, hyperlipidemia, hypoventilation syndrome, CNS lesions, polycystic ovary syndrome, and congestive heart failure. Acanthosis nigricans deserves a brief comment. This is a clinical condition with increased pigmentation in the folds of the neck, along the exterior surface of the distal extremities, and over the knuckles. It may signify increased insulin resistance, which should be evaluated. At each point suggestions for further workup are given when appropriate. Once the workup for etiological and complicating factors is complete, BMI, body fat distribution, and sex and age are noted, and the

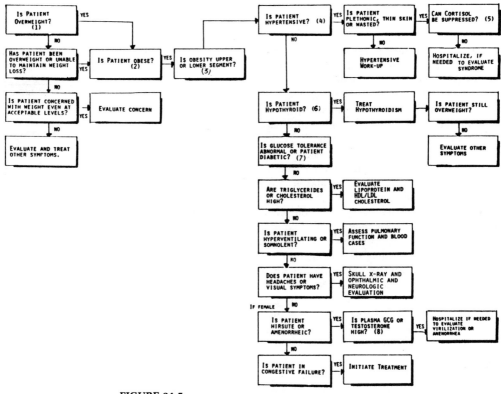

FIGURE 24-5

An algorithm for evaluating the obese individual. (1) Overweight is defined as body mass index above upper limits for age (see Table 24-6). (2) Obesity is defined as a body mass index > 30 kg/m². (3) Upper segment obesity is defined from Figure 24-3 as the top 10th percentile. (4) Blood pressure readings taken with a large cuff that encircles 75% of the arm. (5) Dexamethasone suppression test: Cortisol less than 3 μg/dL (80 nmol/L) at 8:00 A.M., 9 hours after 1 mg of dexamethasone is given orally. (6) Thyroid function:

	T$_4$, Serum thyroxine (corrected) (μg/dl; nmol/L)	TSH, serum thyrotropin (μU/ml = mU/L)
High	12 (154)	7
Normal	5.5–12.0 (71–154)	7
Borderline low	4.0–5.5 (51–71)	7–10
Low	4.0 (51)	10

In the presence of severe illness, a low serum thyroxine level must be interpreted cautiously; it may be a bad prognostic sign but not indicative of hypothyroidism unless TSH is elevated. (7) The diagnosis of diabetes in nonpregnant adults is based on the following: (a) Unequivocal hyperglycemia and classic symptoms of diabetes mellitus; (b) Fasting venous plasma glucose above 140 mg/dl (7.8) mmol/L) on more than one occasion; (c) Fasting plasma glucose below 140 mg/dl (7.8 mmol/L) at some point between 0–2 hours and 2 hours after an oral glucose tolerance test with 75 g glucose (for children, 1.75 g/kg of ideal body weight, not to exceed 75 g).

physician is referred to Figure 24-6 for risk classification.

The algorithm shown in Figure 24-6 is used to determine the degree of risk associated with obesity in individual patients. Those with BMI between 25 and 30 are placed in the low-risk class unless they have android obesity (WHR > 0.95 for males and > 0.80 for females), are less than 40 years old, have medical complications identified in Figure 24-3, or are male. These patients are placed in the moderate-risk class, along with those who have a BMI between 30 and 35. Patients with a BMI between 35 and 40 are also placed in the moderate-risk class unless they have any of the above-mentioned complicating factors, in which case they are placed in the high-risk class along with those whose BMI is greater than 40. Because of increasing complications from obesity, more aggressive therapy should be undertaken at each successively higher risk classification. Based on this assessment of risk, a rational approach to treatment is presented in Table 24-6.

References

1. Bray GA: The Obese Patient: Major Problems in Internal Medicine. Philadelphia, WB Saunders, 1976
2. Hirsch J, Fried SK, Edens NK et al: The fat cell. Med Clin North Am 73:83-96, 1989
3. Björntorp P: Adipose tissue in obesity: Willendorf Lecture. In Hirsch J, Van Itallie JB (eds): Recent

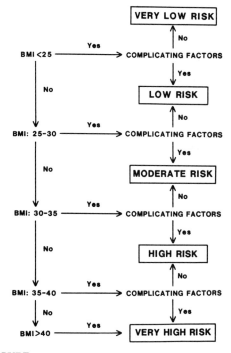

FIGURE 24-6

Risk classification algorithm. The patient is first placed into a category based on body mass index. The presence or absence of complicating factors determines the degree of health risk. Complicating factors include elevated abdominal-gluteal ratio (male, >0.95, female, >0.85), diabetes mellitus, hypertension, hyperlipidemia, male sex, and age less than 40 years. (© George A. Bray, 1987. Used by permission.)

TABLE 24-6

A Classification of Obesity Relating Risk to Choices of Treatment

Risk	Caloric Intake (kcal/d)			Choice of Treatments		
	<200	200–800	>800	Exercise	Drugs	Surgery
Low	NA	3	2	1	NA	NA
Moderate	NA	2	1–2	1	3	NA
High	NA	1	2	3	2	NA
Very high	2	1	1	3	2	1–2

NA, not appropriate; 1, first choice; 2, second choice; 3, third choice.

Advances in Obesity Research V. London, Libbey, 1985

4. Kissebah AH, Vydelingum N, Murray R et al: Relation of body fat distribution to metabolic complications of obesity. J Clin Endocrinol Metab 54:254, 1982

5. Feldman R, Sender AJ, Sieglaub AB: Difference in diabetic and nondiabetic fat distribution patterns by skinfold measurements. Diabetics 18:478, 1969

6. Vague J: The degree of masculine differentiation of obesities: A fact for determining predisposition to diabetes, atherosclerosis, gout and uric calculus disease. Am J Clin Nutr 4:20, 1956

7. Krotkiewski M, Björntorp P, Sjostrom L et al: Impact of obesity on metabolism in men and women. J Clin Invest 72:1150, 1983

8. Stokes J III, Garrison RJ, Kannel WB: The independent contribution of various indices of obesity to the 22-year incidence of coronary heart disease: The Framingham Heart Study. In Vague J, Björntorp P, Vague P (eds): Metabolic Complications of Obesity. Amsterdam, Elsevier Science Publishers, 1985

9. Donahue RP, Abbott RD, Bloom E et al: Lancet 1:820, 1987

10. Mueller WH: The genetics of human fatness. In: Yearbook of Physical Anthropology, vol 2, p 215, 1983

11. Ducimietre P, Richard J, Cambien F: The pattern of subcutaneous fat distribution in middle-aged men and the risk of coronary heart disease: The Paris prospective study. Int J Obes 10:229, 1986

12. Wolff OH: Obesity in childhood: A study of the birth weight, the height and the onset of puberty. Q J Med 24:109, 1955

13. Knittle JL, Timmers K, Ginsberg-Fellner F et al: The growth of adipose tissue in children and adolescents: Cross-sectional and longitudinal studies of adipose cell number and size. J Clin Invest 63:239, 1979

14. Hager A, Sjostrom L, Arvidsson B et al: Body fat and adipose tissue cellularity in infants: A longitudinal study. Metab 26:607, 1977

15. Mossberg HE: Obesity in children: A clinical-prognostical investigation. Acta Paediatr 35:1, 1948

16. Abraham S, Carrol MD, Najjar MF et al: Obese and Overweight Adults in the United States. Vital and Health Statistics, Series 11, No. 230. USDHHS publication (PHS)83-1680. Washington, DC, US Government Printing Office, 1983

17. Braddon FEM, Rodgers B, Wadsworth MEJ et al: Onset of obesity in a 36 year birth cohort study. Br Med J 293:299, 1986

18. McKeown T, Record RG: The influence of reproduction on body weight in women. J Endocrinol 15:393, 1957

19. Naeye RL: Weight gain and the outcome of pregnancy. Am J Obstet Gynecol 135:3, 1979

20. Kannel WB, Gordon T: Physiological and medical concomitants of obesity: The Framingham study. In Bray GA (ed): Obesity in America, pp 125–153. DHEW Publication (NIH)79-249. Washington, DC, US Government Printing Press, 1979

21. Bray GA, York DA: Hypothalamic and genetic obesity in experimental animals: An autonomic and endocrine hypothesis. Physiol Rev 59:719, 1979

22. Bouchard C: Genetic factors in obesity. Med Clin North Am 73:67-81, 1989

23. Glass AR: Endocrine aspects of obesity. Med Clin North Am 73:161-184, 1989

24. Bray GA: Classification and evaluation of the obesities. Med Clin North Am 73:161-184, 1989

25. Stunkard AJ, Sorenson TIA, Hanis C et al: An adoption study of human obesity. N Engl J Med 314:193, 1986

26. Bray GA: Obesity. In King RA, Motulsky A, Rotter J (eds): The Genetic Basis of Common Diseases. New York, Oxford University Press, 1989

27. Stunkard AJ, Foch TT, and Hrubec Z: A twin study of human obesity. JAMA 256:51, 1986

28. Bouchard C, Perusse L, Leblanc C et al: Inheritance of the amount and distribution of human body fat. Int J Obes 12:205, 1988

29. Bray GA: Syndromes of hypothalamic obesity in man. Pediatr Ann 13:525, 1984

30. Goldzieher JW: Polycystic ovarian disease. Fertil Steril 35(4):371, 1981

31. Schemmel R, Mickelson O, Motawi P: Conversion of dietary to body energy in rats as affected by strains, sex and ration. J Nutr 102:1187, 1972

32. Kanarek RB, Hirsch E: Dietary-induced overeating in experimental animals. Fed Proc 36:154, 1977

33. Rothwell NJ, Stock MJ: The development of obesity in animals: The role of dietary factors. Clin Endocrinol Metab 13:437, 1984

34. Fomon SJ, Filer LJ Jr, Thomas LN et al: Relationship between formula concentration and rate of growth of normal infants. J Nutr 98:241, 1969

34a. Fabry P, Fodor J, Hejl Z et al: The frequency of meals: Its relationship to overweight, hypercholesterolemia, and decreased glucose-tolerance. Lancet 2:614, 1964

35. Young CM, Hutter LF, Scanlan SS: Metabolic effects of meal frequency in normal young men. J Am Dietet Assoc 61:391, 1972

36. Bray GA: Lipogenesis in human adipose tissue: Some effects of nibbling and gorging. J Clin Invest 51:537, 1972

37. Romieu I, Willett WC, Stampfer MJ et al: Energy intake and other determinants of relative weight. Am J Clin Nutr 47:406, 1988
38. Wadden TA, Stunkard AJ: Social and psychological consequences of obesity. Ann Intern Med 103:1062, 1985
39. Van Itallie TB: Health implications of overweight and obesity in the United States. The problem of obesity. Ann Intern Med 103(6 pt 2):983, 1985
40. Bruch H: Eating Disorders: Obesity, Anorexia Nervosa and the Person Within. New York, Basic Books, 1973
41. Segal KR, Van Loan M, Fitzgerald PI et al: Lean body mass estimation by bioelectrical impedance analysis: A four-site cross-validation study. Am J Clin Nutr 47:7, 1988
42. Frankel HM: Determination of body mass index (letter). JAMA 255:1292, 1968
43. Haffner SM, Stern MP, Hazuda HP et al: Do upper-body and centralized adiposity measure different aspects of regional body-fat distribution? Relationship to non-insulin-dependent diabetes mellitus, lipids and lipoproteins. Diabetes 36:43, 1987
44. Larsson B, Svardsudd K, Welin L et al: Abdominal adipose tissue distribution, obesity, and risk of cardiovascular disease and death: 13 year follow up of participants in the study of men born in 1913. Br Med J 288:1401, 1984
45. Lapidus L, Bengtsson C, Larsson B et al: Distribution of adipose tissue and risk of cardiovascular disease and death: A 12 year follow up of participants in the population study of women in Gothenburg, Sweden. Br Med J 289:1257, 1984
46. Sjostrom L, Björntorp P: Body composition and adipose tissue cellularity in human obesity. Acta Med Scand 195:201, 1974
47. Drenick EJ, Gurunanjappa SB, Seltzer F et al: Excessive mortality and causes of death in morbidly obese men. JAMA 243:443, 1980
48. Hubert HB, Feinleib M, McNamara PM et al: Obesity as an independent risk factor for cardiovascular disease: A 26-year follow up of participants on the Framingham Heart Study. Circulation 67:968, 1983
49. Rimm AA, Werner LH, Van Yserloo B et al: Relationship of obesity and disease in 73,532 weight-conscious women. Public Health Rep 90:44, 1975
50. Havlik RJ, Hubert HB, Fabsitz RR et al: Weight and hypertension. Ann Intern Med 98:855, 1983
51. Waaler HT: Height, weight and mortality: The Norwegian experience. Acta Med Scand 679:1, 1983
52. National Institutes of Health Consensus Development Panel on the Health Implications of Obesity: Health implications of obesity. Ann Intern Med 103:977, 1985
53. Hartz AJ, Barboriak PN, Wong A et al: The association of obesity with infertility and related menstrual abnormalities in women. Int J Obes 3:57, 1979
54. Engel A: Osteoarthritis and body measurements. Vital Health Stat 11:1–37, 1969
55. Bray GA: Complications of obesity. Ann Intern Med 103:1052, 1985
56. Sharp JT, Barrocas M, Chokroverty S: The cardiorespiratory effects of obesity. Clin Chest Med 1:103, 1980
57. Sonne-Holm S, Sorensen TIA: Prospective study of attainment of social class of severely obese subjects in relation to parental social class, intelligence, and education. Br Med J 292:586, 1986

CHAPTER 25

Characteristics of Obesity

ARTEMIS P. SIMOPOULOS

Obesity is the most common nutritional disorder in the developed world and is assuming significant proportions in the developing world as well.[16] Obesity in the population is associated with increased morbidity and reduced life expectancy. The association of obesity with reduced life expectancy was noted by Hippocrates, who said, "Sudden death is more common in those who are naturally fat than in the lean."[7]

Obesity is a heterogeneous disorder. The development of obesity in humans involves genetic and environmental components that affect endocrine metabolic and regulatory events. However, in the broadest sense, obesity is a disorder of energy balance.

Industrialized societies are characterized by an abundant and palatable food supply and a decrease in physical activity at home, at work, and in transportation as a result of modern technology. Today only 1% of energy used in farm and factory work comes from muscle power, whereas at the beginning of this century 30% of energy in these occupations came from muscle power. Despite several studies on energy expenditure in humans, it is not yet clearly established how much food humans require for weight maintenance. New advances in methods for determining 24-hour energy expenditure in humans using a respiratory chamber indicate the degree of variability of spontaneous physical activity, i.e., fidgeting, to be 100 to 800 kcal·day^{-1} and to be independent of body size.[25] Eighty-one percent of the variance in 24-hour energy expenditure between individuals is explained by differences in fat-free mass. Differences in the thermic effect of food and in spontaneous physical activity contribute significantly to differences in 24-hour energy expenditure in humans.

Roberts et al[26] prospectively studied infants born to overweight mothers. Total energy expenditure at three months of age was 20.7% lower in infants who subsequently became overweight than in those that did not. These findings suggest a genetic susceptibility and that the most appropriate way to prevent this group of infants from becoming obese is by increasing their energy expenditure.

Ravussin and co-workers[24] measured the 24-hour energy expenditure of southwestern American Indians. Results were adjusted for body composition, age, and sex. During a two-year follow-up period, those who had a low adjusted 24-hour energy expenditure had four times the risk of gaining 7.5 kg as compared with persons with a high 24-hour energy expenditure. The resting metabolic rate was also of predictive value. Those with a low metabolic rate were more likely to gain more than 10 kg during a four-year period. This and other studies in white subjects indicate that a low rate of energy expenditure is associated with an increased risk for weight gain. Further, a low rate of energy expenditure and a low metabolic rate contribute to the aggregation of obesity in families.

There is great variation in the rates of energy expenditure among individuals that cannot be accounted for by differences in body size, age, or sex, indicating genetic differences. Therefore, universal recommendations for daily energy needs based on body size, age, and sex will be inappropriate for many individuals. An increase in physical activity along with a decrease in dietary fat are needed to control obesity in sedentary affluent societies.

Overnutrition and a sedentary life-style have led to large numbers in the population becoming overweight or obese, defined as a body mass index (BMI) over 25 and over 30 kg/m^2, respectively. The average American has a BMI of 26.6 kg/m^2, which is equivalent to a body weight 20% above desirable body weight based on the 1959 Metropolitan Life Insurance Company's tables of desirable weight.[19]

In overweight persons the relative risk of diabetes, hypertension, and hypercholesterolemia is greater at ages 20 to 45 years than at ages 47 to 75 years. In addition, body fat distribution appears to influence the risk of disease. For example women with central obesity (android pattern) are more prone to diabetes than women whose obesity is in the lower abdominal and femoral area (gynoid pattern).[4]

The definition of obesity and reference standards used for determining the prevalence of obesity are covered elsewhere in this book. This chapter considers the evidence relating the concept of desirable body weight to health and longevity, the importance of the duration of obesity as it relates to morbidity and mortality, and the relationship of childhood obesity to adult obesity. Data obtained from surveys in the United States on food intake and body weight are presented. The discussion emphasizes the need to consider the effects of obesity on morbidity and mortality in estimating the prevalence of obesity in the population. The data are applicable only to the population under consideration and cannot be extrapolated to other populations.

THE CONCEPT OF DESIRABLE BODY WEIGHT AND ITS HEALTH IMPLICATIONS

Desirable body weight refers to the weight associated with the lowest mortality as determined by the Metropolitan Life Insurance Company in 1959.[19] The table presented a range in weight for a given height based on small, medium, and large frame size.

Garrison et al[12] carried out a study that validated the concept and the range of weight that is desirable in terms of mortality. Further analysis of the data demonstrated rather conclusively that "cigarette smoking is a potential confounder of the relationship between obesity and mortality." Garrison et al examined the data from the Framingham Heart Study using Metropolitan relative weight (MRW), which expresses body weight as a percentage of the desirable weight, as the standard. Minimum mortality occurred at the MRW range 100% to 109%, or a BMI of 21.66 to 23.83 (Tables 25-1 and 25-2). In the Framingham Heart Study, 80% of men whose body weight was under the desirable weight (MRW = 100; BMI = 21.66) were smokers. This analysis suggests that in the U.S. population, the U-shaped or J-shaped univariate relationship between relative weight and mortality results from the mortality risks associated with cigarette smoking. The most common cause of death in these men was cancer. At an MRW of 120% (20% above desirable weight; BMI = 26.0) there was an increased mortality from cardiovascular disease, indicating that even slight increases above desirable weight have dire consequences. Furthermore, the data indicate that the risks associated with excess weight are not confined to subjects who are substantially obese, as was previously thought; in fact, a progressive increase in morbidity and mortality is apparent with even a small increase in weight above the upper limits of the range of the 1959 Metropolitan Life Insurance Company figures.

Hubert et al performed a longitudinal study of coronary risk factors in young adults in the offspring of the Framingham Heart Study.[13] This study showed that

The characteristic most strongly related to lipoprotein and blood pressure changes in both sexes was a change in Quetelet Index (QI). A unit change in QI (<3 kgs), for example, resulted in a change in low density lipoprotein cholesterol of about 3mg/dl in young men. In addition to weight gain, increased cigarette use, decreased alcohol intake and, in women, going on "the pill" were associated with detrimental changes in lipoprotein profiles during follow-up. These findings are among the first to offer prospective evidence which suggests that habits developed during young adulthood, particularly those which influence relative weight, have a substantial effect on lipoprotein cholesterol profiles in both men and women.

TABLE 25-1

Desirable Weight Ranges for Men Ages 25 and Over*

Height (ft, in)	Weight range (lb)	Weight† MRW = 100	Weight‡ MRW = 110	Weight MRW = 120
5'1"	105–134	117	129	140
5'2"	108–137	120	132	144
5'3"	111–141	123	135	148
5'4"	114–145	126	139	151
5'5"	117–149	129	142	155
5'6"	121–154	133	146	160
5'7"	125–159	138	152	166
5'8"	129–163	142	156	170
5'9"	133–167	146	161	175
5'10"	137–172	150	165	180
5'11"	141–177	155	170	186
6'0"	145–182	159	175	191
6'1"	149–187	164	180	197
6'2"	153–192	169	186	203
6'3"	157–197	174	191	209
BMI (all heights):		21.66	23.83	26.00

*From Simopoulos AP: Obesity and body weight standards. Annu Rev Public Health 7:481, 1986. Reproduced by permission. Data are adapted from the 1959 Metropolitan Desirable Weight Table. Weight is given in pounds, without clothing; height without shoes.

†Midpoint of medium frame range, used to compute MRW: MRW = (Actual weight)/(Midpoint of medium frame range) × 100.

‡In the U.S. adult population over 40 years of age, 80% of men and 70% of women have weights that exceed MRW = 110 and, consequently, are at increased risk for cardiovascular disease. The average weight of the adult U.S. population is above MRW = 120; an individual with a weight over MRW = 120 is "obese."

A number of studies have shown a positive relationship between weight gain and increase in blood pressure. In 1974 Ashley and Kamel[3] reported that an increase in MRW from 100% to 110% would predict a rise in systolic blood pressure of 7 mm Hg. Similarly, in 1983 Garrison et al[12] stated, "Adiposity stands out as a major controllable contributor to hypertension. Changes in body fat over 8 years were mirrored by changes in both systolic and diastolic pressure. Markedly obese women in their fourth decade were 7 times more likely to develop hypertension than lean women the same age."

At the workshop on Body Weight, Health, and Longevity, held in January 1982, a number of investigators presented data showing that a weight loss of 10 pounds in overweight individuals improves results on the glucose tolerance test, decreases the insulin requirements of the diabetic,

and significantly lowers the blood pressure of the hypertensive person.[28,29] In 1986 the importance of weight loss in lowering blood pressure was underscored in a study on the effects of weight reduction on left ventricular mass, reported by McMahon et al.[18] These investigators compared the effects of weight loss with those of metoprolol and placebo on blood pressure in young, overweight patients with hypertension. An average weight loss of 8.3 kg was associated with an average drop in blood pressure of 14/13 mm Hg, compared with a decrease of 12/8 mm Hg in the metoprolol group and 9/4 mm Hg in the placebo group.

In 1972 Westlund and Nicholaysen,[34] in a prospective study, showed that in moderate obesity, the risk of diabetes was increased about 10-fold. In subjects whose weights exceeded the standard by 45% or less, the risk increased about 10-fold,

TABLE 25-2

Desirable Weight Ranges for Women Ages 25 and Over*

Height (ft, in)	Weight range (lb)	Weight† MRW = 100	Weight‡ MRW = 110	Weight MRW = 120
4'9"	90–118	100	110	120
4'10"	92–121	103	113	124
4'11"	95–124	106	117	127
5'0"	98–127	109	120	131
5'1"	101–130	112	124	134
5'2"	104–134	116	128	139
5'3"	107–138	120	132	144
5'4"	110–142	124	136	149
5'5"	114–146	128	141	154
5'6"	118–150	132	145	158
5'7"	122–154	136	150	163
5'8"	126–159	140	154	168
5'9"	130–164	144	158	173
5'10"	134–169	148	163	177
BMI (all heights):		21.32	23.47	25.58

*From Simopoulos AP: Obesity and body weight standards. Annu Rev Public Health 7:481, 1986. Reproduced by permission. Data are adapted from the 1959 Metropolitan Desirable Weight Table. Weight is measured in pounds, without clothing; height without shoes.
Note: For women between the ages of 18–25 years, subtract one pound for each year under 25.
†Midpoint of medium frame range—used to compute MRW: MRW = (Actual weight)/(Midpoint of medium frame range) × 100.
‡In the U.S. adult population over 40 years of age, 80% of men and 70% of women have weights that exceed MRW = 110 and, consequently, are at increased risk for cardiovascular disease. The average weight of the adult U.S. population is above MRW = 120; an individual with a weight over MRW = 120 is "obese."

whereas in those whose weights exceeded the standard by more than 45%, the risk increased about 30-fold.

Although it is known that weight loss decreases blood pressure, improves the glucose tolerance of the diabetic, and decreases insulin requirements, it is not known how weight (gain or loss) exerts its effects on human metabolism.

Most of the work on the relationship of obesity to reduced life expectancy has focused on cardiovascular disease. Studies on the relationship of obesity to cancer have not been carried out to the same extent. Certainly no long-term prospective studies comparable in scope to the Framingham Heart Study, which has a 30-year follow-up period, have examined the relationship between obesity and cancer, although the American Cancer Society conducted a long-term prospective

study during the period 1959–1972.[17] Data from the American Cancer Society study show that the risk of cancer increases with weight. Cancer mortality was elevated among those 40% or more overweight. Cancer of the colon and rectum were the principal causes of excess cancer mortality in men, whereas cancer of the gallbladder and biliary passages, breast, cervix, endometrium, uterus, and ovary were the major causes of excess mortality in women.

The mechanism(s) by which overweight increases cancer risk is not known. But a number of studies have implicated estrogen in the development of cancers of the reproductive system such as cancers of the endometrium, cervix, breast, and ovaries.[27] These cancers account for half of all cancers in women. Adipose tissue is the major source of estrogen formation in postmenopausal women, and it is derived by aromatization of androstenedione into estrone.[9] Obese individuals have increased levels of prolactin, androgens, and cortisol, in addition to estrogens.

In order to define precisely the health implications of obesity, and thus begin to formulate the concepts of the relationship among body weight, health, and longevity, and to clarify the terminology used (ideal, desirable, acceptable, MRW) a workshop was held in 1982, sponsored by the National Institutes of Health Nutrition Coordinating Committee and the Centers for Disease Control. The workshop reviewed data developed by the life insurance industry, recent analyses of data from the Framingham Heart Study (5209 subjects),[12,14] and other studies of a variety of populations that examined the relationship of body weight to morbidity and mortality, such as the Build Study 1979[6] and new data from the 1959–1972 American Cancer Society study (755,502 subjects).[17]

Because the risk for most common chronic diseases is multifactorial and overweight most likely contributes in varying degrees to morbidity in different societies, the participants emphasized that the conclusions of the workshop were applicable to the U.S. population only. The data from the Framingham Heart Study were decisive in the conclusions reached by the participants, since the population studied in the Framingham Heart Study does not differ from the U.S. population in terms of morbidity and mortality statistics. Therefore the data from the Framingham Heart Study are considered representative of the U.S. population as a whole.

The workshop participants concluded that in the United States, below-average weights tend to be associated with the greatest longevity, if such weights are not associated with concurrent illness or a history of significant medical impairment. Overweight persons tend to die at a younger age than average-weight persons, particularly those who are overweight at younger ages. The effect of obesity on mortality is delayed, so that it is not seen in short-term studies; the extensive data from the Build Study 1979 show this delayed effect particularly well. The recent analyses of the Framingham Heart Study data emphasize that obesity is a significant independent predictor of cardiovascular disease, with smoking

having a separate effect. Furthermore, the concept of desirable weight developed by the Metropolitan Life Insurance Company in 1959 has been validated by the analyses of the Framingham Heart Study. In addition to the age range of the population studied, the interpretation of studies on body weight, morbidity, and mortality must also carefully consider the definition of obesity used, any pre-existing illnesses, the length of follow-up, and any confounding risk factors. A summary of the workshop's proceedings, including descriptions and critiques of the studies, has been published elsewhere.[28,29]

DURATION OF OBESITY AND ITS RELATION TO MORBIDITY AND MORTALITY

Keys et al[15] considered obesity to be associated with coronary heart disease through its impact on cardiovascular risk factors such as hyperlipidemia and hypertension. Their conclusions were based on short-term studies.

However, the findings from the Manitoba Study[23] and the Provident Mutual Life Study,[5] along with recent analyses of the Framingham Heart Study,[14] suggest that the duration of obesity has an important bearing on the putative relationship of body weight and longevity. Thus the effect of obesity on mortality does not emerge in short-term studies. When the data from the Framingham Heart Study were analyzed using a longer time interval between measurement of obesity and subsequent outcome, it became evident that obesity was a significant independent predictor for cardiovascular disease, independent of age, cholesterol, systolic blood pressure, cigarette smoking, left ventrical hypertrophy, and glucose intolerance. Further, the data indicated that when overweight develops early in adult life and is sustained, the effect on life expectancy is different from the effect caused by obesity that develops in middle age.

PREVALENCE OF OBESITY

Body Weight

In developed countries a trend toward increasing height and weight has been evident as early as the seventh year of life. Similar trends have been noted in adults for several centuries. Millar and Stephens compared the prevalence of overweight and obesity in Britain, Canada, and the United States (Figs. 25-1 and 25-2).[20] All three countries had carried out surveys of their noninstitutionalized populations during the period of 1976–1981, with essentially similar techniques for measuring height and weight. Millar and Stephens defined overweight as a BMI of 25.1 to 30, and obesity as a BMI exceeding 30. Figure 25-1 shows that American men are more likely to be overweight or obese, especially at younger ages. The proportion of excessively heavy men plateaus at about age 50 in all three countries, possibly indicative of a survivor phenomenon. Figure 25-2 shows that the United States has the highest proportion of excessively heavy women at all ages except in the 20- to 24-year-old age range. The difference is greater at ages 45 to 54 years.

There is no evidence that the proportion of overweight or obese women reaches a plateau by age 64, unlike the situation in men.

Estimations on the prevalence of obesity depend not only on the body weight reference standard but also on the type of data used. Data collected by the National Center for Health Statistics (NCHS) are normative data based on a national probability sample. These data are cross-sectional and were generated by three surveys: the National Health Examination Survey (NHES), 1960–1962; and the National Health and Nutrition Examination Surveys (NHANES) I, 1971–1974, and II, 1976–1980.[1,32,33]

A comparison of mean heights and weights of adults ages 18 to 74 years in the three surveys shows that both men and women were taller and heavier in the periods of 1971 to 1974 and 1976 to 1980 than they were in 1960 to 1962 (Table 25-3). The average weight for height of the popu-

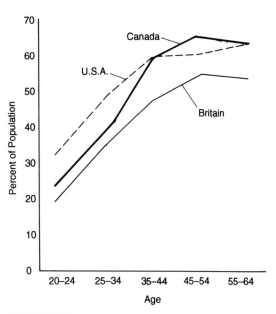

FIGURE 25-1

Prevalence of excessive body weight (BMI) > 25) in men ages 20–64 in Britain (1980), Canada (1981), and the United States (1976–1980). (From Millar WJ, Stephens T: The prevalence of overweight and obesity in Britain, Canada, and the United States. Am J Public Health 77:38, 1987. Reproduced by permission.)

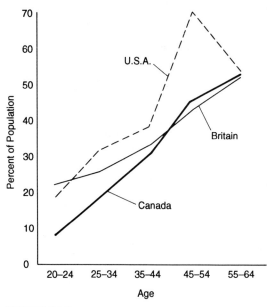

FIGURE 25-2

Prevalence of excessive body weight (BMI > 25) in women ages 20–64 in Britain (1980), Canada (1981), and the United States (1976–1980). (From Millar WJ, Stephens T: The prevalence of overweight and obesity in Britain, Canada, and the United States. Am J Public Health 77:38, 1987. Reproduced by permission.)

TABLE 25-3

Mean Weights and Heights by Age and Sex in Three Populations*

Age Group (yr)	Men			Women		
	NHES	NHANES I	NHANES II	NHES	NHANES I	NHANES II
Weight, kg						
18–24	71.7	74.8	73.9	57.6	59.9	60.8
25–34	76.7	79.8	78.5	60.8	63.5	64.4
35–44	77.1	80.7	80.7	64.4	67.1	67.1
45–54	77.1	79.4	80.7	65.8	67.6	68.0
55–64	74.4	77.6	78.9	68.0	67.6	68.0
65–74	71.7	74.4	74.8	65.3	66.2	66.7
18–74	75.3	78.0	78.0	63.5	64.9	65.3
Height, m						
18–24	1.74	1.77	1.77	1.62	1.63	1.63
25–34	1.76	1.77	1.77	1.62	1.63	1.63
35–44	1.74	1.76	1.76	1.61	1.63	1.63
45–54	1.73	1.75	1.75	1.60	1.62	1.61
55–64	1.71	1.73	1.74	1.58	1.60	1.60
65–74	1.70	1.71	1.71	1.56	1.58	1.58
18–74	1.73	1.75	1.76	1.60	1.62	1.62

Data from Simopoulos AP, Van Itallie TB: Body weight, health, and longevity. Ann Intern Med 100:285, 1984.

*The three populations are those surveyed by the National Health Examination Survey (NHES), 1960–1962, and the National Health and Nutrition Examination Surveys (NHANES) I, 1971–1974, and II, 1976–1980. Two pounds were deducted from NHES data to allow for weight of clothing; total weight of all clothing for NHANES I and II ranged from 0.1 to 0.3 kg and was not deducted from weights in table. Height was measured without shoes.

lation is continuing to increase, which suggests that the population is continuing to become more overweight. Further analyses of these data indicate that the greatest increase in weight occurred in the heavier white and black females, those above the median. Data from these national surveys show that women below the poverty line have a much higher prevalence of overweight between ages 25 and 55 years than women above the poverty line. In multivariate analyses, race and poverty status are independent predictors of overweight in women.

The three NCHS surveys have defined overweight as a condition in which BMI is at or above the 85th percentile of BMI for men (28 kg/m^2) and women ($34 \text{ kg/m}^{1.5}$), ages 20 to 29 years, who were studied between 1976 and 1980.[31] Severe overweight is defined as a BMI (32 kg/m^2 for men and $42 \text{ kg/m}^{1.5}$ for women) at or above the 95th percentile of the same 20- to 29-year-old refer-

ence group. By the NHANES BMI criteria, 32.6 million adult Americans are overweight and 11.5 million are severely overweight. The rationale underlying the use of the 20- to 29-year-old reference population is that young adults are relatively lean, and the increase in body weight that usually occurs as men and women age is due almost entirely to fat accumulation. It is well known, however, that the U.S. population at ages 20 to 29 years is not necessarily lean; therefore, any calculation based on this rationale underestimates the prevalence of obesity. Further, the criteria (85th or 95th percentile) are defined statistically; they are not derived from the morbidity or mortality experience of the survey population. The use of 1.5 instead of 2 as a factor in the calculation of BMI for women underestimates further the prevalence of obesity in women.

Thus, if instead of using normative data generated by cross-sectional surveys, we calculate the prevalence of obesity on the basis of the work of Garrison et al[12] and Hubert et al[14] from long-term prospective studies using criteria that relate obesity to morbidity and mortality from cardiovascular disease, 80% of men and 70% of women over 40 years of age in the Framingham Heart Study are above the desirable weight range (MRW > 110%; kg/m^2 > 24.4) and are at increased risk for cardiovascular disease.[28]

At present we do not have standards for children and adolescents that are based either on morbidity statistics or on data that define obesity as an antecedent to adult disease. Therefore, for these populations, U.S. investigators are using statistical definitions based on normative data.

A large NCHS survey based on a national sample of characteristics of the growth of children in the United States has produced data that led to the development of tables and charts. The children studied represented a cross section of ethnic and socioeconomic groups; as a result, genetic, ethnic, and socioeconomic differences are all part of the final data. For this reason, they are used as reference standards, rather than body weight standards, for the evaluation of growth and development of children in the United States. The charts depict the course of normal growth. Although there is evidence that ethnic differences depend mostly on differences in the prevalence of malnutrition and infectious diseases in various parts of the world, there can be no universal standard.

Food Intake

Not only is the U.S. population getting heavier, but the average energy intake has increased. The most recent survey on food intake was performed by the U.S. Department of Agriculture on 1503 women, 19 to 50 years old, and 548 of their children, one to five years old, in the 48 coterminous states as part of the continuing Survey of Food Intake by Individuals.[22] The data were collected from 1 April 1985 to June 1985, using a one-day recall in the personal interview. These data were compared with data collected in a comparable manner for individuals of the same ages in the Nationwide Food Consumption Survey 1977–78, spring quarter (April through June). Tables 25-4 and 25-5 show a decrease in the mean intake

TABLE 25-4

Mean Intakes of Meat, Poultry, and Fish per Individual in 1977 and 1985, All Income Levels

Age (yr)	Mean Intake (g·day^{-1})	
	1977	1985
Children		
1–3	99	98
4–5	128	114
All	112	104
Women		
19–34	184	179
35–50	188	185
All	186	181

U.S. Department of Agriculture, Nutrition Monitoring Service, NFCS, CSFII Report No. 85-1, 1985. Data collected and compiled by the USDA/NHIS Nationwide Food Consumption Survey. Data collected in the spring of 1977 and 1985.

of meat, poultry and fish by both children and women in 1985 in comparison with 1977, regardless of income, but an increase in total calories over the same time period. Thus, overall energy intake has increased in the past eight years. No data are available on energy expenditure.

THE RELATIONSHIP OF CHILDHOOD OBESITY TO ADULT OBESITY

Obesity in the adult may be preceded by obesity during childhood, but only a few studies of this association[2,8,21] have been reported because reliable longitudinal data from childhood to adulthood are difficult to obtain. Stark et al[30] analyzed data reported in the longitudinal study of obesity in the National Survey of Health and Development in England. They found a positive correlation between relative weight at any two ages covered by the study, which means that the risk of being overweight as an adult is greater for overweight children and adolescents than for those of average or below-average weight. The clinical impression—that most severely overweight children (relative weight >140%) are still overweight in adolescence—was confirmed, but the study

TABLE 25-5

Mean Food Energy Intake per Individual in 1977 and 1985; All Income Levels

Age (yr)	Mean Intake (kcal·day^{-1})	
	1977	1985
Children		
1–3	1210	1372
4–5	1486	1564
All	1335	1446
Women		
19–34	1617	1707
35–50	1514	1602
All	1573	1661

U.S. Department of Agriculture, Nutrition Monitoring Service, NFCS, CSFII Report No. 85-1, 1985. Data collected and compiled by the USDA/NHIS Nationwide Food Consumption Survey. Data collected in the spring of 1977 and 1985.

showed that not all overweight children and adolescents grew into overweight adults. The survey procedure did not allow assessment of the extent to which treatment of severe overweight might have influenced the natural history.

In the United States, Abraham and Nordsieck[2] found that 74% of 11- to 13-year-old overweight boys and 72% of overweight girls in the same age bracket were still overweight as adults, whereas in Stark's study, 40% of the overweight 11-year-old children and 50% of the overweight 14-year-old children were still overweight at 26 years of age. Because of differences in sampling methods and in methods used for assessing overweight, it is difficult to compare the results of these two studies. Stark et al concluded,

> The risk of being overweight in adulthood was related to the degree of overweight in childhood and was about four in ten for overweight 7-year-olds. Analysis of the data in the reverse direction showed that 7% and 13% respectively of the 25-year-old overweight men and women had been overweight at the age of 7. These results suggest that there is no optimal age during childhood for the prediction of overweight in adult life and that excessive weight gain may begin at any time. Overweight children are more likely to remain overweight than their contemporaries of normal weight are to become overweight.[17]

Dietz et al[10] analyzed trends in the prevalence of childhood and adolescent obesity in the United States, using data collected from the NHES Cycles II and III and the NHANES I and II studies in 6- to 11-year-old children and 12- to 17-year-old adolescents. Over the 10- to 15-year periods encompassed by these surveys, obesity and superobesity increased by 54% and 98%, respectively, in 6- to 11-year-olds. In both groups, the increases in prevalence were greater in blacks than in whites. These data indicate that obesity is epidemic in the pediatric population and emphasize the need for more effective therapy and prevention.

Garn and La Velle[11] studied 383 infants and preschool children through early adulthood. Their data show that obese children are more likely to become obese adults. In this study 26% of initially obese preschool children were still obese two decades later, whereas 15% would be expected by chance alone. These investigators used additional data from siblings, parents, and grandparents of the subjects which enabled them to investigate fatness change and fatness continuity in family-line context. The authors state, "At a speculative but probabilistic level, the obese preschool child in a nonobese family may not warrant intervention, especially if reared by a temporary surrogate or day-care sitter. However, an obese child in an obese, weight-gaining family merits far more concern. The family context predicts the future course of obesity, and the family must be fully involved if intervention is to succeed."[11]

The familial aggregation of obesity, diabetes mellitus, coronary artery disease and high blood pressure confers on the offspring of parents (or grandparents) with these conditions an increased risk of developing these same conditions. Particular care, therefore, should be taken to ensure that young adults in these families remain within the range of weights shown in Tables 25-1 and 25-2 and do not gain weight in adult life. It is also true that a substantial proportion of the population without these familial disorders remains at risk of becoming overweight and developing these conditions.

Acknowledgment: This work was supported in part by the Howard Heinz Endowment.

References

1. Abraham S, Johnson CL, Najjar MF: Weight and Height of Adults 18–74 Years of Age, United States, 1971–1974. Vital and Health Statistics, Series 11, No. 211. DHEW publication (PHS) 79-1659. Hyattsville, Md, National Center for Health Statistics, 1979

2. Abraham S, Nordsieck M: Relationship of excess weight in children and adults. Public Health Rep 75:263, 1960

3. Ashley FW Jr, Kamel WB: Relationship of weight change to changes in atherogenic traits: The Framingham Study. J Chronic Dis 27:103, 1974

4. Björntorp P: Classification of obese patients and complications related to the distribution of surplus fat. Am J Clin 45(suppl):1120, 1987

5. Blair BF, Haines LW: Mortality experience according to build at the higher durations. Soc Actuaries Trans 18:35, 1966

6. Build Study 1979. Chicago, Society of Actuaries and Association of Life Insurance Medical Directors, 1979

7. Chadwick J, Mann WN: Medical Works of Hippocrates, p 154. Oxford, England, Blackwell Scientific Publishers, 1950

8. Charney E, Goodman HC, McBride M: Childhood antecedents of adult obesity: Do chubby infants become obese adults? N Engl J Med 295:6, 1976

9. Cleland WH, Mendelson CR, Simpson ER: Effects of aging and obesity on aromatase activity of human adipose tissue. J Clin Endocrinol Metab 60:174, 1985

10. Dietz WH, Gortmaker SL, Sobol AM et al: Trends in the prevalence of childhood and adolescent obesity in the United States (abstr). Pediatr Res 19:527, 1985

11. Garn SM, La Velle M: Two-decade follow-up of fatness in early childhood. Am J Dis Child 139:181, 1985

12. Garrison RJ, Feinleib M, Castelli WP et al: Cigarette smoking as a confounder of the relationship between relative weight and long-term mortality: The Framingham Heart Study. JAMA 249:2199, 1983

13. Hubert HB, Castelli WP, Garrison RJ: Longitudinal study of coronary heart disease risk factors in young adults: The Framingham offspring study. Am J Epidemiol 118:443, 1983

14. Hubert HB, Feinleib M, McNamara PM et al: Obesity as an independent risk factor for cardiovascular disease: A 26-year follow-up of participants in the Framingham Heart Study. Circulation 67:968, 1983

15. Keys A, Aravanis C, Blackburn H et al: Coronary heart disease: Overweight and obesity as risk factors. Ann Intern Med 77:15, 1972

16. Lara-Pantin E: Obesity in developing countries. In Berry E, Blondheim SH, Eliahou HE et al (eds): Recent Advances in Obesity Research. V, pp 5–8. London, John Libbey & Co., 1987

17. Lew EA, Garfinkel L: Variations in mortality by weight among 750,000 men and women. J Chronic Dis 32:563, 1979

18. MacMahon SW, Wilcken DEL, Macdonald GJ: The effects of weight reduction on left ventricular mass: A randomized controlled trial in young, overweight hypertensive patients. N Engl J Med 314:334, 1986

19. Metropolitan Life Insurance Company: New weight standards for men and women. Stat Bull 40:1, 1959

20. Millar WJ, Stephens T: The prevalence of overweight and obesity in Britain, Canada, and the United States. Am J Public Health 77:38, 1987

21. Mullins AG: The prognosis in juvenile obesity. Arch Dis Child 33:307, 1958

22. Nationwide Food Consumption Survey: Continuing Survey of Food Intakes by Individuals. Women 19–50 Years and Their Children 1–5 Years, 1 Day, 1985. CSFII Report No. 85–1. U.S. Department of Agriculture, Nutrition Monitoring Service, NFCS, 1985

23. Rabkin SW, Mathewson FAL, Hsu PH: Relation of body weight to development of ischemic heart disease in a cohort of young North American men after a 25-year observation period. Am J Cardiol 39:452, 1977

24. Ravussin E, Lillioja S, Knowler WC et al: Reduced rate of energy expenditure as a risk factor for body-weight gain. N Engl J Med 318:461, 1988

25. Ravussin E, Lillioja S, Anderson TE et al: Determinants of 24-hour energy expenditure in man: Methods and results using a respiratory chamber. J Clin Invest 78:1568, 1986

26. Roberts SB, Savage J, Coward WA et al: Energy expenditure and intake in infants born to lean and overweight mothers. N Engl J Med 318:461, 1988

27. Simopoulos AP: Fat intake, obesity, and cancer of the breast and endometrium. Med Oncol Tumor Pharmacother 2:125, 1985

28. Simopoulos AP, VanItallie TB: Body weight, health, and longevity. Ann Intern Med 100:285, 1984

29. Body Weight, Health, and Longevity: Conclusions and Recommendations of the Workshop. Nutr Rev 43(2):61, 1985

30. Stark O, Atkins E, Wolff OH et al: Longitudinal study of obesity in the National Survey of Health and Development. Br Med J 283:13, 1981
31. VanItallie TB, Abraham S: Some hazards of obesity and its treatment. In Hirsch J, VanItallie TB (eds): Recent Advances of Obesity Research. IV. Proceedings of the IV International Congress on Obesity. London, John Libbey & Co., 1985
32. Weight by Height and Age of Adults, United States, 1960–1962. Vital and Health Statistics, Series 11, No. 14. Hyattsville, Md, National Center for Health Statistics, 1966
33. Plan and Operation of the National Health and Nutrition Examination Survey, 1976–1980. Vital and Health Statistics, Series 1, No. 15. DHHS publication (PHS) 81-1317. Hyattsville, Md, National Center for Health Statistics, 1981
34. Westlund K, Nicholaysen R: Ten-year mortality and morbidity related to serum cholesterol: A follow-up of 3,751 men aged 40–49. Scand J Clin Lab 127(suppl):1, 1972

CHAPTER 26

The Biocultural Evolution of Obesity:
An Anthropological View

PETER J. BROWN

Throughout most of human history, obesity was never a common health problem, nor was it a realistic possibility for most people. Despite the qualitative adequacy of their diet, most prehistoric and primitive societies were regularly subjected to food shortages. Scarcity has been a powerful agent of natural selection in human biocultural evolution. Both genes and cultural traits that may have been adaptive in the context of past food scarcities today contribute to maladaptive adult obesity in affluent societies.

Anthropology seeks to understand human biology and behavior in the context of two distinct but interacting processes of evolution. Biologic evolution involves changes in the frequency of particular genes over time, primarily because of the action of natural selection on individuals. Cultural evolution involves historical changes in the configurations of cultural systems, that is, the learned patterns of behavior and belief characteristic of social groups, and includes the striking and rapid transformation of human life-styles from small food-foraging societies to large and economically complex states in less than 5,000 years.[1] Humans are distinctive in the emphasis on adaptation through this dual system of inheritance. Natural selection has operated on both genes and culture to generally increase the frequency of traits that enhance an individual's ability to survive and reproduce. In this view, the health and illness of a population can be conceived as measures of biocultural adaptation to a particular ecological setting.[2]

This paper attempts to place human obesity in the context of biologic and cultural evolution. It first examines how the predisposition to obesity so evident in modern societies may have been determined during our species' long evolutionary history as hunter-gatherers. It also explores how variations in the distribution and prevalence of obesity may be related to aspects of culture including economic systems (i.e., modernization), beliefs (i.e., the social symbolism of fatness and cultural ideals of body type), and social organization (i.e., class and ethnicity).

The sources of anthropological data relevant to this evolutionary exploration come from archaeology and ethnography. In both cases the available information is incomplete and its interpretation must be, at times, speculative. Archaeology examines the direct remains of human activities in the 1.6 million years since the appearance of our genus. During most of human history, the exclusive life-style was one of hunting and gathering. Ethnography is the description of the social organization and cultural traditions of other peoples. Cross-cultural ethnographic data can amplify our understanding of prehistoric periods because technologically simple societies provide ethnographic analogies, particularly in terms of economic production and diet. Such analogies can be useful in reconstructing the evolution of obesity. It is imperative, however, that any theory about the origins of obesity help explain what is known about the social distribution of fatness and obesity.

THE SOCIAL DISTRIBUTION OF OBESITY

Humans are among the fattest of all mammals,[3] but this does not imply that obesity is a "natural" condition. In contrast to other mammals, whose fat deposits primarily function as insulation from cold, in humans much (but not all) fat serves as an energy reserve. The nonrandom social distribution of adiposity within and between human populations may provide a key to understanding obesity. Three facts about this social distribution are particularly cogent for an evolutionary reconstruction: (1) a gender difference in the total percent and site distribution of body fat, as well as the prevalence of obesity; (2) a relationship between economic modernization and obesity; and (3) the concentration of obesity in certain ethnic groups or social classes.

Sexual Dimorphism

Differences in fat deposition are an important aspect of sexual dimorphism in *Homo sapiens*.[4] Humans are only mildly dimorphic in morphological variables like stature: males are only 5% to 9% taller than females.[5,6] Dimorphism in soft tissue involves both total body fatness and the site of distribution (e.g., upper versus lower body fat); the clinical importance of this distinction is now widely recognized.[7] On average for young adults in an affluent society, adipose tissue accounts for approximately 15% of body weight in males and about 27% in females.[4]

Fatness, particularly peripheral body fat, is the most dimorphic of the morphological variables (Fig. 26-1). Adult men are larger than women in stature (+8%) and total body mass (+20%), while women have more subcutaneous fat as measured in skin-fold thicknesses in 16 of 17 measurement sites (the exception is the suprailiac site). In general, adult limb fatness is much more dimorphic than trunk fatness, and this pattern appears to be universal.[4,8] It is important that peripheral body fat does not have the same close association with chronic diseases (e.g., non-insulin-dependent diabetes mellitus, hypertension) as trunkal fatness does.[7,9] Thus the sexual dimorphism in fat deposition may be unrelated to the negative health consequences of obesity. The developmental course of this dimorphism occurs at the time of reproductive maturation.[10]

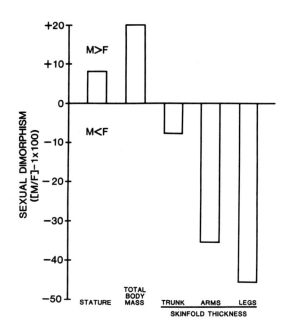

FIGURE 26-1

Sexual dimorphism in stature, body mass, and fat measures among white Americans aged 20 to 70 in Tecumseh, Michigan. Sexual dimorphism was calculated by comparing male versus female means; positive values refer to greater male measures. (Data from Bailey.[64]) Skin-fold thicknesses are the means of four sites (trunk) or five sites (arms and legs); the mean dimorphism in all 17 fat measures is −19%.

Sex differences are also seen in the prevalence of obesity. Despite methodological differences in criteria of obesity, data from the 14 populations shown in Figure 26-2 show that in all of the surveys, females had a higher prevalence of obesity than males. Two points about this figure should be noted: first, it is possible that higher female prevalences are an artifact of sex-specific case definitions for obesity,[11] and second, male-female differences in obesity prevalence vary with age.[12]

Obesity and Modernization

The social distribution of obesity varies between societies depending on their degree of economic

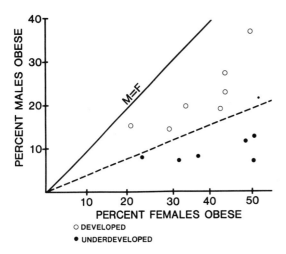

FIGURE 26-2

Gender differences in prevalences of obesity in 14 populations by general economic development. Operational definitions of obesity differ between studies. See Brown and Konner[8] for descriptions of the populations. *Solid line* demarcates equal male-female obesity rates. *Dashed line* indicates an apparent division in the proportion of gender difference in obesity between developed and underdeveloped countries.

modernization. It is significant that anthropometric studies of traditional hunting and gathering populations report no obesity. In contrast, numerous studies of traditional societies undergoing the process of economic modernization (or Westernization) demonstrate rapid increases in the prevalence of obesity.[13-17] Trowell and Burkitt, whose recent volume contains 15 case studies of epidemiological change in modernizing societies, conclude that obesity is the first of these "diseases of civilization" to appear.[18]

Figure 26-2 also suggests that variations in the male-female ratio of obesity prevalence is also related to economic modernization. That is, in less economically modernized populations there is much more female than male obesity, but in more affluent societies the ratio is more nearly equivalent. The reason for this pattern is not completely understood.

Social class (socioeconomic status) can be a powerful predictor of the prevalence of obesity in both modernizing and affluent societies, although the direction of the association varies

with the type of society. It has long been recognized that in heterogeneous and affluent societies like that in the United States, there is a strong inverse correlation between social class and obesity for females.[19,20] In a comprehensive review of the literature, Sobal and Stunkard[21] have demonstrated that in non-Western or developing countries there is a strong and consistent positive association of social class and obesity for men, women, and children; correspondingly, modernizing societies show an inverse correlation between class and protein-calorie malnutrition.[22]

Cultural changes in diet and activity patterns form the link between modernization and obesity. The seemingly invariable pattern of diet modernization includes decreased fiber intake and increased consumption of fat and sugar. The quick shift from "primitive" to high-fat, high-sugar diets with the advent of affluence may be rooted in our evolutionary past.

Obesity and Ethnicity

The idea that particular genotypes predispose individuals to obesity and its related diseases is quite old[23] and is supported by a convincing body of recent research using adoption and twin data[24,25] or focusing on particular obesity-prone populations like the Pima Indians.[26,27] The fact that certain ethnic groups have high rates of obesity is complicated by the entanglement of the effects of genetic heredity and learned culture (environment). It is possible that the role of genetic inheritance is more pronounced in study populations with relatively little cultural heterogeneity (like Denmark or among the Pima). Nevertheless, it is important to recognize that marriage patterns that emphasize ethnic or social class endogamy (for which marriage partner correlations are extremely high[28]) or "assortative mating" by body type may concentrate the genetic predispositions in particular subpopulations.

High prevalences of genetically induced obesity found in certain (non-Athapascan) Amerindian populations may reflect natural selection in particular prehistoric contexts. Wendorf argues that Paleoindian groups who first migrated through the ice-free corridor of Beringa around

12,000 B.C. were ecologically limited to subsisting on large fauna for food and were therefore subjected to strong selective pressure for the "thrifty genotype" that leads to obesity.[29] Later migrations faced more moderate ecological pressures. Similarly, the southwestern United States (home of groups like the Pima) was in the prehistoric past the frequent site of food shortages. Archaeological tree-ring analysis indicates that between 600 and 1249 A.D., rainfall was inadequate every other year and a period of "severe stress" (more than two successive years of total crop failure) occurred at least once every 25 years.[30] The impressive agricultural societies of the prehistoric Southwest had expanded during uncharacteristically good weather and could not be maintained when patterns of lower rainfall resumed.

FOOD SCARCITY AND CULTURAL EVOLUTION

Food shortages have been so common in human history that they could be considered a virtually inevitable fact of life in the past. This fact has shaped the process of cultural evolution from food-foraging group to agrarian state.[31] A cross-cultural ethnographic survey of 118 contemporary nonindustrial societies (with hunting-gathering, pastoral, horticultural, and agricultural economies) found some form of food shortages for all of the societies in the sample.[32] Shortages occur annually or even more frequently for roughly half of the societies, and the shortage is "severe" (i.e., resulting in deaths from starvation) in 29%. Seasonal availability of food results in an annual cycle of weight loss and weight gain in both food-foraging and food-producing societies. Seasonal weight loss is two to three times more severe among African agriculturalists than hunter-gatherers.[33,34]

The hunting-gathering life-style, represented by only a handful of societies today, has been the subject of intensive anthropological research. In general, food foragers live in small, seminomadic bands; experience slow population growth; enjoy high-quality diets; maintain high levels of physical fitness; suffer from periodic food shortages; and are generally healthier than many contemporary Third World populations relying on agriculture. Without romanticizing these societies, the medical evidence is so persuasive that Eaton, Shostak, and Konner have suggested a "paleolithic prescription" of diet and exercise in the view that the current epidemics of chronic diseases are a result of discordance between our ancient genes and modern life-style.[35]

Approximately 12,000 years ago, some human groups shifted from a food-foraging economy to one of food production. This economic transformation allowed population growth and the evolution of complex societies and civilization. Archaeological data suggest that the new agricultural economy was something that people were effectively forced to adopt because of ecological pressures from population growth and food scarcities, or from military coercion.[36] The archaeological record clearly shows that agriculture was associated with osteologic evidence of nutritional stress, poor health, and diminished stature.[37] The beginning of agriculture is also linked to the emergence of social stratification, which had numerous advantages for the ruling class, particularly that of guaranteeing access to food during periods of relative food scarcity.

Humans have also evolved other cultural mechanisms to minimize the effects of food shortages, including (1) economic diversification, (2) storage of foods, (3) knowledge of possible "famine foods," (4) conversion of surplus food into durable valuables to be exchanged for food in emergencies, and (5) cultivation of strong social relations with individuals in other regions.[38] Food shortages are unfortunately not limited to the past. Even in the United States, arguably the richest nation in human history, an estimated 20 million people are hungry.[39]

THE PROBLEM OF PALEOLITHIC VENUS FIGURINES

Given the lack of obesity in contemporary hunter-gatherers and the archaeological evidence of the frequency of food shortages in the past, the Venus figurines of the Upper Paleolithic period are difficult to explain. The best-known of these figurines, like the Venus of Willendorf (Fig. 26-3), are obese (and possibly pregnant). The statuettes most often analyzed by art historians (Fig. 26-4) have a number of recurrent traits: simple treatment of the head, small arms folded over

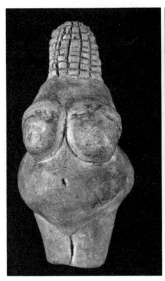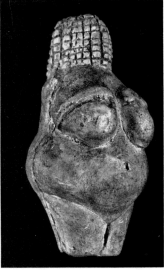

FIGURE 26-3

"Venus" of Willendorf, found in 1908 in Willendorf, Austria; 10.5 cm tall.

the breasts or pointed toward the belly, low breasts extending below the waist, and minuscule or nonexistent feet.[40] Many statuettes have extended buttocks, which may represent steatopygia.[41] The actual archaeological record, however, shows considerably more variation in statuette somatotype. Analysis of 188 extant figurines shows that they depict women from a wide age range, including a large percentage (23%) of thin figurines of prereproductive girls.[42] Using a much smaller sample of figurines (85, overrepresenting mature individuals) Pontius has diagnosed 75% as showing some obesity, and of those, 85% with marked gluteal obesity.[43]

These cultural artifacts are found in sites of a specific archaeological context. In the prehistoric time frame, they are limited to a narrow period, the Gravettian period (27,000 to 19,000 B.C.), which corresponds to the coldest part of the last global glaciation. There is no continuation of the style after the Gravettian. In geographic location, the statuettes have been discovered in Europe from northern Italy to Siberia; they have not been found in Spain.

There is a huge body of literature offering interpretations of these small statues, including treatment of their symbolic functions as mother goddesses, fertility objects, pornography, social alliances, or markers of female power.[44] Irrespec-

tive of their possible symbolic functions, it is not known (and seldom asked) whether the figurines represent actual paleolithic people, and if so, how they could have become obese. Ritenbaugh, pointing out that the very realistic Willendorf figure is characterized by the orthopedic knee abnormalities of the superobese, believes that the figure represents an actual woman.[45]

During the maximum cold period of the Gravettian, the economy of these hunter-gatherer groups in Europe was devoted almost exclusively to cooperative reindeer and mammoth hunting, an economic strategy that also involved the storage of food and the use of permanent settlements; the pattern no longer exists among contemporary hunter-gatherers. This extinct megafauna "specialist" economy produced impressive permanent shelters made of mammoth bones on the central Russian plain.[46] Venus figurines have only been found in the archaeological context of cooperative large mammal hunting; Spain, where no figurines have been found, lacked large herd animals during the Gravettian. It is possible that the people who manufactured the Venus figurines also followed a "specialist" hunting life-style, characterized by an unpredictable but occasionally calorie-rich diet. If certain politically important women were responsible for the food provisions at the permanent shelter,

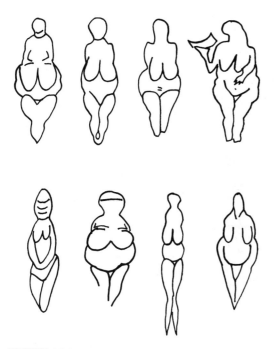

FIGURE 26-4

Outlines of "Venus" figurines from Europe during the Gravettian period showing similarities of design. *Top row, left to right:* Lespugue, Kostienki, Dolni Vestonice, Laussel. *Bottom row:* Parabita, Gagrino I, Gagrino II, Grimaldi. (After Leroi-Gourham, cited in Rice.[42])

then obesity was a possibility. Similarly, lower-body fat deposits may have been a marker of beauty and prestige.

The Social Meaning of Obesity: Cross-Cultural Comparisons

Fatness is symbolically linked to psychological dimensions such as self-worth and sexuality in many societies of the world, including our own, but the nature of that symbolic association is not constant. In mainstream U.S. culture, obesity is socially stigmatized.[47] Most cultures of the world, in contrast, view fatness as a welcome sign of health and prosperity. Given the rarity of obesity in unacculturated preindustrial societies, it is not surprising that many groups have no ethnomedical definition of or concern with obe-

sity. This is the case for food-foragers like the !Kung San, to whom thin people are to be pitied since "thinness" (zham) is viewed as a symptom of starvation.[48]

It may be large body size rather than obesity *per se* that in agricultural societies becomes an admired symbol of health, prestige, prosperity, or maternity. The agricultural Tiv of Nigeria, for example, distinguish between a very positive category "too big" (kehe) and an unpleasant condition "to grow fat" (ahon).[49] The first is a compliment because it is a sign of prosperity (also referring to seasonal weight gain of the dry season); the second term is a rare and undesirable condition.

Even in the industrialized United States, there is ethnic variation in definitions of obesity. Some Mexican-Americans have coined a new term, *gordura mala* ("bad fatness"), because the original term *gordura* continues to have positive cultural connotations.[50] In any case, the definition of obesity is ultimately linked to cultural conceptions of normality, beauty, and health.

Cross-Cultural Variation in Ideal Body Type

Culturally defined standards of beauty may have been a factor in the sexual selection for phenotypes predisposed to obesity. In a classic example, Malcom described the custom of "fattening huts" for elite Efik pubescent girls in traditional Nigeria.[51] A girl spent up to two years in seclusion and at the end of this rite of passage possessed symbols of womanhood and marriagability—a three-tiered hairstyle, clitoridectomy, and fatness. This fatness was a primary criterion of beauty as defined by the elites, who alone had the economic resources to participate in this custom. Similarly, fatter brides (as well as early maturing brides) demand higher bridewealth payments among the Kipsigis of Kenya.[52]

Among the Havasupai of the American Southwest, if a girl at puberty is thin, a fat woman "stands" (places her foot) on the girl's back so that she will become attractively plump. In this society, fat legs, and to a lesser extent fat arms, are considered essential to beauty.[53] Among the Amhara of the Horn of Africa, thin hips are called "dog hips" in a typical insult.[54]

TABLE 26-1

Cross-Cultural Standards of Female Beauty: Ideal Body Characteristics

Characteristic	No. of Societies	% of Category
Overall body		
Extreme obesity	0	0
Plumpness/moderate fat	31	81
Thin/abhorrence of fat	7	19
Breasts		
Large or long	9	50
Small/abhorrence of large	9	50
Hips and legs		
Large or fat	9	90
Slender	1	10
Stature		
Tall	3	30
Moderate	6	60
Small	1	10

A cross-cultural survey of definitions of female ideal body type based on data from the Human Relation Area Files (a cross-indexed compilation of ethnographic information on over 300 of the most thoroughly studied societies) is summarized in Table 26-1. Although these data are weak because of the small number and possibly nonrepresentative nature of the cases,[4] some preliminary generalizations are still possible. Cultural standards of beauty are based on the normal characteristics of the dominant group of a society, and do not refer to physical extremes. No society on record has an ideal of extreme obesity. On the other hand, the desirability of "plumpness" or being "filled out" is found in 81% of the societies. This standard, which probably includes the clinical categories of overweight and mild obesity, apparently refers to the desirability of subcutaneous fat deposits, particularly on the hips and legs. Although there is cross-cultural variation in standards of beauty, this variation falls within a certain range. American ideals of thinness occur in a setting where it is easy to become fat, and preference for plumpness occurs

in settings where it is easy to remain lean. In context, both standards require the investment of individual effort and economic resources; furthermore, each in its context involves a display of wealth. Cultural beliefs about attractive body shape in mainstream American culture place pressure on females to lose weight and are involved in the etiology of anorexia and bulimia.

The Symbolic Meaning of Fatness

Fatness may be a symbol of maternity and nurturance. In traditional societies where women attain status only through motherhood, this symbolic association increases the cultural acceptability of obesity.[55] A fat woman, symbolically, is well taken care of, and she in turn takes good care of her children. Fellahin Arabs in Egypt describe the proper woman as fat because she has more room to bear the child, lactates abundantly, and gives warmth to her children.[56]

The ethnographic record concerning body preferences in males is extremely weak, yet preliminary research suggests a universal expressed preference for a muscular physique and for tall or moderately tall stature.[4] In general, human societies admire large body size as an attribute of attractiveness in men because it symbolizes health, economic success, political power, and social status. "Big Men," political leaders in tribal New Guinea, are described by their constituents in terms of their size and physical well-being: they are men "whose skin swells with 'grease' [or fat] underneath."[57] Large body size may in fact be an index of differential access to food resources. This is seen in chiefdomships, as in ancient Polynesia, where hereditary political leaders sit at the hub of a redistribution system in which chiefly families are assured a portion of each family's harvest. The spiritual power (*mana*) and noble breeding of a Polynesian chief is expected to be seen in his large physical size.

Cultural variation in the meaning of fatness is also found among ethnic groups in the United States. Massara's ethnographic study of the cultural meanings of weight in a Puerto Rican community in Philadelphia[58] documents the positive associations and lack of social stigma of obesity. In addition, quantitative evidence[59] suggests that there are significant differences in ideal body preferences between this ethnic community and mainstream American culture. Positive evaluations of fatness may also occur in lower-class black Americans[60] and Mexican-Americans.[17] These ethnic groups, however, are quite heterogeneous; upwardly mobile ethnics more closely resemble mainstream American culture in attitudes about obesity and ideal body shape.

THE BIOCULTURAL EVOLUTION OF OBESITY

Anthropological information about the frequency of past food shortages, the social distribution of obesity, and the cultural meanings of fatness, when taken together, suggest a biocultural hypothesis of the evolution of obesity. Both genetic and cultural predispositions to obesity may be products of the same evolutionary pressures, involving two related processes: first, genetic traits that cause fatness were selected because they improved the chance of survival in the face of food scarcities, particularly for pregnant and nursing women; second, fatness may have been socially selected because it is a cultural symbol of social prestige and an index of general health.

Since food shortages were ubiquitous for humans under natural conditions, selection favored individuals who could effectively store calories in times of surplus. For most societies, such fat stores would be called on at least every two to three years. Malnutrition from food shortages has a synergistic effect on infectious disease mortality, and decreases birth weights and rates of child growth as well.[61] Females with greater energy reserves in fat would have a selective advantage over their lean counterparts in withstanding the stress of food shortage, not only for themselves but for their fetuses or nursing children. Humans have evolved to "save up" food energy for inevitable food shortages through the synthesis and storage of fat. Females, whose reproductive fitness depends on their ability to withstand the nutritional demands of pregnancy and lactation, appear to have been selected for more slow-releasing peripheral body fat.[62] In addition, a minimal level of female fatness will increase lifetime reproductive success because of its association with regular cycling as well as earlier menarche.[63]

In this evolutionary context the usual range of human metabolic variation must have produced many individuals with a predisposition to become obese; yet they would, in all likelihood, never have had the opportunity to do so. Furthermore, in this context there could be little or no natural selection against such a tendency. Selection could not provide for the eventuality of continuous surplus because it had simply never existed.

SUMMARY

The epidemic of obesity in modern affluent societies has its evolutionary roots in human biologic and cultural traits that had adaptive value in the context of food shortages. Such shortages, particularly disadvantageous to women in their reproductive years, favored individuals who could efficiently store fat during times of food surplus. Not surprisingly, the majority of the world's cultures had or have ideals of feminine beauty that include plumpness. This evolutionary explanation is consistent with the basic facts about the social and epidemiologic distribution of obesity. Under Western conditions of abundance, our biologic tendency to regulate body weight at levels above our ideal cannot be easily controlled, even with a reversal of the widespread cultural ideal of plumpness.

References

1. Wenke RJ: Patterns in Prehistory. New York, Oxford University Press, 1980
2. Brown PJ, Inhorn MC: Disease, ecology and human behavior. In Johnson TM, Sargent CF (eds): Medical Anthropology: Handbook of Theory and Methods. Westport, Conn, Greenwood, 1990
3. Pitts GC, Bullard TR: Some interspecific aspects of body composition in mammals. In: Body Composition in Animals and Man, p 45. Publication No. 1598. Washington, DC, National Academy of Science, 1968
4. Pond CM: Morphological aspects and the ecological and mechanical consequences of fat deposition in wild vertebrates. Annu Rev Ecol Syst 9:519, 1978
5. Stini WA: Malnutrition, body size and proportion. Ecol Food Nutr 1:125, 1978

6. Gaulin S, Boster J: Cross-cultural differences in sexual dimorphism. Ethol Sociobiol 6:219, 1985

7. Kissebah AH, Freedman, DS, Peiris AN: Health risks of obesity. Med Clin North Am 73:11, 1989

8. Brown PJ, Konner M: An anthropological perspective on obesity. Ann NY Acad Sci 499:29, 1987

9. Björntorp P: The associations between obesity, adipose tissue distribution and disease. Acta Med Scand Suppl 723:121, 1987

10. Tanner JM: Growth at Adolescence. Oxford, Blackwell Scientific Publishing, 1962

11. Ritenbaugh C: Obesity as a culture-bound syndrome. Cult Med Psychiatry 6:347, 1982

12. VanItallie TB: Health implications of overweight and obesity in the United States. Ann Intern Med 103:983, 1985

13. Page LB, Damon A, Moellering RC: Antecedents of cardiovascular disease in six Solomon Islands societies. Circulation 49:1132, 1974

14. Zimmet P: Epidemiology of diabetes and its macrovascular manifestations in Pacific populations: The medical effects of social progress. Diabetes Care 2:144, 1979

15. West K: Diabetes in American Indians. In: Advances in Metabolic Disorders. New York, Academic Press, 1978

16. Christakis G: The prevalence of adult obesity. In Bray G (ed): Obesity in perspective, p 209. Fogarty International Center Series on Preventive Medicine, no. 2, 1973

17. Phillips M, Kubisch D: Lifestyle diseases of Aborigines. Med J Aust 143:218, 1985

18. Trowell HC, Burkitt DP: Western Diseases: Their Emergence and Prevention. Cambridge, Mass, Harvard University Press, 1981

19. Goldblatt PB, Moore ME, Stunkard AJ: Social factors in obesity. JAMA 192:1039, 1965

20. Burnight RG, Marden PG: Social correlates of weight in an aging population. Milbank Mem Fund Q 45:75, 1967

21. Sobal J, Stunkard AJ: Socioeconomic status and obesity: A review of the literature. Psychol Bull 105:260, 1989

22. Arteaga P, Dos Santos JE, Dutra de Oliveira JE: Obesity among schoolchildren of different socioeconomic levels in a developing country. Int J Obes 6:291, 1982

23. Neel J: Diabetes mellitus: A "thrifty" genotype rendered detrimental by "progress"? Am J Hum Genet 14:353, 1962

24. Stunkard AJ, Foch TT, Zdenek H: A twin study of human obesity. JAMA 256:51, 1986

25. Stunkard AJ, Sorenson TIAC, Hanis TW et al: An adoption study of obesity. N Engl J Med 314:193, 1986

26. Knowler WC, Pettitt DJ, Savage PJ et al: Diabetes incidence in Pima Indians: Contribution of obesity and parental diabetes. Am J Epidemiol 113:144, 1981

27. Ravussin E, Lillioja S, Knowler WC et al: Reduced rate of energy expenditure as a risk factor for body-weight gain. N Engl J Med 318:467, 1988

28. Carlson EA: Human Genetics. Lexington, Mass, DC Heath, 1984

29. Wendorf M: Diabetes, the ice free corridor, and paleoindian settlement in North America. Am J Phys Anthropol 79:503, 1989

30. Minnis PE: Social Adaptation to Food Stress: A Prehistoric Southwestern Example. Chicago, University of Chicago Press, 1985

31. Johnson AW, Earle T: The Evolution of Human Societies. Palo Alto, Stanford University Press, 1987

32. Whiting MG: A cross-cultural nutrition survey. Doctoral thesis, Harvard School of Public Health, Cambridge, Mass, 1958

33. Wilmsen E: Seasonal effects of dietary intake in the Kalahari San. Fed Proc 37:65, 1978

34. Hunter JM: Seasonal hunger in a part of the West African savanna: A survey of body weights in Nangodi, north-east Ghana. Trans Inst Br Geogr 41:167, 1967

35. Eaton SB, Shostak M, Konner M: The Paleolithic Prescription. New York, Harper & Row, 1988

36. Wenke RJ: Patterns in Prehistory. New York, Oxford University Press, 1980

37. Cohen MN, Armelagos GJ (eds): Paleopathology at the Origins of Agriculture. New York, Academic Press, 1984

38. Colson E: In good years and bad: Food strategies of self-reliant societies. J Anthropol Res 35:18, 1979

39. Physician Task Force on Hunger in America: Hunger in America: The Growing Epidemic. Boston, Mass, Harvard University School of Public Health, 1985

40. Leroi-Gourham A: The Art of Prehistoric Man in Western Europe. London, Thames & Hudson, 1968

41. Gomez-Tabanera JM: Les statuettes féminines paléolithiques dites "Vénus." Asturias, Love-Gijon, 1978

42. Rice P: Prehistoric Venuses: Symbols of motherhood or womanhood. J Anthropol Res 37:402, 1981

43. Pontius AA: Obesity types in Stone Age art. Ann NY Acad Sci 499:331, 1987

44. Gamble C: Interaction and alliance in palaeolithic society. Man 17:92, 1982

45. Ritenbaugh C: New approaches to old problems: Interactions of culture and nutrition. In Chrisman NJ, Maretzki TN (eds): Clinically Applied Anthropology. Dordrecht, Holland, D Reidel, 1982

46. Gladkih MI, Kornietz NL, Soffer O: Mammoth-

bone dwellings on the Russian plain. Sci Am 251:164, 1984

47. Cahnman WJ: The stigma of obesity. Sociol Q 9:294, 1968

48. Lee RB: The !Kung San: Men, Women, and Work in a Foraging Society. Cambridge, Mass, Harvard University Press, 1979

49. Bohannan P, Bohannan L: A source notebook on Tiv religion (5 vols). New Haven, Conn, Human Relations Area Files, 1969

50. Ritenbaugh C: Obesity as a culture-bound syndrome. Cult Med Psychiatry 6:347, 1982

51. Malcom LWG: Note on the seclusion of girls among the Efik at Old Calabar. Man 25:113, 1925

52. Bergerhoff Mulder M: Kipsigis bridewealth payments. In Betzig L, Begerhoff Mulder M, Turke P (eds): Human Reproductive Behaviour. Cambridge, Cambridge University Press, 1988

53. Smithson CL: The Havasupai Woman. Salt Lake City, University of Utah Press, 1959

54. Messing SD: The Highland Plateau Amhara of Ethiopia. Doctoral dissertation, University of Pennsylvania, Philadelphia, 1957

55. Powdermaker H: An anthropological approach to the problem of obesity. Bull NY Acad Sci 36:286, 1960

56. Amnar H: Growing up in an Egyptian Village. London, Routledge & Kegan Paul, 1954

57. Strahern A: The Rope of Moka. New York, Cambridge University Press, 1971

58. Massara EB: Que Gordita! A Study of Weight Among Women in a Puerto Rican Community. New York, AMS Press, 1989

59. Massara EB: Obesity and cultural weight evaluations. Appetite 1:291, 1980

60. Styles MH: Soul, black women and food. In Kaplan JR (ed): A Woman's Conflict: The Special Relationship Between Women and Food. Englewood Cliffs, NJ, Prentice Hall, 1980

61. Stein Z, Susser M: The Dutch famine, 1944–1945, and the reproductive process. Pediatr Res 9:70, 1975

62. Huss-Ashmore R: Fat and fertility: Demographic implications of differential fat storage. Yearbook Phys Anthropol 23:65, 1980

63. Frisch RE: Body fat, menarche, fitness and fertility. Hum Reprod 2:521, 1987

64. Bailey SM: Absolute and relative sex differences in body composition. In Hall R (ed): Sexual Dimorphism in Homo sapiens. New York, Praeger Scientific Publishers, 1982

CHAPTER 27

Epidemiology of Obesity

FREDERICK H. EPSTEIN and MILLICENT HIGGINS

The epidemiology of obesity is concerned with the frequency and distribution of obesity in the population and with its determinants. Ultimately, however, epidemiologic findings must have bearing on individuals and must be based on reasonably representative samples of the population if they are to have general validity. This chapter considers the epidemiology of obesity. The relation of obesity to conditions such as heart disease or diabetes and the prevention of obesity, both aspects of the epidemiology of obesity, are addressed in other chapters.

DEFINITIONS

In recent years, the body mass index (BMI, weight [kg] per height [m²]) has gained recognition as an acceptable surrogate measure of body fatness,[1] especially for epidemiologic purposes, in which ease of measurement and comparability rank high. Its correlation with body fat is of the order of .7 to .8, which compares favorably with other indirect indices of body fat.[2] Nevertheless, persons wtih similar BMI show quite wide variations in body fat.[3] Therefore, it must be kept in mind that the BMI characterizes groups rather than individuals. Measuring obesity in terms of skin-fold thickness, however desirable in principle, suffers from the disadvantages that skin folds are difficult to measure reproducibly, especially in the obese; they reflect subcutaneous fat only; and the measurements are influenced by elasticity of the subcutaneous tissues, which declines in old age. Cross-classification on the sum of triceps plus subscapular skin folds and a weight-height index was proposed by Abraham et al as a method to define categories of leanness-obesity and underweight-overweight with the use of 85th to 95th percentile cut points.[4] Additional information about the distribution of body fat may be obtained from skinfold ratios at different sites, from the waist to hip ratio, and from other measures of regional fat. Assessment of body fat by measuring bioelectric impedance may add useful information in the future.

An international classification of obesity has been proposed by Garrow[5] and endorsed by a panel of the World Health Organization.[6] It is based on the following arbitrary ranges of BMI: below 20, 20–25, 25–30, 30–40, and above 40. In these terms, grade 1 obesity (moderate overweight) is defined as a BMI of 25–29.9 and grades 2 or 3 obesity (severe overweight/obese or morbidly obese) as a BMI of 30–39.9 and 40+, respectively.[2] In comparing the prevalence of obesity in different populations or population groups, it is useful to express it in terms of BMI values of 30 and over.[6,7] In the United States several BMI cut points, including 27.8 and 27.3, have been used to define overweight in men and women respectively. The frequency of a continuous variable like weight or blood pressure should be described not only in terms of the proportion of persons above an arbitrary threshold but also in terms of the entire distribution curve. Nevertheless, a cutoff like a BMI of 30 and over serves a useful purpose, similar to the use of cut points to define hypertension or diabetes.

While the present emphasis is on the BMI, it must be linked to the concept of desirable body weight that has played a decisive part in the development of contemporary views on the health risks of obesity. Desirable weight is based on the Metropolitan relative weight (MRW), derived from the tables of the Metropolitan Life Insurance Company and the Build and Blood Pressure Study. In the past, desirable MRW was not thought to increase with age after the early 20s and, for persons of medium frame, corresponded to a BMI of 22.0 for men and 21.5 for women, but there is current controversy about this issue.[8] The 1983 standards for desirable weight are higher than the 1959 standards as shown in Table 27-1, where BMI values equivalent to selected relative weights are also shown. The correlation between MRW and BMI is very high—greater than .99 in men and women in the Framingham Heart Study aged 30 to 60 years on first examination and greater than .96 in those reexamined at age 60 to 90 years.

Relationships between obesity and mortality or morbidity are relevant to the question of how obesity should be defined. In this connection, the dose-response curve matters because its shape reflects how much health hazard attaches to a given BMI over its entire distribution. Regardless of whether the curve is J-shaped or not, there is no argument that the risk of dying increases with increasing BMI beyond some measure of optimum weight. The relevance of this issue to the prevention of obesity and its ill effects will be discussed in the last section of this chapter.

GEOGRAPHIC PATHOLOGY

"Geographic pathology" is an old-fashioned term used deliberately here to highlight that obesity is a pathologic condition. International comparisons of the frequency of obesity are notoriously difficult to make, largely but not exclusively because the condition has been defined differently in different studies around the world. Therefore, published comparisons usually include only a few countries. The present attempt to present a global picture also falls short of the mark but is more comprehensive than previous summaries. In order to show only comparable data, attention

TABLE 27-1

Body Mass Index (BMI) at Specified Relative Weights in Adults

Metropolitan Relative Weight	BMI	
	Men	Women
Desirable		
1959	22.0	21.5
1983	22.7	22.4
20% overweight		
1959	26.4	25.8
1983	27.2	26.9
40% overweight		
1959	30.8	30.1
1983	31.1	32.3 approx
NCHS NHANES II		
Overweight*	27.8	27.3
Severely overweight†	31.1	32.3

During the period of growth, obesity is defined by weights, specific for height, age, and sex, which exceed the median weight plus 2 SD, derived from a reference population (see text, section on Obesity in Youth and Adolescence).
*≥85th percentile for ages 20–29 years.
†≥95th percentile for ages 20–29 years.

was limited to reports that included obesity defined by the BMI. The corresponding data on prevalence were drawn from eight industrialized and six developing countries, the latter in Latin America (Table 27-2).[1,7,9-12] The prevalence of obesity increases with age but tends to plateau around age 30. There is a tendency toward a higher prevalence in women than men, but the difference is generally not marked except in Finland and in Latin America, where the prevalence in men is much lower than in the developed countries. Obesity is more common in the United States than in the United Kingdom and somewhat more common than in Canada and Australia. The high prevalence in white South Africans is striking. It is not evident why the prevalence is rather low in The Netherlands; the question of the representativeness of the sample arises. The figures from Italy probably are an underestimate, partly explained by the wide age ranges covered. The data from The Netherlands and Italy illus-

TABLE 27-2

Prevalence of Obesity (BMI $\geq$ 30): International Comparisons

Country	Age (yr)	Prevalence (%) Men	Prevalence (%) Women	Reference
Finland	20–29	3.0	3.0	Rissanen et al[9]
	30–39	7.3	6.8	
	40–49	9.8	17.9	
	50–59	12.2	30.2	
	60–69	14.0	26.2	
	70+	13.3	33.1	
	20+	10	18	
Netherlands	20–34	1.9	2.0	Gurney and Gorstein[7]
	35–49	4.2	5.0	
	50–64	5.4	10.3	
United Kingdom	20–24	3	5	Millar and Stephens[10]
	25–34	6	6	
	35–44	8	8	
	45–54	8	12	
	55–64	9	14	
	20–64	8	9	
Italy	15–44	4.8	3.9	Gurney and Gorstein[7]
	45–64	9.9	11.1	
USA	20–24	7	7	Millar and Stephens[10]
	25–34	10	12	
	35–44	12	16	
	45–54	16	18	
	55–64	14	21	
	20–64	12	15	
Canada	25–34	6	4	Millar and Stephens[10]
	35–44	11	8	
	45–54	12	14	
	55–64	14	13	
	25–64	9	8	
Australia	25–34	4.0	5.7	Gurney and Gorstein[7]
	35–44	6.2	7.5	
	45–54	10.2	11.0	
	55–64	9.6	12.5	
	25–64	7	7	Bray[1,11]
South Africa	15–24	3.6	4.6	Jooste et al[12]
	25–34	13.2	10.5	
	35–44	14.3	15.6	
	45–54	20.9	23.8	
	55–64	19.8	31.7	
	15–64	14.7	18.0	
Costa Rica	40–45	5.7	14.4	Gurney and Gorstein[7]
El Salvador	40–45	0.0	1.5	
Guatemala	40–45	0.0	5.6	
Honduras	40–45	2.8	6.0	
Nicaragua	40–45	3.1	16.4	
Panama	40–45	2.3	1.7	

trate the problem of ascertainment, to which reference has already been made.

The data from the Seven-Countries Study are not available in terms of BMI but permit comparisons in terms of overweight, expressed as 10% or more of standard weight or the sum of triceps and subscapular skin folds over 28 mm. The increasing rank order of prevalence according to skin-fold thickness was as follows: Japan, Greece, Finland, Yugoslavia, Italy, The Netherlands, and the United States; the corresponding prevalences were 2%, 11%, 14%, 29%, 28%, 32%, and 63%.[13] In contrast to the prevalence data shown in Table 27-2, Finland ranks low and The Netherlands high. Data from five European regions are reported for women born in 1948.[14] Only mean BMI values are given: those are 23.1 in Sweden, 23.9 in Poland, 23.3 in The Netherlands, 24.1 in northern Italy, and 27.8 in southern Italy.

The data on prevalence just presented are limited to relatively few geographic areas. They may be supplemented by data from the Intersalt[15] and MONICA[16] projects, which are more global in nature but do not use the accepted definition of obesity (Table 27-3). The mean BMI, however, gives a good indication of comparatively large differences in the frequency of obesity, while its value at the 90th percentile point, marking off the 10% of the population with the highest BMI, approximates the information contained in BMI values of 30 or more, which indicate frank obesity. The mean BMI values from the Intersalt study refer to men and women combined. In some countries data were collected in several locations. With regard to mean BMIs, data from Europe are remarkably uniform, with the exception of data from places like Poland or Malta. Values in the United States, referring to both black and white population groups, again tend to be high. Values in Latin America are not particularly low except for one location in Brazil (an Indian tribe). There is much obesity in Trinidad. Markedly low values are consistently found in the Asian-Pacific area, with the exception of Hawaii. BMI values at the 90th percentile point hover around 30 (the threshold value for obesity) in most European locations, indicating the lack of major geographic differences, as did the prevalence data. The value of 27.6 in the People's Re-

public of China is markedly low, reflecting a lower prevalence of obesity.

Obesity is a serious, emerging problem in developing countries, in addition to the continuing problem of undernutrition. The social and economic conditions which lead to the development of obesity in these generally poor countries have been well described by Lara-Pantin.[17] Among the important influences are urbanization, movement of rural inhabitants to cities, migration into developing countries, new eating habits, and a new affluence in some sections of the population. Overnutrition and nutritional imbalance often go hand in hand. It is a great challenge to prevent these trends or to reverse them where they have already taken hold.

PREVALENCE, DETERMINANTS, AND SECULAR TRENDS IN OBESITY: LESSONS FROM THE UNITED STATES

Extensive data on the epidemiology of obesity are available in a number of countries. Data from the United States are particularly comprehensive and accessible and will therefore be used to exemplify the scope and nature of the problem. We recognize that the U.S. experience does not reflect that of the rest of the world; nevertheless, the large amount of available data makes it a useful model to illustrate patterns that are similar in many developed countries.

Prevalence

The prevalence of overweight and obesity depends on their definition. Several criteria were used for the 20- to 74-year-old noninstitutionalized population of the United States examined in the National Health and Nutrition Examination Survey (NHANES II, 1976–80).[18] The 85th and 95th percentile values of BMI distribution at ages 20 to 29 years were selected to identify overweight and severely overweight men with BMI values of 27.8 and 31.1 kg/m² and women with BMI values of 27.3 and 32.3 kg/m² or greater. These values are approximately equivalent to weights 20% and 40% above the midpoint of the recommended weight range for persons of medium build in the 1983 Metropolitan Life Insurance Company tables. Because BMI increases

TABLE 27-3

Mean Body Mass Index (BMI) and Obesity (BMI ≥ 90th Percentile): International Comparisons Based on the Intersalt and Monica Projects

Area	Country	Mean BMI*	BMI at 90th Percentile Point†	
			Men	Women
Northern Europe	Denmark	24.5	30.3	30.0
	Sweden		29.1, 30.4	29.6, 32.0
	Finland	25.4, 25.3	31.6, 31.6, 31.7	32.7, 31.4, 33.0
	Iceland	24.5	30.3	30.5
Western and Central Europe	United Kingdom	25.7, 24.8, 25.2	30.1, 30.2	32.4, 31.4
	Netherlands	24.4		
	Belgium	25.9, 24.9	30.4, 31.5	32.5, 33.6
	France		29.8, 32.5	30.2, 34.2
	Federal Republic of Germany	24.5, 24.5	30.8, 30.9, 31.3, 31.9	31.5, 32.7, 33.2, 32.1
	Switzerland		30.3, 31.8	30.8, 31.2
	Luxemburg		30.8	32.1
Southern Europe	Italy	28.0, 25.4, 25.4, 25.4	30.3, 31.3	31.5, 32.6
	Malta	26.9	32.7	36.5
	Portugal	25.8		
	Spain	25.4, 26.7	30.3	33.4
Eastern Europe	German Democratic Republic	24.9	30.9, 30.6, 31.2	32.0, 33.6, 34.2
	Hungary	26.2	30.8, 31.6	32.4, 33.8
	Poland	26.4, 26.5	31.7	34.3
	Yugoslavia		31.2	34.9
	Czechoslovakia		32.4	34.9
	USSR	25.7	30.6, 30.8, 30.4, 31.1, 30.7	34.5, 36.0, 34.3, 36.1, 36.2
North America	USA	26.4, 30.3, 28.2, 28.0, 25.1	29.9	31.8
	Canada	25.1, 25.2		
South and Central America	Argentina	25.0		
	Brazil	23.4, 21.2		
	Colombia	23.0		
	Mexico	24.4		
	Trinidad	28.2		
Asian-Pacific area	India	20.1, 23.7		
	Japan	21.6, 22.5. 23.1		
	Hawaii	31.2		
	Taiwan	23.1		
	South Korea	22.2		
	Papua, New Guinea	21.7		
	People's Republic of China	22.8, 21.3, 23.8	27.6	29.5
	New Zealand		29.5	29.9
	Australia		29.8, 30.8	30.0, 31.5
Africa	Kenya	20.8		
	Zimbabwe	26.1		

Multiple values within a country refer to different cities.
*Mean BMI refers to age-adjusted values of men and women aged 30–59 years (INTERSALT data).
†The 90th percentile points refer to men and women aged 35–64 years (Monica data).

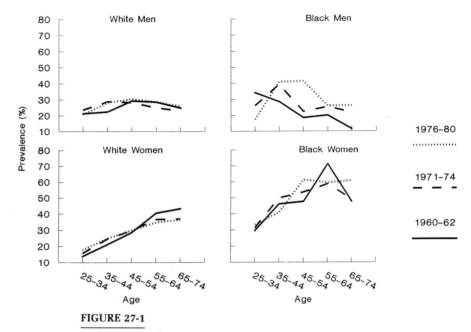

FIGURE 27-1

Prevalence (%) of overweight, United States, 1960–1980. Overweight is defined as a BMI $\geq$ 27.8 kg/m^2 for men and $\geq$ 27.3 kg/m^2 for women. (Source: Division of Health Examination Statistics, National Center for Heath Statistics, Washington, DC.)

with age, more than 15% of the population exceeded the 85th percentile value for 20- to 29-year-olds; in fact, 26%, or about 34 million Americans, were overweight and 9%, or 13 million, were severely overweight. The prevalence of overweight in the period 1976–1980 increased with age in men from age 25 to about age 50, then declined, whereas overweight continued to increase with increasing age to the mid-70s in women (Fig. 27-1). Overweight affected a larger percentage of women than men at ages over 55 in the white population and at ages over 25 years in the black population. In the United States the prevalence of overweight is higher among young white men than young black men, higher in middle-aged black men than middle-aged white men, and about the same in white and black men at ages 55 to 74 years. Among women, overweight is more prevalent among blacks than white at all ages; at ages under 55, the difference is twofold. Approximately 60% of black women aged 45 to 74 years were overweight, and more than 20% were severely overweight.

In the NHANES II study overweight was slightly less frequent in men classified as poor, whereas it was nearly twice as common in poor women compared with women above the poverty level. The excess prevalence of overweight associated with poverty was less in women over 55 and there was virtually no difference at ages under 25.[19,20] In the late 1970s, race and poverty were independently associated with overweight in women. In children, as in men, median BMIs are higher in higher socioeconomic groups; this pattern is also reported for adults from developing countries.[19,21]

Morbidity and mortality data on obesity do not reflect the magnitude of the problem of obesity since statistics usually refer to pathologic conditions associated with obesity rather than to obesity itself. Nevertheless, 232,000 physician office visits were made for obesity or localized adiposity in 1985, and these conditions were listed as the first cause for 32,000 hospital discharges and mentioned as discharge diagnoses for 580,000 hospitalizations in 1987. In 1985, 1042 of a total of approximately 2 million deaths were attributed to obesity as the underlying cause. An alternative measure of the burden of overweight is provided by reports to the National Health Interview Survey which indicate that 27% of males and 46% of females were trying to lose weight. The health consequences of being overweight are discussed in several chapters in this book.

The Distribution and Determinants of Overweight and Obesity

Demographic characteristics, including age, sex, race, and country of residence, are associated with the prevalence of obesity (see Table 27-2 and Fig. 27-1). The experience in the United States will be used to illustrate these and other characteristics that influence the frequency and distribution of overweight (defined as BMI > 27.8 for men and 27.3 for women) and obesity (defined as BMI $\geq$ 30 for both sexes). The arbitrary nature of these or any other cut points is acknowledged, together with the fact that they may not be equally appropriate for men and women or throughout the age range (especially in children and the elderly) or in different subgroups of the population.

Sources of data include the National Center for Health Statistics, principally the NHANES I and II studies,[4,18] and the Framingham Heart Study.[22] Median values of BMI are shown by age and sex in Figure 27-2 for ages 1 to 74 years from NHANES and for ages 60 to 84 years from the Framingham Heart Study. Median BMI is about 15 to 16 from age 2 to 10 years, but it decreases slightly until age 6 and then increases steeply in young men and women to reach levels of about 22 in both sexes at age 19 years. During adult life, BMI values are lower in women than men even though women have a higher percentage of body weight as fat. The sex difference in BMI is less or possibly reversed in the elderly. The survivors of the Framingham cohort who were over 60 years of age when they were reexamined during the same period in which the NHANES II study was conducted had slightly higher BMIs than average for the U.S. noninstitutionalized population. BMIs decreased with increasing age among the oldest old.

Trends in MRW in relation to age in the Framingham population are presented in Figure 27-3. These trends are based on longitudinal observations of men and women examined at two-year intervals and are presented for successive birth cohorts grouped according to age at first

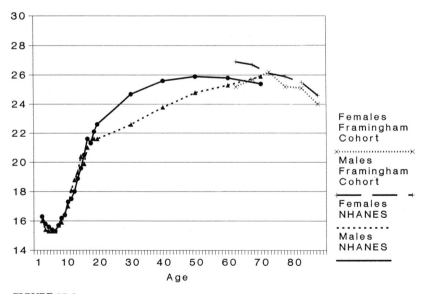

FIGURE 27-2

Median BMI in two populations in the United States.

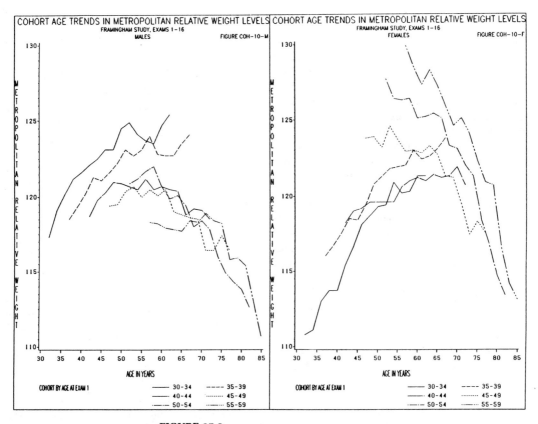

FIGURE 27-3

Cohort age trends in Metropolitan relative weight levels for men and women in the Framingham Heart Study.

examination, beginning in 1948. In men, average MRWs increased with increasing age from age 30 to age 60 or 65 for the most recently born cohorts (aged 30 to 45 years at first examination). Among men aged 45 to 60 years at first examination, relative weights declined steeply with increasing age past 65 or 70 years. There are also differences among the cohorts, with those born more recently having higher MRWs than men born earlier had at the same ages. Thus, both aging and secular trends are apparent among Framingham men; among young adult and middle-aged men they consist of increases in relative weight with age and also over the last 30 years. Relative weights decline with increasing age in elderly men, but there are no clear trends over time. Among women in the younger cohorts (aged 20 to 45 years at first examination), MRI increased

with increasing age to about age 70 and then decreased, but average relative weights appeared to decline after age 55 in the older cohorts (women aged 45 to 60 years at first examination). Secular trends are different from those noted for younger men; in younger women relative weights were lower in more recently born cohorts than they had been when women born in earlier years were of the same ages. Among older women those born more recently (age 50 to 54 years at first examination) also had lower relative weights in old age than elderly women had in the past. Thus, trends with aging are toward increasing relative weight except in old age. Trends in relative weight over time are toward decreasing relative weight among women and increasing relative weight among men; however, there are no clear trends over time among elderly men.

Secular Trends

Trends in the prevalence of overweight during the 20 years from 1960 to 1980 are shown for black and white men and women in the United States in Figure 27-1, where cross-sectional trends with age for ages 25 to 74 are also illustrated. Among white men, neither age trends nor time trends are striking, but the prevalence of overweight appears to increase slightly with increasing age to about age 50, and to decrease with increasing age thereafter. At younger ages overweight was less prevalent in 1960–1962 than in the 1970s, but secular trends are less consistent at older ages. The prevalence of overweight appears to have increased in black men in the past 20 years, and it appears to decrease with increasing age more steeply and beginning at an earlier age than in white men. In both white and black women, the prevalence of overweight increases with increasing age through the age range 25 to 74 years for white women, but it appears to decrease or level off among older black women. Secular trends are toward higher prevalences of overweight over time among younger white women and possibly among older black women, with some inconsistencies. Overweight appears to be less prevalent among older white women than it was in the early 1960s. The final observation from Figure 27-1 is that overweight is more frequent in black women than white women, as discussed above.

Average BMI values and prevalence of overweight show complex patterns varying with sex, age, socioeconomic circumstances, and race, and over time. Summary statistics, generalizations and predictions for total populations, are not possible even within one country; the frequency and distribution of BMI, overweight, and obesity must be considered for defined segments, subgroups, and geographic regions.

OBESITY IN YOUTH AND ADOLESCENCE

Reliable data for cross-cultural comparisons of the prevalence of obesity at younger ages are lacking, even though there has been much attention to the problem of obesity in childhood in a number of countries. The difficulty in obtaining reliable data for comparisons between or even within countries is largely attributable to the lack of a satisfactory measure of obesity during the period of growth. The BMI is considered inappropriate for children and adolescents because of the rapid changes in body shape and composition in the course of development.[23] It is recommended that obesity during this period be defined by weights specific for height, age, and sex that exceed the median weight plus 2 SD, as provided by tables of an international reference population.[23,24] The corresponding weight values at the 97th percentile point can be read off in these tables. The arbitrariness of such a definition of obesity is recognized, but the definition can be used to make population comparisons. The reference population used for this purpose is a U.S. population, based on data from the U.S. National Center for Health Statistics published in 1976.[25]

Using this definition, the prevalence of obesity in preschool children has been estimated in 34 countries.[7] It ranges from values under 1% to around 11%; examples are about 2% in Jordan and Tahiti, 3% in the United Kingdom, 5% in Bolivia and Trinidad, close to 6% in Canada, and 10% to 11% in Jamaica and Chile. Such data cannot be interpreted without additional information on the ways in which the samples were collected, their size, and the socioeconomic groups represented. The data are considered preliminary but they serve a useful purpose in marking the beginning of epidemiologic research in this field.

For schoolchildren and adolescents, there are no similar data available, although data on height and weight were collected in the course of a WHO collaborative study in childhood and youth.[26] They have not been evaluated in terms of standard deviations from the median, but mean BMI values were calculated (Labarthe, unpublished data). Such values are available for boys and girls between the ages of 5 and 20 years in 13 countries, either at selected ages or over consecutive ages from 7 to 15 years. These data permit an assessment of how the BMI matures from childhood into the late teens. In developed countries, the mean BMI reaches values of around 17 at about age 10. This corresponds to data from the United States (see Fig. 27-2). At age 14, mean values have reached 20, being lower in the two developing countries with available data. In France and The Netherlands, continuous data are available up to age 20; mean BMI in the respective countries is 21.9 and 21.5 in young men and 21.3 and 21.5 in young women at age 20. Thus the BMI rises but little in the teen years in these countries. As stated before, a "desirable BMI" is 22.7 for men and 22.4 for women. Therefore, pending further validation, it would seem that the BMI provides useful information starting at puberty. This knowledge should facilitate international comparisons during this crucial period of life in which life-styles are formed.

TRACKING AND CHANGES IN WEIGHT

Many individuals gain or lose weight over time, and some do so repeatedly in a cyclical manner. The trends with aging and over time nevertheless show rather consistent patterns among population groups. Longitudinal patterns can be described with respect to average levels, slope, and variability in a manner comparable to that proposed by Lauer and colleagues[27] to characterize longitudinal patterns of blood pressure. Health consequences of weight gain, weight loss, and persistent obesity are well established, but the adverse consequences of repeated fluctuations in weight have received attention only recently.

Epidemiologic observations from the Framingham Heart Study and a study conducted in Tecumseh, Michigan, will be used to illustrate tracking and changes in weight. Tracking correlation coefficients between weights at repeated examinations over intervals ranging from two years to 30 years are higher when intervals between examinations are shorter.[22] For example, correlations between MRW values measured two years apart are about .95, correlations between MRWs measured 10 years apart are about .85, and they are about .7 when measured 20 years apart. The coefficients were slightly higher in women than in men, and for the longest intervals selective losses from the cohort are likely to have resulted in higher coefficients among survivors. Nevertheless, the magnitude and persistence of these correlations are strong evidence that MRW values "track," that is, individuals tend to maintain their position in the distribution when they are ranked with their peers. Similar patterns were reported for the BMI in the Tecumseh, Michigan, study[28] in which observations were also available for children. Correlations between weight/height^2 measured after a 15-year interval were

lowest in children under two years, being .1 for males and .26 for females. They increased with increasing age in both sexes: from .4 in 3- to 5-year-old boys and to .6 in 15- to 19-year-old boys, and from .5 in 3- to 5-year-old girls to .7 in 15- to 19-year-old girls. Correlations ranged from .7 to .8 in adult men and women.

Changes in weight during two-year intervals ranged from average losses of 15 to 16 pounds in the 10% of the Framingham cohort who lost most weight to average gains of 13 to 14 pounds in the 10% who gained most weight.[29] Garn et al[30] analyzed cross-sectional and longitudinal measurements of fatness in individuals and families in Tecumseh, Michigan, over a period of 20 years and noted that initially lean subjects tended to increase in fatness, whereas initially obese subjects tended to become less fat. These trends were more marked in children and adolescents but were also detected in adults. The trends for change in fatness were more apparent in boys and men than in girls and women. Despite this evidence of regression toward the mean, triceps skin-fold thicknesses and weight at first examination correlated with the same measurements 20 years later. Correlations between weights were higher than those between triceps skin-fold measurements, and both correlations were higher among adults than children. Weight correlations in males and females were similar, whereas triceps correlations were higher in females than males.

Determinants of weight change have received less attention in epidemiologic studies whose major concern is with the influence of weight loss or gain on cardiovascular risk factors such as blood pressure, blood lipids, glucose intolerance, and uric acid. There is undoubtedly useful information on the epidemiology of obesity and weight change awaiting analysis, but studies designed to test specific hypotheses and monitor weight and distribution of body fat at optimum intervals will probably require design of new studies.

FAMILIAL AGGREGATION OF OBESITY

Obesity and leanness run in families. Population-based epidemiologic studies have measured the degree of resemblance among related and unrelated members of families living together or living apart in order to determine the magnitude of genetic and environmental influences on body size, including height, weight, BMI, skin-fold thickness, and other measures of adiposity and obesity. Comparisons have been made of monozygous and dizygous twins, of parents and offspring, among siblings and spouses, and of biologically related and adoptive relatives. New analytic approaches have been used to partition phenotypic variance into components attributable to shared genes and components attributable to shared household environments. Assortative mating contributes to similarity in BMI between spouses.[31] The results of these approaches have been to establish a significant contribution of genes to the determination of body mass, adiposity, and obesity. Longini et al[31] estimated heritability for BMI to be above 30% after adjustment for age, sex, and socioeconomic status. Burns and co-workers[32] detected familial clustering of BMI among relatives of children in Muscatine, Iowa, and estimated that 38% of the variability in BMI was explained by genetic differences and about 15% by shared cultural or environmental exposures. Recent advances in molecular genetics have led to attempts to identify single genes or polygenes that may be implicated, and shared environments or behaviors that may be the result of cultural inheritance. Further advances in understanding the epidemiology of obesity may be expected from better definition of the condition, and identification of more homogeneous phenotypes characterized not only with respect to attributes such as amount and distribution of body fat at one time, but also with respect to changes with aging and susceptibility to gain weight under variable conditions of energy intake and energy expenditure and in relation to a variety of metabolic conditions. It also seems clear that living in the same household contributes to similarities in fatness; Garn et al have reported similar caloric and nutrient intakes resulting from shared family diets.[33,34] Familial resemblance in smoking and drinking habits has been documented in Tecumseh and elsewhere,[35] and these behaviors also influence the amount and distribution of body fat. Other possibly shared behaviors worthy of investigation include patterns of physical activity. Several other possible determinants of body fatness in individuals and in families are considered in the sections on fat and en-

TABLE 27.4

Determinants of and Risk Factors for Obesity

Demographic Factors

Age
Sex
Race
Socioeconomic circumstances
Geography: country of residence, urbanization, industrialization, migration

Familial Factors

Heredity: polygenes; single gene(s) with major effect
Shared environments (cultural inheritance)
Interaction between genetic susceptibility and environmental exposure

Personal Factors

Past or current overweight
Age at onset of obesity
Eating habits
Physical inactivity/sedentary life-style
Metabolic characteristics
Cigarette smoking
Psychological factors
Pregnancy
Concurrent illness or disability

ergy metabolism, regulation of energy intake, and regulation of energy output.

RISK FACTORS FOR OBESITY

Age, sex, race, socioeconomic circumstances, and areas of residence are related to the frequency and distribution of obesity (Table 27-4). Heredity is an important determinant and may act through many genes, each exerting a small effect, or through single genes, which are likely to be rarer but to exert larger effects. Obesity is of multifactorial etiology and interactions among genes as well as between genes and environmental challenges contribute to its development. Unfortunately, methods for measuring potentially important environmental factors and personal characteristics are imprecise and their effects may be exerted over long periods of time, as well as in complex interconnecting relationships. Some environmental factors and personal attributes that merit further investigation include diet, physical activity, cigarette smoking, and alcohol consumption. Patterns of growth, development, and aging provide the background for etiologic factors whose impact may vary over the natural lifetime as well as in response to disease or disability.

NEW DIRECTIONS

New directions are concerned with the acquisition of new knowledge and the more effective application of knowledge already gained. Within the context of needed epidemiologic research, there is no question that more must be learned about population differences in the frequency of obesity between and within countries. In many parts of the world, available data are not representative, and the BMI, however useful, is not an adequate measure of obesity for either clinical or epidemiologic purposes. The more accurately obesity is measured and characterized, the more it will reflect the metabolic and pathologic processes that lead to obesity and the more insight will be gained regarding the causes for inter- and intrapopulation differences. Obesity is not a homogeneous condition and there may well be more to such differences than the mere balance between energy input (caloric intake) and energy output (largely physical activity). It is unlikely that genetic variations account for a major proportion of these differences. However, as one example, genetic differences could certainly exist if there was truth in the existence of a "thrifty genotype" that developed in the course of evolution because of its survival value in periods of famine. Interactions between genetic susceptibility and variable environments may still be important as they might have been in the past. With regard to better measures of obesity, the newer methods available are too complicated and expensive to use in large field studies. What is needed are simplified methods applicable in population surveys. It is likely that better cross-cultural data on the epidemiology of obesity itself, not only its consequences, would provide new etiological leads, giving clues to more effective preventive measures.

Concerning the more effective application of existing knowledge, more needs to be learned about the best ways to motivate people and families, starting in youth, to prevent gain in weight or, if required, to achieve weight loss. In conjunction with this individual, "high-risk" approach to weight control, strategies must be developed to prevent obesity on the population level. The need for such a population strategy becomes apparent if it is realized that most of the excess morbidity and mortality attributable to obesity does not derive from the 10% of the population in the frankly obese range (BMI $\geq$ 30) but the 40% who are slightly or moderately overweight (i.e., the range between the 50th and 90th percentile of the distribution of BMIs). Even though the risk of these persons is not much higher than average, there are so many of them in the population that they account for the majority of the excessive risk associated with obesity. As in the case of other risk factors like elevated serum lipids or blood pressure, the outlook is toward a new generation with a lower population frequency of obesity, implying the need to shift the distribution curve of weight to the left. It is probably relatively easier, assuming new attitudes toward healthy life-styles, to prevent weight gain rather than to lose excessive weight.

References

1. Bray GA: Obesity: Definition, diagnosis and disadvantages. Med J Aust 142:52, 1985
2. Seidell JC, Deurenberg P, Hautvast JGAJ: Obesity and fat distribution in relation to health: Current insights and recommendations. World Rev Nutr Diet 50:57, 1987
3. Durnin JVGA: The prevalence of obesity in the UK. Bibl Nutr Dieta 37:11, 1986
4. Abraham S, National Center for Health Statistics: Obese and Overweight Adults in the United States. Vital and Health Statistics, Series 11, No. 230. DHHS publication (PHS) 83-1680. Washington, DC, US Government Printing Office, 1983
5. Garrow JS: Treat Obesity Seriously: A Clinical Manual. Edinburgh, Churchill Livingstone, 1981
6. World Health Organization: Measuring Obesity: Classification and Description of Anthropometric Data. Report on a WHO Consultation on the Epidemiology of Obesity. Copenhagen, WHO Regional Office for Europe, Nutrition Unit, 1988
7. Gurney M, Gorstein J: The global prevalence of obesity: An initial overview of available data. World Health Stat Q 41:251, 1988
8. Simopoulos AP: Characteristics of obesity: An overview. Ann NY Acad Sci 499:4, 1987
9. Rissanen A, Heliovaara M, Aromaa A: Overweight and anthropometric changes in adulthood: A pro-

spective study of 17000 Finns. Int J Obes 12:391, 1988

10. Millar WJ, Stephens T: The prevalence of overweight and obesity in Britain, Canada, and the United States. Am J Public Health 77:38, 1987

11. Bray GA: Overweight is risking fate: Definition, classification, prevalence, and risks. Ann NY Acad Sci 499:14, 1987

12. Jooste PL, Steenkamp JH, Benade AJS et al: Prevalence of overweight and obesity and its relation to coronary heart disease in the CORIS study. S Afr Med J 74:101, 1988

13. Mancini M, Contaldo F, Farinaro E et al: Medical complications and prevalence of obesity in Italy. Bibl Nutr Dieta 37:1, 1986

14. Cigolini M, Seidel JC, Charzewska J et al: Fat distribution, metabolism and plasma insulin in European women: The European fat distribution study. In Björntorp P, Rossner S (eds): Obesity in Europe 88. London, John Libbey, 1989

15. Intersalt Cooperative Research Group: Intersalt: An international study of electrolyte excretion and blood pressure. Results of 24 hour urinary sodium and potassium excretion. Br Med J 297:319, 1988

16. The WHO MONICA Project: Geographical variation in the major risk factors for coronary heart disease in men and women aged 36–64 years. World Health Stat Q 41:115, 1988

17. Lara-Pantin E: Obesity in developing countries. In Berry EV, Blondheim SH, Eliahou HE et al (eds): Recent Advances in Obesity Research. London, John Libbey, 1987

18. Najjar MF, Rowland M, National Center for Health Statistics: Anthropometric Reference Data and Prevalence of Overweight, United States, 1976–80. Vital and Health Statistics, Series 11, No. 238. DHHS publication (PHS) 87-1688. Washington, DC, US Government Printing Office, October 1987

19. Fulwood R, Abraham S, Johnson C, National Center for Health Statistics: Height and Weight of Adults Ages 18–74 Years by Socio-economic and Geographic Variables. Vital and Health Statistics, Series 11, No. 224. DHHS publication (PHS) 81-1674. Washington, DC, US Government Printing Office, 1981

20. Van Itallie TB: Health implications of overweight and obesity in the United States. Ann Intern Med 103:983, 1987

21. Richards R, De Casseres M: The problem of obesity in developing countries: Its prevalence and morbidity. In Burland WL, Samuel PD, Yudkin J (eds): Obesity Symposium, pp 74–84. New York, Churchill Livingstone, 1974

22. Belanger BA, Cupples LA, D'Agostino RB: The Framingham Study: An Epidemiological Investigation of Cardiovascular Disease. Section 36: Measures at Each Examination and Interexamination Consistency of Specified Characteristics. Framingham Publication No. 88-2970, May 1988

23. Obesity: A Report of the Royal College of Physicians. J R Coll Physicians Lond 17:5, 1983

24. WHO Working Group: Use and interpretation of anthropometric indicators of nutritional status. Bull WHO 64:929, 1986

25. NCHS Growth Charts (HRA 76-1120,25,3). Rockville, Md, Health Resources Administration, Public Health Service, 1976

26. Tell GS, Tuomilehto J, Epstein FH et al: Studies of atherosclerosis precursors and determinants during childhood and adolescence. Bull WHO 64:595, 1986

27. Lauer RM, Clarke WR, Beaglehole R: Level, trend and variability of blood pressure during childhood: The Muscatine study. Circulation 69:242, 1984

28. Higgins MW, Keller JB, Metzner HZ et al: Studies of blood pressure in Tecumseh, Michigan. II. Antecedents in childhood of high blood pressure in young adults. Hypertension 2(suppl 1):1–117, 1980

29. Higgins M, Kannel W, Garrison R et al: Hazards of obesity: The Framingham experience. In Björntorp P, Smith V, Lonnroth (eds): Health Implications of Regional Obesity. Acta Med Scand Suppl 723:23, 1988

30. Garn SM, Pilkington JJ, Lavelle M: Relationship between initial fatness level and long-term fatness change. Ecol Food Nutr 14:85, 1984

31. Longini IM, Higgins MW, Hinton PC et al: Genetic and environmental sources of familial aggregation of body mass in Tecumseh, Michigan. Hum Biol 56:733, 1984

32. Burns TL, Moll PP, Lauer RM: The relation between ponderosity and coronary risk factors in children and their relatives. Am J Epidemiol 129:973, 1989

33. Garn SM, Cole PE, Bailey SM: Living together as a factor in family line resemblances. Hum Biol 51:565, 1979

34. Higgins MW, Kjelsberg M, Metzner H: Characteristics of smokers and nonsmokers in Tecumseh, Michigan. I. The distribution of smoking habits in persons and families and their relationship to social characteristics. Am J Epidemiol 86:45, 1967

CHAPTER 28

Genetic Aspects of Human Obesity

CLAUDE BOUCHARD

This chapter reviews evidence concerning the role of the genotype in human obesity. It deals with the amount of body fat and regional fat distribution, particularly abdominal fat. The influence of inherited factors on various components of energy expenditure is also considered. Results of overfeeding experiments performed with identical twins are briefly highlighted. Because of space limitations, much material cannot be incorporated in this text. The reader is referred to other publications for further information.[4,6,11,16,24]

The role of inherited factors in the development and maintenance of obesity is only partially understood. In contrast, evidence for the contribution of behavioral and life-style factors to the development and maintenance of obesity is abundant and generally clear. However, individual differences are ubiquitous, and it is increasingly recognized that there are inherited differences in the susceptibility to become obese under given behavioral and life-style conditions. These are issues in need of clarification before further progress can be achieved in the understanding of this important health risk factor, particularly as it pertains to abdominal obesity.

OBESITY: A HETEROGENEOUS PHENOTYPE

It has long been recognized that obesity is not a single disorder but rather a heterogeneous group of disorders.[15,18] We are not here referring to the heterogeneity of the clinical manifestations of obesity but to the phenotype of body fat itself. Even if one could define how much fat is involved in obesity and could measure it precisely, there would still exist problems preventing us from considering obesity as a homogeneous phenotype. For instance, one would have to use different phenotypic criteria in males and females, allow for age variation in body fat, and also incorporate differences in fat topography.

Fat topography is defined on at least two axes. The first axis represents individual differences in adipose cell characteristics. It has been suggested, with relatively good supporting evidence, that human obesities can be divided into those with predominantly enlarged fat cells (hypertropic obesity) and those with predominantly increased number of fat cells (hyperplastic obesity).[2] The other axis represents the anatomical distribution of body fat.[30] Thus, excess fat can be stored primarily in the abdominal area (the android or malelike obesity) or in the gluteal and femoral area (the gynoid or femalelike obesity). A subject with excess body fat could have the hypertropic or hyperplastic characteristics and be of the android or gynoid type. Even though other fat topography features may need to be considered for a full description of the obesity phenotype,[15] the two axes defined above are sufficient to show that obesity, or human body fat in general, is a very heterogeneous phenotype. The implication is that a given body fat content may be associated with different phenotypic characteristics and produce different clinical consequences. Yet in most genetic studies, individuals with quite different phenotypic characteristics have been grouped together and studied as if they all had the same trait.

OBESITY: A MULTIFACTORIAL PHENOTYPE

Obesities is a more correct term than *obesity*. But the situation is even more complex, as the phenotypes are not of the simple mendelian kind. Segregation of the genes is not readily perceived, and the influence of the genotype on etiology is generally attenuated or exacerbated by nongenetic factors. Thus, variation in human body fat is attributable to a complex interworking of genetic, nutritional, energy expenditure, psychological, and social variables. In this complex situation, the study of the genetics of the trait must rely primarily on data on relatives by descent or by adoption and the analytic strategies of genetic epidemiology.

An obesity phenotype is therefore a multifactorial trait determined by genetic and nongenetic affectors. Figure 28-1 describes a simple paradigm that integrates general factors affecting body fat and their interactions. Each factor comprises a family of components. *Energy intake* includes not only the total caloric intake but also the macronutrient composition of the intake, the palatability of the diet, its content of various amino acids and other molecules as they influence the metabolic outcomes of the food ingested, and appetite and satiety. *Energy expendi-*

tures include basal and resting metabolism, thermic effect of food, energy expenditure of exercise and work, level of habitual physical activity, temperature-induced thermogenesis, stress-induced thermogenesis, and probably other minor components.

The third component is probably the most complex. It is defined as the interface between energy (nutrient) intake and energy expenditure and reflects the fact that characteristics of the human body have an impact on the outcome of a given set of energy intake and expenditure conditions. Variations in the biologic-behavioral interface can be caused by inherited or acquired conditions. For instance, inherited variants in enzymes of the liver (or other tissues) may influence the efficiency of lipid metabolism in the carrier individuals and alter substrate utilization under certain dietary conditions. This in turn may affect energy balance and influence the body fat phenotype.

These considerations led us to the observation that epidemiologic or population data regarding the role of genes on body fat content or obesity can only be of limited value.[6] It would be more productive in the future to study the primary and secondary affectors of obesity. For instance, genetic analysis of the various components of energy expenditure may yield more conclusive evidence of an inherited susceptibility to be in positive energy balance, or the converse, than if one studied only body fat.

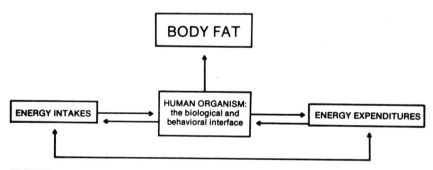

FIGURE 28-1

The major affectors of body fat. (From Bouchard C: Genetics of body fat, energy expenditure and adipose tissue metabolism. In Berry FM, Blondheim SH, Eliahou HE et al (eds): Recent Advances in Obesity Research. V. London, John Libbey & Co, 1987. Reproduced by permission.)

HERITABILITY OF BODY FAT

We will focus on the additive genetic effect (narrow heritability) of three commonly used measurements in obesity: the body mass index (BMI), which is obtained by dividing body weight (kg) by height in (m²), the sum of several skinfold thicknesses (represented by subcutaneous fat), and fat mass, determined by underwater weighing.

In the past half century, it has frequently been observed that obese parents are more likely to have obese children than are lean parents. This does not constitute a clear demonstration that the obesity of the offspring is determined by the so-called obesity genes of the parents, as both generations share not only genes but also the household milieu and many environmental conditions. The results of 11 familial studies of obese children were summarized by Bray[16] and are reproduced in Table 28-1. The data from these early studies are not quite comparable, as obesity was variously defined and methods of ascertainment were not identical across studies. Nonetheless, they clearly suggest that obesity in one parent conferred greater risk of obesity on the offspring. Surprisingly, however, the risk often seemed to be less when both parents were obese. As these data were not fully conclusive, more research with improved design and better assessed obesity phenotype was needed, as suggested by Bray.[16]

The literature on heredity and human obesity is confusing and contradictory. Thus, in various studies the BMI or some other indices of relative weight or skin-fold thicknesses were used, with data gathered on parents and their biologic children, parents and their adopted children, blood-related brothers and sisters, siblings by adoption, and dizygotic and monozygotic twins. With few exceptions, the studies did not distinguish between the effects of genes shared by descent and the effects of household and environmental conditions shared by relatives living together. Only limited research has been reported in which the authors used some of the recent tools of genetic epidemiology.[1,8,12,23] Common conclusions in the literature therefore range from "little genetic effect" to "very high genetic effect" for obesity or body fat.

In clinical settings, the BMI is increasingly used to assess the normality of body weight in

TABLE 28-1

Frequency of Obesity in Parents of Obese Children

Study	No. of Obese Subjects	One or Both Parents Obese (%)	Mother Obese (%)	Father Obese (%)	Both Parents Obese (%)
Dunlop	523	69	39	12	18
Ellis	50	44	26	12	6
Gurney	61	83	43	15	25
Rony	250	69	—	—	—
Bauer	275	73	—	—	—
Mossberg	270	80	36	12	32
Angel	116	78	36	15	25
Iverson	40	77	25	20	32
Withers	100	84	28	13	43
Craddock	78	63	—	—	—
Bray	239	69	33	11	25

From Bray GA: The inheritance of corpulence. In Cioffi LA, James WPT, VanItallie TB (eds): The Body Weight Regulatory System: Normal and Disturbed Mechanisms. New York, Raven Press, 1981. Reproduced by permission. References for the studies cited in the table may be found in the original publication.

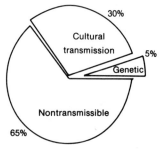

BMI and amount of subcutaneous fat

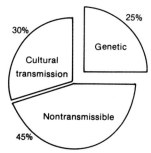

Percent body fat and fat mass.

FIGURE 28-2

Total transmissible variance and its genetic component for indicators of subcutaneous and total body fat. (From Bouchard C et al: Int J Obes 12:205, 1988. (Reproduced by permission.)

individual patients. The correlation between BMI and total body fat (TBF) or percent body fat (%BF) is quite good in large and heterogeneous samples (i.e., about .6 to .8). The predictive value of the BMI is less impressive in an individual subject, especially when the BMI is below 30 kg/m² or so. At higher BMI values, the relationship with body fat is better. It should be kept in mind that the BMI is an indicator of heaviness and only indirectly an indicator of body fat.[6,22] Any estimate of genetic effect on BMI is bound to be influenced by the contribution of the genotype to fat mass, muscle mass, skeletal mass, and other components. Nevertheless, the additive genetic effect on the BMI is worth considering because of the growing popularity of this measure in the clinical assessment of obesity. On theoretical grounds, the proposal that a major gene effect may be present in the distribution of BMI scores is not justified.[32]

Using a model of path analysis,[19] we studied the relative importance of genetic and nongenetic (cultural) components of inheritance as well as the nontransmissible effect in the BMI phenotype after controlling for variations in age and sex.[12] The data were obtained in 1698 members of 409 families that represented nine types of relatives by descent or adoption. Using the correlations computed for each of these kinds of relatives, we reported a total transmissible variance across generations of about 35%, but a genetic effect of only 5% (Fig. 28-2). The nontransmissible variance (about 65%) may in part reflect the fact that several tissues with their own pattern of transmission contribute to the phenotype, or may suggest that the BMI is indeed quite sus-

ceptible to life-style and environmental conditions. The data do indicate that the BMI as an index of heaviness is not characterized by a significant heritability component.

Skin-fold measurements at various sites of the body can be used to estimate the amount of subcutaneous fat. From recent reviews,[11,24] parent-child correlations ranging from .15 to .25 and sibling correlations ranging from .20 to .40 are typical for individual skin-fold measurements. Typically, correlations are higher for dizygotic twins (.4 to .5) and highest for monozygotic twins (.8 to .9).

A more reliable estimate of the amount of subcutaneous fat can be obtained from the sum of several skin folds, particularly if they are equally distributed over the trunk and the upper and lower extremities. Such data (the sum of six skin folds) were available on the familial cohort described above. Using a path analysis procedure, we reported[12] a total transmission effect across generations of about 40%, a transmission effect comparable to that reported by other investigators.[17,20,26] However, the additive genetic component reached only about 5% (see Fig. 28-2), demonstrating that most of the transmission effect had nothing to do with the genotype.[12] In other words, most of the individual differences in skin-fold thicknesses (subcutaneous fat) are independent of the genotype and are associated with the determinants of energy balance, i.e., habitual energy intake and total habitual energy expenditures.

To the best of our knowledge, we have been alone in reporting on the genetic effect in fat mass and %BF measured with one of the accepted direct methods.[12] In this research, we performed underwater weighing measurements of body density in a relatively large number of individuals belonging to the same nine different kinds of relatives. After adjustment for age and sex, about half of the variance in fat mass or %BF was associated with a transmissible effect, and 25% of the variance was an additive genetic effect (see Fig. 28-2). In light of our observations on the low heritability of subcutaneous fat, it is not unreasonable to suggest that the genetic effect seen in fat mass is caused primarily by the deep fat or visceral fat component of fat mass.

Our study was conducted on a sample of normal-weight individuals with only a minority of obese subjects. The genetic epidemiology of human obesity based on large samples of lean and obese subjects, with a valid assessment of body fat, is a task for the future. It should also be recognized that geneticists have not considered to a large extent maternal or paternal effects, X-linked or Y-linked effects, sex-limited effects or major gene effects in the human obesity phenotypes. In one report based largely on normal-weight and moderately overweight subjects, we showed that no specific maternal or paternal effects and no sex-limited effects could be detected for subcutaneous fat or TBF.[12] Unfortunately such data are not available on populations of obese subjects.

Heritability of Abdominal Fat

Excess body fat and obesity have long been recognized as risk factors in the etiology of arteriosclerosis, non-insulin-dependent diabetes, hypertension, and other degenerative conditions associated with a higher death rate. More recently it has been shown that abdominal obesity (the so-called male or android profile of fat deposition) is by itself an independent risk factor that carries an even higher risk than excess body fat per se. Four symposia held in the past few years have been instrumental in bringing together the evidence from five prospective studies and from a score of experimental research studies on the metabolic complications associated with abdominal obesity.[3,10,25,31] The available clinical and experimental data justify the conclusion that abdominal obesity is of particular importance for health and disease.

What do we know about the role of heredity in fat topography in general and abdominal fat in particular? We studied this issue in the cohort of families described above.[5,9,11,12] Figure 28-3 illustrates the results we obtained for two general indicators of regional fat distribution: the ratio of three trunk skin-fold measurements (abdominal, suprailiac, and subscapular) to three extremity skin-fold measurements (biceps, triceps, and medial calf), and the ratio of subcutaneous fat (sum of six skin-fold measurements) to total fat mass (from underwater weighing). The distribution of subcutaneous fat in the trunk relative to the limbs exhibits a genetic effect of about 25%, while the ratio of subcutaneous fat to fat mass is characterized by a heritability coefficient of about 30%.

The most important question is, what is the role of the genotype in abdominal fat accumulation? No data have been reported on the genetics

FIGURE 28-3

Total transmissible variance and its genetic component for indicators of regional fat distribution. (Adapted from Bouchard C et al: Int J Obes 12:205, 1988. Reproduced by permission.)

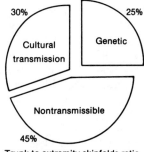

Trunk to extremity skinfolds ratio

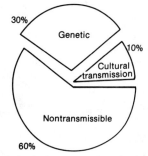

Ratio of subcutaneous fat to fat mass

TABLE 28-2

Total Transmissible Variance Across Generations and Its Heritable Component for Two Indicators of Abdominal Fat Without and with Adjustment for Total Subcutaneous Fat

Variable	Total Transmissible Variance	Biologic Inheritance	Cultural Inheritance	Nontransmissible Variance
Abdominal skin fold	.28	.01	.27	.72
Abdominal + suprailiac skin folds	.36	.10	.26	.64
Scores Adjusted for Sum of Six Skin Folds				
Abdominal skin fold	.33	.20	.13	.67
Abdominal + suprailiac skin folds	.58	.25	.32	.42

Adapted from Bouchard.[5,8] The scores were first adjusted for age and gender and then further adjusted for the sum of six skin-fold measurements representing total subcutaneous fat. Correlations in nine types of relatives by descent or by adoption were analyzed using the BETA path analysis program.

of abdominal visceral fat. However, unpublished material from our laboratory clearly demonstrates that the genotype is the main determinant of individual differences in the amount of visceral fat deposition under chronic long-term overfeeding conditions (Bouchard et al, unpublished results). Even though the amount of subcutaneous fat is primarily influenced by nongenetic factors, there is some evidence that the size of the total abdominal fat depot after adjustment for total fat is significantly affected by genotype.[7,8] This conclusion is supported by the data summarized in Table 28-2. As shown in the table, the amount of subcutaneous abdominal fat exhibits a genetic effect of about 20% and more when the total amount of subcutaneous fat is taken into consideration. These results suggest that for a given level of fatness, the size of the abdominal fat depot varies among individuals, and these variations are significantly influenced by the genotype of the individual. Similar findings were obtained when abdominal fat (abdominal skin fold or the sum of abdominal and suprailiac skin folds) was studied after statistical adjustments for the sum of six skin folds or the densitometrically derived fat mass.

Heritability of Energy Expenditures

Research data are now available on four components of human energy expenditure: habitual

physical activity level, energy cost of submaximal exercise (TEE), resting metabolic rate (RMR), and thermic effect of a meal (TEM). A recent report has suggested that the habitual physical activity level, estimated from a three-day activity record, was significantly influenced by undetermined genetic characteristics, the heritability coefficient reaching about 25% to 30% of the variance.[27] These results were suggestive of inherited differences primarily in the spontaneous level of activity and not for activities of higher energy costs such as exercise and sport participation.

The energy cost of submaximal exercise is an important element in the total energy balance equation, as there are differences in oxygen uptake for a given power output. TEE was studied during submaximal cycle ergometer work loads in 22 pairs of dizygotic twins and 31 pairs of monozygotic twins. Evidence for a rather high ($\geq$45%) genetic effect was found at low power output, but the genetic effect disappeared when the energy expenditure reached about six times the resting metabolic rate level.[14]

RMR[14,21] and TEM[14] were studied in several sets of parent-child pairs and dizygotic and monozygotic twins.[14,21] When RMR was adjusted for differences in body composition, the genetic effect remained significant in all cases. Thus, for RMR per kg of fat-free mass, the genetic effect reached about 40% of the total variance of the phenotype.[14] TEM was studied after a 4.2

TABLE 28-3

Correlation in Various Relatives for the Resting Metabolic Rate (RMR) and Thermic Effect of a 1000 kcal Carbohydrate Meal (TEM)

Variable	Parent-Child (31 pairs)	DZ Twins (21 pairs)	MZ Twins (37 pairs)
RMR (kJ/kg FFM)	.21	.30	.77
TEM (% of intake)	.30	.35	.52

Adapted from Bouchard et al.[14] Interclass correlation for parent-child pairs; intraclass coefficient for the twin samples. When the RMR data were adjusted by regression for the effects of fat-free mass, the correlations were not significantly altered.

MJ (1000 kcal) carbohydrate meal. Our results showed that genetic effect accounted for at least 40% of the variation in the energy expended over RMR during four hours after the meal test. Some of the correlations used for the computation of these heritability estimates in RMR and TEM are summarized in Table 28-3.

It is increasingly clear that there are inherited differences in spontaneous activity level, energy cost of light submaximal exercise, resting metabolic rate, and thermic effect of food. It is not known whether these various genetic effects are generated by the same genetic system or if they arise from independent genetic characteristics. In any case, genetically determined differences in energy expenditure, particularly those close to the resting metabolic rate level, may have considerable significance for understanding the inherited susceptibility to obesity.

Adaptation to Overfeeding in Identical Twins

The low to moderate additive genetic effect (i.e., a range of 5% to about 30%, depending on the phenotype) that we have reported thus far for some of the human body fat components does not imply that genetic factors have little or nothing to do with the development of obesity or with body fat topography. It is generally recognized that some individuals are prone to excessive accumulation of fat, for whom losing weight represents a continuous battle, whereas others seem relatively well protected against such a menace. We have recently tried to test whether such differences could be accounted for by genetic factors. We asked whether there were differences in the sensitivity of individuals to gain fat when chronically exposed to a positive energy balance and whether such differences were dependent or independent of the genotype. If the answer to both of these questions was affirmative, then one would have to conclude that there was a significant genotype-environment interaction effect. The results from one experiment suggest that such an effect exists for body fat.

We submitted both members of monozygotic twin pairs to a similar experimental treatment and compared intrapair (within genotype) and interpair (between genotypes) resemblances in the response.[7] Six pairs of male monozygotic twins ate 4.2 MJ (1000 kal)/day caloric surplus for 22 consecutive days.[13,28] Significant increases in body weight, sum of nine skin-fold measurements, and fat mass were observed after the period of overfeeding. The data showed that there were considerable interindividual differences in the adaptation to excess calories and that the variation observed was not randomly distributed, as indicated by the significant within-pair resemblance in response.

The intrapair resemblance in the response to overfeeding was quite high. For instance, the intraclass correlation of .88 for fat mass indicates that almost 90% of the variance in the response of fat mass to overfeeding is found between genotypes (between pairs), while only about 10% is found within pairs; i.e., members of the same pair tended to gain weight equally. These data indicate that some individuals are more at risk than others to gain fat. In other words, the amount of fat stored in response to a given caloric surplus is probably influenced by the genotype of the individual. These are exciting findings that we recently confirmed in a study using a more prolonged period of overfeeding (Bouchard et al, unpublished).

In these six pairs of overfed twins, RMR, TEM for a 4.2-MJ meal of mixed composition, and TEE were determined before and after the 22-day experimental treatment. Changes in RMR (intrapair resemblance = .63), TEM (intrapair resemblance = .62) and TEE (intrapair resemblance = .78) were also partly genotype dependent.[13,29] Multiple correlation studies indicated that much of the variance in the response of fat mass to overfeeding was accounted for by the changes in RMR, TEM, and TEE (R = .65). This implies that the genotype-overfeeding interaction effect observed in fat mass gain seems to be partly mediated by these three energy expenditure components, themselves characterized by significant genotype-overfeeding interaction effects.[13] These data suggest that chronic overfeeding alters the components of energy expenditure in a manner that differs more between identical twin pairs than among members of the same pairs. The most likely explanation for these observations is that the genotype is an important determinant of the variations encountered in response to given conditions of energy intake. Figure 28-4 illustrates schematically the conclusions that we have reached from this research.

Summary

From the studies reviewed here, we conclude the following points in regard to biologic inheritance in human body fat variation. The additive genetic effect in the amount of subcutaneous fat is quite low, but it is higher (around 25% to 30%) for fat mass and regional fat distribution. These results suggest that visceral fat is perhaps more influenced by the genotype than subcutaneous fat. Body energy gains following overfeeding vary among individuals and are partly genotype dependent. The limited data available suggest that the genotype accounts for a significant proportion ($\geq$40%) of the individual differences in resting metabolic rate, thermic effect of food, and energy cost of light exercise. Individual differences in habitual physical activity level (about 25%) may be characterized by a significant genetic component. The search for genetic markers of the various obesity phenotypes has not been initiated to any extent at this time. However, one can anticipate considerable development in this area in the coming decade.

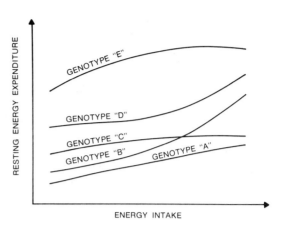

FIGURE 28-4

Variations in energy intake cause changes in energy expenditure which are influenced by the genotype.

Acknowledgment: This work was supported in part by FRSQ of Quebec, FCAR of Quebec, Health and Welfare Canada, Medical Research Council of Canada, NSERC of Canada, and the National Institutes of Health (U.S.A). Drs A. Tremblay, J.P. Després, G. Thériault, L. Pérusse, M.R. Boulay, and C. Leblanc contributed to our research over the years.

References

1. Annest JL, Sing CF, Biron P et al: Familial aggregation of blood pressure and weight in adoptive families. III. Analysis of the role of shared genes and shared household environment in explaining family resemblance for height, weight and selected weight/height indices. Am J Epidemiol 117:492, 1983

2. Björntorp B: Morphological classifications of obesity: What they tell us, what they don't. Int J Obes 8:525, 1984

3. Björntorp P, Smith U, Lönnroth P (eds): Health Implications of Regional Obesity. Proceedings of the

Fourth Acta Medica Scandinavica Symposium, Supplement 723, 1988

4. Bouchard C: Genetic factors in obesity. Med Clin North Am 73:67, 1989

5. Bouchard C: Genetic factors in the regulation of adipose tissue distribution. Acta Med Scand Suppl 723:135, 1988

6. Bouchard C: Genetics of body fat, energy expenditure and adipose tissue metabolism. In Berry EM, Blondheim SH, Eliahou HE et al (eds): Recent Advances in Obesity Research. V. London, John Libbey & Co, 1987

7. Bouchard C: Human adaptability may have a genetic basis. In Landry F (ed): Health Risk Estimation, Risk Reduction and Health Promotion. Ottawa, Canadian Public Health Association, 1983

8. Bouchard C: Inheritance of human fat distribution. In Bouchard C, Johnston FE (eds): Fat Distribution during Growth and Later Health Outcomes. New York, Alan R Liss, 1988

9. Bouchard C: Inheritance of human fat distribution and adipose tissue metabolism. In Vague J, Björntorp B, Guy-Grand B et al (eds): Metabolic Complications of Human Obesities. Amsterdam, Elsevier Science Publishers, 1985

10. Bouchard C, Johnston FE (eds): Fat Distribution during Growth and Later Health Outcomes. Curr Top Nutr Dis 17:374, 1988

11. Bouchard C, Pérusse L: Heredity and body fat. Annu Rev Nutr 8:259, 1988

12. Bouchard C, Pérusse L, Leblanc C et al: Inheritance of the amount and distribution of human body fat. Int J Obes 12:205, 1988

13. Bouchard C, Tremblay A, Després JP et al: Sensitivity to overfeeding: The Québec experiment with identical twins. Prog Food Nutr Sci 12:45, 1988

14. Bouchard C, Tremblay A, Nadeau A et al: Genetic effect in resting and exercise metabolic rates. Metabolism (in press)

15. Bray GA: Definition, measurement, and classification of the syndromes of obesity. In Bray GA (ed): Obesity. Kroc Foundation Symposium on Comparative Methods of Weight Control. London, John Libbey & Co, 1984

16. Bray GA: The inheritance of corpulence. In Cioffi LA, James WPT, VanItallie TB (eds): The Body Weight Regulatory System: Normal and Disturbed Mechanisms. New York, Raven Press, 1981

17. Byard PJ, Sharma K, Russell JM et al: A family study of anthropometric traits in a Punjabi community. Am J Phys Anthropol 64:97, 1984

18. Callaway CW, Greenwood MRC: Introduction to the workshop on methods for characterizing human obesity. Int J Obes 8:477, 1984

19. Cloninger CR, Rice J, Reich T: Multifactorial inheritance with cultural transmission and assortative mating. II. A general model of combined polygenic and cultural inheritance. Am J Hum Genet 31:176, 1979

20. Devor EJ, McGue M, Crawford MH et al: Transmissible and nontransmissible components of anthropometric variation in the Alexanderwohl Mennonites. II. Resolution by path analysis. Am J Phys Anthropol 69:83, 1986

21. Fontaine E, Savard R, Tremblay A et al: Resting metabolic rate in monozygotic and dizygotic twins. Acta Genet Med Gemellol 34:41, 1985

22. Garn SM, Leonard WR, Hawthorne VM: Three limitations of the body mass index. Am J Clin Nutr 44:996, 1986

23. Longini IM, Higgins MW, Hinton PC et al: Genetic and environmental sources of familial aggregation of body mass in Tecumseh, Michigan. Hum Biol 56:733, 1984

24. Mueller WH: The genetics of human fatness. Yearbook Phys Anthropol 26:215, 1983

25. Norgan NG (ed): Human Body Composition and Fat Distribution, p 250. European Nutrition Report 8. Wageningen, Stichting Nederlands Instituut voor de Voeding, 1986

26. Pérusse L, Leblanc C, Bouchard C: Inter-generation transmission of physical fitness in the Canadian population. Can J Sports Sci 13:8, 1988

27. Pérusse L, Tremblay A, Leblanc C et al: Genetic and familial environmental influences in physical activity level. Am J Epidemiol (in press)

28. Poelhman ET, Tremblay A, Després JP et al: Genotype-controlled changes in body composition and fat morphology following overfeeding in twins. Am J Clin Nutr 43:723, 1986

29. Poehlman ET, Tremblay A, Fontaine E et al: Genotype dependency of the thermic effect of a meal and associated hormonal changes following short-term overfeeding. Metabolism 35:30, 1986

30. Vague J: Les obésités: Etude biométrique. Biol Med 36:1, 1947

31. Vague J, Björntorp B, Guy-Grand B et al (eds): Metabolic Complications of Human Obesities. Amsterdam, Elsevier Science Publishers, 1985

32. Zonta LA, Jayakar SD, Bosisio M et al: Genetic analysis of human obesity in an Italian sample. Hum Hered 37:129, 1987

CHAPTER 29

Psychological Aspects
of Human Obesity

ALBERT J. STUNKARD and THOMAS A. WADDEN

This chapter describes recent advances in our understanding of two important psychological aspects of human obesity. The first is the relationship between psychopathology and obesity; the second is the development of the concept of restrained eating. In each case, systematic psychological assessment has moved the field beyond the clinical impressions that had prevailed in the past to new and sometimes revolutionary changes in perspective. Nowhere has such change been more revolutionary than in our views of the relationship between psychopathology and human obesity. Here there has been a 180-degree change in direction in our views of causality during the past two decades. From viewing psychopathology as a (or even the) cause of obesity, we now see it as a result—of living in a society that derogates obesity and obese persons. We have changed from a primarily psychogenic explanation of obesity to a primarily somatogenic one.

THE PSYCHOGENIC THEORY
OF OBESITY

Traditionally, the role of psychological factors in human obesity has been viewed in terms of deviance. For centuries this deviance had been defined by theological norms as sin, the mortal sin of gluttony. More recently the norms have been psychiatric ones, and the deviance has been characterized as emotional disturbance and failed impulse control. Obese persons were viewed as suffering inordinately from such disorders.

The psychogenic theory of obesity, widely accepted for many years, held that obesity resulted from an emotional disorder in which food intake, particularly excessive food intake, relieved the anxiety and depression to which obese persons were unusually susceptible. Psychoanalytic theorists traced the origins of obesity to the oral stage of libidinal development, ascribing problems to a deprivation or an excess of oral supplies.[7,18] The resulting fixation of libido at the oral stage rendered obese persons unusually susceptible to early emotional conflicts and frustrations, which were reactivated in periods of stress in adult life. When faced with these reactivated conflicts, obese persons were regarded as unusually prone to regression to the oral stage of development and thus to excess eating.

These postulated psychodynamics were accepted for many years, in part because they helped to explain five major problems in the treatment of obesity. Three of these problems—not entering treatment, dropping out of treatment, and failing to lose weight—were interpreted as the result of disinclination on the part of obese persons to risk the loss of the oral supplies on which they were dependent. The fourth problem, depression, was attributed to loss of these supplies, and the fifth problem, regaining of weight following treatment, was explained as a result of overeating undertaken in an attempt to restore the supplies.

For many years the psychogenic theory seemed to provide an adequate explanation of these treatment problems. Moreover, it served a useful psychological function for its authors. If the origins of obesity lay in profound psychological disturbances buried deep within the patient, the responsibility for treatment failure similarly lay with the patient.

New explanations of the problems in treating obesity came from two sources. One source was the convincing biologic explanations of the etiology of obesity. The other source was a systematic assessment of the nature and extent of the psychological problems of obese persons. It would be hard to overestimate the importance of the study and measurement of social and psychological variables in contributing to the revolution in our understanding of psychology and obesity. One of the first discoveries, with important implications for this revolution, arose from careful measurement of the extent of psychopathology among obese persons.

MEASUREMENT OF PSYCHOPATHOLOGY AMONG OBESE PERSONS

Population Studies

The long-standing belief that obese persons suffer disproportionately from emotional disturbances has been shown to be incorrect. This belief was first challenged by Moore and her colleagues in a study of 1660 people in midtown Manhattan.[25] They found that obese persons scored somewhat higher than nonobese persons on only three of nine measures of psychopathology. Wadden and Stunkard's review of six subsequent large studies, furthermore, found no difference, and in two of their studies obese persons actually had lower levels of psychopathology than their nonobese counterparts.[50]

The results of studies of obese children parallel those of adults. In the two largest studies of U.S. population samples, those of Sallade[36] and of Wadden et al,[49] levels of self-esteem in obese children and adolescents were similar to those in their nonobese peers, with all scores falling well within normal limits.

Studies of Clinical Populations

In contrast to studies of the obese population as a whole, there have been several reports of increased psychopathology among severely overweight persons seeking dietary or surgical treatment. These studies have typically used the Minnesota Multiphasic Personality Inventory (MMPI) to assess psychopathology,[12] and ten such studies found at least mild elevations in scores for depression, often with elevations on scales measuring hypochondriasis, hysteria, and impulsivity.

By failing to include appropriate control groups, many of these reports overstated the magnitude of psychopathology in obese patients. This is a critical omission, for patients in medical and surgical clinics often display high levels of psychopathology on psychological tests, as demonstrated by Swenson and colleagues in studies of 18,328 patients at the Mayo Clinic.[18] Other studies that have included appropriate control groups have found few differences in psychopathology between obese and nonobese persons in clinical settings.

These findings refuted the age-old belief that overweight persons are more emotionally disabled than persons of normal weight. As such, they went some distance toward dismantling the psychogenic theory of obesity. They did not, however, address the psychological problems that may be specific to obese persons, problems that may not be apparent on the relatively nonspecific rating scales. Recent studies have explored these problems, with results that are important to our understanding of psychological factors in human obesity.

Studies of Psychopathology Specific to Obese Persons

A search for psychological problems specific to obese persons began with clinical assessments of the kind of problems they report. Such problems revolve around weight-specific issues such as dissatisfaction with physical appearance, the stress of dieting, and a sense of isolation due to the failure of family and friends to understand the frustrations of a weight problem in today's society. Once these issues had been identified, more focused clinical and psychometric research was directed toward their elucidation. Three major types of psychological problems specific to obese have been studied: disparagement of the body image, symptoms of dieting, and bulimia.

Disparagement of the Body Image

Some obese persons view their bodies as grotesque and loathesome and believe that others view them with hostility and contempt. Such persons with body image disparagement may be completely preoccupied with their obesity and related feelings of self-loathing.[44,45]

Given the prevalence of prejudice against the obese, one might expect all obese persons to despise their own physical appearance, but such is not the case. Emotionally healthy obese persons show no body image disparagement. The disturbance is most often seen in young women of middle and upper-middle socioeconomic status, groups in which obesity is less prevalent and the sanctions against it are stronger. It seems confined to persons who have been obese since childhood, who have a generalized neurotic disturbance, and whose parents and friends have chided them for their overweight. Adolescence appears to be the period of greatest risk for the development of the disorder.[45]

Symptoms of Dieting

Sanctions against overweight and the prevailing obsession with thinness are powerful incentives for obese persons to diet. Unfortunately, dieting itself may be a source of psychological disturbance. The occurrence of emotional disturbance during dieting was first reported in 1957 when it was noted that more than half of dieters experienced depression, nervousness, weakness, or irritability.[41] Subsequently other adverse emotional reactions have been observed in a variety of reducing regimens.[47] These symptoms resemble those reported by Keys and associates in their study of normal-weight male volunteers on semistarvation diets.[20] In the course of losing one quarter of their body weight, these men experienced depression, weakness, diminished libido, and preoccupation with food. These symptoms have been attributed to a reduction in body weight below a biologic set-point. It is tempting to speculate that the same biologic pressures may

account for the symptoms experienced by obese persons when they diet.[42]

Binge-Eating

In addition to its potential to provoke untoward emotional reactions, dieting may be a precipitating factor in the development of bulimia. This eating disorder is characterized by episodes of binge eating, followed by vomiting or other purging, depressed mood, and self-deprecating thoughts. The disorder occurs in persons of all weights, and it has been estimated that 5% of all obese persons are bulimic. Unlike their nonobese counterparts, obese persons rarely vomit after binging, so they must cope with increased weight in addition to the burden of a distressing pattern of behavior.[41]

The role of dieting in the onset of bulimia has been suggested by both clinical reports and epidemiologic surveys, which indicate that the severe form of the disorder—bulimia nervosa—usually begins during a period of severe dietary restriction. For example, 83% of subjects reported by Fairburn and Cooper[6] and 88% reported by Pyle and associates[30] were dieting at the time of their initial binge-purge episode, even though most subjects were not overweight. Ironically, the role of dieting has not been closely examined in obese persons because it is viewed as appropriate.[51] Nonetheless, severe dietary restriction may have the same negative behavioral consequences in obese persons as it does in both normal-weight and underweight persons.

The desperation and compulsiveness with which many persons seek to lose weight reflect the prevailing climate of intolerance toward obesity. This climate is surely a factor in the recent increase in the prevalence of bulimia and anorexia nervosa. Both disorders represent an intense fear of becoming overweight and thus the object of scorn and ridicule.

Studies of the psychopathology specific to obese persons make it clear that this psychopathology has its origins in strong and pervasive social attitudes that derogate obesity and obese people. These attitudes are widely recognized, yet they have been subjected to only limited investigation. This investigation nevertheless has confirmed the presence of widespread prejudice and discrimination against obese persons.

STUDIES OF PREJUDICE AND DISCRIMINATION

Prejudice and discrimination subject obese persons to severe psychological stress. Contempt for the obese and preoccupation with thinness are everywhere evident. The strong prejudice against the obese cuts across age, sex, race, and socioeconomic status.[1] It begins as early as childhood.

Staffieri has shown that children no more than six years of age describe silhouettes of an obese child as "lazy, dirty, stupid, ugly, cheats, and liars."[40] Goodman, Richardson, and their colleagues showed black-and-white line drawings of a normal-weight child, an obese child, and children with various handicaps, including missing hands and facial disfigurement, to a variety of audiences.[10,23,31] Both children and adults rated the obese child as the least likable. This prejudice extends across races, across rural and urban dwellers, and, saddest of all, even to obese persons themselves.

Obese persons must contend not only with prejudice but also with discrimination, the behavioral enactment of prejudice. Discrimination against obese persons is as widespread as prejudice. Even though discrimination is less readily acknowledged and is harder to document, a surprising amount of evidence has been amassed. One example is college admission. Canning and Mayer found lower acceptance rates into prestigious colleges for obese high school students compared to normal-weight students, even though the two groups did not differ in high school performance, academic qualifications, or application rates to colleges.[3] Similarly, Pargaman found obese students seriously underrepresented in a private college in the Northeast.[28]

The problems do not end with college. Obese persons face discrimination in seeking employment and on the job.[1] Larkin and Pines found that employers rate overweight individuals as less desirable employees than normal-weight individuals, even when they believe the two groups have the same abilities.[22] In one particularly revealing study, Roe and Eickwort found that 16% of employers said they would not hire obese women under any condition, and an additional 44% would not hire them under certain circumstances.[32] Such discrimination is understandable if these employers shared the negative attitudes toward obese job applicants of those studied by Klesges and his colleagues (unpublished findings). Despite comparable qualifications, obese applicants were viewed as having poorer work habits and more likely to have unjustified work absences and to abuse company privileges by feigning illness. An interesting survey published in 1974 in *Industry Week* placed a dollar value on discrimination against obese executives.[16] Only 9% of executives with salaries of $25,000 to $50,000 were more than ten pounds overweight, whereas 39% of those earning $10,000 to $20,000 were comparably overweight. Each pound of fat cost an executive $1,000 a year.

The uniformed services and police and fire departments will not enlist severely overweight persons and often reprimand or discharge persons who fail to maintain an acceptable weight.[1] Even obese persons holding physically nondemanding jobs may experience weight-related discrimination.

Weight-related discrimination may extend to other social institutions, including marriage. For women, weight is a key to social mobility, primarily via marriage. In midtown Manhattan, Goldblatt and his colleagues found that almost twice as many obese women (22%) were downwardly socially mobile as were upwardly socially mobile (12%).[9]

Finally, and painfully, health care providers all too often share the prevailing contempt for the obese. For example, Maddox and Liederman found that one group of 77 physicians described their obese patients as "weak-willed . . . ugly . . . awkward."[24] Keys has confirmed the general antipathy of physicians toward the obese and has suggested that it is based on the belief that obese persons are self-indulgent and "hence at least faintly immoral and inviting retribution."[19] There is no evidence that retribution is of benefit to obese patients.

It is clear that systematic assessment of the mental health of obese persons has advanced our understanding of the relationship between psychopathology and obesity, with a 180-degree change in direction in our idea of causality. In addition, systematic assessment has advanced our understanding of another psychological aspect of obesity—eating behavior.

THE CONCEPT OF RESTRAINED EATING

For the past decade and more, one theory about human eating behavior and its disorders has stood out—the concept of "restrained eating."[14] As the term implies, restrained eating refers to the tendency to restrict food intake in order to control body weight. It is a timely theory in today's climate of widespread preoccupation with body weight.

Historical Perspective

The idea of restrained eating arose during the period when Schachter's "externality" theory of obesity was at the height of its popularity.[38] This theory proposed that obesity arose from a distinctive "external" style of eating, the result of an unusual susceptibility to food cues in the environment. In attempting to elucidate Schachter's theory, Nisbett, one of his students, described "some striking behavioral parallels between obese individuals and hungry individuals."[26] He suggested that obese people "are actually in a chronic state of energy deficit" because of holding their weight below its biologically dictated set-point and are "genuinely hungry." He concluded that this hunger rather than their obesity rendered their eating style "external."

Herman, another student of Schachter, proposed finding out if obese people were "genuinely hungry" because of holding their weight below a set-point simply by asking them. To this end he devised a questionnaire and an ingenious experiment.[13] The striking results of this first experiment triggered a burst of research that continues to the present day.

The experiment involved measurement of the amount of ice cream eaten during a "taste test" that was preceded by either a milkshake preload or no preload.[13] After consuming a milkshake, persons whose eating was judged to be unrestrained ate less during the subsequent ice cream "taste test." "Restrained eaters," defined by high scores on a Restraint Scale, however, behaved very differently. After consuming a milkshake, they ate more!

This paradoxical behavior, termed "counterregulation" by Herman,[13] has been the object of a large amount of research that has replicated it many times among persons of normal weight.[33] Further studies showed that the paradoxical overeating was triggered by the *perception* of the caloric content of the preload rather than by its actual content.[29,39,52] Even the anticipation of a preload had the same effect as an actual preload.[34]

Despite the fact that restraint theory had developed in an effort to understand the eating behavior of obese persons, the original research was carried out largely on persons of normal weight, primarily female college students. This approach seemed reasonable since, following Nisbett, Herman assumed that obese people were restricting their body weight, and the Restraint Scale identified such restriction. In fact, Hibscher and Herman proposed that the "external" and "obese" characteristics of obese people arose from their dieting and not from their obesity; if these characteristics were more common among obese people, it was simply because they dieted more often.[15] Problems with the Restraint Scale, however, began to appear when it was applied to obese persons.

The first problem was the failure of the Restraint Scale to predict the behavior of obese persons, even that most robust of findings, counterregulation, or overeating after a preload. Obese persons did not overeat after a preload; they actually ate less.[33,35]

The second problem with the Restraint Scale lay in its construct validity: it measures not only the dietary restraint or "concern for dieting" for which it had been designed, but also a very different construct—weight fluctuation (in pounds).[4,33] Since weight fluctuation is a characteristic of obesity and is highly correlated with percentage overweight, the Restraint Scale has limited applicability to obese persons.

The problems with the Restraint Scale do not extend to the concept of restrained eating, which remains seminal. For example, a single question about dietary restraint was sufficient to distinguish obese persons who overate in a fast food shop from those who did not.[43] The question was, "Are you the kind of person who eats less than you want to in order to control your weight?"

Development of the Eating Inventory

Problems with the Restraint Scale became apparent about the time that efforts began to develop scales that, although also theoretically informed, were more empirically derived. One such scale was the Eating Inventory, which was developed through repeated testing of persons selected to represent the extremes of dietary restraint and lack of restraint, as well as persons intermediate between the extremes.[46] Factor analysis of the responses of 300 persons yielded three major factors that were refined by successive iteration of the analytic process. The final result was a 51-item scale with three stable, independent factors—cognitive restraint, disinhibition and hunger. Examples of subject statements representing the three factors are: "I do not eat some foods because they make me fat" (cognitive restraint), "Sometimes when I start eating, I just can't seem to stop" (disinhibition), and "I often feel so hungry that I just have to have something to eat" (hunger).

The factor structure of the Eating Inventory has been replicated, most notably by Ganley's study of 442 unselected women.[8] Furthermore, the Eating Inventory appears to measure what it purports to measure. Thus, Laessle and his colleagues measured the daily food intake of 60 healthy young women of normal weight and related it to their scores on the Eating Inventory and the Restraint Scale.[21] The cognitive restraint score of the Eating Inventory correlated $-.46$ ($P < .0001$) with mean daily caloric intake, whereas the Restraint Scale correlated with caloric intake at no more than a nonsignificant $-.04$.

Clinical Applications of the Eating Inventory

Information about the Eating Inventory has been derived largely from clinical applications. It has been used in a number of research projects that have included control groups of persons of normal weight. Measurements obtained in the course of seven studies are listed in Table 29-1, which provides norms for the three factors of the Eating Inventory against which values obtained

TABLE 29-1

Means and Standard Deviations for Normal (Control) Samples

Sample*	N	Factor I: Cognitive Restraint		Factor II: Disinhibition		Factor III: Hunger	
		Mean	(SD)	Mean	(SD)	Mean	(SD)
Unrestrained eaters[46]	62	6.0	(5.5)	5.6	(4.3)	7.0	(4.3)
U.S. control sample (Ganley, unpubl.)	30	11.0	(5.3)	5.2	(2.5)	4.0	(2.6)
Young German women[21]	60	6.6	(4.7)	6.4	(3.5)	4.9	(3.1)
Swedish control group[2]	58	9.8	(4.2)	4.2	(2.8)	2.9	(2.3)
Chilean university students[37]	67	7.7	(5.1)	5.4	(3.1)	4.8	(3.1)
Japanese junior college students[27]	254	5.5	(3.5)	6.9	(2.8)	6.0	(2.9)
Japanese nursing students[27]	270	6.3	(3.6)	6.5	(2.7)	4.9	(2.6)
English control group[6]	35	7.0	(4.7)	—	—	—	—
Pooled estimates		6.6	(4.1)	6.2	(3.0)	5.2	(2.9)

*The first sample in the list included 22 males out of a total of 62 subjects; all other samples were exclusively female.

in studies of clinical conditions can be compared. All but one of these studies dealt exclusively with women, reflecting the strong gender differences in concern with eating behavior.

Obesity

The most important applications of the Eating Inventory have been in the assessment and treatment of obesity. There are major differences between the Eating Inventory scores of obese people who are in treatment and of those who are not. If we consider first obese persons who are not in treatment, scores on cognitive restraint do not differ from those of people of normal weight, whereas the disinhibition and hunger scores are somewhat higher. In marked contrast, obese persons in treatment have greatly elevated cognitive restraint scores[2] (Bjorvell, unpublished findings; Ganley, unpublished findings). Furthermore, an increase in the cognitive restraint score is associated with a favorable outcome. In one study the correlation between cognitive restraint scores and weight loss increased over time.[2]

Just as high scores on cognitive restraint can predict a good outcome, low scores can predict a bad outcome. One particularly bad outcome is dropping out of treatment. In a recent commercial weight loss program involving 94 obese persons, dropping out of treatment was predicted by a combination of low restraint scores and high hunger scores (LaPorte and Stunkard, unpublished findings).

Cognitive restraint scores are becoming a useful tool in the treatment of obesity. They appear able to predict response to treatment and may even be helpful in selecting patients, including particularly the exclusion from treatment of patients whose poor prognosis suggests expensive failures. They may be, as Bjorvell's results suggest,[2] a useful monitor of progress in treatment. They can, for example, supplement information about weight loss with a measure of psychological changes, confirming evident progress or suggesting the need for special treatment measures.

Smoking Cessation

Weight gain is a major problem following smoking cessation. Many people, particularly women, are reluctant to attempt smoking cessation for this reason. Yet some persons gain little or no weight, and it would be helpful if we could tell who they are. The Eating Inventory has permitted a start in this direction. The disinhibition factor not only predicts weight gain following smoking cessation[11] but also overeating on the classic ice cream taste test experiment.[5]

Bulimia

The Eating Inventory has been used to assess bulimia in four studies, the largest of which was Nogami's study of more than 1000 Japanese female students, two groups of which are listed in Table 29-1.[27] The current view that dieting is a risk factor for bulimia was supported by the cognitive restraint scores of 157 of these students who reported that they were binge eaters (8.8 ± 4.2), for they were higher than those of the two samples of junior college (5.5 ± 3.5) and nursing students (6.3 ± 3.6). The disinhibition scores of the binge eaters were also higher.

Studies in England and the United States also found elevations on the cognitive restraint scale, and in one study these scores correlated with the severity of bulimia.[17]

SUMMARY AND CONCLUSIONS

The recent past has seen a 180-degree change in our views on the relationship between psychopathology and obesity. According to the earlier, psychogenic theory of obesity, obese persons suffered inordinately from emotional disturbance and failed impulse control, and had ascribed their obesity to these disorders. Systematic assessment of the nature and extent of the psychological problems of obese persons have contributed greatly to a change from the psychogenic view of obesity to a primarily somatogenic view. Emotional problems specific to obese persons do exist, but they are now seen as consequences of the prejudice and discrimination directed against obese persons.

Systematic assessment has also advanced our understanding of another psychological aspect of human obesity—eating behavior. The concept of restrained eating was introduced by Herman in 1975 to describe the tendency of some persons to restrict their food intake in order to control their body weight. Exploration of the concept led to the discovery of counterregulation—

overeating following a preload by persons defined as restrained eaters by high scores on a restraint scale. A new Eating Inventory that distinguishes cognitive restraint from disinhibition of eating behavior has proved useful in the assessment and treatment of obesity. High cognitive restraint scores predict better outcome of treatment, and the higher the score the better the outcome. Both high cognitive restraint scores and high disinhibition scores are associated with binge eating and bulimia, while high disinhibition scores predict weight gain following smoking cessation.

References

1. Allon N: The stigma of overweight in everyday life. In Wolman B (ed): Psychological Aspects of Obesity: A Handbook, p 130. New York, Van Nostrand Reinhold Co, 1982
2. Bjorvell H, Rossner S, Stunkard AJ: Obesity, weight loss and dietary restraint. Int J Eat Disord 5:727, 1986
3. Canning H, Mayer J: Obesity: Its possible effects on college admissions. N Engl J Med 275:1172, 1966
4. Drewnowski A, Riskey D, Desor JA: Feeling fat yet unconcerned: Self-reported overweight and the restraint scale. Appetite J Intake Res 3:273, 1982
5. Duffy J, Hall SM: Smoking abstinence, eating style, and food intake. J Consult Clin Psychol 56:417, 1988
6. Fairburn CG, Cooper PJ: The clinical features of bulimia nervosa. Br J Psychiatry 144:238, 1984
7. Fenichel O: The Psychoanalytic Theory of Neurosis. New York, WW Norton, 1945
8. Ganley RM: Emotional eating and how it relates to dietary restraint, disinhibition and perceived hunger. Int J Eat Disord 5:635, 1988
9. Goldblatt PB, Moore ME, Stunkard AJ: Obesity, social class, and mental illness. JAMA 192:1039, 1962
10. Goodman N, Dornbusch SM, Richardson SA et al: Variant reactions to physical disabilities. Am Sociol Rev 429, 1963
11. Hall SM, Ginsberg D, Jones RT: Smoking cessation and weight gain. J Consult Clin Psychol 54:342, 1986
12. Hathaway SR, McKinnley JC: Minnesota Multiphasic Personality Inventory. Minneapolis, University of Minnesota, 1982
13. Herman CP, Mack D: Restrained and unrestrained eating. J Pers 43:647, 1975
14. Herman CP, Polivy J: Restrained eating. In

Stunkard AJ (ed): Obesity. Philadelphia, WB Saunders, 1980
15. Hibscher JA, Herman CP: Obesity, dieting, and the expression of "obese" characteristics. J Comp Physiol Psychol 91:374, 1977
16. Industry Week: Fat execs get slimmer paychecks. Industry Week 180:21, 1974
17. Kales EF: Dietary restraint and bulimia (abstr 207). International Conference on Eating Disorders, 1986
18. Kaplan HJ, Kaplan HS: The psychosomatic concept of obesity. J Nerv Ment Dis 125:181, 1957
19. Keys A: Editorial: Obesity and heart disease. J Chronic Dis 1:456, 1955
20. Keys A, Brozek J, Henschel A et al (eds): The Biology of Human Starvation, Vol II. Minneapolis, University of Minnesota Press, 1950
21. Laessle RG, Tuschl RJ, Kotthaus BC et al: Behavioral and biological correlates of dietary restraint in normal life. Appetite J Intake Res (in press)
22. Larkin JE, Pines HA: No fat persons need apply. Sociol Work Occup 6:312, 1979
23. Klesges RC, Klem ML, Hanson CL et al: The effects of applicant's health status and qualification levels on simulated hiring decisions. Int J Obes 14:527, 1990
24. Laessle RG, Tuschl RJ, Kotthaus BC et al: Behavioral and biological correlates of dietary restraint in normal life. Appetite 12:83, 1989
25. LaPorte DJ, Stunkard AJ: Predicting attrition and adherence to a very low calorie diet (VLCD): A prospective investigation of the Eating Inventory. Int J Obes 14:197, 1990.
26. Nisbett RE: Hunger, obesity, and the ventromedial hypothalamus. Psychol Rev 79:433, 1972
27. Nogami Y: A study of binge-eating among female students (in Japanese). Seishingaku 29:155, 1987
28. Pargaman D: The incidence of obesity among college students. J School Health 29:621, 1969
29. Polivy J: Perception of calories and regulation of intake in restrained and unrestrained subjects. Addict Behav 1:237, 1976
30. Pyle RL, Mitchell JE, Eckert ED: Bulimia: A report of 34 cases. J Clin Psychiatry 42:60, 1981
31. Richardson SA, Goodman N, Hastorf AH et al: Cultural uniformity in reaction to physical disabilities. Am Sociol Rev 26:241, 1961
32. Roe DA, Eickwort KR: Relationships between obesity and associated health factors with unemployment among low income women. J Am Med Womens Assoc 31:193, 1976
33. Ruderman AJ: Dietary restraint: A theoretical and empirical review. Psychol Bull 99:247, 1986
34. Ruderman AJ, Belzer LJ, Halperin A: Restraint, anticipated consumption, and overeating. J Abnorm Psychol 94:547–555, 1985

35. Ruderman AJ, Christensen HC: Restraint theory and its applicability to overweight individuals. J Abnorm Psychol 92:210, 1983

36. Sallade J: A comparison of the psychological adjustment of obese vs. non-obese children. J Psychosom Res 17:89–96, 1973

37. Sanfuentes MT, Lolas F: Eating behavior and personality: An exploratory analysis. Pers Individ Diff 9:435, 1988

38. Schachter S: Some extraordinary facts about obese humans and rats. Am Psychol 26:129, 1971

39. Spencer JA, Fremouw WJ: Binge eating as a function of restraint and weight classification. J Abnorm Psychol 88:262, 1979

40. Staffieri JR: A study of social stereotype of body image in children. J Pers Soc Psychol 7:101, 1967

41. Stunkard AJ: The dieting depression: Untoward responses to weight reduction. Am J Med 23:77, 1957

42. Stunkard AJ: Obesity. In Kaplan HI, Freedman AM, Sadock BJ (eds): Comprehensive Textbook of Psychiatry, p 1133. Baltimore, Williams & Wilkins, 1985

43. Stunkard AJ, Coll M, Lundquist S et al: Obesity and eating style. Arch Gen Psychiatry 37:1127, 1980

44. Stunkard AJ, Mendelson M: Obesity and the body image. I. Characteristics of disturbances in the body image of some obese persons. Am J Psychiatry 123:1296, 1967

45. Stunkard AJ, Burt V: Obesity and the body image. II. Age at onset of disturbances in the body image. Am J Psychiatry 123:1443, 1967

46. Stunkard AJ, Messick SM: The three-factor eating questionnaire to measure dietary restraint, disinhibition and hunger. J Psychosom Res 29:71, 1985

47. Stunkard AJ, Rush J: Dieting and depression reexamined: A critical review of reports of untoward responses during weight reduction of obesity. Ann Intern Med 81:526, 1974

48. Swenson WM, Pearson JS, Osborne D: An MMPI Source Book. Minneapolis, University of Minnesota Press, 1973

49. Wadden TA, Foster GD, Brownell KD et al: Self-concept in obese and normal-weight children. J Consult Clin Psychol 52:1104, 1984

50. Wadden TA, Stunkard AJ: Psychopathology and obesity. Ann NY Acad Sci 55, 1987

51. Wardle J, Beinhart H: Binge eating: A theoretical review. Br J Clin Psychol 20:97, 1981

52. Woody EZ, Costanzo PR, Liefer H et al: The effects of task and caloric perceptions on the eating behavior of restrained and unrestrained subjects. Cogn Ther Res 5:381, 1981

CHAPTER 30

Body Weight, Morbidity, and Longevity

THEODORE B. VANITALLIE

The health implications of being obese can be considered from at least four anatomical perspectives: (1) the overall severity of the obesity (how overweight/fat is the individual?); (2) the morphology of the adipose tissue (is it predominantly hypertrophic, hyperplastic, or hyperplastic-hypertrophic?); (3) the pattern of regional subcutaneous fat distribution (does the affected individual exhibit "abdominal" ["upper body"] obesity or "femoral-gluteal" ["lower body"] obesity?); and (4) the relative degree of intra-abdominal fat accumulation, notably within that portion of the visceral adipose tissue drained by the portal venous system.

The present review focuses on the first two anatomical considerations. The issue of regional fat distribution in relation to health risks (items 3 and 4) is taken up elsewhere in this volume.

MEASURES OF OBESITY AND ITS SEVERITY

The severity of obesity is commonly estimated from the body mass index (BMI), an index that attempts to normalize for height, thereby permitting comparison of the transformed weights of individuals of differing statures.[1-3] BMI is determined by dividing weight in kilograms by the square of the height in meters (BMI = weight[kg]/height[m]^2).

It is helpful to have a frame of reference by which to assess degree of overweight. Table 30-1 provides one such framework.[4]

The BMI embodies both the fat and fat-free components of the body; therefore, it is an index of weight (or mass) and not of fatness as such. In the first National Health and Nutrition Examination Survey (NHANES I), conducted during 1971–1974, both BMI and skin-fold thickness (sum of triceps [T] and subscapular [SS] skin-fold thicknesses) were measured in a representative sample of U.S. adults.[5] As shown in Table 30-2, when study subjects were cross-classified according to BMI and T + SS skin-fold thickness, about 6.7% of American men were found to be obese but not overweight, while 10.2% were overweight but not obese.[6] The criteria used by the National Center for Health Statistics to define overweight and obesity are shown in the table. On the other hand, evidence obtained with computed tomography (CT) strongly suggests that measurement of skin-fold ("fat-fold") thickness cannot provide a reliable index of total body fat content. For example, Sjostrom[7] has recently reported CT scan studies indicating that in 19 women (ages 42 ± 9 years and weighing 73 ± 20 kg), subcutaneous fat accounted for 91.6% of body fat mass (BFM). In contrast, in 24 men (ages 40 ± 9 years and weighing 101 ± 25 kg), subcutaneous fat accounted for only 78.7% of BFM. The difference was explained by the fact that 21.3% of BFM was intra-abdominal (visceral) in the male subjects, whereas 8.4% was intra-abdominal in the female subjects.

Although the BMI is a useful measure of obesity, its ability to predict body fat content is limited by the fact that this index is affected by variations in body water, bone mineral mass, and lean tissue mass, notably muscle. Thus, to come to grips with obesity, which refers to body fat

TABLE 30-1

Categories of Severity of Overweight

Category	Body Mass Index (kg/m²)
Acceptable range	20–24.9
Mild overweight	25–27.9
Moderate overweight	28–31.9
Severe overweight	32–41.9
Morbid obesity	42

content, one must measure BFM. In this regard, two recently developed electrical methods, total body electrical conductivity (TOBEC) measurement and bioelectrical impedance analysis (BIA), have been found capable of estimating LBM and BFM rapidly and conveniently.[8,9] In time, methods of this kind may yield new information about the health and mortality risks associated with an enlarged BFM. However, at present it is not clear just how to interpret information about total body fat content in a given individual because not enough is known about the frequency distributions of BFM by sex, age, and race in the U.S. population and about the relation of BFM as such to obesity-associated health risks. Until the newer, "subject-friendly" methods become better established, BMI (which correlates reasonably well with estimated BFM in both population studies and studies of small groups of experimental subjects) is currently the most convenient index available of both relative weight and degree of fatness.[3]

SEVERITY OF OVERWEIGHT (OBESITY) IN RELATION TO HEALTH RISKS

The second National Health and Nutrition Examination Survey (NHANES II), conducted during 1976–1980, clearly revealed that overweight (characterized by a BMI of approximately 28 or higher) is associated with a significantly increased risk of developing hypertension, diabetes, and hypercholesterolemia.[10] As shown in Table 30-3, among young adults who are overweight, the relative risk of developing these potentially dangerous conditions is especially high. As subjects age, these relative risks recede, prob-

TABLE 30-2

Cross-Classification of U.S. Adult Population Aged 20–74 Years According to Distribution of Body Mass Index (W/Hᵖ) and of Triceps Plus Subscapular Skin-Fold Measurements: United States, 1971–1974

	Prevalence (%)	
Categories	Men	Women
Underweight,[a] not obese[b]	18.1	17.8
Normal weight,[c] not obese	52.4	46.7
Normal weight, obese[d]	6.7	6.0
Overweight,[e] not obese	10.2	7.9
Overweight, obese	12.6	21.6

The reference population, on which the percentiles referred to below were based, was made up of a representative sample of civilian noninstitutionalized U.S. men and nonpregnant women, ages 20 to 29 years, who were examined during the first National Health and Nutrition Examination Survey (NHANES I), 1971–1974.

[a]Underweight: <15th percentile of the distribution of BMI (P = 2 for men; 1.5 for women).
[b]Not obese: <85th percentile of the distribution of triceps plus subscapular skin-fold measurements.
[c]Normal weight: ≥15th to <85th percentile of the distribution of the BMI.
[d]Obese: ≥85th percentile of the distribution of triceps plus subscapular skin-fold thicknesses.
[e]Overweight: ≥85th percentile of the distribution of the BMI.

ably because they are increasingly diluted by many other health problems associated with aging.

Apart from its association with an increased relative risk of hypertension, diabetes, and hypercholesterolemia, obesity is thought to cause or exacerbate a great variety of health problems, some of which are listed in Table 30-4.[11]

MORTALITY ASSOCIATED WITH VARIATIONS IN BMI

Many epidemiologic studies, both prospective and retrospective, have shown that as the BMI

TABLE 30-3

Relative Risk Ratios* for Overweight American Adults

Risk Condition	Age Range (yr)		
	20–74	*20–44*	*45–74*
Hypertension	2.9	5.6	1.9
Diabetes mellitus	2.9	3.8	2.1
Hypercholesterolemia	1.5	2.1	1.1

*Prevalence of health problem (%) among overweight persons divided by prevalence of the same problem among nonoverweight persons within the same age range. (Source: Second National Health and Nutrition Examination Survey [NHANES II], 1976–1980.)

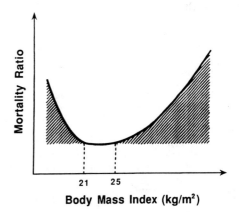

FIGURE 30-1

Generic J- or U-shaped curve describing relationship of body mass index (BMI) to mortality ratio. In this figure, the optimal BMI range is 21 to 25 kg/m². (Adapted from Waaler HT: Height, weight, and mortality: The Norwegian experience. Acta Med Scand Suppl 679:1, 1984.)

increases above a certain "optimal" weight range, so does the mortality ratio (ratio of actual to actuarially expected deaths).[12] The same studies have shown that the mortality ratio also increases as the BMI decreases below the optimal range. These relationships between BMI and mortality ratio are indicated in the generic curve shown in Figure 30-1.

It does not seem necessary to belabor the point that overweight reduces life expectancy; on the other hand, important questions remain about the relationship of overweight to future health status and mortality risk. Some of these questions and brief responses to them follow.

1. *At what point or within what range does overweight (obesity) become discernibly hazardous to health and longevity?*

According to a Norwegian study (one of the largest surveys linking BMI to mortality ratio,[13] the segment of the mortality curve for BMI associated with the lowest mortality lies in the range of 21 to 25 kg/m². In the Build Study 1979 (conducted on 4.2 million policyholders insured by 25 U.S. and Canadian life insurance companies), the most favorable mortality rates were found in men and women who were between 15% below average weight and 5% above average weight.[14] These observations provided the basis for the Metropolitan Life Insurance Company's height and weight tables, published in 1983.[15] If one translates the weights for height recommended in the 1983 tables into BMIs, the resulting opti-

mal BMI range is consonant with that found in the Norwegian study.

2. *Is the mortality ratio lower in overweight women than in comparably overweight men? Are obesity-related health problems less common in overweight women than in comparably overweight men?*

An enhanced tolerance of overweight by women is evident in the 26-year follow-up of female participants in the Framingham Heart Study who at entry were less than 50 years old, were normotensive, did not have elevated cholesterol levels, did not smoke, were not glucose intolerant, and did not have electrocardiographic evidence of left ventricular hypertrophy.[16] The study revealed that aging women in the study who were 10% to 30% above Metropolitan relative weight (MRW, defined as the midpoint of the desirable weight range in the 1959 Metropolitan Life tables of desirable weights[17]) had a much higher probability of remaining free from cardiovascular disease than comparably overweight and aging men.

Among both men and women in the Build Study 1979, relative mortality rose steadily with increasing overweight. Among men, the mortality ratios rose from 117% for those about 20%

TABLE 30-4

Some Health Disorders and Other Problems Thought To Be Caused or Exacerbated By Obesity

Heart
  Premature coronary heart disease
  Left ventricular hypertrophy
  Angina pectoris
  Sudden death (ventricular arrhythmia)
  Congestive heart failure
Vascular system
  Hypertension
  Stroke (cerebral infarction and/or hemorrhage)
  Venous stasis (with lower extremity edema, varicose veins, hemorrhoids, thromboembolic disease involving lower extremities and inferior vena cava)
Respiratory system
  Obstructive sleep apnea
  Pickwickian syndrome (alveolar hypoventilation)
  Secondary polycythemia
  Right ventricular hypertrophy (sometimes leading to failure)
Hepatobiliary system
  Cholelithiasis
  Hepatic steatosis
Hormonal and metabolic functions
  Diabetes mellitus (insulin independent)
  Gout (hyperuricemia)
  Hyperlipidemias (hypertriglyceridemia and hypercholesterolemia)
Kidney
  Proteinuria and, in very severe obesity, nephrosis
  Renal vein thrombosis
Skin
  Striae
  Acanthosis nigricans (benign type)
  Hirsutism
  Intertrigo
  Plantar callus
  Multiple papillomas
Joints, muscles, and connective tissue
  Osteoarthritis of knees
  Bone spurs of the heel
  Osteoarthrosis of spine (in women)
  Aggravation of preexisting postural faults
Neoplasia
  Increased risk of endometrial cancer
  Possibly increased risk of breast cancer
Reproductive and sexual function
  Impaired obstetric performance (increased risk of toxemia, hypertension and diabetes mellitus during pregnancy, prolonged labor, need for cesarean section more frequent)
  Irregular menstruation and frequent anovulatory cycles
  Reduced fertility
Psychosocial function
  Impairment of self-image with feelings of inferiority
  Social isolation
  Subject to social, economic, and other types of discrimination
  Susceptibility to psychoneuroses
  Loss of mobility
  Increased employee absenteeism
Miscellaneous
  Increased surgical and anesthetic risks
  Reduced physical agility and increased accident proneness
  Interference with diagnosis of other disorders

From VanItallie TB: Obesity: Adverse effects on health and longevity. Am J Clin Nutr 32:2723, 1979. Reproduced by permission.

overweight to 139% for those 40% overweight, and to 186% for those about 60% overweight. The corresponding mortality ratios for women 20%, 40%, and 60% overweight were 109%, about 115%, and 140% respectively.[18]

3. *How long does it take for the adverse effect of overweight on health and life expectancy to become manifest?*

The Build Study 1979 showed that the adverse effects on mortality of being overweight tend to be delayed, sometimes for ten years or longer. In contrast, the adverse effects of being underweight appear much sooner. The Manitoba Study of Canadian Air Force recruits first examined at the time of World War II suggested that the latent period between the occurrence of overweight and the subsequent appearance of unfavorable cardiovascular consequences might extend for at least 16 years.[19]

Additional support for the existence of a rather long latent period between the development of overweight or obesity and subsequent mortality risk comes from the Framingham Heart Study's 30-year follow-up, which tabulated the cumulative deaths per 1000 of male nonsmokers of all ages.[20] Figure 30-2 shows deaths per thousand in this cohort plotted against MRW. As the duration of follow-up increases from six to 30 years, the curve that describes the relationship between MRW and mortality takes on a J-shaped configuration. However, it is only after 24 years of follow-up that MRW values ranging from 110 to 130 are found to be associated with an increased mortality risk in this cohort.

4. *In what ways do socioeconomic status, smoking habits, and other variables confound the interpretation of the results of longitudinal studies of the effect of overweight on health and life expectancy?*

It has long been known that social class or socioeconomic status (SES) has pronounced effects on longevity.[18] Death rates observed in overweight persons drawn from the general population may to some extent reflect the higher death rates of persons of low SES as well as the increased mortality associated with being overweight.

As regards cigarette smoking, the Framingham Heart Study found that more than 80% of men in the Framingham study whose BMIs were be-

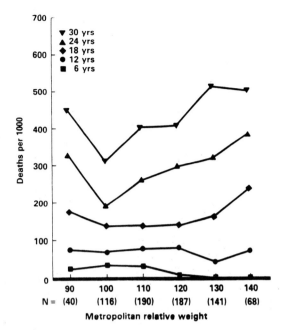

FIGURE 30-2

Cumulative deaths per 1000 over a 30-year follow-up period of nonsmoking male participants in the Framingham Heart Study. Mortality rates are plotted against Metropolitan relative weight (see text for details). (From Feinleib M: Epidemiology of obesity in relation to health hazards. Ann Intern Med 103:1019, 1985. Reproduced by permission.)

low 22 kg/m² were smokers. Only about 55% of the extremely overweight men were smokers. Thus, cigarette smoking was clearly an important confounding factor when it came to interpreting the U-shaped relationship between BMI and mortality risk.[21] As Manson et al[22] put it, "since cigarette smoking is a strong risk factor for mortality and also has an independent inverse association with adiposity, failure to control for its effects will produce an artifactually high mortality in lean subjects."

Other factors that can confound the interpretation of the findings of longitudinal studies include the duration of the study, the health status of the participants at the outset of the study, and the makeup of the population being followed. Thus, if a study is of insufficient duration (i.e., ten years or less), the adverse effects of overweight on health and longevity may not have had time to appear. Also, if the study's participants include individuals who, at the outset, are underweight because of poor health, it will appear as though underweight were a cause rather than an effect of illness. If underweight per se is mistakenly perceived as hazardous to health, the dangers of being overweight will be underestimated. Finally, if the cohort being surveyed is not reasonably representative of the overall population in regard to health status, age distribution, sex distribution, occupation, SES, and diet, then the results simply will not be generalizable.[18-22]

5. *What is the meaning of the J-shaped or U-shaped curve that describes the relationship between BMI and mortality ratio?*

On average, underweight people have a higher risk of dying than do people of average weight. This is partly because a high proportion of underweight people are cigarette smokers.[22] In addition, being underweight (or experiencing recent weight loss) may be symptomatic of a subclinical illness that may later prove fatal. In industrialized societies, underweight people commonly die of lung cancer, obstructive lung disease, and so forth; however, they do not develop these health problems because they are slender. (It must be admitted that people who are underweight because of malnutrition exhibit an increased susceptibility to certain diseases, such as pulmonary tuberculosis. On the other hand, premature coronary heart disease, diabetes, and hypertension—common causes of death among the overweight—can be mitigated or to some extent prevented by long-term weight control.)

For the foregoing reasons, it would seem that a large component of the left limb of the J- or U-shaped curve is artifactual, representing the fact that the increased mortality ratios among the underweight do not result from being slender but rather arise from the adverse effects of a habit (smoking) that is both associated with and tends to promote a low BMI, from malnutrition, or from the presence of a subclinical illness that keeps the body weight low.

When the confounding effects of smoking, undernutrition, and occult illness are controlled for, there remains a direct, positive relationship between increasing BMI and mortality ratio. Indeed, in the Framingham Heart Study, the risk of death within 26 years increased by 1% per extra pound for ages 30 to 42 and by 2% per extra pound for ages 50 to 62.[21]

6. *Is overweight less threatening to health and life expectancy in the elderly? Should there be age-specific height-weight tables?*

Data on the prevalence of diabetes in relation to overweight by age do not support the view that it is safe to be overweight as one gets older. In the U.S. population 65 to 75 years of age, diabetes occurs twice as often among the overweight as among the nonoverweight. Moreover, diabetes occurs twice as often among overweight individuals aged 65 to 75 years as among overweight individuals aged 45 to 55 years.[23] The health hazards of being overweight are less prominent in later life than in earlier adult life, not because the risk has necessarily receded but because other health risks associated with aging have emerged.[10]

Andres[24] used data from the Build Study 1979[14] and from other sources to argue that, as people get older, the best life expectancy occurs at progressively higher relative weights. Thus, Andres has proposed age-specific height-weight tables for men and women which in effect recommend weight ranges for older individuals that are substantially higher than the ranges suggested by Metropolitan Life in its 1959 and 1983 tables.

It is true that the findings of the Build Study 1979 seem to indicate that, in older members of the insured population, weights somewhat above average are associated with optimal life expectancy. However, in evaluating these findings, several important facts have to be borne in mind. First, in the Build Study 1979, the unadjusted published mortality experience for all durations combined understated the long-term mortality among overweight individuals (some of the reasons for this underestimation were discussed earlier in this chapter). This understatement is particularly applicable to individuals 60 years of age and older; hence, conclusions about relative weights associated with the best mortality experience among the elderly should be based on suitably adjusted mortality data.[18] Second, when previously weight-stable older individuals lose an appreciable amount of weight, this loss not infrequently is the harbinger of early death.[25] Thus, when one is examining the relationship of relative weight to longevity, it is important to distinguish older people who are both slender and healthy from those whose declining weight presages a fatal illness.

Finally, and perhaps most important, persons aged 60 or older who have been accepted for life insurance clearly are not at all representative of a cross section of the middle class in that age range. First, they are usually better off financially than the average middle-class individual; of greater importance, they have been carefully screened medically. Thus, their rejection rate for life insurance ranges from 10% to 25%, as compared to about 2% for the insured population overall.[26] It is particularly noteworthy that 65-year-old men accepted for life insurance have recently experienced death rates that are only about 66% of those exhibited by white men of corresponding age in the general population.[27]

Although a case can be made for liberalizing weight standards for people as they age, it must be emphasized that, to the extent that such age-specific standards are based on the mortality experience of affluent elderly people who can pass life insurance medical examinations, they are not really applicable to average Americans in the same age range. Also, life insurance statistics underestimate the long-term mortality among overweight individuals and fail to address the issue of morbidity (for example, the high risk of developing diabetes conferred on older people by a relatively small degree of overweight). For these reasons, it seems prudent to retain the current Metropolitan Life weight-for-height standards until firmer evidence becomes available to justify upward shifts in recommended weights for the elderly.

MORPHOLOGY OF ADIPOSE TISSUE

Because the lipid content of human subcutaneous adipocytes rarely exceeds 1.2 μg/cell (the "normal" lipid content is ca. 0.4–0.6 μg/cell), it is difficult to imagine how people can become severely obese without increasing fat cell number. Indeed, cross-sectional studies that correlated mean fat cell size with severity of obesity have shown that once body fat content increases

beyond a certain point, fat cell size no longer tracks degree of corpulence.[28] Thus, adipocyte hyperplasia must be invoked to account for the continuing expansion of the body's fat mass.

As regards health hazards associated with obesity per se, fat cell hyperplasia without hypertrophy is not clearly associated with impaired glucose tolerance, insulin resistance, hypertension, or hyperlipidemia. On the other hand, fat cell enlargement is believed to be associated with these risk factors, whether or not hyperplasia is present.[28]

Femoral-gluteal (lower body) obesity has sometimes been equated with adipose tissue hyperplasia, and abdominal (upper body) obesity with adipose tissue hypertrophy. Yet, apart from the demonstration that women with abdominal obesity have enlarged fat cells in abdominal subcutaneous adipose tissue, there is little evidence in the literature to substantiate the appealing notion that a particular type of regional fat distribution is consistently associated with a particular pattern of adipose tissue morphology.

Somewhat surprisingly, only a few large-scale surveys have attempted to distinguish between the effects on health and longevity of obesity and those of overweight. Data obtained on a representative sample of the U.S. population during 1971–1974 (NHANES I) showed that individuals overweight by BMI standards but not obese by skin-fold thickness standards (see Table 30-2) were more likely than nonoverweight but obese or nonoverweight and nonobese persons to have high blood pressure.[5] Unfortunately, waist-to-hips circumference ratios were not measured during NHANES I; hence, one cannot rule out a possible association of hypertension with abdominal (and presumably intra-abdominal) fat accumulation in subjects who were classified as overweight but not obese.

Information on the long-term effects on health of obesity vs overweight is available from the Framingham Heart Study.[29] The indices of overweight and obesity that were measured in the Framingham cohort included height; weight; circumferences of waist, upper and lower arms, and wrists; and thicknesses of subscapular, triceps, abdominal, and quadriceps skin folds. The obesity index most predictive of the emerging incidence of coronary heart disease over a 22-year observation period was found to be SS skin-fold thickness (also a marker of upper body obesity). In men, both SS skin-fold thickness and serum total cholesterol contributed more to the risk of coronary heart disease (CHD) than did age. In the Framingham study, "obesity" was found to be a weaker independent risk factor for stroke and other manifestations of cardiovascular disease than it was for coronary heart disease.

Subscapular skin-fold thickness predicted 22-year CHD incidence best for women below age 50 and for men aged 50 to 59 years. Waist circumference and the four skin-fold measurements were generally more predictive of CHD for men than for women and for the young than for the old. Upper body skin-fold measurements generally predicted CHD better than did waist or quadriceps skin-fold measurements.

References

1. Quetelet LAJ: Physique Sociale. Vol 2. Brussels, C Muquardt, 1869
2. Keys A, Fidanza F, Karvonen MJ et al: Indices of relative weight and obesity. J Chronic Dis 25:329, 1972
3. Garrow JS, Webster J: Quetelet's index (W/H²) as a measure of fatness. Int J Obes 9:147, 1985
4. VanItallie TB: Obesity. In Jeejeebhoy KN (ed): Current Therapy in Nutrition, p 314. Burlington, Ontario, BC Decker, 1988
5. VanItallie TB, Abraham S: Some hazards of obesity and its treatment. In Hirsch J, VanItallie TB (eds): Recent Advances in Obesity Research. IV. Proceedings of the 4th International Congress on Obesity, p 1. London, John Libbey & Co, 1985
6. VanItallie TB, Kissileff HR: Human Obesity: A Problem in Body Energy Economics. In Stricker EM (ed): Handbook of Behavioral Neurobiology, Vol 10, Neurobiology of Food and Fluid Intake. New York, Plenum Publishing Corp, 1990
7. Sjostrom L: Total and regional determinations of human adipose tissue (AT) with a multiscan CT technique (abstr). In: Workshop on Basic and Clinical Aspects of Regional Fat Distribution, p 37. Bethesda, Md, National Institutes of Health, September 1989
8. Segal KR, Gutin B, Presta E et al: Estimation of human body composition by electrical impedance methods: A comparative study. J Appl Physiol 58:1565, 1985
9. Lukaski HC, Bolonchuk WW, Hall CB et al: Validation of tetrapolar bioelectrical impedance method to assess human body composition. J Appl Physiol 60:1327, 1986
10. VanItallie TB: Health implications of overweight and obesity in the United States. Ann Intern Med 103:983, 1985
11. VanItallie TB: Obesity: Adverse effects on health and longevity. Am J Clin Nutr 32:2723, 1979
12. Simopoulos AP, VanItallie TB: Body weight, health, and longevity. Ann Intern Med 100:285, 1984
13. Waaler HT: Height, weight, and mortality: The Norwegian experience. Acta Med Scand Suppl 679:1, 1984
14. Build Study 1979. Chicago, Society of Actuaries and Association of Life Insurance Medical Directors of America, 1980
15. Metropolitan Life Insurance Co: 1983 Metropolitan height and weight tables. New York, Metropolitan Life Insurance Co, Statistical Bulletin, Vol 64, pp 2–9, 1983
16. Hubert HB, Feinleib M, McNamara PM et al: Obesity as an independent risk factor for cardiovascular disease: A 26-year follow-up of participants in the Framingham Heart Study. Circulation 67:968, 1983
17. Metropolitan Life Insurance Co: New weight standards for men and women. New York, Metropolitan Life Insurance Co, Statistical Bulletin, Vol 40, pp 1–4, 1959
18. Lew EA: Mortality and weight: Insured lives and the American Cancer Society Studies. Ann Intern Med 103:1024, 1985
19. Rabkin SW, Mathewson FAL, Hsu PH: Relation of body weight to development of ischemic heart disease in a cohort of young North American men after a 26-year observation period: The Manitoba Study. Am J Cardiol 39:452, 1977
20. Feinleib M: Epidemiology of obesity in relation to health hazards. Ann Intern Med 103:1019, 1985
21. Garrison RJ, Feinleib M, Castelli WP et al: Cigarette smoking as a confounder of the relationship between relative weight and long-term mortality: The Framingham Heart Study. JAMA 249:2199, 1983
22. Manson JE, Stampfer MJ, Hennekens CH et al: Body weight and longevity: A reassessment. JAMA 257:353, 1987
23. National Commission on Diabetes: The Scope and Impact of Diabetes. Report of the National Commission on Diabetes to the Congress of the United States. Washington, DC, DHEW publication No. (NIH) 76-1021, 1976
24. Andres R: Mortality and obesity: The rationale for age-specific height-weight tables. In Andres R, Bierman EL, Hazzard WR (eds): Principles of Geriatric Medicine, p 311. New York, McGraw-Hill Book Co, 1985

25. Medical Impairment Study 1983. Vol I. Boston, Society of Actuaries and Association of Life Insurance Medical Directors of America, 1986

26. American Council of Life Insurance: 1984 Life Insurance Fact Book.

27. Society of Actuaries: 1982 Reports of Mortality and Morbidity Experience, p 55. Chicago, Society of Actuaries, 1982

28. Hirsch J, Batchelor B: Adipose tissue cellularity in human obesity. Clin Endocrinol Metabol 5:299, 1976

29. Stokes J III, Garrison RJ, Kannel WB: The independent contributions of various indices of obesity to the 22-year incidence of coronary heart disease. In Vague J, Björntorp P, Guy-Grand B et al (eds): Metabolic Complications of Human Obesities, p 49. Amsterdam, Elsevier, 1985

PART SIX

HUNGER SATIETY AND MOOD

CHAPTER 31

Blood-Brain Barrier Regulation and Diabetes

EAIN M. CORNFORD and MARCIA E. CORNFORD

Brain-barrier membranes are found in all vertebrates. Experimental studies of the mammalian blood-brain barrier (BBB) began in 1889 with the dye-exclusion studies of Paul Ehrlich.[1] Rather than being a passive, relatively immutable mechanical barrier, brain endothelia are now recognized as the dynamic membranous interface between blood and brain that is regulated by the brain itself.[1,2] The functioning BBB has been likened to a gatekeeper,[3] allowing the brain to communicate with the internal plasma environment in a manner analogous to the way in which the five senses permit communication between the brain and the external environment.[4] Anatomically, the BBB capillaries lack fenestrations and interendothelial clefts, show little pinocytosis, and have tight junctions sealing adjacent endothelia.[1] A basement lamella with or without a pericyte surrounds the capillary. One half of the cells are completely tubular or "seamless," highly restrictive, and may be unique to the brain.[5] In BBB capillaries, access to the central nervous system (CNS) is by a transcellular route. In contrast, intercellular clefts or patent fenestrations permit intercellular passage of plasmaborne solutes in many peripheral tissue capillaries. Increased mitochondria, greater electrical resistance, and a number of unique cytoplasmic enzymes also characterize BBB endothelia.[1,6]

INITIATING FORMATION OF BLOOD-BRAIN BARRIER-TYPE CAPILLARIES

Fenestrated capillaries characteristic of the tissue of origin are seen in metastatic brain tumors, but gliomas, originating in the CNS, possess restrictive BBB-type capillaries.[1] In a study using quail chick transplantations, it was demonstrated that abdominal host vessels vascularizing grafted neural tissue formed structural, functional, and histochemical features of BBB capillaries. (The different species of donor and recipient tissues permitted easy identification.) The reverse experiment, in contrast, indicated that brain vessels vascularizing grafted mesodermal tissue were devoid of these characteristics.[7]

Davson and Oldendorf[8] proposed that the nearby astroglial foot processes somehow induced the formation of BBB capillaries. DeBault and Cancilla[9] further demonstrated that γ-glutamyl transpeptidase could be identified in isolated brain capillaries cultured in vitro only if glial cells were present in the media to induce formation of this enzyme. It has subsequently been shown that astrocytes can induce BBB traits in nonneural endothelia in vivo. Ultrastructural studies also indicate that the capillary basal lamina is more distinctly observed when a glial end-foot process is in intimate contact with the endothelium. Thus an increasing body of information[1,10,11] indicates that a stimulus or message originating in the astrocytic foot processes of the glial cells induces the formation of barrier-type endothelial cells in the CNS. Proteins such as basic fibroblast growth factor promote growth of peripheral tissue capillaries,[12] but the unique glial BBB messenger protein awaits definition.

FUNCTIONS OF BLOOD-BRAIN BARRIER CAPILLARIES

Three primary functions can be identified for brain capillary endothelia. In addition to the anatomical barrier, we also recognize an equally important biochemical barrier at this site, and regulatory interface functions in the BBB.[1-4,13,14]

The *anatomical barrier* to the brain, as recognized by Ehrlich, is incomplete. There are small regions in the brain (the circumventricular organs, CVOs) surrounding the ventricles that have porous, non-BBB capillaries; examples are the median eminence, subfornical organ, choroid plexus, and the area postrema.[13] A nonpermeating solute (e.g., inulin, MW = 5000 daltons) may move from the plasma into the cerebrospinal fluid (CSF) via the CVOs; by this mechanism a steady-state plasma-CSF ratio of about 3% is seen for inulin.[2,13,14] It is also known that the extracellular compartment of brain is cerebrospinal fluid (CSF); the so-called blood-CSF barrier is a second (anatomical) brain barrier system. However, because the BBB is some 5000 times larger in surface area than the blood-CSF barrier, it is the BBB capillaries that have regulatory functions.[14] Increased pinocytotic activity (e.g., during seizures) represents another mechanism whereby the anatomical barrier is compromised. Intracarotid injections of hypertonic media with drugs have been used to transiently open the barrier in the treatment of brain tumors. Pioneered by Neuwelt and colleagues,[15] this novel strategy emphasizes the heroic measures taken in clinical circumvention of the anatomical barrier.

The *biochemical barrier* is attributable to the presence of enzymes (e.g., catechol O-methyltransferase, phenol sulfotransferase[16]) in the brain capillary endothelia. Plasma-borne biogenic amines are rapidly metabolized by monoamine oxidase. In this manner, the brain is insulated from systemic bursts of epinephrine. The administration of L-DOPA (dihydroxyphenylalanine) permits significant quantities of the prodrug to penetrate the BBB (via the neutral amino acid transporter) and thus the metabolized dopamine is delivered to treat patients with parkinsonism.[17] Adenosine, a potent neuromodulator, is phosphorylated to adenosine monophosphate (AMP), and free fatty acids are rapidly esterified. Enkephalins are degraded by capillary aminopeptidase and peptidyl dipeptidases; thus the combination of no transport system and this enzymatic barrier precludes any significant distribution of blood-borne enkephalins to the brain.[2] Drug metabolizing enzymes (cytochrome P-450–linked monoxygenase, epioxide hydrolase, NADPH:cytochrome P-450 reductase, and 1-naphthol UDP-gluconosyl transferase) have also been identified in brain capillaries. Their capacity to protect the brain by metabolizing xenobiotics has been recognized, and it was further suggested that CNS-targeted prodrugs might be designed in such a way as to be activated by these BBB-specific enzymes.[18]

Curiously, these enzymes may not always provide a protective function. In Alzheimer's disease, the cerebral (but not the visceral) microvasculature develops amyloid angiopathy (an eosinophilic deposition of beta-pleated sheets of protein). A mechanism has been postulated[19] whereby a circulating amyloid precursor is metabolized by an enzyme unique to the brain capillaries, and thus the depositions characterizing amyloid angiopathy develop solely in the cerebral microvasculature.

The *regulatory interface* collectively describes all of the processes by which the unique functions of the brain are maintained apart from the circulatory system by the BBB capillaries. The evolution of the BBB has provided a fluid environment low in potassium, consistent with the need for reduced potassium levels in order to achieve nerve impulse conduction. Traits such as the increases in BBB capillary mitochondria and electrical resistance,[1] in conjunction with the demonstration of Na^+/K^+-ATPase on the abluminal membranes,[20] all contribute to maintaining the low CNS potassium levels. These endothelia also regulate blood-to-brain nutrient[4,14,21] and peptide[2,13,22] exchange, as well as brain-to-blood movement[1] of acidic compounds.

The complex role of the BBB has been emphasized in conjunction with the disease of this decade, acquired immunodeficiency syndrome (AIDS). Although the exact mechanism is not fully understood, the BBB permits the virus to pass from the bloodstream to brain, but restricts entry of drugs (such as azidothymidine) showing promise of inhibiting the virus in other tissues of the body.[3] The luminal membranes of BBB capillaries contain a protein that is common to T4 helper lymphocytes. Presumably it facilitates adhesion of helper cells to the endothelium and participates in the immune surveillance system. Unfortunately, this protein also acts as a receptor for the AIDS virus. The resultant binding to the endothelial membrane may actually enhance rather than inhibit CNS entry by the virus. Thus the protective function of the BBB is defeated by a virus that attacks neurons and glia, causing memory loss, palsy, dementia, and paralysis.[3,22]

LIPID-MEDIATED BLOOD-BRAIN BARRIER TRANSPORT

Endothelia of the brain, like all proteolipid membranes, restrict the penetration of hydrophilic molecules (e.g., penicillin) but allow the rapid penetration of small lipophilic compounds (e.g., ethanol, caffeine). Brain extraction of many nonnutrients is a function of lipophilic properties.[23] An exception to this generalization is the fungal peptide cyclosporin,[4,13] which is highly lipophilic (log $P_{octanol}$ = 2.9). It does not penetrate the BBB but distributes to the brain much as inulin does.[2] Presumably the hydrophilic portions of this cyclic undecapeptide are conformationally masked in vitro but are sufficiently exposed in vivo to inhibit BBB penetration. However, within the blood, a molecule may have varying degrees of affinity for plasma and endothelial cell components, which will influence its ability to penetrate the capillary and distribute to the brain. In the past decade it was established that many protein-bound ligands can dissociate and traverse the BBB in a single transit. The view that plasma-tissue exchange was primarily a function of that small fraction that was not bound to proteins (i.e., the free, dialyzable ligand) is not supported by in vivo experimental data.[2,4,13] BBB exchange of ligands (anticonvulsant drugs and steroid hormones) bound to albumin, globulin,[1] and even erythrocytes[24] has been demonstrated. Even though the anticonvulsant phenytoin is highly bound (ca. 90%) to plasma proteins, it can be administered for rapid effects in arresting status epilepticus because the amount of drug delivered to the brain is a function of total plasma concentration, and not the freely dialyzable drug level.[1]

REGULATED (CARRIER-MEDIATED) METABOLITE PERMEABILITY

Nutrient Transporters

Blood-to-brain transit of nutrients is accomplished by transporters, proteins present in the capillary membranes that recognize classes of molecules and transfer them from the lumen to brain in milliseconds. Seven major independent transporters are recognized as determinants controlling brain uptake of (1) hexoses, (2) monocarboxylic acids, (3) neutral amino acids, (4) basic amino acids, (5) purine bases, (6) nucleosides, and (7) amines such as choline. These transporters, like enzymes, can be kinetically characterized.[1,4,14,25] Table 31-1 emphasizes the similarity between half-saturation constants for a representative substrate of each of these transporter proteins and the respective normal plasma concentration.[1,4] Because of this similarity, mild increases or decreases in the plasma level of a particular substrate will result in comparable increases or decreases in brain influx. However, after strenuous exercise, plasma lactate levels may increase tenfold. In this situation the BBB monocarboxylic acid transporter is oversupplied with substrate and the transporter actually inhibits blood-to-brain transfer, shielding the brain from a potentially harmful concentration of lactic acid. Thus these transporters function in a manner that promotes brain entry of substrates when plasma concentrations are low but prevents excess brain influx when plasma substrates reach excessive concentrations.

The half-saturation constant for each of the transporters (see Table 31-1) represents that con-

TABLE 31-1

Major Blood-Brain Barrier Nutrient Transporters: Comparison of Plasma Concentrations and Kinetic Constants*

Transporter System	Representative Substrate	Plasma Concentration (mM)	K_m (mM)	V_{max} (nmole · [min − g]$^{-1}$)
Hexose	Glucose	5.5	11.0	1420
Monocarboxylic acid	Lactate	1.1	1.8	91
Neutral amino acid	Phenylalanine	0.05	0.03	14
Neutral AA	Tryptophan	0.07	0.05	18
Neutral AA	Methionine	0.04	0.08	18
Neutral AA	Tyrosine	0.09	0.09	25
Neutral AA	Leucine	0.10	0.09	23
Neutral AA	Isoleucine	0.07	0.14	36
Neutral AA	Histidine	0.05	0.16	33
Neutral AA	Valine	0.14	0.17	14
Basic amino acid	Arginine	0.1	0.09	7.8
Amine	Choline	0.01	0.34	11.3
Nucleoside	Adenosine	0.001	0.025	0.75
Purine	Adenine	0.01	0.011	0.50

Data from Cornford.[1,6]

*K_m = half-saturation constant, V_{max} = transporter maximal velocity. The V_{max} is an indicator of the relative density of the transporter proteins on the capillary membrane: thus, for each nucleoside transporter there are about 10 basic amino acid carriers, 100 monocarboxylic acid transporters, and 1500 glucose transporter proteins. Note that most of the neutral amino acids share, and compete for, a common transporter.

centration of substrate at which one half of the transporter proteins will be bound by their substrate molecules. Note that as in human capillaries,[26] all of the neutral amino acids compete for a common transporter, in contrast to the hexose carrier, where almost exclusively, glucose is the substrate. The maximal velocities represent comparative rates at which these transporters move nutrients across the capillary membranes. The maximal velocities are a function of both the number of transport proteins in the BBB membranes and the rates at which these proteins mobilize the substrate. The point to be emphasized is that the transporters are listed in Table 31-1 in the sequence of greatest to least density. That is, higher maximal velocities are a function of more transporter proteins in the BBB membranes. In keeping with the brain's metabolic requirement for glucose, these data indicate that there are many, many more (about two orders of magni-

tude) glucose transporter proteins in the BBB than any other class of transporter. These transporters can also be rate-limiting for certain metabolic pathways[27-36] in the brain (Table 31-2).

Brain-to-Blood Transporters

The seven transporters listed in Table 31-1 all mediate bidirectional movement of nutrients between the blood and brain and may facilitate brain-to-blood translocation. Functional differences in the brain capillary membrane at the luminal surface as compared to the brain side (i.e., "polarity" of the BBB) are suggested by the observation that the protein composition of the luminal membrane is markedly different from that of the abluminal surface.[37] At least four transporters are believed to be unique to the abluminal BBB surface, and each of the four is an active (energy-dependent) transporter capable of mov-

TABLE 31-2

Rate-Limitation and Blood-Brain Barrier Nutrient Transporters:
Substrate-Limited Pathways of Brain Metabolism

Transporter System	Substrate	Metabolic Pathway	Reference
Hexose	Glucose	Glycolysis (in ischemia)	Drewes and Gilboe[27]
Monocarboxylic acid	Ketone bodies	Oxidation	Hawkins and Biebuyck[28]
Neutral amino acid	Tryptophan	Serotonin synthesis	Fernstrom and Wurtman[29]
Neutral AA	Tyrosine	Catecholamine synthesis	Gibson and Wurtman[30]
Neutral AA	Methionine	S-adenosylmethionine synthesis	Rubin et al[31]
Neutral AA	Histidine	Histamine synthesis	Taylor and Snyder[32]
Neutral AA	Histidine	Carnosine synthesis	Chung-Hwang et al[33]
Nucleoside	Adenosine	ATP synthesis	McIlwain[34]
Amine	Choline	Acetylcholine synthesis	Cohen and Wurtman[35]

From Pardridge WM: Nutr Rev Suppl **44**:15, 1986. Reproduced by permission.

ing substrates against a concentration gradient (Fig. 31-1). These abluminal transporters are (1) a sodium-dependent, insulin-sensitive neutral amino acid A-system, (2) an acidic amino acid transporter, (3) an active anion efflux system capable of transporting probenecid, γ-aminobutyric acid (GABA), and valproate, and (4) Na^+/K^+-ATPase.[1]

Neutral amino acid transport across the BBB from the luminal to abluminal side is generally believed attributable to only a single system, which transports the large neutral amino acids such as phenylalanine, leucine, tryptophan, and methionine. This is the (leucine-preferring) L-system.[36] There is little or no transport of the small neutral amino acids such as glycine, alanine, serine, and proline, suggesting that the (alanine-preferring) A-system is absent on the luminal surface of the BBB capillary.[14] Studies of isolated capillaries, indicated the Na^+-dependent, alanine-preferring A-system was located solely on the abluminal surface of the BBB and was sensitive to ouabain inhibition.[38] Although other interpretations have been proposed (see below), the A-system is hypothesized as an energy-dependent active transport system that pumps amino acids from the brain into the capillary lumen.

It has also been suggested that the acidic amino acid transport system defined in the BBB[39] is an active efflux mechanism that removes both glutamate and aspartate, two putative excitatory neu-

rotransmitters, from the brain interstitial space.[40] The observed uptake of aspartate into circumventricular organs (lacking BBB-type capillaries) but not other regions of the brain[41] is consistent with Pardridge's[40] suggestion.

It has been established that an inequality of blood-to-brain versus brain-to-blood transport of valproic acid exists in BBB capillaries. Valproate is pumped out of the brain by the same anion efflux mechanism that transports GABA acid and probenecid out of the CSF.[42] These anion efflux mechanisms in the CSF-blood barrier are active, energy-dependent systems.[43] A similar active transport of organic acids out of the brain by ATP-dependent mechanisms located on the abluminal capillary membrane has been proposed by Betz and Goldstein[44] and extended to include valproate efflux by the same active mechanism.[45]

The presence of Na^+/K^+-ATPase in brain capillaries has been demonstrated.[46-48] Interestingly, this enzyme (Na^+/K^+-ATPase) is located specifically on the abluminal capillary surface and is not present on the luminal membrane.[49] Presumably this active mechanism maintains the low potassium content required for optimal neural cell function.

On the luminal membrane capillary cell there are at least two sodium ion transport systems. One, the Na^+ pore, can be inhibited by the diuretic amiloride; the other, presumably a coupled Na^+/Cl^- cotransport system, can be inhibited by furosemide.[50] Chloride transport kinetics

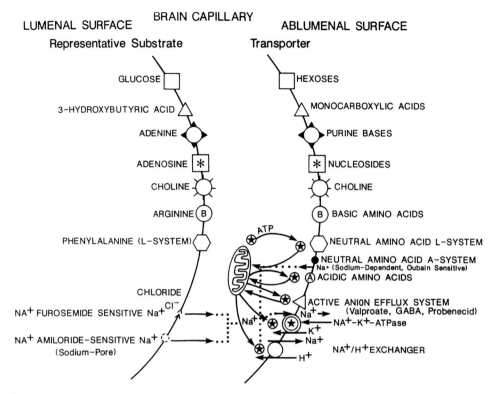

FIGURE 31-1

Differences in the luminal and abluminal surfaces of blood-brain barrier endothelia. The major nutrient transporters (see Table 31-1) are believed to be symmetrically located on the BBB capillaries and to function bidirectionally. In contrast, a group of acidic transporters are believed localized to the abluminal surface and function as energy-dependent, active transporters. Of primary importance is Na^+/K^+-ATPase, a membrane-bound enzyme that effects reduced CNS potassium levels required for impulse conduction. (Adapted from Conford.[1])

are known,[51] but not the inhibition constant of furosemide. In isolated brain capillaries ^{22}Na and ^{86}Rb uptake were furosemide insensitive,[52] indicating that this cotransport system was luminal, and not abluminal. The Na^+/H^+ exchange system is also believed to be abluminal.[52]

Several of these components of the BBB (outlined in Fig. 31-1) display or participate in diabetes-induced alterations[53-75] in function (Table 31-3). Increased nonspecific BBB permeability to tracers such as sucrose has also been reported in experimental diabetes.[76] Diabetic alterations in BBB anatomy are exemplified by a

thickening of the basement membrane[77] and shortened capillary length.[78] Although multiple responses of brain capillary endothelia to diabetic conditions have been reported (see Table 31-3), these responses appear to reflect the complexity of the plasma-brain interface.

Receptors

In addition to transporter proteins, at least seven BBB receptors—atriopeptin, angiotensin II, cationized albumin, insulin, insulin-like growth factors IGF-I and IGF-II, and transferrin—have

TABLE 31-3

Alterations of Blood-Brain Barrier Regulatory Functions in Diabetes

Transporter	Substrate	Modulation	Reference
Hexose	Glucose	20% reduction in BBB glucose transport in diabetic hyperglycemia	Gjedde and Crone[53]
Hexose	Glucose, Mannose, 2-DG, 3-OMG	45% reduction in maximal transport rate of all hexoses examined	McCall et al[54]
Hexose	Glucose	Downregulation in hyperglycemia	Gjedde and Crone[55]
Hexose	Glucose	Downregulation in diabetes restored with both insulin treatment and starvation	McCall et al[56]
		Upregulation in chronic hypoglycemic animals	McCall et al[56]
Hexose	Cytochalasin	Reduced membrane transporter density, reversed with insulin	Matthaei et al[58]
Hexose	Cytochalasin	No decrease in transporters	Harik et al[60]
Hexose	Glucose	Decrease in L-glucose without a decrease in D-glucose influx	Harik and Lamana[59]
Hexose	Glucose	No transporter downregulation in hyperglycemia	Duckrow[61]
Hexose	Glucose, Immunoreactive GLUT-1 isoform	Downregulation of transporter in vivo, and transporter density in isolated BBB capillaries.	Pardridge et al[115]
Hexose	GLUT-1 cDNA	Increased transporter mRNA in BBB capillaries in diabetes.	Choi et al[117]
Hexose	GLUT-1 cDNA, & Immunoreactive GLUT-1	Post-streptozocin insulin therapy normalizes GLUT-1 mRNA, but not BBB glucose transporter protein.	Lutz and Pardridge[118]
Microvessel metabolism	Glucose, 3-OH-butyrate	Oxidation of glucose to CO_2 reduced, 3-OH-butyrate oxidation enhanced in diabetes; in hypoglycemia, oxidation of glucose doubles, 3-OH-butyrate halved	McCall et al[63,64]
Microvessel metabolism	Glucose	Oxidation to CO_2 suppressed in microvessels from alloxan diabetic rabbit brain	Hingorani and Brecher[65]
Monocarboxylic acid	Ketone bodies	Upregulation of transport at 6 and 28 days of diabetes	Mans et al[66]
Monocarboxylic acid	Lactic acid	Unaltered BBB lactate influx	McCall et al[64]
Neutral amino acid	Phenylalanine, tyrosine, and methionine	Reduced influx and reduced brain levels due to altered plasma amino acid levels	Mans et al[67]
Neutral AA	Aromatic and branched-chain acids	Influx is ratio of each acid to sum of plasma amino acid levels	Crandall and Fernstrom[68]
Neutral AA	Tyrosine and leucine	Reduced tyrosine due to high plasma amino acids	Brosnan et al[69]
Neutral AA	Amino acids	Plasma branched-chain amino acids increase in brain; Met, Val increase; Tyr, Trp, Thr decrease	Glanville and Anderson[70]
Basic amino acid	Lysine	Decreased plasma and BBB influx	Mans et al[67]
Amine	Choline	Transporter downregulation	Mooradian[71]
Na/K-ATPase	Sodium	Inhibition (downregulation)	Knudsen,[72] Jakobsen et al[73]
Na^+/H^+ Exchanger		Brain edema of diabetic ketoacidosis postulated to involve brain Na/H function	Van der Meulen et al[74]
Acidic efflux	Aminohippurate	Reduced acidic efflux?	Maepea et al[75]

been demonstrated,[4] and β-adrenoceptors have been identified from dihydroalprenolol-binding studies.[79] Although N-methyl D-aspartate receptors were not found in BBB microvessels,[79] there is little doubt that other receptors are present. (Indirect evidence suggests that a receptor for parathyroid hormone may exist. Brain-derived peptides such as bombesin, neuropeptide Y, neurotensin, somatostatin, substance P, or vasoactive intestinal peptide [VIP] all probably interact with BBB capillaries in some manner.[2,4,6,13,22])

The major differences between receptor-mediated translocation and transporter mechanisms are (1) the way in which molecules are translocated: receptors operate within the cytoplasm; transporter proteins remain within the cell membranes; and (2) the relative time of translocation: transporters on the order of milliseconds; receptors on the order of seconds and perhaps even minutes.[2,4,13]

The BBB receptors are believed to act as transcytosis systems (rather than through a second messenger) and therefore are anticipated to be present on both luminal and abluminal surfaces. The most extensively studied is the insulin receptor, wherein transcytosis is visualized as three sequential steps: (1) endocytosis at the luminal membrane, (2) movement through the endothelial cytoplasm, probably in non-clathrin-containing vesicles, (3) receptor-mediated exocytosis at the abluminal membrane, delivering peptide to the brain interstitium.[2,4] A discussion of BBB transporters (see Table 31-3) and of BBB peptide receptors (Table 31-4)[80-82] in response to the diabetic state is presented below.

NUTRIENT TRANSPORTERS AND BRAIN METABOLISM

Two membrane systems separate plasma nutrients from brain enzymes (BBB and brain cell membranes of neurons or glia). Because the relative surface areas of the smooth-walled BBB capillaries are much smaller than the total brain cell surfaces,[36] the BBB is a potentially rate-limiting step in the translocation of plasma nutrients to their intracellular site of utilization.[4] Many pathways of brain nutrient metabolism are influenced by two regulatory mechanisms—nutrient availability and CNS enzymatic activity.[36] Of the

seven major nutrient transporters defined in the BBB, four are known to directly limit specific pathways of brain metabolism in certain situations (see Table 31-2). When BBB transporter activity is the rate-limiting step, manipulation of the appropriate substrate(s) in the plasma will directly affect the rate of the associated metabolic pathway. Experimental diabetologists have employed this concept in initiating streptozocin diabetes. Animals are typically fasted prior to streptozocin treatment; the fasting causes an increase in plasma ketone bodies and directly enhances brain ketone body oxidation rates. As a consequence of the shift from glucose to ketone body utilization by the brain, side-effects attributable to the rapid streptozocin-induced hyperglycemia are minimized.

The important parameter in recognizing transport-limited metabolic rates is not the plasma nutrient concentration or the rate of BBB translocation, but the concentration of the substrate inside the brain cells. For instance, ketone body levels within the brain are low, at least an order of magnitude lower than that in plasma. Ketone body utilization is always transport-limited.[83] Brain glucose levels are typically 2 to 3 mM in rats,[84] but in pathologic conditions such as hypoglycemia, cerebral anoxia, or seizures, brain glucose levels drop sharply. Under these conditions, a switch from phosphorylation limitation to transport limitation occurs,[84] and BBB glucose transporter activity directly controls brain glucose metabolic rates.[14,36]

The BBB Glucose Transporter

The most abundant glucose transporter protein (MW = 53,000 to 54,000 daltons) may be the GLUT-1 isoform, the facilitative carrier common to human erythrocytes, hepatoma G2 cells, and the brain and BBB. The high glucose utilization rate of the brain has led many workers interested in the study of the transporter protein to isolate and experimentally examine brain and brain microvessel transporters. The high maximal velocity defined for the BBB glucose transporter (see Table 31-1) is indicative of a high density of transporter proteins. Consequently, cytochalasin-B binding studies suggest a tenfold greater concentration of glucose transporter in

TABLE 31-4

Alterations in Blood-Brain Barrier Receptors in Diabetes

Receptor	Modulation	Reference
Insulin	Decreased BBB receptors in diabetes; and increased number with low insulin	Frank et al[80]
Insulin	Downregulation of brain insulin receptor is insulin dose dependent	Devaskar et al[81]
Opiate	Methylnaltrexone (opioid blocker) crosses the BBB in diabetic but not normal mice	Quock et al[82]

BBB capillaries than in brain synaptosomes.[4] The half-saturation constant for the glucose transporter in humans was estimated to be 3 mM, 6 mM, and 9 mM, consistent with estimates from other animals,[85] including the laboratory rat (see Table 31-1). Other kinetic analyses of BBB 3-O-methylglucose transport in humans using positron emission tomography[86] support this concept.

Other distinct glucose transporter proteins have also been identified[62] from other tissues, including: (1) a sodium-dependent, active transporter of kidney and small intestine, (2) a high-capacity facilitative carrier of liver, and (3) an insulin-dependent glucose carrier of muscle and adipose tissue.[87] The human glucose transporter gene is localized to chromosome 1,[88] and a very homologous 2.8-kb glucose transporter mRNA is expressed in both insulin-sensitive and insulin-insensitive tissues in rats and humans.[89] Studies with cDNA to the human rbc transporter further demonstrated that this 2.8-kb mRNA was more abundant in brain capillaries than in any other tissue thus examined.[89] The rat BBB glucose transporter is a 492-amino acid protein that is 98% homologous with the human hepatoma transporter.[90] Homologies between mammalian and bacterial sugar transporters[91] suggest a biologic ubiquity of this protein. Examinations of the sequence of the BBB glucose transporter suggest that it crosses the lipid bilayer 12 times, in the form of alpha-helices,[92] and that both the N- and C-terminal regions, together with a large hydrophilic region near the middle of the sequence, are exposed on the cytoplasmic side of the membrane.[92,93]

In vivo studies demonstrate that the glucose transporter of the BBB is more sensitive to phloretin than phlorizin, is sodium independent, and is insulin insensitive.[14] Mannose and galactose (two other sugars in the diet) may be transported into the brain, in addition to the nonmetabolizable analogues 2-deoxyglucose, 3-O-methylglucose, and 2 fluorodeoxyglucose (FDG).[36] The latter analogue is clinically utilized in metabolic brain mapping of humans injected with ^{18}-F-FDG in positron emission tomography.[94]

Brain Glucose Transport in Diabetes

It is well established that the BBB glucose transporter, unlike that of muscle and adipose tissue, is insulin insensitive in both animals[95] and man.[85] In human diabetic patients, regional cerebral glucose transport has been studied with [^{11}C] 3-O-methylglucose. These five insulin-dependent patients showed no significant alteration in BBB transport of sugar when compared with four normal control subjects.[85]

Gjedde and Crone[53,55] and McCall et al[54] have reported that in chronic hyperglycemia, BBB glucose transport declines. In subsequent studies McCall et al[56] made rats hypoglycemic either by insulinoma implants, an Alzet minipump, or daily injections to produce continual insulin effects. In all three experimental paradigms, increased BBB glucose, mannose, and 2-deoxyglucose transport were observed. The possibility that this could be a consequence of accelerated glucose metabolism was negated in studies showing a similar increase in transport of 3-O-methylglucose, a nonmetabolizable hexose analogue. These studies suggested that the BBB glucose transporter is a functional participant in cerebral glucose homeostasis.[96] This plasticity in the transporter appears to be relatively slow, since the response time is on the order of days, not minutes. (In the intestine, upregulation of the sodium-dependent, active glucose transporter occurs within 24 hours, but downregulation requires three weeks.[97])

In contrast to the above-mentioned studies, Duckrow[61] reported that BBB transport of glucose is not downregulated in hyperglycemic animals. A decrease in permeability times surface area products for glucose was observed in both acute and chronic (streptozocin-induced) hyperglycemia. These decreases were attributed to saturation of the transporter with the elevated plasma glucose levels. Harik and LaManna[59] also reported that glucose transport was unaltered in streptozocin-induced hyperglycemia. These authors also reported an increased L-glucose space in diabetic animals, an observation that might be inconsistent with Lorenzi and associates'[76] report of increased BBB permeability to low molecular weight tracers.

The glucose transporter density has been estimated from in vitro cytochalasin-B binding studies. This ligand reportedly binds to a portion of the glucose transporter, and maximal binding constants are indicative of the relative transporter density. Matthaei et al[58] reported decreased ligand binding to both plasma membranes and microsomes isolated from brain microvessels of animals with streptozocin-induced hyperglycemia. In contrast, Harik et al,[60] in studies of solubilized whole microvessels, reported increased cytochalasin binding in hyperglycemic animals. They noted that downregulation of glucose transporters in chronic hyperglycemia was plausible, and the increased density they found was difficult to explain.[60]

Other studies of microvessels isolated from either diabetic or hypoglycemic animals[63-65] have demonstrated that significant qualitative metabolic changes in BBB capillaries occur in the diabetic and hypoglycemic states. Glucose oxidation and conversion to lactate are diminished in diabetes, but ATP and ATP/ADP ratios are unchanged. Ketone body metabolism is elevated in capillaries from diabetic rats. Similar studies of capillaries from hypoglycemic rats showed a twofold increase in glucose oxidation, while

β-hydroxybutyrate metabolism was halved. In summary, it is apparent that BBB capillaries respond in multiple ways to the spectrum of diabetic changes, and the conflicting reports outlined above require resolution to gain a complete understanding of the BBB glucose transporter responses to altered plasma glucose levels.

Amino Acid Transporters

Three independent transporters in the BBB are responsible for brain uptake of neutral, basic, and acidic amino acids, respectively,[39] from the plasma (see Table 31-1). It has been suggested that the acidic amino acid transporter may also be unique to the abluminal capillary surface, and it may be an energy-dependent, active transporter. Several different neutral amino acid transporters are recognized in cells,[98] and the BBB has been examined for additional systems. As indicated in Figure 31-1, neutral amino acid transport occurs via a sodium-independent, insulin-insensitive (leucine-preferring) L-system. The sodium-dependent and insulin-sensitive (alanine-preferring) A-system is believed to be on the abluminal side of the BBB capillary, although other interpretations exist.[99] No measurable transport of imino-glycine system amino acids occurs at the BBB.[36] On the basis of studies with cysteine as a model substrate, Wade and Brady[100] concluded the alanine-serine-cysteine–preferring system (ASC-system) was not present in the brain. In contrast, evidence of a small but significant ASC transporter in the BBB has been reported by others,[101-103] but the primary role of the L-system in mediating BBB influx of neutral amino acids was noted.[103]

Regulation of these neutral amino acids to the brain is achieved through two mechanisms. First, the relative maximal velocity of the transporter can change either through an increase in the density of transporter proteins or an increase in the rate at which they shuttle substrates (or both). In hepatic encephalopathy, for example, BBB neutral amino acid V_{max} is increased,[104] as are brain tryptophan and serotonin levels; it has been suggested that glutamine or ammonia may induce this change in the neutral amino acid transporter.[36]

A second mechanism by which neutral amino

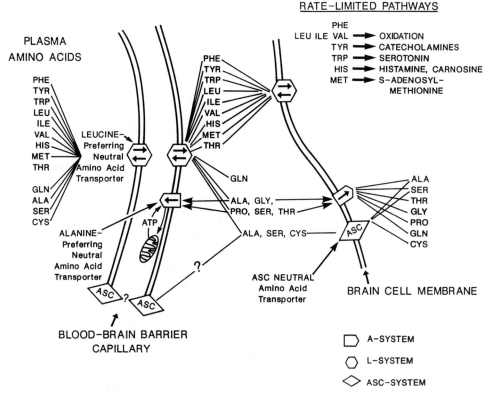

FIGURE 31-2

Plasma neutral amino acids are predominantly translocated to the brain interstitium by a single L-system. In contrast, in brain cell membranes there are at least three neutral amino acid transporters, the leucine-preferring L-system, the alanine-preferring A-system, and the alanine-serine-cysteine–preferring ASC-system. Once inside the brain cells, the large neutral amino acids (LNAAs) are utilized in a variety of substrate-limited pathways of brain metabolism (see Table 31-2). (Modified from Pardridge.[21])

acids are controlled is through competition of the many different substrate amino acids at the BBB site (Fig. 31-2). It has been shown that in normal states and in diabetic animals (Table 31-3), the influx of a single neutral amino acid is a ratio of the concentration of that amino acid compared to the sum total concentrations of all the other competing neutral amino acids. Plasma amino acid profiles are altered with insufficient insulin. Gluconeogenic amino acids are decreased by the liver's use in glucose production, while branched-chain amino acids are increased.[70] While slight qualitative differences exist between reports, alterations in BBB transport of neutral amino acids in diabetes are recognized as a function of the competition between that single, versus the sum total concentration of amino acids, at the BBB.[67-70]

An example of this competition at the BBB can be drawn from the use of tryptophan as a somnolent. The effectiveness of these oral tablets is maximized if they are taken after the postprandial reduction of plasma amino acid levels. Administration of sugar prior to the tryptophan stimulates insulin secretion and activates the A-system transporter in fat and muscle tissue, causing a further reduction in short-chain amino acids and driving the total plasma amino acids lower. Administration of 1000 mg of tryptophan under these conditions results in a sudden, large increase in plasma tryptophan with a concomitantly low sum total concentration of neutral amino acids. Tryptophan transport at the BBB is maximized, and through transport-limited synthesis (as indicated in Table 31-2) an increase in the desired serotonin effector is presumably achieved. Figure 31-2 also emphasizes that several mechanisms function collectively to maintain very low concentrations of neutral amino acids in the brain interstitial space: the L-system, A-system, and ASC-system of brain cells, together with the active A-system on the abluminal border of the BBB capillaries. As a consequence, CSF amino acid levels (CSF amino acids are in equilibrium with brain interstitium) are approximately 10% of plasma levels.[21,36] Low brain interstitial amino acid levels would be expected in the transport-limited metabolic pathways (see Table 31-2).

Many diabetics substitute artificial sweeteners for sugar in their diets. The potential effects of one commonly used sweetener, aspartame, on the brain have been summarized in detail elsewhere.[21] Dietary aspartame (aspartyl-phenylalanine-methyl ester) brings increased quantities of aspartate and phenylalanine into the plasma. The excess aspartate undergoes hepatic metabolism, and phenylalanine levels in the plasma rise significantly. Individuals who are phenylketonuric heterozygotes metabolize phenylalanine at half the rate of controls, and hyperphenylalaninemia is also seen in individuals with liver and renal disease.[21] Untoward potential effects of hyperphenylalaninemia include seizures, hyperactivity, insomnia, and alterations in secretion of growth hormone, prolactin, and gonadotropin. These effects can be attributed in part to competition for the BBB neutral amino acid transporter.[21] Phenylalanine has the highest affinity for this transporter (see Table 31-1; a $K_m = 0.03$ mM concentration means 0.03 mM of this amino acid results in 50% of the transporters being bound with phenylalanine). Increases in plasma phenylalanine and competition for the BBB transporters result in elevated brain phenylalanine levels with a concomitant reduction in brain levels of the competing large neutral amino acids.[21] Since serotonin and catecholamine synthesis are under transporter rate limitation (see Table 31-2), side-effects such as seizures, insomnia, and hyperactivity could be anticipated with reduced inhibitory neurotransmitter (catecholamines and serotonin) synthesis.[21]

Monocarboxylic Acid Transport

Monocarboxylic acid transport is the rate-limiting step in ketone body utilization by the brain. Characteristic of this situation, brain ketone bodies have been found at very low concentrations.[14,28] Monocarboxylic acids are a major source of energy in the brain of the suckling neonate, and elevated BBB transporter activity is observed in neonates.[25] Elevated activity of this transporter has occurred in states of ketosis, such as fasting or a high-fat diet.[36]

This transporter also provides a dramatic illustration of dynamic BBB modulation in selected brain regions. For example, Hawkins and Biebuyck[28] have demonstrated distinct and dramatic differences in the BBB regulation of ketones, particularly in the neocortical regions, indicating that BBB regulation responds to discrete, localized needs. Studies of other BBB transporters also show less dramatic but significant regional differences.[83]

Given that the monocarboxylic acid transporter demonstrates a high degree of physiologic plasticity, changing rapidly in response to nutritional and developmental stimuli, it is not surprising that Mans et al[66] have demonstrated increased activity in diabetic states. Not only is the metabolism of the brain cells altered, but BBB microvessels isolated from diabetic animals display a twofold increase in ketone body oxidation. In microvessels from hypoglycemic animals, ketone oxidation is halved.[63-65] The seemingly inconsistent observation that no alterations in BBB lactate transport were observed in streptozocin-induced hyperglycemia[56] is probably attributable to methodological differences. In the latter study, McCall et al[56] examined whole forebrains; isolated BBB microvessels are typically from the cortical mantles. Furthermore, Mans et al[66] observed diabetically induced increases in ketone body influx only in specific brain regions.

Choline Transport

The BBB amine transporter is somewhat unique in that it appears to significantly facilitate the movement of a single dietary substrate, choline. Analogues such as deanol and hemicholinium can also compete for this transporter locus,[105] but the other major choline-containing compounds in plasma (lecithin and lysolecithin) are excluded by the BBB.[106] Jugular venous blood has a higher choline concentration than the afferent arteries, suggesting a net output of choline from the brain.[107] A possible explanation for this observation is that the brain may synthesize choline *de novo,* and the net release of choline by the brain is equal to the rate of *de novo* synthesis from ethanolamine.[36]

Mooradian[71] reported a decrease in BBB choline transporter kinetics of chronically hyperglycemic, streptozocin-treated rats. Reductions in both the maximal velocity (2.2 vs 0.14, units as in Table 31-1) and the half-saturation constant (0.4 vs 0.12 mM) were in the same direction. The permeability times surface area products are also reduced from 6.4 to 1.67 $\mu l \cdot min^{-1} \cdot g^{-1}$ in these diabetic animals. Possible relationships of this observation to CNS membrane syntheses, neurotransmitter (acetylcholine) synthesis, and alterations in BBB sodium flux (see Table 31-3) await definition, as do the pathophysiologic effects of the observed reduction in BBB transport of choline.

Transport of Nucleic Acid Precursors

As indicated in Table 31-1, there are separate transporters in the BBB for purine bases (adenine and guanine) and nucleosides (adenosine, guanosine, and inosine). Of the pyrimidine bases, uridine is transported by the nucleoside transporter, but not thymine or uracil.[108] Adenosine is a potent neuromodulator and a potent vasodilator in many vascular tissues; it has also been referred to as the endogenous anticonvulsant.[109] Inosine has also been shown to inhibit food intake in animals, presumably through purinergic regulation of food intake.[36] Consequently, it is not surprising that the brain capillaries function as an enzymatic barrier to nucleosides by rapid

conversion to the nucleotide.[110] A function for these nucleotides in the increased mitochondrial content of BBB endothelia remains hypothetical.

Abluminal BBB Transporters

A summary of possible diabetes-induced alterations in the transporters which are believed to be present on the abluminal capillary surface appears in Table 31-3. Reductions in Na^+/K^+-ATPase activity and efflux of acids are based on experimental data, while the possible alterations in the Na^+/H^+ exchanger are hypothesized.

BLOOD-BRAIN BARRIER RECEPTORS

It has been suggested that the BBB insulin receptor system may mediate brain edema in diabetic ketoacidosis patients receiving insulin therapy.[22] No brain edema is seen in these patients when hyperglycemia is normalized by peritoneal dialysis. But with insulin therapy, reductions in brain tonicity lag behind the decrease in plasma osmolarity, and brain edema is seen.[111] These authors suggest that insulin regulates the CNS production of idiogenic osmoles and thus influences brain water balance. Circulating insulin is also believed to regulate the satiety center in the obese patient with type II diabetes,[112] and the BBB receptor would mediate this effect.

The transferrin receptor presumably mediates the distribution of circulating iron into the brain.[4] Some of the BBB peptide receptors may not participate in transcytosis transfer to the brain. Parathyroid hormone and vasoactive intestinal polypeptide activate brain capillary adenyl cyclase, and atriopeptin activates guanyl cyclase.[4] In these situations, the peptides are presumed to act through signal transduction second messengers and induce some other effect on the BBB. Angiotensin II and vasopressin, for example, alter BBB transport of water.[4] Other aspects of BBB receptors and neuropeptide transport in relation to CNS function have been reviewed elsewhere.[2,13,22]

Receptors in Diabetes

Studies of insulin binding to BBB microvessels of rats with streptozocin-induced diabetes[80] have demonstrated that binding of ^{125}I-labeled insulin was highest in control rats (21% per mg protein) and lowest in diabetic animals (15% per mg protein). After the administration of insulin to diabetic rats, binding was increased to 17% per mg protein. These results were also confirmed in studies utilizing cultured brain endothelia; in response to insulin treatment, a downregulation of insulin receptors was observed. When the insulin was removed from the culture medium, insulin receptors returned to control levels. It was concluded that BBB capillaries were involved in the transport of insulin to the brain cells. Furthermore, a defect in BBB response to diabetes may cause a further deficiency in brain insulin when diabetes is poorly controlled.

SUMMARY

Nutrient transporters and other BBB regulatory mechanisms exhibit a series of significant and subtle responses to the diabetic state. The sum of these responses reflects the status of the second century of the BBB: intricate and incompletely defined. A major goal must be to fully understand modulations in glucose and monocarboxylic acid transport and metabolism in the BBB and brain. Modulations in BBB function that limit availability of neurotransmitter precursors in diabetes have been defined: a second critical need is to determine the long-term effects of these changes (and their participation in pathologic, biochemical, and behavioral events) associated with diabetes. A third objective is to define the extent to which other BBB regulatory mechanisms participate in diabetes and diabetic neuropathy. Finally, contemporary and novel approaches must be sought and evaluated for circumvention of the BBB in clinical treatments.

The biologic importance of peptide receptors is apparent when one considers that fully one third of the human genome carries messages for proteins that are found solely in the brain. Some fraction of these proteins no doubt represents peptides with heretofore unappreciated neuromodulatory functions. However, unless these proteins can be delivered to the target site (i.e., across the BBB), their possible clinical uses will not be exploited. The synthesis of chimeric peptides as a vehicle to deliver pharmacologically active peptides to the brain has been proposed. The endogenous opiate β-endorphin is not transported across the BBB. Pardridge and associates[113] have demonstrated that this peptide can be coupled to cationized albumin and the chimeric peptide synthesized. This chimera is taken up and internalized by isolated brain capillaries in vitro, and its brain extraction in vivo is an order of magnitude greater than native endorphin. As yet, cleavage of the chimeric peptide, liberation of the endorphin in the brain interstitium, and biologic activation of the opioid receptors have not been demonstrated. This novel paradigm is of interest for two reasons. First, it emphasizes that current research seems to focus on what the BBB does functionally rather than on what it is. And second, it may represent a rational approach for the development and delivery of peptide neuropharmaceuticals to the CNS and other barrier-protected tissues in disease states such as diabetes.

Recent work seems to support the concept that there is a downregulation of BBB glucose transport in diabetes, as well as a reduction in brain glucose utilization rate.[114] Cerebral blood flow rates also appear to be reduced.[114,115] In vivo studies show a 44% decrease in glucose transporter activity.[115] Analyses of the glucose transporter (GLUT-1) densities in capillaries isolated from streptozocin-treated and control brains indicate a 77% decrease in diabetes, as measured with quantitative Western immunoblots.[115] Continuing work confirms that the BB immunoreactive glucose transporter is downregulated in experimental diabetes, but no normalization of transporter protein was detected in microvessels isolated from streptozocin-treated rats receiving insulin.[116] The mechanism by which this downregulation occurs may be posttranscriptional, because glucose transporter mRNA is not concomitantly decreased. Rather, Choi et al.[117] have shown that BBB glucose transporter mRNA is increased in experimental diabetes, and attribute this to either increased transcription or decreased degradation of the glucose transporter mRNA. Normalization of glucose transporter mRNA is seen after insulin treatment, in contrast to the BBB glucose transporter protein, which was not normalized with exogenous insulin treatment.[116]

Acknowledgment: This work was supported in part by the Veterans Administration and the National Institutes of Health (NS 25554).

References

1. Cornford EM: The blood brain barrier, a dynamic regulatory interface. Mol Physiol 7:219, 1985
2. Pardridge W: Mechanisms of neuropeptide action with the blood-brain barrier. Ann NY Acad Sci 481:231, 1986
3. Pardridge WM: The gatekeeper: How molecules are screened for admission to the brain. Sciences 27:50, 1987
4. Pardridge WM: Recent advances in blood-brain barrier transport. Annu Rev Pharmacol Toxicol 28:25, 1988
5. Wolff JR, Bar T: "Seamless" endothelia in brain capillaries during development of the rat's cerebral cortex. Brain Res 41:17, 1972
6. Cornford EM: Anatomical and developmental aspects of the blood-brain barrier. Sandorama 2:15, 1988
7. Stewart PA, Wiley MJ: Developing nervous tissue induces formation of blood-brain barrier characteristics in invading endothelial cells: A study using quail-chick transplantation chimeras. Dev Biol 84:183, 1981
8. Davson H, Oldendorf WH: Transport in the central nervous system. Proc R Soc Med 60:326, 1967
9. DeBault LE, Cancilla PA: Gamma-glutamyl transpeptidase in isolated brain endothelial cells: Induction by glial cells in vitro. Science 207:653, 1980
10. Cancilla PA: Endothelial and glial cell interactions. In Pardridge WM (moderator): Blood-brain barrier: Interface between internal medicine and the brain. Ann Intern Med 105:82, 1986
11. Janzer JC, Raff MC: Astrocytes induce blood-brain barrier properties in endothelial cells. Nature 325:253, 1987
12. Schweigerer L, Neufeld G, Friedman J et al: Capillary endothelial cells express basic fibroblast growth factor, a mitogen that promotes their own growth. Nature 325:257, 1987
13. Pardridge WM: Receptor mediated peptide transport through the blood brain barrier. Endocrine Rev 7:314, 1986
14. Pardridge WM: Brain metabolism: A perspective from the blood-brain barrier. Physiol Rev 63:1481, 1983
15. Neuwelt EA, Rapoport SI: Modification of the blood-brain barrier in the chemotherapy of malignant tumors. Fed Proc 43:214, 1984
16. Baranczyk-Kuzma A, Audus KL, Borchardt RT: Catecholamine-metabolizing enzymes of bovine brain microvessel endothelial cell monolayers. J Neurochem 46:1956, 1986
17. Gjedde A: The selective barrier between blood and brain. Trends Biochem Sci 11:525, 1986
18. Ghersi-Egea JF, Minn A, Siest G: A new aspect of the protective functions of the blood-brain barrier: Activities of four drug-metabolizing enzymes in isolated rat brain microvessels. Life Sci 42:2515, 1988
19. Vinters HV, Pardridge WM: The blood-brain barrier in Alzheimer's disease. Can J Neurol Sci 13:446, 1986
20. Betz AL: Transport of ions across the blood-brain barrier. Fed Proc 45:2050, 1986
21. Pardridge WM: Potential effects of the dipeptide sweetener aspartame on the blood-brain barrier. In Wurtman RJ, Wurtman JJ (eds): Nutrition and the Brain, vol 7, p 199. New York, Raven Press, 1986
22. Pardridge WM, Oldendorf WM, Cancilla P et al: Blood-brain barrier: Interface between internal medicine and the brain. Ann Intern Med 105:82, 1986
23. Cornford EM, Braun LD, Oldendorf WH et al: Comparison of lipid-mediated blood-brain barrier permeability in neonates and adults. Am J Physiol 243:C161, 1982
24. Cornford EM, Landon KP: Blood-brain barrier transport of CI-912: Single passage equilibration of erythrocyte-borne drug. Ther Drug Monit 7:247, 1985
25. Cornford EM, Cornford ME: Nutrient transport and the blood-brain barrier in developing animals. Fed Proc 45:2065, 1986
26. Choi TB, Pardridge WM: Phenylalanine transport at the human blood brain barrier. J Biol Chem 261:6536, 1986
27. Drewes LR, Gilboe DD: Glycolysis and the permeation of glucose and lactate in the isolated, perfused dog brain during anoxia and postanoxic recovery. J Biol Chem 248:2489, 1973
28. Hawkins RA, Biebuyck JF: Ketone bodies are selectively used by individual brain regions. Science 205:325, 1971
29. Fernstrom JD, Wurtman RJ: Brain serotonin content: Physiological regulation by plasma amino acids. Science 178:414, 1971
30. Gibson CJ, Wurtman RJ: Physiological control of brain norepinephrine synthesis. Life Sci 22:1399, 1978
31. Rubin RA, Ordonez LA, Wurtman RJ: Physiological dependence of brain methionine and S-adenosyl methionine concentrations on serum amino acid patterns. J Neurochem 23:227, 1974

32. Taylor KM, Snyder SH: Dynamics of the regulation of histidine levels in mouse brain. J Neurochem 19:341, 1972

33. Chung-Hwang E, Khurana H, Fisher H: The effect of dietary histidine levels on the carnosine concentration of rat olfactory bulbs. J Neurochem 26:1087, 1976

34. McIlwain H: Transport of adenine derivatives in tissues of the brain. Adv Exp Biol Med 69:253, 1976

35. Cohen EL, Wurtman RJ: Brain acetylcholine: Regulation by dietary choline. Science 191:5661, 1976

36. Pardridge WM: Blood-brain barrier transport of nutrients. Nutr Rev Suppl 44:15, 1986

37. Ladinsky WA, Drewes LR: Characterization of the blood-brain barrier: Composition of the capillary endothelial cell membrane. J Neurochem 41:1341, 1983

38. Betz AL, Goldstein GW: Polarity of the blood-brain barrier: Neutral amino acid transport into isolated brain capillaries. Science 202:225, 1978

39. Oldendorf WH, Szabo J: Amino acid assignment to one of three blood-brain barrier amino acid carriers. Am J Physiol 230:94, 1976

40. Pardridge WM: Regulation of amino acid availability to the brain: Selective control mechanisms for glutamate. In Filer LJ et al (eds): Advances in Biochemistry and Physiology, p. 125. New York, Raven Press, 1979

41. Price MT, Pusateri ME, Crow SE et al: Uptake of exogenous aspartate into circumventricular organs but not other regions of the adult mouse brain. J Neurochem 42:740, 1984

42. Loscher W, Frey HH: Transport of GABA at the blood-CSF interface. J Neurochem 38:1072, 1982

43. Rapoport SI: Blood-Brain Barrier in Physiology and Medicine. New York, Raven Press, 1976

44. Betz AL, Goldstein GW: The basis for active transport at the blood brain barrier. Adv Exp Biol Med 143:5, 1981

45. Cornford EM, Diep CP, Pardridge WM: Blood-brain barrier transport of valproic acid. J Neurochem 44:1541, 1985

46. Goldstein GW: Relation of potassium transport to oxidative metabolism in isolated brain capillaries. J Physiol 286:185, 1979

47. Eisenberg RM, Suddith RL: Cerebral vessels have the capacity to transport sodium and potassium. Science 206:1083, 1979

48. Betz AL, Goldstein GW: Developmental changes in metabolism and transport properties of capillaries isolated from rat brain. J Physiol 312:365, 1981

49. Betz AL, Firth JA, Goldstein GW: Polarity of the blood-brain barrier: Distribution of enzymes between luminal antiluminal membranes of brain capillary endothelial cells. Brain Res 192:17, 1980

50. Betz AL: Sodium transport in capillaries from isolated rat brain. J Neurochem 41:1150, 1983

51. Smith QR, Rapoport SI: Carrier mediated chloride transport across the blood-brain barrier. J Neurochem 42:754, 1984

52. Betz AL: Sodium transport from blood to brain: Inhibition by furosemide and amiloride. J Neurochem 41:1158, 1983

53. Gjedde A, Crone C: Blood-brain glucose transfer: Repression in chronic hyperglycemia. Science 214:456, 1981

54. McCall AL, Millington AR, Wurtman RJ: Metabolic fuel and amino acid transport into the brain in experimental diabetes mellitus. Proc Natl Acad Sci USA 79:5406, 1982

55. Gjedde A, Crone C: Biochemical modulation of blood brain barrier permeability. Acta Neuropathol Suppl 8:59, 1983

56. McCall AL, Fixman LB, Fleming N et al: Chronic hyperglycemia increases glucose transport. Am J Physiol 251:E442, 1986

57. Mooradian AD, Morin AM: Brain uptake of glucose in diabetes mellitus: the role of glucose transporters. Am J Med Sci 301:173–177, 1991

58. Matthaei S, Horuk R, Olefsky JM: Blood-brain glucose transfer in diabetes mellitus: Decreased number of glucose transporters at the blood-brain barrier. Diabetes 35:1181, 1986

59. Harik SI, LaManna JC: Vascular perfusion and blood brain glucose transport in acute and chronic hyperglycemia. J Neurochem 51:1924, 1988

60. Harik SI, Gravina SA, Kalaria RN: Glucose transporter of the blood brain barrier and brain in chronic hyperglycemia. J Neurochem 51:1930, 1988

61. Duckrow RB: Glucose transfer into rat brain during acute and chronic hyperglycemia. Metab Brain Dis 3:201, 1988

62. Bell GI, Kayano T, Buse JB et al: Molecular biology of mammalian glucose transporters. Diab Care 13:198, 1990

63. McCall AL, Sussman I, Tornheim K et al: Effects of hypoglycemia and diabetes on fuel metabolism by rat brain microvessels. Am J Physiol 254:E272, 1988

64. McCall AL, Gould JB, Ruderman NB: Diabetes-induced alterations of glucose metabolism in rat cerebral microvessels. Am J Physiol 247:E462, 1984

65. Hingorani V, Brecher P: Glucose and fatty acid

metabolism in normal and diabetic cerebral microvessels. Am J Physiol 252:E648, 1987

66. Mans AM, Biebuyck JF, Hawkins RA: Regional brain utilization of ketone bodies in starvation and diabetes. J Cereb Blood Flow Metab 1(suppl 1):90, 1981

67. Mans AM, DeJoseph MR, Davis DW et al: Regional amino acid transport into brain during diabetes: Effect of plasma amino acids. Am J Physiol 253:E575, 1987

68. Crandall EA, Fernstrom JD: Effect of experimental diabetes on the levels of aromatic and branched-chain amino acids in rat blood and brain. Diabetes 32:222, 1983

69. Brosnan JT, Forsey RG, Brosnan ME: Uptake of tyrosine and leucine in vivo by brain of diabetic and control rats. Am J Physiol 247:C450, 1984

70. Glanville NT, Anderson GH: The effect of insulin deficiency, dietary protein intake and plasma amino acid concentrations on brain amino acid levels in rats. Can J Physiol Pharmacol 63:487, 1985

71. Mooradian AD: Blood-brain barrier choline transport is reduced in diabetic rats. Diabetes 36:1094, 1987

72. Knudsen GM, Jakobsen J: Blood-brain barrier permeability to sodium: Modification by glucose or insulin? J Neurochem 52:174, 1989

73. Jakobsen J, Knudsen GM, Juhler M: Cation permeability of the blood brain barrier in streptozotocin-diabetic rats. Diabetologia 30:409, 1987

74. Van der Meulen JA, Klip A, Grinstein S: Possible mechanism for cerebral oedema in diabetic ketoacidosis. Lancet 2:306, 1987

75. Maepea O, Karlsson C, Alm A: Blood-ocular and blood-brain barrier function in streptozotocin-induced diabetes in rats. Arch Ophthalmol 102: 1366, 1984

76. Lorenzi M, Healy DP, Hawkins R et al: Studies on the permeability of the blood brain barrier in experimental diabetes. Diabetologia 29:58, 1986

77. Yasuda H, Dyck PJ: Abnormalities of endoneurial microvessels and sural nerve pathology in diabetic neuropathy. Neurology 37:20, 1987

78. Jakobsen J, Sidenous P, Gunderson HJ et al: Quantitative changes of cerebral neocortical structure in insulin-treated long-term streptozotocin-induced diabetes in rats. Diabetes 36:597, 1987

79. Beart PM, Sheehan KAM, Manallack DT: Absence of N-methyl-D-aspartate receptors on ovine cerebral microvessels. J Cereb Blood Flow Metab 8:879, 1988

80. Frank HJ, Pardridge WM, Jankovic-Vokes T et al: Insulin binding to the blood brain barrier in the streptozotocin-diabetic rat. J Neurochem 47:405, 1986

81. Devaskar SU, Karyki L, Devaskar UP: Varying brain insulin concentrations differentially regulate the fetal brain insulin receptor. Biochem Biophys Res Commun 136:208, 1986

82. Quock RM, Ishii MM, Emmanouil DE: Central pharmacological activity of a quaternary ammonium compound in streptozotocin diabetic mice. Life Sci 43:1411, 1988

83. Hawkins RA: Transport of essential nutrients across the blood-brain barrier of individual structures. Fed Proc 45:2055, 1986

84. Crane PD, Pardridge WM, Braun LD et al: The interaction of transport and metabolism on brain glucose utilization: A reevaluation of the lumped constant. J Neurochem 36:1601, 1981

85. Brooks DJ, Gibbs JSR, Sharp P et al: Regional cerebral glucose transport in insulin dependent patients studied using [^{11}C] 3-O-methyl-D-glucose and positron emission tomography. J Cereb Blood Flow Metab 6:240, 1986

86. Vyska K, Magloire JR, Freundlieb C et al: In vivo determination of the kinetic parameters of glucose transport in the human brain using C-11 methyl D-glucose (CMG) and dynamic positron emission tomography. Eur J Nucl Med 11:97, 1985

87. James DE, Brown R, Navarro J et al: Insulin-regulatable tissues express a unique insulin sensitive glucose transport protein. Nature 333:183, 1988

88. Shows TB, Eddy RL, Byers MG et al: Polymorphic human glucose transporter gene (GLUT) is on chromosome 1p31.3-p35. Diabetes 36:546, 1987

89. Flier JS, Mueckler M, McCall AL et al: Distribution of glucose transporter messenger RNA transcripts in tissues of rat and man. J Clin Invest 79:657, 1987

90. Birnbaum MJ, Aspel HC, Rosen OM: Cloning and characterization of a cDNA encoding the rat brain glucose transporter protein. Proc Natl Acad Sci USA 83:5784, 1986

91. Maiden MCJ, Davis EO, Baldwin SA et al: Mammalian and bacterial sugar transport proteins are homologous. Nature 325:641, 1987

92. Mueckler M, Caruso C, Baldwin SA et al: Sequence and structure of a human glucose transporter. Science 229:941, 1985

93. Davies A, Meeran K, Cairns MT et al: Peptide specific antibodies as probes of the orientation of the glucose transporter in the human erythrocyte membrane. J Biol Chem 262:9347, 1985

94. Phelps ME, Mazziotta JC: Positron emission tomography: Human brain function and biochemistry. Science 228:799, 1985

95. Lund-Andersen H: Transport of glucose from blood to brain. Physiol Rev 59:305, 1979

96. Anonymous: Relationship of blood-brain-barrier glucose transport to circulating glucose supply. Nutr Rev 45:218, 1987

97. Diamond JM, Karasov WH: Effect of dietary carbohydrate on monosaccharide uptake by mouse small intestine in vitro. J Physiol 349:419, 1984

98. Christensen HN: On the strategy of kinetic discrimination of amino acid transport systems. J Membr Biol 84:97, 1985

99. Blasberg RG, Fenstermacher JD, Patlak CS: Transport of α-aminobutyric acid across brain capillary and cellular membranes. J Cereb Blood Flow Metab 3:32, 1983

100. Wade LA, Brady HM: Cysteine and cystine transport at the blood brain barrier. J Neurochem 37:730, 1981

101. Sershen H, Lajtha A: Capillary transport of amino acids in the developing brain. Exp Neurol 53:465, 1976

102. Lefauconnier JM, Lacombe P, Bernard G: Cerebral blood flow and blood brain influx of some neutral amino acids in control and hypothyroid 16-day-old rats. J Cereb Blood Flow Metab 5:318, 1985

103. Tovar A, Tews JK, Torres N et al: Some characteristics of threonine transport across the blood brain barrier of the rat. J Neurochem 51:1285, 1988

104. James JH, Escourrou J, Fischer JE: Blood-brain neutral amino acid transport is increased after portacaval anastomosis. Science 200:1395, 1978

105. Cornford EM, Braun LD, Oldendorf WH: Carrier mediated blood-brain barrier transport of choline and choline analogs. J Neurochem 30:299, 1978

106. Pardridge WM, Cornford EM, Braun LD et al: Transport of choline and choline analogs through the blood-brain barrier. In Barbeau A et al (eds): Nutrition and the Brain, vol 5. New York, Raven Press, 1979

107. Aquilonius SM, Ceder G, Lying-Tunell U et al: The arteriovenous difference of choline across the brain of man. Brain Res 99:430, 1975

108. Cornford EM, Oldendorf WH: Independent blood-brain barrier transport mechanisms for nucleic acid precursors. Biochim Biophys Acta 394:211, 1975

109. Williams M: Adenosine—a selective neuromodulator in the mammalian CNS? Trends Neurol Sci 7:164, 1984

110. Wu PH, Phillus JW: Uptake of adenosine by isolated rat brain capillaries. J Neurochem 38:687, 1982

111. Guisado R, Arieff AI: Neurologic manifestations of diabetic comas: Correlation with biochemical alterations in the brain. Metabolism 24:665, 1975

112. Woods SC, Porte D: The role of insulin as a satiety factor in the central nervous system. Adv Metab Dis 10:457, 1983

113. Pardridge WM, Kumagai AK, Eisenberg JB: Chimeric peptides as a vehicle for peptide pharmaceutical delivery to the brain. Biochem Biophys Res Commun 145:307, 1987

114. Jakobsen J, Nedergaard M, Aarslew-Jensen M, Diemer NH: Regional brain glucose metabolism and blood flow in streptozocin-induced diabetic rats. Diabetes 39:437, 1990

115. Pardridge WM, Triguero D, Farrell CR: Downregulation of blood-brain barrier glucose transporter in experimental diabetes. Diabetes 39:1040, 1990

116. Lutz AJ, Pardridge WM: Regulation of the blood-brain barrier glucose transporter in streptozocin diabetes in rats: Insulin therapy normalizes glucose transporter mRNA but not glucose transporter protein in brain capillaries. Diabetes (in press)

117. Choi TB, Boado RJ, Pardridge WM: Blood-brain barrier glucose transporter mRNA is increased in experimental diabetes. Biochem Biophys Res Comm 164:375, 1989

CHAPTER 32

Nutrients and the Biochemical Regulation of Brain Function

CHRISTOPHER J. SCHMIDT and WALTER LOVENBERG

The brain has a major coordinating role in determining the need for and in acquiring nutrients. For this reason, brain function is central to the problem of obesity. However, the brain is such a complex organ that its role in obesity cannot be defined in simple terms. This complexity is achieved by the large number (perhaps as many as 10^{11}) of highly specialized neurons in the brain that communicate with each other through the synthesis, storage, and release of specific neurotransmitter substances. It has been suggested[1,2] that the synthesis of these neurotransmitter substances may in part be dependent on the supply of nutrients to the particular cells. Because the availability of neurotransmitter substances may regulate the overall integral function of the brain, an understanding of the regulation of neurotransmitter synthesis is required for an ultimate understanding of how neurons perform their role. It is therefore possible to construe a relationship between brain function and nutrient intake in man.

The effects of gross malnutrition have been studied in some detail. In general, the brain is fairly well protected from acute dietary deficiencies in the adult, although malnutrition has permanent effects on fetal brain development.[3] The fact that the brain is relatively impervious to acute changes in nutrition may be related to the generous supply of the circulation that it receives. Sokoloff et al[4] have estimated that although the brain accounts for only about 2% of the weight of an adult, it receives 15% of the output of the heart and accounts for 20% to 30% of the resting metabolic rate. This high energy consumption may be necessitated by the nearly continuous electrical activity of the approximately 100 billion neurons of the brain. In addition to the effects of gross malnutrition, it has been suggested by many authors that relatively subtle differences in diet can have a qualitative effect on brain function and consequently on behavior. Although advances in our knowledge of neurochemistry provide a sound foundation for such hypotheses, they remain to be validated by scientific investigation.

This chapter examines the biochemical regulation of synthesis in several neurotransmitter systems and the points where subtle changes in nutrient availability could interact to produce a change in neurochemical function or behavior. Because most normal diets contain sufficient or excess vitamins and minerals and these nutrients form constitutive parts of the macromolecules responsible for neurotransmitter metabolism, they are less likely to be culprits in the subtle effects of diet on behavior. However, there may be conditions under which the availability of the primary precursor of a neurotransmitter may become important. It is the regulatory mechanisms active under these conditions that we will focus on.

NEUROTRANSMITTER SYSTEMS

Neurons in the brain are generally characterized by the type of neurotransmitter substances that they produce and store. As an example, there are three types of catecholamine neurons, depending on the expression of the enzymes tyrosine hydroxylase, dopamine-β-hydroxylase, and phenylethanolamine-N-methyltransferase. Neurons that express only tyrosine hydroxylase are recognized as dopaminergic neurons, while those expressing both tyrosine hydroxylase and dopamine-β-hydroxylase appear as noradrenergic neurons. Neurons expressing all three catecholamine biosynthetic enzymes are adrenergic neurons. In recent years, the situation has become more complex with the recognition that certain neurons express a second or cotransmitter, usually a specific neuropeptide.

Several dozen specific compounds function as neurotransmitters in the brain. The feature common to most of these compounds is that they are nitrogenous and, in general, are derived from dietary protein. This information provides an explanation for how a subtle change in the quality or quantity of dietary protein could affect the synthesis of neurotransmitter and subsequently neurotransmission and behavior.

Figure 32-1 shows schematically how dietary protein is converted into neurotransmitters. In general, the digestion of protein into its component amino acids provides the transmitter directly, or at least the substrates for the neurotransmitter synthesizing enzymes. Amino acids are also the required substrates for the synthesis of numerous neuropeptide precursors, which in turn are degraded by specific proteases to peptide transmitters.

In addition to providing the basic building blocks, the diet must also provide the appropriate vitamins and minerals for the transformations of amino acids into the specific molecules that are the messengers. From the biosynthetic pathways for the biogenic amines (Fig. 32-2, Table 32-1), it is apparent that various vitamins and trace minerals are essential for the enzymic transformation that must take place. Iron appears to be particularly important in this aspect of brain function. Three of the important hydroxylases and monoamine oxidase contain iron. However, iron plays many roles in the neurochemistry of brain, and severe iron deficiency appears to cause disturbances in learning and behavior. This subject has been reviewed recently.[5]

AMINO ACID HYDROXYLASES

The amino acid hydroxylases are the primary regulatory points in the control of biogenic amine biosynthesis. These enzymes constitute a family of enzymes that are mixed-function oxidases. The enzymes of interest here are phenylalanine, tyrosine, and tryptophan hydroxylases. In addition to the amino acid substrate, they each utilize oxygen and tetrahydrobiopterin (BH_4) as cosubstrates. As indicated in Figure 32-2, the products of this reaction are the hydroxylated amino acid, quinoid dihydrobiopterin (BH_2), and water. Although the fundamental reaction mechanism is similar for each enzyme, the regulatory mechanisms are quite distinct, and each enzyme

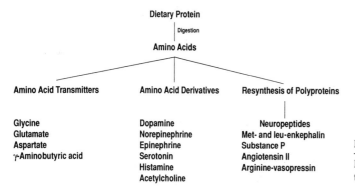

FIGURE 32-1

Dietary protein as a precursor of neurotransmitters.

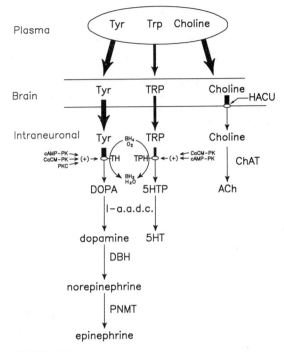

Plasma

Brain

Intraneuronal

FIGURE 32-2

Regulation of catecholamine, 5-HT, and acetylcholine synthesis. (cAMP-PK, cAMP-dependent protein kinase; BH₄, tetrahydrobiopterin; CaCM-PK, calcium-calmodulin–dependent protein kinase; ChAT, choline acetyltransferase; DBH, dopamine-β-hydroxylase; DOPA, dihydroxyphenylalanine; HACU, high-affinity choline uptake; 5-HTP, 5-hydroxytryptophan; PKC, protein kinase C; PNMT, phenylethanolamine-N-methyltransferase; TH, tyrosine hydroxylase; TPH, tryptophan hydroxylase.)

has a characteristic amino acid substrate specificity. Knowledge of the primary structure of these enzymes has increased rapidly. Deduced amino acid sequences for human liver phenylalanine hydroxylase, rat tyrosine hydroxylase, and rabbit tryptophan hydroxylase have been compared.[6] Considerable homology appears to exist in the central portion of the molecules, with very little homology near the amino terminus of the proteins. Analysis of the data[6] on homology of these three enzymes suggests that the catalytic active site is located in the center portion of the molecule, whereas the amino terminal region is involved in regulatory functions. This is consist-

TABLE 32-1

Vitamin and Mineral Content of Enzymes Involved in Biogenic Amine Metabolism

Vitamin or Mineral	Enzyme
Iron	Aromatic amino acid hydroxylases
	Monoamine oxidase
Copper	Dopamine-β-hydroxylase
Pyridoxine	Aromatic-L-amino acid decarboxylase
Riboflavin	Dopamine-β-hydroxylase
Niacin	Quinoid dihydropteridine reductase

ent with the unique regulatory properties of each of these enzymes. Thus, although all three enzymes probably evolved from a common ancestral gene, each has become specialized with regard to substrate specificity and regulatory properties.

Phenylalanine Hydroxylase

The regulation of phenylalanine hydroxylase (PH) is discussed first because of its position in the biochemical pathway leading to catecholamine biosynthesis. The regulation of PH is perhaps the best understood of all the hydroxylases. As such, PH provides a model hydroxylase for examining the types of biochemical regulation that neurotransmitter synthesis may be subject to.

Only a portion of the tyrosine utilized for the formation of brain catecholamines is derived from phenylalanine, since tyrosine is a prevalent amino acid in normal food proteins. However, absence of PH in the liver can lead to phenylketonuria and severe brain dysfunction. Patients with this genetic disease have high circulating levels of phenylalanine. However, it is not known what causes the brain dysfunction. The high circulating levels of phenylalanine clearly play a role, since limiting the amount of phenylalanine in the diet from birth appears to be efficacious in lessening the degree of mental retardation.[7] This is an excellent example of how dietary modification can influence brain function.

PH is subject to a variety of regulatory mechanisms, some of which may be influenced by dietary factors. The enzyme is thought to exist *in vivo* primarily as a tetrameric protein with a molecular weight of about 200,000 daltons. Enzymes isolated from the liver can be activated by the following mechanisms: (1) phosphorylation, (2) phospholipid treatment, (3) limited proteolysis, and (4) allosteric modification by phenylalanine. Two of these modifications may be related to the regulation of this enzyme by dietary factors. The regulation of this important enzyme has been recently reviewed.[8]

PH is normally found in the liver in a low activity state when analyzed using the natural electron donor, BH_4. Of interest, other pterins, such as the 6-methyltetrahydropterins, can serve as electron donors with the unactivated enzyme, but the enzyme activity is much greater with these synthetic pterins. Therefore, in order to study regulation it is essential to use BH_4. It was observed a number of years ago[9] that preincubation of the native unactivated enzyme with the substrate phenylalanine resulted in a large increase in activity, presumably due to a conformational change in the protein. Evidence for this conformational change has been reported from several laboratories.[10-12] Shifts in the native fluorescence of PH show that the substrate can bind to an allosteric site (at least four per tetramer). Whether this regulatory mechanism is of importance for the *in vivo* regulation of the enzyme remains to be proven; logically, however, an excess of substrate would lead to an increase in the activity of the major metabolic enzyme. Thus, nutritional intake of large amounts of phenylalanine would result in increased metabolic capability.

A second mechanism whereby diet could influence the metabolism of phenylalanine and the formation of tyrosine is through the regulation of PH by phosphorylation. Following the observation[13] that tyrosine hydroxylase could be activated by protein phosphorylation, PH was also found to be activated by a cyclic adenosine monophosphate (cAMP)-dependent phosphorylation reaction.[14] Although the characteristics of this activation differ significantly from the activation of tyrosine hydroxylases, it is clear that the activity state of the enzyme can be modified by metabolic factors. In liver cells, this can occur via an action of glucagon. Kaufman and coworkers (see reference 15 for review) have shown that glucagon increases the degree of phosphorylation as well as the specific activity of PH *in vivo*. This response appears to be dependent on the stimulation of cAMP formation. Thus, nutritional factors, including phenylalanine, that stimulate the release of glucagon also serve to enhance the metabolism of phenylalanine and the formation of tyrosine.

Tyrosine Hydroxylase

Tyrosine hydroxylase (TH) is the rate-limiting enzyme in the formation of the catecholamine neurotransmitters: dopamine, norepinephrine, and epinephrine. Enzyme activity appears to be controlled by an elegant regulatory system that may in part be subject to the influence of nutritional factors. TH is composed of four identical subunits, each with a molecular weight of approximately 60,000 daltons. Like PH, TH can be activated by limited proteolysis, which suggests that regulatory and catalytic domains exist on distinct regions of the molecule. The enzyme is also activated by protein phosphorylation,[13] which may have the net effect of altering the intramolecular interaction of the regulatory and catalytic domains. Whereas the regulation of PH can be considered to revolve around the need to avoid excessive accumulation of phenylalanine, the regulation of TH is more closely linked to the supply of its product. Unlike PH, there is no evidence for tyrosine activating TH; however, catecholamines (dopamine, norepinephrine, epinephrine) have been shown to allosterically inhibit TH activity. This allows catecholamine biosynthesis to be regulated directly by its products. However, even this feedback mechanism is subject to further regulation.

Although tyrosine is formed in the liver from the essential amino acid phenylalanine, a large amount comes directly from the diet. As shown in Figure 32-2, TH is dependent on both O_2 and BH_4 for the conversion of tyrosine to dihydroxyphenylalanine (DOPA). This intermediate is present in very small quantities in catecholaminergic neurons, owing to its immediate decarbox-ylation to dopamine by excess L-aromatic amino acid decarboxylase. Further conversion to nor-epinephrine or epinephrine is dependent on the presence of dopamine-β-hydroxylase and phenylethanolamine-N-methyltransferase in the neuron. Since under normal circumstances the concentration of tyrosine in the nerve terminal is not believed to be limiting for enzyme activity, most acute regulation of TH is thought to occur through changes in the affinity of the enzyme for the cofactor, BH_4. In the brain, this regulation occurs through any of three distinct receptor-operated second-messenger systems: the cAMP system, Ca^{2+}-calmodulin system, or the inosi-tol triphosphate-diacylglycerol system. Each of these second messengers has as its effector a unique protein kinase. Phosphorylation of TH by cAMP-dependent protein kinase, Ca^{2+}-calmodulin protein kinase, or protein kinase C reduces the K_m of the enzyme for its cofactor. There is also evidence that phosphorylation of TH reduces its sensitivity to feedback inhibition by catecholamines. An excellent article ad-dressing the interaction of each of the various kinases with TH has recently been published.[16] Changes in the activities of these second-messenger systems thus provide a means whereby catecholamine biosynthesis may be in-fluenced by surrounding neuronal activity. Un-der conditions of normal activity, as little as 20% of TH in the nigrostriatal pathway of the rat is believed to be in the phosphorylated state. Le-vine et al[17] have estimated that cytoplasmic con-centrations of BH_4 are such that only this acti-vated TH is involved in neurotransmitter synthesis. Under these conditions, tyrosine con-centrations are sufficient to produce 75% satura-tion of the enzyme,[18] although this may not hold true under all conditions of neuronal activity. Changes in activity requiring an increase in transmitter synthesis lead to an increase in the percentage of TH in the phosphorylated form. At the point where BH_4 no longer limits enzyme ac-tivity, changes in tyrosine availability may have a significant effect on the rate of transmitter syn-thesis. Changes in neuronal activity and de-mands on the synthetic capacity of the neuron can occur under several conditions. Receptor blockade with the dopamine receptor antagonist

haloperidol increases the firing rate in the nigro-striatal dopaminergic pathway by blocking both inhibitory autoreceptors and postsynaptic recep-tors involved in a polysynaptic feedback loop. An increase in TH phosphorylation has been demonstrated following haloperidol administra-tion.[19] Under these conditions, peripherally ad-ministered tyrosine appears to result in an in-crease in dopamine synthesis.[18] An analogous situation in which tyrosine availability may be-come rate-limiting occurs when the number of functional terminals is insufficient to maintain adequate output of neurotransmitter. Under these conditions the involved neurons attempt to compensate by increasing their firing rate and transmitter synthesis. Tyrosine administration has been reported to increase dopamine turnover in the caudate nucleus following partial unilat-eral lesions of the substantia nigra with 6-hy-droxydopamine, although the amino acid was without effect in the nonlesioned hemisphere.[20] Long-term changes in regulation following such lesions may involve more than allosteric modi-fications of TH activity. Wolf et al[21] have demon-strated an increase in the amount of TH in re-maining dopaminergic terminals following partial lesions of the dopaminergic system. The influence of tyrosine availability under such con-ditions remains to be determined. Such informa-tion would be pertinent to the question of whether tyrosine administration can increase do-pamine synthesis in cases of neuronal degenera-tion such as parkinsonism.

Tryptophan Hydroxylase

The synthesis of serotonin (5-HT) closely paral-lels that of the catecholamines. The hydroxyla-tion of tryptophan by tryptophan hydroxylase (TPH) is rate-limiting and the site of regulation for the entire pathway. The product of the reac-tion, 5-hydroxytryptophan, is decarboxylated to 5-HT by the same L-aromatic amino acid decar-boxylase functioning in catecholamine biosyn-thesis. The biochemical characterization of TPH has lagged behind that of the other hydroxylases, owing to the extreme liability of the purified en-zyme. The enzyme is believed to be composed of multiple identical subunits of approximately 50,000 daltons molecular weight. TPH is also activated by limited proteolysis and phosphorylation (vide infra), suggesting several similarities to the mechanism of regulation of TH. Unlike the situation with catecholaminergic neurons, the concentration of tryptophan in the serotonergic nerve terminal is near the K_m for TPH.[22] Since tryptophan is an essential amino acid, this observation suggests that dietary tryptophan can have a significant effect on 5-HT synthesis. Biopterin cofactor and molecular oxygen are also believed to be present at subsaturating concentrations in the serotonergic terminal, which provides multiple routes for the regulation of this pathway.

There is considerable evidence that TPH activity is acutely regulated by neuronal activity. Several groups have shown that TPH is a substrate for Ca^{2+}-calmodulin protein kinase.[23,24] As described for TH, phosphorylation of the enzyme increases its affinity for BH_4. Thus, increases in the firing rate of serotonergic neurons are closely linked to the rate of transmitter synthesis by the associated increase in intracellular Ca^{2+}. Although not a substrate for cAMP-dependent protein kinase in homogenates, this may be another route for activation of the enzyme in more intact tissue preparations.[25]

Of greater interest to this discussion is the ability of tryptophan availability to influence central 5-HT synthesis. The concentration of tryptophan in the brain is controlled by the plasma ratio of tryptophan to other large neutral amino acids, all of which compete for the same uptake carrier.[26] Tryptophan loading or a high-carbohydrate meal increases this ratio and elevates brain tryptophan concentrations. There are data suggesting that an increase in serotonergic activity mediates the preferential selection of protein-derived calories observed after a carbohydrate snack.[27] Since administration of tryptophan to rats increases central 5-HT concentrations,[18,28] this finding suggests a mechanism whereby nutrient intake could regulate itself via a direct effect on central nervous system function. What remains to be seen is whether increases in the rate of 5-HT synthesis are actually translated into an increase in transmitter release and in those activities mediated by 5-HT. Changes in function are particularly difficult to evaluate for the serotonergic system because of the subtle nature of the behaviors that 5-HT may be involved in. There are contradictory reports of the effects of tryptophan loading on pain sensitivity and locomotion. 5-HT release has been implicated in the control of sleep, and there is some evidence that tryptophan can decrease sleep latency times in some individuals (see reference 26). As with the TH system, it is likely that situations producing an increase in demand for transmitter have the highest probability of displaying a role for precursor availability in the maintenance of serotonergic function.[29]

ACETYLCHOLINE SYNTHESIS

The synthesis of acetylcholine (ACh) differs significantly from the synthesis of the monoaminergic transmitters just discussed. ACh is synthesized from acetyl-coenzyme A and choline by the enzyme choline acetyltransferase (ChAT). Like TPH, the enzyme is not saturated with its substrate choline, yet little more is known about the regulation of the enzyme. The enzyme can be phosphorylated by Ca^{2+}-calmodulin protein kinase,[30] but how this affects the activity of the enzyme is not known. Of the transmitter systems discussed, ACh synthesis is probably the most dependent on the immediate availability of its precursor. A sodium-dependent, high-affinity uptake system unique to cholinergic neurons maintains the supply of choline necessary for transmitter synthesis.[31] A number of studies have shown the activity of this system to be rate-limiting with respect to ACh synthesis.[32] Under normal conditions, the concentration of choline in the synaptic space (1mM) is sufficient to saturate the carrier. Thus, dietary choline generally has little effect on ACh synthesis. However, the uptake system can respond to increases in neuronal firing and demand for transmitter. An increase in high-affinity choline uptake has been observed after treatments that increased the firing rate of cholinergic neurons. Such treatments include the administration of convulsants and electrical stimulation of cholinergic pathways. Perhaps more important is the increase in high-affinity choline uptake measured in residual cholinergic terminals following partial lesions of discrete cholinergic nuclei.[33] Although the exact mechanism responsible for this response is not known, kinetic analysis of such changes has revealed an increase in the number of uptake sites. This effect is Ca^{2+} dependent, as might be ex pected for a link between neuronal activity and transmitter synthesis.

SUMMARY

This chapter has briefly described the synthesis of three neurotransmitters and how the rate of synthesis is precisely controlled. In all cases, the maximum capacity of the biosynthetic pathway far exceeds the actual rates of transmitter synthesis measured in vivo (see Fig. 32-2). This is an indication of the tight regulation under which these systems operate. The biochemical basis for an interaction between substrate availability and neurotransmitter synthesis certainly exists. However, with the possible exception of the serotonergic system, it seems unlikely that supplementation of the discussed transmitter precursors will significantly influence neuronal activity under normal conditions. What remains open to debate is whether these substrates become limiting under conditions that activate the synthetic capability of these systems.

References

1. Lovenberg W: Biochemical regulation of brain function. Nutr Rev 44:6, 1986
2. Anderson GH, Johnston JL: Nutrient control of brain neurotransmitter synthesis and function. Can J Physiol Pharmacol 61:271, 1983
3. Nowak TS, Munro HN: Effects of protein-caloric malnutrition on biochemical aspects of brain development. In Wurtman RJ, Wurtman JJ (eds): Nutrition and the Brain, Vol 2, p 193. New York, Raven Press, 1977
4. Sokoloff L, Fitzgerald GG, Kaufman EE: Cerebral nutrition and energy metabolism. In Wurtman RJ, Wurtman JJ (eds): Nutrition and the Brain, Vol 1, p 87. New York, Raven Press, 1977
5. Youdim MHB, Lovenberg W, Tipton KF: Topics in neurochemistry and neuropharmacology. In Youdim MHB (ed): Brain Iron: Neurochemical and Behavioral Aspects. Taylor and Francis, 1988
6. Grenett HE, Ledley FD, Reed LL et al: Full-length cDNA for rabbit tryptophan hydroxylase: Functional domains and evolution of aromatic amino acid hydroxylase. Proc Natl Acad Sci USA 84: 5530, 1987
7. Armstrong MD, Tyler FH: Studies on phenylketonuria: Restricted phenylalanine intake in phenylketonuria. J Clin Invest 34:565, 1955

8. Kaufman S: Regulation of the activity of phenylalanine hydroxylase. Adv Enzyme Regul 25:37, 1985
9. Tourian A: Activation of phenylalanine hydroxylase by phenylalanine. Biochim Biophys Acta 242:345, 1971
10. Shiman R, Gray DW: Substrate activation of phenylalanine hydroxylase. J Biol Chem 255:4793, 1980
11. Phillips RS, Parniak MA, Kaufman S: Spectroscopic investigation of ligand interaction with hepatic phenylalanine hydroxylase: Evidence for a conformational change associated with activation. Biochemistry 23:3826, 1984
12. Koizumi S, Tanaka F, Kaneda N et al: Nanosecond pulse fluorometry of conformational change in phenylalanine hydroxylase associated with activation. Biochemistry 27:640, 1988
13. Lovenberg W, Bruckwick EA, Hanbauer I: ATP, cyclic AMP, and magnesium increase the affinity of rat striatal tyrosine hydroxylase for its cofactor. Proc Natl Acad Sci USA 72:2955, 1975
14. Abita JP, Milstien S, Chang M et al: In vitro activation of rat liver phenylalanine hydroxylase by phosphorylation. J Biol Chem 251:5310, 1976
15. Kaufman S: The enzymology of aromatic amino acid hydroxylases. In Kaufman S (ed): Health and Disease: New Perspectives, p 205. 1987
16. Zigmond RE, Schwarzschild MA, Rittenhouse AR: Acute regulation of tyrosine hydroxylase by nerve activity and by neurotransmitters via phosphorylation. Annu Rev Neurosci 12:415, 1989
17. Levine RA, Miller LP, Lovenberg W: Tetrahydrobiopterin in the striatum: Localization to dopaminergic nerve terminals and its role in catecholamine synthesis. Science 214:919, 1981
18. Carlsson A, Lindquist M: Dependence of 5-HT and catecholamine biosynthesis on concentrations of precursor amino-acids in rat brain. Naunyn Schmiedebergs Arch Pharmacol 303:157, 1978
19. Lazar MA, Mefford IW, Barchas JD: Tyrosine hydroxylase activation: Comparison of in vitro phosphorylation and in vivo administration of haloperidol. Biochem Pharmacol 31:2599, 1982
20. Melamed E, Hefti F, Wurtman RJ: Tyrosine administration increases striatal dopamine release in rats with partial nigrostriatal lesions. Proc Natl Acad Sci USA 77:4305, 1980
21. Wolf ME, Zigmond MJ, Kapatos G: Tyrosine hydroxylase content of residual striatal dopamine nerve terminals following 6-hydroxydopamine administration: A flow cytometric study. J Neurochem 53:879, 1989
22. Jequier E, Robinson DS, Lovenberg W et al: Further studies on tryptophan hydroxylase in rat brain stem and beef pineal. Biochem Pharmacol 18:1071, 1969

23. Yamauchi T, Fujisawa H: Activation of tryptophan monooxygenase by calcium-dependent regulation protein. Biochem Biophys Res Commun 90:28, 1979

24. Kuhn DM, O'Callaghan JP, Juskevich J et al: Activation of brain tryptophan hydroxylase by ATP-Mg^{2+}-dependence on calmodulin. Proc Natl Acad Sci USA 77:4688, 1980

25. Boadle-Biber MC: Activation of tryptophan hydroxylase from slices of rat brain stem incubated with N_6,O_2-dibutyryladenosine-3',5'-cyclic monophosphate. Biochem Pharmacol 29:669, 1980

26. Wurtman RJ, Hefti F, Melamed E: Precursor control of neurotransmitter synthesis. Pharmacol Rev 32:315, 1981

27. Wurtman RJ: Effects of their nutrient precursors on the synthesis and release of serotonin, the catecholamines, and acetylcholine: Implications for behavioral disorders. Clin Neuropharmacol 11: S187, 1988

28. Curzon G, Marsden CA: Metabolism of tryptophan load in the hypothalamus and other brain regions. J Neurochem 25:251, 1975

29. Marsden CA, Curzon G: Studies on the behavioral effect of tryptophan and p-chlorophenylalanine. Neuropharmacol 15:165, 1976

30. Bruce G, Hersh LB: The phosphorylation of acetylcholine transferase. Neurochem Res 14:613, 1989

31. Yamamura HI, Snyder SH: Choline: High affinity uptake by rat brain synaptosomes. Science 178: 626, 1972

32. Kuhar MJ, Murrin LC: Sodium-dependent, high affinity choline uptake. J Neurochem 30:15, 1978

33. Pedata F, LoConte G, Sorbi S et al: Changes in high affinity choline uptake in rat cortex following lesions of the magnocellular forebrain nuclei. Brain Res 233:359, 1982

CHAPTER 33

Effects of Brain-Gut Peptides on Satiety

JAMES GIBBS and GERARD P. SMITH

Increased food intake can be expressed as an increase in meal size, as a shortening of the intermeal interval, or both, Thus, if increased food intake contributes to the development of obesity, it is essential to understand the normal mechanisms that control the size and frequency of meals. Knowledge of these crucial mechanisms, however, has been surprisingly meager.

Research in this area was sparked by the intuition that the surface of the gastrointestinal tract may be more than the site of absorption of nutrients; rather, the gut itself might be a preabsorptive reservoir of signals that would be released by contact with ingested food. These preabsorptive "satiety signals" would then act to control meal size, to regulate the length of the intermeal interval, or both. This intuition has been fueled by continuing chemical discoveries of neural and hormonal gastrointestinal peptides that might serve as candidate satiety signals. Finally, the fact that many of these same peptides and their receptors are also present in brain tissue has generated enthusiasm for the idea that brain stores of certain peptides might exert direct actions on feeding behavior, unrelated to any peripheral effects. In this chapter, we review the evidence supporting the candidacy of the most prominent peptide satiety signals.

CHOLECYSTOKININ

Of several putative satiety signals (Table 33-1), the classic small-intestinal hormone cholecystokinin (CCK) has received the most attention. Based on our demonstration that the systemic administration of CCK reduced food intake in rats,[36] we proposed in 1973 that this peptide, when it is released by food ingestion, functions as a negative feedback signal to limit meal size (in addition to its other well-known actions on the gastrointestinal tract). Substantial evidence now supports this proposal. The inhibitory action of CCK has been observed in many animal species, including subhuman primates, across a wide variety of test conditions.[92] The action is strongly dose related, and it is behaviorally specific.[93] Administration of the sulfated form of the synthetic C-terminal octapeptide of CCK (CCK-8) evokes satiety, whereas the desulfated form does not[37]; this difference is important because it indicates that exogenous CCK acts at the type A CCK receptor, which predominates in the periphery, and not at the type B receptor, which predominates in brain.

CCK reduces food intake in normal-weight human volunteers after intravenous infusion.[42,98] As in animals, the effect in humans is dose related. Although it has long been known that the rapid bolus administration of CCK can cause discomfort in humans, this consequence cannot account for its ability to reduce food intake: During the slow intravenous infusions used in the double-blind studies of food intake in humans, mild discomfort occurred in less than 15% of subjects,[91] and volunteers were unable to identify days on which they received the peptide.

CCK also reduces food intake at test meals in obese humans.[80] In view of its potential therapeutic use, it is important that repeated administration in animals does not provoke a significant

TABLE 33-1

Peptides That Elicit Satiety After Peripheral Administration

Peptide	Inhibition of Feeding	Inhibition of Sham Feeding	Blockade or Attenuation	Effect in Humans	Antagonism of Exogenous Peptide	Antagonism Increases Feeding
Cholecystokinin	Yes	Yes	Pylorectomy Afferent vagotomy Capsaicin AP-mNTS lesion DMN lesion PVN lesion	Yes	Receptor antagonist	Yes
Glucagon	Yes	No	Vagotomy Hepatic vagotomy Capsaicin Intraportal alloxan AP-mNTS lesion	Yes	—	Yes
Bombesin	Yes	Yes	Visceral disconnection AP-mNTS lesion	Yes	Receptor antagonist Antibody	No

Dashes indicate no study has been published.
(AP-mNTS, area postrema-medial nucleus tractus solitarius; DMN, dorsomedial nucleus; PVN, paraventricular nucleus)

degree of tolerance for its satiating action at an individual meal.[116] Nevertheless, whether repeated administration over time in obese humans can reduce body weight has not been determined.

Although a large amount of evidence has established the fact that exogenous CCK reduces short-term food intake, the importance of endogenous CCK for the normal termination of eating has been a point of frequent dispute. Evidence from studies using the newest generation of highly potent and highly selective CCK receptor antagonists seems to have settled this question. Systemic administration of these agents has now been found to increase food intake in rats,[15,26,81,112] mice,[89] hamsters,[1] and pigs[16] and to increase hunger sensations in humans.[119] Thus, CCK must have a necessary role in controlling food intake. Further experiments will establish the limits under which CCK operates in this manner.

The mechanism of action of CCK is only partially understood. It is thought that CCK that is released by ingested food acts at a peripheral site when it elicits satiety. This conclusion follows from surgical and chemical lesion studies that have demonstrated that afferent[96] capsaicin-sensitive[97] neurons of the abdominal vagus are required for the satiety action of CCK when it is injected peripherally. In addition, removal of the pyloric sphincter of the stomach, an area rich in type A CCK receptors,[69] attenuates the action of high doses of CCK,[70] suggesting that action of the sphincter is necessary for at least a portion of the satiety effect.

How does this peripherally initiated satiety information enter the brain? Afferent neurons of the vagus have their first synaptic relay in the nucleus tractus solitarius of the dorsal hindbrain. Bilateral electrolytic lesions of this region and the neighboring area postrema abolished the satiating effect of low doses of peripherally injected

CCK.[17] (Note that surgical removal of the pyloric sphincter blocked the action of high doses of CCK and that lesions of the dorsal hindbrain blocked the action of low doses. This lack of concordance is one indication that other peripheral sites containing type A CCK receptors—for example, pancreas and afferent fibers of the vagus nerve itself—should be explored for their possible roles in mediating satiety produced by peripheral administration of CCK.[67])

The results of the dorsal hindbrain lesion studies strongly suggest that this region is a relay for CCK-evoked satiety signals. Central projection sites of dorsal hindbrain neurons are logical candidates for further processing of such signals. Unfortunately, experiments with lesions of these projection sites and their ascending pathways have yielded conflicting results; some investigators report large reductions in the satiating potency of peripherally injected CCK after lesions of paraventricular nucleus[9] or after midbrain transections,[10] and others report an intact response to the peptide.[39,95] Much further work is required to identify the brain sites and brain pathways involved in processing the satiety action of peripherally administered CCK.

Although peripherally administered CCK does not penetrate the blood-brain barrier,[77] the brain does contain widely and heterogeneously distributed stores of CCK and CCK receptors. This central system can be activated by direct administration of exogenous CCK. By this route, the peptide has been found to inhibit food intake in a wide variety of animal species.[12,20,59,85] Like peripheral injections, the satiety effect of intracerebroventricular injections is behaviorally specific, and it seems to require action of CCK at type A receptors,[127] which are found in a limited number of locations in brain tissue.[68] To date, only two of these sites, dorsal hindbrain and medial hypothalamus, have been tested for responsivity to direct injections of CCK. Although injections into dorsal hindbrain (nucleus tractus solitarius) were without effect,[8] injections of very low doses of CCK-8 into the paraventricular nucleus of the hypothalamus reduced feeding.[18] Furthermore, administration of the relatively nonspecific CCK antagonists benzotript and proglumide into the paraventricular nucleus reliably increased feeding,[88] suggesting that endogenous CCK in that

site has a role in satiety. How might central neuronal stores of CCK be released in relation to meals? The answer is unknown, but it is of interest that the release of endogenous CCK-8 at hypothalamic sites has been demonstrated after intragastric administration of nutrients in cats[85] and in monkeys[84] but not after intravenous administration of high doses of CCK-8.[85]

In summary, a large, reliable satiety action of exogenous CCK, administered peripherally, has been demonstrated in many species, including humans. Studies using antagonists of CCK receptors strongly indicate that endogenous CCK has a satiety role, although the breadth and importance of such a role have not been systematically explored. Much work remains to be done before an understanding is reached about the mechanism of the satiety action of peripheral CCK and the subsequent processing of this signal, carried by vagal afferent fibers, after its entry into brain tissue. Finally, it remains to be determined how the satiety effect of centrally administered CCK, which models the release of CCK in brain, relates to the satiety effect of peripherally administered CCK.

PANCREATIC GLUCAGON

Pancreatic glucagon was the first peptide tested for a possible effect on satiety. In 1955, within 2 years of the time pure glucagon became available, it was reported to decrease appetite in humans.[105] Two years later, a double-blind trial in humans demonstrated a reduction in food intake and a small but significant decrease in body weight over a 2-week period of repeated intramuscular injections.[87]

A more recent study in humans used an intravenous dose of glucagon small enough (3 ng/kg/min for 10 minutes) to mimic the rise in plasma glucagon that normally follows a meal; this dose reduced test meal size by about 20% and failed to produce any abnormalities on a battery of psychophysical measurements.[28]

An impressive body of subsequent work, reviewed by Geary,[28] has established the efficacy of systemically administered glucagon in producing satiety in a wide variety of mammalian and avian species. Like exogenous CCK, the satiety effect of exogenous glucagon is strongly dose related, rapid in onset, and transient. Un-like CCK, the effect of glucagon appears quite sensitive to environmental conditions, particularly deprivation state and circadian phase: For example, mildly deprived or nondeprived rats are refractory to the satiety influence of glucagon around the time of dark onset but quite responsive 2 or 3 hours later or during the midlight period.[61,115]

In keeping with the fact that glucagon administration to humans failed to produce side-effects, experiments on animals have provided strong convergent evidence that the peptide produces satiety and not some form of sickness, sedation, or competing behavior. Thus, glucagon inhibits liquid food intake in hungry rats but not water intake in thirsty rats, and it fails to produce evidence of aversion in conditioning tests.[62]

All of these results constitute strong evidence that the peripheral administration of exogenous glucagon can, at least under certain experimental conditions, reduce food intake by eliciting a state of satiety in experimental animals and in humans.

Although the mechanism of action of peripherally administered glucagon in producing satiety is not known, some clues have been uncovered. Because the liver is the major target organ for the metabolic actions of glucagon, Novin and his colleagues tested the effects of infusions directly into the hepatic portal vein. By this route, glucagon produced a rapid and dose-related reduction in food intake.[61] The peptide was more potent by this route than when injected intraperitoneally.[115] A total abdominal vagotomy[62] or a selective transection of only the hepatic branch of the vagus[30] produced a complete blockade of intraperitoneally administered glucagon. Because administration of capsaicin,[82] which destroys small-diameter afferent neurons, or electrolytic lesions aimed at the terminal fields of hepatic vagal afferents in the dorsal hindbrain[114] attenuated glucagon-induced satiety, it appears that afferent fibers of the hepatic vagus are the key element supporting this behavioral effect, at least under certain experimental conditions.[113]

The initial intrahepatic target site for glucagon's satiety action remains unknown. The most provocative finding to date is that by Ritter and her colleagues, who showed that injection of al-

loxan into the hepatic portal vein but not into the jugular vein blocked the effect of glucagon under the same experimental conditions as did hepatic vagotomy.[83] Because alloxan is toxic to certain cells bearing glucoreceptors and because intraportal administration of another toxin (furosemide) that produced generalized liver damage failed to have any effect, these results suggest that glucoreceptor cells within the liver are critical for glucagon-induced satiety. Nevertheless, the well-known glycogenolytic function of glucagon does not appear to be involved, because the peptide can inhibit feeding in the absence of significant glycogenolysis or increased blood glucose[107,108]; conversely, glucagon fails to inhibit feeding under conditions in which it provokes marked increases in blood glucose.[29]

In an effort to determine whether endogenous pancreatic glucagon functions normally to limit meal size, Langhans and colleagues used a highly specific antiglucagon antibody. Intraperitoneal administration of the antibody produced a 63% increase in the size of a test meal taken by food-deprived rats; the antibody produced parallel actions (attenuations of meal-induced glycogenolysis and hyperglycemia), which would be expected if the actions of endogenous glucagon were blocked.[52] In another study, direct intraportal infusions of the same antibody increased the size of spontaneous meals by 57% to 73%, depending on the time of day at which rats were feeding.[53] These results constitute persuasive evidence that circulating glucagon has a physiological role in controlling food intake.

BOMBESIN-LIKE PEPTIDES

Bombesin (BBS) is a tetradecapeptide originally isolated from frog skin.[2] Despite these exotic origins, a large family of peptides closely related to amphibian BBS is now known to be widely but heterogeneously distributed in mammalian gastrointestinal tract and brain. In 1979, we found that intraperitoneal injections of BBS produced large, dose-related reductions of food intake in rats.[31] Because the administration of BBS and BBS-like peptides is followed by a wide variety of pharmacologic actions, it was important to determine whether the action on food intake was specific or not (Table 33-2). Several studies sug-

TABLE 33-2

**Peptides That Inhibit Food Intake
After Central Administration**

Peptide	Evidence for Behavioral Specificity
Bombesin	Yes
Calcitonin	No
Calcitonin gene-related peptide	No
Cholecystokinin	Yes
Corticotropin releasing factor	No
Insulin	Yes
Neurotensin	Yes
Oxytocin	Yes
Thyrotropin releasing hormone	No

gested that the inhibition of food intake reflected a true satiety effect of the peptide and was not simply secondary to malaise or some generalized discomfort; the demonstration that systemic BBS inhibited liquid food intake in food-deprived rats but failed to inhibit water intake in water-deprived rats was strong evidence against this possibility.[31,47]

As with CCK, the satiety effect of peripherally administered BBS has been reported in various mammalian and avian species.[4,13,64,106] Based on the apparent safety and efficacy of BBS in subhuman primates,[125] Murrahainen and colleagues tested the effect in nonobese human volunteers. Under double-blind conditions, an intravenous infusion of 4 ng/kg/min produced a significant inhibition of food intake at a test meal without producing significant side-effects.[75]

As might be expected, a number of peptides structurally related to BBS also reduce food intake. Gastrin-releasing peptide, which is found in mammalian stomach, produced a powerful, dose-related, and behaviorally specific inhibition of feeding in rats[33,100] and baboons.[21] The naturally occurring carboxyl-terminal decapeptide of gastrin-releasing peptide (GRP-10, or neuromedin C) had the same action after peripheral administration, but neuromedin B, a related

peptide, was much less potent.[14] Ranatensin, another amphibian peptide that may have a closely related analogue in mammalian tissues, also reduced food intake.[24] All of these peptides, however, were less active than the prototypical amphibian tetradecapeptide.

In an attempt to uncover the mechanism by which systemically administered BBS acted on feeding behavior, we carried out an extensive series of endocrine and neural ablations. In our initial studies, the following lesions all failed to affect BBS-induced satiety: adrenalectomy, hypophysectomy, ventromedial hypothalamic lesions, spinal cord section at the level of the sixth thoracic vertebra, and total subdiaphragmatic vagotomy.[35] Although neither a total subdiaphragmatic vagotomy nor a high thoracic spinal-visceral neural disconnection produced any effect, the combination of both of these lesions—in effect, a neural disconnection of gut from brain—completely blocked BBS-induced satiety.[104] The specific vagal and spinal visceral pathways within the combined lesion that are required for BBS-induced satiety are unknown but should be identifiable by selective lesions. Two reports indicate that either extensive bilateral thoracic dorsal rhizotomies, interrupting afferent information from the upper abdomen,[65] or high dorsal column transection[49] produced a modest attenuation of BBS-induced satiety. The suggestion from these ablation studies is that peripherally administered BBS may act initially at an upper abdominal site, perhaps the stomach,[34] when it elicits satiety (but see Hostetler and colleagues[40]).

As mentioned earlier, satiety can be expressed as a limitation of meal size, as an extension of the intermeal interval, or both. To determine whether exogenous BBS might act to prolong the intermeal interval, in addition to its well-established effect on meal size, we injected it intraperitoneally either before a test meal or during the initial period of satiety after the meal and found that it produced a dose-related extension of the time until a new meal was initiated.[66,117] The dose of BBS required to affect the intermeal interval was lower than the dose required to affect meal size under similar test conditions. It appears that the mechanism of action used by exogenous BBS in extending the intermeal interval is different from the mechanism in reducing meal size, because the combined vagotomy/spinal visceral disconnection that had blocked the action of BBS on meal size (see above) failed to affect the action on the intermeal interval.[104]

Because BBS-like immunoreactivity is present in brain tissue, several groups have studied whether direct central administration affects food intake. Although intracerebroventricular administration of BBS clearly reduced food intake in rats, interpretation of this finding has been clouded by the fact that the peptide caused a parallel marked increase in scratching and stereotyped grooming behavior that appeared to interfere with normal feeding behavior.[48] Two groups, however, have suggested that it is possible to dissociate the two effects: When BBS is administered to the fourth cerebral ventricle, small doses may reduce food intake without causing any detectable alteration in grooming.[23,50] Several studies have examined the effect of direct intracerebral tissue injections of BBS. Positive responses with low doses have been reported in the lateral hypothalamus (50 ng),[103] paraventricular nucleus (100 ng),[118] and nucleus tractus solitarius (1 to 40 ng).[11,41] Each of these studies was notable because it included assessments of the behavioral specificity of the peptide's action, a critical issue for interpreting the results of central manipulations.

An unresolved issue is how the inhibitory action of BBS delivered to the brain relates to the satiety effects achieved with peripheral administration. In a preliminary report that bears on this issue, electrolytic lesions encompassing the area postrema-medial nucleus solitarius of the hindbrain attenuated not only the inhibitory effect of exogenous BBS delivered to the fourth cerebral ventricle, but also the inhibitory effect of intraperitoneal BBS.[51] Furthermore, BBS exerts its satiety action in chronic decerebrate rats, in which all neural connections to forebrain have been eliminated.[22] Thus, the dorsal hindbrain may be necessary and sufficient for satiety evoked by peripherally administered BBS.

Are endogenous BBS-like peptides involved in the regulation of meal size and intermeal interval? Merali and his colleagues have used central and peripheral injections of anti-BBS antiserum and BBS receptor antagonists to investigate this question. Although both treatments attenuated the action of exogenously administered BBS, neither increased food intake by itself.[63] At this point, it is not clear whether the failure of antagonists to increase feeding means that endogenous BBS has no role in the physiology of food intake or simply that the conditions for demonstrating such a function have not been identified. Clearly, the problem merits further work.

OTHER PEPTIDES

Insulin, administered peripherally in large doses, has long been known to provoke feeding in animals and to elicit reports of hunger in humans.[57,58,90] It was not until 1980 that Vander-Weele suggested that smaller doses, closer to the physiologic range, would in fact reduce food intake when delivered chronically to rats.[110] In subsequent studies, this chronic reduction was shown to be due to a decrease in individual meal size. Acute administration of 0.4 to 0.8 U per rat inhibited sham feeding.[76] Because delivery of much smaller doses (1 to 2 mU) directly into the hepatic portal vein produced a potent reduction of meal size but delivery of the same doses into the jugular vein did not, VanderWeele suggested that insulin released by food ingestion may act at the liver, perhaps affecting glycogenolytic processes.[109] The only test of exogenous insulin in humans to date failed to demonstrate any reduction in test meal size, despite a threefold elevation in plasma insulin levels.[120]

Woods and Porte suggested that insulin may have an important inhibitory role in feeding behavior by acting directly on the brain. Their proposal, however, implicates insulin not in the short-term control of individual meal size, but rather as a long-term monitor of the adipose tissue stores of the body. This hypothesis rests on several strong supports: Plasma insulin is well known to vary with the fat mass. In turn, insulin levels in cerebrospinal fluid vary, after a lag period, with plasma levels of insulin.[123] Insulin and insulin receptors can be found within the brain.[5,124] Infusions of small amounts of insulin directly into the cerebrospinal fluid of rats[7] or subhuman primates[122] reduces daily food intake and body weight, without raising plasma insulin levels. Finally, although plasma insulin levels are elevated in obesity, these investigators have found that cerebrospinal fluid levels of insulin, brain levels of insulin,[6] and brain insulin binding[19] all are low in rodent models of obesity, suggesting that the insulin signal from the adipose tissue mass is not reaching its target sites in brain.

It is of interest that this hypothetical mechanism for the regulation of long-term food intake and body weight appears to interact with at least one of the putative short-term satiety signals. In rats and in subhuman primates, although the administration of a very small amount of insulin into the cerebral ventricles failed to affect food intake by itself, it potentiated a subthreshold dose of CCK, and the combination inhibited food intake.[121]

Somatostatin, a tetradecapeptide found in the gastrointestinal tract and brain, appears to act as an inhibitor of multiple pancreatic and gut functions. Administered intraperitoneally to rats and baboons, it produced a dose-dependent and behaviorally specific inhibition of food intake.[56] Intracerebroventricular delivery, however, failed to produce any change in feeding. As found for CCK, total subdiaphragmatic vagotomy blocked the action of somatostatin.[55]

Oxytocin, which is synthesized in cell bodies of intra- and extrahypothalamic neurons, also has binding sites widely distributed in brain tissue. At what appear to be low doses, central administration of this peptide has been reported to have effects on various motivated behaviors, including maternal behavior, sexual behavior, grooming, and foraging. Arletti and colleagues tested the effects of oxytocin on food intake of deprived rats.[3] Although the doses required to reduce feeding after peripheral administration were massive, intracerebroventricular administration of 10 μg per rat produced a marked suppression of food intake, accompanied by increased grooming; this effect was totally reversed by prior intracerebroventricular administration of the equivalent dose of an oxytocin antagonist. Critical additional results were that ventricular administration of the same dose of the antagonist alone produced a doubling of intake without significantly altering normal grooming behavior during the 1-hour period of access to food. Intracerebroventricular oxytocin has also been reported by Olson and associates[78] to reduce food intake.

Calcitonin, which is released postprandially into the circulation, reduced food intake in rats and rhesus monkeys following subcutaneous administration[79] and in rats after intracerebroventricular administration.[25] Maximal inhibition occurred several hours after peripheral injection in rats, suggesting that the peptide is not directly involved in the regulation of meal size. The relationship of calcitonin's peripheral action to its central action was unresolved. In addition, the issue of behavioral specificity after the peripheral injection was unclear, because the synthetic salmon calcitonin used tended to affect water intake as well as food intake in rats and monkeys and because few details were provided about a trial in humans.[79] Mice with genetic diabetes were more sensitive to the anorectic effects of impure salmon calcitonin than their heterozygote littermates.[73]

Calcitonin gene-related peptide (CGRP) is a 37-amino-acid peptide derived through an alternative messenger RNA processing pathway from that of calcitonin itself. CGRP was found to reduce food intake after peripheral and central administration in rats, although less potently than calcitonin.[45] This observation has now been clouded by the finding that the peptide produced results similar to those of aversive agents in conditioned aversion and differential deprivation test paradigms.[46] The behavioral specificity of both calcitonin and CGRP is uncertain.

Corticotropin releasing factor (CRF), a 41-residue peptide that stimulates pituitary adrenocorticotropic hormone and β-endorphin release, also reduced food intake after injection into cerebral ventricles[72] and the paraventricular nucleus of the hypothalamus.[44] Once again, however, the specificity of these actions is in doubt: CRF was not only a potent stimulant of grooming after intracerebroventricular injection, but it also produced a conditioned taste aversion to a taste paired with its administration.[38] Sauvagine, a 40-residue peptide isolated from amphibian skin, with a similar chemical structure and similar biologic functions to CRF, also shares the ability to increase grooming and to produce a conditioned taste aversion.[38] Thyrotropin releasing hormone (TRH), found in brain and gut, reduced both feeding and drinking in rats after intracerebroventricular delivery.[111] The TRH metabolite cyclohistidyl proline diketopiperazine also reduced food intake in rats.[74] TRH reduced food intake in rats[71] and sham feeding in dogs[43] after systemic administration. We found that systemic administration of TRH to rats, although reducing food intake, produced clearly abnormal behaviors at every effective dose.[32] Similar evidence of nonspecific behavioral disruption, rather than a specific satiety action, was noted after peripheral injections of substance P and neurotensin.[32] After central administration, however, neurotensin has been reported to produce behaviorally specific reductions in food intake.[54,99]

Circulating pancreatic polypeptide levels rise dramatically at meals, and this peptide has been shown to reduce food intake and body weight after peripheral administration in lean and obese mice.[27,60] It failed to reduce food intake in rats,[32] and it has not been tested in other species.

Secretin and gastrin, two classic gastrointestinal peptide hormones, had no effect on food intake in rats, even when large doses were given.[36,94]

CONCLUSION

Progress in uncovering the physiological mechanisms of satiety during the past 15 years is evident. Work in this area is accelerating rapidly. The major element in progress to date is the discovery of the key role of a small group of peptides that link the gastrointestinal tract and brain and that support satiety by peripheral and central actions.

Certain themes recur. First, it appears that several peptides have their initial action peripherally. Second, this initial action is relayed centrally by afferent nerves. A major part is played by the abdominal vagus, which is necessary for the satiety action of certain peptides (CCK, glucagon, somatostatin) and important for others (BBS-like peptides). Third, the dorsal hindbrain, specifically the area postrema-nucleus tractus solitarius region, is required for the full expression of peptide-induced satiety. The pivotal role of this region is interesting because it is the site of the first synaptic relay of afferent vagal information and because it is believed to be important

in the integration of visceral and gustatory information.

The development of highly potent and highly specific receptor antagonists and antibodies for several of these peptides has provided indispensable tools for assessing the physiological meaning of effects on food intake produced by the agonists. For CCK and glucagon, the results are already compelling: Endogenous stores of these peptides are important in controlling food intake.

A notable and heartening feature of the research reviewed here has been the consistent concordance of work in experimental animals and in humans. Careful, thorough tests of efficacy and behavioral specificity in rodents have not only repeatedly predicted results in many animal species, including subhuman primates, but have accurately predicted efficacy and the absence of significant side-effects in humans.

What is the promise of this research area for an understanding of obesity? Although the potential is obviously great, much further work is required. It has not been established that alterations in any of the brain-gut peptides discussed here play a part in the development or the maintenance of obesity; this is a topic of current research.[101,102,126] Even if these substances are not involved in the pathophysiology of obesity, their use in treatment bears consideration. It may be possible, for example, to develop releasing agents for particular peptides. Such agents, if calorically trivial, might be used in obese patients to release particular peptides with the aim of limiting meal size or extending the length of the intermeal interval. Exogenous use of the peptides themselves presents several problems, including the lack of orally effective forms and ignorance about their effectiveness in reducing the intake of highly palatable or preferred foods. Because almost all studies to date have examined the effects of the peptides on individual meal size, a major unresolved issue is whether their repeated administration over time would promote weight loss or simply provoke regulatory countermeasures that would neutralize their short-term actions.[116] Finally, of course, the safety of these biologically potent agents when given chronically is unknown and must be unequivocally established.

Acknowledgment: This work was supported in part by U.S. Public Health Service grants NIH DK33248 (JG) and NIMH MH40010 (GPS), and NIMH RSA MK00149 (GPS).

References

1. Adrian TE, Bilchik AJ, Zucker KA et al: CCK receptor blockade increases hamster body weight and food intake. FASEB J 2:A737, 1988

2. Anastasi A, Erspamer V, Bucci M: Isolation and structure of bombesin and alytesin, two analogous active peptides from the skin of the European amphibians Bombina and Alytes. Experientia 27:166, 1971

3. Arletti R, Bennelli A, Bertolini A: Influence of oxytocin on feeding behavior in the rat. Peptides 10:89, 1989

4. Bado A, Lewin MJM, Dubrasquet M: Effects of bombesin on food intake and gastric acid secretion in cats. Am J Physiol 256:R181, 1989

5. Baskin DG, Figlewicz DP, Woods SC et al: Insulin in the brain. Ann Rev Physiol 49:335, 1987

6. Baskin DG, Stein LJ, Ikeda H et al: Genetically obese Zucker rats have abnormally low brain insulin content. Life Sci 36:627, 1985

7. Brief DJ, Davis JD: Reduction of food intake and body weight by chronic intraventricular insulin infusion. Brain Res Bull 12:571, 1984

8. Crawley JN: Neurochemical investigation of the afferent pathway from the vagus nerve to the nucleus tractus solitarius in mediating the "satiety syndrome" induced by systemic cholecystokinin. Peptides (Suppl 1) 6:133, 1985

9. Crawley JN, Kiss JZ: Paraventricular nucleus lesions abolish the inhibition of feeding induced by systemic cholecystokinin. Peptides 6:927, 1985

10. Crawley JN, Kiss JZ, Mezey E: Bilateral midbrain transections block the behavioral effects of cholecystokinin on feeding and exploration in rats. Brain Res 322:316, 1984

11. deBeaurepaire R, Suaudeau C: Anorectic effect of calcitonin, neurotensin and bombesin infused in the area of the rostral part of the nucleus of the tractus solitarius in the rat. Peptides 9:729, 1988

12. Della-Fera M, Baile CA: Cholecystokinin octapeptide: Continuous picomole injections into the cerebral ventricles of sheep suppress feeding. Science 206:471, 1979

13. Denbow DM: Centrally and peripherally administered bombesin decreases food intake in turkeys. Peptides 10:275, 1989

14. DiPoala JA, Gibbs J: Neuromedin C inhibits food intake in rats. Soc Neurosci Abstr 11:38, 1985

15. Dourish CT, Rycroft W, Iversen SD: Postponement of satiety by blockade of brain cholecystokinin (CCK-8) receptors. Science 245:1509, 1989

16. Ebenezer IS, de la Riva C, Baldwin BA: Effects of the CCK receptor antagonist MK-329 on food intake in pigs. Physiol Behav 47:145, 1990

17. Edwards GL, Ladenheim EE, Ritter RC: Dorsal hindbrain participation in cholecystokinin-induced satiety. Am J Physiol 251:R971, 1986

18. Faris PL, Scallet AC, Olney JW et al: Behavioral and immunohistochemical analysis of the function of cholecystokinin in the hypothalamic paraventricular nucleus. Soc Neurosci Abstr 9:184, 1983

19. Figlewicz DP, Dorsa DM, Stein LJ et al: Brain and liver insulin binding is decreased in Zucker rats carrying the 'fa' gene. Endocrinology 117:1537, 1985

20. Figlewicz DP, Sipols AJ, Green P et al: IVT CCK-8 is more effective than IV CCK-8 at decreasing meal size in the baboon. Brain Res Bull 22:849, 1989

21. Figlewicz DP, Stein LJ, Woods SC et al: Acute and chronic gastrin-releasing peptide decreases food intake in baboons. Am J Physiol 248:R578, 1985

22. Flynn FW: Effects of bombesin administration on taste-elicited behaviors of intact and chronic decerebrate rats. Soc Neurosci Abstr 13:881, 1987

23. Flynn FW: Fourth ventricle bombesin injection suppresses ingestive behaviors in rats. Am J Physiol 256:R590, 1989

24. Foelsch PA, Gibbs J, Smith GP: Ranatensin, a bombesin-like peptide, decreases food intake. Proc East Psychol Assoc 58:18, 1987

25. Freed WJ, Perlow MJ, Wyatt RJ: Calcitonin: Inhibitory effect on eating in rats. Science 206:850, 1979

26. Garlicki J, Konturek PK, Majka J et al: Cholecystokinin receptors and vagal nerves in control of food intake in rats. Am J Physiol 258:E40, 1990

27. Gates RJ, Lazarus NR: The ability of pancreatic polypeptide (APP and BPP) to return to normal the hyperglycemia, hyperinsulinemia and weight gain of New Zealand obese mice. Horm Res 8:189, 1977

28. Geary N: Pancreatic glucagon signals postprandial satiety. Neurosci Biobehav Rev 14:323, 1990

29. Geary N, Smith GP: Pancreatic glucagon fails to inhibit sham feeding in the rat. Peptides 3:163, 1982

30. Geary N, Smith GP: Selective hepatic vagotomy blocks pancreatic glucagon's satiety effect. Physiol Behav 31:391, 1983

31. Gibbs J, Fauser DJ, Rowe EA et al: Bombesin suppresses feeding in rats. Nature 282:208, 1979

32. Gibbs J, Gray L, Martin CF et al: Quantitative behavioral analysis of neuropeptides which suppress food intake. Soc Neurosci Abstr 6:182, 1980

33. Gibbs J, Kulkosky PJ, Smith GP: Effects of peripheral and central bombesin on feeding behavior of rats. Peptides (Suppl 2) 2:179, 1981

34. Gibbs J, Smith GP: Gut peptides and food in the gut produce similar satiety effects. Peptides 3: 553, 1982

35. Gibbs J, Smith GP: The actions of bombesin-like peptides on food intake. Ann NY Acad Sci 547:210, 1988

36. Gibbs J, Young RC, Smith GP: Cholecystokinin decreases food intake in rats. J Comp Physiol Psychol 84:488, 1973

37. Gibbs J, Young RC, Smith GP: Cholecystokinin elicits satiety in rats with open gastric fistulas. Nature 245:323, 1973

38. Gosnell BA, Morley JE, Levine AS: A comparison of the effects of corticotropin releasing factor and sauvagine on food intake. Pharmacol Biochem Behav 19:771, 1983

39. Grill HJ, Smith GP: Cholecystokinin decreases sucrose intake in chronic decerebrate rats. Am J Physiol 254:R853, 1988

40. Hostetler AM, McHugh PR, Moran TH: Bombesin affects feeding independent of a gastric mechanism or site of action. Am J Physiol 257:R1219, 1989

41. Johnston SA, Merali Z: Specific neuroanatomical and neurochemical correlates of grooming and satiety effects of bombesin. Peptides (Suppl 1) 9:233, 1988

42. Kissileff HR, Pi-Sunyer FX, Thornton J et al: Cholecystokinin-octapeptide (CCK-8) decreases food intake in man. Am J Clin Nutr 34:154, 1981

43. Konturek SJ, Tasler J, Jaworek J et al: Comparison of TRH and anorexigenic peptide on food intake and gastrointestinal secretions. Peptides (Suppl 2) 2:235, 1981

44. Krahn DD, Gosnell BA, Levine AS et al: Localization of the effects of corticotropin-releasing factor on feeding. Soc Neurosci Abstr 10:300, 1984

45. Krahn DD, Gosnell BA, Levine AS et al: Effects of calcitonin gene-related peptide on food intake. Peptides 5:861, 1984

46. Krahn DD, Gosnell BA, Levine AS et al: The effect of calcitonin gene-related peptide on food intake involves aversive mechanisms. Pharmacol Biochem Behav 24:5, 1986

47. Kulkosky PJ, Gibbs J: Litorin suppresses food intake in rats. Life Sci 31:685, 1982

48. Kulkosky PJ, Gibbs J, Smith GP: Behavioral effects of bombesin administration in rats. Physiol Behav 28:505, 1982

49. Ladenheim EE, Ritter RC: High dorsal column transection attentuates bombesin-induced suppression of food intake. Soc Neurosci Abstr 14:1108, 1988

50. Ladenheim EE, Ritter RC: Low-dose fourth ventricular bombesin selectively suppresses food intake. Am J Physiol 255:R988, 1988

51. Ladenheim EE, Ritter RC: Caudal hindbrain participation in suppression of feeding by central and peripheral bombesin. Soc Neurosci Abstr 15:964, 1989

52. Langhans W, Zieger U, Scharrer E et al: Stimulation of feeding in rats by intraperitoneal injection of antibodies to glucagon. Science 218:894, 1982

53. LeSauter J, Geary N: Hepatic portal infusion of glucagon antibody increases spontaneous meal size in rats. Soc Neurosci Abstr 15:656, 1989

54. Levine AS, Kneip J, Grace M et al: Effect of centrally administered neurotensin on multiple feeding paradigms. Pharmacol Biochem Behav 18:19, 1983

55. Levine AS, Morley JE: Peripherally administered somatostatin reduces feeding by a vagally mediated mechanism. Pharmacol Biochem Behav 16:897, 1982

56. Lotter EC, Krinsky R, McKay JM et al: Somatostatin decreases food intake of rats and baboons. J Comp Physiol Psychol 95:278, 1981

57. Lovett D, Booth DA: Four effects of exogenous insulin on food intake. Q J Exp Psychol 22:406, 1970

58. MacKay EM, Calloway JW, Barnes RH: Hyperalimentation in normal animals produced by protamine insulin. J Nutr 20:59, 1940

59. Maddison S: Intraperitoneal and intracranial cholecystokinin depress operant responding for food. Physiol Behav 19:819, 1977

60. Malaisse-Legae F, Carpentier JL, Patel YC et al: Pancreatic polypeptide: A possible role in the regulation of food intake in the mouse. Experientia 33:915, 1977

61. Martin JR, Novin D: Decreased feeding in rats following hepatic-portal infusion of glucagon. Physiol Behav 19:461, 1977

62. Martin JR, Novin D, VanderWeele DA: Loss of glucagon suppression of feeding after vagotomy in rats. Am J Physiol 234:E314, 1978

63. Merali Z, Moody T, Kateb P et al: Antagonism of satiety and grooming effects of bombesin by antiserum to bombesin and by [Tyr[4], D-Phe[12]] bombesin: Central versus peripheral effects. Ann NY Acad Sci 547:489, 1988

64. Miceli MO, Malsbury CW: Effects of putative satiety peptides on feeding and drinking behavior in golden hamsters. Behav Neurosci 99:1192, 1985

65. Mindell S, DiPoala J, Wiener S et al: Satiety effect of bombesin is attenuated by dorsal rhizotomy and spinal cord transection. Proc East Psychol Assoc 57:11, 1986

66. Mindell S, DiPoala JA, Wiener S et al: Bombesin increases postprandial intermeal interval. Soc Neurosci Abstr 11:38, 1985

67. Moran TH, McHugh PR: Gastric and nongastric mechanisms for satiety action of cholecystokinin. Am J Physiol 254:R628, 1988

68. Moran TH, Robinson PH, Goldrich MS et al: Two brain cholecystokinin receptors: Implications for behavioral actions. Brain Res 362:175, 1986

69. Moran TH, Robinson PH, McHugh PR: Pyloric CCK receptors: Site of mediation for satiety? Ann NY Acad Sci 448:621, 1985

70. Moran TH, Shnayder L, Hostetler AM et al: Pylorectomy reduces the satiety action of cholecystokinin. Am J Physiol 255:R1059, 1988

71. Morley JE, Levine AS: Thyrotropin releasing hormone suppresses stress-induced eating. Life Sci 27:1259, 1980

72. Morley JE, Levine AS: Corticotropin releasing factor, grooming and ingestive behaviors. Life Sci 31:1459, 1982

73. Morley JE, Levine AS, Brown DM et al: The effect of calcitonin on food intake in diabetic mice. Peptides 3:17, 1982

74. Morley JE, Levine AS, Prasad C: Histidyl-proline diketopiperazine decreases food intake in rats. Brain Res 210:475, 1981

75. Muurahainen NE, Kissileff HR, Thornton J et al: Bombesin: Another peptide that inhibits feeding in man. Soc Neurosci Abstr 9:183, 1983

76. Oetting RL, VanderWeele DA: Insulin suppresses intake without producing illness in sham feeding rats. Physiol Behav 2:557, 1985

77. Oldendorf WH: Blood-brain barrier permeability to peptides: Pitfalls in measurement. Peptides (Suppl 2) 2:109, 1981

78. Olson BR, Chow M-S, Hruby VJ et al: Oxytocin infused intracerebroventricularly inhibits food intake in rats. Appetite 12:227, 1989

79. Perlow MJ, Freed WJ, Carman JS et al: Calcitonin reduces feeding in man, monkey and rat. Pharmacol Biochem Behav 12:609, 1980

80. Pi-Sunyer X, Kissileff HR, Thornton J et al: C-terminal octapeptide of cholecystokinin decreases food intake in obese men. Physiol Behav 29:627, 1982

81. Reidelberger RD, O'Rourke MF: Potent cholecystokinin antagonist L-364,718 stimulates food intake in rats. Am J Physiol 257:R1512, 1989

82. Ritter S, Weatherford SC: Capsaicin pretreatment blocks glucagon-induced suppression of food intake. Appetite 7:291, 1986

83. Ritter S, Weatherford SC, Stone SL: Glucagon-induced inhibition of feeding is impaired by hepatic portal alloxan injection. Am J Physiol 250: R682, 1986

84. Schick RR, Reilly WM, Roddy DR et al: Neuronal cholecystokinin-like immunoreactivity is postprandially released from primate hypothalamus. Brain Res 418:20, 1987

85. Schick RR, Yaksh TL, Go VLW: Intracerebroventricular injections of cholecystokinin octapeptide suppress feeding in rats: Pharmacological characterization of this action. Regul Pept 14:277, 1986

86. Schick RR, Yaksh TL, Go VLW: An intragastric meal releases the putative satiety factor cholecystokinin from hypothalamic neurons in cats. Brain Res 370:349, 1986

87. Schulman JL, Carleton JL, Whitney G et al: Effect of glucagon on food intake and body weight in man. J Appl Physiol 11:419, 1957

88. Schwartz DH, Dorfman DB, Hernandez L et al: Cholecystokinin. 1. CCK antagonists in the PVN induce feeding. 2. Effects of CCK in the nucleus accumbens on extracellular dopamine turnover. In Wang RY, Schoenfeld R (eds): Cholecystokinin Antagonists, p 285. New York, Alan R Liss, 1988

89. Silver AJ, Flood JF, Song AM et al: Evidence for a physiological role for CCK in the regulation of food intake in mice. Am J Physiol 256:R646, 1989

90. Silverstone JT, Besser M: Insulin, blood sugar and hunger. Postgrad Med J 47:427, 1971

91. Smith GP, Gibbs J: The effect of gut peptides on hunger, satiety, and food intake in humans. Ann NY Acad Sci 499:132, 1987

92. Smith GP, Gibbs J, Jerome C et al: The satiety effect of cholecystokinin: A progress report. Peptides 2:57, 1981

93. Smith GP, Gibbs J, Kulkosky PJ: Relationships between brain-gut peptides and neurons in the control of food intake. In Hoebel BG, Novin D (eds): The Neural Basis of Feeding and Reward, p 149. Brunswick, ME, Haer Institute, 1982

94. Smith GP, Gibbs J, Young RC: Cholecystokinin and intestinal satiety in the rat. Fed Proc 33:1146, 1974

95. Smith GP, Jerome C, Cushin BJ et al: Abdominal vagotomy blocks the satiety effect of cholecystokinin in the rat. Science 213:1036, 1981

96. Smith GP, Jerome C, Norgren R: Afferent axons in abdominal vagus mediate satiety effect of cholecystokinin in rats. Am J Physiol 249:R638, 1985

97. South EH, Ritter RC: Capsaicin application to central or peripheral vagal fibers attenuates CCK satiety. Peptides 9:601, 1988

98. Stacher G, Steinringer H, Schmierer G et al: Cholecystokinin octapeptide decreases intake of solid food in man. Peptides 3:133, 1982

99. Stanley BG, Hoebel BG, Leibowitz SF: Neurotensin: Effects of hypothalamic and intravenous injections on eating and drinking in rats. Peptides 4:493, 1983

100. Stein LJ, Woods SC: Gastrin releasing peptide reduces meal size in rats. Peptides 3:833, 1982

101. Strohmayer A, von Heyn R, Dornstein L et al: CCK receptor blockade by L-364,718 increases food intake and meal taking behavior in lean but not obese Zucker rats. Appetite 12:240, 1989

102. Strohmayer AJ, Greenberg D, von Heyn R et al: Blockade of cholecystokinin (CCK) satiety in genetically obese Zucker rats. Soc Neurosci Abstr 14:1196, 1988

103. Stuckey JA, Gibbs J: Lateral hypothalamic injection of bombesin decreases food intake in rats. Brain Res Bull 8:617, 1982

104. Stuckey JA, Gibbs J, Smith GP: Neural disconnection of gut from brain blocks bombesin-induced satiety. Peptides 6:1249, 1985

105. Stunkard AJ, Van Itallie TB, Reis BB: The mechanism of satiety: Effect of glucagon on gastric hunger contractions in man. Proc Soc Exp Biol Med 89:258, 1955

106. Taylor IL, Elashoff J, Garcia R: Effects of pancreatic polypeptide, caerulein, and bombesin in obese mice. Am J Physiol 248:G277, 1985

107. VanderWeele DA, Geiselman PJ, Novin D: Pancreatic glucagon, food deprivation and feeding in intact and vagotomized rabbits. Physiol Behav 23:155, 1979

108. VanderWeele DA, Haraczkiewicz E, DiConti MA: Pancreatic glucagon administration, feeding, glycemia, and liver glycogen in rats. Brain Res Bull (Suppl 4) 5:17, 1980

109. VanderWeele DA, Haraczkiewicz E, Van Itallie TB: Insulin and satiety in obese and normal-weight rats. Soc Neurosci Abstr 5:225, 1979

110. VanderWeele DA, Pi-Sunyer FX, Novin D et al: Chronic insulin infusion suppresses food ingestion and body weight gain in rats. Brain Res Bull (Suppl 4) 5:7, 1980

111. Vijayan E, McCann SM: Suppression of feeding and drinking activity in rats following intraventricular injection of thyrotropin releasing hormone (TRH). Endocrinology 100:1727, 1977

112. Watson CA, Schneider LH, Corp ES et al: The effects of chronic and acute treatment with the potent peripheral cholecystokinin antagonist L-364,718 on food and water intake in the rat. Soc Neurosci Abstr 14:1196, 1988

113. Weatherford SC, Ritter S: Glucagon satiety: Diurnal variation after hepatic branch vagotomy or intraportal alloxan. Brain Res Bull 17:545, 1986

114. Weatherford SC, Ritter S: Lesion of vagal afferent terminals impairs glucagon-induced suppression of food intake. Physiol Behav 43:645, 1988

115. Weick BG, Ritter S: Dose-related suppression of feeding by intraportal glucagon infusion in the rat. Am J Physiol 250:R676, 1986

116. West DB, Fey D, Woods SC: Cholecystokinin persistently suppresses meal size but not food intake in free-feeding rats. Am J Physiol 246:R776, 1984

117. Wiener SM, Gibbs J, Smith GP: Prolonged satiating effects of cholecystokinin and bombesin in rats. Soc Neurosci Abstr 10:553, 1984

118. Willis GL, Hansky J, Smith GC: Ventricular, paraventricular and circumventricular structures involved in peptide-induced satiety. Regul Pept 9:87, 1984

119. Wolkowitz OM, Gertz B, Weingartner H et al: Hunger in humans induced by MK-329, a specific peripheral-type cholecystokinin receptor antagonist. Biol Psychiatry 28:169, 1990

120. Woo R, Kissileff HR, Pi-Sunyer FX: Elevated postprandial insulin levels do not induce satiety in normal-weight humans. Am J Physiol 247:R745, 1984

121. Woods SC, Gibbs J: The regulation of food intake by peptides. Ann NY Acad Sci 575:236, 1989

122. Woods SC, Lotter EC, McKay LD et al: Chronic intracerebroventricular infusion of insulin reduced food intake and body weight of baboons. Nature 282:503, 1979

123. Woods SC, Porte D Jr: Relationship between plasma and cerebrospinal fluid insulin levels of dogs. Am J Physiol 233:E331, 1977

124. Woods SC, Porte D Jr, Strubbe JH et al: The relationships among body fat, feeding, and insulin. In Ritter RC, Ritter S, Barnes CD (eds): Feeding Behavior: Neural and Humoral Controls, p 315. New York, Academic Press, 1986

125. Woods SC, Stein LJ, Figlewicz DP et al: Bombesin stimulates insulin secretion and reduces food intake in the baboon. Peptides 4:687, 1983

126. Woolf GM, Howard JM, Flower MA et al: Postprandial plasma cholecystokinin (CCK) and food intake in lean and obese subjects. Gastroenterology 94:A502, 1988

127. Zhang D-M, Bula W, Stellar E: Brain cholecystokinin as a satiety peptide. Physiol Behav 36:1183, 1986

CHAPTER 34

Brain Serotonin, Food Intake Regulation, and Obesity

JOHN D. FERNSTROM

Serotonin (5-HT) neurons in the brain are thought to participate in the regulation of food intake and appetite. Pharmacologic studies, for example, suggest that when 5-HT receptors are stimulated, food intake is suppressed. Nutritional studies also reveal that the ingestion of particular macronutrients can alter 5-HT synthesis (and presumably release) by modifying the brain uptake and levels of the 5-HT precursor, tryptophan (TRP). The 5-HT neuron therefore appears to be strongly involved in the governing of appetite, both influencing and being influenced by food intake. In the review that follows, each of these relationships is examined, as well as a model that postulates the regulation of carbohydrate appetite by meal-induced changes in 5-HT synthesis and release. This model has been used as a basis for postulating the existence of a subgroup of obese patients who gain weight because of an uncontrolled urge to consume carbohydrates ("carbohydrate cravers"). The overall conclusion is that this model is not sufficiently validated to be useful in understanding food intake regulation by 5-HT neurons and that carbohydrate cravers, though appealing in concept, probably do not exist in reality. However, it will also be emphasized that, as their pharmacology becomes better defined, 5-HT drugs appear to be becoming more and more useful as agents for controlling appetite.

SEROTONIN PHARMACOLOGY, APPETITE, AND OBESITY

Drugs That Modify Serotonin Synaptic Transmission

To appreciate how drugs alter food intake by modifying 5-HT synaptic transmission, it is useful first to consider the known mechanisms by which drugs affect the 5-HT neuron (Fig. 34-1). Two broad classes of 5-HT drugs can be distinguished—those that increase and those that decrease 5-HT transmission.

The drugs that increase 5-HT transmission include precursors, releasers, reuptake blockers, blockers of 5-HT metabolism, and 5-HT agonists (see Fig. 34-1). Typically, 5-hydroxytryptophan (5-HTP) has been the precursor administered to stimulate 5-HT synthesis (and presumably release). Administration of 5-HTP stimulates 5-HT formation because the enzyme that decarboxylates 5-HTP to 5-HT (aromatic-L-amino acid decarboxylase [AAAD]) is unsaturated with substrate. Hence, an increase in tissue 5-HTP levels causes an immediate increase in 5-HT production. The use of 5-HTP, however, imparts a degree of nonspecificity, because AAAD is a ubiquitous enzyme. Serotonin is thus made in all cells when 5-HTP is given[49] and can lead to effects not involving 5-HT neurons.[54] In contrast, TRP shows great specificity as a substrate, caus-

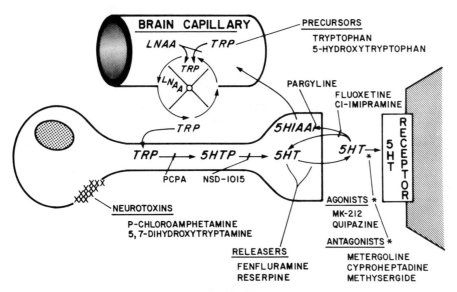

FIGURE 34-1

Neuropharmacologic agents that affect the serotonin neuron in brain. Shown
are the competitive mechanism for TRP transport into brain, the 5-HT biosynthetic pathway, and the processes of 5-HT release, interaction with receptors,
and presynaptic reuptake. Specidfic drugs and/or amino acids are known to
affect each of these processes. The 5-HT synthetic pathway involves TRP hydroxylation to 5-HTP, catalyzed by TRP hydroxylase, and subsequent 5-HTP
decarboxylation to 5-HT, catalyzed by the enzyme AAAD. Serotonin is metabolized to 5-HIAA in reactions mediated sequentially by MAO and aldehyde
dehydrogenase. The 5-HT agonists and antagonists shown are probably not selective for particular 5-HT receptor subtypes but are (or have been) widely
used. (NSD-1015, m-hydroxybenzylhydrazine; MK-212, 6-chloro-2-[1-
piperazinyl]-pyrazine)

ing 5-HT synthesis to be stimulated only in those
cells normally producing it. The reason for this
difference is that TRP must first be hydroxylated,
and then decarboxylated to form 5-HT (see Fig.
34-1). The hydroxylating enzyme TRP hydroxylase is only found in 5-HT-producing cells (it is
not ubiquitous). Tryptophan administration
stimulates 5-HT formation for the same reason
that 5-HTP does. TRP hydroxylase is unsaturated
at normal brain TRP concentrations, such that
increasing brain TRP level increases the enzyme's saturation with substrate and thus the
rate of the reaction.[25] However, TRP is not as
pharmacologically potent as 5-HTP, probably because the neuron's TRP hydroxylating capacity
is normally only a fraction of its 5-HTP decarbox-

ylating capacity. Potency is therefore sacrificed
for specificity.

Serotonin releasers cause 5-HT to be disgorged
from synaptic nerve endings, typically by deplet-
ing storage vesicles or proteins. Reserpine is
the classic 5-HT releaser, but it is not specific,
causing the release of all the known biogenic
amines.[16] A more interesting 5-HT releaser is fenfluramine, which is currently used widely as an
anorectic agent. The 5-HT reuptake blocker takes
advantage of the fact that the principal route of
5-HT removal from the synapse is through presynaptic reuptake. Various drugs are now available for blocking this process (e.g., chlorimipra-
mine, fluoxetine). Blockers of 5-HT metabolism
are principally inhibitors of monoamine oxidase

(MAO), the enzyme that initiates the conversion of 5-HT to its principal metabolite, 5-hydroxyindoleacetic acid (5-HIAA). Because MAO (even its subtypes) is responsible for catabolizing more than a single biogenic amine, MAO inhibitors cannot be agents that produce changes specific to 5-HT.

Serotonin precursors, releasers, reuptake blockers, and inhibitors of 5-HT metabolism all increase 5-HT neurotransmission by enhancing the amount of 5-HT available in the synaptic cleft for interacting with 5-HT receptors. In contrast, 5-HT agonists act directly to stimulate 5-HT receptors. Serotonin receptors are not a single entity; like receptors for other amine transmitters, there are several subtypes.[15] Two broad classes are generally distinguished, 5-HT$_1$ and 5-HT$_2$, based on their affinities for different receptor ligands. There appears to be no clear anatomical distinction between these two subclasses (at least at present): Either receptor subtype can apparently occur on presynaptic 5-HT nerve terminals (where they may act as autoreceptors) or on postsynaptic effector cells.[15]

The drugs that decrease 5-HT transmission include 5-HT synthesis inhibitors, large neutral amino acids (LNAA) *other* than TRP, 5-HT neurotoxins, and 5-HT antagonists. Serotonin synthesis inhibitors typically have not been useful clinically. The most common is parachlorophenylalanine (PCPA), which is an inhibitor of TRP hydroxylase. However, PCPA also inhibits phenylalanine hydroxylase and is thus not specific. Inhibitors of AAAD are not of much use either, because they inhibit the synthesis of almost all decarboxylated biogenic amines. Administration of LNAA other than TRP can inhibit 5-HT synthesis by blocking TRP uptake into brain, thus lowering brain TRP levels.[25] The LNAA have this effect because TRP and the other LNAA share a saturable, competitive transport carrier across the blood-brain barrier. Increasing the blood level of one or more LNAA therefore has the effect of inhibiting competitively the transport of the remaining LNAA into brain.[58]

Serotonin neurotoxins (e.g., 5,7-dihydroxytryptamine) cause a selective destruction of 5-HT neurons. They are therefore useful experimentally but not clinically.

Finally, 5-HT antagonists block 5-HT transmission by directly blocking postsynaptic 5-HT receptors. Several antagonists exist, including some that are subtype selective and some that are not. The antagonists most commonly used, both experimentally and clinically, are not subtype specific (e.g., methysergide, metergoline, cyproheptadine).

Effects of Serotonin Drugs on Food Intake

Serotonin Agonists

Several 5-HT drugs have been tested on appetite and food intake in rats and in humans, and a fairly consistent set of data has emerged. Considering first drugs that *stimulate* transmission across 5-HT synapses, the most potent would be 5-HT agonists. Quipazine and several other, structurally related 5-HT agonists, for example, inhibit food intake when administered systemically.[64,72] This action is blocked by the coadministration of 5-HT antagonists (e.g., metergoline), affirming that the effect is mediated by a 5-HT receptor. Serotonin itself, when microinjected directly into the brain, also reduces food intake,[39] suggesting that peripherally administered 5-HT agonists may suppress appetite by an action mediated *within* the brain. However, peripheral administration of 5-HT *also* suppresses food intake [and the effect can be blocked by a 5-HT antagonist].[30,61] Because 5-HT cannot cross the blood-brain barrier (in adult mammals),[56] these results suggest that the effect is mediated peripherally. Moreover, the effect is selective; it is not simply due to malaise induced by the amine.[61] This peripheral action of 5-HT does not negate the likelihood that 5-HT agonists act within the brain to reduce food intake. It simply indicates that peripherally administered 5-HT agents can influence food intake by way of peripheral as well as central actions. This view seems underscored by the results of other studies (see below) using different classes of 5-HT drugs.

Studies with 5-HT agonists in the past treated the 5-HT receptor as a single entity. It is now apparent that like other transmitter receptors, the 5-HT receptor has several subtypes. Two main classes are now recognized, 5-HT$_1$ and 5-HT$_2$ receptors. The 5-HT$_2$ receptor appears (so far) to be a single entity, but three subtypes of the 5-HT_1 receptor are currently accepted: 5-HT_{1a}, 5-HT_{1b}, and 5-HT_{1c}. A number of drugs that show agonist specificity for the 5-HT_{1a} and 5-HT_{1b} receptors are now available. Not surprisingly, these drugs have been tested for their effects on food intake. For example, Dourish and colleagues[19] observed that the administration of 8-hydroxy-2-(di-n-propylamino)tetralin (8-OH-DPAT), an agonist selective for the 5-HT_{1a} receptor, *stimulates* food intake in rats. Other 5-HT_{1a} agonists produce the same effect.[20,72,73] In contrast, 5-HT_{1b} agonists inhibit food intake.[20,37] The explanation offered for these opposite effects is that the 5-HT_{1a} receptor is a presynaptic autoreceptor, which inhibits the firing of 5-HT neurons; the 5-HT_{1b} receptor is presumed to be postsynaptic.[19,20] Accordingly, the 5-HT_{1a} agonist indirectly reduces postsynaptic effects of 5-HT, which should (and apparently does) produce effects on feeding opposite to those of postsynaptic 5-HT agonists (like the 5-HT_{1b} agonists). From other experiments, Kennett and colleagues[37] suggest that the appetite-suppressing effects of the 5-HT_{1b} agonists are not mediated at 5-HT_2 receptors. However, additional work is required to clarify whether and how agonists that act at the 5-HT_{1c} and 5-HT_2 receptors influence food intake.[72] At present, though it is clear that 5-HT receptor subtypes exist and when stimulated produce different effects on food intake, the relationships among the various 5-HT receptor subtypes and appetite are only beginning to be studied.

Fenfluramine

Another class of 5-HT drug causing 5-HT receptor stimulation is the 5-HT releasing agent. Fenfluramine is the example in this class most typically associated with appetite effects (though fenfluramine not only releases 5-HT but also blocks its reuptake[31]). Fenfluramine has probably also been the 5-HT agent most studied, because it is used clinically to reduce appetite and weight. Fenfluramine is structurally related to amphetamine, a potent anorectic agent, but does not act at catecholamine synapses and is not a stimulant.[64] Various studies in both rats and humans have shown fenfluramine to be a potent suppressor of food intake[6,11,67,68] and to exert its effects

by way of 5-HT receptor stimulation.[14] In addition, the study of fenfluramine anorexia has led to specific notions about how 5-HT agents can influence appetite and food intake.

First, the drug is acknowledged to have an effect within the brain: When injected directly into the brain, fenfluramine reduces food intake.[6,42] This effect may be purely behavioral. In general, the drug is said to diminish intake by shortening meals rather than by reducing their frequency. Accordingly, the drug is said to work by a meal satiety mechanism rather than by a meal initiation mechanism.[6,11] However, the effect may instead (or in addition) be primarily physiological and only indirectly behavioral. That is, some data suggest that central administration of fenfluramine activates central autonomic circuits that slow gastric emptying.[62] Such an effect should report a feeling of stomach fullness to the brain and thus lead indirectly to a behavioral response—reduced eating.[65] Second, fenfluramine is believed by some to have a purely *peripheral* locus of action, acting either through a physiological (inhibition of gastric emptying[18]) or a metabolic mechanism (promotion of lipolysis[22]). In this case, the reduction of food intake would also be an *indirect* behavioral effect.

The metabolic issue has become interesting from a new perspective. Fenfluramine has been known for some time to influence carbohydrate and lipid metabolism,[60] which, as indicated earlier, could indirectly alter caloric intake. In 1986, however, Even and Nicolaidis[23] reported that fenfluramine could also act to modify caloric *expenditure* as well. Their notion is that the drug makes caloric utilization less efficient.[23] In particular, they noted that physical activity in rats treated with fenfluramine was associated with a greater caloric expenditure than in vehicle-treated animals.[23] This observation is appealing because it could explain why, for example, after chronic drug treatment, food intake returns to predrug values even though lost weight is not regained.[23] Levitsky and Stallone[44] embraced a similar model, though they believe that fenfluramine promotes the inefficient use of calories during eating (diet-induced thermogenesis). Though this latter notion is disputed,[22] there is agreement that anorectic agents like fenfluramine should be studied as much for their effects on caloric expenditure as for their actions on caloric acquisition.

Finally, fenfluramine has been the 5-HT drug of choice for studying whether such agents influence macronutrient intake, as well as generally reducing caloric intake. Several early studies suggested that fenfluramine administration would selectively suppress appetite for carbohydrates but not for protein or fat.[75,76] These studies have led to a model (discussed later) in which 5-HT neurons are viewed as a central feature of a brain mechanism regulating appetite for carbohydrates. They have also precipitated the notion that this mechanism is faulty in some obese individuals and accounts for their obese state.[79,80] However, several studies now dispute the notion that fenfluramine selectively suppresses carbohydrate consumption.[47,57] This issue is still not fully resolved, because Shor-Posner and colleagues[66] reported that nor-fenfluramine selectively reduces carbohydrate intake when administered directly into the hypothalamus. The effect is obtained only at a time of day when animals are normally selecting high levels of carbohydrate: dark onset (when rats normally begin their main period of daily eating). If this observation is correct, then perhaps the 5-HT neuron can influence carbohydrate intake at some meals. This issue is later discussed further.

Serotonin Precursors

Both 5-HT precursors, TRP and 5-HTP, have been studied for their effects on food intake. Early work focused on 5-HTP: Its peripheral administration to rats reduced food intake.[9,36] This effect was independent of water intake and was not associated with lethargy (i.e., it was not a nonspecific effect).[36] It could also be related to a central nervous system action, because the coadministration of a drug that blocks 5-HTP decarboxylation, but only *outside* the brain, did not prevent the anorectic effect.[8]

The natural 5-HT precursor TRP has also been studied, but its administration does not produce effects as potent as those with 5-HTP. This is perhaps not surprising, for two reasons. First, TRP is a natural constituent of food but 5-HTP is not, and one would not *a priori* expect normal

food constituents to be potent pharmacologically. Second, less 5-HT is formed when TRP is administered than when 5-HTP is injected. This is because the activity of TRP hydroxylase is small in comparison with that of AAAD, and TRP hydroxylase is present in relatively few cells and neurons whereas AAAD is ubiquitous. In rats, TRP injection has been reported by some[40,50] but not other laboratories[59] to reduce food intake. In one of the positive studies,[50] however, the effect of TRP could not be convincingly linked to a central nervous system action. In general, because the effects of TRP are small, they may be missed if sufficient attention is not paid to experimental conditions.[40,50] Effects have also been observed in humans: Silverstone and Goodall,[68] for example, observed a small but significant reduction in the caloric content of meals in subjects given TRP (0.5, 1, or 2 g) in a double-blind cross-over study. Similar observations have also been made by others,[7,35] though in the study by Hrboticky and colleagues,[35] the side-effects associated with TRP use may have suppressed food intake nonselectively. Finally, as in studies with fenfluramine, effects of TRP have been sought on macronutrient selection. These have not been found in several studies[35,59,79]; in others, the reported effects are not impressive[50] or are difficult to interpret.[7] Overall, if TRP has effects, they appear to be small.

Serotonin Reuptake Blockers

Serotonin reuptake blockers offer a new and interesting neuropharmacologic approach to the control of food intake. These agents produce relatively few side-effects and are very specific, because their biochemical mechanism of action focuses their effects on genuine 5-HT synapses (they enhance 5-HT interactions indirectly, by blocking presynaptic reuptake of released 5-HT [see Fig. 34-1]). The reuptake blocker of greatest current interest is fluoxetine (Prozac; LY110140). Soon after its discovery as a specific 5-HT reuptake blocker, Goudie and colleagues[32] observed that peripheral injections of the drug reduced food intake in rats. Moreover, the effect was found to be additive with that of 5-HTP, as it should be: 5-HTP injection should increase 5-HT formation and thus presumably release, whereas fluoxetine should block the uptake of the 5-HT. Much more amine should thus be in the synapse after both compounds are given than after either is given alone. A reduction in feeding was also observed when fluoxetine was administered directly into the hypothalamus, a known center of feeding control that receives 5-HT nerve terminals.[42] Though this observation does not exclude a peripheral site of fluoxetine action, it suggests that a central site of action participates in the anorectic effects of the drug. Fluoxetine appears not to have been tested in combination with TRP. Nevertheless, its synergism with 5-HTP to reduce food intake at least supports the notion that its effects on food intake are mediated through a 5-HT synapse.

Fluoxetine has also been found to reduce food intake in humans. Levine and colleagues[43] administered the drug to obese patients for 5 weeks and noted much greater weight reduction in these subjects than in those given the drug vehicle. A similar study in obese subjects[24] was conducted for 8 weeks, and it also showed fluoxetine to be efficacious in lowering body weight. The subjects also reported diminished interest in eating following the initiation of a meal, a sign consistent with the view that 5-HT neurons are most important in satiety mechanisms.[6] Other 5-HT reuptake blockers have also been studied (e.g., zimelidine, indalpine, paroxetine) and are reported to cause similar effects.[70,72] Finally, Wurtman and others have reported fluoxetine and another 5-HT reuptake inhibitor (CGS 10686B) not only to reduce food intake in rats but also to reduce selectively the intake of carbohydrates.[38,75] If as much dispute over such macronutrient-specific effects occurs for 5-HT reuptake blockers when others test them as has arisen after the study of fenfluramine, it is unclear at present if such effects will stand the test of time. Until then, they should be viewed as tentative.

Drugs That Inhibit Serotonin Transmission

From the preceding discussion, it seems clear that stimulating 5-HT receptors causes an inhibition of feeding and leads to weight reduction. Accordingly, one might imagine that reducing 5-HT transmission would have the opposite behavioral action (i.e., to stimulate food intake and

weight gain). Three classes of 5-HT drugs have been used to address this notion: 5-HT receptor antagonists, 5-HT neurotoxins, and TRP hydroxylase inhibitors. Of these, the 5-HT antagonists have provided the most reliable information. Cyproheptadine appears to be the 5-HT antagonist most studied. This drug causes an increase in food intake in rats[4] and cats.[13] It also increases appetite and food consumption in normal and underweight adult humans,[48,69] children,[5,55] and patients with anorexia.[34] These effects are not attributable to the antihistaminic action of cyproheptadine[68] or to changes in fluid intake or peripheral metabolic effects (e.g., a change in carbohydrate metabolism[69]; a change in thyroid function[48]). Other antagonists have also been tested and found to increase appetite[68] and also to antagonize fenfluramine-induced anorexia.[12]

An increase in weight has also been recorded in rats treated with neurotoxins that destroy 5-HT neurons,[63] though this appears not be a uniform finding.[2] Injection of the TRP hydroxylase inhibitor PCPA was also reputed to stimulate food intake and weight gain[10]; however, this effect was subsequently found to be nonspecific.[46] In general, studies using neurotoxins and enzyme inhibitors have been less than satisfying, probably because their pharmacologic specificity is far from perfect.

In summary, studies using drugs that alter 5-HT transmission indicate that 5-HT release inhibits food intake and reduces body weight. As a body of psychopharmacologic literature, the results are remarkably consistent across drug class and across laboratories. In contrast, it is not clear whether these drugs selectively modify appetite for or intake of one particular macronutrient (e.g., carbohydrate).

EFFECTS OF FOOD INTAKE ON SEROTONIN SYNTHESIS: RELEVANCE TO CARBOHYDRATE APPETITE AND OBESITY

Serotonin neurons not only influence food intake (as evidenced by the earlier pharmacologic studies); they are also influenced by food intake. This latter relationship has been suggested to be important in the control of appetite and to have an etiologic role in certain forms of obesity (discussed later).

The biochemical basis for effects of food intake on 5-HT synthesis appears to be primarily that 5-HT synthesis is tied directly to local TRP concentration. Brain TRP concentration can influence 5-HT synthesis, because the enzyme catalyzing the first and rate-limiting step in the pathway, TRP hydroxylase (see Fig. 34-1), is normally unsaturated with substrate. Changes in brain TRP level thus alter enzyme saturation and consequently the rate of TRP hydroxylation and 5-HT synthesis overall. Brain TRP levels, in turn, respond rapidly to changes in TRP uptake from the circulation. Accordingly, brain TRP level and 5-HT synthesis are sensitive to phenomena that alter brain TRP uptake. One such phenomenon is food-related changes in serum amino acid levels.

Originally, food-induced effects on TRP availability and 5-HT synthesis were viewed in the context of the chronic diet: Increases or decreases in dietary TRP intake over a several-week period, by raising or lowering the *overall* availability of amino acids (including TRP) to the organism, would correspondingly increase or decrease brain 5-HT levels or synthesis.[17,28,33] However, the dietary conditions required to produce these effects could only be labeled as extreme and thus of limited physiologic interest (at least in developed countries; they remain a significant concern in underdeveloped nations). Dietary effects on 5-HT synthesis have now been identified following the ingestion of single meals by well-nourished experimental animals. In particular, the ingestion of a carbohydrate (protein-free) meal has been shown rapidly to increase brain TRP uptake and 5-HT synthesis, whereas consumption of a protein-containing meal does not.[25] The basis for these different effects derives from the manner in which TRP is transferred from blood to brain. TRP is taken up into brain by a transport carrier located at the blood-brain barrier.[56] This carrier transports not only TRP but also several other LNAA (*e.g.*, tyrosine, phenylalanine, leucine, isoleucine, and valine). The transport carrier is saturable and competitive[58]; hence, the uptake of TRP depends not only on its own blood level but also on the blood concentrations of the other LNAA. For example, brain TRP uptake and levels increase either when

blood TRP concentrations rise or when the blood levels of the other LNAA fall.

The competitive transport model can explain the increase in brain TRP level induced by carbohydrate consumption and the absence of such changes when the ingested meal contains protein. In a fasting rat, carbohydrate ingestion induces insulin secretion, which raises blood TRP levels and lowers the blood concentrations of the other LNAA, particularly the branched-chain amino acids.[29] The result is to increase TRP's competitive advantage for brain uptake and consequently brain TRP level. The ingestion of a protein-containing meal also induces insulin secretion, which raises blood TRP level and lowers the blood levels of the other LNAA. But this meal also adds dietary amino acids to the circulation, thus raising the blood levels of all the LNAA. The net result is to raise by proportionally similar amounts the blood levels of *both* TRP *and* the combined blood levels of the other LNAA. To the competitive transport carrier, such changes signal no net alteration in competition. Consequently, neither brain TRP uptake nor its levels are changed after ingestion of a protein-containing meal.

A model for the meal-to-meal regulation of carbohydrate intake has been advanced. It includes as a biochemical mechanism "sensing" the changes in brain TRP level and 5-HT synthesis induced by carbohydrate ingestion. The model is constructed from three experimental observations: first, the report that over time, rats maintain their daily carbohydrate intake at a constant level[76] (apparently, in such a model, the continual meal-to-meal adjustment of carbohydrate intake would maintain constancy of carbohydrate intake over long periods); second, the observation that ingesting a carbohydrate meal increases brain 5-HT synthesis (whereas ingesting a protein-containing meal does not); and third, the results of pharmacologic studies (cited earlier) purporting to show that the administration of drugs that enhance transmission across 5-HT synapses (*e.g.*, fluoxetine and fenfluramine) selectively suppresses carbohydrate intake.[38,76] Together, these findings have been synthesized into the following model to describe the meal-to-meal regulation of carbohydrate intake (Fig. 34-2): When a carbohydrate meal is ingested, the blood

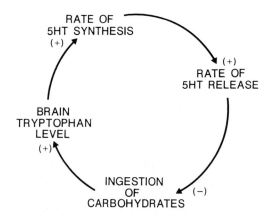

FIGURE 34-2

Putative model of carbohydrate intake regulation. Portions of this model are now disputed. The ingestion of carbohydrates by fasting rats is known to raise brain TRP levels and to stimulate 5-HT synthesis. The increase in synthesis may cause increased 5-HT release from nerve terminals, though this is at present unproven. Based on the interpretation of pharmacologic studies, which are controversial, the increased release of 5-HT has been postulated to inhibit specifically the subsequent appetite for carbohydrates.

levels of TRP rise and those of the other LNAA fall, brain TRP level rises, and 5-HT synthesis is stimulated. This sequence leads to enhanced release of 5-HT from brain neurons, in turn reducing the intake of carbohydrates (and raising the relative intake of protein). As carbohydrate intake declines (relative to protein intake), the serum level of TRP relative to those of the other LNAA falls, and thus brain TRP uptake and levels and 5-HT synthesis and release decline. As a result, the inhibition of carbohydrate intake (appetite) moderates, and the animal resumes eating carbohydrates.

Though this model is attractive, it is flawed. First, there is evidence that the chronic level of carbohydrate intake is actually not tightly controlled. There appears to be considerable variability in the amount of carbohydrate that individual rats elect to eat over extended periods,[1,41,83] suggesting the *absence* of a control system. Second, animals will not maintain an elected level of carbohydrate intake when they must press a bar an ever increasing number of times to obtain carbohydrate food pellets. In con-

trast, they *will* defend their preferred level of total calorie intake or their intake of a nutritionally adequate basal level of protein when such bar-pressing demands are made.[2] If carbohydrate intake were a regulated commodity, the animals should defend their level of carbohydrate intake (i.e., maintain the "set-point" for carbohydrate intake), but they do not. Third, there is no known nutritional requirement for carbohydrate in rats or humans as there is for total calories and for protein.[52,53] In the absence of such a requirement, it is difficult to imagine the need for a control system to regulate carbohydrate intake. Fourth, the pharmacologic studies in rats and humans purporting to show selective suppression of carbohydrate intake by drugs that stimulate 5-HT transmission do not present a clear, selective suppression of carbohydrate intake. For example, macronutrient effects of fenfluramine interpreted as showing a selective suppression of carbohydrate intake actually show a suppression of fat intake as well.[26,76,78] Similarly, studies conducted in other laboratories reveal that fenfluramine produces an anorectic effect that is *not* macronutrient selective.[47,57] Findings by Shor-Posner and colleagues[66] (namely, that the microinjection of norfenfluramine directly into the hypothalamus at one time of day, but not others, reduces carbohydrate intake selectively) do not remedy the problem, because the model requires an effect to be *continuously* present. Consequently, one is left with the overall impression that fenfluramine does not selectively suppress appetite for or intake of carbohydrates, at least at most times of the day and night (if Shor-Posner and associates[66] are right). This conclusion for fenfluramine is important, because the fenfluramine findings have been the principal pharmacologic data base cited to support the putative, selective inhibitory effect of 5-HT release on carbohydrate intake[74,77-79] and because the selective inhibitory effect of fenfluramine (i.e., of enhanced 5-HT release) on carbohydrate intake is required in order for the regulatory loop to exist. For if fenfluramine (i.e., 5-HT release) suppresses carbohydrate *and* protein *and* fat intakes, as appears likely, then the result of administering this drug would be to lower plasma levels of *both* TRP and the other LNAA together as the intake of all macronutrients fell, leading to no net change in the competitive uptake of TRP into brain and hence no net change in 5-HT synthesis or release. Consequently, there would be no modified signal in brain to change the ingestive behavior induced initially by the drug (i.e., increased 5-HT release), one way or the other. Therefore, in the absence of a selective inhibitory effect of 5-HT release on carbohydrate intake, the carbohydrate regulatory loop cannot exist. Together, all of the previous considerations suggest that the proposed model (see Fig. 34-2) for regulating carbohydrate intake is likely not to be generally valid.

This conclusion also casts doubt on a particular etiology for obesity, postulated to occur based on the earlier idea that carbohydrate intake is regulated.[79,81] The contention was that obesity could follow in some individuals from a malfunction of the regulatory loop, leading them to overeat carbohydrate-rich snacks. Such individuals have been dubbed carbohydrate cravers.[81] They are reputed to be quite sensitive to the effects of fenfluramine on carbohydrate snack intake, whereas noncravers are not.

Aside from the fact that such individuals probably do not exist because the regulatory loop (faulty or not) does not exist, studies offered in support of carbohydrate cravers have not been generally convincing, for several reasons. First, a careful definition of the carbohydrate craver has never been made. In published studies, such individuals have been selected through advertisements specifically seeking carbohydrate cravers. The self-styled carbohydrate cravers who respond are then screened using a snack selection test in which the successful subject is observed to choose carbohydrate-rich, protein-poor snacks almost exclusively.[81] All such carbohydrate snacks, however, contained considerable amounts of fat, and almost all were sweet, complicating a clean interpretation of the true features of the snacks favored by the subjects. Moreover, the general appeal of the carbohydrate snacks was probably much greater than that of the protein snacks offered (e.g., Pepperidge Farm granola cookies versus Slim Jim beef jerky). Hence, hedonistic and sensory qualities undoubtedly entered into the selection as uncontrolled variables, making the labeling of individuals who select the carbohydrate snacks as carbohydrate cravers at best a debatable point. Perhaps an indication of the inadequacy of this

definition procedure is the fact that using it, non-carbohydrate cravers were apparently quite hard to find.[45,81] The definition and selection criteria are clearly too weak to pick out the real carbohydrate cravers among us, should they exist.

Second, a clear definition of the carbohydrate food craved by the carbohydrate craver has never been made. Must it be pure carbohydrate? Must it be sweet? Can it contain fat? Can it contain protein, and if so, how much? This latter consideration is important, given the knowledge that in rats, even a few percent (around 5%) protein added to a carbohydrate meal can suppress the meal's ability to raise brain TRP levels.[84] That should also be true in humans. If so, then almost all of the carbohydrate-rich foods and snacks used in the human studies published to date contained a level of protein sufficient to block any carbohydrate-induced rise in brain TRP level and 5-HT formation.[80] The subjects craving these foods were therefore presumably not motivated to eat them because they affected brain 5-HT. In general, the lack of precision in defining and formulating the test foods seriously compromises the investigators' ability to draw convincing conclusions from their studies.

Third, data indicate that fenfluramine administration suppresses both carbohydrate and protein intakes in humans,[81] thus undermining the dietary-amino acid-transmitter rationale (see Fig. 34-2) that generated the present incarnation of the carbohydrate craver idea in the first place.

For all of these reasons, there is little justification to embrace the notion of a carbohydrate regulatory loop, much less of a carbohydrate-craving obese patient. It would undoubtedly turn out to be the case, if a sampling of carbohydrate cravers were carefully examined, that their craving would actually be found to be for fat or for sweetness, not for carbohydrate per se.[21]

As a final point related to carbohydrate intake regulation and obesity, the model in Figure 34-2 has been invoked to raise concern about a putative, counterintuitive effect of ingesting the artificial sweetener aspartame (APM). Aspartame is a phenylalanine (PHE)-containing dipeptide. Its ingestion raises blood PHE and tyrosine levels.[71] PHE and tyrosine are LNAA and thus compete with TRP for brain transport. The notion is that if APM is consumed with carbohydrates, the expected rise in brain TRP uptake and 5-HT synthesis will be blocked: The APM-induced increase in serum PHE and tyrosine levels would prevent the carbohydrate-induced increase in TRP transport into brain. As a result, 5-HT synthesis/release would not increase, and (to complete the loop) the appetite for carbohydrate would not be suppressed. Hence, an unusual effect would occur: An individual consuming a piece of cake, say, and some APM-sweetened soda would be compelled to eat more, not less, cake by virtue of having consumed the low-calorie, APM-sweetened soda. The APM would block the feedback signal (the rise in 5-HT release) needed to suppress carbohydrate appetite.

In fact, there is little cause for concern about this issue for two reasons. First, as discussed earlier, the carbohydrate regulatory loop probably does not exist. Second, though APM ingestion can indeed block TRP uptake and 5-HT synthesis following carbohydrate ingestion,[27,82] the threshold dose required to produce this effect is quite large (>500 mg/kg in rats) and must be administered as a single dose.[27] A conservative calculation of the dose-equivalent for humans is 100 mg/kg, based on a fivefold difference in amino acid metabolizing capacity between humans and rats.[51] This dose of aspartame has the sweetness equivalent of about 3 pounds of sugar for a 70-kg person (aspartame is 200 times sweeter than sugar by weight) and would have to be consumed all at once even to hypothesize any effects on brain TRP uptake and 5-HT synthesis in humans. This amount of sweetness is indeed extreme. Moreover, if the person just mentioned, eating cake and drinking APM-containing soda, consumed this dose of APM in the beverage, he or she would have to consume at least 3.25 gallons all at once before a 5-HT-related effect on cake-eating behavior could even be imagined (a 12-ounce can of soda contains 180 mg of APM[71]). This is indeed an immense volume. Therefore, concern about APM stimulation of carbohydrate appetite, at least based on these considerations, seems overdrawn and unjustifiable.

CONCLUSION

This chapter has reviewed the evidence that 5-HT neurons influence and are in turn biochemically influenced by food intake. First, it is clear that various pharmacologic agents, focused on the 5-HT synapse, are efficacious in increasing or decreasing food intake and appetite in humans. Such agents have been and will undoubtedly continue to be clinically useful in the control of appetite and body weight. Second, it is also clear that food can alter brain 5-HT synthesis under certain dietary conditions, based on how its ingestion alters the brain uptake of TRP: The consumption of carbohydrates following a fast stimulates brain TRP uptake and 5-HT synthesis, whereas protein consumption under the same conditions blocks carbohydrate-induced increases in brain TRP and 5-HT. Third, however, a model developed from these biochemical and pharmacologic findings that purports to show a regulatory loop controlling carbohydrate intake is probably not valid. Accordingly, predictions from it regarding the existence of individuals who become obese because of a craving for carbohydrates and the attendant recommendations regarding pharmacologic and other treatments to control their carbohydrate craving are probably incorrect.

Acknowledgment: Some of the studies described in this review from the author's laboratory were supported in part by a grant from the National Institutes of Health (HD24730).

References

1. Ackroff K, Schwartz D, Collier G: Macronutrient selection by foraging rats. Physiol Behav 38:71, 1986
2. Ashley DVM: Factors affecting the selection of protein and carbohydrate from a dietary choice. Nutr Res 5:555, 1985
3. Ashley DVM, Coscina DV, Anderson GH: Selective decrease in protein intake following brain serotonin depletion. Life Sci 24:973, 1979
4. Baxter MG, Miller AA, Soroko FE: The effect of cyproheptadine on food consumption in the fasted rat. Br J Pharmacol 39:229P, 1970
5. Bergen SS: Appetite stimulating properties of cyproheptadine. Am J Dis Child 108:270, 1964
6. Blundell JE: Serotonin and appetite. Neuropharmacology 23:1537, 1984
7. Blundell JE, Hill AJ: Serotoninergic modulation of the pattern of eating and the profile of hunger-satiety in humans. Int J Obes (Suppl 3) 11:141, 1987

8. Blundell JE, Lathem CJ: Serotonergic influences on food intake: Effect of 5-hydroxytryptophan on parameters of feeding behavior in deprived and free-feeding rats. Pharmacol Biochem Behav 11:431, 1979

9. Blundell JE, Leshem MB: The effect of 5-hydroxytryptophan on food intake and on the anorexic action of amphetamine and fenfluramine. J Pharm Pharmacol 27:31, 1975

10. Breisch ST, Zemlan FP, Hoebel BG: Hyperphagia and obesity following serotonin depletion by intraventricular p-chlorophenylalanine. Science 192:382, 1976

11. Burton MJ, Cooper SJ, Popplewell DA: The effect of fenfluramine on the microstructure of feeding and drinking in the rat. Br J Pharmacol 72:621, 1981

12. Clineschmidt BV, Bunting PR: Differential effects of pharmacological agents acting on monoaminergic systems on drug-induced anorexia. Prog Neuropsychopharmacol Biol Psychiatry 4:327, 1980

13. Clineschmidt BV, Hanson HM, McGuffin JC et al: Appetite stimulant activity of 3-carboxy-10,11-dihydroxyproheptadine. Arch Int Pharmacodyn Ther 223:287, 1976

14. Clineschmidt BV, McGuffin JC, Werner AB: Role of monoamines in the anorexigenic actions of fenfluramine, amphetamine, and p-chloromethamphetamine. Eur J Pharmacol 27:313, 1974

15. Conn PJ, Sanders-Bush E: Central serotonin receptors: Effector systems, physiological roles and regulation. Psychopharmacology 92:267, 1987

16. Cooper JR, Bloom FE, Roth RH: The Biochemical Basis of Neuropharmacology, 5th ed. New York, Oxford University Press, 1986

17. Culley WJ, Saunders RN, Mertz ET et al: Effect of a tryptophan deficient diet on brain serotonin and plasma tryptophan level. Proc Soc Exp Biol Med 113:645, 1963

18. Davies RF, Rossi J, Panksepp J et al: Fenfluramine anorexia: A peripheral locus of action. Physiol Behav 30:723, 1983

19. Dourish CT, Hutson PH, Curzon G: Low doses of the putative serotonin agonist 8-hydroxy-2-(di-n-propylamino) tetralin (8-OH-DPAT) elicit feeding in the rat. Psychopharmacology 86:197, 1985

20. Dourish CT, Hutson PH, Kennett GA et al: 8-OH-DPAT-induced hyperphagia: Its neural basis and possible therapeutic relevance. Appetite (Suppl) 7:127, 1986

21. Drewnowski A: Letter to the editor. Changes in mood after carbohydrate consumption. Am J Clin Nutr 46:703, 1987

22. Even P, Couland H, Aucouturier JL et al: Correlation between metabolic and behavioral effects of

dexfenfluramine tratment. Clin Neuropharmacol (Suppl 1) 11:S93, 1988

23. Even P, Nicolaidis S: Metabolic mechanism of the anorectic and leptogenic effects of the serotonin agonist fenfluramine. Appetite (Suppl) 7:141, 1986

24. Ferguson JM, Feighner JP: Fluoxetine-induced weight loss in overweight non-depressed humans. Int J Obes (Suppl 3) 11:163, 1987

25. Fernstrom JD: Role of precursor availability in the control of monoamine biosynthesis in brain. Physiol Rev 63:484, 1983

26. Fernstrom JD: Food-induced changes in brain serotonin synthesis: Is there a relationship to appetite for specific macronutrients? Appetite 8:163, 1987

27. Fernstrom JD, Fernstrom MH, Grubb PE: Effects of aspartame ingestion on the carbohydrate-induced rise in tryptophan hydroxylation rate in rat brain. Am J Clin Nutr 44:195, 1986

28. Fernstrom JD, Hirsch MJ: Brain serotonin synthesis: Reduction in corn-malnourished rats. J Neurochem 28:877, 1977

29. Fernstrom JD, Wurtman RJ: Elevation of plasma tryptophan by insulin in the rat. Metabolism 21:337, 1972

30. Fletcher PJ, Burton MJ: Effects of manipulations of peripheral serotonin on feeding and drinking in the rat. Pharmacol Biochem Behav 20:835, 1984

31. Garattini S, Jori A, Buczko W et al: The mechanism of action of fenfluramine. Postgrad Med J (Suppl 1) 51:27, 1975

32. Goudie AJ, Thornton EW, Wheeler TJ: Effects of Lilly 110140, a specific inhibitor of 5-hydroxytryptamine uptake, on food intake and on 5-hydroxytryptophan-induced anorexia. Evidence for serotoninergic inhibition of feeding. J Pharm Pharmacol 28:318, 1976

33. Green H, Greenberg SM, Erickson RW et al: Effect of dietary phenylalanine and tryptophan upon rat brain amine levels. J Pharmacol Exp Ther 136:174, 1962

34. Halmi KA, Eckert E, LaDu TJ et al: Anorexia nervosa: Treatment efficacy of cyproheptadine and amitriptyline. Arch Gen Psychiatry 43:177, 1986

35. Hrboticky N, Leiter LA, Anderson GH: Effects of L-tryptophan on short term food intake in lean men. Nutr Res 5:595, 1985

36. Joyce D, Mrosovsky N: Eating, drinking and activity in rats following 5-hydroxytryptophan (5-HTP) administration. Psychopharmacologia 5:417, 1964

37. Kennett GA, Dourish CT, Curzon G: 5-HT$_{1b}$ agonists induce anorexia at a postsynaptic site. Eur J Pharmacol 141:429, 1987

38. Kim S-H, Wurtman RJ: Selective effects of CGS 10686B, dl-fenfluramine or fluoxetine on nutrient selection. Physiol Behav 42:319, 1988

39. Kruk ZL: Dopamine and 5-hydroxytryptamine inhibit feeding in rats. Nature 246:52, 1973

40. Lathem CJ, Blundell JE: Evidence for the effect of tryptophan on the pattern of food consumption in free feeding and food deprived rats. Life Sci 24:1971, 1979

41. Leathwood PD, Ashley DVM: Strategies of protein selection by weanling and adult rats. Appetite 4:97, 1983

42. Leibowitz SF, Weiss GF, Shor-Posner G: Medial hypothalamic serotonin in the control of eating behavior. Int J Obes (Suppl 3) 11:109, 1987

43. Levine LR, Rosenblatt S, Bosomworth J: Use of a serotonin re-uptake inhibitor, fluoxetine, in the treatment of obesity. Int J Obes (Suppl 3) 11:185, 1987

44. Levitsky DA, Stallone D: Enhancement of the thermic effect of food by D-fenfluramine. Clin Neuropharmacol (Suppl 1) 11:S90, 1988

45. Lieberman HR, Wurtman JJ, Chew B: Changes in mood after carbohydrate consumption among obese individuals. Am J Clin Nutr 44:772, 1986

46. MacKenzie RG, Hoebel BG, Ducret RP et al: Hyperphagia following intraventricular p-chlorophenylalanine-, leucine-, or tryptophan-methyl esters: Lack of correlation with whole brain serotonin levels. Pharmacol Biochem Behav 10:951, 1979

47. McArthur RA, Blundell JE: Protein and carbohydrate self-selection: Modification of the effects of fenfluramine and amphetamine by age and feeding regimen. Appetite 4:113, 1983

48. Mertz DP, Stelzer M: Zum mechanismus der appetit- un gewichtsteigernden wirkung von cyproheptadin. I. Klinische erfahrungen und hormonjodstudien. Klin Wochenschr 47:1189, 1969

49. Moir ATB, Eccleston D: The effects of precursor loading in the cerebral metabolism of 5-hydroxyindoles. J Neurochem 15:1093, 1968

50. Morris P, Li ETS, MacMillan ML et al: Food intake and selection after peripheral tryptophan. Physiol Behav 40:155, 1987

51. Munro HN: Evolution of protein metabolism in mammals. In Munro HN (ed): Mammalian Protein Metabolism, Vol III, p 133. New York, Academic Press, 1969

52. National Academy of Sciences: Nutrient Requirements of Domestic Animals, Number 10: Nutrient Requirements of Laboratory Animals, 3rd rev ed, p 7. Washington, DC, National Academy of Sciences, 1978

53. National Academy of Sciences: Recommended Dietary Allowances, 9th rev ed, p 33. Committee on Dietary Allowances, Food and Nutrition Board, National Research Council. Washington, DC, National Academy of Sciences, 1980

54. Ng LKY, Chase TN, Colburn RW et al: Release of [³H]dopamine by L-5-hydroxytryptophan. Brain Res 45:499, 1972

55. Noble RE: Effect of cyproheptadine on appetite and weight gain in adults. JAMA 209:2054, 1969

56. Oldendorf WH: Brain uptake of radiolabeled amino acids, amines, and hexoses after arterial injection. Am J Physiol 221:1629, 1971

57. Orthen-Gambill N, Kanarek RB: Differential effects of amphetamine and fenfluramine on dietary self-selection in rats. Pharmacol Biochem Behav 16:303, 1982

58. Pardridge WM, Oldendorf WH: Kinetic analysis of blood brain barrier transport of amino acids. Biochim Biophys Acta 401:128, 1975

59. Peters JC, Bellissimo DB, Harper AE: L-tryptophan injection fails to alter nutrient selection by rats. Physiol Behav 32:253, 1984

60. Pinder RM, Brogden RN, Sawyer PR et al: Fenfluramine: A review of its pharmacological properties and therapeutic efficacy in obesity. Drugs 10:241, 1975

61. Pollack JD, Rowland N: Peripherally administered serotonin decreases food intake in rats. Pharmacol Biochem Behav 15:179, 1981

62. Rowland N, Carlton J: Inhibition of gastric emptying by peripheral and central fenfluramine in rats: Correlation with anorexia. Life Sci 34:2495, 1984

63. Saller CF, Stricker EM: Hyperphagia and increased growth in rats after intraventricular injection of 5,7-dihydroxytryptamine. Science 192:385, 1976

64. Samanin R, Mennini T, Garattini S: Evidence that it is possible to cause anorexia by increasing release and/or directly stimulating postsynaptic serotonin receptors in the brain. Prog Neuropsychopharmacol Biol Psychiatry 4:363, 1980

65. Share I, Martyniuk E, Grossman MI: Effect of prolonged gastric feeding on oral food intake in dogs. Am J Physiol 169:229, 1952

66. Shor-Posner G, Grinker JA, Marinescu C et al: Hypothalamic serotonin in the control of meal patterns and macronutrient selection. Brain Res Bull 17:663, 1986

67. Shoulson I, Chase TN: Fenfluramine in man: Hypophagia associated with diminished serotonin turnover. Clin Pharmacol Ther 17:616, 1975

68. Silverstone T, Goodall E: Serotoninergic mechanisms in human feeding: The pharmacological evidence. Appetite (Suppl) 7:85, 1986

69. Silverstone T, Schuyler D: The effect of cyproheptadine on hunger, caloric intake and body weight in man. Psychopharmacologia 40:335, 1975

70. Simpson RJ, Lawton DJ, Watt MH et al: Effects of zimelidine, a new antidepressant, on appetite and body weight. Br J Clin Pharmacol 11:96, 1981

71. Stegink LD, Filer LJ (eds): Asparyytame: Physiology and Biochemistry. New York, Marcel Dekker, 1984

72. Wong DT, Fuller RW: Serotonergic mechanisms in feeding. Int J Obes (Suppl 3) 11:125, 1987

73. Wong DT, Reid LR: Fenfluramine antagonizes the stimulation of food intake induced by the putative 5-hydroxytryptamine$_{1a}$ agonist, isapirone, in non-fasted rats. J Pharm Pharmacol 39:570, 1987

74. Wurtman JJ, Moses PL, Wurtman RJ: Prior carbohydrate consumption affects the amount of carbohydrates that rats choose to eat. J Nutr 113:70, 1983

75. Wurtman JJ, Wurtman RJ: Fenfluramine and fluoxetine spare protein consumption while suppressing caloric intake by rats. Science 198:1178, 1977

76. Wurtman JJ, Wurtman RJ: Drugs that enhance central serotoninergic transmission diminish elective carbohydrate consumption by rats. Life Sci 24:895, 1979

77. Wurtman JJ, Wurtman RJ: Studies on the appetite for carbohydrates in rats and humans. J Psychiat Res 17:213, 1982/83

78. Wurtman JJ, Wurtman RJ: D-fenfluramine selectively decreases carbohydrate but not protein intake in obese subjects. Int J Obes (Suppl 1) 8:79, 1984

79. Wurtman JJ, Wurtman RJ, Growdon JH et al: Carbohydrate craving in obese people: Suppression by treatments affecting serotoninergic transmission. Int J Eating Disord 1:2, 1981

80. Wurtman J, Wurtman RJ, Mark S et al: D-Fenfluramine selectively suppresses carbohydrate snacking by obese subjects. Int J Eating Disord 4:89, 1985

81. Wurtman JJ, Wurtman RJ, Reynolds S et al: Fenfluramine suppresses snack intake among carbohydrate cravers but not among noncarbohydrate cravers. Int J Eating Disord 6:687, 1987

82. Yokogoshi H, Roberts CH, Caballero B et al: Effects of aspartame and glucose administration on brain and plasma levels of large neutral amino acids and brain 5-hydroxyindoles. Am J Clin Nutr 40:1, 1984

83. Yokogoshi H, Theall CL, Wurtman RJ: Selection of dietary protein and carbohydrate by rats: Changes with maturation. Physiol Behav 36:979, 1986

84. Yokogoshi H, Wurtman RJ: Meal composition and plasma amino acid ratios: Effects of various proteins or carbohydrates, and of various protein concentrations. Metabolism 35:837, 1986

CHAPTER 35

Environmental Light, Mood, and Seasonal Affective Disorder

DAN A. OREN and NORMAN E. ROSENTHAL

"When the winter sets in, darkness does not begin suddenly; for about two months there is first a disappearance of the sun for only a few minutes, the next day it is double that time, and the next day it is double that time. . . . It takes two months before it entirely disappears. Then the gloom of the Arctic night sets in, and although the Eskimos spent their time telling stories and legends and tried hard to amuse us, I could notice a depression among ourselves, as well as among the people . . . that reached its climax about Christmas. . . . Although we had a very good Christmas dinner and everything we could wish for in the way of food, we were all very blue."

Frederick A. Cook, M.D., 1894
Surgeon to the Peary Arctic Expedition[1]

The idea that light could have a role in our moods or appetite must date back to humankind's first awareness of emotions. In a world where the sun was once the central deity and today remains a powerful regulator of human behavior, only recently has a scientific appreciation of the impact of environmental light on mood emerged. Recognizing the still dawning history of the impact of surrounding light on psychopathology, in this chapter we illuminate the beginnings and current status of this fertile field of inquiry.

Although seasonally distributed influences on affective illness have been recorded by physicians as ancient as Hippocrates (circa 400 B.C.E.),[2] Cook's observations are the earliest we have found specifically linking seasonal loss of sunlight to a mood disorder. Accompanying United States Naval Lieutenant Robert E. Peary on one of his early Arctic expeditions, Cook noted the profound influences of light on the voyagers and on the Eskimos themselves. Such symptoms as loss of sexual desire, fatigue, loss of energy, and profoundly depressed mood were noted by Cook to be manifested not just in the observed Eskimos, but in the observers as well. The lack of light, not the winter cold, was perceived as the cause of the syndrome, given Cook's estimation that the Eskimos kept their igloos well heated. As for the explorers, Cook noted that he "never suffered from the cold and none of our party did."[1,3] On an Antarctic expedition in 1898, he found the crew of the *Belgica* to become "affected, body and soul, with languor," only to find some relief with bright artificial light or heat from an open fire.[4] In later years, other individuals would pick up Cook's theme. Hasselbalch reported in 1905 that a "light bath" including ultraviolet radiation produced feelings of increased energy, exhilaration, and hypomania.[5] Specifically reviewing the incidence of suicide in both the Northern and Southern Hemispheres, Gaedeken in 1911 drew a direct connection between sunshine and mood.[6] Drawing on Cook's observations, Llewellyn in 1932 suggested that visual pathways were linked to the powerful phenomenon of environmental light having an impact on mood.[7]

Surprisingly, in a century whose earliest decades saw humanity making great strides toward understanding the influence of environmental nutrients and pathogens on our health, significant interest in light and mood disorders lay dormant until the late 1970s. One patient in particular was a catalyst for the resurgent interest in light. Complaining of a 13-year history of fall-winter depressive episodes and spring-summer mood elevations, attributing the changes to altered periods of environmental light, scientist-patient Herbert E. Kern piqued the interest of several researchers at the National Institute of Mental Health.[8] Lewy and his colleagues, speculating that exposing a patient to two periods of bright lights extending normal daylight hours would improve mood, found a dramatic improvement in the patient's affect.[9] The next winter, 11 patients underwent light therapy, and Rosenthal and colleagues dubbed the winter-depression syndrome *seasonal affective disorder* (SAD).[10] Though some within the psychiatric community have been hesitant to recognize seasonally mediated and light-alleviated mood swings without further evidence, confirmatory studies involving hundreds of patients treated by other independent groups continue to support the basic findings of the original reports.[8] In recognition of the apparently solid nature of the syndrome and the creative opportunities for further research that it offers, the most recent psychiatric diagnostic guidebook, the *Diagnostic and Statistical Manual of Mental Disorders* (DSM-III-R), calls for noting the presence of seasonality in cases of recurrent mood disorders.[11]

PHENOMENOLOGY

In our clinic, we have defined SAD as occurring in patients with a history of at least one incident of major affective disorder, depressed,[12] and regularly occurring fall-winter depressions remitting during spring or summer. Initial criteria required that at least two winter-depressive episodes be consecutive and that the winter timing be unaccounted for by psychosocial variables. DSM-III-R narrowed the category of patients with SAD by requiring that they have more than two episodes of fall-winter depression and that these seasonal episodes take place more than

three times as often as spring-summer depressions.[11] In order to focus on the pure syndrome, the data that follow apply solely to those SAD patients we have studied who also gave no evidence of any other major psychiatric disorder.

The almost universal symptoms of winter depression noted in patients with SAD are dysphoria and decreased activity. Concomitant symptoms of irritability, anxiety, decreased libido, and social withdrawal are usually noted. Unlike classically depressed patients, most patients with SAD find themselves with "atypical depressed"[13] symptoms of increased appetite and weight and increased fatigue in winter, despite their increased quantities of sleep.[14] Some patients with SAD are more disturbed by these vegetative symptoms than by the mood changes themselves. Because these physical manifestations of the disorder frequently precede the psychological changes and prove disturbing to patients, patients with SAD often consult their internists or family physicians before seeking psychiatric assistance. The depressions are usually mild to moderate, but 6% of the patients we have seen have needed to be hospitalized, and 1% have required electroconvulsive treatments.[15]

More than 80% of the nearly 300 patients with SAD seen in the clinic at the National Institute of Mental Health (NIMH) have been women. Given potential selection biases, this figure may overstate the true relative prevalence of the disorder among women.[16] The average onset of the disorder in our population has been at approximately age 22, with the depressive episodes lasting about 5 months.[15] These figures are nearly identical to those of the New York State Psychiatric Institute group.[16] SAD depressive episodes typically begin in November for patients residing near the 38.9° N latitude of Washington, DC.[14] This corresponds to the period when total hours of daylight in Washington decrease to less than 10.[17] Retrospective data inform us that untreated SAD depressive episodes generally resolve by springtime, although some individuals do not fully recover before the early summer. Many have reported that travel to latitudes nearer the equator resulted in remission or diminution of their symptoms.[15] In Washington, DC, the depression typically has ended by April, when total hours of daylight exceed 13.[17] Many of our patients have reported a history of briefly depressed moods recurring even in spring and midsummer if the weather is cloudy or if they spend time in a dimly lit area.[10] Many patients with SAD have experienced summertime reversal of their winter symptoms. Mild hypomania with elation, increased libido, social activity, increased energy, diminished sleep requirements, reduced appetite, and loss of winter weight commonly appeared during the summers.[18]

EPIDEMIOLOGY

The epidemiologic understanding of SAD is in its infancy. Nevertheless, certain patterns have prevailed in our population of patients.[19] Diagnostically, 59% of patients at NIMH had histories of bipolar II disorder[12] (depressive and hypomanic episodes), 8% had bipolar I disorder (depressive and full manic episodes), and 33% had a history of unipolar depression. Familial factors may be involved in the disorder, given that more than half of the patients studied have reported a history of major affective disorder in at least one first-degree relative.[16,18] SAD has also been encountered in children, who present with fatigue, irritability, difficulty getting out of bed in the morning, and school problems.[20] Rather than perceiving an internal change in their mood, children with SAD described to date have noted their symptoms in the context of the external world (of parents and teachers) treating them harshly. These symptoms appear to be winter-linked phenomena that reflect an underlying depressed mood instead of manifestations of school phobia that may reflect separation anxiety.

Though rigorous epidemiologic studies have yet to be carried out, mail and newspaper surveys indicate that the prevalence of SAD increases with increasing latitude.[21-24] The diminished sunlight available in the latitudes more distant from the equator likely accounts for this pattern. Clinical studies have documented the presence of the syndrome in North America, Europe, and Australia.[16,25-27] Subclinical *forme fruste* versions of the syndrome (S-SAD) appear as well.[28] One canvass in Maryland found approximately 4% of the population to have SAD and greater than 10% more to have subsyndromal

SAD.[29] Many more people among the general population may have mild seasonal symptoms as well. In one random survey of New Yorkers, for example, 50% of respondents reported increased wintertime fatigue, 47% reported increased wintertime weight, 42% reported increased wintertime sleep, and 31% reported depressed wintertime mood.[23,30]

BIOLOGY

Certain biologic parameters have been found to be abnormal in patients with seasonal winter depressions. Hormonal profiles, biochemical challenges, immune responses, and visual evoked phenomena all yield data that help define the phenomena associated with seasonal changes in light patterns and replacement with bright artificial light.

Sleep studies reveal significant differences between persons with winter depressions and normal individuals. In consonance with patients' own reports, winter sleep in patients with SAD is increased in duration. Although slow-wave (delta) sleep is decreased in winter, patients with SAD have more rapid-eye-movement (REM) and non-REM sleep. Light therapy partially counters these distortions in sleep architecture.[31]

It is not clear how the reported winter weight gain[32] can be reconciled with patients' increased levels of the thyroid hormone T_4 in winter. Thyroid-stimulating hormone (TSH), perhaps suppressed by the T_4, has been reported to be reduced in patients with SAD.[32] Other thyroid parameters studied to date (free T_4, T_3, and thyroid releasing hormone [TRH] stimulation), however, have been within normal limits.[10]

Measurement of core body temperature promises to reveal certain elements of the pathophysiology of SAD. Twenty-four-hour core temperature measurements of patients as a group showed no significant difference from those of normal persons. Nevertheless, light treatment significantly enhanced the amplitude of the patients' circadian variation.[33]

Additional hormonal profiles noted in patients with SAD are recorded in Table 35-1.[31] In contrast to the immunobiologic status of many depressed patients who manifest decreased response of peripheral blood lymphocytes to

TABLE 35-1

Hormonal Profiles in Seasonal Affective Disorder

	Substance	Change Relative to Normals
Plasma	Growth hormone	Reduced
	Melatonin	Reduced (Rosenthal NE, Skwerer RG, Kasper S et al: Personal communication)
	P.M. prolactin	Reduced
Cerebrospinal fluid	Homovanillic acid	Unchanged
	Methylhydroxyphenylglycol	Unchanged
	5-Hydroxyindoleacetic acid	Unchanged
Challenges	m-CPP	Greater mood lability, cortisol and prolactin (Jacobsen FM, Joseph-Vanderpool JR, Rosenthal NE: Personal communication)
	DST	Unchanged[34]
	Corticotropin releasing hormone	Adrenocorticotrophic hormone response blunted (Joseph-Vanderpool JR, Rosenthal NE: Personal communication)

mitogen stimulation,[35] depressed patients with SAD have been observed to have an abnormally increased response to the mitogens phytohemagglutinin and concanavalin A.[31] Whereas eye exposure to bright white light enhanced lymphocyte blastogenesis in normal persons, in patients with SAD the overresponsiveness was normalized (Skwerer RG, Rosenthal NE, Fleisher TA et al: Personal communication). Further in vivo studies are required to determine the clinical significance of these findings; these in vitro studies of altered response to mitogens could serve as a potential SAD trait marker.

Preliminary data from our group indicate that several parameters of eye function examined in summer and winter, including visual acuity, visual field measurements, and dark adaptation thresholds of rods and cones all have been within normal limits. There is no evidence yet that the cortical visual pathway is disturbed in SAD (Murphy DGM, Abas M, Winton F et al: Personal communication). Further investigation of these areas, however, will be useful. Findings of general physical examinations and routine blood chemistries have also been normal in this population.[10]

MECHANISM

The task of identifying the etiology of SAD has been challenging. Two clues offer promise for revealing the mechanism of the disorder. One is that SAD is linked to a time of year when people are exposed to less sunlight than at other times. The second is that the alteration of ambient light in winter can effectively treat the depression. From these observations, however, the possible lines of reasoning diverge. Though all the theories that follow are based on potentially faulty post hoc ergo propter hoc reasoning, they are the best we have so far.

One possible explanation for the disorder is that the short days of winter deprive susceptible patients of sufficient quanta of light for maintenance of affective stability and a euthymic state. By replacing the relative deficiency of light in winter, perhaps, the possible photon-deficient depression is treated. Rosenthal and colleagues' initial report documenting that bright light acted as an antidepressant in patients with SAD whereas dim light did not forms the cornerstone of this hypothesis.[10] The failure of ordinary light to prevent winter depressions in this population indicated that some aspect of delivering a large quantity of photons to patients was intrinsic to the antidepressant response.

Site of action also seems crucial to the antidepressant effect. In an elaborate schema designed to tease out the antidepressant mechanism of light, Wehr and colleagues[36] found that the eyes and not the skin appeared to mediate the effects of light treatment in patients with SAD. Comparing bright light exposure to the face, neck, arms, and legs versus the eyes, the NIMH group demonstrated much greater antidepressant effects of phototherapy when light was applied to the eyes. Duncan and others have shown in patients with SAD that visual P300s (a dynamic brain event-related potential measuring the amount of brain attention or processing committed to a stimulus[37]) are enhanced by light in direct proportion to its antidepressant effects. This phenomenon was not noted with auditory P300s (Duncan CC, Deldin PJ, Skwerer RG et al: Personal communication). A comparative study of red, blue, and white lights has not defined a specific part of the spectrum as having antidepressant properties.[38] Further studies examining light in the green region of the spectrum may clarify whether SAD is somehow linked to the eye's rods or cones, given that the maximal response to light for these types of receptors is about 510 and 550 nm, respectively.[39,40] Because retinal illumination increases turnover of photoreceptor disks,[41] perhaps this turnover is linked to the antidepressant effect. One unconfirmed report that indirect bright lights are sufficient for an antidepressant response suggests that the effects of the light may be mediated by the retinal periphery, composed predominantly of rods.[42]

For some time, variations of the melatonin hypothesis of SAD have seemed attractive to investigators, but no study has provided a definitive confirmation or disavowal of the idea.[19] The potential importance of melatonin in SAD was suggested by the superior antidepressant effects of bright versus dim light, given Lewy's finding that bright light suppresses melatonin blood levels in humans.[43] The theory conjectured that perhaps light's suppression of melatonin induced an antidepressant effect. This would be consistent with the idea that the antidepressant effect of light is mediated through the rods, because the rod photoreceptors are most sensitive to light at virtually the same wavelength at which nocturnal melatonin is highly suppressed.[44] Arguments against the melatonin hypothesis were encountered when the administration of melatonin to successfully treated patients with SAD did not blunt the antidepressant effect of light therapy. Nevertheless, symptoms characteristic of SAD, such as fatigue, increased appetite, carbohydrate craving, and social withdrawal, were exacerbated to a greater extent than in patients receiving placebo.[45] When depressed SAD patients in a second study were treated with atenolol—a β-adrenergic blocker that can reduce nighttime melatonin levels—and failed to improve, it became clear that there were limits to the melatonin hypothesis. If an alternative means of suppressing melatonin failed to have an antidepressant effect, it seemed unlikely that the suppression of melatonin by bright light was specifically responsible for the antidepressant effect.[46] At most, the suppression of pineal melatonin may account for some of the symptoms that resolve during light therapy, but there is no convincing evidence yet that it is central to the disorder.

The phase-shift hypothesis has been attractive to some SAD researchers.[47] Lewy and colleagues built this theory (linked to the circadian rhythm of melatonin that peaks in the dark hours of night)[48] on their ability to delay the nocturnal rise of melatonin with evening bright light exposure and, conversely, to advance the rhythm with bright light in the morning.[49-51] Two groups have suggested that their patients with SAD had abnormally delayed melatonin rhythms. These were advanced by bright light therapy in the morning. The association between the phase-advancing and antidepressant effects of light suggested a connection between delayed circadian rhythms and depression.[52,53] Neither group, however, has yet shown a statistical difference between patients and normal persons. With regard to circadian phase markers, other studies have shown no alterations in timing of melatonin secretion before or after treatment[54] (Rosenthal NE, Sack DA, Skwerer RG: Personal communication). A number of studies documenting the effectiveness of light treatment at different times of the day and evening are not consistent with the phase-shift theory.[55-58]

Depue and colleagues have proposed that dopamine might also have a key role in SAD.[59] They found evidence of reduced prolactin secretion in patients with SAD but not in normal volunteers in winter and summer.[60] Because low basal prolactin secretion may result from compensatory up-regulation of D_2 receptors in the anterior pituitary gland associated with low functional activity of dopamine,[61] Depue hypothesized that their finding may indicate a dopaminergic deficiency in SAD. His group also identified an increased frequency of eye blinks in depressed patients with SAD.[62] Because spontaneous eye blink rates may reflect dopaminergic function in the nigrostriatal tract,[63] they suggested a hypodopaminergic state in the nigrostriatal system associated with an up-regulation of dopamine receptors in the prefrontal cortex. The group also suggested that SAD patients have less efficient heat loss responses in winter than normal controls and that this response is normalized during light treatment and during summer. Because this response is partially dependent on dopaminergic activity in the hypothalamic and nigrostriatal tracts, according to the dopamine hypothesis, blunted thermoregulatory heat loss in SAD may represent another manifestation of a dopaminergic deficiency.[64]

Finally, serotonin deficiency has been suggested as a cause of winter depressions. As early as 1967, Coppen nominated this neurotransmitter as one whose functional deficiency might be responsible for depressive disorders.[65] Wurtman and colleagues have postulated that carbohydrate craving may reflect a functional serotonin deficiency.[66] That this craving is a prominent symptom in SAD is consistent with the theory. Additionally, seasonal variations of serotonin metabolism have been observed in human platelets[67,68] and in postmortem brains.[69] Preliminary work demonstrating the exaggerated effect on mood of the postsynaptic serotonin agonist m-CPP suggests the value of pursuing this hypothesis (Jacobsen FM, Joseph-Vanderpool JR, Rosenthal NE: Personal communication). Reports that light exposure may alter serotonin re-

TABLE 35-2

Guidelines for Phototherapy

1. A full-spectrum light source of 2500 lux is placed 3 feet from the patient.
2. Patients face the lights and glance at them at least once a minute.
3. Patients start with 4 hours a day (at convenient times) in front of the lights. If that fails after 5 days, they try the lights at different times. If that works, they reduce the light treatment period to the minimum needed daily to prevent relapse.
4. Maintain treatment until daily sunlight is sufficient for a patient to be euthymic.

ceptor sensitivity in rat neurons tie light treatment to this hypothesis.[70,71]

TREATMENT

Though bright light has been the treatment of choice for winter depressions (Table 35-2), alteration of environmental light is but one viable treatment approach. Although there are few clinical trials of antidepressant medications specifically for SAD, our clinical experience suggests that patients with SAD can be successfully treated with polycyclic antidepressants, monoamine oxidase inhibitors, or lithium.[72] The use of fluoxetine in our clinic has also appeared helpful in several cases. Many patients with SAD turn to phototherapy in order to avoid the well-known side-effects of the standard pharmaceutical agents.

As with other treatments in psychiatric illness, we do not understand how light therapy works. The earliest recorded description and successful treatment of an apparent case of SAD was by Esquirol, who in the early 19th century advised his patient to travel from Belgium to Italy during the winter. Esquirol viewed the success not in terms of light, but as a matter of moving the patient out of a cold and moist climate.[73] As noted earlier, Cook foreshadowed modern research by using bright artificial light to combat the sadness and anergy of his crew when they sailed through an Antarctic winter.[4] Marx also noted that winter depression responded to treatment with bright light.[74] Lewy and colleagues, as noted previously, began the modern use of phototherapy as an effective treatment modality for winter depressive conditions.[9] Shortly afterward, Kripke proposed the use of light therapy for nonseasonal depressions.[75]

Illuminance, measured in terms of quanta of light sensed over time by a certain surface area,[40] has been the first treatment variable studied systematically.[8] Critical to this point is the distance of the subject from the light source. Typically researchers have used a set of Vita-Lites situated 90 cm from the subject in order to achieve an illuminance of 2500 lux.[10] The light was initially delivered from a metal box containing eight of the fluorescent lamps. The box was covered by a neutral Plexiglas diffuser. We have obtained 2500 lux with six Power-Twist Vita-Lite lamps in the box. The NIMH group has asked patients to sit facing the lights and glance briefly at them approximately once a minute. They have been encouraged to engage in other activities while seated.[18] Given the cumbersome and commercially expensive nature of these light boxes, simplification of the treatment devices would be welcome. Therefore, our group has also designed a portable light helmet to facilitate further research.

We cannot say with certainty when the "best" time for daily light treatment is. The phase-shift theory of light treatment suggests that morning light, by advancing circadian rhythms, evokes its antidepressant effect.[50] Several studies seem to confirm this hypothesis[51,76,77] (Avery DH, Khan A, Dunner DL: Personal communication). Other carefully conducted studies, however, have shown that evening light exposure, alone or in combination with morning light treatments, induces significant antidepressant effects.[36,55] Early morning lights in combination with afternoon or nighttime lights have also had antidepressant effects.[55,56] The ideal duration of light treatment has yet to emerge as well. On a simple level, a few studies indicate that the greater the daily duration, the greater their antidepressant effect.[8,52,75,78,79] Duration may interact with intensity in the delivery of a total quantity of light for successful treatment. Such an interaction is supported by Terman's report of successful treatment with very high illuminance light delivery

(10,000 lux) over a short 30-minute interval (as opposed to 2 hours of evening light of conventional intensity).[30] This report holds promise of more convenient therapies. Greater levels of intensity, however, may be harmful to the retina.[80] At least one study indicates no added efficacy of greater than 2-hour light periods.[79] In our view, a reasonable treatment approach begins with 4 hours of daily light at convenient hours. If this regimen fails to trigger an antidepressant response within the typical 2- to 5-day interval noted for patients with SAD,[81,82] then using the lights for the first 4 hours of the day or dividing exposure between morning and afternoon may be considered. The discovery and validation of a reliable method to determine the ideal timing and duration of light treatment for a particular individual would represent a major therapeutic advance.

Our own longitudinal experience suggests that the two thirds of patients with SAD who respond to phototherapy should be maintained on the treatment until they gain sufficient daily bright exposure from other sources, typically in the spring. Premature withdrawal from phototherapy usually results in a return of the depressive syndrome. After the summer, it is often appropriate to resume phototherapy prophylactically near the calendar date when the patient's depressive episodes have begun historically.[18]

In order to reproduce the qualities of bright sunlight as closely as possible, most investigators have used full-spectrum fluorescent lighting for treatment of SAD. Because a significant portion of the sun's radiation reaches the earth as ultraviolet light (300 to 400 nm wavelength), initial researchers in this area did not wish to ignore this form of light. Full-spectrum fluorescent lights closely resemble the spectral distribution of natural outdoor light. On the other hand, the standard fluorescent light sources of "warm white" and "cool white" provide far more yellow and orange light and significantly less red, green, blue, violet, and ultraviolet light than natural outdoor light of similar illuminance. Preliminary studies using nonultraviolet light sources hint that the ultraviolet part of the spectrum may be unnecessary for a significant therapeutic response[8,42] (Yerevanian BJ, Grota LJ: Personal communication), but atypical depressive symptoms of SAD may still respond more favorably to ultraviolet light (Frank A, Docherty J, Welch B et al: Personal communication). This point is of concern because of the theoretical possibility that the ultraviolet light exposure might adversely affect the eyes or the skin. A formal short-term study[10] and several years of clinical experience with light treatment have not revealed any changes in eye function or anatomy with recurrent full-spectrum light use under our direction, but study of greater numbers of patients is still required.

Use of the bright white light treatment has been a benign experience for most patients. Side-effects are few, though some patients complain about eye strain, headaches, irritability, fatigue, or nausea. Eye strain and headaches often diminish after a few days of treatment, and they may be minimized by decreasing the duration of therapy or increasing distance from the light.[8,18] Light administered too late in the evening may sometimes result in difficulty falling asleep. Similarly, some patients exposed to more light than they need become excessively "activated" or hypomanic.[10]

CURRENT CONTROVERSIES

Researchers of environmental light-related mood disorders have the privilege of an effective treatment for a disorder that is poorly understood. Physicians often understand the subtle mechanisms of an illness but are powerless to stop it. In yet other circumstances, physicians stand ignorant of both disease process and treatment. In the quest to replace ignorance with discovered knowledge, controversy frequently reigns. Two areas of SAD research in particular have aroused dissonance between various well-respected groups of clinical investigators.

Our experience has been that the majority of patients with SAD have had winter depressions and summertime manic or hypomanic episodes[10,15]; other research groups have found their patients to have predominantly unipolar depressions.[16,83] Unfortunately, different diagnostic standards for a hypomanic episode influence the results found in different centers. Until this semantic issue is resolved, precise description of the syndrome will suffer. One respected research

group has further clouded the description of the syndrome by broadening its definition of SAD to include patients who meet criteria for RDC minor depression without necessarily having a major depression.[16] This expansion of the definition may be valid, given that the minor depressive response to light therapy is indistinguishable from that in major depression; nevertheless, boundaries for comparative research are blurred. If different groups are comparing unlike populations, their arguments over discrepancies may be furious but signify nothing.

Some of the most impassioned debate has concerned the phase-shift hypothesis regarding the mechanism of phototherapy.[30,51-53,84,85] Well-planned studies have failed to resolve whether abnormal circadian rhythms in fact do lie at the core of SAD. As interest in this field grows and distinct research groups attempt to replicate one another's work by following identical research protocols, some consensus should be achieved. Perhaps by narrowing research diagnostic criteria to examine subgroups of SAD, investigators will determine if phase shifts are at the core of some patients' winter depressions. If this were true, phase typing might provide some therapeutic guidelines.[47,51]

One further controversy that attracts skeptics unfamiliar with the effects of phototherapy is the suggestion that phototherapy succeeds only as a placebo. Although it is difficult to rule out any involvement of the placebo effect, several arguments suggest that placebo effects alone do not account for the efficacy of phototherapy. These arguments include the demonstration of light's efficacy by several groups, the repeated responses within some individual patients, the characteristic time course of response to treatment and relapse following treatment withdrawal, the existence of a dose-response curve for light intensity, and the suggestion of a circadian rhythm of treatment sensitivity.[8]

NONSEASONAL DEPRESSION

Kripke and his group have pioneered the research in treatment of nonseasonal depression by increasing environmental light. Their initial studies testing 1 hour of bright light failed to show more than a trivial antidepressant response. A follow-up study using 1 hour of bright light (producing at least 1500 lux) from 5:00 A.M. to 6:00 A.M. and another hour of bright light from 9:00 P.M. to 10:00 P.M. was similarly unsuccessful in inducing an antidepressant response.[86,87] Use of inadequate illuminance for inadequate intervals may have contributed to these failures.[88,89] Yerevanian's group found bright incandescent light unhelpful in nonseasonally depressed patients.[42] Nevertheless, Kripke's modest but significant antidepressant responses using 3 hours of evening bright lights offer hope that different treatment paradigms might prove beneficial in nonseasonally depressed patients.[90,91] The implication of such a finding could have further significance in tying the environmental variable of light to a wide range of psychiatric illness.

BRIGHT LIGHT AND NORMAL PEOPLE

What is the effect of environmental light on normal people? At least three reports indicate that bright light benefits subjects with mild winter depression, as in subsyndromal seasonal depressions.[79,92,93] Common experience suggests that many of us will choose to be in a brightly lit room rather than a dim one; however, there are limits to normal preference for bright lights on all occasions. Those who read in bed at night may prefer an adequate bedside lamp to a bright ceiling fixture, to ease them into the dark world of sleep. On our research ward, several of the staff enjoy the bright outdoors and prefer bright fluorescent lighting to incandescent lamps but have found the lights used for treatment of SAD to be uncomfortable. Genhart and others found that elderly persons living in residential housing complexes had little tolerance of the bright lights commonly used for phototherapy (Genhart M, Kelly KA, Coursey RD et al: Personal communication). Two formal studies of light exposure to normal people have now demonstrated no mood-altering effects.[28,94] Light, therefore, is not a universal euphoriant.

CONCLUSION

From a public health perspective, research on light, mood, and appetite does not yet offer crisp guidelines. It seems as though environmental light has a critical role in maintaining a euthymic state for many people. Most people, however, have evolved so that their moods are tolerably stable within the environment in which they live. Given cost and some people's lack of reaction or adverse reactions to high-intensity lamps, installation of a set of Vita-Lites at every desk or work station does not seem wise. Nevertheless, workplaces and schools accommodating the needs of those who are sensitive to dim light may improve the mood and productivity of many adults and children by enhancing their lighting environment.[93,95,96] If shorter periods of light of higher intensity than has been used to date prove helpful to people, then light treatment before going to work or school may become less onerous. In the meantime, architects and urban planners may wish to consider the idea of preserving environmental light as a factor in their design of our future homes, schools, and workplaces.

If we return to the subject of Arctic night, where this chapter began, we may note a small irony of history. Dr. Frederick A. Cook, perhaps the first author specifically to link seasonal sunlight changes to mood, was a man obsessed by his quest for fame. In the early years of this century, he deceptively contended that he had beaten Lieutenant Peary in the race to the North Pole.[97] His latter years were spent in jail for mail fraud after failure of oil well claims he had made.[98] Had the surgeon appreciated that his connection of environmental light to mood would blossom in the many ways this chapter has outlined, he might have pursued his early findings and avoided prison. Whether SAD would subsequently have been named *Cook's disease* we cannot say, but observations linking light to mood will keep many psychiatrists and scientists busy for years to come and, we hope, many patients satisfied through what would have been their winters of discontent.

References

1. Cook FA: Gynecology and obstetrics among the Eskimos. Brooklyn Med J 8:154, 1894
2. Hippocrates: Aphorisms. In Hippocrates, Vol iv, p 129. Cambridge, Harvard University Press, 1931
3. Cook FA: Medical observations among the Esquimaux. N Y J Gyn Ob 4:282, 1894

4. Cameron I: Antarctica: The Last Continent. London, Cassell & Co, 1974
5. Hasselbalch KA: Die wirkungen des chemischen lichtbades auf respiration und blutruck. Skan Arch Physiologie 17:431, 1905
6. Gaedeken P: Uber die psycho-physiologische bedeutung der atmosphärischen verhältnisse, insbesondere des lichts. Z Psychotherapie Med Psychologie 3:129, 1911
7. Llewellyn LJ: Light and sexual periodicity. Nature 129:868, 1932
8. Rosenthal NE, Sack DA, Skwerer RG et al: Phototherapy for seasonal affective disorder. J Biol Rhyth 3:101, 1988
9. Lewy AH, Kern HA, Rosenthal NE et al: Bright artificial light treatment of a manic-depressive patient with a seasonal mood cycle. Am J Psychiatry 139:1496, 1982
10. Rosenthal NE, Sack DA, Gillin JC et al: Seasonal affective disorder: A description of the syndrome and preliminary findings with light therapy. Arch Gen Psychiatry 41:72, 1984
11. Spitzer RL, Williams JBW (eds): Diagnostic and Statistical Manual of Mental Disorders, 3rd rev ed. Washington, DC, American Psychiatric Association, 1987
12. Spitzer RL, Endicott J, Robins E: Research diagnostic criteria: Rationale and reliability. Arch Gen Psychiatry 35:773, 1978
13. Liebowitz MR, Quitkin FM, Stewart JW et al. Phenelzine vs. imipramine in atypical depression. Arch Gen Psychiatry 41:669, 1984
14. Garvey MJ, Wesner R, Godes M: Comparison of seasonal and nonseasonal affective disorders. Am J Psychiatry 145:100, 1988
15. Rosenthal NE, Wehr TA: Seasonal affective disorders. Psychiatr Ann 17:670, 1987
16. Terman M, Botticelli SR, Link BG et al: Seasonal symptom patterns in New York: Patients and population. In Thompson C, Silverstone T (eds): Seasonal Affective Disorder. London, CNS Publishers, 1989
17. United States Naval Observatory, Nautical Almanac Office: Table of sunrise and sunset no. 1061. Washington, DC, US Govt Printing Office, 1965
18. Jacobsen FM, Rosenthal NE: Seasonal affective disorder. In Georgotas A, Cancro R (eds): Depression and Mania: A Comprehensive Textbook, pp 104–116. New York, Elsevier Science, 1988
19. Rosenthal NE, Sack DA, James SP et al: Seasonal affective disorder and phototherapy. Ann N Y Acad Sci 453:260, 1985
20. Rosenthal NE, Carpenter CJ, James SP et al: Seasonal affective disorder in children and adolescents. Am J Psychiatry 143:356, 1986
21. Potkin S, Zetin M, Stamenkovic V et al: Seasonal affective disorder: prevalence varies with latitude and climate. Clin Neuropharmacol (Suppl 4)9:181, 1986
22. Lingjaerde O, Bratlin T, Hansen T et al: Seasonal affective disorder and midwinter insomnia in the far north: Studies on two related chronobiological disorders in Norway. Clin Neuropharmacol (Suppl 4)9:187, 1986
23. Rosenthal NE, Terman M, Targum SD et al: Prevalence of SAD and S-SAD by latitude in continental United States. Presented at the 141st meeting of the American Psychiatric Association, Montreal, Quebec, 1988
24. Rosen LN, Targum SD, Terman M et al: Prevalence of seasonal affective disorder at four latitudes. Psychiatry Res 31:131, 1990
25. Thompson C: Seasonal affective disorder and phototherapy: Experience in Britain. (Suppl 4)9:190, 1986
26. Wirz-Justice A, Graw P, Bucheli C et al: Seasonal affective disorder in Switzerland: A clinical perspective. In Thompson C, Silverstone T (eds): Seasonal affective disorder. CNS Publishers, 1989, pp 69–76
27. Boyce P, Parker G: Seasonal affective disorder in the southern hemisphere. Am J Psychiatry 145:96, 1988
28. Kasper S, Rogers SLB, Yancey A et al: Phototherapy in individuals with and without subsyndromal seasonal affective disorder. Arch Gen Psychiatry 46:837, 1989
29. Kasper S, Wehr TA, Bartko JJ et al: Epidemiological findings of seasonal changes in mood and behavior. Arch Gen Psychiatry 46:823, 1989
30. Terman M: On the question of mechanism in phototherapy for seasonal affective disorder: considerations of clinical efficacy. J Biol Rhyth 3:155, 1988
31. Skwerer RG, Jacobsen FM, Duncan CC et al: Neurobiology of seasonal affective disorder and phototherapy. J Biol Rhyth 3:135, 1988
32. Rosenthal NE, Genhart M, Jacobsen FM et al: Disturbances of appetite and weight regulation in seasonal affective disorder. Ann N Y Acad Sci 499:216, 1987
33. Rosenthal NE, Levendosky AA, Skwerer RG et al: Effects of light treatment on core body temperature in seasonal affective disorder. Biol Psychiatry 27:39, 1990
34. James SP, Wehr TA, Sack DA et al: The dexamethasone suppression test in seasonal affective disorder. Compr Psychiatry 27:224, 1986
35. Kronfol Z, Silva J, Greden J et al: Impaired lymphocyte function in depressive illness. Life Sci 33:241, 1983

36. Wehr TA, Skwerer RG, Jacobsen FM et al: Eye versus skin phototherapy of seasonal affective disorder. Am J Psychiatry 144:753, 1987

37. Duncan-Johnson CC, Donchin E: The p300 component of the event-related potential as an index of information processing. Biol Psychiatry 14:1, 1982

38. Brainard GC, Sherry D, Skwerer RG et al: Effects of different wavelengths in seasonal affective disorder. J Affective Disord 20:209, 1990

39. Fein A, Szuts EZ: Photoreceptors: Their Role in Vision. Cambridge, Cambridge University Press, 1982

40. Records RE: Physiology of the Human Eye and Visual System. Hagerstown, Harper & Row, 1979

41. Spalton DJ: Pigmentary retinopathies. In Rose FC (ed): The Eye in General Medicine, pp 121–122. Baltimore, University Park Press, 1983

42. Yerevanian BI, Anderson JL, Grota LJ et al: Effects of bright incandescent light on seasonal and nonseasonal major depressive disorder. Psychiatry Res 18:355, 1986

43. Lewy AJ, Wehr TA, Goodwin FK et al: Light suppresses melatonin secretion in humans. Science 210:1267, 1980

44. Brainard GC, Lewy AJ, Menaker M et al: Effect of light wavelength on the suppression of nocturnal plasma melatonin in normal volunteers. Ann N Y Acad Sci 453:376, 1985

45. Rosenthal NE, Sack DA, Jacobsen FM et al: Melatonin in seasonal affective disorder and phototherapy. J Neural Transm Suppl 21:257, 1986

46. Rosenthal NE, Jacobsen FM, Sack DA et al: Atenolol in seasonal affective disorder: A test of the melatonin hypothesis. Am J Psychiatry 145:52, 1988

47. Lewy AJ, Sack RL: Light therapy and psychiatry. Proc Soc Exp Biol Med 183:11, 1986

48. Illnerová H, Zvolsky P, Vaněček J: The circadian rhythm in plasma melatonin concentration of the urbanized man: The effect of summer and winter time. Brain Res 328:186, 1985

49. Lewy AJ, Sack RL, Singer CM: Immediate and delayed effects of bright light on human melatonin production: Shifting "dawn" and "dusk" shifts the dim light melatonin onset (dlmo). Ann N Y Acad Sci 453:253, 1985

50. Lewy AJ, Sack RL, Singer CM: Assessment and treatment of chronobiologic disorders using plasma melatonin levels and bright light exposure: The clock-gate model and the phase response curve. Psychopharmacol Bull 20:561, 1984

51. Lewy AJ, Sack RL, Singer CM: Treating phase typed chronobiologic sleep and mood disorders using appropriately timed bright artificial light. Psychopharmacol Bull 21:368, 1985

52. Terman M, Terman JS, Quitkin FM et al: Response

53. Lewy AJ, Sack RL, Miller LS et al: Antidepressant and circadian phase-shifting effects of light. Science 235:352, 1987

54. Thompson C, Franey C, Arendt J et al: A comparison of melatonin secretion in depressed patients and normal subjects. Br J Psychiatry 152:260, 1988

55. James SP, Wehr TA, Sack DA et al: Treatment of seasonal affective disorder with light in the evening. Br J Psychiatry 147:424, 1985

56. Wehr TA, Jacobsen FM, Sack DA et al: Phototherapy of seasonal affective disorder: Time of day and suppression of melatonin are not critical for antidepressant effects. Arch Gen Psychiatry 43:870, 1986

57. Jacobsen FM, Wehr TA, Skwerer RA et al: Morning versus midday phototherapy of seasonal affective disorder. Am J Psychiatry 144:1301, 1987

58. Isaacs G, Stainer DS, Sensky TE et al: Phototherapy and its mechanisms of action in seasonal affective disorder. J Affective Disord 14:13, 1988

59. Depue RA, Arbisi P, Spoont MR et al: Dopamine functioning in the behavioral facilitation system and seasonal variation in behavior: Normal population and clinical studies. In Rosenthal NE, Blehar MC (eds): Seasonal Affective Disorders and Phototherapy, pp 230–259. New York, Guilford Press, 1989

60. Depue RA, Arbisi P, Spoont MR et al: Seasonal and mood independence of low basal prolactin secretion in premenopausal women with seasonal affective disorder. Am J Psychiatry 146:989, 1989

61. Jimerson DC, Post RM: Psychomotor stimulants and dopamine agonists in depression. In Post RM, Ballenger JC (eds): Neurobiology of Mood Disorders, Vol 1, pp 619–628. Baltimore, Williams & Wilkins, 1984

62. Depue RA, Iacono WG, Muir R et al: Effects of phototherapy on spontaneous eye-blink rate in seasonal affective disorder. Am J Psychiatry 145:1457, 1988

63. Karson CN: Spontaneous eye-blink rates and dopaminergic systems. Brain 106:643, 1983

64. Arbisi PA, Depue RA, Spoont MR et al: Thermoregulatory response to thermal challenge in seasonal affective disorder: A preliminary report. Psychiatry Res 28:323, 1989

65. Coppen A: The biochemistry of affective disorders. Br J Psychiatry 113:1237, 1967

66. Wurtman JJ, Wurtman RJ, Growdon JH et al: Carbohydrate craving in obese people: Suppression by treatments affecting serotonergic transmission. Int J Eating Disord 1:2, 1981

67. Arora RC, Kregel L, Meltzer HY: Seasonal variation

of serotonin uptake in normal controls and depressed patients. Biol Psychiatry 19:795, 1984

68. Wirz-Justice A, Richter P: Seasonality in biochemical determinations: A source of variance and a clue to the temporal incidence of affective illness. Psychiatry Res 1:53, 1979

69. Carlsson A, Svennerholm L, Winblad B: Seasonal and circadian monoamine variations in human brains examined post-mortem. Acta Psychiatr Scand (Suppl 280)61:75, 1980

70. Mason R: Effects of chronic constant illumination on the responsiveness of rat suprachiasmatic, lateral geniculate and hippocampal neurons to ionophoresed 5-HT. J Physiol 357:13P, 1984

71. Cox CM, Mason R, Meal A et al: Altered 5-HT sensitivity and synaptic morphology in rat CNS induced by long-term exposure to continuous light. Br J Pharmacol 89:528P, 1986

72. Joseph-Vanderpool JR, Rosenthal NE: Phototherapy for seasonal affective disorder. Drug Ther 18:57, 1988

73. Esquirol E: Des Maladies Mentales. Paris, J-B Baillière, 1838

74. Marx H: "Hypophysäre insuffizienz," bei lichtmangel. Klin Wochenschr 24/25:18, 1946

75. Kripke DF: Photoperiodic mechanisms for depression and its treatment. In Perris C, Struwe G, Jansson B (eds): Biological Psychiatry 1981, pp. 1249–1252. Elsevier, North Holland Biomedical Press, 1981

76. Terman M, Quitkin FM, Terman JS et al: The timing of phototherapy: Effects on clinical response and the melatonin cycle. Psychopharmacol Bull 23:354, 1987

77. Lewy AJ, Sack RL, Singer CM et al: The phase shift hypothesis for bright light's therapeutic mechanism of action: theoretical considerations and experimental evidence. Psychopharmacol Bull 23:349, 1987

78. Wirz-Justice A, Bucheli C, Schmid AC et al: A dose relationship in bright white light treatment of seasonal depression. Am J Psychiatry 143:932, 1986

79. Terman M, Terman JS, Quitkin FM et al: Dosing dimensions of light therapy: Duration and time of day. In Thompson C, Silverstone T (eds): Seasonal Affective Disorder. London, CNS Publishers, 1989, pp 187–204

80. Sykes SM, Robison WG Jr, Waxler M et al: Damage to the monkey retina by broad-spectrum fluorescent light. Invest Ophthalmol Vis Sci 20:425, 1981

81. Lewy AJ: Treating chronobiologic sleep and mood disorders with bright light. Psychiatr Ann 17:664, 1987

82. Byerley WF, Brown J, Lebegue B: Treatment of seasonal affective disorder with morning light. J Clin Psychiatry 48:447, 1987

83. Hellekson C: Phenomenology of seasonal affective disorder: An Alaskan perspective. In Rosenthal NE, Blehar M (eds): Seasonal Affective Disorders and Phototherapy, pp 33–45. New York, Guilford Press, 1989

84. Lewy AJ, Sack RL: The phase-shift hypothesis of seasonal affective disorder. Am J Psychiatry 145:1041, 1988

85. Jacobsen FM, Wehr TA, Rosenthal NE: Dr. Jacobsen and associates reply. Am J Psychiatry 145:1042, 1988

86. Kripke DF: Therapeutic effects of bright light in depressed patients. Ann N Y Acad Sci 453:270, 1985

87. Kripke DF, Mullaney DJ, Gillin JC et al: Phototherapy of non-seasonal depression. Biol Psychiatry 20:993, 1985

88. Kripke DF, Risch SC, Janowsky D: Bright white light alleviates depression. Psychiatry Res 10:105, 1983

89. Kripke DF, Risch SC, Janowsky D: Lighting up depression. Psychopharmacol Bull 19:526, 1983

90. Kripke DF, Mullaney DJ, Savides TJ et al: Phototherapy for nonseasonal major depressive disorders. In Rosenthal NE, Blehar M (eds): Seasonal Affective Disorders and Phototherapy, pp 342–356. New York, Guilford Press, 1989

91. Kripke DF, Gillin JC, Mullaney DJ et al: Treatment of major depressive disorders by bright white light for 5 days. In Halaris A (ed): Chronobiology and Psychiatric Disorders, pp 207–239. New York, Elsevier, 1987

92. Rosenthal NE, Sack DA, Carpenter CJ et al: Antidepressant effects of light in seasonal affective disorder. Am J Psychiatry 142:163, 1985

93. Kasper S, Rogers SLB, Madden PA et al: The effects of phototherapy in the general population. J Affective Disord 18:211, 1990

94. Rosenthal NE, Rotter A, Jacobsen FM et al: No mood-altering effects found after treatment of normal subjects with bright light in the morning. Psychiatry Res 22:1, 1987

95. Jacobsen FM, Wehr TA, Sack DA et al: Seasonal affective disorder: A review of the syndrome and its public health implications. Am J Public Health 77:57, 1987

96. London WP: Full-spectrum classroom light and sickness in pupils. Lancet 2:1205, 1987

97. Peary E: In Encyclopedia Americana, Vol 21, pp 584–585. 1987

98. Cook FA: In Encyclopedia Americana, Vol 7, p 714. 1987

CHAPTER 36

Anorexia Nervosa and Bulimia Nervosa

MICHAEL J. DEVLIN and B. TIMOTHY WALSH

Obesity is not a psychiatric diagnosis. Although there is ample evidence of the medical and social costs of obesity, community surveys have generally not found obese persons to be any more psychologically disturbed than their normal-weight counterparts.[46] Therefore, when psychiatrists use the term *eating disorders*, they refer not to obesity but to the syndromes of anorexia nervosa and bulimia nervosa. This chapter reviews the clinical features of these two syndromes

ANOREXIA NERVOSA

History

Although eating disorders in general and anorexia nervosa in particular have attracted great popular attention in the past half of this century, anorexia nervosa is an illness with a much longer history. It has been suggested that the fasting and asceticism of several Italian saints of the Middle Ages might today be interpreted as symptoms of anorexia nervosa.[2] The first case in the medical literature of what is thought to be anorexia nervosa was described 300 years ago by Richard Morton in a *Treatise of Consumption*. In that volume, he described an 18-year-old girl with "nervous consumption," an illness marked by studiousness, weight loss, and amenorrhea. A series of cases was reported more than a century ago by Sir William Gull, who named the syndrome *anorexia nervosa*. Thus, although the current cultural emphasis on dieting and thinness probably plays a part in the high frequency of eating disorders, anorexia nervosa is an illness to which

humanity has been susceptible for hundreds of years. It is not simply a product of 20th century cultural mores.

Diagnostic Criteria

The diagnostic criteria for anorexia nervosa are presented in Table 36-1.[1] The first criterion requires that patients refuse to maintain a weight above a minimal normal weight for age and height. Although the diagnostic criteria suggest that 85% of expected weight is a reasonable guideline for the degree of underweight necessary for the diagnosis, most clinicians agree that normal thinness gradually overlaps with underweight, which in turn overlaps with emaciation; no sharp dividing line separates these degrees of weight loss. Despite being underweight, patients with anorexia nervosa are intensely afraid of becoming fat and typically become more afraid as they lose weight. Patients also display a distortion of body image—they view with great displeasure either their weight or some particular part of their body that they believe to be unattractive. Finally, the current diagnostic criteria require that women with anorexia nervosa be amenorrheic.

Clinical Characteristics

Anorexia nervosa usually begins in midadolescence, with a peak age of onset around 16 years. Rarely, cases begin before menarche. New cases occur with some frequency in the third decade

TABLE 36-1

Diagnostic Criteria for Anorexia Nervosa

Refusal to maintain body weight over a minimal normal weight for age and height, e.g., weight loss leading to maintenance of body weight 15% below that expected; or failure to make expected weight gain during period of growth, leading to body weight 15% below that expected.

Intense fear of gaining weight or becoming fat, even though underweight.

Disturbance in the way in which one's body weight, size, or shape is experienced, e.g., the person claims to "feel fat" even when emaciated, believes that one area of the body is "too fat" even when obviously underweight.

In females, absence of at least three consecutive menstrual cycles when otherwise expected to occur (primary or secondary amenorrhea). (A woman is considered to have amenorrhea if her periods occur only following hormone, e.g., estrogen, administration.)

(American Psychiatric Association Committee on Nomenclature and Statistics: Diagnostic and Statistical Manual of Mental Disorders, 3rd ed, rev. Washington, DC, American Psychiatric Association, 1987)

of life and rarely in the fourth. The onset of anorexia nervosa after the age of 40 is an extreme rarity and should prompt consideration of other diagnoses.

Anorexia nervosa occurs primarily in females, who make up about 90% of the cases. However, the illness does occur in males and in all major respects is identical to that in females, with the obvious exception of the amenorrhea. Anorexia nervosa has a long-documented tendency to occur more frequently in the upper socioeconomic classes and in this century has been described in virtually all industrialized nations including Europe, South Africa, Australia, and Japan.

There is probably some tendency for children who eventually develop anorexia nervosa to be somewhat obsessional and shy premorbidly.[15] However, most patients show little or no serious psychopathology until the development of anorexia nervosa. The onset of illness frequently seems precipitated by one of the minor traumas that characterize adolescence, such as leaving home for school or camp, the beginning of heterosexual dating, or a casual unflattering remark. Patients begin to diet in an apparent attempt to restore their self-esteem, and their dieting initially does not obviously differ from that of many other young people who never develop psychological problems. However, in those who develop anorexia nervosa, the obsession with food and dieting seems to accelerate so that the more weight that is lost, the more patients wish to lose. They typically become socially isolated and withdrawn, assume a moralistic demeanor, and become stubborn and intent on losing weight. Throughout the illness they exhibit an impressive denial of physical or psychological problems; this denial is often the most difficult aspect of initiating treatment.

As the illness develops, patients with anorexia nervosa exhibit a number of peculiar psychological and behavioral symptoms. They become obsessed with food and its preparation, may collect diet books and recipes, and even spend long periods of time cooking meals for others that they themselves will not eat. Many patients develop peculiar eating habits, such as an inability to eat in the presence of others, the prolongation of meals, and a penchant for peculiar food combinations. In fact, the use of the term *anorexia* to describe this syndrome is, strictly speaking, inappropriate, because patients retain some sensation of hunger until very late in the illness. One apparent manifestation of a drive to eat is the frequent occurrence of uncontrollable binge eating among patients with anorexia nervosa who may therefore also meet diagnostic criteria for bulimia nervosa (discussed later). At some point during the evolution of the illness, most patients with anorexia nervosa engage in increased physical activity, which serves both their intense drive for accomplishment and their desire to expend calories.

Physical Findings

Table 36-2 lists a number of the common physical findings and laboratory abnormalities observed in patients with anorexia nervosa.[19,20,51] It should be noted that patients with anorexia nervosa and bulimia nervosa are susceptible to the physical complications of both syndromes.

TABLE 36-2

Medical Complications of Anorexia Nervosa and Bulimia Nervosa

Anorexia Nervosa	Bulimia Nervosa
Physical Signs and Symptoms	
Cachexia, body fat depletion	Ulceration or scarring of dorsal surface of
Bradycardia, hypotension, hypothermia	the hand
Salivary gland hypertrophy	Salivary gland hypertrophy
Lanugo hair	Dental enamel erosion
Amenorrhea	Oligomenorrhea or amenorrhea
Edema	
Constipation	
Polyuria	
Laboratory Findings	
Anemia, leukopenia	Electrolyte abnormalities (hypokalemic
Elevated liver enzymes	alkalosis)
Low fasting glucose	Elevated serum amylase
Increased serum cholesterol	
Hypothalamic/pituitary/endocrine gland	
abnormalities	
Delayed gastric emptying	
Cortical atrophy on computed tomography	
Complications	
Sudden death possibly related to the	Ipecac-induced cardiomyopathy
presence of prolonged QT interval	Esophageal or gastric rupture
Acute gastric dilatation	Pneumomediastinum
Osteoporosis	"Cathartic colon"

Changes in vital signs can be quite impressive, with pulses often 50 beats per minute or lower. Peripheral edema is only occasionally observed and, when it does develop, is usually a transient phenomenon during the early stage of refeeding. Lanugo, fine body hair that is normally seen only in infants, sometimes develops during anorexia nervosa.

Anorexia nervosa is characterized by a multitude of endocrine abnormalities.[5] One of the most striking is the diminished production of gonadal steroids in both women and men. This disturbance is secondary to diminished pituitary gonadotrophin secretion, which in turn appears secondary to diminished hypothalamic secretion of gonadotropin releasing hormone. Thus, the amenorrhea of anorexia nervosa is a form of hypothalamic amenorrhea. Although patients with anorexia nervosa may exhibit the lowered body temperatures, cold intolerance, bradycardia, and

"hung" reflexes associated with hypothyroidism, serum thyroxine levels are in the low normal range and levels of thyroid-stimulating hormone are usually normal. Although 30 years ago patients with anorexia nervosa were believed to have diminished adrenocortical steroid production, studies have now established that plasma cortisol levels and adrenal steroid production tend to be elevated in this illness.

Gastric emptying is slowed so that some of the patients' complaints of bloating and fullness for prolonged periods of time after normal-sized meals may have an objective basis.[9] Mild elevation of the serum levels of hepatic enzymes (e.g., serum glutamic-oxaloacetic transaminase, serum glutamic-pyruvic transaminase) occurs occasionally, particularly during the initial phase of weight gain. Serum cholesterol level is sometimes elevated but normalizes as weight is regained.

Prolonged QT interval has been noted in several patients with anorexia nervosa, and it has been suggested that this electrocardiographic abnormality may be associated with sudden death.[25] Significant fluid and electrolyte disturbances are primarily encountered in patients who induce vomiting or abuse laxatives or diuretics. Partial diabetes insipidus has also been described,[18] and patients with anorexia nervosa may exhibit impressive polyuria.

A documented and potentially important abnormality in anorexia nervosa is reduced bone density.[39,40] It may be secondary to both diminished dietary calcium intake and reduced estrogen production. Pathologic fractures at a young age have been reported, raising concern about the long-term effects of this illness on the risk for osteoporosis.

Importance of Nutrition

With few exceptions, the physical and laboratory abnormalities observed in anorexia nervosa are secondary to malnutrition and normalize with restoration of body weight.[19,51] However, as noted earlier, there is concern that the decrease in bone density may increase the risk of developing osteoporosis later in life. Also, factors other than nutrition may be important in the development and persistence of the amenorrhea. One third to one half of patients who develop anorexia nervosa cease menstruating before serious weight loss has occurred, and conversely, menstruation is more likely to resume in individuals who have made full psychological as well as physical recovery.[12]

There is also compelling evidence that in addition to its physical effects, the emaciation of anorexia nervosa plays a major part in the development of a number of the psychological and behavioral characteristics of this syndrome. Studies of prisoners of war and of volunteers who participated in an experiment on the effects of starvation conducted at the University of Minnesota during World War II indicate that normal individuals, under conditions of starvation, become preoccupied with food and develop many of the strange dietary patterns observed in patients with anorexia nervosa.[13,44] They are also prone to develop disturbances of mood and to become socially isolated. This observation is important because it suggests that many of the psychological aberrations noted in underweight patients with anorexia nervosa reflect not only the patients' intrinsic psychopathology but also the serious effects of malnutrition on psychological state. Thus, full psychological recovery may be impossible without weight restoration.

Course

The course of anorexia nervosa is enormously variable.[22] In a significant fraction of patients, anorexia nervosa is a fatal illness, with death resulting from either inanition or suicide. The mortality rate of patients once hospitalized for anorexia nervosa is probably between 5% and 20% if patients are monitored for extended periods such as 20 or 30 years. This finding emphasizes that anorexia nervosa has one of the highest mortalities of any psychiatric illness and that in some patients it is a chronic illness. At the other extreme, approximately 50% of hospitalized patients make a full psychological and physical recovery. Between these two extremes lies a wide range of outcomes, with some patients leading a marginal existence in terms of both weight and psychological function and other patients only mildly impaired. It is impossible at present to predict with any certainty the course of anorexia nervosa at the time of presentation, although several studies have suggested that an early age of onset is a relatively favorable prognostic factor.

Treatment

The first priority in the care of patients with anorexia nervosa is the treatment of acute medical problems such as electrolyte disturbances, which may require intravenous therapy. Once any acute problems are resolved, the focus turns to weight restoration. On units experienced in the care of anorexia nervosa, most patients can be convinced to consume sufficient food or caloric supplements (e.g., Ensure or Sustacal) to produce adequate weight gain. Physical techniques such as nasogastric tubes or intravenous hyperalimentation are only rarely required. Daily caloric intake should be gradually raised to achieve a weight gain of 2 to 5 pounds a week, which usually requires the consumption of 2500 to 4000 calories/day.

The psychological treatment of patients with anorexia nervosa is typically multifaceted.[15] In experienced units, patients usually receive individual therapy and participate in group treatment with other patients with eating disorders. Particularly for younger patients, the involvement of the family is mandatory. A wide variety of medications have been advocated as being potentially useful in the treatment of anorexia nervosa, but the few controlled studies conducted to date do not indicate that medication has a major impact on the treatment response of hospitalized patients.[31]

BULIMIA NERVOSA

Diagnostic Criteria

The term *bulimia* has come to refer to a pattern of binge eating associated with some form of purging or other deliberate means of weight control. Although occasional reports of such behavior had appeared in the psychiatric literature,[3,37] it was not until the late 1970s that this eating disorder was recognized as a discrete syndrome, first as an "ominous variant of anorexia nervosa"[43] and later as an illness that could occur independently of anorexia nervosa.[16]

As currently defined (Table 36-3),[1] the syndrome is termed *bulimia nervosa*, suggesting a parallel with anorexia nervosa. Although most patients with bulimia nervosa are of normal weight, an anorectic-like drive for thinness, here defined as "a persistent overconcern with body shape and weight," is required for the diagnosis. Although some of the behavioral features of the syndrome, including the methods used to prevent weight gain and the minimum binge frequency, are clearly specified in these criteria, other aspects of the diagnosis, such as the definition of a binge ("rapid consumption of a large amount of food in a discrete period of time") are problematic.

Clinical Characteristics

Demographics

Bulimia nervosa has been identified primarily in women in their teens and 20s, although men also develop the illness at a rate about one tenth that of women.[45] Patients are primarily Caucasian, al-

TABLE 36-3

Diagnostic Criteria for Bulimia Nervosa

Recurrent episodes of binge eating (rapid consumption of a large amount of food in a discrete period of time).

A feeling of lack of control over eating behavior during the eating binges.

The person regularly engages in either self-induced vomiting, use of laxatives or diuretics, strict dieting or fasting, or vigorous exercise in order to prevent weight gain.

A minimum average of two binge eating episodes a week for at least 3 months.

Persistent overconcern with body shape and weight.

(American Psychiatric Association Committee on Nomenclature and Statistics: Diagnostic and Statistical Manual of Mental Disorders, 3rd ed, rev. Washington, DC, American Psychiatric Association, 1987)

though not exclusively so, and they represent various socioeconomic backgrounds.[26] Studies using rigorous diagnostic criteria suggest that the prevalence of bulimia nervosa is approximately 1% to 2% among precollege and college women,[8,27,45] although transient subthreshold bulimic behavior appears to be much more common. Although the majority of patients who are currently diagnosed as bulimic are of normal weight,[32] bulimia nervosa may be underrecognized in obese persons.[24]

Binge Eating

The cardinal feature of a bulimic patient's eating pattern is a binge, which consists of a large amount of food eaten rapidly, usually with a sense of loss of control. Typical binge frequencies of patients presenting to eating disorders clinics range from 2 to 20 binges per week. The most precise information about the actual content of a binge has come from studies in which bulimic patients are asked to binge in a monitored laboratory setting. One such study carried out by our own group found that in a binge meal, patients consumed more than 3000 calories, over twice the amount consumed by controls asked to overeat. However, the macronutrient compositions of the patients' and the controls' meals were surprisingly similar.[49]

Purging

Although the current diagnostic criteria for bulimia nervosa require only that patients regularly engage in some behavior designed to prevent weight gain, including fasting or vigorous exercise, most patients who receive the diagnosis engage in some form of active purging. Of purging methods, vomiting is the most common, occurring in 88.1% in one series, followed by laxative abuse (60.6%) and diuretic abuse (33.1%).[32] Diet pill abuse is also commonly reported as a method of weight control among bulimic patients.

Overconcern with Body Shape and Weight

Thinness has become an increasingly important goal, both in society and for individuals, particularly for women. Some clinicians believe that the overvaluing of ideals of thinness and a tendency to evaluate one's overall worth in terms of weight and shape are the core psychopathological features of bulimia nervosa. This position has been cogently presented by Fairburn and Garner,[10] who argue that this overriding concern with weight is common to both bulimia nervosa and anorexia nervosa and that effective and lasting treatments must be aimed toward altering these concerns. The differential efficacy of treatments that actively address these issues and those that do not has not yet been established (discussed later).

Medical Complications

The usual physical sequelae and possible serious complications of bulimia nervosa are outlined in Table 36-2. Outward signs of repeated self-induced vomiting include calluses on the back of the hand and fingers, salivary gland enlargement, and erosion of dental enamel. Elevations of serum amylase are routinely observed in bulimic patients who vomit and are generally not clinically significant. Fluid and electrolyte abnormalities, including dehydration, hypokalemia, hypochloremia, hyponatremia, and metabolic alkalosis, occur frequently and can, when sufficiently severe, lead to disturbances of cardiac conduction and rhythm. Bulimic patients who use ipecac to induce vomiting can develop a potentially lethal cardiomyopathy. Infrequent serious complications of repeated vomiting include esophageal or gastric rupture and pneumomedi-astinum. Long-standing laxative abuse can lead to laxative dependence and severe constipation.[35]

Neuroendocrine Abnormalities

As in anorexia nervosa, the study of neuroendocrine abnormalities in bulimia nervosa has yielded results that are interesting, if not always readily interpretable. Several groups have reported dexamethasone suppression test (DST) abnormalities in more than one third of normal-weight bulimic patients.[5] Although this evidence was initially interpreted as linking bulimia with depression, other studies have suggested that DST nonsuppression may result from abnormally low dexamethasone levels in these patients, indicating that factors other than abnormal hypothalamic-pituitary-adrenal axis function may contribute to DST abnormalities in these patients.[50] The menstrual disturbances that often afflict even normal-weight bulimic patients are accompanied by gonadotropin abnormalities, which in some cases resemble those in underweight anorectic patients.[6] Low T_3 levels in bulimic patients[29,38] provide an additional suggestion that despite being at a statistically normal weight, these patients may show physiological similarities to underweight anorectic patients.

Clinical Course

Because bulimia nervosa has been recognized as a clinical entity for only about a decade, more is known about the onset of the illness than about its long-term outcome. Concerning the onset of the syndrome, it is of note that the vast majority of patients (85%) begin binge eating during a period of dieting.[33] Although the natural course of untreated bulimia nervosa is yet unknown, treatment studies have begun to report follow-up data on patients who have completed various treatment programs. The most encouraging reports derive from psychotherapeutic treatment studies that report continued improvement in most patients at 1 year after treatment.[11,14,30] Follow-up data from medication studies, when provided, are somewhat less favorable,[48] with many patients relapsing after discontinuation of medication. Although naturalistic outcome studies, not restricted to any particular form of treatment, are beginning to appear,[21,23] more data are clearly needed before conclusions can be drawn about the prognosis of bulimia nervosa.

Treatment

Currently accepted treatments for bulimia nervosa can be categorized into two basic approaches: the use of medications, most notably antidepressants, and the use of structured forms of psychotherapy. Treatments differ importantly in their structure as well as in their underlying philosophy, with some focusing more on binge/ purge behavior and others targeting body weight preoccupation and dissatisfaction. Although several approaches have proved to be beneficial in the treatment of bulimia nervosa, their mechanisms of therapeutic action are much less clear.

Pharmacologic Treatments

In the early 1980s, clinical investigators, impressed by the frequent occurrence of depressive symptoms in their bulimic patients, began to conduct trials of antidepressant medications. Several placebo-controlled double-blind studies have clearly demonstrated a beneficial effect of antidepressant medication over placebo in reduction in binge frequency.[47] Interestingly, the beneficial effects of antidepressants in bulimic patients do not seem to be restricted to those patients who are simultaneously depressed,[48] and the mechanism by which these medications lead to clinical improvement are unclear. Questions concerning the optimal length of drug treatment for bulimic patients and the outcome of patients following medication discontinuation remain for the most part still unanswered and are the subjects of ongoing investigations.

Psychotherapeutic Treatments

Psychotherapy for patients with bulimia nervosa has been conducted on both an individual and group basis and has followed various treatment models. Two of the best studied of these treatments are cognitive/behavioral therapy and exposure with response prevention. Cognitive/ behavioral programs[11,14,30] incorporate self-monitoring of intake and dietary counseling along with cognitive restructuring aimed at modifying patients' maladaptive thinking about food, weight, and self-esteem. These treatment regi-

mens typically last for several months and involve one or more sessions per week. Exposure and response prevention (ERP) programs[41,42] require repeated sessions in which patients are asked to eat anxiety-provoking foods without vomiting. The goal of ERP is that patients will be able to eat increasing amounts of an increasing variety of foods with less anxiety, leading to a reduction in the temptation to purge. Systematic trials of these techniques have thus far yielded promising results. An important challenge at this point is to identify the specific components of these often intensive and time-consuming programs that are most beneficial to patients.

A key issue in the treatment of bulimia is the differential effectiveness of treatment modalities: Are some of the treatments more effective than others, and are there factors that predict a specific patient's likelihood of responding to a particular treatment? Only one study has thus far compared medication with structured psychotherapy in the treatment of bulimia. Mitchell and colleagues[34] have reported preliminary results suggesting that although both forms of treatment were effective, a very intensive cognitive/behavioral group treatment was superior to antidepressant (imipramine) treatment on most outcome measures, and the combination of medication and group treatment was not significantly more effective than group treatment without medication. It is not clear that these results can be extrapolated to other forms of psychotherapy, and further studies are needed to provide a scientific basis for treatment planning.

CURRENT RESEARCH

At present, anorexia nervosa and bulimia nervosa remain enigmatic disorders. Although much has been learned about their clinical features and symptomatic treatment, detailed etiologic mechanisms are obscure. Two areas of current research interest that may yield results also relevant to our understanding of obesity involve studies of metabolism and of the psychobiology of hunger and satiety.

Two studies have suggested that caloric requirements for weight maintenance may vary systematically among different subgroups of patients with eating disorders.[28,36] Patients with the bulimic subtype of anorexia nervosa appear to require fewer calories for weight maintenance than do nonbulimic patients.[28] Other studies have indicated that normal-weight patients with bulimia require fewer calories to maintain than do other eating disorder patients[36] and have lower resting energy expenditures than do controls.[7] In view of suggestions that weight cycling can bring about an increase in metabolic efficiency,[4] it is conceivable that bulimic patients' repeated attempts at weight loss induce an energy-conserving state that promotes weight gain, leading to further attempts at dieting.

Another area of inquiry focuses on disturbances in hunger and satiety. Geracioti and Liddle[17] monitored the postingestive release of cholecystokinin (CCK) in a group of normal-weight bulimic patients. CCK is a peptide hormone whose release may be part of the physiological mechanisms responsible for the development of satiety. Levels of CCK following a standard meal were significantly reduced in bulimic patients compared with controls, paralleling a blunting in their postprandial satiety. These responses tended to normalize in a subgroup of patients who were restudied after antidepressant treatment. The significance of this intriguing preliminary finding in the pathophysiology of bulimia nervosa is not yet clear. However, it is conceivable that patients with this illness have a deficit—presumably an acquired one—in satiety that serves to perpetuate their eating disturbance.

Other investigations have been and are being carried out with the ultimate aim of identifying the factors that trigger and maintain eating disorders. It is unlikely that a single level of analysis will be sufficient to explain the occurrence of these illnesses. Rather, processes occurring at cultural, familial, psychological, and biologic levels must be integrated as we attempt to develop a fuller understanding of these serious illnesses.

References

1. American Psychiatric Association Committee on Nomenclature and Statistics: Diagnostic and Statistical Manual of Mental Disorders, 3rd ed, rev. Washington, DC, American Psychiatric Association, 1987

2. Bell RM: Holy Anorexia. Chicago, University of Chicago Press, 1985

3. Binswanger L: The case of Ellen West. In May R (ed): Existence, pp 237–364. New York, Simon & Schuster, 1958

4. Brownell KD, Greenwood MRC, Stellar E et al: The effects of repeated cycles of weight loss and regain in rats. Physiol Behav 38:459, 1986

5. Devlin MJ, Walsh BT: The neuroendocrinology of anorexia nervosa. In Current Topics in Neuroendocrinology, Vol 8, pp 291–307. Berlin, Springer-Verlag, 1988

6. Devlin MJ, Walsh BT, Katz JL et al: Hypothalamic-pituitary-gonadal function in anorexia nervosa and bulimia. Psychiatry Res 28:11, 1989

7. Devlin MJ, Walsh BT, Kral JG et al: Metabolic abnormalities in bulimia nervosa. Arch Gen Psychiatry 47:144, 1990

8. Drewnowski A, Hopkins SA, Kessler RC: The prevalence of bulimia nervosa in the U.S. college student population. Am J Public Health 78:1322, 1988

9. Dubois A, Gross HA, Ebert MH et al: Altered gastric emptying and secretion in primary anorexia nervosa. Gastroenterology 77:319, 1979

10. Fairburn CG, Garner DM: The diagnosis of bulimia nervosa. Int J Eating Disord 5:403, 1986

11. Fairburn CG, Kirk J, O'Connor M et al: A comparison of two psychological treatments for bulimia nervosa. Behav Res Ther 24:629, 1986

12. Falk JR, Halmi KA: Amenorrhea in anorexia nervosa: Examination of the critical body weight hypothesis. Biol Psychiatry 17:799, 1982

13. Franklin JC, Schiele BC, Brozek J et al: Observations on human behavior in experimental semistarvation and rehabilitation. J Clin Psychol 4:28, 1948

14. Freeman CPL, Barry F, Dunkeld-Turnbull J et al: Controlled trial of psychotherapy for bulimia nervosa. Br Med J 296:521, 1988

15. Garfinkel PE, Garner DM: Anorexia Nervosa. A Multidimensional Perspective. New York, Brunner/Mazel, 1982

16. Garner DM, Garfinkel PE, O'Shaughnessy M: Validity of the distinction between bulimia with and without anorexia nervosa. Am J Psychiatry 142:581, 1985

17. Geracioti TD, Liddle RA: Impaired cholecystokinin secretion in bulimia nervosa. N Engl J Med 319:683, 1988

18. Gold PW, Kaye W, Robertson GL et al: Abnormalities in plasma and cerebrospinal-fluid arginine vasopressin in patients with anorexia nervosa. N Engl J Med 308:1117, 1983

19. Halmi KA, Falk JR: Common physiological changes in anorexia nervosa. Int J Eating Disord 1:16, 1981

20. Herzog DB, Copeland PM: Eating disorders. N Engl J Med 313:295, 1985

21. Herzog DB, Keller MB, Lavori PM et al: A 30-month follow-up study of bulimia nervosa. Presented at the 141st annual meeting of the American Psychiatric Association, 1988

22. Herzog DB, Keller MB, Lavori PW: Outcome in anorexia nervosa and bulimia nervosa. J Nerv Ment Dis 176:131, 1988

23. Herzog DB, Keller MB, Lavori PW et al: Short-term prospective study of recovery in bulimia nervosa. Psychiatry Res 23:45, 1988

24. Hudson JI, Pope HG, Wurtman J et al: Bulimia in obese individuals: Relationship to normal-weight bulimia. J Nerv Ment Dis 176:144, 1988

25. Isner JM, Roberts WC, Heymsfield SB et al: Anorexia nervosa and sudden death. Ann Intern Med 102:49, 1985

26. Johnson C, Lewis C, Hagman J: The syndrome of bulimia: Review and synthesis. Psychiatr Clin North Am 7:247, 1984

27. Johnson-Sabine E, Wood K, Patton G et al: Abnormal eating attitudes in London schoolgirls—a prospective epidemiological study: Factors associated with abnormal response on screening questionnaires. Psychol Med 18:615, 1988

28. Kaye WH, Gwirtsman HE, Obarzanek E et al: Caloric intake necessary for weight maintenance in anorexia nervosa: Nonbulimics require greater caloric intake than bulimics. Am J Clin Nutr 44:410, 1986

29. Kiyohara K, Tamai H, Kobayashi N et al: Hypothalamic-pituitary-thyroidal axis alterations in bulimic patients. Am J Clin Nutr 47:805, 1988

30. Lacey JH: Bulimia nervosa, binge eating, and psychogenic vomiting: A controlled treatment study and long term outcome. Br Med J 286:1609, 1983

31. Mitchell JE: Psychopharmacology of anorexia nervosa. In Meltzer HY (ed): Psychopharmacology. The Third Generation of Progress, pp 1273–1276. New York, Raven Press, 1987

32. Mitchell JE, Hatsukami D, Eckert ED et al: Characteristics of 275 patients with bulimia. Am J Psychiatry 142:482, 1985

33. Mitchell JE, Hatsukami D, Pyle RI et al: The bulimia syndrome: Course of the illness and associated problems. Compr Psychiatry 27:165, 1986

34. Mitchell JE, Pyle RL, Eckert ED et al: Preliminary results of a comparison treatment trial of bulimia nervosa. In Pirke KM, Vandereycken W, Ploog D (eds): The Psychopharmacology of Bulimia Nervosa, pp 152–157. New York, Springer-Verlag, 1988

35. Mitchell JE, Seim HC, Colon E et al: Medical complications and medical management of bulimia. Ann Intern Med 107:71, 1987

36. Newman MM, Halmi KA, Marchi P: Relationship of clinical factors to calorie requirements in subtypes of eating disorders. Biol Psychiatry 22:1253, 1987

37. Nogami Y: On the "binge eating" in adolescence. Nichidai Igaku Zasshi 32:218, 1973

38. Pirke KM, Pahl J, Schweiger U et al: Metabolic and endocrine indices of starvation in bulimia: A comparison with anorexia nervosa. Psychiatry Res 15:33, 1985

39. Rigotti NA, Neer RM, Jameson L: Osteopenia and bone fractures in a man with anorexia nervosa and hypogonadism. JAMA 256:385, 1986

40. Rigotti NA, Nussbaum SR, Herzog DB et al: Osteoporosis in women with anorexia nervosa. N Engl J Med 311:1601, 1984

41. Rosen JC, Leitenberg H: Bulimia nervosa: Treatment with exposure and response prevention. Behav Res Ther 13:117, 1982

42. Rossiter EM, Wilson GT: Cognitive restructuring and response prevention in the treatment of bulimia nervosa. Behav Res Ther 23:349, 1985

43. Russell G: Bulimia nervosa: An ominous variant of anorexia nervosa. Psychol Med 9:429, 1979

44. Schiele BC, Brozek J: Experimental neurosis: Resulting from semistarvation in man. Psychosom Med 10:31, 1948

45. Schotte DE, Stunkard AJ: Bulimia vs bulimic behaviors on a college campus. JAMA 258:1213, 1987

46. Striegel-Moore R, Rodin J: The influence of psychological variables in obesity. In Brownell KD, Foreyt JP (eds): Handbook of Eating Disorders, pp 99–121. New York, Basic Books, 1986

47. Walsh BT: Pharmacotherapy of eating disorders. In Blinder BJ, Chaitin BF, Goldstein R (eds): The Eating Disorders, pp 469–476. PMA Publishing, 1989

48. Walsh BT, Gladis M, Roose SP et al: Phenelzine vs placebo in 50 patients with bulimia. Arch Gen Psychiatry 45:471, 1988

49. Walsh BT, Kissileff HR, Cassidy SM et al: Eating behavior of women with bulimia. Arch Gen Psychiatry 46:54, 1989

50. Walsh BT, Lo ES, Cooper T et al: Dexamethasone suppression test and plasma dexamethasone levels in bulimia. Arch Gen Psychiatry 44:797, 1987

51. Warren MP, Vande Wiele RL: Clinical and metabolic features of anorexia nervosa. Am J Obstet Gynecol 117:435, 1973

CHAPTER 37

Management of Psychotropic Drug-Induced Obesity

JERROLD G. BERNSTEIN

Obesity is one of the most frequently encountered conditions in medical practice and one of the most difficult to treat. Although increased caloric consumption is the most prevalent etiologic factor in the development of obesity, many medications can alter eating patterns and cause significant weight gain. Drugs capable of influencing food preference and satiety, particularly if they must be administered during a period of many months or years, such as the psychotropic agents, present a particular risk for the development of pharmacologically induced obesity.

Psychotherapeutic drugs, which include antianxiety agents, antipsychotic drugs, antidepressants, and lithium carbonate, have revolutionized the practice of psychiatry since the mid-1950s and yielded the most promising therapeutic outcomes for various mental disorders. As with all other categories of pharmaceutical agents, these medications unfortunately carry with them many side-effects. Drowsiness, dry mouth, constipation, dizziness, and tremor are among the most commonly recognized side-effects of psychotherapeutic medications. Carbohydrate craving, increased hunger and thirst, and significant weight gain are becoming increasingly recognized complications of psychotropic drug treatment. Indeed, it is not uncommon for a patient to gain as much as 20 to 40 pounds during the course of 1 to 2 years of treatment with antidepressant medication. Unfortunately, many people prematurely discontinue the use of psychotropic medication or unilaterally decrease the dosage to inadequate levels in an attempt to cope with intolerable weight gain.

Greater awareness of the potential risk of drug-induced obesity, prescription of alternative medications, and proper attention to dietary considerations all can contribute to eliminating therapeutically induced weight gain, and in some cases, many patients who have become obese during previous treatment can lose weight effectively. This chapter reviews current thinking about the mechanisms of drug-induced weight gain and evidence for potential appetite reduction by some of the newer psychotropic medications. The problem of weight gain during psychopharmacologic treatment primarily relates to antidepressants, lithium, and antipsychotic drugs, which are the focus of this chapter. There is no evidence that any of the antianxiety agents of the benzodiazepine class such as alprazolam, diazepam, or lorazepam have any influence on appetite or body weight. Likewise, the nonbenzodiazepine antianxiety agent buspirone has not been implicated as a source of appetite stimulation or weight gain. Thus, the antianxiety agents are not discussed further in this chapter.

CYCLIC ANTIDEPRESSANTS

Tricyclic and heterocyclic antidepressants inhibit nerve reuptake mechanisms for serotonin, norepinephrine, and dopamine.[1,2] Inhibition of neurotransmitter uptake increases neurotransmitter availability in the brain and is the apparent mechanism of their antidepressant action.[1] Cyclic antidepressants also block various neurotransmitter receptors, which may contribute to both their therapeutic effects and unwanted side-effects.[1-3] Chronic administration of antidepressants produce variable down-regulation of β-adrenergic and serotonin S_2 receptors.[4,5] Most cyclic antidepressants block histamine H_1 receptors and cholinergic receptors. Some antidepressants block dopamine and β-base adrenergic receptor sites.[5] Some of these drugs possess significant affinity for serotonin S_2 receptors.[5] Thus, the pharmacologic action of cyclic antidepressants is more complicated than is indicated by their ability to inhibit nerve uptake mechanisms.

Most of the currently marketed tricyclic and heterocyclic antidepressants stimulate appetite and create cravings for both complex carbohydrates and sweets.[1,4] As a consequence of their effects on appetite, considerable weight gain is noted in association with prolonged use of these medications. The anticholinergic action of these drugs produces dry mouth and increased thirst, which may lead to the frequent use of candy and chewing gum and the consumption of large volumes of high-calorie beverages.[1] In clinical practice, patients being maintained on tricyclic antidepressants often report the consumption of large volumes of fluid (Table 37-1).

Paykel and colleagues investigated weight gain in 51 depressed women who had responded favorably to initial treatment with amitriptyline.[6] Of those patients, 19 were maintained on the drug for 9 months and 32 were withdrawn from medication after 3 months. During the first 3 months of treatment with amitriptyline, the 32 patients who were to have their medication withdrawn at the 3-month point in treatment experienced a mean weight gain of 4.59 kg, whereas those 19 patients who were to be maintained for an additional 6 months on active medication experienced a mean weight gain of 3.33 kg.[6] During the subsequent 6 months of amitriptyline maintenance, patients gained a mean of 2.50 kg, whereas those patients who were maintained on placebo for the remaining 6 months gained a mean of 0.20 kg.[6] Eighty-seven percent of the maintenance amitriptyline patients reported persistent craving for carbohydrates, compared with 29% of the non–drug-maintained patients.[6] Car-

TABLE 37-1

Antidepressant Drugs and Body Weight

Tendency to Increase Appetite and Body Weight

Greatest	Intermediate	Least
Amitriptyline	Imipramine	Amoxapine
	Trimipramine	Desipramine
	Nortriptyline	Trazodone
	Doxepin	
	Phenelzine	Tranylcypromine
	(MAO inhibitor)	(MAO inhibitor)

May Decrease Appetite and Facilitate Weight Loss

Fluoxetine
Bupropion

bohydrate craving correlated with the dose of amitriptyline, although the amount of weight gain was not related significantly to drug dose.[6]

Berken and colleagues[7] examined the effects of amitriptyline, nortriptyline, and imipramine on appetite and weight gain in 40 depressed outpatients. This study found a mean weight increase of 1.3 to 2.9 pounds/month during 6 months of treatment, yielding a total weight gain of 3 to 16 pounds during the period of the study.[7] Increase in weight paralleled preference for sweets and caused some patients to discontinue antidepressant drug treatment. Weight loss was observed after discontinuing medication. Weight gain occurred with amitriptyline or nortriptyline even at doses of 25 mg/day and was more marked at higher doses. Patients on standard therapeutic doses of amitriptyline gained an average of 4 pounds/month.[7] Thirty-five percent of the patients in that study reported hyperphagia, and 73% experienced carbohydrate cravings and a preference for sweets.[7] Amitriptyline administration in a dose of 50 mg twice daily to six normal volunteers during a period of 28 days failed to produce weight gain, although two subjects noted increased appetite.[8] These normal volunteers showed no significant abnormalities in glucose tolerance curves or peak insulin levels during the course of drug administration.[8] Paykel's study noted no abnormalities in fasting glucose, plasma insulin, or glucose tolerance. However, patients on amitriptyline had more carbohydrate craving and a more robust growth hormone response to exogenous insulin.[6]

Studies of the effect of amitriptyline on appetite and weight gain have generally found both to begin to increase between the first and second month of drug treatment.[6,9] In clinical practice, a similar time course of the onset of appetite stimulation and weight gain is observed. In the clinical use of antidepressants, amitriptyline is the drug most frequently associated with carbohydrate craving and weight gain. When patients experience these side-effects during amitriptyline treatment, change to a different antidepressant frequently produces some reduction in carbohydrate craving and reduces or stops weight gain.

Doxepin, trimipramine, and imipramine stimulate appetite and weight gain slightly less than does amitriptyline. Amoxapine has much less tendency to increase appetite, thirst, and body weight than does amitriptyline. Amoxapine has minimal effect on either serotonin reuptake or serotonin receptors.[1] Its lesser likelihood to provoke weight gain may also be related to the fact that its antagonism of histamine H_1 and acetylcholine receptors is considerably weaker than many other antidepressants.[5]

Desipramine has minimal antihistaminic, anticholinergic, and antiserotonin activity and primarily exerts its antidepressant action by inhibiting nerve reuptake of norepinephrine rather than serotonin.[1,5] Patients experience less dry mouth, thirst, and appetite stimulation with desipramine than with many other antidepressants. Stern and colleagues studied desipramine in 17 female and 14 male depressed patients.[10] They found that during a 5-week period of treatment with desipramine patients were able to lose a mean of just over 2 pounds.[10] In that study, 24 of 31 patients lost weight, 6 patients gained some weight, and 1 patient experienced no weight change. Appetite and weight increases with psychotropic drugs seem very likely linked to actions at the serotonin receptor site. Compounds that increase serotonergic activity may decrease appetite and facilitate weight loss, whereas those that antagonize serotonin receptors may increase appetite and stimulate weight gain.[11] Desipramine is essentially devoid of both serotonergic and serotonin antagonist effects.[1] Anticholinergic induced thirst, which is minimal with desipramine, may also partially explain its lesser ability to produce weight gain.

Histamine antagonism by psychotropic drugs may be another mechanism by which these compounds increase appetite and weight, and thus the very weak histamine antagonism of desipramine may further explain its favorable profile from the standpoint of appetite and weight.[4,5]

Robinson and colleagues compared trazodone, amoxapine, and maprotiline in a multicenter study of 243 endogenously depressed outpatients.[12] In that 4-week double-blind trial, they observed significantly smaller weight gains in patients treated with trazodone (0.9 pounds) than with amoxapine (1.6 pounds) or maprotiline (4 pounds).

Fluoxetine is an antidepressant that is a potent inhibitor of serotonin reuptake mechanisms.[11,13] This drug has minimal effects on either norepinephrine or dopamine uptake.[5] Fluoxetine is essentially devoid of antihistaminic activity and anticholinergic effects.[5] Numerous studies in both depressed and nondepressed individuals have documented fluoxetine's ability to decrease appetite, reduce carbohydrate craving, and facilitate significant weight loss.[11,14] The serotonergic action of fluoxetine appears to explain both its ability to reduce carbohydrate craving and its antidepressant effect.[14] Generally, larger doses of fluoxetine (40 to 60 mg/day) are required to suppress carbohydrate craving, but many patients achieve a satisfactory antidepressant response at 20 mg/day and experience anxiety, insomnia, and excessive sweating at higher doses of this drug.[13]

Bupropion is a weak inhibitor of dopamine reuptake, but it does not alter uptake of norepinephrine or serotonin. It appears that its antidepressant action is related to dopaminergic effect, which may also account for its ability to reduce appetite and facilitate weight loss. One study found a mean 3.3-pound weight loss during 13 weeks of treatment with bupropion.[15] Another study, which is yet unpublished, found a mean weight loss of 1.6 pounds after 6 weeks of bupropion treatment at daily doses of 300 mg. The appetite-suppressant effect of this drug may prove to be analogous to that of the amphetamines, which also possess weak dopaminergic activity. The major disadvantage of bupropion is that it is somewhat more likely than other antidepressants to lower seizure threshold in bulimic patients, patients with convulsive disorders, and individuals receiving daily doses in excess of 450 mg. Current experience suggests that fluoxetine and bupropion would be appropriate therapeutic agents in persons who have gained weight on other antidepressants.

MONOAMINE OXIDASE INHIBITORS

Monoamine oxidase (MAO) inhibitors, including phenelzine, isocarboxazid, and tranylcypromine, may produce carbohydrate craving, increased appetite, and weight gain.[1] Phenelzine has not infrequently been associated with increased appetite, carbohydrate craving, and weight gain.[9] Its ability to stimulate appetite and weight gain is less than that with amitriptyline. Most often, weight increases with phenelzine are in the range of 5 to 10 pounds, whereas patients on amitriptyline may not uncommonly gain 10 to 20 pounds during a year of therapy. Isocarboxazid may also increase appetite, stimulate carbohydrate craving, and cause weight gain.[16]

Tranylcypromine produces less appetite stimulation and weight gain and may be useful in patients who have previously responded to phenelzine but have experienced intolerable appetite stimulation and weight gain.[1] In several patients whom I have changed from phenelzine to tranylcypromine, comparable levels of control of both depressive and panic symptoms have been maintained, concurrently with decreased appetite, carbohydrate craving, and weight. Patients who are overweight when they start on MAO inhibitor antidepressants or those who have previously gained weight on antidepressants may best be treated with tranylcypromine. Although patients may generally be switched from a tricyclic to an MAO inhibitor without a drug-free interval, changing therapy from phenelzine to tranylcypromine is best accomplished after a 7- to 14-day phenelzine-free period, because maximal levels of MAO inhibition before instituting tranylcypromine may predispose patients to an initial hypertensive response to tran-

ylcypromine. At least 4 weeks should elapse after discontinuation of fluoxetine before initiating MAO inhibitor antidepressants.

Van Praag and Leijnse found a significant decline in fasting blood glucose levels after oral glucose tolerance tests in patients treated with hydrazine-type MAO inhibitors.[17] They suggested an association between reduced blood glucose levels and the appetite-stimulating effect of these agents.[17] Studies by Cooper and Ashcroft found that phenelzine increased insulin-induced hypoglycemia, whereas tranylcypromine did not.[18] Gander found that appetite stimulation, carbohydrate craving, and weight gain were greater in a series of patients receiving combined MAO inhibitors and tricyclic antidepressants.[19]

One advantage of MAO inhibitor antidepressants is that they produce considerably less dry mouth and thirst than do tricyclic antidepressants, thus lessening the contribution of excessive fluid consumption as a potential source of weight gain.

LITHIUM

Because lithium is generally administered for long periods of time, its ability to stimulate appetite and weight gain is extremely important.[20] Vendsborg and colleagues found a mean weight gain of 10 kg in 45 of 70 patients who had been receiving lithium for a period of 2 to 6 years.[21] Most of these patients experienced increased thirst, and a correlation was noted between fluid intake and the amount of weight gain. That study found that when lithium was administered in conjunction with other psychotropic medications, weight gain was enhanced. They noted that patients who were overweight at the start of the study were more likely to experience weight gain while receiving lithium. O'Connell reported a mean weight gain of 8.9 pounds in 44 patients who received lithium for a 30-month period.[22] Studies of long-term lithium maintenance therapy have found increased thirst in association with lithium and have attributed a portion of the weight gain to the consumption of high-calorie beverages.[23] Many lithium-treated patients complain of excessive hunger and food cravings, particularly for carbohydrates.

Lithium increases brain concentrations of tryptophan, the precursor of serotonin, and also is capable of stimulating serotonin synthesis; however, in some studies, lithium has been shown to either inhibit or have no effect on serotonin turnover.[20] Lithium has been demonstrated to reduce brain serotonin receptors in rats.[24] It is possible that the reduction in brain serotonin receptors may, at least in part, account for appetite stimulation and weight gain associated with lithium therapy. The findings of reduced serotonin receptor site sensitivity in association with neuroleptic drugs, antidepressant drugs, and lithium may help to explain the appetite stimulation, carbohydrate craving, and weight gain that accompany this chemically diverse group of drugs.

Although changes in glucose tolerance have been invoked to explain the influence of lithium on body weight, studies in humans and animals have not found consistent increases or decreases in glucose tolerance during short- or long-term lithium administration.[25] Some studies have suggested that lithium-induced metabolic changes including stimulation of glycogen synthesis may explain its weight-promoting action, though the data are neither consistent nor convincing for these mechanisms.[26] Shortly after initiating lithium therapy, many patients experience fluid retention and some develop mild peripheral edema.[1,21] Many lithium-maintained patients may retain as much as 5 to 7 pounds of fluid. In these individuals, diuretics, either thiazides or spironolactone, in conjunction with regularly measured serum electrolytes and lithium concentrations, may be a safe and effective means to minimize weight gain secondary to fluid retention.[1,23]

In patients whose affective illness requires maintenance treatment with lithium but in whom weight gain is excessive, the alternative of carbamazepine or valproate maintenance may be considered. Numerous studies have documented an acute antimanic effect of carbamazepine and sodium valproate, and several investigators have found these compounds to be useful in the prophylaxis against recurrent affective episodes.[13] Carbamazepine and valproate are much less likely than lithium to promote weight gain, and I and other investigators have successfully used them in the maintenance of patients who previously gained excessive amounts of weight during lithium therapy.[1,13]

Several studies and extensive clinical experience indicate that lithium may have a significant effect on thyroid function. Mild hypothyroidism is not uncommon in patients maintained for prolonged periods of time with lithium.[20,23] Also, many patients remain clinically euthyroid with normal blood thyroid indices but develop goitrous enlargement of the thyroid gland during long-term lithium administration.[20] Decreased thyroid function or the development of goiter may contribute to lithium-associated weight gain and may require the coadministration of thyroid hormone, along with continuing lithium therapy.[1]

ANTIPSYCHOTIC DRUGS

Although the antipsychotic action of neuroleptic drugs is linked to their ability to block dopamine receptors, these compounds have an affinity for various receptors, including α-adrenergic sites, histamine receptors, and acetylcholine receptors.[1,2] Some neuroleptic drugs inhibit serotonergic receptors and block reuptake mechanisms for norepinephrine, dopamine, and serotonin.[2,3] Molindone, the only neuroleptic that decreases appetite and body weight, has an indole nucleus, as does serotonin.[1] Because serotonin has been implicated as a potential central mediator of appetite mechanisms and food choice, the possibility that differential actions of the various antipsychotic drugs in stimulating appetite mechanisms may be related to actions at the serotonin receptor site is enticing.[11,12] Studies using fenfluramine-induced facilitation of the hind limb withdrawal reflex in spinal rats indicate that chlorpromazine, thioridazine, and mesoridazine antagonize the serotonin receptor peripherally.[29] Using that experimental technique, trifluoperazine, haloperidol, pimozide, and molindone all failed to block serotonin receptors.[29] It is possible that the inhibitory effect of the low-potency neuroleptic drugs on serotonin receptors may explain their greater ability to increase appetite and body weight. The failure of molindone to block serotonin sites may account for its ability to decrease appetite and weight in patients.

The low-potency neuroleptic drugs, which are

stronger appetite stimulants, also possess greater ability to block histamine receptor sites than do the higher-potency neuroleptics.

Virtually all published studies of the obesity-inducing potential of antipsychotic drugs have cited chlorpromazine as the agent most likely to induce weight gain (Table 37-2).[9] One study of male schizophrenic patients revealed a weight gain of 8 to 9 pounds during 12 weeks of chlorpromazine administration.[30] Patients receiving other phenothiazines, including promazine, mepazine, perphenazine, prochlorperazine, and triflupromazine, all experienced weight gain, but less than the chlorpromazine-treated patients.[20] The greatest weight gain took place in the early weeks of treatment, and patients tended to return to premedication levels after discontinuing medication.[30] In that study, the investigators were unable to correlate changes in appetite with dosage of medication or the amount of weight increase. A retrospective study of weight changes in male and female patients in state hospitals revealed an average weight increase of 15.9% of maximal ideal body weight in chlorpromazine-treated patients compared with 8% in those taking perphenazine and 6.7% in those receiving clopenthixol.[31] That study noted a positive correlation of weight gain with chlorpromazine doses exceeding 400 mg/day. Fifty percent of patients who were switched from chlorpromazine to perphenazine in a therapeutically equivalent dose experienced weight loss and in some cases reached pretreatment weight. Of the patients changing from chlorpromazine to perphenazine, 25% continued gaining weight, and the remaining 25% remained at the increased body weight without any further gain or loss after a change in medication.[31] Clinical experience with haloperidol reveals a considerably lower potential to stimulate appetite and promote weight gain than with chlorpromazine and other phenothiazines.[1] Perhaps the failure of haloperidol to block central serotonergic receptors accounts for its lesser ability to stimulate appetite and weight gain.[1,29] Molindone appears neither to stimulate appetite nor induce significant weight gain. In an 11-week study in which molindone was compared with trifluoperazine, patients receiving molindone gained an average of 0.9 pounds and those receiving trifluoperazine gained an average

TABLE 37-2

Antipsychotic Drugs and Body Weight

Tendency to Increase Appetite and Body Weight

Greatest	Intermediate	Least
Chlorpromazine	Trifluoperazine	Haloperidol
Thioridazine	Perphenazine	Loxapine
Mesoridazine	Thiothixene	

May Decrease Appetite and Facilitate Weight Loss

Molindone

of 4.1 pounds.[32] Another study of 23 patients treated with molindone for a period of 6 to 19 months revealed a mean weight loss of 6.5 pounds.[33] However, five patients in that study did gain some weight. Gardos and Cole studied nine chronic schizophrenic patients and found a mean weight loss of 7.6 kg (range 0.9 to 16.8 kg) during three months of treatment with molindone.[34] After the course of molindone treatment, patients were returned to their previous neuroleptic therapy; some continued to lose weight, and others resumed their premolindone pattern of weight gain.[34] The extent of weight loss reported with molindone was dramatic and may reflect the fact that patients had been receiving other neuroleptics before starting molindone; thus, the weight loss may have resulted from both discontinuation of the previous neuroleptic and the administration of molindone.

In addition to invoking a mechanism of serotonin antagonism to explain neuroleptic-induced appetite stimulation and weight gain, other mechanisms must also be considered. One of the most frequently noted side-effects of psychotropic medication is the ability of both neuroleptics and tricyclic antidepressants to block acetylcholine receptors, both centrally and peripherally.[1] The peripheral anticholinergic effect gives rise to increased heart rate, decreased sweating, blurred vision, constipation, urinary retention, and dry mouth, with associated increased thirst.[1] It is very likely that the ability of psychotropic drugs to produce dry mouth and thereby stimulate thirst plays a part in their ability to facilitate weight gain.[9,13] Patients with drug-induced dry mouth tend to consume large quantities of fluid in an attempt to quench their thirst. Consumption of large volumes of high-calorie soft drinks, as well as sweetened coffee and tea, can add considerably to patients' daily caloric intake.[13]

Experimental studies in rats treated with phenothiazine compounds revealed increased food intake and greater utilization of calories.[35] Some studies in both humans and animals have found a rise in serum glucose levels during chlorpromazine treatment.[36] One study using animals found that chlorpromazine directly decreased glucose-induced insulin release from pancreatic beta cells in vitro and decreased glucose oxidation in the pentose-phosphate shunt and Embden-Meyerhof pathway in vitro.[37] Various endocrine changes have been found in patients receiving neuroleptic drugs, including increased serum prolactin levels and variable changes in serum cortisol concentration.[38] Although some investigators have attempted to link the neuroleptic-induced weight gain to changes in glucose metabolism and serum cortisol concentrations, there is little evidence to support this belief. Persistently abnormal serum glucose or insulin values are seldom noted, even in the course of long-term high-dose neuroleptic treatment. Likewise, extended administration of neuroleptic drugs in several studies has failed to produce serum cortisol concentrations significantly different from those in normal controls.[38] Although various metabolic changes may, on occasion, occur in patients receiving neuroleptic medications, the tendency of these changes to be inconsistent and indeed to return toward normal with continuing long-term treatment fails to support these mechanisms as important for neuroleptic-induced weight gain.[38]

Because increased consumption of high-calorie beverages is almost universal in patients experiencing dry mouth secondary to psychotropic medications, it is advisable, whenever possible, to prescribe those neuroleptic drugs with the lowest anticholinergic potency and to minimize the use of antiparkinsonian medications in conjunction with prolonged neuroleptic therapy, because these compounds also increase thirst.[1] The use of molindone or haloperidol by psychotic patients who are obese or in whom weight gain has occurred during previous antipsychotic chemotherapy would be the most appropriate therapeutic alternative.

DIETARY MANAGEMENT

There is considerable risk of patients developing obesity during the course of psychotropic drug therapy. It is the responsibility of the physician to alert patients to the possibility of this problem and to advise them of ways to minimize it. In many instances, the most appropriate management is for a physician to prescribe those therapeutic agents that have less potential of inducing carbohydrate craving and weight gain. In some cases, medications that have less propensity for appetite stimulation do not provide a satisfactory therapeutic response in the management of psychiatric disorders. In those instances, a physician must at times prescribe drugs that are more potent inducers of carbohydrate craving and weight gain. When these latter medications must be used for an optimal therapeutic response, it is recommended that patients be instructed about healthy eating habits and appropriate dietary restrictions, which may minimize the development of obesity. It is generally more appropriate and easier to prophylactically prescribe dietary limitations than to achieve weight loss by dietary restriction once a patient has become obese.

Although the major effect of psychotropic drugs on appetite is to increase patients' consumption of starches and sweet foods, many patients treated with these medications consume larger than normal quantities of all foods during treatment. Because foods rich in fats provide patients with the most concentrated source of calories, it is my practice and general clinical recommendation to advise patients to eliminate fried foods, potato chips, and salted nuts from their diet. I also recommend that patients minimize their consumption of cheese, ice cream, and red meat. Restriction of these foods in the diet lessens caloric intake and allows a bit of a cushion against the calories of the increased carbohydrates that patients may be consuming. I recommend that patients be aware of the tendency to consume more sweets and other carbohydrate foods and that they use sugar-containing hard candy and tea or coffee sweetened with 1 teaspoonful of sugar per cup as between-meal and nighttime snacks. I also recommend the use of crispbread crackers with low fat content as a snack food because they provide crunchiness and chewability at a lower caloric cost than chips and nuts. Advise patients that when using hard candy as a snack food, the candy should be allowed to dissolve slowly in the mouth rather than chewed, because prolonging the snacking process in this way may reduce caloric consumption. I advise patients to avoid sugar-containing soft drinks and fruit juices because increased thirst with psychotropic drugs may lead to prodigious consumption of these beverages. Candy bars, a source of concentrated calories, should generally be eliminated from the diet during psychotropic drug therapy. These limitations allow many of my patients to reduce or eliminate drug-induced weight gain. Neither clinical studies nor my own experience has found exercise programs to be particularly beneficial in eliminating psychotropic drug-induced weight gain.

Some patients do not achieve a satisfactory therapeutic response when treated with those psychotropic agents less likely to induce carbohydrate craving or weight gain. In those individuals, treatment may have to continue with amitriptyline, imipramine, or hunger-inducing phenothiazines. In those individuals, the previously outlined dietary restrictions should be repeatedly emphasized during the course of drug therapy. Furthermore, in some of those individuals, the coadministration of fenfluramine, along with psychotropic medication, may suppress carbohydrate craving, appetite stimulation, and weight gain.[1,13] Fenfluramine is a direct-acting serotonin receptor stimulant. Several studies have found this compound capable of reducing carbohydrate craving and consumption, thereby facilitating weight loss in obese patients who are carbohydrate cravers.[1] This drug also has an antidepressant action and may in some cases enhance the efficacy of other antidepressants. On rare occasions, particularly in those individuals with a pervasive psychotic disorder, fenfluramine may enhance psychotic symptoms. Thus, its use needs to be considered individually on a patient-by-patient basis. When higher doses of fenfluramine are used for a prolonged period of time, patients may become dependent on this medication; therefore, long-term or high-dose administration is generally not appropriate, and after several months of therapy, the dose should be gradually tapered rather than abruptly discontinued. In the United States, only dl-fenfluramine is available for clinical use. This compound is associated with some drowsiness and dizziness as side-effects. In Europe, d-fenfluramine is commercially available and has been found to produce minimal side-effects with much less dizziness and drowsiness than does the dl isomer. Although weight gain associated with psychotropic drug therapy continues to be a significant clinical problem, creative approaches to altering the pharmacologic regimen and diet are highly effective management techniques.

References

1. Bernstein JG: Induction of obesity by psychotropic drugs. Ann N Y Acad Science 499:203, 1987
2. Richelson E, Pfenning M: Blockade by antidepressants and related compounds of biogenic amine uptake into rat brain synaptosomes: Most antidepressants selectively block norepinephrine uptake. Eur J Pharmacol 104:277, 1984
3. Hall H, Ogren SO: Effects of antidepressant drugs on different receptors in the brain. Eur J Pharmacol 70:393, 1984
4. Richardson JW, Richelson E: Antidepressants: A clinical update for medical practitioners. Mayo Clinic Proc 59:330, 1984
5. Richelson E, Nelson A: Antagonism by antidepressants of neurotransmitter receptors of normal human brain in vitro. J Pharmacol Exp Ther 230:94, 1984
6. Paykel ES, Mueller PS, De La Vergne PM: Amitriptyline, weight gain and carbohydrate craving: A side effect. Br J Psychiatry 123:501, 1973
7. Berken GH, Weinstein DO, Stern WC: Weight gain: A side effect of tricyclic antidepressants. J Affective Disord 7:133, 1984
8. Nakra BRS, Rutland P, Verma S et al: Amitriptyline and weight gain: A biochemical and endocrinological study. Current Medical Research and Opinion 4:602, 1977
9. Rockwell WJK, Ellinwood EH, Trader DW: Psychotropic drugs promoting weight gain: Health risks and treatment implications. Sout Med J 76:1407, 1983
10. Stern SL, Cooper TB, Johnson MH et al: Lack of weight gain under desipramine. Biol Psychiatry 22:796, 1987
11. Asberg M, Eriksson B, Martensson B et al: Thera-

peutic effects of serotonin uptake inhibitors in depression. J Clin Psychiatry (Suppl 4) 47:23, 1986

12. Robinson DS, Corcella J, Feighner JP et al: A comparison of trazodone, amoxapine, and maprotiline in the treatment of endogenous depression: Results of a multicenter study. Curr Ther Res 35:549, 1984

13. Bernstein JG: Handbook of Drug Therapy in Psychiatry, 2nd ed. Littleton, MA, PSG Publishing, 1988

14. Hartó NE, Spera KF, Branconnier RJ: Fluoxetine-induced reduction of body mass in patients with major depressive disorder. Psychopharmacol Bull 24:220, 1988

15. Feighner J, Hendrickson G, Miller L et al: Double-blind comparison of doxepin versus bupropion in outpatients with a major depressive disorder. J Clin Psychopharmacol 6:27, 1986

16. Harris B, Young J, Hughes B: Comparative effects of seven antidepressant regimes on appetite, weight, and carbohydrate preference. Br J Psychiatry 148:590, 1986

17. Van Praag HM, Leijnse B: The influence of some antidepressives of the hydrazine type on the glucose metabolism in depressed patients. Clin Chim Acta 8:466, 1963

18. Cooper AJ, Ashcroft G: Potentiation of insulin hypoglycemia by MAOI antidepressant drugs. Lancet 1:407, 1966

19. Gander DR: The clinical value of monoamine oxidase inhibitors and tricyclic antidepressants in combination. International Congress Series No. 122. Amsterdam, Excerpta Medica, 1966

20. Ortiz A, Dabbagh M, Gershon S: Lithium: Clinical use, toxicology and mode of action. In Bernstein JG (ed): Clinical Psychopharmacology, pp 111–144. Littleton, MA, John Wright-PSG Publishing, 1984

21. Vendsborg PB, Bech P, Rafaelsen OJ: Lithium treatment and weight gain. Acta Psychiatr Scand 53:139, 1976

22. O'Connell RA: Lithium's site of action: Clues from side effects. Compr Psychiatry 12:224, 1971

23. Vestergaard P, Amdisen A, Schou M: Clinically significant side effects of lithium treatment. Acta Psychiatr Scand 62:193, 1980

24. Treiser S, Kellar KJ: Lithium: Effects on serotonin receptors in rat brain. Eur J Pharmacol 64:183, 1980

25. Shopsin B, Stern S, Gershon S: Altered carbohydrate metabolism during treatment with lithium carbonate. Arch Gen Psychiatry 26:566, 1972

26. Plenge P, Mellerup ET, Rafaelson OJ: Lithium action on glycogen synthesis in rat brain, liver, and diaphragm. J Psychiatr Res 8:29, 1970

27. Selverstone T: Mood and food: A psychopharmacological enquiry. Ann N Y Acad Sci 499:321, 1987

28. Goodall E, Selverstone T: The effect of the 5-HT releasing drug D-fenfluramine and the 5-HT receptor blocker, metergolone on food intake in human subjects. Ann N Y Acad Sci 499:321, 1987

29. Weidley EF, Setler PE, Rush JA: The serotonin blocking properties of antipsychotic drugs. Pharmacologist 22:279, 1980

30. Klett CJ, Caffey EM Jr: Weight changes during treatment with phenothiazine derivatives. J Neuropsychiatry 2:102, 1960

31. Amdisen A: Drug-produced obesity: Experiences with chlorpromazine, perphenazine and clopenthixol. Dan Med Bull 11:182, 1964

32. Gallant DM, Bishop MP: Molindone: A controlled evaluation in chronic schizophrenic patients. Curr Ther Res 10:441, 1968

33. Kellner R, Rada RT, Egelman A et al: Long-term study of molindone hydrochloride in chronic schizophrenics. Curr Ther Res 20:686, 1976

34. Gardos G, Cole JO: Weight reduction in schizophrenics by molindone. Am J Psychiatry 134:302, 1977

35. Greenberg SM, Ellison T, Mathues JK: Comparative studies of growth stimulating properties of phenothiazine analogs in the rat. J Nutr 76:302, 1962

36. Erle G, Basso M, Federspil G et al: Effect of chlorpromazine on blood glucose and plasma insulin in man. Eur J Clin Pharmacol 11:15, 1977

37. Ammon HPT, Orci L, Steinke J: Effect of chlorpromazine (CPZ) on insulin release in vivo and in vitro in the rat. J Pharmacol Exp Ther 187:423, 1973

38. Hippius H, Ackenheil M, Muller-Spahn F: Neuroendocrinological and biochemical effects of chronic neuroleptic treatment. In Kemali D, Racagui G (eds): Chronic Treatment in Neuropsychiatry. New York, Raven Press, 1985

CHAPTER 38

Effect of Exercise on Food Intake

F. XAVIER PI-SUNYER

Epidemiologic data from the United States have shown that the prevalence of obesity among Americans is about double today what it was in 1900. It is also known that Americans are consuming about 5% fewer calories today than they were then.[11] If they are consuming less and are fatter, it stands to reason that they must be expending less energy. Americans have become inactive. This inactivity seems to be the price of technologically advanced societies, given all the mechanical help at our disposal. Definitive figures comparing 1900 with today are not available. A humorous but telling small example of energy savings has been reported by the Illinois Bell Telephone Company, which has estimated that in the course of 1 year an extension phone saves a person approximately 70 miles of walking. This could be translated to as much as 7000 to 10,000 kcal/year, which is the caloric equivalent of 2 to 3 pounds of fat.[30]

How important our inactivity is to the increasing prevalence of obesity is unclear. There have been few studies relating inactivity to obesity. Obese children have been found to be less active than lean children in four reports.[5,12,28,29] However, other studies have not been able to document such a difference.[3,31,33] In adults, also, a number of investigators have concluded that obese persons are less active than lean ones.[1,4,6,19] Again, others have not found such a difference.[18,20] All the investigations just cited have been by questionnaire or relatively crude measures of activity; energy expenditure has not actually been measured. Also, studies have generally been inadequate in defining levels of obesity in the subjects studied and for the lengths of time the subjects were observed. Thus, whether obese individuals are actually less active than lean persons is unclear, though the data are suggestive. More importantly, because obese individuals generally expend more energy per given activity, one cannot simply measure the amount of time spent in activity. Careful measurements of energy expenditure for long periods of time are necessary, including both activity and rest, to resolve whether obese persons in a free-living state actually expend less total energy per 24-hour period. These are difficult studies to carry out, and it is not surprising that we do not have the data in hand.

STUDIES IN FREE-LIVING VOLUNTEERS

Because extended energy expenditure measurement for prolonged periods of time is so difficult and so confining, observers have devised other strategies. The simplest is to take a group of individuals, exercise them, and see if they lose weight.

Results of studies of obese volunteers have been conflicting, some showing weight loss, some showing no change, and some showing an actual weight increase. Such inconsistency suggests that intake is not tightly coupled to expenditure in obese persons. Because food intake has not been measured in these studies, however, it is unclear whether the results support the existence of an anorectic response. When analyzing the weight changes, various theoretically calculated intake responses are found.

Two studies, one in which obese men were exercised by Dempsey[7] and the other in which obese women were exercised by Dudleston and Bennion,[8] reported weight loss, but the weight loss was attributed to the increased energy expenditure created by the exercise rather than to decreased food intake. In the first study, the exercise was calisthenics, running, weight training, and isometrics for 8 weeks, and the individuals lost 4.7 kg, made up of 5.8 kg lost as fat and 1.1 kg gained as lean tissue. Their records showed no change in food intake. In the second study, the young women exercised on treadmills and bicycles for one hour four times per week. The amount of weight they lost could be accounted for by the extra energy expended. Thus, these two studies suggest that exercise has no effect on food intake, neither increasing nor decreasing it.

Other exercise studies have suggested a decrease in weight with the exercise, which has been attributed to decreased food intake. Oscai and Williams[21] studied 5 obese men who ran 30 min/day 3 days/week for 4 months. They lost 4.5 kg in weight and 3.6 kg in fat. Although no food intake data were collected, the energy costs of exercise and the body composition changes suggest decreased food intake as a factor in the weight loss. A similar report was published by Boileau and colleagues.[2] One of the problems with studies of weight loss associated with exercise is that often only "finishers" are counted. If a study is long and arduous, such as that by Gwinup,[13] in which patients exercised 120 minutes a day, 7 days/week for 1 year, only very motivated subjects will continue to the end (11 of 34 in this study). Furthermore, they may also be motivated to diet consciously as well as to run, even though they have been told that they can eat freely. The decrease in food intake may be due to a change in life-style that includes not just exercise, but also decreased dietary and alcohol intake, rather than being due to an effect of the exercise itself on food intake. In other words, the two behavior changes of increased exercise and decreased calorie intake may occur in parallel rather than as a cause-and-effect phenomenon.

Two studies showed little effect of exercise matched to a free diet on weight loss.[16,34] Weltman and colleagues[34] divided 58 mildly obese men into exercise alone, diet alone, exercise plus diet, or control groups and found that diet caused a loss of 5 to 9.5 kg over 10 weeks, whereas exercise alone only caused a weight loss of 0.9 kg. Exercise and diet together, causing a weight loss of 5.4 kg, was no more effective than diet alone. The exercise consisted of walking at 3.5 miles per hour (mph) 4 times per week for 45 min/day. Since the subjects signed up for this study because they wanted to lose weight, and they were not randomized into the different groups, it is difficult to know what motives and goals were involved in their choices. Therefore, it is very difficult to draw conclusions from the study.

In another study, Heymsfield and associates[14] examined the weight loss in obese women ingesting 900 kcal/day for 5 weeks. The patients were assigned to a sedentary group or a group that exercised an average of 346 kcal/day. The exercise did not hasten weight loss, which was essentially identical in the two groups.

Hill and co-workers,[15] on the other hand, in a study in which subjects were given an average of 1200 kcal/day for a 12-week period, with or without exercise, found that the exercised subjects had a greater reduction in body weight and body fat percentage than did the nonexercised subjects.

Leon and colleagues[17] carried out the most successful study of weight loss with exercise. They reported on ten healthy overweight young men 19 to 31 years old who volunteered for an exercise study. The only dietary advice was to eat whatever they wanted. The subjects walked 5 days/week for 16 weeks for 90 min/day, expending between 1000 and 1200 kcal/day (very strenuous exercise). The volunteers lost 5.7 kg of weight, 5.9 kg of body fat, and no lean body mass. In this case, vigorous regular walking for long periods of time, expending more than 1000 kcal/day, did have an effect on body weight and body fat reduction. Again, however, it is unclear whether these obese young men, investing a great amount of time and effort into this protocol for 16 weeks, did not also consciously diminish their food intake, even though they were told they could eat freely.

The inability to lose weight with relatively low levels of activity is clearly shown by the studies by Krotkiewsky and colleagues.[16] These investigators developed a protocol that was amenable to severely overweight women. It consisted of a 30-minute program including warm-up, calisthenics, and jogging. The program was scheduled for 3 days/week for 6 months. A beneficial effect on glucose tolerance and a lowering of insulin levels were noted, but no effect on weight or body fat. This study demonstrated two things: First, the insulin resistance and hyperinsulinemia of severe obesity can be improved by exercise independent of weight loss; second, the level of exercise expenditure must be quite substantial before weight is lost. The outpatient studies just reviewed demonstrate that at exercise levels that are realistic for adult obese patients to sustain—that is, approximately 2 to 4 kcal/min above rest—the effect on weight is very small. This finding gives little support to the idea that moderate exercise has an inhibitory effect on food intake.

METABOLIC WARD STUDIES

Studies that have exercised individuals and actually have measured food intake are rare. This is because accurately measuring food intake in people is very difficult. Thus, although it is commonly believed that food intake is inhibited by exercise, there are very few data available to confirm this.

Three studies done in a metabolic ward setting carefully measured food intake in response to exercise, but they were of very short duration.[9,22,32] Exercise was prescribed, but food intake was left *ad libitum*. However, the test periods were very short (5 to 7 days), and no cross-over studies to control for time effect were conducted. In an interesting but also short study by Edholm,[10] 12 lean young men varied their exercise while their food intake was being monitored. Although no correlation could be found between their energy expenditure and their food intake on a given day, there was some correlation with food intake 2 days later.

Studies of Obese Women

Because of the paucity of reasonably long studies on the effect of exercise on food intake in a controlled environment, we proceeded to carry out a longer exercise study in obese women in a metabolic ward setting. It is clear that a hospital setting presents some problems. It is not equivalent to living at home with the strains and stresses of everyday life, it presents food prepared by others, and the act of measuring food intake in itself may affect the intake. However, we believed that only in such a controlled setting could food intake be accurately measured, and accurate food intake measurement is essential in such a study.

We chose obese female volunteers whose weights had been stable for 6 months. They were asked to join a protein metabolism study and were told they might gain or lose weight. This was done to prevent enrollment of women seeking to lose weight, because they might consciously limit their intake. Our method of measuring food intake was covert. We used a platter method of presenting food in which individual items are presented in large excess, each on its own platter, and the volunteer is asked to take and eat as much as she wants. The food is covertly weighed before and after eating.[24]

Six obese women were selected. Their subject profiles are presented in Table 38-1. The women spent 57 days on the metabolic unit. The results have been published.[35] They underwent a 5-day evaluation period and three 19-day study periods. During the initial evaluation period, mean energy expenditure was measured using the factorial method.[35] Subjects recorded the nature and duration of all their activities on a diary card. The energy cost of eight activities (sleeping, lying down, sitting quietly, sitting talking, sitting knitting, standing, up and about, and treadmill walking at their chosen speed) was measured by indirect calorimetry. For each day, the amount of time spent in each activity was multiplied by the energy cost of that activity to determine the total 24-hour expenditure. Body composition changes were calculated according to the energy-nitrogen balance method as well as the total body water-nitrogen balance method.[35]

After the initial sedentary baseline period, during which they ate freely and their weight remained stable, the volunteers were assigned to three 19-day periods: one sedentary, one doing mild exercise, and one doing moderate exercise. The mild exercise was calculated to expend the

TABLE 38-1

Subject Profile

Subject	Age (years)	Height (cm)	Weight (kg)	% Ideal Weight	% Fat*
A1	32	164.4	101.70	183.2	45.2
A2	61	155.1	86.50	173.9	40.5
A3	42	169.7	98.35	165.3	42.6
A4	46	161.4	79.10	150.7	42.5
A5	53	172.6	113.10	183.9	50.0
A6	22	158.2	74.00	144.4	39.7
Mean	42.6	163.5	92.10	166.9	43.4
SEM	5.3	2.5	5.5	6.2	1.5

*% Fat was calculated using total body potassium determinations of body composition.

(Woo R, Garrow JS, Pi-Sunyer FX: Effect of exercise on spontaneous calorie intake in obesity. Am J Clin Nutr 36:470, 1982)

equivalent of 10% of each individual's 24-hour energy expenditure during the baseline sedentary period; the moderate exercise was 25% of 24-hour energy expenditure. Exercise was done on a treadmill set at 2.5% grade, with subjects choosing their own comfortable speed of walking, which averaged about 3 mph. The exercise periods were assigned using a Latin square design to control for period effects. The energy cost of all the activities previously described was measured by indirect calorimetry twice a week. Results are shown in Figure 38-1. It may be seen that we were successful in increasing energy expenditure appropriately with the exercise periods but that the food intake did not keep up. The women's intake was fixed from period to period and was not significantly different. Because of the increase in expenditure and the lack of change in intake, caloric balance was negative in both of the exercise periods. The changes in weight, fat, and lean body mass in the different periods are shown in Figure 38-2.

These studies in obese women showed a dissociation between exercise and food intake. As exercise effort increased, food intake remained fixed, suggesting an uncoupling of the energy intake from the energy expenditure in these women. The exercise required an average of 39 min/day of brisk walking at mild and 96 min/day at moderate levels. There are two possible interpretations of the results. It can be concluded

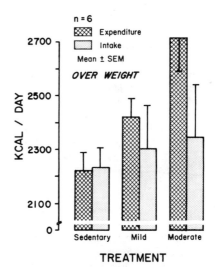

FIGURE 38-1

Energy expenditure and energy intake (mean ± in six obese women during three 19-day periods. The women were sedentary for one period and for the other two periods exercised on a treadmill at a mild degree (raising expenditure to 110% of sedentary daily expenditure) and at a moderate degree (raising expenditure to 125% of sedentary daily expenditure). (Woo R, Pi-Sunyer FX: Effect of increased physical activity on voluntary intake in lean women. Metabolism 34:836, 1985)

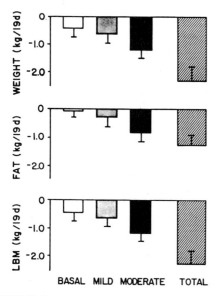

FIGURE 38-2

Weight and body composition changes with treatment (n = 6) (mean ± SEM). Fat changes were obtained from the average of E-N balance and total body weight (TBW)-N balance estimates. Lean body mass (LBM) changes were obtained from the average of TBW and TBW-N balance methods. (Woo R, Garrow JS, Pi-Sunyer FX: Effect of exercise on spontaneous calorie intake in obesity. J Clin Nutr 36:470, 1982)

that an inhibiting effect on food intake occurred because calorie intake stayed the same and it would be expected to increase and keep pace with expenditure, or it can be concluded that obese subjects demonstrate a fixed energy intake that is unaffected by exercise.

We then proceeded to see if a more prolonged period of the moderate exercise would show similar results. A full 57 days of moderate exercise at 25% above 24-hour expenditure were tested using the same protocol in three obese women.[36] As in the first study, the obese women maintained their food intake fixed at a level considerably below their expenditure. Mean daily intake was 1903 kcal/day, and mean daily expenditure was 2882 kcal/day over the 57-day period and did not change with time. As a result, the women lost weight at a consistent rate of 0.12 kg/day. As in the initial study, their food intake did not

change from the initial baseline sedentary period to their exercise periods and did not correlate with their energy expenditure. Intake seemed to be regulated by factors other than energy expenditure, so that there was an uncoupling of energy intake from energy expenditure.

Studies of Lean Women

Because of the intriguing effect of exercise on food intake in obese women, we then wished to determine the role of exercise-related factors on the food intake of normal-weight persons. Lean women volunteers were studied using exactly the same protocol as for the obese women. The characteristics of these women are shown in Table 38-2. The results of the study have been reported previously.[37] Because these lean women were much more efficient at exercising than the obese women had been, however, they had to spend more time on the treadmill to expend 10% and 25% above their 24-hour energy expenditure. Thus they spent an average of 139 minutes on the treadmill during the mild exercise period and 250 minutes during the moderate exercise period. Their energy expenditure and intake are presented in Figure 38-3. The women significantly increased energy intake as energy expenditure increased. In other words, the normal-weight women responded to the increased exercise by increasing their intake appropriately and thus maintained their weight. The proportion of calories coming from protein, fat, and carbohydrate did not change during the three different periods. They were in caloric balance, and their weight and body composition did not change. There was no indication of an inhibitory effect of exercise on food intake.

STUDIES CHANGING THE PALATABILITY OF THE DIET

Because the overweight individuals we studied ate at a caloric level that seemed to be set by factors other than physical activity, we thought we would investigate this further. We postulated that factors that might be important included palatability, variety, and availability of food or other sensory and psychological factors. We therefore studied obese persons using gourmet food that

TABLE 38-2

Subject Characteristics

Subject	Age (years)	Height (cm)	Weight (kg)	% Ideal* Weight	% Fat†
1	21	157.5	47.3	87.1	27.9
2	34	168.0	55.0	89.3	22.8
3	51	160.0	60.9	108.9	41.9
4	33	159.0	51.1	91.4	18.0
5	48	158.5	59.6	109.7	31.7
Mean	37	160.6	54.8	97.3	28.5
SEM	6	2.1	2.8	5.5	4.5

*Midpoint of medium frame, Metropolitan Life Insurance Tables.
†Determined by total body potassium using 60 mEq/kg lean body mass (Fat = weight − lean body mass)

(Woo R, Pi-Sunyer FX: Effect of increased physical activity on voluntary intake in lean women. Metabolism 34:836, 1985)

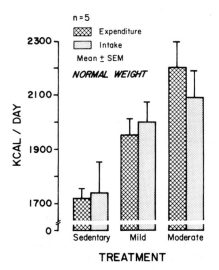

FIGURE 38-3

Energy expenditure and energy intake (mean ± SEM) in five lean women during three 19-day periods. The women were sedentary for one period and for the other two periods exercised on a treadmill at a mild degree (raising expenditure to 110% of sedentary daily expenditure) and at a moderate degree (raising expenditure to 125% of sedentary daily expenditure). (Woo R, Pi-Sunyer FX: Effect of increased physical activity on voluntary intake in lean women. Metabolism 34:836, 1985

was considerably tastier. A similar protocol of measurement of energy expenditure and energy intake was followed. Four obese young men were asked to exercise at four levels: (1) baseline or normal activity (calculated from pedometer data), (2) walking on a treadmill for a period of time calculated to increase the 24-hour energy expenditure 10% above the baseline period, (3) walking to increase energy expenditure 40% above the baseline period, and (4) back to baseline. The results are shown in Figure 38-4.[23] Although expenditure was increased with increasing exercise as planned, intake remained fixed, much as it had in the earlier study on obese women. However, the fixed intake was at a much higher level than in the previous study, and the volunteers did not reach balance until period three, when they were expending 40% above their usual. It therefore seems that although exercise had little effect on their food intake, the palatability of the diet exerted a powerful effect. The plentiful gourmet foods that were used seemed to drive the intake to a point considerably higher than was the case in the women who ate much plainer fare.

A persuasive body of literature suggests that the sensory characteristics of food affect the amount eaten. It has been proposed in a series of studies[26,27] that the calories that an individual

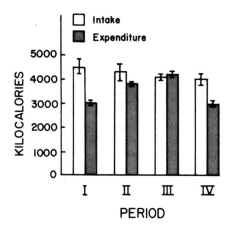

FIGURE 38-4

Energy expenditure and energy intake (mean ± SEM) in four obese men during four 10-day periods (1 to 4). The subjects were either at a basal level of activity (which included their usual walking—periods 1 and 4), or their activity was increased by further walking on a treadmill to a mild degree (100% of basal daily activity—period 2) or a moderate degree (140% of basal activity—period 3). (Woo R, Pi-Sunyer FX: Effect of increased physical activity on voluntary intake in lean women. Metabolism 34:836, 1985)

ingests may be manipulated by changing the taste, look, and variability of the food presented. The hypothesis is that satiety is not a fixed physiological point but that it fluctuates according to the sensory qualities of the foods ingested. The studies I have described are in agreement with such a hypothesis.

CONCLUSION

The inhibitory properties of exercise on food intake have been acclaimed by many enthusiasts. However, the data from human studies are very scarce. This is because accurately measuring food intake in people over a prolonged period is very difficult. In addition, measuring energy expenditure for an extended time has been problematic and intrusive. The doubly labeled water method of measuring energy expenditure in free-living persons may make the measurement of "energy out" much easier, but its accuracy still leaves something to be desired. Given the prob-

lems of measuring energy taken in and energy produced, it is clear that balance studies will be sparse. Because of these difficulties, other strategies have been tried, the simplest being to exercise people and to determine whether they lose weight or change body composition. At exercise levels that are realistic for obese people, the changes in weight and the loss of body fat are usually modest. The studies available generally have been flawed by poor design, including nonrandomized groups of study subjects, lack of controls, and not counting dropouts. Most studies have been conducted outside of a metabolic ward setting, despite the fact that measurements of energy intake and energy expenditure are more precisely made in a laboratory or metabolic ward.

We have carried out a series of careful studies to try to clarify the question of the effect of exercise on food intake. The response was decidedly different in a group of lean women than in a group of obese women. The lean women were exposed to a protocol that allowed for voluntary food intake but prescribed a set physical activity. During an inactive period, the women freely ate an amount of food that matched their energy expenditure. This coupling of intake with expenditure was sustained during all three treatment periods in the study. Regardless of whether treadmill walking was added to or subtracted from daily activity, subjects adjusted their intake to their expenditure. Thus, these lean individuals maintained weight and body composition by accurately adjusting their intake to their expenditure.

In contrast, the obese women did not adjust intake. The caloric intake remained fixed throughout the sedentary and exercise periods. Therefore, when exercise was added to the regimen, because no compensatory increase in energy expenditure occurred, a significant negative energy balance was obtained. These results suggest that in obese women, exercise at moderate, realistic levels does not regulate intake, at least within 19-day periods. Because other studies of food intake had suggested that obese persons undereat monotonous, less palatable diets and overeat gourmet foods,[25] we decided to study the effect of exercise on food intake using much more palatable, gourmet foods. With such a paradigm in obese young men, we found that their intake was still fixed and unresponsive to exercise cues, but they ate much more food so that they only came into caloric balance during their heaviest exercise period.

Some form of regulation of caloric intake to match expenditure is necessary to maintain body weight. Lean individuals seem to be able to maintain this energy equilibrium. Obese individuals, however, seem to be insensitive to this matching system. There does not seem to be an immediate physiological drive in obese persons to replace calories expended in physical activity. Their intake seems to be determined more by other factors, such as palatability, than by cues that they receive from their activity pattern. These obese individuals have a great reserve of body fat. It is possible that they also have a lesser sensitivity to internal signals of hunger and satiety. Therefore, whatever signals are generated in obese subjects by exercise alone may be attenuated or overwhelmed by other cues that are generated by the foods to be eaten. This possibility supports a stronger role for food-derived signals than for those from exercise in regulating calorie intake in obese people. Whether eating behavior would revert to a normal lean pattern with weight loss and approximation of body weight and body fat toward normal needs to be investigated. It is unclear whether the insensitivity to exercise cues in obese people is due to body compositional factors (such as excess body fat) or to an inherent difference in behavioral response to food that would persist after weight loss. More research into this question needs to be pursued.

Exercise does cause weight loss.[35,36] The calorie deficit created is directly accountable to the number of calories expended, because no special effect on food intake occurs in obese persons. Therefore, exercise can be useful for weight reduction, but it must be coupled to a dietary regimen to have a major impact on weight.

References

1. Bloom WL, Eidex MF: Inactivity as a major factor in adult obesity. Metabolism 16:679, 1967
2. Boileau RA, Buskirk ER, Horstman DH et al: Body compositional changes in obese and lean men during physical conditioning. Med Sci Sports Exerc 3:183, 1971
3. Bradfield RB, Paulos J, Grossman L: Energy expenditure and heart rate of obese high school girls. Am J Clin Nutr 24:1482, 1971
4. Brownell KD, Stunkard AJ, Albaum JM: Evaluation and modification of exercise patterns in the natural environment. Am J Psychiatry 137:1540, 1980
5. Bullen BA, Reed RB, Mayer J: Physical activity of obese and non-obese adolescent girls appraised by motion picture sampling. Am J Clin Nutr 14:211, 1974
6. Chirico A, Stunkard AJ: Physical activity and human obesity. N Engl J Med 263:935, 1960
7. Dempsey JA: Anthropometrical observations on obese and non-obese young men undergoing a program of vigorous physical exercise. Res Q Exerc Sport 35:275, 1964
8. Dudleston AK, Bennion M: Effect of diet and/or exercise on obese college women. J Am Diet Assoc 56:126, 1970
9. Durrant ML, Roystron JP, Wloch RT: Effect of exercise on energy intake and eating patterns in lean and obese humans. Physiol Behav 29:449, 1982
10. Edholm OG: Energy balance in man—studies carried out by the Division of Human Physiology, National Institute of Medical Research. J Hum Nutr 31:413, 1977
11. Friend B: Changes in Nutrients in the U.S. Diet Caused by Alterations in Food Intake Patterns. Prepared for The Changing Food Supply in America Conference, May 22, 1974, sponsored by the Food and Drug Administration
12. Johnson ML, Burke MS, Mayer J: Relative importance of inactivity and overeating in the energy balance of obese high school girls. Am J Clin Nutr 4:37, 1956
13. Gwinup G: Effect of exercise alone on the weight of obese women. Arch Intern Med 135:676, 1975
14. Heymsfield SB, Casper K, Hearn J et al: Rate of weight loss during underfeeding: Relation to level of physical activity. Metabolism 38:215, 1989
15. Hill JO, Schlundt DG, Sbrocco T et al: Evaluation of an alternating-calorie diet with and without exercise in the treatment of obesity. Am J Clin Nutr 50:248, 1989
16. Krotkiewsky M, Mandroukas K, Sjostrom L et al: Effects of long-term physical training on body fat, metabolism and blood pressure in obesity. Metabolism 28:650, 1979
17. Leon AS, Conrad J, Hunninghake DB et al: Effects of a vigorous walking program on body composition and lipid metabolism of obese young men. Am J Clin Nutr 33:1776, 1979
18. Lincoln JE: Caloric intake, obesity, and physical activity. Am J Clin Nutr 25:390, 1972
19. Mayer J, Roy P, Mitra KP: Relation between caloric intake, body weight, and physical work. Am J Clin Nutr 4:169, 1956

20. Maxfield E, Konishi F: Patterns of food intake and physical activity in obesity. J Am Diet Assoc 49:406, 1966

21. Oscai LB, Williams BT: Effect of exercise on overweight middle-aged males. J Am Geriatr Soc 16:794, 1968

22. Passmore R, Thomson JG, Warnock GM: A balance sheet of the estimation of energy intake and energy expenditure as measured by indirect calorimetry using the Kofranyi-Michaelis calorimeter. Br J Nutr 6:253, 1952

23. Pi-Sunyer FX: Effect of exercise on food intake. In Hirsch J, Van Itallie TB (eds): Recent Advances in Obesity Research IV, pp 368–373. London, John Libbey & Co, 1985

24. Porikos KP, Booth G, Van Itallie TB: Effect of covert nutritive dilution on the spontaneous food intake of obese individuals: A pilot study. Am J Clin Nutr 30:1638, 1977

25. Porikos KP, Pi-Sunyer FX: Regulation of food intake in human obesity: Studies with caloric dilution and exercise. Clin Endocrinol Metab 13:547, 1984

26. Rolls BJ, Rowe EA, Rolls ET: How sensory properties of food affect human feeding behavior. Physiol Behav 29:409, 1982

27. Rolls BJ, Rowe ET, Rolls ET et al: Variety in a meal enhances food intake in man. Physiol Behav 26:215, 1981

28. Rose HE, Mayer J: Activity, caloric intake, and the energy balance of infants. Pediatrics 41:18, 1968

29. Stefanik PA, Heald FL, Mayer J: Caloric intake in relation to energy output of obese and non obese adolescent boys. Am J Clin Nutr 7:55, 1959

30. Stern JS: Is obesity a disease of inactivity? In Stunkard A, Stellar E (eds): Eating and Its Disorders. New York, Raven Press, 1984

31. Stunkard AJ, Pestka J: The physical activity of obese girls. Am J Dis Chil 103:812, 1962

32. Warnold E, Lenner RA: Evaluation of the heart rate method to determine the daily energy expenditure in disease: A study in juvenile diabetics. Am J Clin Nutr 30:304, 1977

33. Wilkinson PW, Parkin JM, Pearlson G et al: Energy intake and physical activity in obese children. Br Med J 1:756, 1977

34. Weltman A, Matter S, Stamford BA: Caloric restriction and/or mild exercise: effects on serum lipids and body composition. Am J Clin Nutr 33:1002, 1980

35. Woo R, Garrow JS, Pi-Sunyer FX: Effect of exercise on spontaneous calorie intake in obesity. Am J Clin Nutr 36:470, 1982

36. Woo R, Garrow JS, Pi-Sunyer FX: Voluntary food intake during prolonged exercise in obese women. Am J Clin Nutr 36:478, 1982

37. Woo R, Pi-Sunyer FX: Effect of increased physical activity on voluntary intake in lean women. Metabolism 34:836, 1985

PART SEVEN

ASSOCIATED HEALTH IMPAIRMENTS

CHAPTER 39

Obesity and Disease

KEAVEN M. ANDERSON and WILLIAM B. KANNEL

DEFINITION AND PREVALENCE OF OBESITY

Obesity may be defined as the storage of excess calories in fat. For practical purposes, it has been measured in various ways such as percent of body fat, skin-fold thicknesses, waist:hip circumference ratio, and weight adjusted for height. Two commonly used weight for height measures are Metropolitan relative weight (MRW)[35,36] and body mass index (BMI = weight in kilograms divided by the square of height in meters).

The second National Health and Nutrition Survey (NHANES II, 1976–1980)[37] defined the cutoff for obesity to be the 85th percentile of BMI among 20- to 29-year-olds (27.8 for men and 27.3 for women). This is approximately 20% overweight by the 1983 MRW tables.[43] By this definition, it was estimated that approximately 34 million people in the United States were obese.[37] The prevalence was affected by factors such as sex, age, economic status, and race (black versus white). Obesity was more prevalent in lower- than in higher-income women. It was also more prevalent among blacks than whites, especially among black women. Just over 60% of black women age 45 to 55 years were obese, whereas only 30% of white women in this age-group were obese.[43] Among men, obesity prevalence increased until age 55 and then decreased. No such decrease was noted in women, although there was still a big increase from age 20 to 55 years.

OBESITY AND LONGEVITY

In the short term, there is little relationship between obesity and morbidity/mortality, whereas longer term there is a strong relationship. Figure 39-1 shows age-adjusted all-cause mortality by 1959 MRW for various lengths of follow-up for men from the Framingham Heart Study.[12,35] The figures are based on age-adjusted rates (direct method) for 2219 men who at the beginning of the follow-up period were from 29 to 62 years of age, free of coronary heart diseae (CHD) and cancer, and for whom weight, height, and smoking information were available. The relationship is J shaped, with lowest mortality occurring around the "desirable" value of 100. For six and 12 years of follow-up there is excess mortality only in very obese men. The longer the follow-up, the stronger the association between obesity and mortality in both smokers and nonsmokers.

Separating these analyses by smoking habit considerably affects the strength of the association uncovered.[16] In 1959, among men under MRW of 100, 80% were smokers. For MRW of 140% or more, only 55% were smokers. Thus if the data in Figure 39-1 are combined, the rates for lower weights are closer to the smokers' curve whereas the rates for the higher weights are closer to the nonsmokers' curve. The curve is thus flattened, disguising the actual positive association between MRW and long-term mortality that exists for both smokers and nonsmokers.

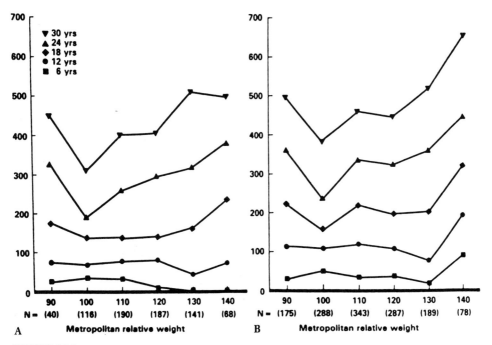

FIGURE 39-1

Cumulative deaths per 1000 male nonsmokers **(A)** and smokers **(B)** of all ages.
(Reprinted with permission from Ann Intern Med 103:1020, 1985.)

Figure 39-2 shows age-specific 26-year mortality by smoking status for men.[16] This is still the cohort members free of CHD and cancer at the beginning of follow-up. With one minor exception, for each age–smoking habit combination, the lowest mortality was in the 100% to 109% MRW category. Higher mortality occurred in both lower- and higher-weight groups. Although *relative* increases in mortality occur in the youngest group, *absolute* differences are somewhat similar for all age-groups. When investigators say the relationship is stronger in younger age-groups, they are often referring to *relative* rather than *absolute* differences in mortality. Relative changes are the easiest changes to evaluate when applying commonly used analytic methods such as logistic regression.

The Metropolitan Life Insurance Company[35] has published desirable weight tables that do not depend on age. Andres and colleagues[3] have argued that weight goals for greatest longevity should be age specific. They argue that insurance data show lowest mortality at higher weight lev-els as age increases. The Build Study[8] data they cite do not adjust for smoking status.

It is important to note that a history of obesity is associated with increased mortality in individuals over age 65 in the Framingham study.[18]

In a cohort of nearly 80,000 Dutch men weighed at age 18 and observed for 32 years, minimum mortality was found in a very lean group with BMI from 19 to 19.99, with higher mortality in lower and higher BMI categories.[22] The 32-year mortality ranged from about 4% to 5.5% in the different weight categories. No smoking information was available for this study.

It is widely agreed that weight loss associated with diagnosed illness or even subclinical illness is associated with mortality. Thus it has been argued that people with pre-existing medical conditions should not be considered in analyses studying optimal weights.[30] Not accounting for prevalent disease can have the same dampening effect on the relation between obesity and morbidity/mortality that not accounting for smoking habit does. In this case, a disproportionate num-

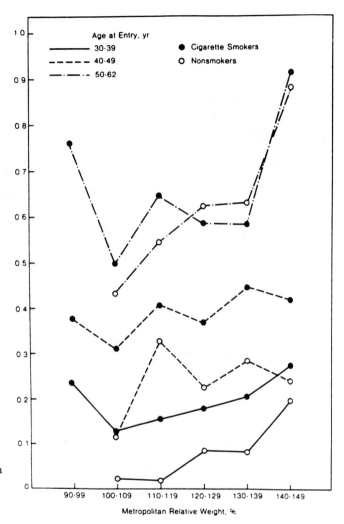

FIGURE 39-2

Proportion of men dying in 26 years for each MRW class by 10-year age-group and cigarette smoking at the first Framingham Heart Study examination. Men with a history of cardiovascular disease were excluded. (Garrison RJ et al: Cigarette smoking. JAMA 249:2201, 1983)

ber of low-weight individuals have some prevalent condition putting them at increased risk for mortality.

OBESITY AND MORBIDITY

Coronary Heart Disease

The long-term relationship between obesity—as measured by 1959 MRW—and risk of cardiovascular disease is strong for both men and women.[23] The association between MRW and CHD using 26 years of follow-up from the Framingham Study is shown in Figure 39-3. Multi-

variate models discussed by Hubert and colleagues[23] included covariates for age, cholesterol level, systolic blood pressure, cigarette smoking, left ventricular hypertrophy, and glucose intolerance. In men and women, MRW was significantly associated with the development of CHD and congestive heart failure. In women, MRW was also associated with elevated risk of stroke.

It has been argued that in the absence of other cardiovascular risk factors, obesity is not a risk factor for CHD.[25,31] Long-term follow-up of men and women under 50 years old from the Framingham Study without known risk factors did show an association with disease, however.[23]

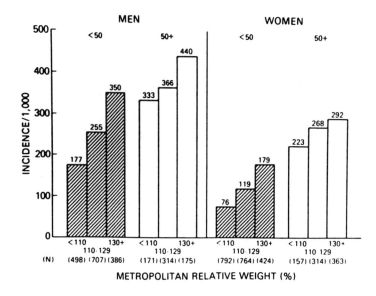

FIGURE 39-3

Twenty-six-year incidence of CHD by MRW at entry among Framingham men and women younger than age 50 years and age 50 years or older. N = the number at risk for an event. Numbers above the bars give the actual incidence rates per 1000. (Hubert HB, Feinleib M, McNamara PM et al: Obesity as an independent risk factor for cardiovascular disease: A 26-year follow-up of participants in the Framingham Heart Study. Circulation 67:971, 1983)

Central obesity has been shown to be related to CHD incidence in several studies.[10,28,29,42] Subscapular skin folds (SSF) were more strongly associated with 13-year CHD incidence than BMI in 7692 men from the Honolulu Heart Study. The trend by tertile of SSF within each tertile of BMI was nearly as strong as the trend with no adjustment for BMI (Figs. 39-1 and 39-4). The opposite was not true: there was no significant association between BMI and CHD incidence after adjusting for tertile of SSF (Figs. 39-2 and 39-5). The skinfold relationship was maintained in a multivariate model adjusting for age, BMI, total cholesterol, glucose, triglycerides, hypertensive status, and cigarette smoking.

Among Framingham men and women ages 36 to 68 years, SSF was found to be a stronger predictor of 22-year CHD incidence than BMI in both sexes.[42] This comparison was made using logistic models adjusting for multiple risk factors.

In a study of 792 54-year-old men from Gothenburg, Sweden, with 13 years of follow-up, the waist:hip circumference ratio was used as a measure of central adiposity.[28] This measure was found to be more strongly associated with heart disease and stroke than BMI, the sum of three skin folds (subscapular, triceps, parathoracic), waist circumference, or hip circumference. The

association was not statistically significant after adjusting for other risk factors, but given the results of Framingham and Honolulu, this is probably attributable to the small size of the study. The authors concluded that weight distribution may be a better predictor of cardiovascular disease than degree of adiposity.

Measures of obesity were studied in 1462 women from Gothenburg, Sweden, ages 30 to 60 years, with 12 years of follow-up.[29] Waist:hip ratio was found to be more strongly associated with CHD, stroke, and death than other measures of obesity. This relationship remained significant or borderline significant when adjusting for age, BMI, cholesterol level, triglyceride level, and systolic blood pressure.

Diabetes

Diabetes occurs in obese persons at three times the rate in nonobese.[43] As noted earlier, central adiposity is associated with the development of cardiovascular disease. Upper body obesity differs from lower body obesity in that the former is apparently primarily hypertrophic whereas the latter is hyperplastic.[26,27] Hypertrophic cells have been found to be insulin resistant,[38,39] and individuals with upper body obesity have been found to be more insulin resistant than other

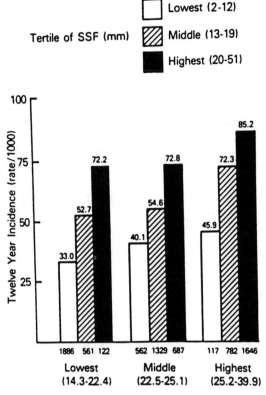

FIGURE 39-4

Age-adjusted 12-year incidence of definite CHD in tertiles of SSF within each tertile of BMI. Significant effect of SSF within lowest and highest ($P < 0.01$), and within middle ($P < 0.05$) tertiles of BMI. Figures along the x axis are numbers at risk. (Donahue RP, Abbott RD, Bloom E et al: Central obesity and coronary heart disease in men. Lancet 1987)

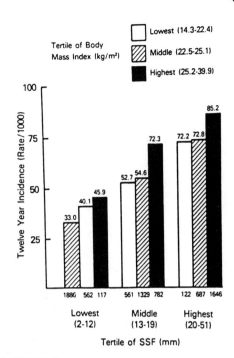

FIGURE 39-5

Age-adjusted 12-year incidence of definite CHD in tertiles of BMI within each tertile of SSF. Effect of BMI is not significant within any tertile of SSF. Figures along the x axis are numbers at risk. (Donahue RP, Abbott RD, Bloom E et al: Central obesity and coronary heart disease in men. Lancet 1987)

obese individuals.[11,26,27,44] Diabetic individuals, especially women, often have central or upper body fat distribution.[13,19,20,24,26,34,41]

Other Morbidity and Mortality

The American Cancer Society observed men and women over age 30 for 13 years.[15] A study included 336,442 men and 419,060 women free of cancer, CHD, stroke, and no 4.5 kg weight loss in the preceding 12 months. Relative weight was computed using age- and sex-specific average weight for each given height. Prostate and colorectal cancer mortality were increased in obese men. Cancer of the endometrium, uterus, cervix, ovary, gallbladder, and breast were increased in obese women. This study also found excess mortality from digestive disease (mainly gallbladder).

Gout, hyperuricemia, gallstone disease, and osteoarthrities have been linked with obesity.[6,7,14] Obese persons tend to have reduced pulmonary function compared with nonobese. Hormonal abnormalities tend to occur in both obese men and women.[7] Men have decreased serum levels of testosterone, whereas estradiol and estrone are increased. Obese women have menstrual irregularities more often than nonobese.

CHANGE IN WEIGHT AND ITS HEALTH CONSEQUENCES

Involuntary weight loss as diagnosed at a hospital on an in- or outpatient basis is an ominous sign.[33] Note that two thirds of the patients in that study did not have involuntary weight loss as their chief complaint. The authors of this study were able to diagnose a physical cause of weight loss in 59 (65%) of the 91 patients studied. There was a wide range of physical causes, including cancer or cardiovascular disease in 26 (29%) of the 91 studied. Comparing people who lost weight and kept it off versus those who regained some or all of their weight showed that those who did not regain weight had a worse prognosis. These results are the opposite of what one would hope to find in a healthy population. That is, weight loss (among the obese) is thought to improve health, and a cycle of weight loss and gain is thought to be deleterious to health.

It is difficult in a study such as the Framingham Study to exclude subjects, such as those just mentioned, on the basis of a diffuse set of diagnoses. One reason for this is a lack of a concise, accessible list of diagnoses made. Another reason is that it is difficult to decide exactly what set of diagnoses is justifiably excluded. Apparently there is no epidemiologic study of weight loss among certified healthy subjects. The closest thing to this is perhaps from the Build and Blood Pressure Study.[9] Men initially issued rated life insurance policies because of overweight were later given standard policies; they were found to have lower mortality than those who did not later receive standard policies. The obvious methodologic criticism of this study is that the men not later issued standard policies may have been disqualified at later dates for reasons other than being overweight.

Hubert and colleagues[23] found an association between weight gain since age 25 and cardiovascular disease in both men and women. Hamm and colleagues[17] have shown that reported variation in weight is associated with elevated risk of mortality due to CHD. More specifically, those who reportedly both lost and gained substantial amounts of weight between the ages of 20 and 40 years were at higher risk than those who reported neither. This study uses a long-term (25 year) follow-up starting at ages 40 to 56 years. Unfortunately, this report did not include separate information on those who lost and did not regain significant amounts of weight after significant loss. This is because of a small sample size (personal communication). Also, the group with variable weights included individuals with a single gain and loss cycle. It would be of great interest to determine if those who failed to regain after losing weight had a prognosis closer to the group with stable weight or the group with weight variability.

THE ASSOCIATION OF OBESITY WITH RISK FACTORS

Epidemiologic studies have found associations between obesity and worsened values of many risk factors for cardiovascular disease. These risk factors include cholesterol and its subfractions low-density lipoprotein (LDL), very low density lipoprotein (VLDL), and high-density lipoprotein (HDL), blood pressure, uric acid, blood glucose, diabetes, and vital capacity. Because weight loss often improves many of these risk factors, it would appear to be a useful measure for preventing cardiovascular disease.

Both cross-sectional and longitudinal studies have been used to examine the relationship between obesity and risk factors. Cross-sectional studies give a snapshot in time of which risk factors are elevated in obese people, whereas longitudinal studies show which risk factors are elevated as people gain weight.

Ashley and Kannel[4] compared changes in weight in the first nine biennial Framingham examination cycles with changes in total cholesterol, systolic blood pressure, uric acid, and blood glucose. Subjects were not fasting for these examinations. Weight gain was significantly correlated with deleterious changes in each of the variables studied in both men and women. Regression lines were computed associating each of these changes with weight. Using a risk factor model with these presumed changes suggests that weight is an important risk determinant. For instance, a 25- to 44-year-old man who gains 10% (relative) weight increases his CHD risk factors (on average) consistent with a 38% increase in 2-year CHD risk.

These Framingham Study results have been extended using data from the Framingham Offspring Study, in which fasting blood specimens and lipoprotein fractions were studied.[2] Weight gain was associated with higher total, LDL, and VLDL cholesterol. Weight gain was associated with lower HDL cholesterol. All of these results held for both men and women.

Borkan and colleagues[5] studied change in weight and its association with changes in risk factors in men frm 21 to 81 years of age at study entry in the Normative Aging Study. Changes in weight were found to be associated with changes in blood pressure, cholesterol, triglycerides, fasting and 2-hour postprandial blood glucose, uric acid, and vital capacity.

The waist to hip circumference measure of central adiposity has been found to be associated with increased age, blood pressure, cholesterol, triglycerides, cigarette smoking, and blood glucose in women.[29] In a smaller study of men, this ratio was also found to be associated with blood pressure.[28]

PREVENTIVE IMPLICATIONS

The high and increasing prevalence of obesity in affluent countries, its multiple atherogenic concomitants, and its demonstrated association with cardiovascular morbidity and mortality make obesity a major health hazard. Because of this, a substantial amount of cardiovascular and other disease is attributable to unrestrained weight gain. Controversy about the relation of body weight to morbidity and mortality has been generated by confounding effects of smoking, coexistent subclinical disease, and short duration of follow-up. Obesity is a major contributor to the high prevalence of hypertension, dyslipidemia, diabetes, and hyperuricemia in the general population. Weight reduction has been shown to produce an improvement of all these components of the cardiovascular risk profile. Obesity also appears to be a contributor to cancers of the colon, prostate, and rectum in men and of the breast, ovary, uterus, and biliary tract in women. It also predisposes to arthritis.

Body weights exceeding 20% above median or desirable weights constitute an established hazard to health. Central or abdominal patterns of obesity appear to have more deleterious metabolic effects. Weight control through diet and exercise clearly constitutes a major hygienic means for avoiding or correcting the major atherogenic contributors to cardiovascular disease.

Although there are many unresolved issues, obesity control holds great promise for avoiding many of the leading disabling and lethal illnesses. Weight control by itself in some cases can correct hypertension, diabetes, and dyslipidemia, whereas in other cases it can reduce the drug dose needed to treat these conditions. Although the rationale is sound and the potential benefits great, it must be admitted that convincing demonstration of the efficacy of correcting obesity is unlikely to be forthcoming because of the difficulty in achieving sustained weight loss for long periods.

The continued high prevalence of obesity and inefficacy of treatment indicate a need to avoid substantial weight gain and to maintain a greater sense of urgency about moderate weight increases. More information is needed about possible hazards of repeated unsuccessful attempts to lose weight. Further progress in controlling obesity and its metabolic and disease consequences must await further insights into the pathogenesis of the condition and the life-styles that promote it.

References

1. Abraham S, Johnson CL: Prevalence of obesity in adults in the United States. Am J Clin Nutr 33:364, 1980
2. Anderson KM, Wilson PWF, Garrison RJ et al: Longitudinal and secular trends in lipoprotein cholesterol measurements in a general population sample. Atherosclerosis 68:59, 1987
3. Andres R, Elahi D, Tobin JD et al: Impact of age on weight goals. Ann Intern Med 103:1030, 1985
4. Ashley FW Jr, Kannel WB: Relation of weight change to changes in atherogenic traits: The Framingham Study. J Chronic Dis 27:103, 1974
5. Borkan GA, Sparrow D, Wisniewski C et al: Body weight and coronary disease risk: Patterns of risk factor change associated with long-term weight change. Am J Epidemiol 124:410, 1986
6. Bray GA (ed): Obesity in America. NIH Publication 4:79–359. Bethesda, MD, National Institutes of Health, 1979

7. Bray GA: Complications of obesity. Ann Intern Med 103:1052, 1985

8. Build Study 1979. Chicago, Society of Actuaries and Association of Life Insurance Medical Directors of America, 1980

9. Build and Blood Pressure Study. Chicago, Society of Actuaries and Association of Life Insurance Medical Directors of America, 1959

10. Donahue RP, Abbott RD, Bloom E et al: Central obesity and coronary heart disease in men. Lancet 284:821, 1987

11. Evans DJ, Hoffman RG, Kalkhoff RK et al: Relationship of body fat topography to insulin sensitivity and metabolic profiles in premenopausal women. Metabolism 33:68, 1984

12. Feinleib M: Epidemiology of obesity in relation to health hazards. Ann Intern Med 103:1019, 1985

13. Feldman R, Sender AJ, Siegelaub AB: Difference in diabetic and nondiabetic fat distribution patterns by skinfold measurements. Diabetes 18:478, 1969

14. Friedman GD, Kannel WB, Dawber TR: The epidemiology of gall-bladder disease: Observations in the Framingham study. J Chronic Dis 19:273, 1966

15. Garfinkel L: Overweight and cancer. Ann Intern Med 103:1034, 1985

16. Garrison RJ, Feinleib M, Castelli WP et al: Cigarette smoking as a confounder of the relationship between relative weight and long-term mortality: The Framingham Heart Study. JAMA 249:2199, 1983

17. Hamm P, Shekelle RB, Stamler J: Large fluctuations in body weight during young adulthood and twenty-five-year risk of coronary death in men. Am J Epidemiol 129:312, 1989

18. Harris T, Cook EF, Garrison RJ et al: Body mass index and mortality among nonsmoking older persons. JAMA 259:1520, 1988

19. Hartz AJ, Rupley DC, Kalkhoff RK et al: Relationship of obesity to diabetes: Influence of obesity level and body fat distribution. Prev Med 12:351, 1983

20. Hartz AJ, Rupley DC, Rimm AA: The association of growth measurements with disease in 32,856 women. Am J Epidemiol 119:71, 1984

21. Health implications of obesity. National Institutes of Health consensus development conference statement. Ann Intern Med 103:1073, 1985

22. Hoffmans MDA, Kromhout D, de Lezenne Coulander C: The impact of body mass index of 78,612 18-year-old Dutch men on 32-year mortality from all causes. J Clin Epidemiol 41:749, 1988

23. Hubert HB, Feinleib M, McNamara PM et al: Obesity as an independent risk factor for cardiovascular disease. A 26-year follow-up of participants in the Framingham Heart Study. Circulation 67:968, 1983

24. Joos SK, Mueller WH, Hanis CL et al: Diabetes alert study: Weight history and upper body obesity in diabetic and nondiabetic Mexican American adults. Ann Hum Biol 11:167, 1984

25. Keys A: Overweight, obesity, coronary heart disease and mortality. Nutr Rev 38:297, 1980

26. Kissebah AH, Vydelingum N, Murray R et al: Relationship of body fat distribution to metabolic complications of obesity. J Clin Endocrinol Metab 54:254, 1982

27. Krotkiewski M, Björntorp P, Shostrom L et al: Impact of obesity on metabolism in men and women: Importance of regional adipose tissue distribution. J Clin Invest 72:1150, 1983

28. Larsson B, Svärdsudd K, Welin L et al: Abdominal adipose tissue distribution, obesity, and risk of cardiovascular disease and death: 13-year follow-up of participants in the study of men born in 1913. Br Med J 288:1401, 1984

29. Lapidus L, Bengtsson C, Larsson B et al: Distribution of adipose tissue and risk of cardiovascular disease and death: A 12-year follow-up of participants in the population study of women in Gothenburg, Sweden. Br Med J 289:1257, 1984

30. Lew EA: Mortality and weight: Insured lives and the American Cancer Society Studies. Ann Intern Med 103:1024, 1985

31. Mann GV: The influence of obesity on health. N Engl J Med 291:178; 291:226, 1974

32. Manson JE, Stampfer MJ, Hennekens CH et al: Body weight and longevity. JAMA 257:353, 1987

33. Marton KI, Sox HC Jr, Krupp JR: Involuntary weight loss: Diagnostic and prognostic significance. Ann Intern Med 95:568, 1981

34. Mueller WH, Joos SK, Hanis CL et al: The diabetes alert study: Growth, fatness and fat patterning, adolescence through adulthood in Mexican Americans. Am J Physiol Anthropol 64:389, 1984

35. New weight standards for men and women. Statistical Bulletin. Metropolitan Life Insurance Company 40:1, 1959

36. 1983 Metropolitan Height and Weight Tables. Statistical Bulletin. Metropolitan Life Insurance Company 64:1, 1983

37. National Center for Health Statistics: Plan and Operation of the National Health and Nutrition Examination Survey, 1976–80. DHHS publication (PHS) 81-1317. (Vital and Health Statistics, series 1, no 15). Washington, DC, US Public Health Service, 1981

38. Olefsky JM: The insulin receptor: Its role in insulin resistance of obesity and diabetes. Diabetes 25:1154, 1976

39. Salans LB, Knittle JL, Hirsch J: The role of adipose cell size and adipose tissue insulin sensitivity in

the carbohydrate intolerance of human obesity. J Clin Invest 47:53, 1968

40. Simopoulos AP, Van Itallie TB: Body weight, health, and longevity. Ann Intern Med 100:285, 1984

41. Sims EAH: Definitions, criteria and prevalence of obesity. In Bray GA (ed.): Obesity in America, pp 20–36. NIH Publication 4:79–359. Bethesda, MD, National Institutes of Health, 1979

42. Stokes J III, Garrison RJ, Kannel WB: The independent contributions of various indices of obesity to

the 22-year incidence of coronary heart disease: The Framingham Study. In Vague J (ed): Metabolic Complications of Human Obesity, pp 49–57. Amsterdam, Elsevier, 1987

43. Van Itallie TB: Health implications of overweight and obesity in the United States. Ann Intern Med 103:983, 1985

44. Ward WK, Johnston C, Beard JC et al: Abnormal fat distribution in subjects predisposed to NIDDM. Clin Res 33:67A, 1985

CHAPTER 40

Glucose Metabolism in Obesity and Type II Diabetes

RICCARDO C. BONADONNA and RALPH A. DEFRONZO

Obesity and type II (non–insulin-dependent) diabetes (NIDDM) frequently occur together.[46,118,180] A number of studies have shown that obesity is a strong risk factor for the later development of NIDDM[6,97,118,221] and shares with it the syndrome of insulin resistance.* Both conditions are at least in part genetically determined, as shown in several family studies.[6,26,118,153,206,208-210] Moreover, insulin resistance also appears to be a familial trait.[96,132] Summing up, obese individuals and 80%–90% of non–insulin-dependent diabetic (NIDD) patients have altered body composition, insulin resistance, and a genetic background predisposing to their disease.

From these observations stems the long-held hypothesis that obesity may be considered a prediabetic state and that much can be learned from similarities and dissimilarities between the two diseases, in an effort to elucidate the natural history of NIDDM in humans.

This chapter focuses on our current knowledge and concepts regarding glucose metabolism in type II diabetes and obesity. In order to fully understand the specific features characterizing glucose metabolism in obesity and NIDDM, it is necessary to be conversant with some basic concepts of normal glucose metabolism. For the sake of simplicity, we recapitulate only those essential characteristics that are germane to our topic.

---

* 15-17,22,29,31,46,49,50,57,61,62,73,91,100,119,160,161,172,173,180

GLUCOSE METABOLISM AND INSULIN: AN INTEGRATED OVERVIEW

Organ Classification and Glucose Metabolism

Throughout the entire life span, glucose is taken up from the circulation by several body tissues and supplied to the plasma pool by the liver in the postabsorptive state and by the gut after being absorbed from the intestinal lumen in the fed state.

Two cell systems, the brain and the red blood cells (RBCs), are strictly glucose dependent for their metabolism under normal circumstances and require approximately 556 μmol (~100 mg) of glucose per minute. Brain glucose uptake displays a zero-order (concentration-independent) kinetics—that is, an acute increase in blood glucose concentration above the normal postabsorptive values does not elicit any change in brain glucose metabolism.[54,79,87,144] However, this relation is lost when the blood glucose concentration declines significantly below the postabsorptive values, when brain glucose utilization is an approximately linear function of arterial glucose concentration. In the low range of blood glucose levels, the lower the glucose concentration, the less is brain glucose disposal.[54,87,203] As a corollary, in order to supply neurons with an adequate flux of glucose, the circulating glucose concentration must be greater than 3.6 mmol/liter (65 mg/dl); at glucose levels below this, neuroglucopenia ensues.[54,203] This is a life-threatening situation, and complex homeostatic mechanisms are readily activated as the glucose concentration reaches this threshold.[20,42,45,79,86,144,184,203]

Brain tissue and RBCs use 140 to 150 g of glucose per day, or about half of the carbohydrate content in a 2200-kcal diet containing 50% carbohydrate. Moreover, brain and RBC glucose utilization is constant over time, whereas feeding and consequent exogenous glucose availability are phasic. At times in the day, glucose availability greatly exceeds the needs of the glucose-dependent organs, and because glucose is not allowed to accumulate in the extracellular space, the glucidic "leftovers" must be disposed of by other organs. An important point is that the amount of these leftovers is highly variable between individuals and between days, ranging from 50 to 250 g of carbohydrate on any given day.

In sharp contrast to the glucose-dependent organs, whose glucose utilization is fixed, the organs that dispose of the dietary carbohydrate intake that exceeds the needs of the brain/RBCs must be able to time and tailor their glucose uptake to the effective glucose availability. Two of these organs, skeletal muscle and adipose tissue, possess this capability, but are dependent on acute changes in circulating insulin concentration, and therefore they are called insulin dependent.[31,47,73,74,143,166,173]

In the postabsorptive state, when the insulin concentration is low, muscle and adipose tissue, although they represent about 60% of the body weight, consume only approximately 167 μmol (30 mg) of glucose per minute (i.e., barely 20% of whole body glucose uptake).[31,47,173] However, in the fed state, when insulin secretion is stimulated, they greatly increase their glucose uptake, even though the glucose concentration rises no more than 30% to 40%.[47,68,105,106,116,176] From a quantitative standpoint, skeletal muscle has the greater impact on whole body glucose economy, accounting for 60% to 70% of glucose disposal in the fed state. Adipose tissue, although sensitive to insulin, plays a minor part in overall glucose utilization.[13] This should not be surprising, because the fat-free cytoplasm (i.e., the glucose-metabolizing mass) of adipose tissue is only 0.7 to 0.8 kg, much less than the 28 kg of muscle mass in a 70-kg person.

In summary, we have outlined two opposite situations: In the glucose-dependent organs (brain and RBCs), utilization is fixed and constant and a readily available source of glucose must be present to match utilization; in the insulin-dependent organs, availability is phasic and independently determined, and utilization must be regulated by insulin to match availability.

A third organ involved in the disposal of the carbohydrate excess is the liver itself. Of the three major monosaccharides normally present in the diet, fructose and galactose are taken up so avidly by the liver that only negligible quantities are presented to the peripheral tissues for metabolism. On the contrary, only a fraction (<30%; see below) of a glucose meal is metabolized by the liver.[68,106,116,177] The factors regulating liver glucose uptake have proved difficult to investigate in humans. At our present state of knowledge, it seems possible to state that hyperglycemia stimulates liver glucose uptake in an approximately linear fashion, whereas hyperinsulinemia has little or no effect at all during intravenous glucose administration.[48,49,65,70] On these grounds, if one assumes that the hepatic fractional glucose extraction measured in the postabsorptive state (3.6%) remains unchanged during the day, an average 70-kg person eating a 2200-kcal/50% carbohydrate diet between 8 A.M. and midnight would have a net hepatic glycogen accrual of at most 12.9 g.[106,117,177] Conversely, between midnight and 8 A.M., hepatic glycogen has a net negative balance of at least 26.9 g. After approximately 1 week, liver glycogen stores would be completely depleted. Clearly, factors other than insulin and glucose may have an important role.

Several studies of animals have provided compelling evidence that the route of administration of glucose may have a significant impact on hepatic glucose disposal. If the gut (portal vein) is the site of glucose administration (entry), hepatic glucose uptake is enhanced, both in the presence and in the absence of hyperinsulinemia. Studies have indicated that a positive portal-arterial glucose gradient is responsible for the greater hepatic glucose uptake observed with oral versus intravenous glucose administration.[1,2,103]

In humans, earlier studies provided evidence

in favor of a putative gut factor, which for the same levels of glucose and insulin concentrations would magnify hepatic glucose uptake if the load were administered enterally rather than parenterally.[48] Identification of the gut factor, however, has been elusive.[10] Furthermore, in humans, precise quantitation of the contribution of the gut factor to liver glucose uptake has never been made. The experimental evidence obtained in dogs speaks clearly in favor of a portal factor and is now compelling.[1,2,103] Its existence in humans needs still to be proved and its quantitative role measured.

Another factor that might explain the discrepancy between hepatic glucose uptake and glycogen breakdown over 24 hours is the possibility that in the fed state, glycogen may be formed starting from three-carbon precursors (lactate-alanine) through the gluconeogenic pathway.[146] This route that channels carbon skeletons into glycogen has been named the *indirect pathway*, as opposed to the *direct pathway*, which goes from glucose to glucose-6-phosphate to uridine diphosphate (UDP)-glucose to glycogen.[123,151] Extensive evidence has been provided that the indirect pathway is operative in rats[151,152,200] and, in specific dietary states, can account for more than 50% of liver glycogen accrual.[200] In humans, the experimental data are much less abundant and conclusive, because the investigators generally have been able to set only an upper boundary for the direct pathway and a lower boundary for the indirect pathway.[63,139,140] In one study, these limitations were circumvented by an ingenious multi-isotope technique and the relative proportions of the direct and indirect pathways in accounting for total hepatic glycogen synthesis were calculated. In the most common dietary state, the direct pathway has the dominant role in humans, accounting for 69% of glycogen synthesis in the liver.[199]

A third class of organs, which include the liver and pancreatic beta cells, can be defined as glucose sensors. Although this function is readily appreciated for beta cells, whose insulin secretion is finely regulated by the ambient glucose concentration,[15,33,51,94] it is commonly overlooked that hepatic glucose production also is influenced by the plasma glucose level. Indeed,

hyperglycemia *per se* has an inhibitory effect on liver glucose output.[129] Conversely, during profound insulin-induced hypoglycemia, the liver delivers glucose to the circulation even in the absence of any hormonal counterregulatory signal (liver autoregulation).[20]

Therefore, both beta cells and the liver perceive glucose concentration as an input and deliver an appropriate output, insulin and glucose, respectively, according to their specialized function. For both organs, the output also is self-regulatory, because hyperinsulinemia inhibits insulin secretion[55] and hyperglycemia inhibits glucose production.[129] Moreover, the output of each organ modulates the output of the other organ. Insulin inhibits hepatic glucose output[22,29,91,172]; glucose stimulates the output of insulin by the beta cell.[15,33,51,94]

A caveat that should be borne in mind is that in this qualitative description, little regard has been given to the hierarchy of the different signals. For instance, in the liver, during insulin-induced hypoglycemia, very low glucose levels must be reached before the glucose signal can "escape" and override the insulin signal, thereby stimulating hepatic glucose output.[20] As a general rule, the hormonal regulation (insulin and insulin-antagonist hormones) has a much greater influence than the glucose-mediated regulation on liver glucose output. Moreover, in normal life, glucose concentration varies within a relatively narrow range, thus dictating that the role of glucose in turning on and off hepatic glucose production must be minor when compared with insulin.

A fourth class of organs, the gut and the kidneys, also have an essential role in normal glucose homeostasis. These organs mediate the entry (gut) or re-entry (kidney) of glucose into the internal milieu. Owing to their remarkable ability to absorb (or reabsorb) completely and to transfer glucose to the circulation, these organs could be described as "glucovorous." The task of the gut is to completely absorb the glucose that is present in the diet with extreme efficiency, because under normal circumstances all the glucose present in a meal is absorbed in the first 100 cm distal to the pylorus. The task of the kidneys is to completely reabsorb all of the glucose that is present in the glomerular ultrafiltrate, a load of about 1240 g/day.

Two important points need emphasis: First, only the gut provides a net supply of new glucose to the body. Second, above a plasma glucose concentration of approximately 10 mmol/liter (180 mg/dl), the kidneys do not reabsorb all of the filtered glucose and function as an effective "sink," protecting the body and the brain in particular from the deleterious effects of hyperglycemia.[89,145,146]

Glucose Homeostasis in the Postabsorptive and Fed States

By synthesizing all of this information, a global, integrated picture of glucose metabolism can be formulated. In the postabsorptive state, the glucose-dependent organs impose an obligatory rate of glucose utilization by the body and dictate that plasma glucose concentration be maintained above a minimal level of approximately 3.6 mmol/liter (65 mg/dl). A glucose sensor, the liver, provides the glucose input necessary to maintain the fasting plasma glucose between 3.9 and 5 mmol/liter (70 to 90 mg/dl), while the other glucose sensor, the beta cells, maintains a minimal rate of glucose metabolism by the insulin-dependent organs. During the fed state, a glucovorous organ, the gut, supplies the body with a net addition of glucose. Beta cells, glucose sensors, regulate the metabolism of the insulin-dependent organs by increasing their rate of glucose utilization to precisely dispose of the glucose that is in excess of the immediate needs of the glucose-dependent organs and of the liver glucose uptake. At the same time, hyperinsulinemia restrains the hepatic glucose production. In both the fed and postabsorptive state, the other glucovorous organs, the kidneys, salvage all the glucose present in the renal ultrafiltrate.

Biochemical Correlates of Organ Specialization

Despite their apparent diversity, the four different classes of organs described earlier share a single common function. All of them transfer glucose in an irreversible net fashion from one physioanatomical space to another. In the glucose-dependent (brain and RBCs) and insulin-dependent (muscle and adipose tissue) organs, as well as in the glucose sensors (beta cells and liver), glucose is transferred from the extracellular space to the intracellular hexose-phosphate pool by transmembrane transport and phosphorylation. In the liver, during the postabsorptive state, this sequence is reversed and substituted with dephosphorylation of glucose-6-phosphate by glucose-6-phosphatase and net transport of free glucose outside the cell through a glucose transporter. In the glucovorous organs (gut and kidneys), this sequence is substituted by glucose transport from the lumen to the cell (mucosal membrane) to the interstitial fluid (basolateral membrane).

A number of different glucose carrier proteins have now been identified and their tissue distribution characterized.[12,34,72,81,107,114,136,150,216] It should be emphasized that each different glucose carrier protein possesses a unique molecular structure that corresponds to a specific functional behavior. This wealth of information can be combined with the current notions on the tissue distribution of the hexokinase isozymes.[39,137,138,154,196] Table 40-1 lists for each class of organs the protein carrier and the hexokinase that are most abundant and responsible for the net transfer of glucose (carrier-enzyme or symporter-carrier). There is a close correspondence between our descriptive macroscopic classification and the biochemical functional couple of proteins (glucose carrier and hexokinase) present in each organ class. For instance, the glucose-dependent organs are characterized by the couple Glut 1-hexokinase I, whereas in the glucose sensors the couple Glut 2-hexokinase IV (glucokinase) predominates.

It is tempting to speculate that the expression of the individual glucose carrier protein and hexokinase is linked and that the functional protein couple is, to a large extent, responsible for the functional specialization of each organ. If this proposition were to receive experimental validation in the future, a corollary of it would be that if a specific organ displays an abnormal functional behavior, its specific functional protein couple should be affected to a relevant extent.

TABLE 40-1

Protein Carriers and Hexokinases Responsible for Net Transfer of Glucose

Organ	Proposed Class	Protein Carrier	Hexokinase Coupler
Brain	Glucose dependent	Glut 1 (and 3)	HK I
Erythrocyte	Glucose dependent	Glut 1	HK I
Adipose tissue	Insulin dependent	Glut 4 (and 1)	HK II
Skeletal muscle	Insulin dependent	Glut 4 (and 1)	HK II
Liver	Glucose sensor	Glut 2	HK IV$_L$
Beta cell	Glucose sensor	Glut 2	HK IV$_P$
Gut	Glucovorous	Symporter—Glut 3 (Glut 2 and 5)	
Kidney	Glucovorous	Symporter—Glut 3 (Glut 2 and 5)	

The Roman numeral indicates the isozyme class, and the subscripts L and P define the subspecies of hexokinase (HK) typical of liver and pancreatic beta cell, respectively. Symporter indicates the Na$^+$-glucose symporter.

INSULIN ACTION AND SECRETION IN OBESITY AND TYPE II DIABETES

Insulin Resistance: Definition

The organ classification that we proposed earlier should allow classification of any disorder of glucose metabolism as a pathologic process that affects one or more of the specific organ classes and, in all likelihood, the particular biochemical machinery that serves the typical function of that organ.

Obesity and diabetes share the characteristic of insulin resistance,[180] but diabetes adds to it the presence of overt hyperglycemia, (i.e., the breakage of normal glucose homeostasis).[46]

Insulin resistance can be operatively defined as a less than expected biologic response to the hormone. It follows from this definition that there can be as many cellular insulin resistances as there are biologic effects of the hormone, including also lipid and amino acid metabolism. From the standpoint of organ physiology, there can be as many insulin resistances as there are organs that the hormone is able to influence. Within the context of insulin-stimulated glucose metabolism, however, our attention should focus on the insulin-dependent organs (especially skeletal muscle) and on the liver, because the liver

is the only site of the endogenous glucose production.

On the other hand, the presence of hyperglycemia calls our attention to any organ whose functional alteration can potentially disrupt glucose homeostasis. In NIDDM, the functions of the glucose-dependent (brain and RBCs) and of the glucovorous (gut and kidneys) organs are preserved and unaltered by the disease. In particular, this leads us to focus on the pancreatic beta cells as an important pathogenic factor in the development of hyperglycemia.

The Oral Glucose Load: An Overlooked Lesson

Despite its simplicity, the oral glucose load, if carried out in obese and nonobese subjects (Table 40-2) who are matched for their degree of glucose tolerance (Fig. 40-1), reveals that (1) for the same degree of glucose tolerance, obesity is associated with postprandial hyperinsulinemia, irrespective of the presence of diabetes; and that (2) for the same degree of obesity, overt type II diabetes mellitus is characterized by postprandial hypoinsulinemia (see Fig. 40-1).

Hyperinsulinemia in the presence of comparable ambient glucose concentration is a character-

TABLE 40-2

The Oral Glucose Load

	Lean	Obese	Lean NIDD	Obese NIDD
N (Females/males)	14 (9/5)	17 (8/9)	8 (5/3)	8 (5/3)
Age (years)	48 ± 5	53 ± 3	62 ± 2	57 ± 2
Body weight (kg)	68 ± 2	90 ± 3*	69 ± 4	87 ± 4
Lean body mass (kg)	50 ± 3	56 ± 3	52 ± 4	54 ± 3
Fat mass (kg)	25 ± 2	38 ± 2*	26 ± 2	38 ± 3*
BMI (kg/sm)	23 ± .6	31 ± 1	23 ± .8	33 ± 1.3
FPG (mg/dl)	88 ± 2	90 ± 2	171 ± 18*	164 ± 11*
FPI (mU/l)	8 ± 1	14 ± 2*	8 ± 1	19 ± 4*

*Characteristics of the study population relative to the data presented in Figures 40-1, 40-4, and 40-7.

istic marker of and (presumably) a compensatory mechanism for insulin resistance.

Hypoinsulinemia in the presence of an increased ambient glucose concentration points out that a beta-cell defect plays a major part in sustaining the hyperglycemia.

Thus, the following scenario emerges: Obesity affects the response of target organs to insulin, whereas diabetes strikes the ability of the pilot gland (glucose sensor) to cope with a glucose challenge. It is therefore evident that NIDDM is a disease that impairs the function of at

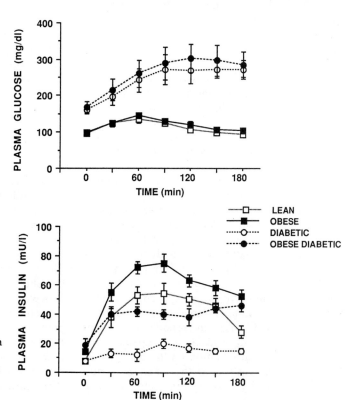

FIGURE 40-1

Plasma glucose (*upper panel*) and insulin (*lower panel*) concentrations in the lean normotolerant, obese normotolerant, lean diabetic, and obese diabetic subjects described in Table 40-2.

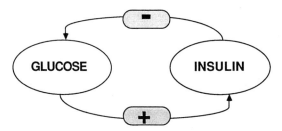

FIGURE 40-2

The homeostatic loop that links plasma glucose and plasma insulin. Insulin causes a decrease in plasma glucose; glucose is a secretagogue for insulin.

least one of the glucose sensors, the beta cells.[28,33,90,94,99,171,226]

Surprisingly, the standard interpretation of the oral glucose load segregates the two entities (obesity and diabetes) from a metabolic viewpoint and strongly suggests that in the passage from normal to abnormal glucose tolerance, an important role must be attributed to a beta-cell failure.[46,171,226] In humans, however, the clinical and epidemiologic overlap between the two syndromes remains relatively unexplained. Investigation of the complex interplay between obesity and diabetes, therefore, warrants the use of more sophisticated technologies than the standard oral glucose load, during which the system glucose-insulin works as an effective, homeostatic closed loop (Fig. 40-2). Only by experimentally breaking the insulin-glucose feedback system can one examine the individual contributions of insulin secretion and insulin sensitivity and delineate the specific metabolic features of diabetes and obesity. To the unwary reader, suffice it to say that in humans the standard tool used to transform the insulin-glucose system into an open-loop structure is the so-called clamp technique, by which an investigator can fix both the insulin and glucose concentrations at a predetermined level and measure the metabolic responses of the body to a constant glycemic or hyperinsulinemic stimulus. The technique also allows one to measure the pancreatic insulin response to a fixed hyperglycemic stimulus.[51] In this chapter, we primarily focus our attention on the biologic effects caused by insulin in the body. Such response is typically multifactorial and involves many various biochemical events in different organs. As outlined earlier, two of these are important target organs for insulin action and are relevant to the whole body glucose homeostasis: the liver, on the supply side, and the skeletal muscle, on the removal side. A concise discussion is also devoted to some specific features of insulin secretion in obesity and NIDDM.

The Liver

It was previously held that the liver is insulin resistant in obesity but not in type II diabetes mellitus. More detailed studies performed in our laboratory using the insulin clamp technique have shown that in the low range of insulin concentrations, lean NIDD subjects show a defective hepatic response to insulin, manifesting itself as excessive glucose output from the liver in the presence of hyperinsulinemia.[91] An analogous defect has been documented in obesity.[22]

Hepatic insulin resistance is of special importance in diabetic subjects,[29] who differ from normotolerant obese people in that they do not secrete enough insulin to maintain normal glucose homeostasis. When fasting plasma glucose concentrations exceed 11 mmol/liter (200 mg/dl), NIDD patients as a rule have abnormally increased glucose output from the liver in the postabsorptive state, and this increase has a key role in perpetuating the hyperglycemia.[46] Two biochemical pathways sustain hepatic glucose production: glycogenolysis and gluconeogenesis. As shown in Figure 40-3, Consoli and colleagues, using an elegant and ingenious isotopic technique,[40] have measured gluconeogenesis in humans and shown that the excess of hepatic glucose production observed in diabetic patients is almost entirely accounted for by increased rate of gluconeogenesis.[41] Such results are consistent with previous data, showing that in nonketotic diabetic patients the net splanchnic, and presumably liver, uptake of gluconeogenic precursors was increased.[222]

An increased flux through the gluconeogenetic pathway can be due to increased supply of three-carbon precursors for glucose synthesis or increased efficiency in the conversion of three-carbon compounds to glucose within the liver. If the former hypothesis were true, one should

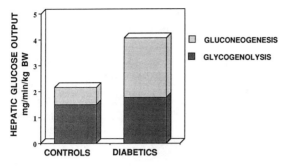

FIGURE 40-3

Components (glycogenolysis and gluconeogenesis of hepatic glucose output in controls and type II diabetic persons. (Consoli A, Nurjhan N, Capani F et al: Predominant role of gluconeogenesis in increased hepatic glucose production in NIDDM. Diabetes 38:550, 1989)

observe in diabetic patients an augmented output of lactate/alanine from the peripheral tissues (skeletal muscle). If the latter hypothesis were true, one should observe in diabetic patients an increased fractional conversion of three-carbon compounds to glucose. Studies have shown that both pathogenetic mechanisms are operative in NIDD subjects.[30,155,156] It seems reasonable to postulate that the same mechanism responsible for increased hepatic glucose output in the basal state is also responsible for hepatic insulin resistance in NIDDM—namely, that increased rate of gluconeogenesis underlies the excessive hepatic glucose production during hyperinsulinemia.[29,91] It should be noted, however, that gluconeogenesis has never been measured in diabetic persons during low-dose insulin clamp studies.

Much less information is available about which biochemical pathway is responsible for hepatic insulin resistance in normotolerant obese subjects. Based on the general concept that gluconeogenesis is less insulin sensitive than glycogenolysis even in normal humans,[79] a reasonable working hypothesis is that gluconeogenesis is the main abnormality responsible for hepatic insulin resistance in obesity. In support of this hypothesis, in an earlier study using the splanchnic balance technique, it was shown that splanchnic (liver) uptake of gluconeogenic precursors is increased in obesity and that during a

low-rate glucose infusion that caused a mild rise in insulin concentration, net splanchnic glucose output and uptake of gluconeogenic precursors were greater in the obese than in the control subjects.[64]

Hyperinsulinemia in the normal daily life fully compensates for the hepatic insulin resistance observed in obese subjects in the postabsorptive state.[170] Whether hyperinsulinemia also can completely offset the decrease in hepatic sensitivity to insulin in the fed state is still unknown, because no tracer studies of glucose dynamics after a meal have been performed in obese subjects.

A hotly debated issue is whether obesity worsens the hepatic insulin resistance already found in diabetes. Stated otherwise, is the liver of the obese diabetic patients more insulin resistant than the liver of the lean diabetics? In Figure 40-4 we present our personal data retrieved from the study population described in Table 40-2, and it can be easily appreciated that this is indeed the case. These observations are in agreement with the data published by other groups.[100,119]

Thus, there is a spectrum of liver derangements in hepatic insulin resistance in which opposite extremes are represented by lean normotolerant individuals and obese diabetic persons; normotolerant obese subjects and the lean diabetic individuals occupy an intermediate position.

Earlier in this chapter we highlighted the point that the liver can be thought of as a glucose sensor and that included among the regulators of hepatic glucose output is the ambient glucose concentration. A question that logically follows from this is whether the liver is "blind" to glucose in obesity or diabetes in analogy to what occurs to the beta cell in diabetes. This is not an easy question to answer. To better clarify the potential conundrum that we are faced with, let us assume for a moment what the hepatic response would be if there were normal insulin sensitivity but an abnormal (decreased) glucose-restraining effect on liver glucose output. For the same insulin/glucose levels, more glucose would be delivered to the circulation by the liver. This is the kind of result that is obtained during a classic insulin clamp experiment, and it is tradi-

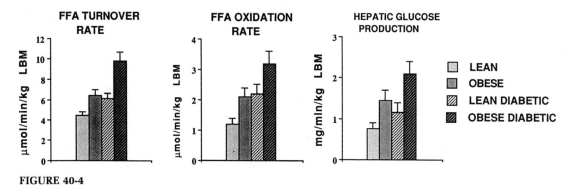

FIGURE 40-4

Plasma FFA fluxes and hepatic glucose production in the study population described in Table 40-2 at a plasma insulin concentration of 25 mU/liter and euglycemia. All three parameters are greater in obese normotolerant individuals and in lean diabetic persons than in lean controls. Obese diabetic individuals display greater fluxes than the other three groups.

tionally considered indicative of insulin resistance; strictly speaking, however, one cannot differentiate the specific contributions of glucose and insulin in the pathogenesis of an abnormal hepatic response. The only way to answer this question is to perform the experiment in the complete absence of either insulin or glucose and to examine the effects of increasing levels of the other parameter on liver glucose output. Obviously, in an intact organism only the former possibility (absence of insulin) can be pursued, by suppressing insulin secretion with either somatostatin or galanin. Such a study has actually been performed in controls and NIDD subjects, but because the focus was on the effects of hyperglycemia and insulinopenia on whole body glucose disposal, the data relative to hepatic glucose production were not reported.[7]

The liver contributes to the maintenance of normal glucose tolerance in two ways. First, as discussed earlier, the liver must respond to the combined effects of hyperinsulinemia and hyperglycemia and suppress the endogenous production of glucose. Second, during a meal, not only must the liver shut off its glucose production, but it must take up and dispose of the dietary glucose by converting it to its storage form of glycogen.[68,106,116,139,140,174,175,177,199] By using a double tracer technique, several groups have shown that during an oral glucose load, the

suppression of hepatic glucose production is less complete in NIDDM, and this abnormality plays an important part in determining postmeal glucose intolerance.[69,71] Similar studies have yet to be performed on obese subjects.

The glucose-storing function of the liver is very difficult to quantitate in humans because it is necessary to measure the glucose balance between the portal vein and the hepatic veins or, alternatively, perform serial liver biopsies to quantitate the increase over time of hepatic glycogen content. These technical as well as ethical difficulties justify the paucity of the existing data. Therefore, the possibility should be kept in mind that owing to the limits of our current techniques, we may underestimate the true impact that the liver has on postmeal hyperglycemia in diabetes.

Skeletal Muscle

Within the physiologic range of plasma insulin concentration, both obesity and NIDDM are characterized by decreased whole body glucose uptake.[180] Because under these experimental conditions approximately 70% to 80% of glucose is metabolized in skeletal muscle, it follows that skeletal muscle, an insulin-dependent organ, must be insulin resistant in both obesity and NIDDM. These extrapolations have been con-

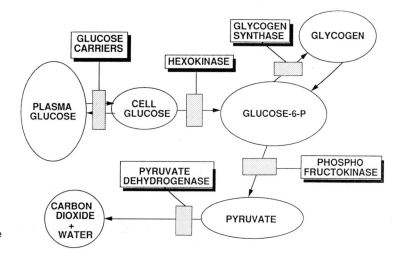

FIGURE 40-5

Potential pacemakers of glucose metabolism in skeletal muscle.

firmed by studies in which limb (forearm or leg) glucose uptake has been measured directly under both euglycemia and hyperinsulinemia.[31,49,122,173] It should be noted that under these experimental conditions of constant glycemia, glucose uptake equals (and is a measure of) glucose phosphorylation. In Figure 40-5, the biochemical steps that can potentially influence glucose metabolism in skeletal muscle are presented.

As outlined earlier in this chapter, the net, irreversible removal (phosphorylation) of glucose from the extracellular pool by the insulin-dependent organs is served by the functional couple Glut 4-hexokinase II. It is therefore reasonable to hypothesize that if phosphorylation is impaired, one or both components of the functional couple should display a decreased response to insulin. This conceptual background has given momentum to a proliferation of investigations about glucose transport in normal humans and in various insulin-resistant states. Because of technical difficulties in examining glucose transport in muscle, most studies have been performed on adipocytes.[17,35,36,73,74,83,111,112,166,237] However, one study has examined glucose transport *in vitro* in a skeletal muscle preparation from morbidly obese individuals with and without NIDDM. Glucose transport was found to be resistant to insulin in both obese normotolerant and obese diabetic subjects.[53] In order to study glucose transport *in vivo*

in muscle, we developed a multiple tracer technique for the quantitation of transmembrane glucose transport in the forearm skeletal muscle and have demonstrated that glucose transport is markedly resistant to the action of insulin in lean NIDD patients under conditions of both euglycemia and hyperinsulinemia.[22]

The insulin-mediated stimulation of glucose transport in the insulin-dependent tissues is mechanistically caused by the translocation of Glut 4 carriers from an intracellular (microsomal) pool to the plasma membrane and by an increased intrinsic activity of the transporter.[5,43,109,110,212,217] Several studies have examined the possibility that in skeletal muscle of NIDD patients the transcription or the translation of the genetic message encoding the Glut 4 protein is decreased. In contrast to what had been found in animal models of insulinopenic diabetes,[9,82,205] no changes in the specific mRNA or Glut 4 protein content have been detected in obese and NIDD patients.[92,95,165] Therefore, other possibilities should be taken into consideration to explain the decrease in glucose transport in skeletal muscle.

Thus far the activity of hexokinase II in insulin-resistant syndromes has received very little attention. After glucose has entered the cell and been phosphorylated, two main metabolic fates are available (Figure 40-6): irreversible loss through either oxidation to carbon dioxide/water

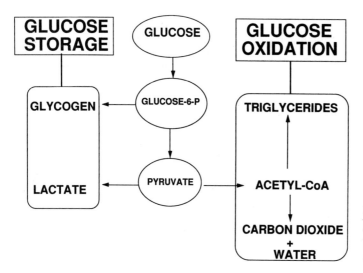

FIGURE 40-6

Glucose metabolic fluxes as measured by the combination of the tracer glucose and indirect calorimetry techniques.

or through conversion to lipids; or "storage" as glycogen or three-carbon compounds (*i.e.*, nonoxidative glucose disposal). Each biochemical pathway, if impaired, would cause a buildup of glucose-6-phosphate, the product of the hexokinase reaction, and this increase would in turn decrease hexokinase activity and limit glucose phosphorylation rate. Both the oxidative and nonoxidative pathways of glucose disposal can be quantitated by indirect calorimetry, both at the whole body and at the regional (limb) level.[66,75] As shown in Figure 40-7, both obese and NIDD subjects display insulin resistance in both the oxidative and nonoxidative routes of glucose metabolism. These results are in agreement with previously published studies.[14,61,62,91,130,131] As was previously described for hepatic glucose production, we can define a spectrum of insulin resistance for muscle glucose uptake. At the two extremes lie lean normotolerant individuals and obese diabetic persons with obese nondiabetic persons and lean diabetic subjects in between.

As stated before, the ability of insulin to stimulate both glucose oxidation and glucose storage is impaired in obesity and NIDDM: At high insulin concentrations, when glucose metabolism is enhanced, glucose storage (*i.e.*, glycogen formation) plays the dominant part in accounting for insulin resistance.[131] Furthermore, by using nuclear magnetic spectroscopy, Shulman and colleagues

have shown that glycogen synthesis in skeletal muscle during hyperglycemia/hyperinsulinemia is depressed in NIDD patients and accounts for almost all of the defect in glucose storage as simultaneously quantitated by indirect calorimetry.[201] Similar studies have yet to be carried out on obese nondiabetic individuals.

The identification of decreased nonoxidative and oxidative fluxes has paved the way to the direct investigation of the two enzymes glycogen synthase and pyruvate dehydrogenase (PDH), which are believed to be rate limiting for glycogen synthesis (glucose storage) and glucose oxidation, respectively.[18,143] A substantial body of evidence has shown that glycogen synthase activity is defective in skeletal muscle biopsy specimens obtained from both nondiabetic obese and NIDD subjects.[57,233] Somewhat less information has been collected about PDH, but the available evidence suggests that its activity also is depressed in skeletal muscle of diabetic patients. Decreased PDH activity has also been documented in adipocytes of obese subjects.[142]

The regulation of glycogen synthase and PDH is similar in many ways. Dephosphorylation activates both enzymes, whereas phosphorylation inhibits them. For both enzymes, the degree of phosphorylation is under the control of a system of specific kinase(s)/phosphatase(s). For both, cell exposure to insulin causes dephosphorylation and covalent activation of the en-

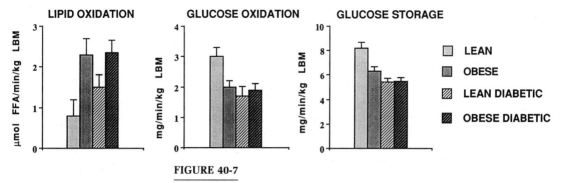

FIGURE 40-7

Lipid oxidation, glucose oxidation, and glucose storage in the study population described in Table 40-2, at a plasma insulin concentration of 200 mU/liter and euglycemia. Lipid oxidation is greater in the obese individuals than in the lean normotolerant controls. Glucose fluxes are uniformly decreased in the obese and diabetic individuals.

zyme.[37,38,101,159,164,231] Because nonoxidative glucose disposal (*i.e.*, glycogen formation) has been shown to be impaired in obesity and NIDDM, several investigators have turned their attention to the study of the regulation of glycogen synthase in skeletal muscle. The protein phosphatase activity specific for glycogen synthase has been studied in muscle biopsy samples and found to be defective in obesity.[76,115] The protein phosphatase has not yet been examined in NIDDM. Very little is known about the PDH kinase/phosphatase system in the muscle of either obese or diabetic people.

An additional mechanism of cellular insulin resistance has been searched in the muscle fiber composition. It is well known that type 1 (slow-twitch oxidative) fibers are markedly more sensitive to insulin action than type 2B (fast-twitch glycolytic) fibers. An increased proportion of type 2B fibers could, therefore, induce a state of insulin resistance.[134,135] In insulin-resistant Pima Indians, the proportion of type 2B fibers was, indeed, increased, and the percent of type 1 fibers was decreased. Both proportions were significantly correlated with the whole body insulin-mediated glucose metabolism, although the association was somewhat weaker than one would expect for a primary factor of insulin resistance.[133] Clearly, more studies are needed to clarify the exact role of muscle fiber composition in determining insulin sensitivity.

In summary, defects in at least three potential rate-limiting steps for glucose metabolism (see Fig. 40-5) have been identified in both obesity and diabetes: glucose transport, glycogen synthase, and PDH. It is noteworthy that glucose transport lies proximally in the sequence to glycogen synthase and PDH, whereas glycogen synthase and PDH are distal to glucose transport but parallel to each other. In such a situation, it is an intricate matter to establish which defect, if any, is primary or, alternatively, whether all defects are necessary for the full expression of insulin resistance in skeletal muscle. Moreover, the diversity of these cellular defects raises the possibility that diabetes and obesity are characterized by a defective metabolic network. This could result from multiple distinct metabolic loci of insulin resistance in skeletal muscle. Alternatively, a very early and proximal step (e.g., transduction of the signal after insulin binds to its own receptor) in the cascade of events triggered by insulin could be abnormal and lead to impaired activation of glucose transport and the glucose-metabolizing enzymes.[32,78,204,213]

The studies discussed earlier reflect the basic assumption that the causes of insulin resistance are to be sought in skeletal muscle at the level of the myocyte. In the past few years, some investigators have explored the possibility that important correlates (and perhaps causes) of insulin resistance may be found in the characteristics of the connective tissue present in skeletal muscle.

Of the multiple functions performed by connective tissue in skeletal muscle, the one that is germane to our topic is the delivery of substrates and hormones, in particular glucose and insulin, to the cell surface. The amount of glucose supplied to the skeletal muscle equals the arterial glucose concentration multiplied by the blood flow. It has long been held that changes in blood flow do not affect the amount of glucose metabolized in muscle, the latter being determined essentially by cellular metabolic activity. Data have now provided evidence that at high physiologic insulin concentrations, leg blood flow covaries with the metabolic response of the leg to insulin—that is, a stimulation of glucose uptake is accompanied by increased blood flow. In several insulin-resistant states, including obesity, the ability of insulin to increase leg blood flow has been shown to be markedly impaired, and this has been suggested to account for more than half of the insulin resistance.[121,122] Whether the decrease in blood flow is an epiphenomenon that results from insulin resistance or whether it has true pathophysiologic relevance, in that the decreased blood flow limits glucose disposal, is not known at present.

A possible anatomical counterpart of decreased muscular blood flow in insulin-resistant states may be the observation that impaired insulin action in obesity is associated with decreased capillary density in skeletal muscle.[133] This phenomenon would delay the diffusion-mediated transfer of substrate and hormones to the cell and impose steeper gradients in the interstitial fluid, resulting in decreased glucose concentrations at the cell surface. Moreover, fewer capillaries per unit of tissue weight also mean less surface area available for exchange. Both factors would concur to cause a lower insulin concentration at the surface of the target cell, as suggested by earlier kinetic studies.[102,198] The endothelial barrier itself has been proposed as a possible rate-limiting step of insulin action in peripheral tissues. In this scheme, impaired insulin diffusion out of the vascular bed would decrease the interstitial insulin concentration to which the cell is exposed, leading to a diminution of the biologic response to the hormone.[235] Although these studies are far from conclusive, they have the merit of reminding us that an organ is more than just the sum of the cells that compose it and that its global metabolic response can be influenced by factors other than cellular biochemical events.

Insulin Secretion in Obesity and Type II Diabetes

Since the early 1960s, it has been known that hyperinsulinemia is a characteristic feature of obesity.[55,173] Several important questions are raised as a consequence of this finding: Is hyperinsulinemia secondary to beta-cell hypersecretion or decreased clearance of circulating insulin? Does hyperinsulinemia precede or follow the onset of insulin resistance? Does hyperinsulinemia compensate for insulin resistance? Is hyperinsulinemia per se an inducer of insulin resistance?

As for the first question, a number of studies using quite heterogeneous techniques have shown that hypersecretion plays a major part in determining hyperinsulinemia in human obesity.[25,148,170,195] A measurable but less evident factor is decreased removal of the hormone across the splanchnic area, more precisely in the liver, the organ that accounts for about 80% of the body's capability of degrading insulin.[44,59,149] As for the second question, prospective studies in cohorts of subjects at high risk of becoming obese later in life should be undertaken, in order to monitor both the development of hyperinsulinemia and the concomitant insulin sensitivity by an independent standard technique to assess insulin action, like the insulin clamp. Insulin concentration is now used in epidemiologic studies as an accepted index of insulin sensitivity in glucose-tolerant subjects. This approach, by itself, precludes determining whether hyperinsulinemia predicts the future development of insulin resistance or just accompanies it.

It is inherent in the definition of simple obesity as a glucose-tolerant state that hyperinsulinemia must be able to compensate for insulin resistance and ensure normal glucose homeostasis in normal daily life, when normal glucose homeostasis means plasma glucose concentration and fluxes that are superimposable to nonobese persons. However, even in glucose-tolerant obese persons, this may not hold true under an experimental situation of an exaggerated secretory stimulus for the beta cell. We have shown that during a hyperglycemic clamp, glucose-tolerant obese subjects metabolize less glucose than lean controls despite marked hyperinsulinemia. Therefore, in relatively unphysiologic conditions, such as a 120′ hyperglycemic clamp at a glucose concentration of approximately 12 mmol/liter, it is possible to document a less than adequate hypersecretory response of the beta cells to compensate peripheral insulin resistance in glucose-tolerant obese individuals.[22]

Hyperinsulinemia has long been suspected to cause insulin resistance. The available experimental evidence, however, is far from clear. Acute studies performed in humans suggest that hyperinsulinemia can cause insulin resistance,[4,141] whereas chronic studies in rats seem to indicate that hyperinsulinemia paradoxically can increase insulin sensitivity.[218,227] At this time, therefore, this debate is far from settled.

Insulin secretion in human NIDDM is a complex function. Earlier studies provided the entire spectrum of possible answers to the question: What is insulin secretion like in NIDD patients[60]? These findings have led investigators to realize that insulin secretion in NIDDM is truly heterogeneous and that several factors (e.g., obesity, duration of the disease, degree of metabolic control) underlie this heterogeneity. More carefully conducted studies have documented that the beta-cell secretory capacity for both glucose and nonglucose secretagogues is decreased in NIDD individuals.[33,94,171,181,219,225,226,229] Moreover, there is some evidence that beta-cell mass also is decreased by about 30% to 40% in NIDDM. This beta-cell loss is not sufficient per se to explain the breakage of glucose homeostasis, however, and an additional specific defect of beta cells needs to be postulated in NIDDM.[27,192,228,230] Interestingly, in relatives of NIDD patients, who are at high risk for developing the disease later in life, subtle defects in insulin secretion that have been found may be an index of a specific functional abnormality.[162] This finding also points out that the beta cells can have an important pathogenetic role in the development of NIDDM. Further details on this topic are given in a subsequent section.

OBESITY: FROM INSULIN RESISTANCE TO TYPE II DIABETES

Insulin Resistance and Development of Type II Diabetes

Obesity and diabetes appear to affect muscle glucose metabolism in a strikingly similar fashion. Nonetheless, most of the available evidence leans toward the additivity (although to a partial degree) of the two syndromes in determining insulin resistance.[46,180] This phenomenon can be due to exceedingly increased risk of developing diabetes in that subset of the obese normotolerant population characterized by the most severe degree of insulin resistance, the exacerbation of insulin resistance during the natural history preceding and following the onset of the overt disease, and a combination of these possibilities.

In Pima Indians, Nauruans, and Mexican Americans, hyperinsulinemia, an accepted marker for insulin resistance, is a strong predictor of the development of diabetes.[97,202] This evidence is still lacking for Caucasians. However, Caucasian subjects with a positive family history of NIDDM and therefore at high risk for developing the disease later in life have been reported to be insulin resistant, even when studied in a phase of preserved glucose tolerance.[56] Similar evidence has been found in Mexican Americans.[93] These data support the hypothesis that no further significant deterioration of insulin sensitivity occurs when an individual passes from normal glucose tolerance to NIDDM. Rather, beta-cell failure appears to be the key event that causes the emergence of hyperglycemia.

Although this body of evidence indicates that deterioration of beta-cell function may play a pivotal part in the emergence of NIDDM, a role for progressive deterioration of insulin sensitivity cannot be ruled out.

In the next two sections, we discuss two potential factors that are capable of inducing a progressive impairment in insulin sensitivity.

Free Fatty Acids: A Metabolic Antagonist

Circulating free fatty acids (FFA) have been the object of thorough investigation in the past de-

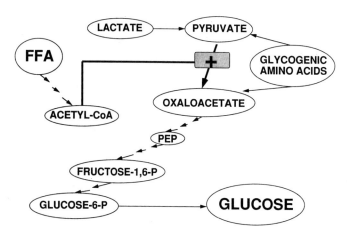

FIGURE 40-8

Operation of Randle's cycle in the liver. Increased FFA supply/oxidation leads to a buildup in acetyl-CoA, which in turn stimulates pyruvate carboxylase to form oxaloacetate from pyruvate in the first committed step of gluconeogenesis. (PEP, phosphoenolpyruvate)

cade, because, by a substrate competition mechanism, proposed by Randle and Newsholme about 30 years ago, they can potentially increase liver glucose output and impair glucose removal by the peripheral tissues.[178,179] The putative mechanisms responsible for these FFA-mediated effects on liver and muscle are depicted in Figures 40-8 and 40-9. Briefly, a high rate of hepatic FFA oxidation would increase intracellular acetyl-CoA levels, which in turn stimulate pyruvate carboxylase, the first committed enzyme in the gluconeogenetic pathway. Therefore, gluconeogenesis, which in itself is a relatively insulin-resistant biochemical pathway, would be increased and more glucose would be supplied by the liver to the systemic circulation.[58,77,207,232] One study suggests that elevated FFA concentrations can also impair the interaction of insulin with its own receptor and some of the postbinding events involved in the transduction of the signal from the receptor to the effectors.[211] In muscle tissues, the increase in acetyl-CoA that results from high FFA oxidation, in the presence of a constant cellular energy demand, would inhibit PDH (by stimulating PDH-kinase, which induces the phosphorylation of PDH) and, as a consequence, glucose oxidation. Furthermore, the excess of acetyl-CoA would lead to an increased formation and concentration of citrate, which in turn inhibits phosphofructokinase (PFK).[179,231] The inhibition of glycolysis leads to the buildup of substrate in the hexose-phosphate pool, including glucose-6-phosphate, which is a powerful inhibi-

tor of hexokinase, and uridine diphosphoglucose (UDPG), which is the substrate for glycogen synthase. Glucose phosphorylation would eventually be directly inhibited. The same substrate, glucose-6-phosphate, that is responsible for hexokinase inhibition also is an allosteric activator of glycogen synthase, which at the same time should undergo an increased "push" action from its substrate, UDPG. Therefore, the net effect of elevated FFA on glycogen synthesis depends on the balance of these diverse and opposite effects. As a general rule, glucose oxidation should be decreased, whereas glycogen synthesis may be inhibited to a variable extent.

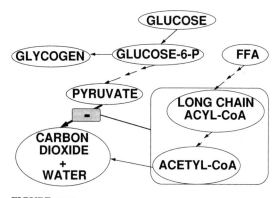

FIGURE 40-9

Operation of Randle's cycle in the skeletel muscle. Increased FFA supply/oxidation causes a buildup of long-chain acyl-CoA and acetyl-CoA, which in turn inhibit PDH and glucose oxidation.

A number of studies have shown that it is possible to induce substrate competition between FFA and glucose in humans in the peripheral tissues, during hyperinsulinemia, and that both glucose oxidation and storage, although the latter to a later time and to a lesser extent, are inhibited by an exaggerated lipid oxidation rate.[21,67,215] The effects on the liver have been documented under conditions of hypoinsulinemia and hyperglycemia.

If the substrate competition has any role in the pathogenesis of the metabolic deterioration in the peripheral tissues in patients with NIDDM, one should observe the following pattern of phenomena:

1. Increased FFA disposal/oxidation is paralleled by an increased rate of lipid oxidation.
2. Increased FFA/lipid oxidation is concomitant with and paralleled by a decrease in glucose oxidation and, possibly, in glucose storage.
3. As the glucose tolerance worsens, more and more lipids are oxidized and less and less glucose is oxidized and stored.

In nonobese diabetic persons, however, although the antilipolytic effect of insulin is impaired and increased rates of FFA disposal/oxidation can be shown, total lipid oxidation does not appear to be sufficiently elevated to account for impaired muscular glucose disposal during hyperinsulinemia (see Fig. 40-7). As a consequence, substrate competition does not seem to be a primary cause of decreased glucose metabolism.

In normotolerant obese subjects, FFA disposal/oxidation rates are increased in the lean (muscle) tissues and are paralleled by augmented total lipid oxidation. This phenomenon is particularly evident in the low range of physiologic hyperinsulinemia. At the same time, a decrease in glucose oxidation is observed. At higher insulin concentrations, glucose storage plays the dominant role in determining insulin resistance and is accompanied by increased lipid oxidation rates, despite the fact that FFA disposal/oxidation rates reach a plateau (data not shown). Therefore, in uncomplicated obesity, there are grounds to believe that increased FFA/lipid oxidation plays a part in determining insulin resistance, at least in

the glucose oxidative pathways and perhaps in glucose storage.

In obese diabetic persons there is a further decrease of glucose oxidation and storage, but it is not paralleled by a proportional increase of lipid oxidation. This experimental evidence suggests that substrate competition has relatively little to do with the further metabolic derangement that occurs when an obese normotolerant person progresses to an overtly obese diabetic individual.

Taken together, these data suggest that substrate competition might have a role in causing and sustaining peripheral (skeletal muscle) insulin resistance in uncomplicated obesity but has a minor role, if any, in mediating the metabolic derangement that characterizes overt diabetes.

The other potential interaction betweeen FFA and glucose metabolism involves the liver. If substrate competition plays a significant part in the passage from normal glucose tolerance to NIDDM, the following phenomena should be observed in NIDD patients:

1. An increased FFA disposal/oxidation.
2. The increase in FFA oxidation should be paralleled by an impairment in insulin-mediated inhibition of hepatic glucose production.
3. As glucose tolerance worsens, a parallel deterioration of hepatic insulin sensitivity and increase in FFA disposal/oxidation should take place.

As shown in Figure 40-4, this is exactly the pattern that is observed. A spectrum of hepatic insulin resistance is closely mirrored by an increasing rate of FFA disposal/oxidation.

It is important to note that both lean and obese NIDD patients have increased FFA oxidation when compared with their weight-matched normotolerant counterparts. In the obese subjects, the artificial increment of circulating FFA by Intralipid infusion causes an increase in liver glucose output even in the presence of hyperinsulinemia.[11] In NIDDM, hepatic glucose output is exaggerated, and this increase is accounted for by gluconeogenesis,[41] which represents that pathway of glucose production that is lipid sensitive, being driven by FFA oxidation. Although these data are not to be considered proof of a cause-and-effect relationship, they are entirely consistent with the possibility that FFA has a role in causing hepatic insulin resistance and contributes to the deterioration in glucose tolerance.

Glucose: A Metabolic Toxin

Since it was first proposed by Unger and Grundy a few years ago,[220] the hypothesis that hyperglycemia *per se* causes peripheral insulin resistance and impairs the ability of the beta cells to respond to a hyperglycemic stimulus (Fig. 40-10) has been substantiated by a compelling body of experimental evidence. In rats made diabetic with partial pancreatectomy, phlorhizin treatment, which restores euglycemia completely by inducing glucosuria, prevents the onset of peripheral insulin resistance[187] and beta cells' blindness to a hyperglycemic stimulus.[186] The response to other nonglucose secretagogues is either normal or paradoxically increased. The mechanism by which hyperglycemia *per se* causes insulin resistance seems to be related to down-regulation of glucose transport in the insulin-dependent tissues.[193,194] With respect to the beta cells, the *in vivo* findings closely mirror the *in vitro* results obtained in the perfused pancreas and isolated islets.[23,99,124-128,238] Importantly, the reduction of beta-cell mass is not sufficient *per se* to create the functional abnormalities of insulin secretion typical of this animal model of diabetes. Even modest hyperglycemia is *conditio sine qua non* to induce beta-cell blindness to the stimulatory effect of glucose on insulin secretion.[125]

The concept of glucose toxicity has been well documented in animal models of diabetes and in *in vitro* systems and undoubtedly in these models rests on solid ground. The available evidence in humans is somewhat less abundant.[183,236] With respect to tissue sensitivity to insulin, Yki-Jarvinen and colleagues have shown that in insulin-dependent diabetic persons, 24 hours of hyperglycemia (~16 mM) leads to a 20% decrease in insulin-mediated glucose disposal.[236] We documented a similar impairment in insulin action in healthy volunteers after only a small increment (+2.2 mM) in plasma glucose concentration for 72 hours.[52] With regard to insulin se-

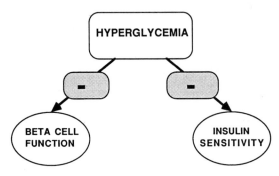

FIGURE 40-10

The postulate of glucose toxicity: Hyperglycemia impairs insulin secretion and deteriorates insulin sensitivity.

cretion, only some indirect evidence is available. It is well documented that NIDD subjects have a specific defect in the ability of the beta cells to respond to glucose, whereas the response to nonglucose stimuli is relatively intact. Effective lowering of the plasma glucose concentration, regardless of the therapy, leads to amelioration of the beta cells' ability to respond to the hyperglycemic stimuli.[46]

Despite the paucity of experimental data in humans, glucose toxicity should now be considered an important factor in any attempt to explain the pathogenesis of NIDDM. An excessive review of this issue has been published.

A Path from Obesity to Type II Diabetes

As discussed in detail earlier, a triad of metabolic disturbances characterizes obese NIDD subjects when compared with normotolerant obese individuals:

1. A decrease in glucose-stimulated insulin secretion
2. An increase in hepatic glucose production, both in the basal state and in the low range of physiologic hyperinsulinemia
3. A decrease in insulin-mediated glucose uptake

Any hypothetical pathogenetic sequence leading from obesity to NIDDM should be able to account for the generation of this metabolic-hormonal triad and be compatible with the temporal sequence of events that accompanies the onset of overt diabetes. In Pima Indians, this sequence is known in some detail[189,190] and resembles very closely the pattern of events described in a primate model of obese NIDDM.[98] According to these models of NIDDM, normotolerant obese individuals are insulin-resistant but maintain normal glucose tolerance because their beta cells are able to compensate for insulin resistance. With increasing duration or severity of obesity, there may be a further deterioration in insulin sensitivity. Nonetheless, glucose tolerance is only mildly impaired because the beta cells are able to further augment their secretion of insulin, although this increase does not completely restore glucose tolerance to normal. The next step is the development of frank diabetes mellitus. It is heralded by a decline in insulin secretion from its markedly augmented levels. Although the plasma insulin response still remains high when compared with normal-weight controls, it is insufficient to compensate completely for the insulin resistance. With time, severe glucose intolerance ensues as a result of progressive decline in insulin secretion and resultant insulinopenia.

The data that we reviewed earlier can help us to clarify further the steps underlying this chain of events. Normotolerant obese persons are insulin resistant and force their beta cells to secrete more insulin in order to compensate for insulin resistance. We have shown, however, that hyperinsulinemia in obese persons is not fully compensatory and that after a hyperglycemic stimulus, beta cells in obese persons are unable to secrete enough insulin to maintain the same glucose disposal rate as in lean controls.[22] Any event deteriorating glucose homeostasis, therefore, as a rule causes a more sustained hyperglycemia in obese persons than in normal-weight individuals. If, moreover, for either genetic or environmental reasons, a modest loss of beta-cell mass (e.g., 30% to 40%, the amount of beta-cell loss that can be documented in NIDDM) occurs, the remnant pancreas, which under normal circumstances should still be able to guarantee glucose homeostasis, in obese persons fails to maintain glucose concentration within the narrow physiologic range. Episodic hyperglycemia is

first observed, and later prolonged mild hyperglycemia. According to the glucose toxicity hypothesis, even this mild hyperglycemia further impairs insulin secretion and aggravates peripheral insulin resistance. The deterioration of insulin secretory capacity induces greater hyperglycemia but also releases the antilipolytic control on the adipose tissue. More FFA is made available for oxidation in the liver, and gluconeogenesis and total glucose output are stimulated beyond the physiologic limits. In contrast to the lean controls, in fact, the liver of normotolerant obese persons, if exposed to a lipid load, increases glucose output even in the presence of hyperinsulinemia. Therefore, slight hyperglycemia and increased FFA supply/oxidation may account for the presence of the metabolic/hormonal triad that differentiates obese NIDD patients from normotolerant obese individuals. Once started, this pathogenetic cascade (Fig. 40-11) has the potential to "feed forward" and become a vicious cycle that eventually leads to overt hyperglycemia. If these mechanisms are in fact responsible for the passage from normal glucose tolerance to NIDDM, and given their intrinsic feed-forward nature, one would expect the progression from preserved glucose tolerance to NIDDM to take place in a relatively narrow time frame. Prospective studies are needed to either confirm or disprove this conceptual scheme.

Central Distribution of Fat: A Diabetogenic Obesity?

A large body of data shows that within the wide, heterogeneous spectrum of human obesity, it is possible to identify a specific phenotype that is associated with insulin resistance and a propensity to develop NIDDM.[221] Epidemiologic studies have documented that a central pattern of fat distribution, as characterized by an increased ratio of the waist to hip circumference (W:H ratio), is a strong, independent predictor for the later development of NIDDM.[97] The W:H ratio is a compounded index of several fat depots. A high W:H ratio is dependent on both the distribution between central (abdominal) and peripheral fat, as well as the distribution within the abdominal area (i.e., intra-abdominal versus subcutaneous). The same amount of fat mass, if located within

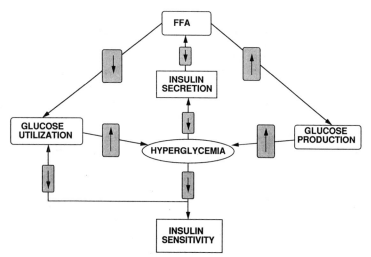

FIGURE 40-11

The pathogenetic cascade that leads to and sustains hyperglycemia in obese diabetic individuals. Hyperglycemia impairs insulin secretion and insulin sensitivity. Decreased insulin secretion causes increased FFA output, on which insulin exerts an inhibitory effect. Increased FFA levels decrease glucose utilization and stimulate glucose production. Both these effects cause greater hyperglycemia.

the abdomen (central region), contributes to a higher W:H ratio than if located in the abdominal subcutaneous depots. In one study, homozygous twins were overfed and the distribution of the newly formed fat studied by computed tomography (CT) scans. The distribution of the newly formed fat, as visualized by CT scans, was to a much larger extent influenced by some inheritable factor (i.e., by being a member of a specific pair of twins) than any other index.[26] Thus, the genome apparently plays an important part in the control of fat distribution.

A high W:H ratio has been shown to be an important correlate of glucose metabolism. Subjects with a preponderance of central fat are characterized by hepatic insulin resistance and increased FFA turnover and, presumably, oxidation[108] (Fig. 40-12). A more profound degree of insulin resistance, affecting both oxidative and nonoxidative pathways of glucose metabolism, also has been demonstrated in subjects with high W:H ratio as opposed to patients with the same fat mass but a peripheral distribution of the adipose tissue[57,117,120,169] (Fig. 40-13). Moreover,

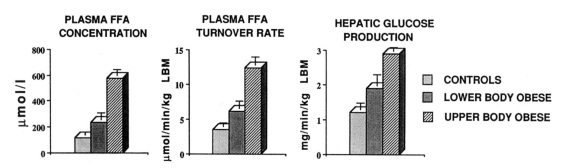

FIGURE 40-12

Plasma FFA concentration and turnover and hepatic glucose production in controls and obese individuals of different body fat distribution, at plasma insulin concentration of mU/liter and euglycemia. (Jensen MD, Haymond MW, Rizza RA et al: Influence of body fat distribution on free fatty acid metabolism in obesity. J Clin Invest 83:1168, 1989)

FIGURE 40-13

Whole body glucose disposal in controls
and obese individuals of different body
fat distribution, at plasma insulin concentration of 70 mU/liter and euglycemia. (Peiris AN, Struve MF, Mueller
RA et al: Glucose metabolism in obesity:
Influence of body fat distribution. J Clin
Endocrinol Metab 67:760, 1988)

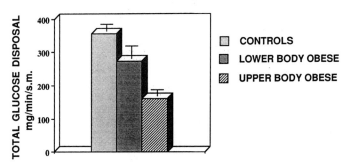

we have observed that an increase in intra-
abdominal fat, as quantitated by magnetic resonance imaging, is associated with an increased
severity of insulin resistance that affects primarily the nonoxidative metabolic pathways.[24] This
is analogous to the situation observed in the
normoglucose tolerant relatives of NIDD patients.[56,93] However, this correlation between fat
topography and insulin action was present only
within the obese subset of patients and was not
observed in lean subjects. In the lean group, total
body fat content, not fat topography, was a major
determinant of tissue sensitivity to insulin. To
the extent that nonoxidative glucose disposal can
be equated with peripheral glycogen formation,
central adiposity appears to determine or to be
associated with a defect in glycogen synthesis in
skeletal muscle. These obese subjects with a high
W:H ratio have indeed been shown to have a
decreased activity of the enzyme glycogen synthase.[57] Central obesity also is associated with
more conspicuous hyperinsulinemia, reduced
insulin clearance,[167,168] and reduced capillary
density and altered muscular fiber composition
in skeletal muscle.[133] Last but not least, increased
levels of testosterone and catecholamines,
insulin-antagonistic hormones, have also been
observed in obese subjects with a central pattern
of obesity.

In summary, a specific constellation of epidemiologic, metabolic, morphological, and hormonal features distinguish obese persons with a
central distribution of fat apart from obese individuals with a peripheral pattern of fat localization. In the pathway that we have hypothesized
from normal glucose tolerance to NIDDM, obese
persons with high W:H ratio have many pathoge-

netic factors that contribute to the disruption of
normal glucose homeostasis (high plasma FFA,
increased hepatic glucose production, peripheral
insulin resistance). Whether central obesity is
etiologically responsible for these diabetogenic
factors, whether these factors are causally related
to central obesity, or whether these diabetogenic
factors and central obesity are unrelated (i.e., this
subset of patients is "enriched" with genes that
cause or favor beta-cell failure) remains to be determined.

CONCLUSIONS

At the end of this overview of glucose metabolism in obesity and NIDDM, it is legitimate to
wonder how far we still are from unfolding and
explaining the relationship between these two
conditions and how close we are to elevating our
descriptions and observations to the level of
cause-and-effect relationships. Although much
indeed has been learned, important break-
throughs are eagerly awaited in this field. Major
difficulties obviously are present in the study of
diseases, such as obesity and NIDDM, that take
decades to fully evolve into the clinical syndrome, are highly heterogeneous, and are determined by multiple genetic and environmental
factors. Today we still are far from obtaining a
comprehensive, mechanistic understanding of
the etiology, pathogenesis, and natural history of
these two diseases.

However, among the scholars of glucose metabolism, an infectious confidence has enveloped
the field. Extensive epidemiologic projects have
moved from the cross-sectional to the prospective phase of study, and this advance should

allow investigators to select with unprecedented accuracy those groups of obese subjects who are at very high risk to develop NIDDM. The genome is no longer an inaccessible, treasured vault of mysterious knowledge; slowly, painstakingly, but steadily its secrets are beginning to be unraveled.

Although obesity and NIDDM continue to impose a high toll on Westernized societies, optimism is warranted, because researchers today have the expertise to ask the right questions and the appropriate tools to answer them.

References

1. Adkins BA, Myers SR, Hendrick GK et al: Importance of the route of intravenous glucose delivery on hepatic glucose balance in the conscious dog. J Clin Invest 79:557, 1987

2. Adkins-Marshall BA, Myers SR, Hendrick GK et al: Interaction between insulin and glucose-delivery route in regulation of net hepatic glucose uptake in conscious dogs. Diabetes 39:87, 1989

3. Andreone TL, Printz RL, Pilkis SJ et al: The amino acid sequence of rat liver glucokinase deduced from cloned cDNA. J Biol Chem 263:363, 1989

4. Baker B, Mandarino LJ, Brick B et al: Influence of changes in insulin receptor binding during insulin infusions on the shape of the insulin dose-response curve for glucose disposal in man. J Clin Endocrinol Metab 58:392, 1984

5. Baly DL, Horuk R: Dissociation of insulin-stimulated glucose transport from the translocation of glucose carriers in rat adipose cells. J Biol Chem 262:21, 1987

6. Barner AH, Eff C, Leslie RD et al: Diabetes in identical twins: A study of two pairs. Diabetologia 20:87, 1981

7. Baron AD, Kolterman OG, Bell J et al: Rates of noninsulin-mediated glucose uptake are elevated in type II diabetic subjects. J Clin Invest 76:1782, 1985

8. Baron AD, Schaeffer L, Shragg P et al: Role of hyperglucegonemia in maintenance of increased rates of hepatic glucose output in type II diabetics. Diabetes 36:274, 1987

9. Berger J, Biswas C, Vicario PP et al: Decreased expression of the insulin-responsive glucose transporter in diabetes and fasting. Nature 340:70, 1989

10. Bergman R, Bier J, Hourigan P: Intraportal glucose infusion matched to oral glucose absorption: Lack of evidence for "gut factor" involvement in hepatic glucose storage. Diabetes 31:27, 1982

11. Bevilacqua S, Bonadonna RC, Buzzigoli G et al: Acute elevation of free fatty acid levels leads to hepatic insulin resistance in obese subjects. Metabol Clin Exp 36:502, 1987

12. Birnbaum MJ: Identification of a novel gene encoding an insulin-responsive glucose transporter protein. Cell 57:305, 1989

13. Björntorp P, Sjostrom L: Carbohydrate storage in man: speculations and some quantitative considerations. Metab Clin Exp (Suppl 2)27:1853, 1978

14. Boden G, Ray TK, Smith PH et al: Carbohydrate oxidation and storage in obese non-insulin-dependent diabetic patients: Effects of improved glycemic control. Diabetes 32:982, 1983

15. Bogardus C, Lillioja S, Howard BV et al: Relationships between insulin secretion, insulin action, and fasting plasma glucose concentration in nondiabetic and non-insulin-dependent diabetic subjects. J Clin Invest 74:1238, 1984

16. Bogardus C, Lillioja S, Mott D et al: Relationship between degree of obesity and in vivo insulin action in man. Am J Physiol 248:E286, 1985

17. Bogardus C, Lillioja S, Mott D et al: Relationship between obesity and maximal insulin-stimulated glucose uptake in vivo and in vitro in Pima Indians. J Clin Invest 73:800, 1984

18. Bogardus C, Lillioja S, Stone K et al: Correlation between muscle glycogen synthase activity and in vivo insulin action in man. J Clin Invest 73:1185, 1984

19. Bolaffi JL, Heldt A, Lewis LD et al: The third phase of in vitro insulin secretion: Evidence for glucose insensitivity. Diabetes 35:370, 1986

20. Bolli G, De Feo P, Perriello G et al: Role of hepatic autoregulation in defense against hypoglycemia in humans. J Clin Invest 75:1623, 1985

21. Bonadonna RC, Zych K, Boni C et al: Time dependence of the interaction between lipid and glucose in humans. Am J Physiol 257:E49, 1989

22. Bonadonna RC, Del Prato S, Cobelli C et al: Glucose transport in skeletal muscle is insulin-resistant in type 2 diabetes. Diabetologia (Suppl) 33:A23, 1990

23. Bonner-Weir S, Trent DF, Weir GC: Partial pancreatectomy in the rat and subsequent defects in glucose-induced insulin release. J Clin Invest 71:1544, 1983

24. Bonora E, Del Prato S, Ghiatas A et al: Total body fat content and its topography exert differential effects on glucose metabolism in normal weight and obese nondiabetic women. Diabetes (Suppl 1):39:115A, 1990

25. Bonora E, Zavaroni I, Bruschi F et al: Peripheral hyperinsulinemia of simple obesity: pancreatic hypersecretion or impaired insulin metabolism? J Clin Endocrinol Metab 59:1121, 1984

26. Bouchard C, Tremblay A, Despres JP et al: The response to long-term overfeeding in identical twins. N Engl J Med 322:1477, 1990

27. Brooks JR: Operative approach to pancreatic carcinoma. Semin Oncol 6:357, 1979

28. Brunzell JD, Robertson RP, Lerner RL et al: Relationships between fasting plasma glucose levels and insulin secretion during intravenous glucose tolerance tests. J Clin Endocrinol Metab 42:222, 1976

29. Campbell PJ, Mandarino LJ, Gerich J: Quantification of the relative impairment in actions of insulin on hepatic glucose production and peripheral glucose uptake in non-insulin-dependent diabetes mellitus. Metab Clin Exp 37:15, 1988

30. Capaldo B, Napoli R, Di Bonito P et al: Glucose and gluconeogenic substrate exchange by the forearm skeletal muscle in hyperglycemic and insulin-treated type II diabetic patients. Diabetologia (Suppl)33:A211, 1990

31. Capaldo B, Napoli R, Di Marino L et al: Quantitation of forearm glucose and free fatty acid (FFA) disposal in normal subjects and type II diabetic patients: Evidence against an essential role for FFA in the pathogenesis of insulin resistance. J Clin Endocrinol Metab 67:893, 1988

32. Caro JF, Sinha MK, Raju SM et al: Insulin receptor kinase in human skeletal muscle from obese subjects with and without non-insulin-dependent diabetes. J Clin Invest 79:1330, 1987

33. Cerasi E, Luft R, Efendic S: Decreased sensitivity of the pancreatic beta-cells to glucose in prediabetic and diabetic subjects: A glucose dose-response study. Diabetes 21:224, 1972

34. Charron MJ, Brosius FC, Alper SL et al: A glucose transport protein expressed predominantly in insulin-responsive tissues. Proc Natl Acad Sci USA 86:2535, 1989

35. Ciaraldi TP, Kolterman OG, Olefsku JM: Mechanisms of the postreceptor defect in insulin action in human obesity: Decrease in glucose transport system activity. J Clin Invest 68:875, 1981

36. Ciaraldi TP, Kolterman OG, Scarlett JA et al: Role of glucose transport in the post-receptor defect of non-insulin-dependent diabetes mellitus. Diabetes 31:1016, 1982

37. Cohen P: Protein phosphorylation and the control of glycogen metabolism in skeletal muscle. Philos Trans R Soc Lond [Biol] B302:13, 1983

38. Cohen P: Muscle glycogen synthase. In Boyer PD, Krebs EG (eds): The Enzymes, Vol 17, pp 461–497. Orlando, FL, Academic Press, 1986

39. Colowick SP: The hexokinases. In Boyer PD (ed): The Enzymes, Vol 9, pp 1–48. New York, Academic Press, 1973

40. Consoli A, Kennedy F, Miles J et al: Determina-
tion of Krebs cycle metabolic carbon exchange in vivo and its use to estimate gluconeogenesis in man. J Clin Invest 80:1303, 1987

41. Consoli A, Nurjhan N, Capani F et al: Predominant role of gluconeogenesis in increased hepatic glucose production in NIDDM. Diabetes 38:550, 1989

42. Cryer P, Gerich JE: Glucose counterregulation, hypoglycemia, and intensive therapy in diabetes mellitus. N Engl J Med 313:232, 1985

43. Cushman S, Wardzala L: Potential mechanism of insulin action on glucose transport in the isolated rat adipose cell: Apparent translocation of intracellular transport system to the plasma membrane. J Biol Chem 255:4758, 1980

44. Davidson MB, Harris MD, Rosenberg CS: Inverse relationship of metabolic clearance rate of insulin to body mass index. Metab Clin Exp 36:219, 1987

45. De Feo P, Perriello G, De Cosmo S et al: Comparison of glucose counterregulation during short-term and prolonged hypoglycemia in normal humans. Diabetes 35:563, 1986

46. DeFronzo RA: The triumvirate: β-cell, muscle, liver: A collusion responsible for NIDDM. Diabetes 37:667, 1988

47. DeFronzo RA, Ferrannini E, Hendler R et al: Regulation of splanchnic and peripheral glucose uptake by insulin and hyperglycemia in man. Diabetes 32:35, 1983

48. DeFronzo RA, Ferrannini E, Hendler R et al: Influence of hyperinsulinemia, hyperglycemia, and the route of glucose administration on splanchnic glucose exchange. Proc Natl Acad Sci USA 75:5173, 1978

49. DeFronzo RA, Gunnarsson R, Bjorkman O et al: Effects of insulin on peripheral and splanchnic glucose metabolism in non-insulin-dependent (type II) diabetes mellitus. J Clin Invest 76:149, 1985

50. DeFronzo RA, Soman V, Sherwin RS et al: Insulin binding to monocytes and insulin action in human obesity, starvation, and refeeding. J Clin Invest 62:204, 1978

51. DeFronzo RA, Tobin JD, Andres R: Glucose clamp technique: A method for quantifying insulin secretion and resistance. Am J Physiol 237:E214, 1979

52. Del Prato S, Sheehan P, Leonetti F et al: Effect of chronic hyperglycemia on insulin secretion and glucose metabolism. Diabetes (Suppl 1):35:196A, 1986

53. Dohm GL, Tapscott EB, Pories WJ et al: An in vitro human muscle preparation suitable for metabolic studies: Decreased insulin stimulation of glucose transport in muscle from morbidly obese and diabetic subjects. J Clin Invest 82:486, 1988

54. Editorial: Hypoglycemia and the nervous system. Lancet 2:759, 1985

55. Elahi D, Nagulesparan M, Herscopf RJ et al: Feedback inhibition of insulin secretion by insulin: Relation the hyperinsulinemia of obesity. N Engl J Med 306:1196, 1982

56. Eriksson J, Franssila-Kallunki A, Edstrand A et al: Early metabolic defects in persons at increased risk of non-insulin-dependent diabetes mellitus. N Engl J Med 321:337, 1989

57. Evans DJ, Murray R, Kissebah AH: Relationship between skeletal muscle insulin resistance, insulin-mediated glucose disposal, and insulin binding: Effects of obesity and body fat topography. J Clin Invest 74:1515, 1984

58. Exton JH, Corbin JG, Park CR: Control of gluconeogenesis in liver. IV. Differential effects of fatty acids and glucagon on ketogenesis and gluconeogenesis in the perfused rat liver. J Biol Chem 244:4095, 1969

59. Faber OK, Christensen K, Kehlet H et al: Decreased insulin removal contributes to hyperinsulinemia in obesity. J Clin Endocrinol Metab 53:618, 1981

60. Fajans SS: Heterogeneity of insulin secretion in type II diabetes. Diabetes Metab Rev 2:347, 1986

61. Felber JP, Ferrannini E, Golay A et al: Role of lipid oxidation in the pathogenesis of insulin resistance of obesity and type II diabetes. Diabetes 36:1341, 1987

62. Felber JP, Meyer HU, Curchod B et al: Glucose storage and oxidation in different degrees of human obesity measured by continuous indirect calorimetry. Diabetologia 20:39, 1981

63. Felig P, Wahren J, Hendler R: Influence of oral glucose ingestion on splanchnic glucose and gluconeogenic substrate metabolism in man. Diabetes 24:468, 1975

64. Felig P, Wahren J, Hendler R et al: Splanchnic glucose and amino acid metabolism in obesity. J Clin Invest 53:582, 1974

65. Felig P, Wahren J: Influence of endogenous insulin secretion on splanchnic glucose and amino acid metabolism. J Clin Invest 50:1702, 1971

66. Ferrannini E: The theoretical basis for indirect calorimetry: A review. Metab Clin Exp 37:287, 1988

67. Ferrannini E, Barrett EJ, Bevilacqua S et al: Effect of fatty acids on glucose production and utilization in man. J Clin Invest 72:1737, 1983

68. Ferrannini E, Bjorkman O, Reichard G et al: The disposal of an oral glucose load in healthy subjects: A quantitative study. Diabetes 34:580, 1985

69. Ferrannini E, Simonson DC, Katz LD et al: The disposal of an oral glucose load in patients with non-insulin-dependent diabetes. Metab Clin Exp 37:79, 1988

70. Ferrannini E, Wahren J, Felig P et al: The role of fractional glucose extraction in the regulation of splanchnic glucose metabolism in normal and diabetic man. Metab Clin Exp 29:28, 1980

71. Firth R, Bell P, Marsh H et al: Postprandial hyperglycemia in patients with noninsulin-dependent diabetes mellitus: Roles of hepatic and extrahepatic tissues. J Clin Invest 77:1525, 1986

72. Flier JS, Mueckler M, McCall AL et al: Distribution of glucose transporter messenger RNA transcripts in tissues of rat and man. J Clin Invest 79:657, 1987

73. Foley JE, Kashiwagi A, Lillioja S et al: Sensitivity of glucose uptake in insulin in vitro and in vivo in obese Pima Indians. Int J Obes 9:151, 1985

74. Foley JE, Thuillez P, Lillioja S et al: Insulin sensitivity in adipocytes from subjects with varying degrees of glucose tolerance. Am J Physiol 251:E306, 1986

75. Frayn K: Calculation of substrate oxidation rates in vivo from gaseous exchange. J Appl Physiol 55:628, 1983

76. Freymond D, Bogardus C, Okubo M et al: Impaired insulin-stimulated muscle glycogen synthase activation in vivo in man is related to low fasting glycogen synthase phosphatase activity. J Clin Invest 82:1503, 1988

77. Friedman B, Goodman EH Jr, Weinhouse S: Effects of insulin and fatty acids on gluconeogenesis in the rat. J Biol Chem 242:3620, 1967

78. Freidenberg GR, Henry RR, Klein HH et al: Decreased kinase activity of insulin receptors from adipocytes of non-insulin-dependent diabetic subjects. J Clin Invest 79:240, 1987

79. Frizzell R, Campbell P, Cherrington A: Gluconeogenesis and hypoglycemia. Diabetes Metab Rev 4:51, 1988

80. Fukumoto H, Kayano T, Buse JB et al: Cloning and characterization of the major insulin-responsive glucose transporter expressed in human skeletal muscle and other insulin-responsive tissues. J Biol Chem 264:7776, 1989

81. Fukumoto H, Seino S, Imura H et al: Sequence, tissue distribution, and chromosomal localization of mRNA encoding a human glucose transporter-like protein. Proc Natl Acad Sci USA 85:5434, 1988

82. Garvey TW, Hueckstadt TP, Birnbaum MJ: Pretranslational suppression of an insulin-responsive glucose transporter in rats with diabetes mellitus. Science 245:60, 1989

83. Garvey TW, Hueckstadt TP, Matthaei S et al: Role of glucose transporters in the cellular insulin re-

sistance of type II non-insulin-dependent diabetes mellitus. J Clin Invest 81:1528, 1988

84. Garvey WT, Olefsky JM, Matthaei S et al: Glucose and insulin co-regulate the glucose transport system in primary cultured adipocytes. J Biol Chem 262:189, 1987

85. Gepts W, Lecompte PM: The pancreatic islets in diabetes. Am J Med 70:105, 1981

86. Gerich J, Cryer P, Rizza R: Hormonal mechanisms in acute glucose counterregulation: The relative roles of glucagon, epinephrine, norepinephrine, growth hormone and cortisol. Metab Clin Exp 29:1164, 1980

87. Gerich JE: Glucose counterregulation and its impact on diabetes mellitus. Diabetes 37:1608, 1988

88. Giroix MH, Portha B, Kergoat M et al: Glucose insensitivity and amino acid hypersensitivity of insulin release in rats with non-insulin-dependent diabetes: A study with the perfused pancreas. Diabetes 32:445, 1983

89. Gjedde A, Crone C: Blood-brain glucose transfer: Repression in chronic hyperglycemia. Science 214:456, 1981

90. Grill V, Westberg M, Ostenson CG: Beta cell insensitivity in a rat model of non-insulin-dependent diabetes. J Clin Invest 80:664, 1987

91. Groop LC, Bonadonna RC, Del Prato S et al: Glucose and free fatty acid metabolism in non-insulin-dependent diabetes mellitus: Evidence for multiple sites of insulin resistance. J Clin Invest 84:205, 1989

92. Groop LC, Koranyi L, Eriksson J et al: Expression of insulin-responsive glucose transporter mRNA in skeletal muscle of patients with type 2 diabetes. Diabetologia (Suppl)33:A23, 1990

93. Gulli G, Haffner S, Ferrannini E et al: What is inherited in NIDD? Diabetes (Suppl 1)39:116A, 1990

94. Halter JB, Graf RJ, Porte D Jr: Potentiation of insulin secretory responses by plasma glucose levels in man: Evidence that hyperglycemia in diabetes compensates for impaired glucose potentiation. J Clin Endocrinol Metab 48:946, 1979

95. Handberg AA, Vaag A, Damsbo P et al: Expression of insulin regulatable glucose transporters in skeletal muscle is not affected by type II diabetes. Diabetologia (Suppl)33:A10, 1990

96. Haffner SM, Stern MP, Hazuda HP et al: Increased insulin concentrations in nondiabetic offspring of diabetic parents. N Engl J Med 319:1297, 1988

97. Haffner SM, Stern MP, Mitchell BD et al: Incidence of type II diabetes mellitus in Mexican Americans predicted by fasting insulin and glucose levels, obesity, and body fat distribution. Diabetes 39:283, 1990

98. Hansen BC, Bodkin NL: Heterogeneity of insulin responses: Phases in the continuum leading to non-insulin-dependent diabetes mellitus. Diabetologia 29:713, 1986

99. Hoenig M, MacGregor LC, Matschinsky FM: In vitro exhaustion of pancreatic beta cells. Am J Physiol 250:E502, 1986

100. Hollenbeck CB, Chen Y, Reaven GM: A comparison of the relative effects of obesity and non-insulin-dependent diabetes mellitus on in vivo insulin-stimulated glucose utilization. Diabetes 33:622, 1984

101. Ingebritsen TS, Cohen P: Protein phosphatase: Properties and role in cellular regulation. Science 221:331, 1983

102. Insel PA, Liljenquist JE, Tobin JD et al: Insulin control of glucose metabolism in man. J Clin Invest 55:1057, 1975

103. Ishida T, Chap Z, Chen J et al: Differential effects of oral, peripheral intravenous, and intraportal glucose on hepatic glucose uptake and insulin and glucagon extraction in conscious dogs. J Clin Invest 72:590, 1983

104. Iynedjian PB, Pilot P-R, Nouspikel T et al: Differential expression and regulation of the glucokinase gene in liver and islet of Langerhans. Proc Natl Acad Sci USA 86:7837, 1989

105. Jackson R, Peters N, Advani U et al: Forearm glucose uptake during the oral glucose tolerance test in normal subjects. Diabetes 22:442, 1973

106. Jackson R, Roshania R, Hawa M et al: Impact of glucose ingestion on hepatic and peripheral glucose metabolism in man: An analysis based on simultaneous use of the forearm and double isotope techniques. J Clin Endocrinol Metab 63:541, 1986

107. James DE, Strube M, Mueckler M: Molecular cloning and characterization of an insulin-regulatable glucose transporter. Nature 33:83, 1989

108. Jensen MD, Haymond MW, Rizza RA et al: Influence of body fat distribution on free fatty acid metabolism in obesity. J Clin Invest 83:1168, 1989

109. Joost HG, Weber TM, Cushman SW: Qualitative and quantitative comparison of glucose transport activity and glucose transporter concentration in plasma membranes from basal and insulin-stimulated rat adipose cells. Biochem J 249:155, 1988

110. Joost HG, Weber TM, Cushman SW et al: Insulin-stimulated glucose transport in rat adipose cells: Modulation of transporter intrinsic activity by isoproterenol and adenosine. J Biol Chem 261:10033, 1986

111. Kashiwagi A, Bogardus C, Lillioja S et al: In vitro insensitivity of glucose transport and antilipoly-

sis to insulin due to receptor and postreceptor abnormalities in obese Pima Indians with normal glucose tolerance. Metab Clin Exp 33:772, 1984

112. Kashiwagi A, Verso MA, Andrews J et al: In vitro insulin resistance of human adipocytes isolated from subjects with non-insulin-dependent diabetes mellitus. J Clin Invest 72:1246, 1983

113. Katz L, Glickman M, Rapoport S et al: Splanchnic and peripheral disposal of oral glucose in man. Diabetes 32:675, 1983

114. Kayano T, Fukumoto H, Eddy RL et al: Evidence for a family of human glucose transporter-like proteins. J Biol Chem 263:15245, 1988

115. Kida Y, Esposito-Del Puente A, Bogardus C et al: Insulin resistance is associated with reduced fasting and insulin-stimulated glycogen synthase phosphatase activity in human skeletal muscle. J Clin Invest 85:476, 1990

116. Kelley D, Mitrakou A, Marsh H et al: Skeletal muscle glycolysis, oxidation, and storage of an oral glucose load. J Clin Invest 81:1563, 1988

117. Kissebah AH, Wydelingum N, Murray R et al: Relation of body fat distribution to metabolic complications of obesity. J Endocrinol Metab 54:254, 1982

118. Knowler WC, Pettitt DJ, Savage PJ et al: Diabetes incidence in Pima Indians: Contributions of obesity and parental diabetes. Am J Epidemiol 113:144, 1981

119. Kolterman OB, Insel J, Saekow M et al: Mechanisms of insulin resistance in human obesity: Evidence for receptor and postreceptor defects. J Clin Invest 65:1272, 1980

120. Krotkiewski M, Björntorp P, Sjostrom L et al: Impact of obesity on metabolism in man and women. Importance of regional adipose tissue distribution. J Clin Invest 72:1150, 1983

121. Laakso M, Edelman SV, Brechtel G et al: Decreased effect of insulin to stimulate skeletal muscle blood flow in obese man: A novel mechanism for insulin resistance. J Clin Invest 85:1844, 1990

122. Laakso M, Edelman SV, Olefsky JM et al: Kinetics of in vivo muscle insulin-mediated glucose uptake in human obesity. Diabetes 39:965, 1990

123. Landau BR, Wahren J: Quantification of the pathways followed in hepatic glycogen formation from glucose. FASEB J 2:2368, 1988

124. Leahy JL, Bonner-Weir S, and Weir GC: Abnormal glucose regulation of insulin secretion in models of reduced β-cell mass. Diabetes 33:667, 1984

125. Leahy JL, Bonner-Weir S, Weir GC: Minimal chronic hyperglycemia is a critical determinant of impaired insulin secretion after an incomplete pancreatectomy. J Clin Invest 81:1407, 1988

126. Leahy JL, Cooper HE, Deal DA et al: Chronic hyperglycemia is associated with impaired glucose

influence on insulin secretion. J Clin Invest 77:908, 1986

127. Leahy JL, Cooper HE, Weir GC: Impaired insulin secretion associated with near normoglycemia: study in normal rats with 96-h in vivo glucose infusion. Diabetes 36:459, 1987

128. Leahy JL, Weir GC: Evolution of abnormal insulin secretory responses during 48-h in vivo hyperglycemia. Diabetes 37:217, 1988

129. Liljenquist J, Mueller G, Cherrington A et al: Hyperglycemia per se (insulin and glucagon withdrawn) can inhibit hepatic glucose production in man. J Clin Endocrinol Metab 48:171, 1979

130. Lillioja S, Bogardus C, Mott DM et al: Relationship between insulin-mediated glucose metabolism and lipid metabolism in man. J Clin Invest 75:1106, 1985

131. Lillioja S, Mott DM, Zawadzki JK et al: Glucose storage is a major determinant of in vivo "insulin resistance" in subjects with normal glucose tolerance. J Clin Endocrinol Metab 62:922, 1986

132. Lillioja S, Mott DM, Zawadzki JK et al: In vivo insulin action is a familial characteristic in nondiabetic Pima Indians. Diabetes 36:1329, 1987

133. Lillioja S, Young AA, Culter CL et al: Skeletal muscle capillary density and fiber type are possible determinants of in vivo insulin resistance in man. J Clin Invest 80:415, 1987

134. Lindgarde E, Erickson K-F, Lithell H et al: Coupling between dietary changes, reduced body weight, muscle fiber size and improved glucose tolerance in middle-aged men with impaired glucose tolerance. Acta Med Scand 212:99, 1982

135. Lithell H, Lindgarde F, Hellsing K et al: Body weight, skeletal muscle morphology and enzyme activities in relation to fasting serum insulin concentration and glucose tolerance in 48-year-old men. Diabetes 30:19, 1981

136. Maenz DD, Cheeseman CI: The Na^+-dependent D-glucose transporter in the enterocyte basolateral membrane: Orientation and cytochalasin B binding characteristics. J Membr Biol 97:259, 1987

137. Magnuson MA, Andreone TL, Printz RL et al: The glucokinase gene: Structure and regulation by insulin. Proc Natl Acad Sci USA 86:4838, 1989

138. Magnuson MA, Shelton KD: An alternate promoter in the glucokinase gene is active in the pancreatic β-cell. J Biol Chem 264:15936, 1989

139. Magnusson I, Chandramouli V, Schumann WC et al: Quantitation of the pathways of hepatic glycogen formation on ingesting a glucose load. J Clin Invest 80:1748, 1987

140. Magnusson I, Chandramouli V, Schumann WC et al: Pathways of hepatic glycogen formation in humans following ingestion of a glucose load in the fed state. Metab Clin Exp 38:583, 1989

141. Mandarino LJ, Baker B, Rizza R et al: Infusion of insulin impairs human adipocyte glucose metabolism in vitro without decreasing adipocyte insulin receptor binding. Diabetologia 27:358, 1984

142. Mandarino LJ, Madar Z, Kolterman OG et al: Adipocyte glycogen synthase and pyruvate dehydrogenase in obese and type II diabetic subjects. Am J Physiol 251:E489, 1986

143. Mandarino L, Wright K, Verity L et al: Effects of insulin infusion on human skeletal muscle pyruvate dehydrogenase, phosphofructokinase, and glycogen synthase. J Clin Invest 80:655, 1987

144. Marks V, Rose F: Physiologic responses to hypoglycemia. In Hypoglycemia, 2nd ed, New York, Blackwell Scientific Publications, pp 69–89, 1981

145. Matthaei S, Horuk R, Olefsky JM: Blood-brain glucose transfer in diabetes mellitus: Decreased number of glucose transporters at blood-brain barrier. Diabetes 35:1181, 1986

146. McCall AL, Millington WR, Wurtman RJ: Metabolic fuel and amino acid transport into the brain in experimental diabetes mellitus. Proc Natl Acad Sci USA 79:5406, 1982

147. McGarry JD, Kuwajima M, Newgard CB et al: From dietary glucose to liver glycogen: The full circle round. Ann Rev Nutr 7:51, 1987

148. McGuire EA, Tobin JD, Berman M et al: Kinetics of native insulin in diabetic, obese and aged men. Diabetes 28:110, 1979

149. Meistas MT, Margolis S, Kowarski AA: Hyperinsulinemia of obesity is due to decreased clearance of insulin. Am J Physiol 245:E155, 1983

150. Mueckler M, Caruso C, Baldwin S et al: Sequence and structure of a human glucose transporter. Science 229:941, 1985

151. Newgard CB, Hirsch LJ, Foster DW et al: Studies on the mechanism by which exogenous glucose is converted into liver glycogen in the rat: A direct or an indirect pathway? J Biol Chem 258:8046, 1983

152. Newgard CB, Moore SV, Foster DW et al: Efficient hepatic glycogen synthesis in refeeding rats requires continued carbon flow through the gluconeogenic pathway. J Biol Chem 259:6958, 1984

153. Newman B, Selby JV, King MC et al: Concordance for type 2 (non-insulin-dependent) diabetes mellitus in male twins. Diabetologia 30:763, 1987

154. Nishi S, Susumu S, Bell GI: Human hexokinase: Sequences of amino- and carboxyl-terminal halves are homologous. Biochem Biophys Res Commun 157:937, 1988

155. Nurjhan N, Consoli A: Evidence that intrahepatic mechanisms are primarily responsible for increased gluconeogenesis in non–insulin-dependent diabetes mellitus (NIDDM). Diabetes (Suppl 1)39:4A, 1990

156. Nurjhan N, Consoli A, Gerich J: Important contribution of gluconeogenesis for increased postprandial hepatic glucose output in type 2 diabetes. Diabetologia (Suppl 33):A58, 1990

157. Nuttall FQ, Ganon MC, Corbett VA et al: Insulin stimulation of heart glycogen synthase D phosphatase (protein phosphatase). J Biol Chem 251:6724, 1976

158. Ohlson L-O, Larsson B, Svarsudd K et al: The influence of body fat distribution on the incidence of diabetes mellitus: 13.5 years of follow-up of the participants in the study of men born in 1913. Diabetes 34:1055, 1985

159. Okubo M, Bogardus C, Lillioja S et al: Glucose-6-phosphate stimulation of human glycogen synthase phosphatase. Metab Clin Exp 37:1171, 1988

160. Olefsky JM, Kolterman OG: Mechanisms of insulin resistance in obesity and non-insulin-dependent (type II) diabetes. Am J Med 70:151, 1981

161. Olefsky JM, Kolterman OG, Scarlett JA: Insulin action and resistance in obesity and non-insulin-dependent type II diabetes mellitus. Am J Physiol 243:E15, 1982

162. O'Rahilly S, Turner RC, Matthews DR: Impaired pulsatile secretion of insulin in relatives of patients with non-insulin-dependent diabetes. N Engl J Med 318:1225, 1988

163. Orci L, Thorens B, Ravazzola M et al: Localization of the pancreatic beta cell glucose transporter to specific plasma membrane domains. Science 245:295, 1989

164. Parker PJ, Caudwell FB, Cohen P: Glycogen synthase from rabbit skeletal muscle: Effect of insulin on the state of phosphorylation of seven phosphoserine residues in vivo. Eur J Biochem 130:227, 1983

165. Pedersen O, Bak JF, Andersen PH et al: Evidence against altered expresson of GLUT1 or GLUT4 in skeletal muscle of patients with obesity or NIDDM. Diabetes 39:865, 1990

166. Pedersen O, Hjollund E, Sprensen NS: Insulin receptor binding and insulin action in human fat cells: Effects of obesity and fasting. Metab Clin Exp 9:884, 1982

167. Peiris AN, Mueller RA, Struve MF et al: Splanchnic insulin metabolism in obesity: Influence of body fat distribution. J Clin Invest 78:1648, 1986

168. Peiris AN, Mueller RA, Struve MF et al: Relationship of androgenic activity to splanchnic insulin metabolism and peripheral glucose utilization in premenopausal women. J Clin Endocrinol Metab 64:162, 1987

169. Peiris AN, Struve MF, Mueller RA et al: Glucose

metabolism in obesity: Influence of body fat distribution. J Clin Endocrinol Metab 67:760, 1988

170. Polonsky KS, Given BD, Hirsch L et al: Quantitative study of insulin secretion and clearance in normal and obese subjects. J Clin Invest 81:435, 1988

171. Polonsky KS, Given BD, Hirsch LJ et al: Abnormal patterns of insulin secretion in non-insulin-dependent diabetes mellitus. N Engl J Med 318:1231, 1988

172. Prager R, Wallace P, Olefsky JM: In vivo kinetics of insulin action on peripheral glucose disposal and hepatic glucose output in normal and obese subjects. J Clin Invest 78:472, 1986

183. Richter EA, Hansen BF, Hansen SA: Glucose-induced insulin resistance of skeletal muscle glucose transport and uptake. Biochem J 252:733, 1988

184. Rizza R, Cryer P, Gerich J: Role of glucagon, catecholamines, and growth hormone in human glucose counterregulation: Effects of somatostatin and combined alpha- and beta-adrenergic blockade on plasma glucose recovery and glucose flux rates following insulin-induced hypoglycemia. J Clin Invest 64:62, 1979

185. Rossetti L, Giaccari A, DeFronzo RA: Glucose toxicity. Diabetes Care 13:610, 1990

186. Rossetti L, Shulman GI, Zawalich W et al: Effect of chronic hyperglycemia on in vivo insulin secretion in partially pancreatectomized rats. J Clin Invest 80:1037, 1987

187. Rossetti L, Smith D, Shulman GI et al: Correction of hyperglycemia with phloridzin normalizes tissue sensitivity to insulin in diabetic rats. J Clin Invest 79:1510, 1987

188. Ruderman NB, Toews CJ, Shafrir E: Role of free fatty acids in glucose homeostasis. Arch Intern Med 123:299, 1969

189. Saad MF, Knowler WC, Pettitt DJ et al: The natural history of impaired glucose tolerance in Pima Indians. N Engl J Med 319:1500, 1988

190. Saad MF, Pettit DJ, Mott DM et al: Sequential changes in serum insulin concentration during development of non-insulin-dependent diabetes. Lancet I:1356, 1989

191. Saccà L, Sherwin RS, Hendler R et al: Influence of continuous physiologic hyperinsulinemia on glucose kinetics and counterregulatory hormones in normal and diabetic humans. J Clin Invest 63:849, 1979

192. Saito K, Yaginuma N, Takahashi T: Differential volumetry of A, B, and D cells in the pancreatic islets of diabetic and non-diabetic subjects. Tohoku J Exp Med 129:273, 1979

193. Sasson S, Cerasi E: Substrate regulation of the glucose transport system in rat skeletal muscle. J Biol Chem 261:16827, 1986

194. Sasson S, Edelson D, Cerasi E: In vitro autoregulation of glucose utilization in rat soleus muscle. Diabetes 36:1041, 1987

195. Savage PJ, Flock EV, Mako ME et al: C-peptide and insulin secretion in Pima Indians and Caucasians: Constant fractional hepatic extraction over a wide range of insulin concentration and in obesity. J Clin Endocrinol Metab 48:594, 1979

196. Schwab DA, Wilson JE: Complete amino acid sequence of rat brain hexokinase, deduced from the cloned cDNA, and proposed structure of a mammalian hexokinase. Proc Natl Acad Sci USA 86:2563, 1989

197. Scofield RF, Kosugi K, Schumann WC et al: Quantitative estimation of the pathways followed in the conversion of glucose administered to the fasted rat. J Biol Chem 260:8777, 1985

198. Sherwin RS, Kramer KJ, Tobin JD et al: A model of the kinetics of insulin in man. J Clin Invest 53:1481, 1974

199. Shulman GI, Cline G, Schumann WC et al: Quantitative comparison of pathways of hepatic glycogen repletion in fed and fasted humans. Am J Physiol 259:E335, 1990

200. Shulman GI, Rossetti L, Rothman DL et al: Quantitative analysis of glycogen repletion by nuclear magnetic resonance spectroscopy in the conscious rat. J Clin Invest 80:387, 1987

201. Shulman GI, Rothman DL, Jue T et al: Quantitation of muscle glycogen synthesis in normal subjects and subjects with non-insulin-dependent diabetes by ^{13}C nuclear magnetic resonance spectroscopy. N Engl J Med 322:223, 1990

202. Sicree RA, Zimmet PZ, King HOM et al: Plasma insulin response among Nauruans: Prediction of deterioration in glucose tolerance over six years. Diabetes 36:179, 1987

203. Siesjo B: Hypoglycemia, brain metabolism and brain damage. Diabetes Metab Rev 4:113, 1988

204. Sinha MK, Pories WJ, Flickinger EG et al: Insulin-receptor kinase activity of adipose tissue from morbidly obese humans with and without NIDDM. Diabetes 36:20, 1987

205. Sivitz WI, DeSautel SL, Kayano T et al: Regulation of glucose transporter messenger RNA in insulin-deficient states. Nature 340:72, 1989

206. Sörensen TIA, Price RA, Stunkard AJ et al: Genetics of obesity in adult adoptees and their biological siblings. Br Med J 298:87, 1989

207. Struck E, Ashmore J, Wieland O: Effects of glucagon and long chain fatty acids on glucose production by isolated perfused rat liver. Adv Enzyme Regul 4:219, 1966

208. Stunkard AJ, Foch TT, Hrubec Z: A twin study of human obesity. JAMA 256:51, 1986

209. Stunkard AJ, Harris JR, Pedersen NL et al: The

body-mass index of twins who have been reared apart. N Engl J Med 322:1483, 1990

210. Stunkard AJ, Sörensen TIA, Hanis C: An adoption study of human obesity. N Engl J Med 314:193, 1986

211. Svedberg J, Björntorp P, Smith U et al: Free-fatty acid inhibition of insulin binding, degradation, and action in isolated rat hepatocytes. Diabetes 39:570, 1990

212. Suzuki K, Kono T: Evidence that insulin causes translocation of glucose transport activity to the plasma membrane from an intracellular storage site. Proc Natl Acad Sci USA 77:2542, 1980

213. Takayama S, Kahn CR, Kubo K et al: Alteration in insulin receptor autophosphorylation in insulin resistance: Correlation with altered sensitivity to glucose transport and antilipolysis to insulin. J Clin Endocrinol Metab 66:992, 1988

214. Taskinen MR, Bogardus C, Kennedy A et al: Multiple disturbances of free fatty acid metabolism in non-insulin-dependent diabetes: Effect of oral hypoglycemic therapy. J Clin Invest 76:637, 1985

215. Thiebaud D, DeFronzo RA, Jacot E et al: Effect of long chain triglyceride infusion on glucose metabolism in man. Metab Clin Exp 31:1128, 1982

216. Thorens B, Sarker HK, Kaback HR et al: Cloning and functional expression in bacteria of a novel glucose transporter present in liver, intestine, kidney, and β-pancreatic islet cells. Cell 55:281, 1988

217. Toyoda N, Flanagan JE, Kono T: Reassessment of insulin effects on the V_{max} and K_m values of hexose transport in isolated rat epididymal adipocytes. J Biol Chem 262:2737, 1987

218. Trimble ER, Wier GC, Gjinovci A et al: Increased insulin responsiveness in vivo and in vitro consequent to induced hyperinsulinemia in the rat. Diabetes 33:444, 1984

219. Turner RC, McCarthy ST, Holman RR et al: Beta-cell function improved by supplementary basal insulin secretion in mild diabetes. Br Med J 1:1252, 1976

220. Unger RH, Grundy S: Hyperglycemia as an inducer as well as a consequence of impaired islet function and insulin resistance: Implications for the management of diabetes. Diabetologia 28:119, 1985

221. Vague J: The degree of masculine differentiation of obesities: A factor determining predisposition to diabetes, atherosclerosis, gout and uric calculous disease. Am J Clin Nutr 4:20, 1956

222. Wahren J, Felig P, Cerasi E et al: Splanchnic and peripheral glucose and amino acid metabolism in diabetes mellitus. J Clin Invest 51:1870, 1972

223. Waldhausl W, Gasic S, Bratusch-Marrain P et al: The 75-g oral glucose tolerance test: Effect on splanchnic metabolism of substrates and pancreatic hormones release in healthy man. Diabetologia 25:489, 1983

224. Walkenbach RJ, Hazen R, Larner J: Reversible inhibition of cyclic AMP-dependent protein kinase by insulin. Mol Cell Biochem 19:31, 1978

225. Ward WKI, Beard JC, Porte D: Clinical aspects of islet beta-cell function in non-insulin-dependent diabetes mellitus. Diabetes Metab Rev 2:297, 1986

226. Ward WK, Bolgiano DC, McKnight B et al: Diminished B-cell secretory capacity in patients with noninsulin dependent diabetes mellitus. J Clin Invest 74:1318, 1984

227. Wardzala LA, Hieshman M, Pofcher E et al: Regulation of glucose utilization in adipose cells and muscle after long-term experimental hyperinsulinemia in rats. J Clin Invest 76:460, 1985

228. Warren KW, Braasch JW, Thurn CW: Diagnosis and surgical treatment of carcinoma of the pancreas. Curr Probl Surg 132:3, 1968

229. Welborn TA, Stenhouse NS, Johnson CJ: Factors determining serum insulin response in a population sample. Diabetologia 5:263, 1969

230. Westermark P, Wilander E: The influence of amyloid deposits on the islet volume in maturity-onset diabetes mellitus. Diabetologia 15:417, 1978

231. Wieland O: The mammalian pyruvate dehydrogenase complex: Structure and regulation. Rev Physiol Biochem Pharmacol 96:124, 1983

232. Williamson JR, Kreisberg RA, Felts PW: Mechanism for the simulation of gluconeogenesis by fatty acids in perfused rat liver. Proc Natl Acad Sci USA 56:247, 1966

233. Wright KS, Beck-Nielsen H, Kolterman OG et al: Decreased activation of skeletal muscle glycogen synthase by mixed-meal ingestion in NIDDM. Diabetes 37:436, 1988

234. Wright JK, Seckler R, Overath P: Molecular aspects of sugar ion cotransport. Annu Rev Biochem 55:225, 1986

235. Yang YJ, Hope ID, Bergman RN: Insulin transport across the capillaries is a rate limiting step of insulin action in dogs. J Clin Invest 84:1620, 1989

236. Yki-Jarvinen H, Helve E, Koivisto VA: Hyperglycemia decreases glucose uptake in type I diabetes. Diabetes 36:892, 1987

237. Yki-Jarvinen H, Kubo K, Zawadzki J et al: Dissociation of in vitro sensitivities of glucose transport and antilipolysis to insulin in NIDDM. Am J Physiol 253:E1, 1987

238. Zawalich WS, Zawalich KC, Shulman GI et al: Chronic in vivo hyperglycemia impairs phosphoinositide hydrolysis and insulin release in isolated perfused rat islets. Endocrinology 126:253, 1990

Obesity and Hyperlipidemia: Results from the Prospective Cardiovascular Münster (PROCAM) Study

GERD ASSMANN and HELMUT SCHULTE

The European Atherosclerosis Society (AES) emphasized in a policy statement[1] about strategies for the prevention of coronary heart disease (CHD) that "overweight confers an increased risk of CHD, and more pronounced obesity is a risk factor of other risk-related variables. The control of overweight of all degrees is justified in its own right; in addition, weight reduction is important in ameliorating abnormal lipid and lipoprotein levels, hypertension, hyperuricemia and non-insulin dependent diabetes." To demonstrate the relationship between obesity and hyperlipidemia, some results of the Prospective Cardiovascular Münster (PROCAM) study are shown.

DESCRIPTION OF THE PROCAM STUDY

In the PROCAM study, employees of 52 companies and authorities are examined for cardiovascular risk factors and then kept under observation to record all deaths as well as new myocardial infarctions and strokes. The examination at the beginning of the observation period comprises an anamnesis using standardized questionnaires, measurement of the blood pressure and anthropometric data, a resting electrocardiographic tracing (ECG), and collection of a blood sample after a 12-hour fast for the determination of more than 20 laboratory parameters. The methods used for the examinations[2] and the laboratory tests[3] are described in detail elsewhere. The examination is carried out in a converted former x-ray bus on the employer's site during paid working hours. Any employee may participate in the study. Participation is voluntary (between 40% and 80% take part, average 60%) and is free of charge both to the volunteers and to their employers (apart from loss of work). About 20 people are examined each day. All findings are reported to the person's general practitioner, and the volunteer is told whether the results of the examination are normal or whether a checkup by his or her general practitioner is necessary. We ourselves neither carry out nor arrange for any intervention but leave this to the individual's general practitioner.

Questionnaires are then sent to the participants every 2 years to record any myocardial infarctions or strokes that have occurred in the meantime and to find out about any deaths. At the initial examination, the participants were told to expect a questionnaire every 2 years. The response rate was 96% after two reminders by mail and phone if necessary. For all deaths and any other incidents suspected from the information in the questionnaire, we request hospital records and records from the attending physician in order to verify the diagnosis or the cause of death. Surviving patients are first asked for their permission. The initial examination is repeated after 6 to 7 years.

TABLE 41-1

**Mean Value and SD of BMI
According to Age**

Age (years)	Men	Women
20–29	23.5 ± 3.5	21.9 ± 3.0
30–39	25.2 ± 3.1	24.0 ± 3.9
40–49	26.2 ± 3.0	25.4 ± 4.2
50–59	26.6 ± 3.0	26.5 ± 4.3
20–59	25.0 ± 3.7	24.0 ± 4.2

The study began in 1979, and the recruitment phase was completed at the end of 1985. Full data records are held on a total of 19,698 participants in the PROCAM study. The ages range from 16 to 65 years. The 13,737 men had an average age of 41.4 years, with a standard deviation of 11.2 years. The 5961 women had a distinctly lower age of 36.6 ± 12.5 years.

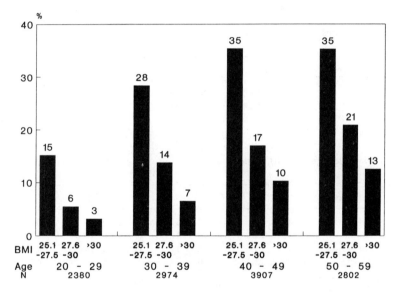

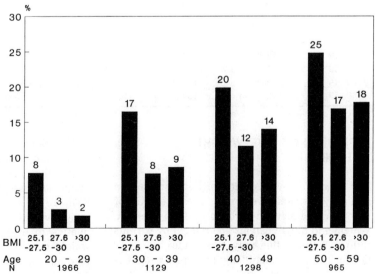

FIGURE 41-1

Prevalence of overweight men **(A)** and women **(B)**.

TABLE 41-2

Lipids and Lipoproteins in Relation to Age and BMI in Men

Cholesterol (mg/dl), mean ± SD

	BMI			
Age (years)	*<25*	*25.1–27.5*	*27.6–30*	*>30*
20–29	180 ± 35	191 ± 37	201 ± 34	208 ± 42
30–39	202 ± 38	210 ± 43	216 ± 41	217 ± 39
40–49	217 ± 42	224 ± 42	230 ± 45	226 ± 41
50–59	222 ± 40	232 ± 42	229 ± 42	234 ± 45

Triglycerides (mg/dl), mean ± SD

	BMI			
Age (years)	*<25*	*25.1–27.5*	*27.6–30*	*>30*
20–29	98 ± 65	136 ± 104	156 ± 88	202 ± 158
30–39	121 ± 83	157 ± 209	195 ± 166	206 ± 155
40–49	136 ± 121	168 ± 145	200 ± 163	243 ± 196
50–59	128 ± 87	154 ± 105	178 ± 131	202 ± 162

HDL cholesterol (mg/dl), mean ± SD

	BMI			
Age (years)	*<25*	*25.1–27.5*	*27.6–30*	*>30*
20–29	47 ± 11	43 ± 11	41 ± 8	38 ± 8
30–39	48 ± 12	44 ± 12	41 ± 10	40 ± 10
40–49	48 ± 12	45 ± 11	43 ± 14	40 ± 10
50–59	49 ± 13	46 ± 12	44 ± 11	41 ± 10

LDL cholesterol (mg/dl), mean ± SD

	BMI			
Age (years)	*<25*	*25.1–27.5*	*27.6–30*	*>30*
20–29	113 ± 31	121 ± 31	130 ± 33	131 ± 34
30–39	131 ± 34	136 ± 35	138 ± 35	138 ± 34
40–49	143 ± 37	147 ± 36	150 ± 38	146 ± 36
50–59	148 ± 36	157 ± 36	151 ± 37	155 ± 39

DEFINITION OF OVERWEIGHT AND OBESITY

The degree of overweight can be expressed in several ways. Relative weight uses the ratio or percentage of actual weight to desirable weight. Weight and height can also be related by various ratios. Of these, the body mass index (BMI) or Quetelet index (weight/height,[2] where weight is in kilograms and height in meters) has the best correlation with body fat and is thus preferred.[4] In practice, methods involving measurement of height and weight, preferably expressed as the BMI, are the best approaches to determining who is overweight (*i.e.*, has an elevated body weight relative to height) and distinguishing an overweight person from a person who is obese (*i.e.*, who has too much fat). Overweight is arbitrarily

TABLE 41-3

Lipids and Lipoproteins in Relation to Age and BMI in Women

Cholesterol (mg/dl), mean ± SD

Age (years)	BMI			
	<25	25.1–27.5	27.6–30	>30
20–29	183 ± 32	184 ± 35	184 ± 42	180 ± 32
30–39	193 ± 36	199 ± 39	194 ± 34	205 ± 40
40–49	210 ± 41	216 ± 38	215 ± 42	216 ± 37
50–59	243 ± 44	241 ± 40	244 ± 42	238 ± 40

Triglycerides (mg/dl), mean ± SD

Age (years)	BMI			
	<25	25.1–27.5	27.6–30	>30
20–29	84 ± 40	99 ± 78	112 ± 63	100 ± 41
30–39	85 ± 45	101 ± 53	108 ± 56	134 ± 104
40–49	85 ± 38	100 ± 61	120 ± 76	127 ± 61
50–59	101 ± 50	113 ± 55	127 ± 90	127 ± 73

HDL cholesterol (mg/dl), mean ± SD

Age (years)	BMI			
	<25	25.1–27.5	27.6–30	>30
20–29	57 ± 12	53 ± 14	48 ± 12	46 ± 11
30–39	58 ± 14	52 ± 14	49 ± 11	46 ± 12
40–49	60 ± 14	55 ± 13	53 ± 13	47 ± 13
50–59	62 ± 15	57 ± 13	56 ± 14	53 ± 13

LDL cholesterol (mg/dl), mean ± SD

Age (years)	BMI			
	<25	25.1–27.5	27.6–30	>30
20–29	108 ± 29	112 ± 30	113 ± 35	113 ± 35
30–39	118 ± 32	127 ± 36	126 ± 32	131 ± 38
40–49	134 ± 38	141 ± 35	139 ± 36	143 ± 33
50–59	161 ± 41	162 ± 39	164 ± 37	161 ± 35

defined as a BMI between 25 and 30. Obese is defined as a BMI above 30.[4] In the following evaluations, the participants of the PROCAM study are divided into persons with acceptable relative body weight (BMI < = 25), with overweight up to 10% (BMI 25.1 to 27.5), with overweight of more than 10% to 20% (BMI 27.6 to 30), and obese persons (BMI > 30).

RESULTS

Prevalence of Overweight and Obesity

The following evaluations are restricted to 12,063 male and 5358 female participants of the PROCAM study ages 20 to 59 years and free of myocardial infarction and stroke. Next to age,

TABLE 41-4

Action Limits According to Recommendations of the EAS

Treatment Group	Cholesterol (mg/dl)		Triglycerides, Fasted (mg/dl)
A	200–250		<200
B	250–300		<200
C	<200		200–500
D	200–300		200–500
E	>300	and/or	>500

relative body weight shows the most immediate connection to nearly all the risk factors, and because of the positive correlation between age and relative body weight (Table 41-1), these two factors reinforce each other. To eliminate the "competing" effects of age and relative body weight, the following analyses were done in different age subgroups (20 to 29 years, 30 to 39 years, 40 to 49 years, and 50 to 59 years).

In all age subgroups, the mean value of the BMI in men was higher than in women. Figure 41-1 shows the prevalence of overweight and

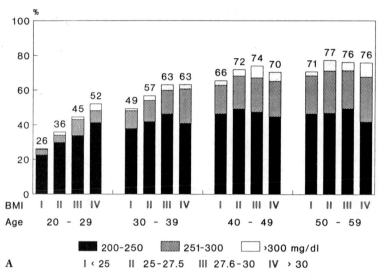

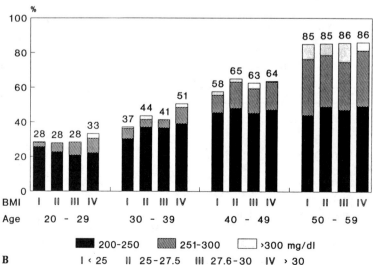

FIGURE 41-2

Prevalence of elevated cholesterol levels in men **(A)** and in women **(B)**.

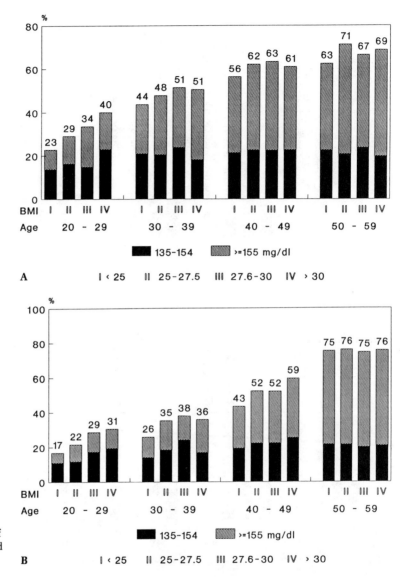

FIGURE 41-3

Prevalence of elevated levels of LDL cholesterol in men **(A)** and in women **(B)**.

obesity in age subgroups. The frequency of overweight and obesity increases with age in both sexes, in women more so than in men. In men age 40 and older and in women age 50 and older, more than one in two shows excess body weight.

Lipids and Lipoproteins in Relation to Body Weight

Cholesterol, triglycerides, and high-density lipoprotein (HDL) cholesterol were determined in the serum, whereas low-density lipoprotein (LDL) cholesterol was calculated by the Friedewald formula,[5] in cases where triglyceride values of less than 400 mg/dl were found:

$$\text{LDL cholesterol} = \text{cholesterol} - \text{triglycerides}/5 - \text{HDL cholesterol}$$

In Tables 41-2 and 41-3, the mean values of lipids and lipoproteins broken down by age and BMI are given in men and women, respectively.

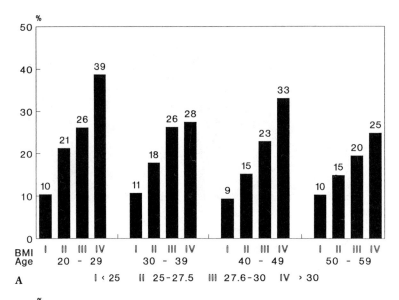

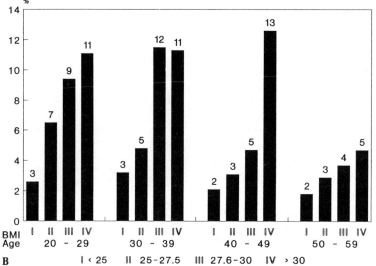

FIGURE 41-4

Prevalence of HDL cholesterol levels < 35 mg/dl in men **(A)** and in women **(B)**.

Total cholesterol increases slightly with BMI, in younger men more so than in the elderly. In women there is no correlation between cholesterol and BMI in the age subgroups. Triglycerides show a strong direct correlation, whereas HDL cholesterol shows a strong inverse relation with BMI in all age subgroups in both sexes. LDL cholesterol is higher in individuals with excess BMI than in persons with acceptable relative body weight. The differences decrease with increasing age. A correlation between the degree of overweight and LDL cholesterol is found in younger men only.

Hyperlipidemia and Excess Body Weight

The EAS has established simplified action limits for plasma lipids and lipoproteins in adults as guidelines for choosing suitable levels of ther-

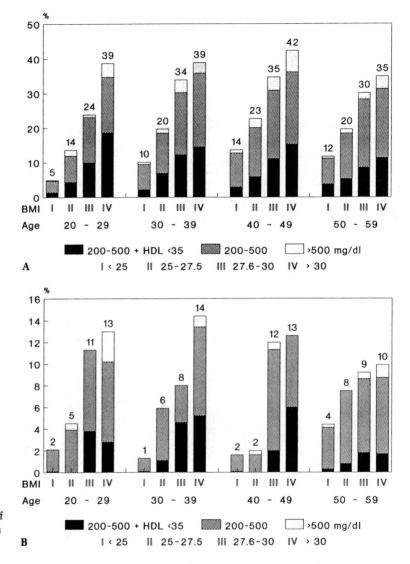

FIGURE 41-5

Prevalence of elevated levels of triglycerides in men **(A)** and in women **(B).**

apy.[1,6] According to the type and severity of the hyperlipidemia, five treatment groups (A through E) may be distinguished (Table 41-4).

When possible, a level of LDL cholesterol of 135 mg/dl is the aim in hypercholesterolemic patients with multiple or severe risk factors and of 155 mg/dl in the absence of other risk factors.[6] The cutoff point for HDL cholesterol of 35 mg/dl should be regarded as a provisional guideline.[1] The groups A through E and the underlying cut-

off points of the recommendation of the EAS are used to determine hyperlipidemia in the following evaluations. Figures 41-2 to 41-6 show the prevalence of hyperlipidemia in the subgroups of persons with acceptable weight, moderate and severe overweight, and obesity in the four age subgroups under consideration.

Only in younger persons is there a linear relationship between the prevalence of hypercholesterolemia and the BMI. Neither the prevalence

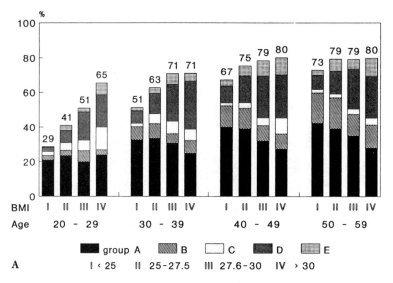

A

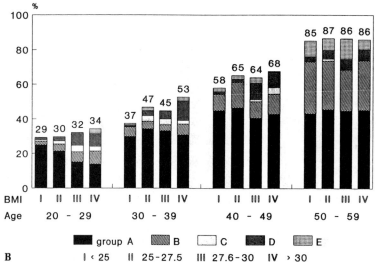

B

FIGURE 41-6

Prevalence of hyperlipidemia in men **(A)** and in women **(B)**.

nor the degree of hypercholesterolemia increases with relative body weight in older individuals (Fig. 41-2).

Nearly the same situation can be observed with LDL cholesterol (Fig. 41-3). The relative frequency of slightly elevated LDL cholesterol concentrations is constant for all age and BMI subgroups. The increased prevalence of elevated LDL cholesterol values in older persons and in young individuals with overweight and obesity depends on a higher percentage of markedly elevated LDL cholesterol concentration.

In contrast, a strong linear correlation is noted between the BMI and the prevalence of low HDL cholesterol concentration in all age-groups in both sexes. Obese persons have about a threefold risk of low HDL cholesterol levels compared with age-matched individuals with acceptable body weight. Men have lower HDL cholesterol values than women. Therefore, the prevalence of low HDL cholesterol levels is much higher in men.

Triglyceride concentrations also differ between men and women. Elevated triglyceride values were found four times more frequently in men than in women. There is a strong direct relation between elevated triglyceride levels and the BMI. Especially, the particularly atherogenic combination of raised triglyceride level and reduced HDL cholesterol increases markedly with the degree of overweight (Fig. 41-5). If the BMI was taken into consideration, the percentage of individuals with elevated triglyceride values did not depend on age.

The frequencies of groups A through E of hyperlipidemia according to the recommendations of the EAS are shown in Figure 41-6. In women, the prevalence of hyperlipidemia depends markedly on age (Fig. 41-6B). Within the subgroups of age up to 50 years, only a slight direct relation between increasing BMI and the prevalence of hyperlipidemia can be observed, caused by higher proportion of group D (combined hyperlipidemia). In men, the dependency of hyperlipidemia on the BMI within age subgroups is more pronounced. Two in three obese young men suffer from hyperlipidemia—more than twice as many as men of the same age with acceptable body weight. The difference in the frequency of hyperlipidemia between men of normal and high weight becomes markedly smaller with increasing age. As in women, the difference is caused by a higher proportion of group D, above all. Therefore, the major lipid problem in obese people compared with persons of normal weight is not so much isolated hypercholesterolemia but mixed hyperlipidemia and hypertriglyceridemia associated with or complicated by low levels of HDL cholesterol.

Acknowledgment: This work was supported by the Bundesministerium für Forschung und Technologie, Ministerium für Wissenschaft und Forschung NRW, Deutsche Forschungsgemeinschaft, and Landesversicherungsanstalt (LVA) Westfalen.

References

1. Study Group, European Atherosclerosis Society: Strategies for the prevention of coronary heart disease: A policy statement of the European Atherosclerosis Society. Eur Heart J 8:77, 1987
2. Assmann G, Schulte H: Procam-Studie. Hedingen Zürich, Panscientia Verlag, 1986
3. Assmann G, Oberwittler W, Schulte H et al: Prädiktion und Früherkennung der koronaren Herzkrankheit. Internist 21:446, 1980
4. Bray GA: Obesity. In Kaplan NM, Stamler J (eds): Prevention of Coronary Heart Disease—Practical Management of the Risk Factors, pp 73–85. Philadelphia, WB Saunders, 1983
5. Friedewald WT, Levy RJ, Fredrickson DS: Estimation of the concentration of low-density-lipoprotein cholesterol in plasma, without use of the preparative ultracentrifuge. Clin Chem 18:499, 1972
6. Study Group, European Atherosclerosis Society: The recognition and management of hyperlipidaemia in adults: A policy statement of the European Atherosclerosis Society. Eur Heart J 9:571, 1988

CHAPTER 42

Obesity and Atherosclerosis

EDWIN L. BIERMAN and JOHN D. BRUNZELL

Evidence has accumulated to suggest that obesity has a role in the pathogenesis of atherosclerotic cardiovascular disease (ASCVD). This conclusion is derived from several lines of evidence:

1. Retrospective and prospective epidemiologic studies that show a relationship between obesity, particularly abdominal adiposity, and the emergence of premature coronary heart disease (CHD)
2. The known association between obesity and weight gain and metabolic risk factors for ASCVD, particularly those related to altered lipid and carbohydrate metabolism
3. The familial clustering of obesity with specific genetic disorders that lead to premature atherosclerosis, such as non–insulin-dependent diabetes mellitus (NIDDM) and familial combined hyperlipidemia (FCHL)

POPULATION STUDIES

Retrospective life insurance data on total mortality as a function of increasing body weight are reviewed elsewhere. Much of this mortality results from ASCVD. By simple univariate analysis, there appears to be a uniform relationship between degree of overweight and ASCVD.[1] However, when subjected to multivariate analysis, obesity often fails to emerge as an "independent" risk factor.[2-4] Because the effect of obesity on atherogenesis is likely to be mediated by alterations in metabolic risk factors (Table 42-1), which in themselves have a direct role in the pathogenesis of atherosclerosis, it is not surprising that when one statistically "corrects" for the other factors, the relation between obesity and CHD is attenuated or disappears. Further, obesity is not independently associated with the severity of atherosclerotic lesions.[5] It is difficult to interpret multivariate analyses of risk factors, which assume independence of variables, when many of these risk factors are obviously interdependent. However, in individual patients, obesity does not exist independently but usually in conjunction with hypertension and the array of metabolic abnormalities listed in Table 42-1. As discussed later, this link is largely due to abdominal, or central, adiposity.

Examples of prospective studies underscore the nature of the link between obesity, particularly abdominal adiposity, and the emergence of premature atherosclerotic disease. In the pooling project, data from five prospective studies of factors involved in the development of CHD were pooled for analytic purposes.[4] These studies spanned three occupation-based populations (Albany Civil Servants, Chicago Gas Company, Chicago Western Electric Company) and two community-based populations (Framingham, MA, and Tecumseh, MI) and included approximately 8400 white men ages 40 to 64 years. The mean length of follow-up was 8.6 years. A high relative weight was associated with an increased risk of a first major coronary event only for men in their 40s. For older groups, no effect of age on the risk of developing CHD has been noted.[1] Thus, it appears that the risk for ASCVD with obesity relates specifically to premature CHD (*i.e.*, before age 50 in men).

TABLE 42-1

Alterations in Risk Factors Associated With Abdominal Adiposity

Hypercholesterolemia
Hypertriglyceridemia
Low levels of high-density lipoprotein (HDL)
   cholesterol
Hyperglycemia
Hyperinsulinemia
Hypertension

The Framingham Study[3,6,7] included more than 5000 men and women living in Framingham, MA. Participants were initially examined between 1948 and 1950 and re-examined at 2-year intervals thereafter. Weight gain was associated with an increase in serum levels of cholesterol, uric acid, glucose, and blood pressure. Overweight was also associated with an increased risk of sudden death, presumably from CHD. Analysis after 26 years indicated that relative weight at entry into the study was an independent predictor of development of cardiovascular diseases, particularly in women. The 26-year incidence of CHD (including angina pectoris) and death from CHD was predicted from the initial degree of overweight using multiple logistic regression analysis. The predictive power for the relative degree of overweight was independent of age, plasma cholesterol levels, systolic blood pressure, cigarette smoking, or glucose intolerance[7] (of note, analyses did not include triglyceride or HDL cholesterol levels). Relative body weight of the women also was independently predictive of the likelihood for developing ASCVD. Weight gain after the young adult years increased the risk of cardiovascular disease in both sexes.

The Seven Countries Study[8] involved an international collaborative examination of risk factors for development of CHD in 16 cohorts of men in the United States, Europe, and Japan. Men at entry into this prospective study were between 40 and 59 years old. Among the men from the United States and southern Europe, few if any significant relationships were found between body weight, the risk of myocardial infarction,

and death due to CHD, but overweight was found to be correlated with angina pectoris. Among the men from northern Europe, statistically significant correlations were noted between all measures of body weight (body mass index [BMI] and skin-fold thicknesses) and coronary events. Overall, in the 15-year follow-up of these groups, relative body weight did not predict the risk of death from CHD. These findings contradict the conclusions based on life insurance statistics.

The American Cancer Society studied the association of mortality with body weight in more than 750,000 people followed prospectively between 1959 and 1972.[9] Relative death rates among subgroups that deviated above or below the average body weight were compared with the death rate for the group with weights that were between 90% and 109% of the group mean. The overall mortality rate increased with increasing body weight, largely as a result of cardiovascular disease. No increase in mortality was observed until the BMI exceeded 25 kg/m², at which point the increase in relative mortality was almost linear for both sexes. These findings are similar to the increases observed both in the Build and Blood Pressure Study of 1979 and in the Framingham Study.

In the Norwegian prospective study,[11] height and weight measurements were obtained for most of that country's population (1.7 million men and women ages 15 to 90) during the course of mass x-ray screenings conducted between 1963 and 1975. Relative mortality increased in curvilinear fashion as the BMI increased above 27 kg/m².

In prospective studies, the relation between cardiovascular disease and obesity seems mediated by body fat distribution. The waist-to-hip ratio was found to be a predictor of myocardial infarction and angina in a prospective study in men[12] and in women[13] in Sweden. Subscapular skin-fold measurements were found to be a better predictor than BMI of subsequent cardiovascular disease in men in Hawaii[14] and in Paris.[15]

ALTERED METABOLIC RISK FACTORS FOR ATHEROSCLEROSIS

Associations of obesity with alterations in lipoprotein metabolism may be related to the risk of developing coronary atherosclerosis. Total plasma cholesterol levels are related to premature CHD, with a fivefold increase in morbidity in those who were 30 to 39 years of age at entry into the Framingham Study,[16] as compared with a 0.6-fold increase in those who were 40 to 49 and 50 to 59 years of age at entry. A similar increase in CHD events as a function of plasma cholesterol was seen in younger individuals in the MRFIT trial as compared with the older individuals.[17] Obesity is associated with elevated total plasma cholesterol levels. This effect is due to elevations of both triglyceride-rich very low density lipoprotein (VLDL) cholesterol and intermediate-density lipoprotein (IDL) cholesterol.[18,19] Even if total cholesterol level in obesity is normal or only slightly elevated, the transport of low-density-lipoprotein (LDL) cholesterol through the plasma compartment increases.[20] This increased transport is consistent with the correlation between increased cholesterol production and obesity, which amounts to approximately 20 more milligrams of cholesterol for each extra kilogram of body fat. Furthermore, this increase in LDL transport and in cholesterol synthesis may be related to the production of VLDL triglyceride and VLDL apoprotein B, which tends to increase in relation to the degree of obesity. Triglyceride levels are increased as reported in many studies, and hypertriglyceridemia is associated with premature CHD in most but not all studies.[21]

Decreased HDL cholesterol levels are associated with increased risk of CHD in older and younger individuals.[22,23] HDL cholesterol levels are decreased in obese men and women,[24] as well as in those with elevated glucose levels[25] and with elevated triglyceride levels.[26]

Elevated fasting plasma glucose levels are also associated with premature CHD. Diabetic individuals, particularly those with NIDDM, also have low HDL cholesterol levels, higher blood pressure, and higher plasma triglyceride and cholesterol levels.[27]

Hyperinsulinemia, whether in studies of whole populations[28-30] or of individuals with NIDDM,[31] appears to be a significant risk factor for the development of CHD. Hyperinsulinemia is a known compensatory consequence of the insulin resistance associated with obesity.[32]

Various tenable potential biologic explanations describe why each of these metabolic risk factors associated with obesity, either alone or in combination, can be involved in atherogenesis. Evidence suggests a common denominator that explains their frequent coexistence, with central obesity, leading to insulin resistance and hyperinsulinemia, being the prime factor.

Adiposity distributed centrally in the abdominal region ("hypertrophic," "upper body," or "android" obesity), usually associated with weight gain in adult years, appears to be distinctly associated with insulin resistance, hyperinsulinemia, and consequent hyperglycemia, hyperlipidemia, and hypertension, compared with generalized distributions of body fat.[33-37] The lipoprotein abnormalities are characterized by elevated VLDL and IDL levels, small dense LDL with elevated apolipoprotein B levels, and decreased HDL 2b levels.[18,19] Some evidence suggests even more precise localization of risk-related adiposity to visceral compared with subcutaneous abdominal adipose tissue.[38-39] The metabolic effects of variation of total body fat compared with subcutaneous and visceral abdominal fat have been summarized elsewhere.[40]

FAMILIAL CLUSTERING OF OBESITY AND ATHEROSCLEROSIS

Several genetic disorders occur on a population background of the syndrome of central obesity, insulin resistance, hypertension, hyperlipidemia, and hyperglycemia. Two inherited disorders, FCHL and NIDDM, contain the various components of this syndrome,[41] with an emphasis on hyperlipidemia and hyperglycemia, respectively. The hyperlipidemia of the central obesity syndrome (increased small VLDL, increased IDL, small dense LDL with elevated apolipoprotein B, and decreased HDL 2b) is the hyperlipidemia noted in both familial combined hyperlipidemia[42,43] and NIDDM.[44] How these two genetic disorders (FCHL and NIDDM), which form the extremes of this syndrome and are inherited separately, are related to the milder expression of the syndrome is unknown. Whether or not other individuals with central obesity have hypertension, hyperglycemia, hyperlipid-

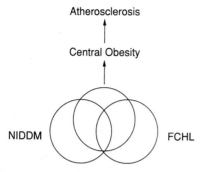

Atherosclerosis

Central Obesity

NIDDM

FCHL

FIGURE 42-1

The manifestations of the central obesity syndrome are seen in NIDDM and FCHL. The third circle contains "others" with central obesity. Whether or not the circles overlap or are entirely separate is unknown; this is a critical question, the answer to which will greatly help in understanding the role of obesity in atherosclerosis.

emia, and an increased risk of premature atherosclerosis remains to be determined.

References

1. Larsson B, Björntorp P, Tibblin G: The health consequences of moderate obesity. Int J Obes 5:97, 1981

2. Bray GA, Davidson MB, Drenick EJ: Obesity: A serious symptom. Ann Intern Med 77:779, 1972

3. Shurtleff D: In Kannel WB, Gordon T (eds): Some Characteristics Related to the Incidence of Cardiovascular Disease and Death: The Framingham Study 18-Year Follow-Up. DHEW Publication (NIH) 74-599. Washington, DC, US Govt Printing Office, 1974

4. The Pooling Project Research Group: Relationship of blood pressure, serum cholesterol, smoking habit, relative weight and ECG abnormalities to incidence of major coronary events: Final report of the Pooling Project. J Chronic Dis 31:201, 1978

5. Solberg LA, Strong JP: Risk factors and atherosclerotic lesions: A review of autopsy studies. Arteriosclerosis 3:187, 1983

6. Sorlie P, Gordon T, Kannel WB: Body build and mortality: The Framingham Study. JAMA 243:1828, 1980

7. Hubert HB, Feinleib M, McNamara PM et al: Obesity as an independent risk factor for cardiovascular disease: A 26-year follow-up of participants in the Framingham Heart Study. Circulation 7:968, 1983

8. Keys A: Overweight, obesity, coronary heart disease and mortality. Nutr Rev 38:297, 1980

9. Lew EA, Garfinkel L: Variations in mortality by weight among 750,000 men and women. J Chronic Dis 32:563, 1979

10. Society of Actuaries: Build and Blood Pressure Study, 1959, Vol I, pp 1–268. Chicago, Study of Actuaries, 1960

11. Waaler HT: Height, weight and mortality: The Norwegian experience. Acta Med Scand (Suppl) 679:1, 1984

12. Larsson B, Svardsudd K, Welin L et al: Abdominal adipose distribution, obesity, and risk of cardiovascular disease and death: 13-year follow up of participants in the study of men born in 1913. Br Med J 288:1401, 1984

13. Lapidus L, Bengtsson C, Larsson B et al: Distribution of adipose tissue and risk of cardiovascular disease and death: A 12-year follow-up of participants in the population study of women in Gothenburg. Br Med J 289:1257, 1984

14. Donahue RP, Abbott RD, Bloom E et al: Central obesity and coronary heart disease in men. Lancet 1:882, 1987

15. Ducimetier P, Richard J, Cambien F: The pattern of subcutaneous fat distribution in middle-aged men and the risk of coronary heart disease. Int J Obes 10:229, 1986

16. Dawber TR: Risk factors for atherosclerotic disease. In Current Concepts, pp 5–36. Kalamazoo, MI, Upjohn, 1975

17. Martin MJ, Hulley SB, Browner WS et al: Serum cholesterol, blood pressure, and mortality: Implications from a cohort of 361,662 men. Lancet 2:933, 1986

18. Peeples LH, Carpenter JW, Israel RG et al: Alterations in low-density lipoproteins in subjects with abdominal adiposity. Metabolism 38:1029, 1989

19. Terry RB, Wood PD, Haskell WL et al: Regional adiposity patterns in relation to lipids, lipoprotein cholesterol, and lipoprotein subfraction mass in man. J Clin Endocrinol Metab 68:191, 1989

20. Grundy SM, Mok HY, Zech L et al: Transport of very low density lipoprotein triglycerides in varying degrees of obesity and hypertriglyceridemia. J Clin Invest 63:1274, 1979

21. Brunzell JD, Austin MA: Plasma triglyceride and coronary disease. N Engl J Med 320:1273, 1989

22. Castelli WY, Doyle JP, Gordon T et al: HDL cholesterol and other lipids in coronary heart disease: The Cooperative Lipoprotein Phenotyping Study. Circulation 55:767, 1977

23. Miller NE, Forde OH, Thelle DS et al: High-density lipoprotein and coronary heart disease: A prospective case-control study. Lancet 1:965, 1977

24. Garrison RJ, Kannel WB, Feinleib M, et al: Cigarette smoking and HDL cholesterol: The Framingham offspring study. Atherosclerosis 30:17, 1978

25. Lopez-Virella MFL, Stone PG, Colwell JA: Serum high density lipoprotein in diabetic patients. Diabetologia 13:285, 1977

26. Schaeffer EJ, Anderson DW, Danner RN et al: Plasma triglycerides in regulation of HDL cholesterol levels. Lancet 2:391, 1978

27. Bierman EL, Brunzell JD: Interrelation of atherosclerosis, abnormal lipid metabolism, and diabetes mellitus. In Katzen HM, Mahler RJ (eds): Diabetes, Obesity and Vascular Disease, pp 187–210. New York, Halsted Press, 1978

28. Pyörälä K, Savolainen E, Kaukola S et al: Plasma insulin as coronary heart disease factor: Relationship to other risk factors and predictive value during 9.5-year follow-up of the Helsinki Policemen Study population. Acta Med Scand (Suppl) 701:38, 1985

29. Dulcimetiere P, Eschwege E, Papoz L et al: Relationship of plasma insulin levels to the incidence of myocardial infarction and coronary heart disease mortality in a middle-aged population. J Diabetologia 19:205, 1980

30. Welborne TA, Wearne K: Coronary heart disease incidence and cardiovascular mortality in Busselton with reference to glucose and insulin concentrations. Diabetes Care 2:154, 1979

31. Standl E, Janka HU: High serum insulin concentrations in relation to other cardiovascular risk factors in macrovascular disease of type 2 diabetes. Horm Metab Res Suppl 15:46, 1985

32. Bierman EL, Bagdade JD, Porte D Jr: Obesity and diabetes: The odd couple. Am J Clin Nutr 21:1434, 1968

33. Hirsch J: Adipose cellularity in relation to human obesity. Adv Intern Med 17:289, 1971

34. Kissebah AH, Peiris AN: Biology of regional body fat distribution: Relationship to non–insulin-dependent diabetes mellitus. Diabetes Metab Rev 5:83, 1989

35. Krotkiewski M, Björntorp P, Sjöström L et al: Impact of obesity on metabolism in men and women: Importance of regional adipose tissue distribution. J Clin Invest 72:1150, 1983

36. Reaven G: Role of Insulin Resistance in Human Disease: Banting Lecture 1988. Diabetes 37:1595, 1988

37. Stern MP, Haffner SM: Body fat distribution and hyperinsulinemia as risk factors for diabetes and cardiovascular disease. Arteriosclerosis 6:123, 1986

38. Fujioka S, Matsuzawa Y, Tokunaga K et al: Contribution of intraabdominal fat accumulation to the impairment of glucose and lipid metabolism in human obesity. Metabolism 36:54, 1987

39. Shuman WP, Newell Morris LL, Leonetti DL et al: Abnormal body fat distribution detected by computed tomography in diabetic men. Invest Radiol 21:483, 1986

40. Bouchard C, Bray GA, Hubbard VS: Basic and clinical aspects of regional fat distribution. Am J Clin Nutr 52:946, 1990

41. Brunzell JB: Obesity and coronary heart disease: A targeted approach. Arteriosclerosis 4:180, 1984

42. Brunzell JD, Albers JJ, Chait A et al: Plasma lipoproteins in familial combined hyperlipidemia and monogenic familial hypertriglyceridemia. J Lipid Res 24:147, 1983

43. Krauss RM, Albers JJ, Brunzell JD: An apolipoprotein B-enriched low density lipoprotein subspecies in familial combined hyperlipidemia. Clin Res 31:503, 1983

44. Brunzell JD, Chait A, Bierman EL: Plasma lipoproteins in human diabetes mellitus. In Alberti KGM, Krall LP (eds): The Diabetes Annual I, pp 323–348. Amsterdam, Elsevier Medical Publishers, 1985

CHAPTER 43

Obesity and the Heart

VICKI SARA BLUMBERG and JONATHAN ALEXANDER

Cardiovascular disease has been the leading cause of death in the United States for several decades. Research efforts to identify those modifiable risk factors have resulted in a significant decline in the cardiovascular mortality rate since the mid-1960s. Although the observation that cardiac dysfunction exists commonly in obese persons has been long-standing, it has now been shown that obesity alone independently increases one's risk of cardiovascular morbidity and mortality. Clinical researchers spent years accruing epidemiologic and pathologic data in an effort to demystify this decisive link, bringing the importance of obesity as a significant health hazard to the forefront. This chapter reviews several subjects relating to obesity and the heart, beginning with cardiac pathology and pathophysiology. Arrhythmias, because they predispose obese patients to sudden death, are discussed, followed by the more controversial topic of the link between obesity and coronary artery disease. For clinicians, a section describing testing and screening procedures follows a brief review of preoperative evaluation. Finally, the effects of obesity treatment on cardiac parameters are elucidated.

CARDIAC PATHOLOGY

In his extensive 1980 review *Obesity and the Heart*, James K. Alexander details the history of the study of cardiac pathology in obesity, which is briefly summarized here.[1] More than 50 years ago, Smith and Willius evaluated gross and microscopic specimens of the cardiovascular system in obese subjects at autopsy.[2] They observed clinical circulatory dysfunction in morbidly obese patients and were the first to systematically study cardiac anatomy in this group. They reported postmortem studies of 136 patients with an average excess body weight of 45% (32.3 kg). They found that heart weight increased with increasing body weight. Furthermore, absolute cardiac weight was considerably greater in overweight subjects than in persons of ideal body weight. Finding an excess of epicardial fat in 95% of specimens, they concentrated on what they called "adiposity of the heart." Epicardial fat was found to penetrate only the right ventricle and to varying degrees. The authors cited nine patients in whom congestive symptoms developed independent of other primary cardiac disease seen at autopsy. Three of these patients actually died of congestive heart failure. They concluded that fatty infiltration of the heart, as it is called today, impaired cardiac function enough for the heart to fail and even cause death. This entity was again studied in the 1930s and was found by no means to be limited to hearts of obese persons. Peers of Smith and Willius, Saphir and Corrigan, reviewed 58 autopsy cases[3] and recorded only 18 as obese. Nine of the total number of patients were actually emaciated, having various acute and chronic illnesses. In two of the obese individuals, however, fatty infiltration was the only obvious cause of death. Furthermore, both of these deaths were sudden. Appreciating the fact that very obese individuals tend to float in water more easily than nonobese individuals, W. C. Roberts and J. D. Roberts studied the "floating heart," or hearts so laden with fat that they did not sink in water.[4] They found the amount of fat in the atrial septum to be increased in all of their 55 subjects at autopsy. Criteria for "lipomatous hypertrophy of the atrial septum" were recognized in 25%, and of the 29% of these patients who died of acute myocardial infarction, nearly half had rupture of the left ventricular free wall or ventricular septum. The researchers concluded that cardiac rupture during acute myocardial infarction is much more common in a fat-laden heart than in a nonfatty heart. Other case histories in which severe fatty infiltration led to a decrease in myocardial function have since been cited. Arrhythmias were also recognized, possibly resulting from significant fat infiltration in regions of the sinoatrial node, atrioventricular node, and His bundle.[1] The functional significance of lesser degrees of myocardial fatty infiltration was either inconsequential or difficult to assess. Because in various clinical settings the incidence at autopsy of fatty infiltration of the heart is only 3%,[5] unlike the conclusions of earlier 20th century pathologists, this finding is now believed to be quite rare, even in obesity.

Further clarification was sought in the mid 1960s by Alexander and his colleagues after observing severe cardiac hypertrophy in grossly obese patients. They studied 12 autopsy cases of long-standing, severe obesity in patients who had been free of hypertension or other possible associated cardiac disease.[6] Increased heart weight was observed in each case, and increased left ventricular wall thickness was seen in all 11 cases cited. None had isolated right ventricular hypertrophy. Biventricular hypertrophy was seen in one. Diffuse muscular hypertrophy was seen in all cases, whereas gross infiltration of the myocardium by fat was not. Although two of four hearts weighing in excess of 600 g had an increase in epicardial fat, it was not enough to account for the marked increase in cardiac weight. It was thus concluded that the most specific and significant anatomic alteration in hearts of very obese persons is left ventricular hypertrophy.

MYOCARDIAL PATHOPHYSIOLOGY

Much is now known about the myocardial pathophysiology of obesity. Early recognition that obe-sity causes cardiac enlargement, specifically left ventricular hypertrophy, prompted investigators to compare the cardiomyopathy of obesity with that of essential hypertension. The fact that the two disorders frequently coexist in an individual made it necessary to determine whether this association additionally harms a patient or perhaps even mitigates against detrimental cardiovascular effects. The hemodynamics of *essential hypertension* in the *nonobese* population have now been well elucidated. In the early stages of this disorder, cardiac output is elevated and peripheral resistance is abnormally high. This inappropriate elevation in resistance raises blood pressure. Further increases in peripheral resistance occur with excesses in smooth-muscle contraction. As total peripheral resistance increases, cardiac output falls and intravascular volume becomes progressively contracted. As blood pressure elevation progresses, the heart adapts to compensate for an increased afterload. Afterload reflects the wall tension that the ventricle must generate to eject blood into the aorta. This increase in wall tension generated by a higher left ventricular pressure is a potent stimulus for myocyte thickening and lengthening. Compensatory *concentric* left ventricular hypertrophy develops and normalizes wall stress without changing the internal dimensions of the cardiac chambers. This phase of adaptation may remain clinically and electrocardiographically silent.[7]

Through the work of Alexander, Messerli, and others, a different hemodynamic profile is found to characterize *obese* patients. As a result of the increase in adipose tissue stores, an increment in total body oxidative requirements occurs at rest and with exercise. Adipose tissue is metabolically active and from it are derived free fatty acids important for the metabolism of skeletal and cardiac muscle. The adipose tissue bed may represent an important volume reservoir as blood flow to subcutaneous adipose tissue increases up to sevenfold with exercise.[8] As a result of weight loss, decrements in cardiac output have been shown to reflect a reduction in adipose tissue blood flow due to smaller adipocyte volume.[9] The increased body surface area in obese persons represents an additional increase in skin and lean body mass. Because the arteriovenous oxygen difference is normal or only slightly increased, the cardiac output must increase proportionally to the increase in minute volume oxygen consumption. The resting heart rate in obesity has been observed to remain essentially within the normal range, hence this increase in cardiac output must be due to an increase in stroke volume. Total blood volume and plasma volume are expanded, in contrast to that of nonobese individuals with essential hypertension. Nonhypertensive obese patients must then experience a decrement in total peripheral resistance for arterial pressure to remain within the normal range. To accommodate the volume expansion and stroke volume increase, left ventricular enddiastolic volume must therefore increase. Thus, obesity represents a volume-expanded state resulting in an increase in preload. The resulting left ventricular chamber dilatation increases wall stress and therefore afterload. As in hypertension, cardiovascular reserve is preserved by a

compensatory hypertrophy of the left ventricle. However, unlike hypertension, in which the ratio between wall thickness and internal cavitary radius is increased, in obesity this ratio remains essentially normal and the compensatory left ventricular hypertrophy is *eccentric* (Fig. 43-1).[10] These differences in components of left ventricular function are summarized in Table 43-1.[11] In a study of 171 patients, body weight and body surface area were shown to be the most powerful determinants of left ventricular wall thickness, chamber size, and left ventricular muscle mass.[12] As a rule of thumb, the investigators suggest that left ventricular hypertrophy can be anticipated in more than 50% of patients who are more than 50% overweight.[10]

More data now confirm earlier observations that isolated *right* ventricular hypertrophy has not been a finding in the obese population. Right ventricular abnormalities may be encountered,

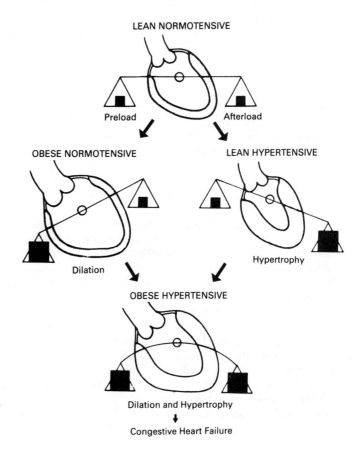

FIGURE 43-1

Adaptation of the heart to obesity and hypertension. (Messerli FH: Cardiovascular effects of obesity and hypertension. Lancet 1:1165, 1982)

TABLE 43-1

Left Ventricular Function

	Obesity	Hypertension
Cardiac output	↑	—
Contractility	↓	↑
Preload	↑ ↑	—
Afterload	↑	↑ ↑
Stroke work	↑	↑

however, in obese patients with pulmonary disease. Obesity hypoventilation is noted in less than 5% of morbidly obese patients[13] and is characterized by episodes of apnea during sleep. These episodes result in hypoxemia, increased pulmonary resistance due to hypoxic vasoconstriction, and hypercapnea. In a study of patients with this entity, it was shown that many develop pulmonary hypertension secondary to left ventricular dysfunction as well as hypoxic pulmonary vasoconstriction.[14] Elevated left atrial and pulmonary venous pressures result from increased left ventricular end-diastolic pressure. The high cardiac output affects the pulmonary circulation as well by causing right ventricular hypertrophy. Necropsy studies of patients with obesity hypoventilation consistently demonstrate biventricular hypertrophy.[1] Just as severe lung disease poses an additional burden on the heart, so does the coupling of hypertension with obesity. When the two diseases are superimposed, right ventricular dilatation can be encountered.[15]

Systemic vascular resistance has been found to be a reliable indicator of systemic hypertensive vascular disease. Previous investigators have suggested that obese hypertensive patients may be protected from end-organ damage by virtue of the fact that systemic vascular resistance is lowered.[16] Perrera and Damon showed that accelerated hypertension with papilledema and arteriolar necrosis in renal biopsy specimens was more prevalent in lean than in obese hypertensive women.[17] However, left ventricular stroke work has been shown to be more than 60% higher in obese hypertensive patients than in corresponding lean normotensive subjects.[18] Indeed, the Honolulu Heart Program challenged

previous suggestions of a possible "protective mechanism" and concluded from a 12-year study that hypertension is associated with an increased risk of cardiovascular disease in both obese and nonobese men and that the relationship of blood pressure to cardiovascular disease incidence does not vary with the level of body mass index.[19] Hypertension, as it relates to obesity, is examined in detail by another contributor to this anthology. Suffice it to say that the superimposition of these two disorders, especially when untreated, certainly puts a patient at increased risk for congestive heart failure.[18] It can result from a combination of left ventricular systolic (impaired contraction) and diastolic (decreased compliance) dysfunction.

Several studies have sought to identify preclinical heart disease in obese subjects. Carabello's group studied 14 asymptomatic obese patients free of hypertension and angiographic coronary narrowing.[20] The degree of obesity was considered moderate, with an average increase over ideal body weight of 50% and a lower limit for inclusion of 25%. Load-independent indices were used to evaluate ventricular function. Concordant with earlier studies, increases in cardiac output, stroke work, cardiac hypertrophy, and left ventricular filling pressure were seen. Unexpectedly, however, there was an inverse correlation between obesity and wall stress and a positive correlation between the degree of obesity and ejection fraction. In other words, enhanced cardiac performance was noted in moderately obese subjects free of hypertension and coronary artery disease. Garavaglia and Messerli studied mild to moderately obese, asymptomatic, hypertensive subjects. When a load-independent ratio of end-systolic wall stress to end-systolic volume index was examined, myocardial contractility was found to be depressed despite overall well-preserved pump function.[21] In what was originally believed to be a study with results contradicting these, DeDivitiis studied ten young subjects who had various degrees of obesity and were also free of other pathologic disease. They underwent left and right heart catheterization, and various hemodynamic variables were calculated. Left ventricular function was estimated by a ratio of stroke work index (SWI) to left ventricular end-diastolic pressure (LVEDP) (Fig. 43-2).[22]

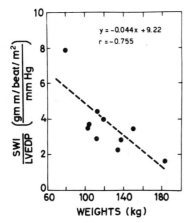

FIGURE 43-2

The significant negative correlation between the ratio of the SWI to the left ventricular LVEDP and weight, showing that the higher the degree of obesity, the greater the impairment of left ventricular function. (DeDivitiis D, Fazio S, Petitto M et al: Obesity and cardiac function. Circulation 64:3, 1981)

Eight of the heaviest subjects were found to have impaired left ventricular function despite an increase in filling pressure and volume. Hence, even in young, asymptomatic subjects free of hypertension or coronary artery disease, left ventricular impairment correlated positively with the degree of obesity. In a noninvasive study by Romano and colleagues, systolic time intervals and the ratio of pre-ejection period (PEP) to left ventricular ejection time (LVET) were used to represent a means of detecting early left ventricular systolic dysfunction. This group also showed a correlation between the amount of overweight, transverse cardiac diameter as seen on chest x-ray, and left ventricular dysfunction, despite a young age, lack of additional cardiac risk factors, and a lack of symptoms.[23] Comparisons of these studies have prompted several researchers to point out a common factor: the subjects found to have preclinical left ventricular systolic dysfunction have a higher degree of obesity than those obese patients in whom left ventricular systolic function is preserved.

Diastolic dysfunction of the left ventricle, as demonstrated by electrocardiographic evidence of left atrial abnormality and the reduction of the left atrial emptying index, is encountered in hypertensive patients before the development of electrocardiographic evidence of left ventricular hypertrophy.[24] This has now been demonstrated to occur early in obesity as well. The left atrial emptying index was actually reduced more in obese patients than in lean hypertensive persons and reduced most in obese hypertensive patients. Electrocardiographic evidence of left atrial abnormality correlated best with reduced ventricular diastolic performance and may also provide early noninvasive evidence of changes in cardiac structure and function.[24]

Alexander describes two scenarios in which clinical symptoms may become apparent.[1] A congestive circulatory state is noted when chronic volume overload due to long-standing obesity increases to the point where distensibility of the vascular bed and diastolic compliance decline despite well-preserved pump function. In this group, it may be said that myocardial hypertrophy has kept up with chamber dilatation. Ejection fraction, as shown by echocardiography or radionuclide ventriculography, remains within the normal range (normal systolic function). The second setting represents the more classic form of congestive heart failure due to abnormal myocardial systolic function. Wall stress increases when ventricular hypertrophy has not kept up with chamber dilatation, and left ventricular systolic function deteriorates. In obesity, the adverse prognosis of congestive heart failure due to impaired ventricular systolic performance is similar, at best, to that in nonobese patients and may indeed be worse. Mortality may exceed 50% per year when compensation is not accomplished by treatment (Benotti JR: Lecture notes of October of Harvard Continuing Medical Education Conference on Obesity. Boston, MA, 1988).

ARRHYTHMIAS/SUDDEN DEATH

Even in ancient times, obesity was recognized as a significant obstacle in the pursuit of longevity. Hippocrates stated that "sudden death is more common in those who are naturally fat than in the lean."[25] In the Framingham Heart Study, obesity was found to be a strong predictor of sudden death. The study further demonstrates that independent of blood pressure, evidence of left ventricular hypertrophy on a resting electrocardiogram is a particularly dangerous finding. It increased the risk of subsequent cardiovascular disease more than threefold and significantly raised cardiovascular mortality statistics.[26] Several studies have shown an increase in ventricular ectopy in hypertensive patients with left ventricular hypertrophy, independent of obesity. One study has shown this to be the case even in treated hypertensive patients with left ventricular hypertrophy.[27] The investigators demonstrated an increase not only in isolated ventricular extrasystoles but in complex ventricular ectopy as well. There was no evidence that the results were due to either hypokalemia alone or diuretic therapy. They also point out that complex ventricular arrhythmias have been shown to predict cardiovascular mortality more accurately in other cardiac conditions as well, such as ischemic heart disease and hypertrophic cardiomyopathy. In their investigation of sudden death in obesity, Messerli and colleagues studied lean and obese subjects matched for arterial blood pressure.[28] Obese subjects without eccentric left ventricular hypertrophy (as determined by echocardiography) had ten times the prevalence of premature ventricular contractions than their lean counterparts. Notably, in the obese patients *with* eccentric left ventricular hypertrophy, the prevalence of premature ventricular contractions was three times higher than this, or 30 times higher than in their lean counterparts (Fig. 43-3).[28] Most importantly, when subdivided according to the Lown and Wolf classification of increasing complexity of ectopy, those with higher left ventricular diastolic diameter as well as left ventricular mass scored higher. In other words, obese patients with eccentric left ventricular hypertrophy are more prone to complex ventricular ectopy (Table 43-2).[28] Messerli offers that although a firm causal relationship between ventricular ectopy and sudden death has not been shown, common sense would dictate that those patients with a higher degree of electrical instability are the most vulnerable. In Drenick and Fisler's study of sudden cardiac arrest in morbidly obese surgical patients,[29] the patients had been clinically stable and free of evident acute stress or intercurrent illness at the time of death. Whenever the terminal events were monitored,

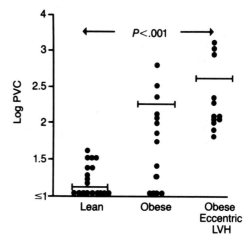

FIGURE 43-3

Prevalence of premature ventricular contractions (PVCs) expressed on a logarithmic scale in lean subjects and obese patients with and without eccentric left ventricular hypertrophy (LVH). (Messerli FH, Nunez BD, Ventura HO et al: Overweight and sudden death: Increased ventricular ectopy in cardiopathy of obesity. Arch Intern Med 147:1727, 1987)

either ventricular tachycardia or ventricular fibrillation was seen. The predisposition to malignant arrhythmias noted in these patients may have been directly related to a prolongation of the QT interval as seen on electrocardiogram. This point will be elaborated on later. Several explanations have been proposed for the observation that an increase in myocardial mass may give rise to increased ventricular irritability. Although it has been suggested that left ventricular hypertrophy is a silent marker for coronary artery disease, pathologic, experimental, and clinical evidence do not substantiate this. It has been shown that afterpotentials, which may predispose to ventricular arrhythmias, can be induced in hypertrophic rat myocardium but not in normal rat myocardium.[30] A clinical study involving patients with hypertrophic cardiomyopathy revealed induction of ventricular tachycardia by electrical stimulation in 82% of subjects.[31] In none of the patients in a "control" group with severe coronary artery disease but normal left ventricular function and no previous infarction was ventricular tachycardia inducible. Electro-

TABLE 43-2

Classification (of Lown and Wolf) of Lean and Obese Patients With and Without Left Ventricular Hypertrophy

Maximal Classification of Lown and Wolf	Lean	Obese	
		Without Eccentric LVH	With Eccentric LVH*
0	19	7	1
I	4	4	3
II	0	4	2
III	1	0	4
IV	0	0	4

*$P < .005$ between obese patients with eccentric left ventricular hypertrophy (LVH) and both other groups.

physiologic mechanisms have been considered and summarized by Messerli and colleagues[28]:

First, enlarged myocytes, multiple intercalated disks, and electrically silent (i.e. fibrotic) areas in fibrotic regions disturb intercellular current flow and wave propagation, thereby giving rise to reentry mechanisms. Second, mechanical stretching of isolated myocytes has been shown to increase excitability threshold. Volume overload states such as seen in obesity produce chamber dilatation and increase ventricular wall stress [as in the present study] thereby possibly enhancing the arrhythmogenic potential by this mechanism. Third, the increased wall stress and stroke work of the left ventricle in obesity increases myocardial oxygen requirements and could lead to subendocardial ischemia. Experimental and clinical data indicate that ectopic activity increases with progressive underperfusion of the myocardium. Although none of our patients had clinical evidence of coronary artery disease, it must be remembered that left ventricular hypertrophy by itself diminishes coronary reserve and may give rise to relative ischemia. Thus, the hypertrophied myocardium, whether the result of chronic volume or pressure overload, provides a fertile soil for the sprouting of ventricular arrhythmias.

CORONARY ARTERY DISEASE

The fact that obesity poses an increased hazard for the development of coronary heart disease has long been recognized. Many studies using univariate analysis have shown increased morbidity and mortality in obese patients, attribut-able to coronary heart disease. In an American Cancer Society study of approximately 750,000 men and women in the general population,[32] mortality due to coronary artery disease among those persons 30% to 40% heavier than average was nearly 50% higher than among those of average weight. Furthermore, a linear dose-response relationship was found, as exhibited by a risk 90% higher than average for those individuals more than 40% overweight. There is little debate that obesity is related to a disadvantageous coronary risk profile.[33] Data from the two National Health and Nutrition Examination Surveys (NHANES I and II) is extensive. NHANES II in particular showed a strong association between the prevalence of obesity and cardiovascular disease risk factors.[34] Hypertension (as defined by blood pressure greater than 160/95) was 2.9 times higher for overweight persons compared with nonoverweight. Many studies corroborate the observation that the young are particularly at risk, and this study was no exception. In those persons ages 20 to 44, the prevalence of hypertension was 5.6 times higher. In this young group, the prevalence of hypercholesterolemia (total cholesterol over 250 mg/dl) was shown to be approximately twice that of nonoverweight persons. Because data have now shown an adverse coronary risk associated with levels less than this, the risk of hypercholesterolemia is probably underestimated in the NHANES study. The prevalence of diabetes was nearly three times greater in overweight than nonoverweight persons. In addition to the fact that non–insulin-dependent diabetes mellitus (NIDDM) is now known to be inherited,[35] individuals with NIDDM are more obese than the nondiabetic population. Despite this genetic predisposition, weight loss improves hyperinsulinemia, peripheral insulin resistance, and the glucose intolerance associated with obesity.

Because obesity often begins in early life, the Bogalusa Heart Study helps to clarify the influence of persistent obesity in childhood on cardiovascular risk factors.[36] Epidemiologists studied the relationship between changes in triceps skin-fold thickness and level of serum lipids in a biracial group of 1598 children in Bogalusa, LA. At entry, the children were 5 to 12 years of age and were restudied 5 years later. The investigators noted that 20% to 30% of children, especially among whites, were obese. A close interrelationship between obesity and hyperlipidemia, accompanied by hyperinsulinemia, was noted in those children even without morbid obesity. Risk factors seemed to reach a threshold level near the 70th percentile of skin-fold thickness, a level not believed to be extreme in the general population. They also concluded that the effect of persistent obesity is likely to be expressed as higher cardiovascular morbidity as adults.

Whether obesity alone, independent of associated adverse cardiovascular risk factors, is associated with a higher incidence of coronary artery disease has been an issue of much more controversy. Alexander points out that autopsy studies "must be interpreted with the reservation that the nutritional status of the individual at postmortem examination may not reflect that existing during the development of atheromatous lesions."[1] To obviate this limitation he quotes a study by Montenegro and Solberg from 1968 assessing the extent of coronary disease versus obesity in 350 accidental deaths.[37] There was no obvious correlation between fatty streaks or raised atheromatous lesions and any of the indices of obesity for any of the varied ethnic and geographic groups of individuals. Similar conclusions were drawn from examination of coronary angiograms in relation to height/weight index.[38] A small but interesting study by Warnes and Roberts examined 12 cases at autopsy. Patients

died between the ages of 25 and 59 years, and all weighed more than 300 pounds.[39] Each had been severely obese for several years before death, usually from puberty. Only two patients (ages 42 and 59 years) had one or more epicardial coronary arteries narrowed more than 75% in cross-sectional area by atherosclerotic plaque. The investigators concluded that these extremely obese patients who died prematurely did not have more coronary atherosclerosis than might be expected at their ages. Epidemiologic studies provide another means of assessing the importance of obesity on coronary disease. In her review, Hubert recognizes this epidemiologic controversy, pointing out the problem with comparing results from studies often conducted in dissimilar populations, having differences in the length of follow-up, or using very different methodologies.[33] She therefore reviews prospective studies in North American populations in which longitudinal observation was continued for a minimum of 4 to 5 years.

Multivariate analyses adjust for the influence of other coronary heart disease risk factors and reveal significant independent relationships between obesity and disease. The eight cohort studies of the Pooling Project Research Group[40] revealed discrepant results when analyzed separately, but when the data from all the studies were combined, obesity was associated positively with the risk of coronary artery disease. Significant results were especially found in the younger cohorts studied. The obesity index used to characterize the populations was Metropolitan Relative Weight (MRW), or the percentage of desirable weight (the ratio of actual weight to desirable weight × 100). "Desirable weight" was derived from the 1959 Metropolitan Life Insurance Company tables. In 40- to 49-year-old men, a 10% increase in MRW was associated with a 13% to 19% increase in disease incidence. In the Manitoba Study of nearly 4000 men monitored for 26 years, there was a linear increase of cardiovascular risk with body mass index.[41] This impact was most evident in those who were studied before middle age. Another more well-known study is the Framingham Heart Study.[26] Earlier data suggesting that obesity per se was not an independent risk factor were based on shorter periods of follow-up, and this has now been re-evaluated after 26 years. At entry to the study the disease-free Framingham cohort appeared to be considerably overweight. Cardiovascular disease was manifested by coronary artery disease, congestive heart failure, stroke, and intermittent claudication. In summary, the study reveals that MRW predicted the 26-year incidence of angina, coronary disease other than angina, and coronary death in men, *independent* of age, cholesterol, systolic blood pressure, smoking, left ventricular hypertrophy, and glucose intolerance (Fig. 43-4).[26] Relative weight in women was a particularly significant predictor of coronary disease, coronary death, and stroke.

In both sexes, weight gain after the young adult years conveyed an increased risk of cardiovascular disease that could not be attributed either to the initial weight or levels of risk factors that may have resulted from the weight gain. Of note

is that a strong and significant association between weight and coronary disease did not evolve until the 8-year follow-up. Probably because of the small number of events in this group, it took 14 years to prove significance for women. This hiatus suggests that the discrepancies in other studies may, at least in part, be due to the shorter periods of observation.

Data now show that the fat distribution pattern in obesity may be a better predictor of cardiovascular risk than just the degree of adiposity. Two patterns of fat distribution may be identified. Android obesity is typical in men and is defined by fat cell deposits in the central abdominal region. Gynecoid obesity is more common in women, with fat cell deposits predominately in the legs and buttocks. Abdominal obesity is characterized by having a high waist-to-hip (W:H) ratio. Two studies in Sweden revealed an increase in

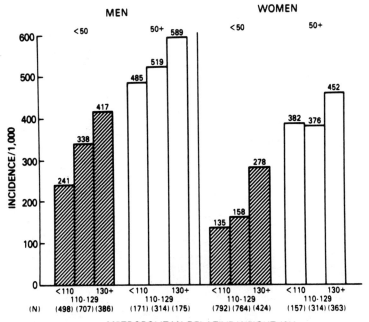

FIGURE 43-4

Correlation between the 26-year incidence of cardiovascular disease by MRW at entry among Framingham patients younger/older than age 50. N = the number at risk for an event. Numbers above the bars give the actual incidence rates per 1000. (Hubert HB, Feinleib M, McNamara PM et al: Obesity as an independent risk factor for cardiovascular disease: A 26-year follow-up of participants in the Framingham Heart Study. Circulation 67:970, 1983)

cardiovascular risk when the W:H ratio exceeded 1 in men and 0.8 in women. Specifically, in a 13-year follow-up of 792 male residents of Gothenburg, the W:H ratio was significantly associated with stroke, ischemic heart disease, and total cardiovascular death.[42] Another study in women from the same town reveals a significant positive correlation of the W:H ratio to the 12-year incidence of myocardial infarction, angina, stroke, and death.[43] The investigators believe that abdominal fat cells are more metabolically active than those of the periphery and release more fatty acid. Increased fatty acid release elevates hepatic formation of triglycerides and interferes with insulin kinetics, thus confirming another study revealing higher lipid and blood glucose levels in those with greater abdominal obesity. Increased circulating fatty acids have also been implicated as being arrhythmogenic.

Data now also support the clinical observation that thromboembolic disease is increased in the obese population.[44] Fibrinolytic activity has been shown to play a protective role in ischemic heart disease and has now been demonstrated to vary inversely with excessive body weight.[45] When weight reduction occurs, fibrinolytic activity has been shown to increase.[46] It has been suggested that this may be mediated by varying levels of plasminogen activator.[47] It has additionally been shown that antithrombin III, the principal endogenous circulating anticoagulant, is diminished in morbidly obese patients and may be restored to normal with weight loss.[48,49]

CARDIOVASCULAR TESTING/SCREENING

For clinicians, great reliance must be placed on the noninvasive cardiovascular evaluation of an obese patient because of the difficulty encountered in performing a meaningful physical examination. This is especially true in trying to detect preclinical abnormalities of cardiac function in an asymptomatic and otherwise healthy individual. In Romano and colleagues' study of 17 severely obese young subjects without clinical cardiovascular disease, the workers examined the chest x-ray film, evaluating cardiac size in two different ways.[23] Measurement of the transverse diameter of the cardiac silhouette has been suggested as a satisfactory index of cardiac size in

obese persons, as well as calculation of the cardiothoracic ratio, where 0.5 is considered the upper limit of normal. Romano and associates found the transverse cardiac diameter to be greater in obese subjects than in the control group, and each obese patient had a greater diameter than that expected for sex, age, and body composition. In addition, the transverse cardiac diameter was significantly correlated with the degree of overweight. Although this linear relationship to degree of overweight was not found with the cardiothoracic ratio, almost 59% showed a cardiothoracic ratio greater than 0.5.

Because of its relatively low cost and lack of invasiveness, the electrocardiogram is often used in evaluating obese patients. As previously mentioned, Lavie and co-workers stated that evidence of left atrial abnormality on electrocardiogram correlated well with a reduced left atrial emptying index.[24] This observation is believed to be a reflection of reduced left ventricular diastolic function. Frank's group investigated the electrocardiogram in 1029 patients with various degrees of obesity.[50] The data were controlled for age, sex, and blood pressure, and subjects were free of cardioactive medications. Normal sinus rhythm was found to be overwhelmingly present, in 73.5% of the patients. Of those remaining, 19% were bradycardic and only 0.5% exhibited sinus tachycardia. Despite heart rate remaining within the normal range for the majority, a trend was noted toward increasing heart rate with increasing percent overweight. Repolarization abnormalities were present in 11% of patients; however, these nonspecific ST- and T-wave changes were thought to be independent of the degree of obesity and correlated more with an increase in age and blood pressure. Significant conduction abnormalities were infrequent, and there was only a slight but statistically significant increase in the PR interval and QRS duration with increasing obesity. However, as with heart rate, these increases remained within the range of normal. Previous studies have demonstrated a tendency toward left-axis deviation in obesity. However, as in this study, the mean QRS frontal plane vector remains within the normal range. Only 0.7% had left-axis deviation beyond $-30°$. This is clearly in agreement with Zack and colleagues' study of left-axis deviation and adiposity using data from the U.S. NHANES I.[51] They similarly found that with increasing adiposity, a leftward shift of the mean QRS axis occurs in both men and women; however, this association is lost as the QRS axis becomes abnormally deviated to the left. Therefore, left-axis deviation within the normal range may be attributed to adiposity itself, whereas abnormal left-axis deviation likely represents a true cardiac abnormality. Perhaps the most important electrocardiographic abnormality found commonly in obesity is a prolongation of the QT interval. In Frank and co-workers' study, a mild increase was found in 28.3% and a markedly prolonged QT interval in 4% of their obese subjects.[50] The abnormality could not be attributed to electrolyte abnormalities or drug effects. This observation may have profound clinical consequences. In the previously mentioned study by Drenick and Fisler, who investigated sudden cardiac arrest in morbidly obese surgical patients,[29] 29 of 38 were found to have a prolonged QT interval on electrocardiogram, indicating a predisposition to malignant arrhythmias. Significantly, only 9 of 38 patients who suddenly died had normal QT intervals when all tracings were re-examined. It is especially noted that of 45 preoperative baseline electrocardiograms, 39 were originally interpreted as being normal. Clearly, when interpreting an electrocardiogram in an obese subject, a precise measurement of the QT interval must be routine.

Data regarding interpretation of QRS voltage on an electrocardiogram from an obese patient remain inconclusive. Various researchers have commented on the low voltage noted and explain it as the attenuation of voltage by its passage through a thickened, fat-laden chest wall. Other investigators have found, as in Frank's large study,[29] an increasing amplitude of QRS voltage with increasing percent overweight. Alexander found that in his patients with circulatory congestion, despite impressive degrees of left ventricular hypertrophy on anatomical examination, evidence of hypertrophy on electrocardiogram was usually absent.[1] In one study and review of this issue, Nath's group examined the sensitivity and specificity of electrocardiographic criteria for left and right ventricular hypertrophy in morbidly obese persons.[52] Their study compares electrocardiographic voltage with echocardio-

graphic data. In all categories, a high value of specificity was found along with an extremely low value of sensitivity. This observation appears to corroborate the conflicting results of the other studies reviewed and allows the researchers to conclude that electrocardiography is very limited in its ability to detect ventricular hypertrophy and enlargement in extreme obesity.

This limitation may motivate clinicians to recommend *echocardiography* for obese patients. Two-dimensional studies in particular may be invaluable in assessing ventricular performance and valvular function or in screening for previous ischemic injury by assessing regional wall motion abnormalities. The significance of detecting left ventricular hypertrophy in an obese patient has been previously emphasized, and the echocardiogram has been shown to reliably detect mild degrees of left ventricular hypertrophy,[52] especially when compared with the electrocardiogram, which may poorly correlate.

If left ventricular hypertrophy is found by echocardiogram, it may be prudent to consider *ambulatory electrocardiographic monitoring* for the detection of arrhythmias. This is especially important because the sensitivity of a routine electrocardiogram has been even more reduced by the new multichannel recorders, which provide less than half a minute of monitoring in a resting subject. Detection of ventricular ectopy, especially repetitive or sustained, warrants close monitoring of the QT interval. If QT interval is prolonged, a thorough investigation including measurement of serum electrolytes, monitoring of diuretic therapy, or a complete cardiac consultation may be warranted.

Radionuclide ventriculography may provide additional data in patients with overt congestive heart failure or myocardial infarction, allowing a more precise quantitative evaluation of ventricular systolic performance.

In obese patients in whom coronary disease is clinically suspected, an *exercise test* (sometimes performed in conjunction with thallium imaging) may be useful. A routine test may be physically difficult to accomplish in an obese patient, and hence, Persantine may be used as a pharmacologic stressor. If these tests demonstrate stress-induced regions of inadequate myocardial perfusion that reperfuse on the redistribution phase, angiography may be necessary in symptomatic individuals to determine the extent and severity of coronary lesions.

In patients with biventricular hypertrophy and clinical signs of obesity hypoventilation, arterial blood gas determination is crucial. Pulmonary function tests as well as a sleep study in a fully specialized sleep laboratory may be warranted. This is especially true if a patient is found to be hypoxemic, because bradycardia has been documented to occur with oxygen desaturation.

EFFECT OF TREATMENT

The vast number of patients requesting assistance with this devastating disease and the increased availability of noninvasive cardiovascular tests for evaluation and follow-up have significantly helped to increase our knowledge about the effects of weight loss on cardiac structure and function.

Alexander demonstrated a decrease with weight loss in circulating blood volume, plasma volume, cardiac output, and stroke volume.[1] Despite this observation, he reported that in those very obese initially, there was a persistent elevation in left ventricular filling pressure with exercise. He concluded that the myocardial hypertrophy responsible for diminished left ventricular compliance does not regress with weight loss. Several studies have questioned this conclusion. Kaltman and Goldring also demonstrated improvement in hemodynamic parameters with weight loss.[53] In their study, weight reduction in three of four patients did result in a restoration of normal left ventricular response with exercise. Clinical relief of edema and dyspnea and an objective reduction in the cardiac silhouette on chest x-ray film were also observed. Reversibility of left ventricular dysfunction with weight loss has been shown by Alpert and colleagues.[54] A group of 62 patients who were at least twice their ideal weight were studied for approximately 4 months after gastric restrictive surgery. There was a significant decrease in body weight, arterial blood pressure, and left ventricular chamber size and a significant improvement in left ventricular function. Despite these clinical results, no significant change in ventricular septal thickness, posterior wall thickness, or mean left ventricular dimension was noted. In contrast, MacMahon and colleagues studied 56 patients before and after dietary weight loss.[55] They did find a significant decrease in interventricular septal thickness, posterior wall thickness, and left ventricular mass. Not only were their findings independent of blood pressure, but the subjects had lost only a moderate amount of weight (an average of 8.3 kg) compared with a much larger amount (an average of 55 kg) in Alpert and coworkers'[54] study. The discrepancies among these studies are obvious and may demonstrate that there are varying degrees of cardiac damage with weight gain that may not be completely or even partially reversible once a critical point has been reached.[56] Nevertheless, all of these studies demonstrate a reduction in blood pressure and a clinical improvement in symptoms and exercise tolerance with weight loss. The decrease in arterial blood pressure with weight loss can be partially explained hemodynamically by the reduction in total circulating and central blood volumes that consequently reduce the venous return and cardiac output. It has been previously suggested that arterial blood pressure declines in patients on weight-reduction diets as a result of a decrease in dietary sodium intake, thus accomplishing the reduction in blood volumes. However, Reisin's group showed a reduction in resting circulating levels of plasma norepinephrine with weight loss while dietary sodium levels were held normal, suggesting an additional mechanism by which a reduction in arterial pressure is accomplished.[57]

SURGICAL/ANESTHETIC IMPLICATIONS

Preoperative cardiac evaluation of obese patients is imperative to decrease perioperative risk. Argarwal and co-workers[58] have shown that massively obese patients have significant intraoperative elevations in filling pressures and, compared with nonobese subjects, greater depressions of cardiac index and left and right ventricular stroke work. In nonobese persons, cardiac index is also depressed intraoperatively but should return to the preoperative level. In contrast, the immediate postoperative cardiac index of an obese patient remains abnormally depressed. Thus, as summarized by Pasulka's group, "morbidly obese patients have abnormal cardiac parameters, significant deterioration of cardiac function intraoperatively and delayed cardiac recuperation compared with that of nonobese subjects."[44] When it has been determined that a patient is at high risk, invasive monitoring by Swan-Ganz catheterization or arterial line placement may be particularly helpful.[59]

Even in the obese young population without evidence of cardiopulmonary disease, Vaughn and associates[60] found lower than normal preoperative values for arterial oxygenation, intraoperative hypoxemia, and several days of postoperative hypoxemia. Patients with the obesity-hypoventilation syndrome may be unable to tolerate such pulmonary changes, and preoperative weight loss and control of edema may be essential before elective surgery.[59]

CONCLUSION

The etiology of obesity in any given individual usually involves a myriad of factors. Despite the many treatment approaches, obesity remains a chronic relapsing disease yet without a clear cure. For most patients, it is important to develop management strategies in which personal responsibility for life-style changes are emphasized. There is overwhelming evidence that obesity has serious adverse effects on the cardiovascular system. Weight loss and its maintenance clearly can reduce the health risks of cardiomyopathy and coronary artery disease. Whether this is accomplished independently or by a reduction in cardiac risk factors, a sensible and medically supervised weight management program ought to be considered a fundamental ingredient in the prevention of serious cardiovascular disease.

References

1. Alexander JK: Obesity and the heart. Curr Probl Cardiol 5:1, 1980
2. Smith HL, Willius FA: Adiposity of the heart. Arch Intern Med 52:911, 1933
3. Saphir O, Corrigan M: Fatty infiltration of the myocardium. Arch Intern Med 52:410, 1933
4. Roberts WC, Roberts JD: The floating heart or the heart too fat to sink: Analysis of 55 necropsy patients. Am J Cardiol 52:1286, 1983
5. Carpenter HM: Myocardial fat infiltration. Am Heart J 63:491, 1962
6. Amad KH, Brennan JC, Alexander JK: The cardiac pathology of obesity. Circulation 32:740, 1965
7. Messerli FH: Obesity in hypertension: How innocent a bystander? Am J Med 77:1077, 1984
8. Kovach AG, Rosell S, Sandar P et al: Blood flow, oxygen consumption and free fatty acid release in subcutaneous adipose tissue during hemorrhagic shock in control and phenoxybensamine treated dogs. Circ Res (Suppl 6) 26:733, 1970
9. Alexander JK, Peterson KL: Cardiovascular effects of weight reduction. Circulation 45:310, 1972
10. Messerli FH: Cardiovascular effects of obesity and hypertension. Lancet 1:1165, 1982
11. Messerli FH: Cardiovascular adaptations to obesity and arterial hypertension: Detrimental or beneficial? Int J Cardiol 3:94, 1983
12. Messerli FH, Sundgaard-Riise K, Ventura HO et al: Clinical and hemodynamic determinants of left ventricular dimensions. Arch Intern Med 144:477, 1984
13. Alexander JK, Amad KH, Cole VW: Observations on some clinical features of extreme obesity with particular reference to cardiorespiratory effects. Am J Med 32:512, 1962
14. Sugerman HJ, Baron PL, Fairman RP et al: Hemodynamic dysfunction in obesity hypoventilation syndrome and the effects of treatment with surgically induced weight loss. Ann Surg 207:604, 1988
15. Lavie CJ, Ventura HO, Messerli FH: Cardiopathy of obesity. IM 9:57, 1988
16. Barrett-Connor E, Khaw K: Is hypertension more benign when associated with obesity? Circulation 72:53, 1985
17. Perrera GA, Damon A: Height, weight and their ratio in the accelerated form of hypertension. Arch Intern Med 100:263, 1957
18. Messerli FH, Sundgaard-Riise K, Reisin E et al: Disparate cardiovascular effects of obesity and arterial hypertension. Am J Med 74:808, 1983
19. Bloom E, Reed D, Yano K et al: Does obesity protect hypertensives against cardiovascular disease? JAMA 256:2972, 1986
20. Carabello BA, Gittens L: Cardiac mechanics and function in obese normotensive persons with normal coronary arteries. Am J Cardiol 59:469, 1987
21. Garavaglia GE, Messerli FH, Nunez BD et al: Myocardial contractility and left ventricular function in obese patients with essential hypertension. Am J Cardiol 62:594, 1988
22. DeDivitiis O, Fazio S, Petitto M et al: Obesity and cardiac function. Circulation 64:477, 1981
23. Romano M, Carella G, Cotecchia MR et al: Abnormal systolic time intervals in obesity and their re-

lationship with the amount of overweight. Am Heart J 112:356, 1986

24. Lavie CJ, Amodeo C, Ventura HO et al: Left atrial abnormalities indicating diastolic ventricular dysfunction in the cardiopathy of obesity. Chest 92:1042, 1987

25. Chadwick J, Mann WN: The Medical Works of Hippocrates. Aphorisms, Sect II, p 44. Springfield, IL, Charles C Thomas, 1950

26. Hubert HB, Feinleib M, McNamara PM et al: Obesity as an independent risk factor for cardiovascular disease: A 26-year follow-up of participants in the Framingham Heart Study. Circulation 67:968, 1983

27. McLenachan JM, Henderson E, Morris KI et al: Ventricular arrhythmias in patients with hypertensive left ventricular hypertrophy. N Engl J Med 317:787, 1987

28. Messerli FH, Nunez BD, Ventura HO et al: Overweight and sudden death: Increased ventricular ectopy in cardiopathy of obesity. Arch Intern Med 147:1725, 1987

29. Drenick EJ, Fisler JS: Sudden cardiac arrest in morbidly obese surgical patients unexplained after autopsy. Am J Surg 155:720, 1988

30. Aronson RS: Afterpotentials and triggered activity in hypertrophied myocardium from rats with renal hypertension. Circ Res 48:720, 1981

31. Anderson KP, Stinson EB, Derby GC et al: Vulnerability of patients with obstructive hypertrophic cardiomyopathy to ventricular arrhythmia induction in the operating room: Analysis of 17 patients. Am J Cardiol 51:811, 1983

32. Lew EA, Garfinkel L: Variations in mortality by weight among 750,000 men and women. J Chronic Dis 32:563, 1979

33. Hubert HB: The importance of obesity in the development of coronary risk factors and disease: The epidemiologic evidence. Ann Rev Public Health 7:493, 1986

34. National Center of Health Statistics (NHANES II): Vital and Health Statistics, Series I, No. 15, 1981

35. Barnett AH, Eff C, Leslie RDG et al: Diabetes in identical twins: A study of 200 pairs. Diabetologia 20:87, 1981

36. Aristimuno GG, Foster TA, Voors AW et al: Influence of persistent obesity in children with cardiovascular risk factors: The Bogalusa heart study. Circulation 69:895, 1984

37. Montenegro MR, Solberg LA: Obesity, body weight, body length and atherosclerosis. Lab Invest 18:594, 1968

38. Cramerk K, Paulin S, Werko L: Coronary angiographic findings in correlation with age, body

weight, blood pressure, serum lipids and Smoking Habits. Circ Res 33:888, 1966

39. Warnes CA, Roberts WC: The heart in massive (more than 300 pounds or 136 kilograms) obesity: Analysis of 12 patients studied at necropsy. Am J Cardiol 54:1087, 1984

40. Pooling Project Research Group: Relationship of blood pressure, serum cholesterol, smoking habit, relative weight and ECG abnormalities to incidence of major coronary events: Final report of the Pooling Project. J Chronic Dis 31:201, 1978

41. Rabkin SW, Mathewson FAL, Hsu PH: Relation of body weight to development of ischemic heart disease in a cohort of young North American men after a 26 year observation period: The Manitoba Study. Am J Cardiol 39:452, 1977

42. Larsson B, Svardsudd K, Welin L et al: Abdominal adipose tissue distribution, obesity and risk of cardiovascular disease and death: 13-year follow-up of participants in the study of men born in 1913. Br Med J 288:1401, 1984

43. Lapidus L, Bengtsson C, Larsson B et al: Distribution of adipose tissue and risk of cardiovascular disease and death: A 12-year follow-up of participants in the population study of women in Gothenburg, Sweden. Br Med J 289:1257, 1984

44. Pasulka PS, Bistrian BR, Benotti PN et al: The risks of surgery in obese patients. Ann Intern Med 104:540, 1986

45. Ogston D, McAndrew GM: Fibrinolysis in obesity. Lancet 2:1205, 1964

46. Grace CS: Fibrinolysis and obesity: The effect of weight reduction. Australas Ann Med 18:32, 1969

47. Almer L, Janzon L: Low vascular fibrinolytic activity in obesity. Thromb Res 6:171, 1975

48. Bern MM, Bothe A Jr, Bistrian B et al: Effects of low-dose warfarin on antithrombin III levels in morbidly obese patients. Surgery 94:78, 1983

49. Batist G, Bothe A Jr, Bern M et al: Low antithrombin III in morbid obesity: Return to normal with weight reduction. JPEN 7:447, 1983

50. Frank S, Colliver JA, Frank A: The electrocardiogram in obesity: Statistical analysis of 1029 patients. J Am Coll Cardiol 7:295, 1986

51. Zack PM, Wiens RD, Kennedy HL: Left-axis deviation and adiposity: The United States health and nutrition examination survey. Am J Cardiol 53:1129, 1984

52. Nath A, Alpert MA, Terry BE et al: Sensitivity and specificity of electrocardiographic criteria for left and right ventricular hypertrophy in morbid obesity. Am J Cardiol 62:126, 1988

53. Kaltman AJ, Goldring RM: Role of circulatory con-

gestion in the cardiorespiratory failure of obesity. Am J Med 60:645, 1976

54. Alpert MA, Terry BE, Kelly DL: Effect of weight loss on cardiac chamber size, wall thickness and left ventricular function in morbid obesity. Am J Cardiol 55:783, 1985

55. MacMahon SW, Wilcken DEL, MacDonald GJ: The effect of weight reduction on left ventricular mass. N Engl J Med 314:334, 1986

56. Messerli FH: Cardiopathy of obesity: A not-so-Victorian disease. N Engl J Med 314:378, 1986

57. Reisin E, Frohlich ED, Messerli FH et al: Cardio-vascular changes after weight reduction in obesity hypertension. Ann Intern Med 98:315, 1983

58. Agarwal N, Shibutani K, SanFilippo JA et al: Hemodynamic and respiratory changes in surgery of the morbidly obese. Surgery 92:226, 1982

59. Terry BE: Morbid obesity: Cardiac evaluation and function. Gastroenterol Clin North Am 16:215, 1987

60. Vaughn RW, Englehardt RC, Wise L: Postoperative hypoxemia in obese patients. Ann Surg 180:877, 1974

CHAPTER 44

Hypertension in Obesity

H. E. ELIAHOU, P. SHECHTER, and A. BLAU

The association of hypertension with obesity has been recognized for many years.[20] The close relation between body weight and blood pressure (BP) is true not only in children[34] but also in adults.[39] Population studies show that a rise in BP is associated with an increase in body weight.[6] Community screening showed that the prevalence of hypertension doubled in overweight young persons ages 20 to 39 years and is at least 50% more prevalent in overweight persons in the 40- to 64-year-old age-group than in nonoverweight individuals.[46] The Framingham Study showed that an excess of only 20% in body weight over ideal weight is associated with an eightfold increase in the incidence of hypertension later on.[21]

A rise in BP is associated with an increase in body weight or adiposity.[6] It seems that the type of fat distribution pattern has an important relevance to complications, such as hypertension, hyperlipidemia, decreased glucose tolerance, and hyperinsulinemia.[2,22] Abdominal obesity typical of the male fat distribution pattern (androgenic or apple type) is considered to be associated with hypertension, whereas the female type of distribution, the so-called gynecoid or pear type, is not.[25] Women with android obesity have other aberrant endocrine features, which include elevated levels of free testosterone in plasma and low sex hormone binding globulin as well as a resistance to insulin.[15] Thus it seems that the basic endocrine status is more important than the obesity itself in the development of those complications usually associated with obesity.[3]

The practical question whether it is the overweight or the excess body fat that is responsible for the development of hypertension is answered by the National Health and Nutrition Examination Survey (NHANES) II in 1980.[32] Obesity is defined as a body mass index (BMI) in excess of 28, when the BMI is measured by weight in kilograms divided by the square of the height in meters or an excess body fat equal to or greater than 38 mm, as measured by the sum of the triceps plus subscapular skin-fold thickness.[49] It is clearly established that it is not the excess body fat but rather the abnormal BMI that is associated with hypertension.[42] Schneider and Messerli[43] conclude from these findings that overweight and not just excess fat may be linked to hypertension.

Though a significant proportion of hypertensive persons are overweight, not all who are hypertensive are obese and not all obese patients are hypertensive. Thus, the association between hypertension and obesity does not directly apply to all obese or overweight individuals. This observation seems to explain the disappearance of this correlation when a whole population is studied. For example, in a large group of mildly hypertensive patients there was no correlation between BMI and BP. Similarly, the Tecumseh Study showed a correlation of a very low order between body weight and BP in a whole population.[14]

A study of the general population found that for every 10-kg rise in body weight there is an increase of only 3 and 2 mm Hg in the systolic and diastolic BP, respectively.[4] Thus, between the two disorders there must be a linking factor that is not present in all the patients who gain weight.

However, the association becomes obvious when the reverse is considered—that is, if an overweight hypertensive patient loses weight, then his or her hypertension is ameliorated and often is reduced to the accepted normal limits.[17,48]

A controlled study of 121 overweight patients with uncomplicated essential hypertension noted a definite and marked improvement in BP following body weight reduction.[35] Three groups of patients were studied: I, those with body weight reduction alone without drugs; IIA, those with body weight reduction with regular and steady antihypertensive therapy; and IIB, those with regular antihypertensive therapy but without dietary therapy. Patients in all groups had initial BP greater than 140 mm Hg systolic and 90 mm Hg diastolic. There was a follow-up period of 6 months (three 2-month phases): phase 1, 2 months to establish a baseline without intervention; phase 2, 2 months on weight reduction program; and phase 3, maintenance of the re-

duced body weight. Urine was collected for 24 hours to test for sodium at the end of phase 2.

The diet consisted of 1200 calories for men and 1000 calories for women and contained 35% protein, 35% carbohydrate, and 30% lipids. The patients were encouraged to eat salty foods.

Table 44-1 shows the initial data in the three groups. Combined BP categories were as follows:

Normal: systolic $\leq$ 140 mm Hg and diastolic $\leq$ 90 mm Hg

Mild: systolic 141 to 160 or diastolic 91 to 104 mm Hg (or both)

Moderate: systolic 161 to 180 or diastolic 105 to 114 mm Hg (or both)

Severe: systolic > 180 or diastolic > 114 mm Hg (or both)

Table 44-2 shows the reduction in BP in the groups and Table 44-3 shows the reduction in body weight and BP according to the initial weight.

The sodium excretion in the urine during phase 2 was as follows: group I 165.3 $\pm$ 51.7, group IIA 184.7 $\pm$ 42.8, and group IIB 154.8 $\pm$ 79.0 mEq/24 hours. These values definitely in-

TABLE 44-1

Comparison of the Three Study Groups According to Sex, Age, Initial Weight, and Initial Blood Pressure

Datum Studied	Group I	Group IIA	Group IIB
Total group	24	57	26
Males	16	42	10
Females	8	15	16
< 45 years old	17	26	12
45 + years old	7	31	14
Age (years)	37.9 $\pm$ 13.3*	46.3 $\pm$ 10.9	47.0 $\pm$ 13
Initial weight (kg)	85.5 $\pm$ 12.9	84.7 $\pm$ 9.2	80.9 $\pm$ 9.2
Initial % overweight	30.0 $\pm$ 14.4	29.5 $\pm$ 11.5	34.4 $\pm$ 14.4
Initial systolic blood pressure (mm Hg)	157 $\pm$ 13.9	171.7 $\pm$ 27.4	170.8 $\pm$ 27.5
Initial diastolic blood pressure (mm Hg)	105.9 $\pm$ 10.7	112.9 $\pm$ 11	108.6 $\pm$ 10
Combined initial blood pressure categories†:			
Normal	—	—	—
Mild	14 (58%)	13 (23%)	7 (27%)
Moderate	6 (25%)	21 (37%)	8 (31%)
Severe	4 (17%)	23 (40%)	11 (42%)

*Mean $\pm$ SD.
†For definitions see text.

TABLE 44-2

Reduction (Mean and SD) in Blood Pressure (mm Hg) from Phase I to Phase III According to Age and Sex

	Group I	Group IIA	Group IIB
Systolic			
Total group	25.7 ± 16.8	37.4 ± 21.3	6.9 ± 23.2
< 44 years old	23.5 ± 16.1	32.1 ± 21.1	5.9 ± 19.6
45 + years old	30.9 ± 18.6	41.6 ± 21.6	7.7 ± 26.7
Males	26.3 ± 14.4	32.7 ± 20.3	0.4 ± 10
Females	24.3 ± 22	49.9 ± 21.2	10.9 ± 28.1
Diastolic			
Total group	20 ± 10.5	23.3 ± 11.6	2.5 ± 10.4
< 44 years old	18.9 ± 11.1	22.8 ± 11.6	2.9 ± 11.9
45 + years old	22.6 ± 9.5	23.7 ± 11.7	2.1 ± 9.5
Males	21.2 ± 9.3	21.5 ± 11.5	3.2 ± 3.8
Females	17.6 ± 13.1	28.2 ± 10.6	1.9 ± 13.2

dicate that urine sodium was increased at all stages and that there was definitely no difference in salt intake in the different groups of patients in phase 2 of the study.

BP returned to normal in no less than 75% of the patients in group I (weight reduction alone) and in 61% in group IIA (weight reduction plus antihypertensive therapy). This effect was present in both sexes, at all ages, at all levels of BP, and in the moderately and severely obese persons, without any salt restriction. In contrast, the group that was not placed on a dietary regimen did not lose weight and did not have a significant change in BP. The researchers concluded that weight control is an important tool in the control of hypertension in overweight subjects. This reduction in BP occurred despite an unrestricted salt intake, which was kept at a rather high level.

More than two thirds of the overweight hypertensive patients were observed to achieve normal BP with a loss of only one half of the excess weight.[11] This occurred despite the fact that

TABLE 44-3

Mean (± SD) Reduction in Weight and Blood Pressure from Phase I to Phase III, According to Initial Weight,* in Patients Who Were on the Dietary Program

Initial Weight Category	No. of Patients	Reduction in Group I			No. of Patients	Reduction in Group IIA		
		Weight (kg)	Systolic Blood Pressure (mm Hg)	Diastolic Blood Pressure (mm Hg)		Weight (kg)	Systolic Blood Pressure (mm Hg)	Diastolic Blood Pressure (mm Hg)
Moderately overweight	8	6.7 ± 2.8	28.1 ± 13.1	19.4 ± 9	13	8.2 ± 2.9	28.1 ± 18.1	20.7 ± 8.5
Obese	8	10.3 ± 3.7	20.6 ± 9.4	18 ± 6.7	25	10.3 ± 4.1	34.6 ± 23.1	24.2 ± 13.1
Very obese	8	9.5 ± 5.5	28.2 ± 24.9	22.6 ± 15.2	19	10.3 ± 3.5	47.8 ± 19.5	23.9 ± 11.7

*Initial weight categories according to % overweight: moderately overweight, 11%–20%; obese, 21%–35%; very obese, > 36%.

there was no salt restriction and the 24-hour urine sodium excretion was not different from that obtained before the onset of dietary therapy. The mean BP reduction for a 1% reduction in overweight was 1.9 ± 0.9 mm Hg for the systolic and 1.3 ± 0.8 mm Hg for the diastolic. Another important clinical observation was that many of the overweight patients reached normotension long before achieving ideal body weight. In fact 31 of 38 such patients who reached the limits of normotension still were overweight in excess of 10% of their ideal body weight.[11] Using individual regression equations during the follow-up, no correlation was found between the individual slopes (of BP reduction against body weight) and the initial percent overweight. However, the individual slopes correlated highly with the initial BP.[11]

Adlersberg and colleagues[1] as early as 1946 achieved an average reduction of 32 mm Hg in systolic and 16 mm Hg in diastolic BP after an average loss of 10.5 kg in body weight by dietary therapy for an average of 8.2 months.

Nevertheless, the compliance failure is very high because of the inability of many of the overweight individuals to adhere to their diet. It is not enough to rationally explain to patients the importance of weight reduction and the prevention of obesity. Patients have to accept this behavioral change emotionally as well and to overcome the emotional and personality problems that led them to establish overeating as a habit or a compensatory mechanism for other problems. In 1981, we reported compliance failure to be as high as 89 of 212 (i.e., 42%).[11]

Furthermore, long-term follow-up showed that many of the patients who successfully lost weight initially and reduced their BP returned to values close to their initial body weight after 5 to 11 years (mean $\pm$ SD = 6.7 ± 2.1 years).[13] These patients showed somewhat lower BP at the end of follow-up despite the fact that their body weight returned to the initial level. Thus, successful dietary therapy in body weight reduction requires strong motivation, which needs to be renewed because it usually wanes with time.

Large errors can be made in the measurement of BP in obese individuals when the measurement is made with a regular cuff 15 cm long, which is too small for a thick arm. The error can

be as large as 10 to 15 mm Hg if the arm circumference is disproportionately large.[27,28] Thus it is advisable to use an 18-cm cuff for patients with a large arm circumference. The measurement must also be made with the arm at rest for at least 3 minutes, because a measurement taken with the arm unsupported can give a falsely high reading.

PATHOGENESIS

Although the association between obesity and hypertension is well established, the underlying mechanisms are still obscure. A few changes that might be responsible for this association are discussed next.

Glomerular Filtration Surface Area

The hypothesis put forward by Brenner and colleagues[5] claiming that hypertension develops when the renal filtration surface is decreased seems attractive and may explain the finding that certain obese patients are hypertensive whereas others are normotensive, as well as the fact that reducing body weight in obese hypertensive patients is always associated with some decrease in BP. The hypothesis claims that the major abnormality in the initiation of high BP in essential hypertension is in the kidneys. The postulate is that a decreased filtration surface area results from a reduced number of nephrons or a decrease in filtration surface area in the glomerulus itself. This deficit may contribute to renal sodium retention and thus to systemic hypertension. Thus if a person has a congenitally reduced filtration surface area, any gain in body weight results in a discrepancy between the increased body mass and the unchanged filtration surface area, which will lead to the development of hypertension. Conversely, any obese person with hypertension, by reducing body weight, is actually adjusting his or her body mass to the filtration surface area in the kidneys, thus relieving hypertension.

Arterial pressure and body weight are closely related in children as well as in adults. An increase in body mass is attended by a concomitant rise in arterial pressure, as noted in populations in which hypertension frequently develops when there is weight gain with age.[33,47]

Nevertheless, there is surprisingly no change

in BP in children between the ages of 2 and 6 years, despite a considerable weight gain.[33] Is this because there is at this age a parallel growth of the kidneys, allowing for an increase in filtration surface area at the same time? Animals born with a complete set of glomeruli continue to increase their glomerular filtration rate (GFR) after birth. In the beginning, SNGFR rises till it reaches the adult values. This is followed by an increase in total kidney GFR, probably as a result of the addition of functional nephrons as well as an increase in the rate of filtration in the individual nephrons.[18,45]

Hemodynamic Changes

Several investigators found an increase in cardiac output and blood volume in obesity.[37,52] Reisin and colleagues[38] found that in obese versus lean essential hypertensive patients, when the results are given in absolute values there is a definite increase in cardiac output and total blood volume (cardiac output, 6.1 ± 0.3 versus 5.1 ± 0.3 liters/min, respectively [$P < 0.05$]; blood volume, 5171 ± 380 versus 3913 ± 213 ml, respectively [$P < 0.01$]). The data presented by Messerli and associates[29] also show a marked increase in cardiac output and in total blood volume. However, when the results are expressed per kilogram of body weight, this difference disappears and is even reversed. This observation is strengthened by the findings by Mujais and Tarazi,[31] who noted no difference in cardiac index between 50 obese and 59 nonobese essential hypertensive patients and between them and 25 normal subjects. The figures were as follows: cardiac index, 2.8 ± 0.1 versus 2.8 ± 0.09 liters/min/m^2 in men and 2.9 ± 0.1 versus 2.8 ± 0.1 in women in the obese and nonobese hypertensive patients, respectively, and 2.9 ± 0.09 in men and 3.4 ± 0.2 liters/min/m^2 in the normal subjects. Their total peripheral resistances were also similar. They concluded that the hemodynamic profile of obese hypertensive patients is not different from that of nonobese hypertensive patients. It is important to mention here that because fat tissue has a lower metabolism than other tissue, it would seem that factoring the results by the actual body weight of the obese person would cause loss of significance (e.g., of the differences in cardiac output or blood volume), which is not

valid. Thus, the absolute increases of these parameters are real and seem to influence the outcome in an obese patient. To this information we can add that the stroke volume in essential hypertension is high: 101 ± 5 in obese patients versus 74 ± 4 ml in lean individuals.[28]

Forearm hemodynamics in obese and nonobese hypertensive patients were studied using pulsed Doppler velocimetry.[41] This was done to avoid comparing hemodynamic parameters in absolute values for obese and nonobese patients, in whom it is not appropriate to use such absolute values because of the marked differences in body weight and surface area. Reference values as per kilogram of body weight or per lean body weight are also disputable because of these marked changes. The patients studied were not under any medicinal therapy and had repeated diastolic BP measurements exceeding 95 mm Hg. Obesity was diagnosed when the BMI (weight/height^2 in kg/m^2) exceeded 27.2 kg/m^2.

The normotensive obese and hypertensive obese patients showed higher brachial artery blood velocity and forearm volume than the normotensive nonobese subjects. They were not different from the hypertensive nonobese subjects. Comparing the hypertensive patients only, the obese patients had a much higher blood flow velocity and blood flow, as well as lower vascular resistance. The researchers conclude that the obese hypertensive patients are characterized by a hyperkinetic forearm circulation in comparison with nonobese hypertensive patients.[34]

Reisin and colleagues[38] studied the hemodynamic characteristics of obese hypertensive patients. They defined obese persons as those with a body weight 20% greater than the ideal body weight. Established hypertension was diagnosed when outpatient systolic and diastolic BP exceeded 140 and 90 mm Hg, respectively, on at least three successive occasions. They found that for any measurement of BP, obese patients had greater total blood volume, cardiac output, and renal blood flow. Calculated total peripheral resistance and renal vascular resistances were less than in lean hypertensive or normotensive patients. In summary, obese hypertensive patients have an elevated cardiac output and stroke volume and an expanded absolute blood volume but a normal corrected blood volume, body weight, and cardiac index, when compared with lean

TABLE 44-4

Clinical Characteristics, Systemic and Renal Hemodynamic Measurements in Lean and Obese Hypertensive Patients

	Lean Hypertensive Patients	Obese Hypertensive Patients	P
Number	14	42	
Age (years)	43.7 ± 2	41.1 ± 1	
Weight (kg)	63 ± 3	90 ± 2	
Height (cm)	1.70 ± 2	1.70 ± 2	
% Desirable weight	-2 ± 1	$+42 \pm 3$	
Mean arterial pressure (mm Hg)	114 ± 4	115 ± 2	
Cardiac output (liters/min)	5.35 ± 0.2	6.15 ± 0.2	< 0.05
Total peripheral resistance (units)	21 ± 0.8	18 ± 0.6	< 0.01
Renal blood flow (ml/min)	898 ± 53	1119 ± 34	< 0.01
Renal blood flow (ml/min/cm)	5.3 ± 0.3	6.6 ± 0.2	< 0.05
Renal vascular resistance (units)	126 ± 1	102 ± 0.4	< 0.01
Total blood volume (ml)	4141 ± 206	5039 ± 145	< 0.01

Values are expressed as the mean $\pm$ SEM, (NS, not significant)

hypertensive patients. They also have lower peripheral resistance at all levels of hypertension,[16,29] as well as lower renovascular resistance[36,38] (Table 44-4).

Insulin and Carbohydrate Intolerance

Obesity is associated with hyperinsulinemia and glucose intolerance.[30] Insulin was shown to have an antinatriuretic effect.[7] DeFronzo and colleagues[8] and Kolanowsky and associates[23] found that insulin increases sodium reabsorption in the renal tubules. DeFronzo[9] suggested that the development of hypertension in obesity may be due to renal sodium retention, secondary to the high insulin levels found in obesity. This idea was also supported by Krotkiewski and co-workers.[24] Furthermore, insulin was found to increase plasma norepinephrine levels.[51]

Catecholamines

In a study of normotensive obese women, it was found that a low-energy diet, achieved by decreasing carbohydrates only, containing an average of 9.2 kcal/kg ideal body weight, decreased plasma noradrenaline concentrations (in the supine position from 0.17 ± 0.04 ng/ml to 0.07 ± 0.02 ng/ml by the 11th day), together with a

prompt reduction in BP. The urinary metabolite 4-hydroxy-3-methoxymandalate was promptly reduced as well. There was no change in the plasma adrenaline concentration. The investigators think that this is a possible mechanism by which weight reduction reduces the high BP in obese hypertensive patients.[19]

Landsberg[26] found that the turnover rate of ³H.norepinephrine in sympathetic nerve endings in small animals is markedly decreased during fasting and is increased after sucrose feeding.

Glucose injection in humans was found to be associated with an increase in plasma norepinephrine levels.[40]

Sowers and colleagues concluded that obese hypertensive patients had a higher supine plasma norepinephrine, epinephrine and plasma renin activity (PRA) levels and a higher norepinephrine response to upright posture and isometric grip contraction.[44]

High Plasma Renin Activity

PRA was found to be high in obese hypertensive patients. The mean PRA was as follows: at rest, in normotensive controls, 0.64 ± 0.33; in nonoverweight hypertensive patients, 1.06 ± 0.07; and in overweight hypertensive patients, 1.45 ± 0.19 ng/ml/hour. The respective values after ambulation were 1.6 ± 0.8, 2.4 ± 0.16, and 3.38

± 0.39 ng/ml/hour.[12] Weight reduction was accompanied by at least 50% reduction in PRA levels, which were independent of sodium intake.[10]

The link between obesity and the development of essential hypertension is still unknown. It seems that hypertension in obese subjects is a state of maladaption of hemodynamic homeostatic mechanisms, the primary event being a relative or absolute rise in cardiac output or blood volume or both. In normal persons, however, this is usually accompanied by a decrease in the total peripheral resistance, diuresis, and natriuresis. For some yet unknown reason, in obese persons, these defensive mechanisms are not operating adequately, resulting in a rise in BP.

The importance of the factors mentioned in the development of hypertension is not clear. It is possible that their interactions are important; e.g., excess food stimulating an increase in insulin, the latter activating the sympathetic nervous system. Alternatively, a common denominator that has not yet been elucidated may be operative in causing these factors, which are thought to lead to the resultant hypertension.

References

1. Adlersberg D, Coler HR, Laval J: Effect of weight reduction on course of arterial hypertension. Mt Sinai J Med (NY) 12:984, 1946
2. Björntorp P: Hypertension and other complications in human obesity. J Clin Hypertens 2:163, 1986
3. Björntorp P: Adipose tissue distribution and morbidity. In Berry EM, Blondheim SH, Eliahou HE et al (eds): Recent Advances in Obesity Research V, pp 60–65. London, John Libbey & Co, 1986
4. Boe J, Humerfelt S, Wedervang G: The blood pressure in a population: Blood pressure readings and height and weight determinations in the adult population of the city of Bergen. Acta Med Scand (Suppl 321) 157:1, 1957
5. Brenner BM, Garcia DL, Anderson S: Glomeruli and blood pressure: Less of one, more of the other. Am J Hypertens 1:335, 1988
6. Chiang BN, Perlman LV, Epstein FH: Overweight and hypertension. Circulation 39:403, 1969
7. DeFronzo RA, Cooke CR, Andres R et al: The effect of insulin on renal handling of sodium potassium and calcium and phosphate in man. J Clin Invest 55:845, 1975
8. DeFronzo RA, Robin J, Andres R: The glucose clamp technique: A method for the quantification of beta cell sensitivity to glucose and of tissue sensitivity to insulin. Am J Physiol 237a:E214, 1979
9. DeFronzo RA: Effect of insulin and glucagon on electrolytes and blood pressure in experimental animals: Obesity and hypertension. Proceedings of the Satellite Symposium to the 3rd International Congress on Obesity, Florence, Italy, Oct 6–7, 1980
10. Dornfeld LP, Maxwell MH, Waks A et al: Mechanisms of hypertension in obesity. Kidney Int (Suppl 22) 32:S-254, 1987
11. Eliahou HE, Iaina A, Gaon T: Body weight reduction necessary to attain normotension in the overweight hypertensive patient. Int J Obes (Suppl 1) 5:157, 1981
12. Eliahou HE: Role of obesity in the pathogenesis of primary hypertension. In Amery A (ed): Cardiovascular Disease: Pathophysiology and Treatment. The Hague, Martin Nijhoff Publishers, 1982
13. Eliahou HE, Cohen D, Herzog D: Obesity and Hypertension: What correlation at long-term follow-up? In Berry E, Blondheim H, Eliahou HE et al (eds): Recent Advances in Obesity Research V. London, John Libbey & Co, 1986
14. Epstein FH, Francis T, Hayner NS et al: Prevalence of chronic diseases and distribution of selected physiologic variables in a total community. Tecumseh, Michigan. Am J Epidemiol 81:307, 1965
15. Evans PJ, Hoffman RG, Kalkhoff RK et al: Relationship of androgenic activity to body fat typography, fat cell morphology and metabolic aberrations in premenopausal women. J Clin Endocrinol Metab 57:304, 1983
16. Frohlich ED, Messerli FH, Reisin ED et al: The problem of obesity and hypertension. Hypertension 5:71, 1983
17. Heyden S: The working man's diet. II. Effect of weight reduction in obese patients with hypertension, diabetes, hyperuricemia and hyperlipidemia. Nutr Metab 22:14, 1978
18. Horster M, Valtin H: Postnatal development of renal function: Micropuncture and clearance studies in the dog. J Clin Invest 50:779, 1971
19. Jung RT, Shetty PS, Barrand M et al: Role of catecholamines in hypotensive response to dieting. Br Med J 1:12, 1979
20. Kannel WE, Brand N, Skinner J et al: The relation of obesity to blood pressure and development of hypertension. The Framingham Study. Ann Intern Med 67:48, 1967
21. Kannel WB, Gordon T, Offutt D: Left ventricular hypertrophy by electrocardiogram: Prevalence, incidence and mortality in the Framingham Study. Ann Intern Med 71:89, 1969
22. Kissebah AH, Evans DJ, Peiris A et al: Endocrine characteristics in human obesities: Role of sex steroids. In Vague J, Björntorp P, Guy-Grand P et al

(eds): Metabolic Complications of Human Obesities, pp 115–130. Amsterdam, Elsevier, 1983

23. Kolanowsky J, Salvador G, Desmecht P et al: Influence of glucagon on natriuresis and glucose-induced sodium retention in the fasting obese subject. Eur J Clin Invest 7:167, 1977

24. Krotkiewski M, Mandroukas M, Sjostrom L et al: Effects of long-term physical training on body fat, metabolism and blood pressure in obesity. Metabolism 28:649, 1979

25. Krotkiewski M, Björntorp P, Sjostrom L et al: Impact of obesity on metabolism in men and women: Importance of regional adipose tissue distribution. J Clin Invest 72:1150, 1983

26. Landsberg L: Nutrition and regulation of the sympathetic nervous system and its relation to hypertension: Obesity and hypertension. Proceedings of the Satellite Symposium to the 3rd International Congress on Obesity, Florence, Italy, October 6–7, 1980

27. Maxwell MH,, Schroth PC, Waks AU et al: Error in blood pressure measurement due to incorrect cuff size in obese patients. Lancet ii:33, 1982

28. Messerli FH, Christie B, deCarvalho JGR et al: Obesity and essential hypertension: Hemodynamics, intravascular volume sodium excretion and plasma renin activity. Arch Intern Med 141:81, 1981

29. Messerli FH, Sundgaard-Riise K, Reisin ED: Disparate cardiovascular effects of obesity and arterial hypertension. Am J Med 74:808, 1983

30. Modan M, Halkin H, Almog S et al: Hyperinsulinemia: A link between hypertension obesity and glucose intolerance. J Clin Invest 75:809, 1985

31. Mujais SK, Tarazi RC, Dustan HP et al: Hypertension in obese patients: Hemodynamic and volume studies. Hypertension 4:84, 1982

32. National Center of Health Statistics: Plan and operation of the National Health and Nutrition Examination Survey, 1976–1980. Department of Health and Human Services Publication (PHS) 15,81; Vital and Health Statistics Series I. Washington, DC, US Public Health Service, 1981

33. NHLBI Task Force on blood pressure control in children: Pediatrics 59:797, 1077

34. Raison JM, Safar ME, Cambien FA et al: Forearm hemodynamics in obese normotensive and hypertensive subjects. J Hypertens 6:299, 1988

35. Reisin E, Abel R, Modan M et al: Effect of weight loss without salt restriction on the reduction of blood pressure in overweight hypertensive patients. N Engl J Med 298:1, 1978

36. Reisin ED, Ventura HO, Messerli FH et al: Renal and systemic hemodynamics correlate with body weight in established hypertensive patients (abstract). Kidney 23:175, 1983

37. Reisin E, Messerli FH, Ventura HO et al: Renal hemodynamics in obese and lean essential hypertensive patients. In Messerli FH (ed): Kidney in Essential Hypertension, pp 125–130. Boston, Martinus Nijhoff Publishers, 1983

38. Reisin E, Messerli FG, Ventura HO: Renal hemodynamic studies in obesity hypertension. J Hypertens 5:397, 1987

39. Report of the Hypertension Task Force: Vol 9. NIH Publication 79-1631:59-77. Washington, DC, US Department of Health, Education and Welfare, 1979

40. Robertson D, Garland GS, Robertson RM et al: Comparative assessment of stimuli that release neuronal and adrenomedullary catecholamines in man. Circulation (Suppl 4) 59:637, 1949

41. Safar M, Peronneau J, Levenson J et al: Pulse Doppler: Diameter, velocity and flow of brachial artery in sustained essential hypertension. Circulation 63:393, 1981

42. Salans LB, Cushman SW, Weismann RE: Studies of human adipose tissue: Adipose cell size and number in nonobese and obese patients. J Clin Invest 52:929, 1973

43. Schnieder RE, Messerli FH: Obesity hypertension. Med Clin North Am 71:991, 1987

44. Sowers R, Whitfield LA, Catania RA et al: Role of the sympathetic nervous system in blood pressure maintenance in obesity. J Clin Endocrinol Metab 54:1181, 1982

45. Spitzer A, Brandis M: Functional and morphologic maturation of superficial nephrons: Relationship to total kidney function. J Clin Invest 53:279, 1974

46. Stamler R, Stamler J, Riedlinger WE et al: Weight and blood pressure: Findings in hypertension screening in one million Americans. JAMA 240:1607, 1978

47. Symonds B: The blood pressure in healthy men and women. JAMA 80:232, 1923. (Cited by Dustan H: Ann Intern Med 193:1047, 1985)

48. Tyroler HA, Heyden S, Hames CG: Weight and hypertension. In Paul O (ed): Evans County Study of Blacks and Whites, Epidemiology and Control of Hypertension, pp 177–202. New York, Stratton Intercontinental

49. Van Itallie TB: Health implications of overweight and obesity in the United States. Ann Intern Med 103:983, 1985

50. Velasquez MT, Hoffmann RG: Overweight and obesity in hypertension. Q J Med 54:205, 1985

51. Well S, Lilavivathana U, Campbell G: Increased plasma norepinephrine concentrations and metabolic rates following glucose ingestion in man. Acta Endocrinol (Copenh) 29:806, 1982

52. Whyte HM: Blood pressure and obesity. Circulation 19:511, 1959

CHAPTER 45

Reproductive and Hormonal Alterations in Obesity

JAMES R. GIVENS

During the past three decades there has been considerable progress in documenting and understanding the various alterations in hormone secretion in obesity. An important factor responsible for the advancement of knowledge in this area has been the development of methods for measuring physiologic quantities of hormones in body fluids and in fat and determining the dynamics of their secretion and metabolism. The aim of this chapter is to provide an overview of the obesity-related clinical alterations in reproduction and a description of some of the specific hormonal changes associated with obesity. The putative role of hyperinsulinemia in the genesis of the hormonal changes in obesity is emphasized in this chapter.

The hormonal changes associated with obesity are not necessarily abnormal or even dysfunctional; many are compensatory and physiologic. For example, the hyperinsulinemia of obesity compensates for the insulin resistance, thereby maintaining euglycemia.[1] Diabetes mellitus (type II) develops if a compensated state of euglycemia is not initiated and properly sustained. Likewise, the decrease in total serum testosterone observed in moderately obese males, caused by a decrease in the circulating level of the testosterone-estradiol binding globulin (TeBG), is compensated by an increase in the percentage of testosterone not bound to TeBG.[2] This response permits maintenance of a normal circulating free testosterone level and normal androgenic activity (Fig. 45-1). However, some of the hormone changes in obesity that have a primary compensatory function may also have an undesirable secondary effect. For example, although the hyperinsulinemia of obesity usually overcomes the insulin resistance, the increased insulin may enhance renal retention of sodium and possibly cause hypertension as an undesirable secondary effect.[1]

OVARIAN FUNCTION IN OBESITY

Abnormal Menses

The incidence of obesity in women with menstrual disorders was reported in 1952 by Rogers and Mitchell.[3] These Boston physicians determined that menstrual disorders were related to obesity. They found that 43% of women with abnormal menses were obese, compared with only 13% of the control group of women with normal menstrual cycles. The two most common menstrual disorders were secondary amenorrhea and dysfunctional uterine bleeding. The incidence of obesity in these two conditions was 48% and 58%, respectively.

A large clinical study was conducted by Hartz and colleagues,[4] who interviewed more than 26,000 obese women enrolled in a weight-reduction program. The incidence of abnormalities of menstruation was directly related to the degree of obesity. For example, the incidence of menstrual disorders was 2.6% in those who were less than 20% above ideal body weight and was

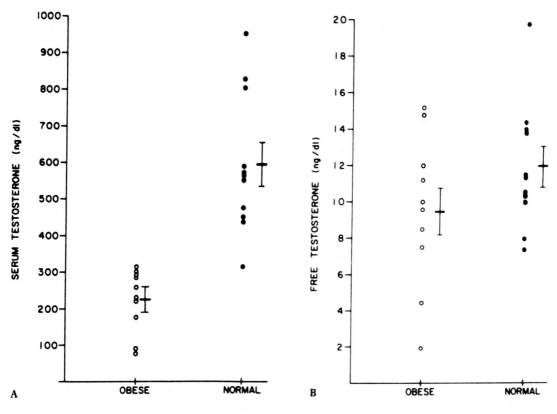

FIGURE 45-1

(A) Percent free testosterone in normal and obese men. Mean value is significantly higher in obese men ($P < 0.001$). Error bars show mean ± SEM. (B) Free testosterone concentration in normal and obese men. Mean values are not significantly different. Error bars show mean ± SEM. (Glass AR et al: Low serum testosterone and sex-hormone-binding globulin in massively obese men. J Clin Endocrinol Metab 45:1211, 1977)

8.4% in those who were more than 74% above ideal body weight. Women with menorrhagia or facial hirsutism were also significantly more obese than the women who had normal menstrual flow. The presence of hirsutism was related to the duration of obesity. These data suggest that hyperandrogenism is a correlate of obesity.

Oligo-Ovulation

A common organic cause of chronic oligo-ovulation is hyperandrogenism.[5] The source of the excessive androgens is the ovaries or the ad-

renals or both. The most frequent cause of ovarian hypersecretion of androgens is polycystic ovarian syndrome (PCOS). Obesity is a common feature of PCOS, which is a nontumorous, dysfunctional condition of the ovary with luteinizing hormone (LH)-dependent hypersecretion of androgens from hyperplastic theca and stromal cells.[6] A polycystic ovary is the final common expression of several specific entities. The ovarian histologic findings reflect chronic oligo-ovulation due to delayed or deranged follicular maturation. The clinical expression of PCOS includes hyperandrogenism, relative sterility, and obesity.[7] Follicular maturation is normally a finely balanced physiological event controlled by inhibitory and stimulatory factors, including LH, follicle-stimulatory hormone (FSH), estrogens, androgens, and insulin. The pathogenesis, therefore, is variable, because any one of a number of abnormal events or conditions may disrupt folliculogenesis.

The onset of the clinical expression of PCOS is perimenarchal. Obese girls usually have early menarche.[8] It is not unusual for menarche to occur by 10 years of age. The initiation of menstruation requires the attainment of a certain body mass and percent body fat.[8,9] If this critical mass is obtained early, then menarche may occur at an earlier age than in normal-weight individuals. According to the data of Frisch, menstruation usually begins when the body weight reaches 106 pounds with approximately 22% body fat.[9] Growth rate may also be excessive, with early completion of growth in obese girls.

Obesity is usually present before menarche (90 of 98 cases),[10] suggesting that obesity may be the proximate or initiating event in the pathogenesis of some cases of PCOS. To determine the contribution of obesity to the abnormal menses, Mitchell and Rogers[11] determined the response of the amenorrhea in their obese women to a low-calorie diet and weight reduction. Thirty-two obese, amenorrheic women participated in the study; each received 1200 calories/day. Fifteen of the 32 women who lost weight had resumption of cyclic menses; four became pregnant. Those who failed to lose weight did not have resumption of menses. Bates and Whitworth[12] also reported successful treatment of infertility by weight loss in 18 obese, anovulatory, hyperandrogenic women who met the broad criteria for the diagnosis of PCOS. Each had increased serum levels of androstenedione and testosterone that were reduced to normal with dietary restriction of calories and weight loss. All had spontaneous resumption of menses, and 77% conceived without additional therapy. Clearly, weight reduction was a valuable therapeutic modality for correcting the reproductive derangements due to abnormalities in sex hormone dynamics in these obese women.

The concept that the ovaries may be a source of excess androgens in some patients who have obesity as their primary disorder remains contro-versial. The effect of caloric restriction and weight loss on PCOS needs further study. An androgenic multicystic ovary may occur in obese women through the development of an abnormal gonadotropin secretory pattern—that is, a predominance of LH over FSH that develops secondary to the noncylic estrogen produced in peripheral tissues, such as in fat. This imbalance may produce a clinical and biochemical state that is characterized by oligo-ovulation due to improper folliculogenesis in the ovary. These changes that are characteristic of PCOS, however, may have an unknown molecular defect that is unmasked and expressed as a result of the obesity.

Hyperinsulinemia and Ovarian Function

The most common cause of hyperinsulinemia is the insulin resistance of obesity. Women with upper body obesity have enlarged adipocytes that are associated with hyperinsulinemia and hyperandrogenemia; those with lower segment obesity do not have insulin resistance and hyperinsulinemia to the same degree.[13] It is now clear that the high insulin levels that are present in upper body obesity are responsible for the increased synthesis and secretion of certain steroids, particularly androgens, from the ovary. Evidence from in vitro studies indicates that insulin enhances the stimulatory action of LH on ovarian theca and stroma cells.[14] The result is an increased production rate of androgens, forming the basis for the development of androgenic polycystic ovaries in insulin-resistant states characterized by acanthosis nigricans and ovarian theca/stroma cell hyperplasia.[13,14] Affected women form a subset of patients with PCOS and are described as having PCOS-acanthosis nigricans (PCOS-AN). Their unique features are very high fasting insulin (>40 μ/ml) and testosterone levels (>100 ng/ml) and normal LH and FSH levels.

There is indirect evidence that insulin also modulates (enhances) the metabolic clearance of the nonpolar steroids, possibly by promoting their uptake in fat or by increasing their renal clearance.[15] Data indicate that insulin directly inhibits TeBG synthesis,[16,17] thus increasing the metabolic clearance rate of those steroids bound to this protein and enhancing *in vivo* androgenicity by increasing the availability of androgens to the responsive tissues.

Luteal Phase Defect

A relatively common reproductive disturbance causing infertility and recurrent abortion in obese women is luteal phase deficiency.[18,19] In this disorder, minimal or only subtle alterations may be noted in the character of the menses. Menstruation may be cyclic, but with a variable interval between menses. The primary hormonal derangement is inadequate secretion of progesterone by the corpus luteum, resulting in insufficient preparation of the endometrium for implantation of the embryo. Progesterone stimulates the maturation of the endometrial glands and induces the decidual changes in the stroma that are necessary for normal implantation and survival of the embryro. The etiology of luteal phase deficiency is multifactoral. Normal corpus luteum function requires proper cycling of circulating LH and FSH during the follicular phase. A common feature of the disorder is dysgenesis of gonadotropin secretion—namely, a subnormal rise of FSH in the follicular phase and a subnormal response of progesterone during the luteal phase. The estradiol and LH levels are usually normal.

The low circulating level of progesterone in luteal insufficiency associated with obesity could be the result of a dilution effect due to the uptake of progesterone from the circulation into the enlarged fat mass rather than to subnormal production. This possibility has not been addressed experimentally. Progesterone is nonpolar and thus freely enters fat.[20]

Diagnosis of a luteal phase defect requires documentation by timed biopsy of an out-of-phase endometrial histology of more than 2 days, a subnormal midluteal serum progesterone level, or both.[18,19] This disorder, which should be considered a syndrome because of its diverse etiology, is responsible for 10% to 30% of infertility in women and is likely one of the most common causes of infertility in obese women.

It must be emphasized that a significant number of obese women have normal ovulatory menstrual cycles and are fertile, suggesting that the quantity of fat is not the only factor influencing reproduction. It is now clear that the body location of the excess fat is also a determining factor.[21] The endocrine-metabolic alterations characteristic of obesity are highly correlated with the body distribution of the excess fat. Hyperandrogenism and insulin resistance, with the resultant hyperinsulinemia, are strongly positively correlated with the degree of fat accumulation in the abdominal area as determined by a high waist:hip (W:H) circumference ratio. It is assumed that the endocrine-metabolic alterations observed in women with abdominal obesity are the cause of their oligo-ovulation and relative infertility and that women with excess fat in the gluteo-femoral region do not have these derangements and therefore are more likely to have normal cyclic menses. However, endocrine studies of eumenorrheic obese women are limited in scope and number. Data from several laboratories document that significant hormonal changes occur even in eumenorrheic, nonhirsute obese women.

In summary, obese women may have disordered ovarian function, which causes oligo-ovulation and produces amenorrhea or dysfunctional uterine bleeding. The most common cause of this scenario is PCOS. A subset of PCOS is due to insulin enhancement of ovarian androgen production. Obesity may cause infertility due to ovarian dysfunction in the absence of grossly abnormal menses, such as may occur in luteal phase insufficiency.

ADRENAL FUNCTION IN OBESITY

Increased Cortisol Secretion Rate

The cortisol secretion rate is directly proportional to body weight.[22] The increased cortisol production observed in obesity has been reproduced in normal humans made obese by overfeeding.[23] The caloric content and composition of the diet also affect cortisol secretion.[24] Starvation decreases the cortisol secretion rate, and a high-protein diet and a diet with a high carbohydrate/fat content increases the cortisol secretion rate.[25] An increase in the metabolism of cortisol in obesity is evidenced by a shortened plasma half-life.[26,27] This observation confirms the earlier findings of increased urinary excretion of 17-hydroxycorticosteroids (17-OHCS) with normal serum cortisol levels. Migeon and colleagues[26] postulated that the increased rate of clearance of cortisol from the circulation increases gluconeogenesis by the liver. This concept is supported by the finding of a significant correlation between the cortisol production rate and insulin resistance.[26] The magnitude of the decrease in the blood glucose after exogenous insulin administration was inversely correlated with the cortisol secretion rate ($r = -0.63$; $P = < 0.01$).[24] Migeon and associates postulated that the increased adrenal activity in obesity is due to hyperinsulinemia.[26]

There is evidence of renal and dietary protein effects on the turnover rate of cortisol in obesity. Schteingart and Conn[24] reported that a direct correlation exists between creatinine clearance and urinary levels of 17-OHCS. These two entities increase and decrease together with similar changes in protein or caloric intake. In addition, dietary protein induces and fasting apparently reduces the activity of the steroid-metabolizing liver enzyme Δ^4-ketosteroid hydrogenase. Thus, the metabolic clearance rate of the steroids with this structural configuration is enhanced by increased protein intake.[24]

Increased Adrenal Androgens

Kurtz and colleagues[28] in our laboratory measured the metabolic clearance rate (MCR) and plasma concentration and calculated the blood production rate of dehydroepiandrosterone (DHEA) and androstenedione in 27 eumenorrheic, nonhirsute women (8 normal weight, 19 obese > 125% ideal body weight). The data are depicted in Figure 45-2. Compared with the normal-weight women, in the obese women, the MCRs of DHEA and androstenedione were increased 81% and 74%, respectively, and were not different in the two groups. The mean production rate of androstenedione and DHEA was increased in the obese women 94% and 53%, respectively, above the normal values.

The increased MCRs of DHEA and androstene-

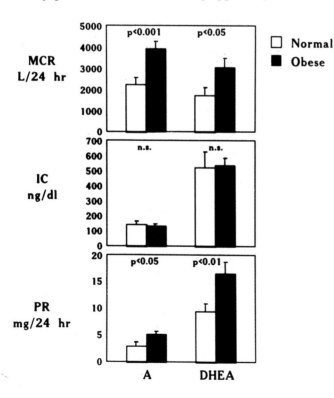

FIGURE 45-2

Mean (SEM) MCRs, 24-hour integrated serum concentration (IC) and PR of DHEA in normal and obese groups (Kurtz BR et al: Maintenance of normal circulating levels of androstenedione and dehydroepiandrosterone in obesity despite increased metabolic clearance rates: Evidence for a servo-control mechanism. J Clin Endocrinol Metab 64:1261, 1987)

dione in the obese women were associated with an increased production rate such that the serum concentration of the two hormones was not different from those of the normal-weight women (see Fig. 45-2). These data confirm those of Kirschner and colleagues,[29] who found an increased MCR and production rate of androstenedione in young obese women but normal serum levels of androstenedione. This laboratory also documented an increased production rate and MCR with normal plasma levels of testosterone, dihydrotestosterone, and 3-α-androstanediol in eumenorrheic, nonhirsute obese women.[29]

These data suggest that a control mechanism operational in nonhirsute, eumenorrheic, obese women adjusts the production rate to the MCR so that the plasma concentration remains normal. Kirschner and associates[29] proposed that this is a finely balanced system that becomes dysfunctional when the MCR of a steroid cannot increase proportionately to a change in its production rate, or vice versa.

The production rate and the MCR of DHEA were each positively correlated with the circulating level of insulin (r = 0.84 and 0.73, respectively).[15] Thus, the MCR and the production rate of DHEA were coupled (r = 0.84) through a common relationship to insulin (Figs. 45-3, 45-4, and

45-5). These data are compatible with the concept of a cause-and-effect relationship between insulin and the MCR and the production rate of DHEA of equal magnitude in eumenorrheic, nonhirsute obese women. Thus, the MCR and the production rate are coupled through a common functional attachment to insulin. The hyperinsulinemia that characterizes obesity is responsible for the concordant increase in the MCR and the production rate of DHEA in obese women.

The increased production rate of DHEA and androstenedione in eumenorrheic, nonhirsute obese females may be accomplished by increased sensitivity or responsivity of the steroids to adrenocorticotropic hormone (ACTH). The data documenting these findings were derived from a continuous infusion of physiologic doses of ACTH in normal-weight and age-matched, nonhirsute, eumenorrheic women[30] (Fig. 45-6). The dose range of ACTH extended from below threshold through threshold. The threshold dose of ACTH for androstenedione was lower (increased sensitivity) and the slope of the DHEA response was greater (increased responsivity) in the obese women than in the normal-weight women.[30]

There is indirect evidence that the increased response to ACTH in obesity is due to the enhancing influence of the hyperinsulinemia of

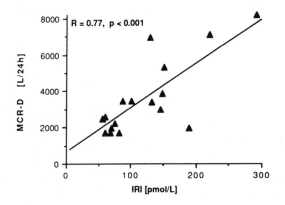 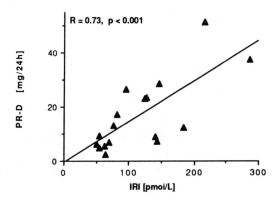

FIGURE 45-3

Linear regression analysis of basal peripheral circulating IRI versus the MCR-D and PR-D in the control women. (Farah MJ et al: Biomodal correlation between the circulating insulin level and the production rate of dehydroepiandrosterone: Positive correlation in normal and obese controls and negative correlation in polycystic ovarian disease with acanthosis nigricans. J Clin Endocrinol Metab 70:1075, 1990)

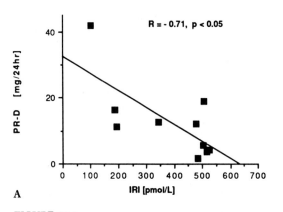
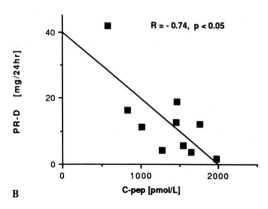

FIGURE 45-4

Linear regression analysis of the basal peripheral circulating IRI **(A)** versus the 24-hour PR-D **(B)** in women with PCOS-AN. (Farah MJ et al: Biomodal correlation between the circulating insulin level and the production rate of dehydroepiandrosterone: Positive correlations in normal and obese controls and negative correlation in polycystic ovarian disease with acanthosis nigricans. J Clin Endocrinol Metab 70:1075, 1990)

obesity.[31] The first line of evidence for this is the positive correlation between the insulin level and the MCR and the production rate of DHEA (see Figs. 45-3, 45-4, and 45-5). A second line of evidence that insulin is functionally involved in the MCR and the production rate of DHEA is the documentation by in vitro studies of the enhancement of the responses of DHEA and androstenedione to ACTH in primary monolayer cultures of bovine adrenal cells to which graded physiologic doses of insulin were added.[31] These data suggest that at normal concentrations, insulin modulates the action of ACTH to preferentially enhance androgen secretion from the adrenal cortex. The most likely effect of insulin is to increase 17,20-lyase activity coupled with a promotion of substrate flux. The increased MCR of nonpolar steroids such as DHEA is due, at

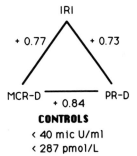
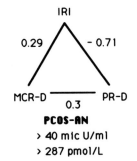

FIGURE 45-5

Comparison of the coefficients of correlation of the peripheral circulating IRI concentration, 24-hour MCR-D, and 24-hour PR-D in controls and women with PCOS-AN. (Farah MJ et al: Biomodal correlation between the circulating insulin level and the production rate of dehydroepiandrosterone: Positive correlation in normal and obese controls and negative correlation in polycystic ovarian disease with acanthosis nigricans. J Clin Endocrinol Metab 70:1075, 1990)

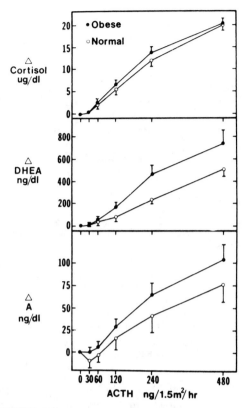

FIGURE 45-6

Mean (± SEM) incremental (Δ) responses of serum F, DHEA, and A to the continuous infusion of α-ACTH-(1-24) in normal and obese, nonhirsute, eumenorrheic women. The ACTH dose was doubled every hour, and samples were obtained at the end of each hour. (Komindr S et al: Relative sensitivity and responsivity of serum cortisol and two adrenal androgens to ∂-adrenocorticotropin-[1-24] in normal and obese, nonhirsute, eumenorrheic women. J Clin Endocrinol Metab 63:860, 1986)

least in part, to the increased fat volume because they are freely diffusible into fat.

EXTRAGLANDULAR STEROID METABOLISM IN OBESITY

The mechanism responsible for the increased androgen activity in obese women is multifaceted. In addition to increased glandular secretion, a state of hyperandrogenemia is produced in sim-

ple obesity by the decreased binding capacity of TeBG. This reduces the bound fraction of testosterone and increases the percentage free fraction through the dynamics of binding to TeBG, which determines the rate of transfer of a bound steroid from the circulation into the tissues. Therefore, the MCR of a steroid bound to TeBG is inversely related to the level of TeBG.[32] Obesity results in the suppression of TeBG, and weight loss raises the level. The control of TeBG synthesis is based on the degree of androgenicity; androgens inhibit and estrogen stimulate. Studies now indicate that insulin also inhibits the synthesis of TeBG.[17]

The stroma of the enlarged fat mass has the enzymatic machinery for converting androgens to estrogens, especially androstenedione to estrone. Obesity is therefore characterized as producing excessive estrogens, especially estrone.[1]

REPRODUCTIVE FUNCTION IN OBESE MEN

Most obese men have normal reproductive function despite a decrease in serum testosterone level. Libido and potency are normal. The external genitalia are normal, although the penis may appear small because it recedes into the increased fat. The testes are normal in size and consistency. The decreased circulating total testosterone level is due to an equivalent decrease in TeBG.[2] However, the percentages of free or unbound testosterone is increased, thus compensating for the depressed total level. The normal basal LH levels, a normal LH response to LH releasing hormone, and the normal percentage rise in testosterone following administration of human chorionic gonadotropin or clomiphene[2] support the concept of hormonal compensation of the hypothalamic-pituitary-testes axis. Thus, there is no objective evidence of hypogonadism from either the clinical or laboratory standpoint in most obese men.

Some massively obese men (those with >200% ideal body weight) have a decrease in the free as well as total testosterone. This decrement may be due to enhanced peripheral conversion of testosterone to estradiol, which is directly related to the degree of obesity[33] (Figs. 45-7 and 45-8). Obesity is likely at least in part the result of associated hyperinsulinemia. Thus, the increase in

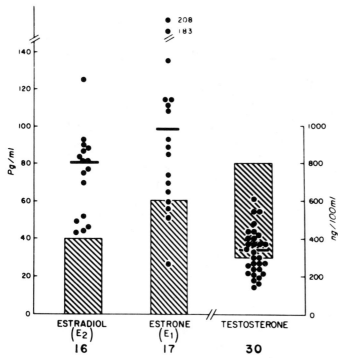

FIGURE 45-7

Serum E_2, E_1, and testosterone levels in obese men compared with normal controls, normal range. Values in obese men are plotted as individual points with the horizontal line representing their mean. The number of obese subjects included for each hormone measurement is represented by the number under each bar graph. (Schneider G et al: Increased estrogen production in obese men. J Clin Endocrinol Metab 48:633, 1979)

TeBG with weight loss in obesity is at least partially secondary to correction of the hyperinsulinemia.

Acknowledgment: The original studies of the author were conducted in the Clinical Research Center of the University of Tennessee, Memphis, which is supported by Grant RR-211 from the General Clinical Research Center Program of the NIH. This study was also supported in part by USPHS Grant AM-31312-02.

References

1. Bray GA: Obesity: An endocrine perspective. In DeGroot LJ (ed): Endocrinology, 2nd ed, p 2320. Philadelphia, WB Saunders, 1989
2. Glass AR, Swerdloff RS, Bray GA et al: Low serum testosterone and sex-hormone-binding-globulin in massively obese men. J Clin Endocrinol Metab 45:1211, 1977
3. Rogers J, Mitchell GW Jr: The relation of obesity to menstrual disturbances. N Engl J Med 247:53, 1952
4. Hartz AJ, Barboriak PN, Wong A et al: The association of obesity with infertility and related menstrual abnormalities in women. Int J Obes 3:57, 1979

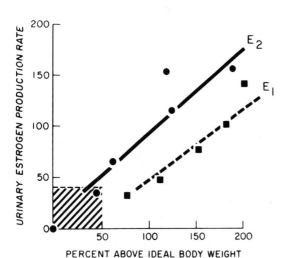

FIGURE 45-8

Urinary E_2 and E_1 production rates, expressed as micrograms per day, are plotted against the percentage above ideal body weight for 10 obese men. (Schneider G et al: Increased estrogen production in obese men. J Clin Endocrinol Metab 48:633, 1979)

5. Glass AR, Dahms WT, Abraham G et al: Secondary amenorrhea in obesity: Etiologic role of weight-related androgen excess. Fertil Steril 30:243, 1978

6. Givens JR: Polycystic ovaries: A sign, not a diagnosis. Semin Reprod Endocrinol 2:271, 1984

7. Yen SS: The polycystic ovary syndrome. Clin Endocrinol 12:177, 1980

8. Crawford JD, Osler DC: Body composition at menarche: The Frisch-Revelle hypothesis revisited. Pediatrics 56:449, 1975

9. Frisch RE: Body fat, puberty and fertility. Biol Rev 59:161, 1984

10. Yen SS, Chaney C, Judd HL: Functional aberrations of the hypothalamic-pituitary system in polycystic ovary syndrome: A consideration of the pathogenesis. In James VH, Serio M, Guisti G (eds): The Endocrine Function of the Human Ovary. New York, Academic Press, 373, 1976

11. Mitchell GW Jr, Rogers J: The influence of weight reduction on amenorrhea in obese women. N Engl J Med 249:835, 1953

12. Bates GW, Whitworth NS: Effects of obesity on sex steroid metabolism. J Chronic Dis 35:893, 1982

13. Barbieri RL, Ryan KJ: Hyperandrogenism, insulin resistance, and acanthosis nigricans syndrome: A common endocrinopathy with distinct pathophysiologic features. Am J Obstet Gynecol 147:90, 1983

14. Barbieri RL, Makris A, Ryan KJ: Effects of insulin on steroidogenesis in cultured porcine ovarian theca. Fertil Steril 40:237, 1983

15. Farah MJ, Givens JR, Kitabchi AE: Bimodal correlation between the circulating insulin level and the production rate of dehydroepiandrosterone: Positive correlation in normal and obese controls and negative correlation in polycystic ovarian disease with acanthosis nigricans. J Clin Endocrinol Metab 70:1075, 1990

16. Peiris AN, Sothmann MS, Aiman EJ et al: The relationship of insulin to sex hormone-binding globulin: Role of adiposity. Fertil Steril 52:69, 1989

17. Plymate SR, Matej LA, Jones RE et al: Inhibition of sex hormone-binding globulin production in the human hepatoma (Hep G2) cell line by insulin and prolactin. J Clin Endocrinol Metab 67:460, 1988

18. Soules MR, McLachlan RI, Ek M et al: Luteal phase deficiency: Characterization of reproductive hormones over the menstrual cycle. J Clin Endocrinol Metab 69:804, 1989

19. Sherman BM, Korenman SG: Measurement of serum LH, FSH, estradiol and progesterone in disorders of the human menstrual cycle: The inadequate luteal phase. J Clin Endocrinol Metab 39:145, 1974

20. Evans DJ, Hoffmann RG, Kalkhoff RK et al: Relationship of androgenic activity to body fat topography, fat cell morphology, and metabolic aberrations in premenopausal women. J Clin Endocrinol Metab 57:304, 1983

21. Kissebah AH, Vydelingum N, Murray R et al: Relation of body fat distribution to metabolic complications of obesity. J Clin Endocrinol Metab 54:254, 1982

22. Jackson IM, Mowat JI: Hypothalamic-pituitary-adrenal function in obesity and the cortisol secretion rate following prolonged starvation. Acta Endocrinol 63:415, 1970

23. Sims EA, Danforth E Jr, Horton ES et al: Endocrine and metabolic effects of experimental obesity in man. Recent Prog Horm Res 29:457, 1973

24. Schteingart DE, Conn JW: Dietary protein and corticosteroid secretion. Acta Diabetol Lat (Suppl 1) 9:328, 1972

25. Anderson KE, Rosner W, New MI et al: Dietary protein-carbohydrate ratio alters reciprocally plasma testosterone and cortisol levels in normal subjects (abstr). Hepatology 6:1177, 1986

26. Migeon CJ, Green OC, Eckert JP: Study of adrenocortical function in obesity. Metabolism 12:718, 1963

27. Prezio JA, Carreon G, Clerkin E et al: Influence of body composition on adrenal function in obesity. J Clin Endocrinol Metab 24:481, 1964

28. Kurtz BR, Givens JR, Komindr S et al: Maintenance of normal circulating levels of Δ^4-androstenedione and dehydroepiandrosterone in simple obesity despite increased metabolic clearance rates: Evidence for a servo-control mechanism. J Clin Endocrinol Metab 64:1261, 1987

29. Kirschner MA, Samojlik E, Silber D: A comparison of androgen production and clearance in hirsute and obese women. J Steroid Biochem 19:607, 1983

30. Komindr S, Kurtz BR, Stevens MD et al: Relative sensitivity and responsivity of serum cortisol and two adrenal androgens to α-adrenocorticotropin-(1-24) in normal and obese, nonhirsute, eumenorrheic women. J Clin Endocrinol Metab 63:860, 1986

31. Kramer RE, Hubert GD, Buster JE et al: Interactions between insulin and ACTH in the control of adrenal cortisol and androstenedione production in primary cultures of bovine adrenocortical cells (abstr). Proceedings of the 71st annual meeting of the Endocrine Society, 1989, p 1435

32. Rosenfield RL, Maudelonde T, Moll GW Jr: Biologic effects of hyperandrogenemia in polycystic ovary syndrome. Sem Reprod Endocrinol 2:281, 1984

33. Pasquali R, Casimirri F, Melchionda N et al: Weight loss and sex steroid metabolism in massively obese men. J Endocrinol Invest 11:205, 1988

CHAPTER 46

Obesity in Pregnancy

RONALD K. KALKHOFF

In the United States, the prevalence of obesity among adult women is approximately 24%, and severe obesity is estimated to represent one third of this 24%, or 8% in this population.[1] During the reproductive years, the incidence of morbid obesity in pregnancy is as high as 10% in all pregnancies.[2] In a retrospective study of 9667 pregnancies, about 5% of women were over 150% of ideal prepregnancy weight and nearly 20% weighed more than 120% of ideal values.[3] Thus, it would appear that the incidence and severity of obesity among pregnant women are not too different from what exists generally in nonpregnant adult women in America.

This review initially focuses on metabolic differences that exist between nonobese and obese gravid women. The discussion proceeds to what impact obesity may have on maternal and fetal morbidity and mortality. From this information, certain diagnostic and therapeutic strategies are developed and discussed in the closing section.

METABOLIC DIFFERENCES BETWEEN OBESE AND NONOBESE PREGNANT WOMEN

Carbohydrate Tolerance

Serial measurements of fasting plasma glucose concentrations in nonobese healthy women throughout pregnancy reveal a significant reduction as early as the tenth week of gestation.[4] Levels may continue to fall or remain relatively fixed at this lower level until term. Fasting plasma insulin concentrations also steadily rise throughout pregnancy after the tenth week,[5] whereas basal plasma glucagon levels show little change of physiological significance.[6]

According to prospective studies of results of oral glucose tolerance tests (OGTT) in normal nonobese pregnant women, the glucose response curves are significantly higher after the 20th week and insulin responses begin to rise after the 11th week and steadily increase thereafter.[5] A more exaggerated suppression of plasma glucagon during OGTT during pregnancy has been observed.[6] In early to midgestation, heightened plasma insulin concentrations may be attributed to trophic effects of key hormones such as progesterone on pancreatic islets in concert with the development of beta-cell hyperplasia and maternal tissue anabolism (e.g., body fat deposition). In late pregnancy, insulin resistance emerges as a consequence of increasing plasma titers of contrainsulin hormones, including free cortisol, progesterone, placental lactogen, and prolactin. This catabolic change meets the need for transferring stored nutrients from the maternal host to the rapidly growing fetus and explains the slight deterioration of OGTT results in late pregnancy.[7]

In healthy, obese, premenopausal women, insulin resistance is well documented in the nonpregnant state. Reduced insulin sensitivity in adipose tissue, liver, and peripheral tissues (skeletal muscle) is well documented.[8] Defects in both insulin receptor binding and postinsulin receptor events have been reported.[8] Pancreatic beta-cell compensation characterized by heightened basal as well as postprandial plasma insulin concentrations parallels degrees of overweight.

Some major metabolic changes from normal are anticipated in obese pregnant women because they are challenged by the insulin resistance of late pregnancy superimposed on resistance already associated with their obese state *per se*. Although it is true that obese women are more vulnerable to gestational diabetes (see later discussion), truly nondiabetic obese women with negative family histories of diabetes demonstrate very few metabolic differences from nonobese women during pregnancy.

In a sequential study of women who were more than 150% of ideal prepregnancy weight, the same patterns of change were observed in plasma glucose and insulin concentrations in early, mid-, and late gestation as compared with a nonobese group.[9] No significant differences in hemoglobin A1$_c$ or average plasma glucose concentrations were derived from values obtained at four different time intervals throughout the day. Unpublished studies of these same two groups of women also revealed no significant differences in plasma glucose responses during OGTT throughout gestation. Only basal plasma glucose was slightly, though significantly, higher in the obese women in late pregnancy. On the other hand, fasting as well as postchallenge plasma insulin responses during OGTT progressively rose and were consistently higher than in the nonobese group (Table 46-1).

It is concluded that although substantially more insulin resistance attends obesity in pregnancy, obese, nondiabetic expectant mothers are capable of boosting insulin secretion and plasma insulin concentrations sufficiently to maintain plasma glucose profiles that are not different from nonobese control subjects.

Plasma Lipids

During normal human gestation, median total plasma triglyceride concentrations rise steadily throughout advancing pregnancy and are 3.6-fold greater at term than in nonpregnant women. Most of the lipoprotein fractions carrying triglycerides also rise proportionally.[10] Total plasma levels of cholesterol and phospholipids rise to a much lesser extent. Most of the cholesterol elevation can be attributed to increased low-density (49%) and high-density (23%) lipoprotein cholesterol.[10] Free fatty acids and glycerol in plasma change little during the first two trimesters of normal gestation but rise significantly in the prepartum period.[11]

How obesity might influence plasma lipids

TABLE 46-1

Metabolic Changes in Obese Pregnant Women Relative to Nonobese Pregnant Women

Parameter	Early Gestation	Midgestation	Late Gestation	Postpartum
Fasting plasma glucose	NS	NS	↑	NS
Fasting plasma insulin	↑	↑	↑	↑
GTT glucose response	NS	NS	NS	NS
GTT insulin response	↑	↑	↑	↑
Hemoglobin A1$_c$	NS	NS	NS	NS
Fasting plasma triglyceride	NS	NS	NS	NS
Fasting plasma cholesterol	NS	NS	NS	NS
Fasting total plasma amino acid	NS	↓	NS	NS

Statistical comparisons were made between nine healthy nonobese and ten healthy obese pregnant women whose respective average prepregnancy weights (± SEM) were 111 ± 4% and 171 ± 10% of ideal body weight. (GTT, 50 g oral glucose tolerance test; NS, no significant difference; arrows indicate a significant change from nonobese mean values) (Kalkhoff RK, Kandaraki E, Morrow PG et al: Relationship between neonatal birthweight and maternal plasma amino acid profiles in lean and obese nondiabetic women and in type I diabetic pregnant women. Metabolism 37:234, 1988. Also from unpublished observations) during gestation is not entirely clear because most studies that address this question have been done on patients with coexisting type II diabetes or gestational diabetes mellitus. In these two combined disorders, the principal changes are significantly higher levels of total triglycerides and very low density lipoprotein triglyceride.[12,13]

In our own unpublished observations of very obese nondiabetic women and nonobese control women throughout pregnancy, we found no significant differences between the two groups with respect to fasting and 24-hour profile concentrations of total triglycerides and cholesterol. These observations collectively suggest that there is a normal increment of most lipid fractions in the plasma of normal nonobese pregnant women. Obesity, in the absence of diabetes and other complications, does not appear to alter this pattern or the actual plasma levels (see Table 46-1).

Plasma Amino Acids

Total plasma amino acids concentrations decrease in early normal pregnancy relative to values in nonpregnant women. They remain at this level only to rise again shortly after delivery. In our studies of obese pregnant women, total plasma amino acid profiles were not significantly different from those in the nonobese women except at midgestation, when they were 12% lower.[9]

When profiles of 18 individual amino acids were obtained in the two groups, very few differences existed. The only consistent changes in the obese women were significantly lower alanine levels during early and midgestation and a depressed histidine concentration throughout pregnancy. The latter finding most likely represents greater histidine catabolism in obese gravid subjects. When type I and gestational diabetes are studied in a similar fashion, significant disturbances in plasma amino acids are observed.[9,14]

It is of interest that in severe obesity in the nonpregnant state, insulin resistance is often expressed by significant elevations of branched-chain amino acids.[15] This was not observed in our pregnant obese women.[9] However, 6 to 8 weeks postpartum, the five branched-chain amino acids—valine, leucine, isoleucine, tyrosine and phenylalanine—were higher in the obese women, and tyrosine and phenylalanine

elevations achieved significance relative to values in postpartum nonobese subjects.[9] Because insulin resistance in the obese state in late gestation is more intense than that after delivery, one might anticipate greater elevations of prepartum levels of these specific amino acids. Reasons for the lack of this change remain unclear.

Table 46-1 summarizes the results of prospective studies of our nonobese and obese pregnant women. The only major difference between the two groups was the significantly higher plasma insulin concentration in the fasting state and following an oral glucose load. Thus, we conclude that few disturbances in carbohydrate, lipid, and amino acid metabolism occur in healthy obese women throughout gestation. It should be emphasized, however, that such data derived from plasma concentration measurements indicate nothing about fluxes of substrate into and out of the maternal plasma compartment or into the placental-fetal unit.

Body Composition

Surveys conducted in the United States reveal that nonobese women gain approximately 10.9 to 12.3 kg (24 to 27 pounds) during a 40-week gestation. The preponderance of total maternal weight gain is body fat and other tissue accretion (e.g., breasts, blood elements, lean body mass). The weight gain that takes place during the latter half of pregnancy mostly relates to uterine, placental, and fetal growth.[16]

Studies now suggest that weight gain and body fat accumulation during pregnancy in regions like Western Europe may be decidedly higher than in chiefly agrarian countries like The Gambia, where long hours of physical exertion are common.[17] Thus, it appears that environment has a major influence on these parameters.

Energy Balance

Total caloric cost of normal pregnancy beyond that needed for nonpregnancy weight maintenance was estimated by Hytten and Chamberlain[16] to be 80,000 kcal, or approximately 300 additional kcal/day. About one half of this caloric expenditure is devoted to deposition of more body fat; the other half relates to energy needs to increase maternal cardiac output and support growth of the developing conceptus. Indirect calorimetry and doubly labeled water ($^2H_2^{18}O$) techniques have been used to estimate resting metabolic rate (RMR) and thermic effects of food (TEF) and exercise (TEE). RMR accounts for more than 60% of the total energy expenditure per day. Prospective studies of normal women throughout pregnancy show a high degreee of variability in TEE.[18] RMR may actually decline in early pregnancy and then rise in some women. In others, a steady increment in RMR is observed throughout gestation. This same prospective investigation found little impact of TEF on overall energy economy during gestation. On the other hand, there appears to be mounting evidence that variations in physical activity (i.e., TEE) have an important role in variations of the overall caloric cost of pregnancy.[17,18]

According to Durnin's review,[19] the additional energy needs during a typical Western European pregnancy are closer to 60,000 kcal than to the 80,000 kcal value estimated by Hytten and Chamberlain.[16] Because the increment in food intake was only in the range of 20,000 kcal (100 kcal/day), two thirds of the increased energy needs were not accounted for. They concluded that reduced physical exertion, especially in the late stages of pregnancy, conserved substantial amounts of energy to offset the increased caloric demands of gestation. Additional food intake in the range of 100 kcal/day is considerably less than extra food intakes (about 300 additional kcal/day) recommended by the various international health agencies.

When caloric intake is subnormal in pregnancy, both RMR and TEE may decrease in association with little or no body fat accumulation, often conserving sufficient energy to allow for acceptable fetal development and lactation postpartum.[17]

In obesity, RMR among age- and sex-matched individuals is frequently higher than in normal-weight women. This difference relates most closely to greater body size and lean body mass in obese persons. According to J.C. King (Written communication, University of California–Berkeley, December, 1989), RMR in obese pregnant women exceeds values in obese nonpregnant women. Nonresting metabolic rates in obese pregnant women, however, are lower than in nonpregnant obese women. A similar relationship is observed in nonobese pregnant and nonpregnant individuals, but resting and nonresting energy expenditures are proportionally lower than corresponding values in obese persons.

In summary, studies now suggest that both lean and obese pregnant women meet the increased energy needs of pregnancy by increasing food intake slightly and by reducing physical exertion. The total additional energy needs of pregnancy in the Western world are probably less than 300 additional kcal/day and closer to 100 kcal/day.[19]

MATERNAL COMPLICATIONS

It is difficult to compare the large number of surveys on obesity in pregnancy because of the great variability in definitions of obesity and its complications, selection of control patients, study design, and depth of statistical analyses. For example, some investigations are limited to morbidly obese expectant mothers, and mild to moderately overweight individuals are included in the control group. Degrees of obesity are defined during pregnancy rather than before conception. Others define and subdivide degrees of obesity in terms of prepregnancy body mass index or percent of ideal body weight. Some series do not separate complications present before conception from similar pregnancy-onset problems. In others, specific complications are selected for analyses and all others are ignored. Despite these difficulties, enough information about maternal complications is available to provide a general consensus and highlight the controversies. For purposes of discussion, they are classified into antepartum, intrapartum, and postpartum events.

The Antepartum Period

According to one review of the literature between 1960 and 1982, 143 publications were devoted to obesity and pregnancy.[20] Of these, only 26 that involved 10,440 cases were relevant to maternal morbidity in this condition. In the opinion of the reviewers, only a few antenatal problems were sufficiently prevalent to regard them as more frequent among obese pregnant women. The selection of these problems, however, was somewhat arbitrary. They included

TABLE 46-2

Prevalence (%) of Antepartum Complications in Obese Pregnant Women

Parameter	Underweight < 85% IBW	Normal Weight 85–120% IBW	Moderately Obese 120–150% IBW	Severely Obese > 150% IBW	P Value*
Number of subjects	607	7170	1445	444	
Hypertensive disease	0.9%	1.9%	7.0%	17.2%	< .05
Pre-eclampsia–eclampsia	3.8%	4.4%	6.6%	6.9%	< .05
Diabetes	1.2%	1.4%	3.9%	10.4%	< .05
Anemia	5.4%	4.3%	3.2%	2.4%	< .05
Thrombophlebitis	0.3%	0.1%	0.4%	0.4%	< .05
Urinary tract infection	5.9%	5.8%	8.0%	9.4%	< .05

*P values calculated from chi-square analysis. (IBW, ideal body weight)

(From Garbaciak JA, Richter M, Miller S et al: Maternal weight and pregnancy complications. Am J Obstet Gynecol 152:238, 1985)

pre-eclampsia and the separate elements of this disorder, diabetes mellitus, varicose veins, subnormal weight gain, and the need for cesarean section.

Several additional published studies have now confirmed these earlier findings and have placed the relative risks of each in better perspective. Table 46-2 summarizes the study by Garbaciak and colleagues,[3] who categorized 10,000 pregnancies according to percent of ideal prepregnancy weight (underweight, normal weight, obese, and severely obese). All complications, with the exception of anemia, were significantly higher in the obese groups. Generally, there was a continuum of prevalence as the degree of obesity increased. This trend was most apparent with respect to hypertension, diabetes mellitus, and urinary tract infections (UTIs). The results of this study are in close agreement with another comprehensive evaluation of 4100 pregnancies subsequently published by Abrams and Parker,[21] who used a similar study design.

Hypertension and Pregnancy-Induced Hypertension

It is well established that essential hypertension is more common among obese persons and that its severity parallels the degree of overweight.[22] The prevalence of hypertension in representative studies of pregnant, morbidly obese subjects varies between 5% and 66%.[3,21-26] In those series in which the degree of obesity is carefully defined

and a nonobese control group is used, the prevalence also varies greatly, between 5.3% and 22.6%,[3,21,23] but it is of interest that hypertension in the control groups also has a widely differing prevalence.

Table 46-3 summarizes the relative risks of hypertension in three well-controlled studies in which obesity was defined as greater than 135% of ideal weight in one and less than 150% in the remaining two. Relative risks were 4.49,[21] 8.70,[3] and 2.42,[23] respectively. A simple average of the three reports would place relative risk at about 5.2.

In a similar fashion, the three studies had a prevalence of pregnancy-onset hypertension (i.e., pre-eclampsia or eclampsia) of 9.1%, 6.9%, and 14.0%, respectively, in severely obese subjects.[3,21,23] Table 46-3 summarizes the individual and collective relative risk of this disorder as compared with a nonobese population of pregnant women. Thus, the prevalence of pregnancy-induced hypertension among severely obese women was 1.9-fold greater.

Diabetes Mellitus

Diabetes mellitus occurs much more frequently among obese than nonobese pregnant women. The reported overall incidence is between 4% and 18% among overweight gravid women as compared with a 1% to 3% incidence among nonobese. Unfortunately, very few studies distinguish between type I insulin-dependent

TABLE 46-3

Relative Risk of Antenatal Complications in Severely Obese Pregnant Women

Parameter	Relative Risk*	P Value
Anemia	0.63	< .001
Diabetes mellitus	6.57	< .001
Hypertension	2.42 to 8.70 (mean = 5.2)	< .001
Pregnancy-induced hypertension	1.91	< .001
Urinary tract infection	1.42	< .001

*Mantel Haenzel relative risk estimate was calculated from combined data of Garbaciak and colleagues,[3] Abrams and Parker,[21] and Edwards and co-workers.[23] Nonobese pregnant women (N = 10,789) were compared with obese pregnant women (N = 994) whose prepregnancy weight was at least 135% of ideal body weight.

(Abrams BF, Parker J: Overweight and pregnancy complications. Int J Obes 12:293, 1987)

diabetes and type II non–insulin-dependent diabetes that predated pregnancy versus pregnancy-onset or true gestational diabetes mellitus.

In the three comprehensive studies analyzed by Abrams and Parker,[21] the relative risk for all types of diabetes mellitus in obese pregnant women who are at least 135% above ideal weight is 6.57, as compared with nonobese women (see Table 46-3). In one of the three surveys by Edwards and colleagues, the majority of diabetic patients had gestational diabetes and the incidence in obese women (10.6%) exceeded that in the nonobese women (2.8%) by 3.8-fold.[23]

Two studies that examined the impact of mild to moderate obesity on the prevalence of all types of diabetes during pregnancy reported an incidence that was also significantly higher than in nonobese subjects but lower than in severely obese women.[3,21] One can conclude from these data that the risk for developing gestational or pregnancy-onset diabetes in severely obese women is about four or more times greater than in nonobese subjects. All forms of diabetes observed in severe obesity and pregnancy, whether prepregnancy or pregnancy-onset, exceed the occurrence in nonobese subjects by more than six

times. The relative risks in lesser degrees of obesity are intermediate between those of severely obese and nonobese women.

A relationship between obesity and diabetes is emphasized in the pregnant state, in which the development of increasing insulin resistance of advancing pregnancy is superimposed on the pre-existing insulin resistance of obesity. This double stress undoubtedly accounts for the more frequent emergence of impaired carbohydrate tolerance in this group of patients.

Urinary Tract Infections

UTI includes pyelonephritis, cystitis, and urethral infections. According to the reports by Garbaciak and colleagues,[3] Abrams and Parker,[21] and Edwards and associates,[23] the incidences of UTI among their control nonobese populations were 5.8%, 4.2%, and 10.6%, respectively. In the first two studies in which mild to moderate obesity was studied, the incidence of UTI was 8.0% and 5.8%, which significantly exceeded that in the control group with a relative risk of about 1.4. Among severely obese patients, the UTI in all three studies was observed in 9.4%, 5.3%, and 10.1%, respectively. Thus, Edwards and co-workers found no increase in UTI in their severely obese population,[23] whereas Garbaciak and colleagues[3] and Abrams and Parker[23] reported significantly increased prevalence, with relative reported risks of 1.62 and 1.39, respectively. According to Abrams and Parker's combined analysis of the three studies,[3,21,23] the relative risk for UTI was significant at 1.42 (see Table 46-3).

Some previously published reports of 100 obese pregnant women or less also report an increased incidence of UTI. According to the review by Ruge and Andersen,[20] seven studies investigated UTI between the years 1960 and 1982. Two of seven reported an increased incidence.

Anemia

Anemia among severely obese pregnant women is significantly less common than in a nonobese pregnant population.[3,21,23] The relative risk ranges between 0.56 and 0.72, with an average of 0.63 (Table 46-3).

The reasons for lower prevalence of anemia in obesity and pregnancy are not clear. However, anemia is also less common among nonpregnant obese women[22] and presumably relates to a higher frequency of amenorrhea and oligomenorrhea and less menstrual blood and iron losses. This advantageous effect on iron balance may be carried into pregnancy.

Subnormal Maternal Weight Gain

Very few investigations have examined subnormal weight gain in obese pregnant women. Gross and co-workers define inadequate weight gain as averaging less than 224 g/week.[25] In their series, which compared women weighing 90 kg (200 pounds) or more at any time during pregnancy with other women who weighed less than 90 kg, the relative incidence of inadequate weight gain among the obese (9.7%) and less obese women (3.9%) were significantly different.

Edwards and co-workers found a much higher percentage of severely obese women (>150% ideal prepregnancy weight) who gained less than 12 pounds (31.2%) relative to a truly nonobese control group (4.3%).[23] Excessive weight gain among the two groups did not differ significantly from their control groups and was observed in 5.2% and 7.2% of the two populations, respectively.

Thus, it would appear that subnormal weight gain, as opposed to excessive weight accumulation, can occur as much as eight times more often among women who are morbidly obese during gestation.

Venous Disease

Most publications on maternal complications in obesity do not dwell on venous diseases such as varicose veins, thrombophlebitis, or thromboembolic disease. A review of past literature suggests that varicose veins are more common among obese gravid subjects.[20] Surveys now find an overall incidence of venous disease of less than 1% regardless of degree of obesity,[23,24,26] indicating that a very large population must be studied to identify accurate trends and significance. In one study involving nearly 10,000 subjects, the relative risk for developing thrombophlebitis in moderate and severely obese patients was about 1.33 and was significant relative to nonobese control subjects (see Table 46-2).[3] However, the number of afflicted women was very small, and the researchers hesitated to draw any firm conclusions.

It is concluded that venous disease as an antepartum complication of obesity in pregnancy is marginally greater than in nonobese pregnant women. Only one study[3] found the prevalence and relative risk to be greater in overweight gravid subjects.

Gallbladder Disease

Obesity *per se* poses a significant risk for developing symptomatic gallstones and gallbladder disease. The prevalence of the problem rises steadily with degree of overweight.[22] Some studies report that parity also increases gallbladder disease risk. In a comprehensive analysis of nearly 90,000 middle-aged women, obesity was found to be a most important risk factor, but relative parity did not significantly modify the prevalence of gallbladder disease in this population.[27]

The Intrapartum Period

Primary cesarean section in the United States has increased from 5.5% of all pregnancies in 1970 to 15.2% in 1978. In Sweden, between the years 1973 and 1979, the cesarean section rate rose from 5.5% to 11.9%.[28] This procedure is more commonly done in obese pregnant women.[20] Table 46-4 shows the percentage of cesarean sections performed in nonobese and obese populations in three representative studies.[3,21,23] Two of three studies with a combined total of 14,000 subjects found a significant increase in cesarean section procedures with increasing degree of obesity.[3,21] In one study, the incidence was even higher among obese women if antepartum complications (e.g., diabetes, hypertension) coexisted.[3] In the third study,[23] involving approximately 400 subjects, the prevalence of cesarean section delivery was no higher in very obese subjects. However, when the three studies were statistically analyzed together,[21] the relative risk of primary cesarean section intervention was significantly higher in the severely obese group (1.6). Some but not all studies that do not include a homogeneous nonobese control group also support this conclusion.[24,25]

Although primary cesarean section is more commonly performed in obese women, the reasons are not entirely clear. Large fetuses with cephalopelvic disproportion, prolonged gestation, sluggish responses to medical induction of

TABLE 46-4

Prevalence (%) of Primary Cesarean Section in Nonobese and Obese Pregnant Women

Study	Nonobese	Moderately Obese	Severely Obese
Garbaciak et al[3]	10.4%	12.4%	19.6%*
Abrams and Parker[21]	13.3%	16.9%	21.5%*
Edwards et al[23]	8.6%	—	11.0%

*Asterisk denotes a significant difference among the three weight categories.

labor, and a higher prevalence of antenatal complications that might necessitate cesarean section are contributing factors.

Morbidity from primary cesarean section also has been investigated in studies of obese women.[28] The most common complication is infection involving wounds, the urinary tract, or the endometrium. Although some studies uncover a trend toward higher morbidity after cesarean section in obese women,[24] the great majority fail to find obesity as a significant factor in the development of complications after primary procedures.[28,29] Obesity, however, may be an important factor in the development of infection after emergency cesarean sections as opposed to elective procedures.[28] Factors that more closely relate to this postoperative complication include duration of ruptured membranes and duration of labor before cesarean section, as well as severity of anemia.[28]

Other potential complications of labor and delivery have been examined, and there appear to be no important differences between obese and control groups.[25] The only major difference in the intrapartum state in obese women is the greater incidence of primary cesarean sections. Different factors that may be responsible for the higher cesarean section rate in obese women are reviewed.

The Postpartum Period

Potentiation of Obesity by Pregnancy

Progressive heaviness among women is often observed after successive pregnancies. To quantify these changes, Greene and co-workers[30] analyzed data obtained from more than 7000 women who had two pregnancies within 6 years. After ad-

justing for several variables known to affect body weight during gestation, it was shown that weight gain of 20 pounds or more during the first gestation had a statistically significant effect on ultimate weight before the second pregnancy. Thus, the more weight a gravid woman gains in excess of 20 pounds, the more weight she retains after delivery (Table 46-5).

TABLE 46-5

Influence of Maternal Weight Gain During a Pregnancy on Weight Retention Before a Second Pregnancy Within 6 Months

Prenatal Weight Gain (pounds)	Number of Women	Adjusted Interpregnancy Weight Gain (lbs)
> 40	304	+ 17.7 ± 0.6*
36–40	287	+ 10.9 ± 0.64*
31–35	567	+ 8.0 ± 0.44*
26–30	1100	+ 5.6 ± 0.33*
22.6–25	890	+ 4.5 ± 0.36*
20.1–22.5	596	+ 3.3 ± 0.43*
17.6–20	886	+ 2.1 ± 0.36 (NS)
16–17.5	490	+ 1.0 ± 0.47 (NS)
11–15	979	+ 0.6 ± 0.34 (NS)
5–10	579	− 1.7 ± 0.44 (NS)
< 5	438	− 2.0 ± 0.42 (NS)

Values are mean ± SEM.
*Asterisk indicates a significant interpregnancy weight gain.
(NS, not significant)
(From Greene GW, Smicklas-Wright H, Scholl TO et al: Postpartum weight change: How much of the weight gained in pregnancy will be lost after delivery? Obstet Gynecol 71:701, 1988)

These observations are somewhat in conflict with recommended weight gain of 22 pounds or more to support normal fetal growth, because that amount would guarantee some weight retention. Although gestational weight gain is one of the most important indices in prognosticating future body weights, other factors have some influence on degree of obesity during and after pregnancy. They include marital status, cigarette smoking, prepregnancy weight, race, socioeconomic status, complications during gestation, and ultimate duration of breast-feeding.[30] The researchers emphasize the need for individual balance between controlling pregnancy weight gain and assuring optimal maternal and fetal well-being.

PERINATAL MORTALITY AND COMPLICATIONS

Perinatal Mortality

Table 46-6 records perinatal mortality rates for infants born of normal-weight and obese mothers in three studies for which there was an adequate nonobese control group.[3,21,23] Perinatal mortality for the nonobese group ranged between 0.67% and 1.9%. Only one of the three studies showed a significant increase in overall neonatal deaths among moderately and severely obese mothers (see Table 46-6).[3] When their groups were further subdivided into those without and those with maternal antenatal complications, neonatal mortality rates in moderately and severely obese mothers with no antenatal complications did not

have increased neonatal mortality. However, those obese mothers with antenatal complications had three times more neonatal mortality than nonobese mothers with antenatal complications.

The results of these studies suggest that maternal obesity has no major effect on neonatal death rates. However, when maternal antenatal complications are superimposed on obesity, death rates may be significantly higher than in nonobese groups.

Additional studies have assessed the effects of maternal obesity on the outcome of preterm as opposed to full-term deliveries. In a report by Lucas and colleagues,[31] mean gestational age of 771 early deliveries was 31 months and birth weight was less than 1850 g. Maternal obesity level, defined by Quetelet index, categorized the preterm deliveries according to mother's weight in the first trimester (thin, normal, mild obesity, and moderate to severe obesity). After excluding congenital anomalies and deaths within the first 48 hours of birth, they found that apart from gestational age, maternal fatness had a significant negative effect on infant survival up to 18 months of age. Both factors were separate and distinct from other antenatal complications. The relative risk of death was four times greater among the heaviest women than among the nonobese women.

Although the reasons for these differences require clarification and more study, the findings suggest that maternal obesity may have a greater deleterious effect on the outcome of preterm deliveries than on full-term parturition.

TABLE 46-6

Perinatal Mortality (%) in Nonobese and Obese Pregnant Women

Study	Nonobese	Moderate Obesity	Severe Obesity
Abrams and Parker[21]	1.8	1.7	2.3
Edwards et al[23]	1.9	—	2.4
Garbaciak et al[3]			
No antenatal complications	0.5	0.93	1.16
With antenatal complications	1.19	3.15	3.76*
Overall perinatal mortality	0.67	1.66	2.25*

*Asterisk denotes significant differences among the three weight categories.

Neonatal Birth Weight and Macrosomia

For several years, it has been known that both maternal prepregnancy weight and weight gain during gestation have a significant influence on neonatal weight.[32,33] Obese pregnant women have heavier babies, and several studies have shown that this outcome is independent of, though additive to, other factors known to promote heavy birth weights, including diabetes and prolonged gestation.[25,34]

Macrosomia (birth weights >4000 to 4500 g) occurs in approximately 1.3% to 1.7% of all pregnancies.[35] Nevertheless, when a retrospective analysis of macrosomic births is performed, mothers were significantly more obese, were older with higher parity, and were more frequently diabetic and postmature (>42 weeks gestation) than a control group of 19,000 women bearing normal-weight infants. Further analysis revealed that relative prevalence of maternal obesity at term (>90 kg) was 77%, whereas the prevalence of postmaturity (10.8%) and diabetes (8%) were considerably lower.[35] It is also of interest that macrosomic newborns were more often boys, by a ratio of approximately 2:1. From these data, it appears that heavier babies and fetal macrosomia are more common among obese women and that prevalence rises as degree of obesity increases.[3,21,24,35]

One study also has focused on the relationship between weight gain during gestation and birth weight in 3000 deliveries in which mothers were carefully stratified according to prepregnancy body mass index and percent deviation from ideal weight.[36] These investigators found a close relationship between maternal weight gain and birth weight among mothers who were underweight, normal weight, and mildly obese (up to 135% of ideal weight). However, those mothers whose prepregnancy weight exceeded 135% of ideal weight gave birth to heavier babies whose weight was approximately the same despite a wide range of maternal weight gain between 0 and 15 kg. This finding confirms other studies that also have suggested that weight gain among more severely obese women during full-term gestations has little influence on birth-weight outcome.[25,34] These studies also show that severely

obese mothers are less likely to give birth to small-for-gestational-age babies than are nonobese or mildly obese women.[25,34] Although there is no specific explanation for this phenomenon, some speculate that abundance of fat stores in very overweight mothers guarantees substrate for fetal growth independent of differing levels of food intake and weight gain in this group.

A primary reason for understanding the link between fetal macrosomia and maternal obesity is the potential for serious birth trauma and other complications if vaginal delivery is attempted in this situation. Difficult delivery due to shoulder dystocia may result in intracranial, intraocular, and abdominal organ hemorrhage as well as clavicular fracture and facial and brachial plexus nerve injuries. In addition, the more difficult, prolonged delivery can be complicated by newborn asphyxia with depressed Apgar scores.[37]

Obesity in Offspring of Obese Mothers

Both environmental and genetic factors have a role in the perpetuation of obesity in families. The importance of heredity was documented in Stunkard and colleagues' study of adopted children, whose weight was more closely related to that of their natural parents than to that of their foster parents.[38] In another investigation, infants of obese mothers were found to be significantly more obese than infants of nonobese mothers at 12 months of age.[23]

Measurements of energy balance using the doubly labeled water technique have been applied to studies of infants born to lean and obese mothers.[39] In those babies of heavy mothers who became obese after 6 months of age (6 of 12 offspring), all had a 21% lower total energy expenditure, which could account for their heavier weight. Because food intake was approximately the same in all infants, the implications of this study are that reduced energy expenditure rather than increased food intake was responsible.

Calorimetry also has been used to assess energy balance in a 2-year prospective study of adults. In those subjects who gained the most weight during this period, both resting energy expenditure and TEE were significantly lower than average. This trait also was found to cluster within families, suggesting that it may be an inherited factor responsible for the susceptibility to obesity in certain family groups.[40]

To summarize, these data suggest that offspring of obese mothers are also prone to become obese, and this tendency may relate more to reduced energy expenditure by some mechanism that may, in part, be inherited.

DIAGNOSTIC AND THERAPEUTIC STRATEGIES

From the foregoing discussion, it is obvious that obese pregnant women and their offspring are at higher risk for certain complications. For this reason, every effort should be made to reduce body weight to as close to normal as possible before conception occurs. If pregnancy is already established and obesity coexists, careful screening and ongoing maternal surveillance are indicated to prevent the emergence of significant hypertension and pre-eclampsia–eclampsia. If these problems are present, adequate medical control and continued monitoring of blood pressure are indicated.

The American Diabetes Association and the Second International Workshop-Conference on Gestational Diabetes also recommend that all pregnant women should be screened for pregnancy-onset diabetes mellitus between the 24th and 28th week of gestation.[41] Because obese gravid women are at higher risk for developing gestational diabetes, it is especially important to rule out this problem. A 50-g oral glucose load is administered without regard to time of day or time of last meal. A 1-hour venous plasma level of 140 mg/dl or greater is positive and requires a complete OGTT to establish the diagnosis.[41] If diabetes is diagnosed, strict plasma glucose control with diet alone or diet with insulin therapy, if necessary, is suggested.[41]

Quality obstetric care also dictates repeated searches for underlying asymptomatic or minor UTIs in obese pregnant women in order to prevent a more serious UTI that may significantly increase morbidity as an antenatal complication.[42] Early eradication with appropriate antibiotic therapy is indicated.

Because macrosomic neonates are more frequently born to obese pregnant women, prepartum surveillance should include ultrasonogra-phy at appropriate time intervals. Cesarean section is recommended in those instances in which vaginal delivery may result in birth trauma and asphyxia because of large fetal size.

It is difficult to make specific recommendations about diet for obese expectant mothers, because TEE, as discussed earlier, may vary a great deal in different individuals. In the Western world, a conservative approach is to prescribe 30 kcal/kg prepregnancy weight with a total weight gain goal in the range of 20 pounds.[43] This recommendation is supported to some extent by the findings of optimal perinatal survival with weight gain of this magnitude among women who are over 135% of ideal weight.[44] Weight is closely monitored and adjustments are made in the diet, if necessary, to achieve the desired goal. It is of great importance to arrange ongoing interactions between obese women and a registered dietician so that nutritional guidelines are understood. It is undesirable for obese pregnant women to gain excessive weight, which might increase susceptibility to pregnancy-onset diabetes, hypertension–pre-eclampsia, and edema, as well as advance postpartum obesity.

After delivery, continuing efforts to reduce maternal body weight to an acceptable level are emphasized. Infants also should be monitored for excessive weight gain, and steps should be taken to contain it without jeopardizing adequate nutrition. Weight control for both mother and child may be helped by a reasonable increase of physical activity.

Acknowledgment: Research performed by the author and cited in this review was supported by NIH grants AM 22105 and RR 00058 and by a grant from TOPS Club, Inc., Obesity and Metabolic Research Program. Assistance from Ann Schwoerer in preparation of this chapter is also gratefully acknowledged.

References

1. Abraham S, Carroll M, Naijar MF: Trends in obesity and overweight among adults age 20–74 years: United States 1960–1962, 1971–1974, 1976–1980. In Vital and Health Statistics, Series 11. Hyattsville, MD, National Center for Health Statistics, 1985
2. Gross T, Sokal RJ, King KC: Obesity in pregnancy:

Risks and outcome. Obstet Gynecol 56:446, 1980

3. Garbaciak JA, Richter M, Miller S et al: Maternal weight and pregnancy complications. Am J Obstet Gynecol 152:238, 1985

4. Victor A: Normal blood sugar variation during pregnancy. Acta Obstet Gynecol Scand 53:37, 1974

5. Kuhl C: Glucose metabolism during and after pregnancy in normal and gestational diabetic women, Part 1. Influence of normal pregnancy on serum glucose and insulin concentrations during basal fasting conditions and after a challenge with glucose. Acta Endocrinol 75:709, 1975

6. Luyckx AS, Gerard J, Gaspard U et al: Plasma glucagon levels in normal women during pregnancy. Diabetologia 11:549, 1975

7. Kalkhoff RK, Kissebah AH, Kim HJ: Carbohydrate and lipid metabolism during normal pregnancy: Relationship to gestational hormone action. Semin Perinatol 2:291, 1978

8. Kolterman OG, Insel J, Saekow M et al: Mechanisms of insulin resistance in human obesity: Evidence for receptor and postreceptor defects. J Clin Invest 65:1272, 1980

9. Kalkhoff RK, Kandaraki E, Morrow PG et al: Relationship between neonatal birthweight and maternal plasma amino acid profiles in lean and obese nondiabetic women and in type I diabetic pregnant women. Metabolism 37:234, 1988

10. Knopp RH, Bergelin RO, Wahl PW et al: Population-based lipoprotein lipid reference values for pregnant women compared to nonpregnant women classified by sex hormone usage. Am J Obstet Gynecol 143:626, 1982

11. McDonald-Gibson RG, Young M, Hytten FE: Changes in nonesterified fatty acids and glycerol in pregnancy. Br J Obstet Gynaecol 82:460, 1975

12. Knopp RH, Chapman M, Bergelin R et al: Relationships of lipoprotein lipids to mild fasting hyperglycemia and diabetes in pregnancy. Diabetes Care 3:416, 1980

13. Hollingsworth DL, Grundy SM: Pregnancy-associated hypertriglyceridemia in normal and diabetic women: Differences in insulin-dependent, non-insulin-dependent, and gestational diabetes. Diabetes 31:1092, 1982

14. Metzger BE, Phelps RL, Freinkel N et al: Effects of gestational diabetes on diurnal profiles of plasma glucose, lipids and individual amino acids. Diabetes Care 3:402, 1980

15. Felig P, Marliss E, Cahill G Jr: Plasma amino acid levels and insulin secretion in obesity. N Engl J Med 281:811, 1969

16. Hytten F, Chamberlain G (eds): Clinical Physiology in Obstetrics, p 163. New York, Blackwell Scientific Publications, 1980

17. Lawrence M, Whitehead RG: Physical activity and total energy expenditure of child-bearing Gambian village women. Eur J Clin Nutr 42:145, 1987

18. Prentice AM, Whitehead RG, Coward WA et al: Correspondence: Reduction in postprandial energy expenditure during pregnancy. Br Med J 295:266, 1987

19. Durnin JVGA: Energy requirements of pregnancy: An integration of the longitudinal data from the five-country study. Lancet 2:1131, 1987

20. Ruge S, Andersen T: Obstetric risks in obesity: An analysis of the literature. Obstet Gynecol Surv 40:57, 1985

21. Abrams BF, Parker J: Overweight and pregnancy complications. Int J Obes 12:293, 1987

22. Rimm AA, Werner LH, Van Yserloo B et al: Relationship of obesity and disease in 73,532 weight-conscious women. Public Health Serv Rep 90:44, 1975

23. Edwards LE, Dickes WF, Alton IR et al: Pregnancy in the massively obese: Course, outcome, and obesity prognosis of the infant. Am J Obstet Gynecol 131:479, 1978

24. Johnson SR, Kolberg BH, Varner MW: Maternal obesity and pregnancy. Surg Gynecol Obstet 164:431, 1987

25. Gross T, Sokal RJ, King KC: Obesity in pregnancy: Risks and outcome. Obstet Gynecol 56:446, 1980

26. Calandra C, Bell DA, Beischer NA: Maternal obesity in pregnancy. Obstet Gynecol 57:8, 1981

27. MacClure KM, Hayes KC, Colditz GA et al: Weight, diet, and the risk for symptomatic gallstones in middle-aged women. N Engl J Med 321:563, 1989

28. Nielsen TF, Hokegard KH: Postoperative caesarean section morbidity: A prospective study. Am J Obstet Gynecol 146:911, 1983

29. Wolf HN, Gross TL, Sokol RJ et al: Determinants of morbidity in obese women delivered by cesarean. Obstet Gynecol 71:691, 1988

30. Greene GW, Smicklas-Wright H, Scholl TO et al: Postpartum weight change: How much of the weight gained in pregnancy will be lost after delivery? Obstet Gynecol 71:701, 1988

31. Lucas A, Morley R, Cole TJ et al: Maternal fatness and viability of preterm infants. Br Med J 296:1495, 1988

32. Eastman NJ, Jackson E: Weight relationships in pregnancy. Obstet Gynecol Surv 23:1003, 1968

33. Niswander KR, Singer J, Westphal M et al: Weight gain during pregnancy and prepregnancy weight. Obstet Gynecol 33:482, 1969

34. Kliegman RM, Gross T: Perinatal problems of the obese mother and her infant. Obstet Gynecol 66:299, 1985

35. Spellacy WN, Miller S, Winegar A et al: Mac-

rosomia: Maternal characteristics and infant complications. Obstet Gynecol 66:158, 1985

36. Abrams BF, Laros RK Jr: Prepregnancy weight, weight gain, and birthweight. Am J Obstet Gynecol 154:503, 1986

37. Schwartz R: The infant of the diabetic mother. In Davidson, JK (ed): Clinical Diabetes Mellitus: A Problem-Oriented Approach, p 500. New York, Thieme, 1986:500.

38. Stunkard AJ, Sorensen TIA, Hanis C et al: An adoption study of human obesity. N Engl J Med 314:193, 1986

39. Roberts SB, Savage J, Coward WA et al: Energy expenditure and intake in infants born to lean and overweight mothers. N Engl J Med 318:461, 1988

40. Ravussin E, Lillioja S, Knowler WC et al: Reduced energy expenditure as a risk factor for body-weight gain. N Engl J Med 318:467, 1988

41. Freinkel N (Chairman): Summary and recommendations of the Second International Workshop-Conference on Gestational Diabetes Mellitus. Diabetes (Suppl 2) 34:123, 1985

42. Naeye RL: Causes of the excessive rates of perinatal mortality and prematurity in pregnancies complicated by maternal urinary-tract infections. N Engl J Med 300:819, 1979

43. Schulman PK, Gyves MT, Merkatz IR: Role of nutrition in the management of the pregnant diabetic patient. Semin Perinatol 2:353, 1978

44. Naeye RL: Weight gain and the outcome of pregnancy. Am J Obstet Gynecol 135:3, 1979

CHAPTER 47

Obesity and Musculoskeletal Disease

ALFRED JAY BOLLET

Weight-bearing stresses on bones and joints are affected by body weight; therefore, obesity would be expected to have a role in the pathogenesis, clinical manifestations, and course of musculoskeletal disease. In addition, the metabolic influence of adipose tissue, particularly on estrogen metabolism, can influence skeletal metabolism. The clinical relevance of these phenomena has been established primarily by epidemiologic studies, and this evidence is reviewed in this chapter.

OBESITY AND ARTHRITIS

The most common form of arthritis, osteoarthritis, primarily results from wear of the surfaces of articular cartilage, a consequence of physical stresses that produce metabolic changes that lead to alterations in the structure of the articular cartilage. As the disease process progresses, the surface of the cartilage becomes roughened and cracked, then thins as wear causes loss of cartilage substance. The resulting decreased thickness of the articular cartilage produces the narrowing of the space between the bony joint surfaces, which can be visualized on x-ray films as narrowing of the joint space. Secondary changes are also seen, such as proliferation of bone and cartilage at the joint margins (osteophyte formation), as well as increased density of the underlying bone, now subject to more physical stress because of loss of the protective effect of the articular cartilage. Because physical stresses on joint surfaces can be affected by the weight borne by those surfaces, obesity can be

expected to influence the incidence or at least the severity of osteoarthritis.

In obese individuals, increased weight can exacerbate stress on joints and thus the amount of wear that occurs in joints subject to weight-bearing stress. A direct correlation between weight and physical stress on joint surfaces is not expected because of variations in the amount of joint protection offered by muscle function and the damaging effect of influences such as abnormalities in posture, occupational stresses, and other factors that ameliorate or magnify the stresses. Distortions of joint alignment are frequent in obese people, altering the physical stresses in joints. For example, most obese individuals have a varus deformity of the knees, an attempt to bring the feet under the center of gravity made necessary by the separation of the thighs due to adiposity. Extra stress is therefore placed on the medial compartment of the knee, which shows the earliest and most severe osteoarthritic alteration in these patients.

Early studies of this subject showed that symptomatic osteoarthritis of the knees is more common in obese patients[1] than in the general population, but hip disease is not increased,[2] and there is no definite evidence of an increased frequency of osteoarthritis in non–weight-bearing joints.

In a large epidemiologic study in northern England, Kellgren and Lawrence[3,4] found generalized osteoarthritis twice as frequently in people classified as obese (weighing more than 10% above standards for sex, age, and height) as in nonobese people. The incidence of osteoarthritis was increased even in finger joints, clearly not subject to weight-bearing stress. Acheson and Collart[5] found a similar pattern in New Haven, CT, suggesting a generalized metabolic abnormality affecting cartilage metabolism and not simply an effect of weight bearing. Another study[6] failed to find increased radiologic evidence of osteoarthritis in obese men who had carried more than twice their ideal weight for many years, but these patients were almost all younger than 45 years, and only three were older than 50 years.

Genetic factors could play a part in the osteoarthritis associated with obesity, and the discovery of a strain of mice with genetically determined obesity as well as osteoarthritis, primarily of the shoulder, permitted study of the linkage between these two phenomena. In these obese mice, the genetics of the obesity and the osteoarthritis were clearly separate,[7] establishing that there was a dominant influence of hereditary factors producing the osteoarthritis rather than the obesity. In two studies of nonobese mice that were fed high-fat diets to produce obesity, conflicting results were obtained; in one study using saturated fat (lard), an increased incidence of osteoarthritis was observed,[8] but in another study using unsaturated vegetable fat, no increase in osteoarthritis occurred despite the development of obesity.[9]

In an epidemiologic study of the population of Framingham, the risk of osteoarthritis of the knee was increased in those in the heaviest quintile of weight at the first examination, compared with those in the lightest three quintiles; the risk was not increased for those in the second heaviest quintile. The association between weight and knee osteoarthritis was stronger in women than in men.[10]

In the U.S. National Health and Nutrition Examination Survey (NHANES I), a significant association was found between osteoarthritis of the knee and overweight, as well as a correlation with race and occupation. A key observation in this study was a dose-response effect between obesity and osteoarthritis of the knee, not established in previous studies. The survey also found an association between knee-bending demands and osteoarthritis of the knee for persons ages 55 to 64 years. Such occupational stresses are

another important factor in the development of osteoarthritis of the knee.[11]

In a similar epidemiologic study in Britain, obesity correlated with radiographic osteoarthritis of the knees in women, whereas clinical and radiographic osteoarthritis of the fingers and knees did not correlate with previous strenuous occupations.[12]

There was no evidence, however, of rheumatic disease in weight-bearing joints being more common in overweight individuals, contrary to the "wear-and-tear" hypothesis. In a 10-year follow-up, neither baseline weights nor weight change was a significant predictor of change in the other scores. No association was observed between overweight and lumbosacral disorders, either in the cross-sectional study or in the 10-year follow-up.[13]

Obesity can affect the therapy as well as the pathogenesis of osteoarthritis. One possible therapeutic implication of obesity is the role of body weight in drug dose. Because most antirheumatic drugs are tightly protein bound, the volume of distribution (Vd) of the drugs is determined primarily by the size of the extracellular fluid space, and dose may have to be adjusted in large people in order to achieve a satisfactory therapeutic concentration of the drug. Obesity can result in high body weight without a proportionate increase in extravascular volume and thus can influence the distribution and toxicity of antirheumatic drugs in an unexpected manner. Two studies of nonsteroidal anti-inflammatory agents have addressed this issue. Analysis of salicylate kinetics revealed small differences between obese and control groups in the Vd, unbound Vd, and mean clearance of total or unbound salicylate. Following normalization for total weight, however, values of total Vd and mean clearance were significantly smaller in obese subjects than in those of normal weight, implying the possibility of increased accumulation of the salicylate and toxicity unless doses are appropriately adjusted downward. The investigators concluded that during long-term therapy, salicylate dose for obese individuals should not be adjusted upward in proportion to total weight.[14]

On the other hand, in a study of ibuprofen kinetics, peak ibuprofen concentration was significantly decreased in obese subjects. The Vd of ibuprofen was increased in obese subjects, and this increased distribution correlated positively with body weight. The Vd corrected for body weight was decreased in obese subjects, and this decrease correlated negatively with body weight. Ibuprofen clearance was also increased in obese subjects, and the increase correlated positively with body weight. Because the independent variables, Vd and clearance, were increased in parallel in the obese subjects, the dependent variable, elimination half-life, was unchanged. Clinically, these data indicate that in obese patients, the ibuprofen dose may be increased in order to achieve adequate therapeutic plasma concentrations.[15]

Because surgical replacement of severely damaged osteoarthritic joints has become a major aspect of the therapy of this disease, the influence of obesity on the outcome of surgery is a relevant consideration in both osteoarthritis and rheumatoid arthritis. One study that addressed this issue consisted of 53 knees replaced for osteoarthritis and 18 for rheumatoid arthritis. The prognosis was adversely affected by obesity, although the overall results were excellent or good in 76% of cases.[16]

Influence of Obesity on Other Types of Arthritis

Rheumatoid arthritis, the most common form of chronic inflammatory arthritis, is primarily due to altered immune processes. The joint changes consist of inflammation, thickening of synovial tissues, and in some cases destructive and deforming changes, along with inflammatory systemic disease. Obesity would not be expected to affect the pathogenetic mechanisms in this disease, and epidemiologic studies have failed to show any correlation between body weight and severity or rate of progression of the disease in patients with rheumatoid arthritis.

Obesity has been indirectly responsible for the development of a form of inflammatory arthritis. Patients who were given jejunoileal bypass surgery as treatment for obesity developed arthritis, presumably the result of bacterial overgrowth in the blind loop of the small bowel created surgically. It also occurred in patients with naturally occurring blind loops of small bowel.[17]

A study of the mechanism of the effect of intestinal bypass surgery on bone dynamics was performed. Iliac bone histomorphometry was studied after in vivo double tetracycline labeling 3 to 14 years after intestinal bypass surgery for obesity in 21 patients, selected because of clinical suspicion of metabolic bone disease. Results were compared with those of 40 age-matched normal control subjects.

It was found that clinically significant bone loss after intestinal shunt surgery results from the combined effects of an unsustained increase in bone resorption and a sustained decrease in bone formation.[18]

OBESITY AND GOUT

Gout, another form of joint disease, is influenced by obesity. The incidence of gout is proportional to the degree of hyperuricemia in various populations. In a large epidemiologic study in Tecumseh, MI, hyperuricemia was found in 11.4% of individuals with a relative weight at or above the 80th percentile, whereas only 5.7% of those between the 21st and 79th percentile of relative weight had hyperuricemia, and 3.4% of those below the 21st percentile.[19]

EFFECT OF OBESITY ON BONE

An effect of obesity on the skeleton and on the frequency and severity of osteoporosis has also been established. Increased weight bearing can result in an augmented skeletal mass, primarily through increased remodeling and a net decrease in bone removal. The effects of obesity are more complex than that, however, particularly in the group most susceptible to clinically significant osteoporosis—postmenopausal women. Newer techniques to measure bone mineral density have confirmed clinical impressions that the incidence of osteoporosis and fractures of the hip is diminished in obese subjects. A number of studies have shown that obese women have greater bone mass, at least in weight-bearing sites, than postmenopausal women of normal body weight.

One study determined bone mineral density of the lumbar spine, trochanter, and femoral neck, measured by dual photon absorptiometry, in premenopausal women who were within 30% of their ideal body weight. They were compared with women of similar age all of whom weighed at least 30% more than their ideal body weight. Positive correlations between body weight and bone mineral density were found at each of the three weight-bearing sites but not at the mid-radius (measured by single photon absorptiometry).[20]

A French study measured bone mineral density by dual photon absorptiometry of the lumbar spine, as well as serum osteocalcin and various gonadal hormone levels. Women were categorized into four groups according to their menopausal status and their weight. Comparison between groups revealed significant effects of menopausal status and obesity on bone mineral density and bone turnover; even moderate obesity decreased postmenopausal bone loss.[21]

In another study of postmenopausal women ages 40 to 70 years, bone mineral density of the spine (L2–4), hip (at the femoral neck, Ward's triangle, and greater trochanter sites, determined by dual photon absorptiometry), and radius (measured by single photon absorptiometry) showed that the heavier women had significantly greater bone mineral density at each site than did the normal-weight women.

In normal-weight women, there was a significant negative correlation between bone mineral density and years since menopause at each measurement site (except the greater trochanter); in the obese women, bone mineral density decreased with increasing years since menopause at the radius site only, and bone mineral content at the hip (femoral neck and Ward's triangle region) as well as the radius declined with increasing years after menopause. Thus, body size is a significant determinant of bone mineral density in this population. The pattern of loss of bone mineral density from Ward's triangle and femoral neck regions of hip are similar to that of the spine. The bone mineral content and bone mineral density findings in the hip suggest that remodeling occurs at this weight-bearing site, producing a favorable effect on bone strength.[22]

A study of the risk factors for vertebral fractures due to osteoporosis in 105 male patients during a 4-year period revealed that obesity was protective, whereas the relative risk for osteoporosis was increased among those who smoked cigarettes, drank alcoholic beverages, or had an associated medical disease known to affect calcium or bone metabolism.[23]

References

1. Kellgren JH, Lawrence JS, Bier F: Genetic factors in generalized osteoarthritis. Ann Rheum Dis 22:237, 1963
2. Saville PD, Dickson J: Age and weight in osteoarthritis of the hip. Arthritis Rheum 11:635, 1968
3. Kellgren JH, Lawrence JS: Osteo-arthrosis and disc degeneration in an urban population. Ann Rheum Dis 17:388, 1958
4. Kellgren JH: Osteoarthritis in patients and populations. Br Med J 2:1, 1961
5. Acheson RM, Collart AB: New Haven survey of joint diseases. XVII. Relationship between some characteristics and osteoarthrosis in a general population. Ann Rheum Dis 34:349, 1975
6. Goldin RH, McAdam L, Louie JS et al: Clinical and radiological survey of the incidence of osteoarthrosis among obese patients. Ann Rheum Dis 35:349, 1976
7. Sokoloff L, Crittenden LB, Yamamoto RS et al: The genetics of degenerative joint disease in mice. Arthritis Rheum 5:531, 1962
8. Silberberg M, Silberberg R: Osteoarthrosis in mice fed diets enriched with animal or vegetable fat. Arch Pathol 70:385, 1960
9. Sokoloff L, Mickelsen O: Dietary fat supplements, body weight and osteoarthritis in BDA/2JN mice. J Nutr 85:117, 1965
10. Felson DT, Anderson JJ, Naimark A et al: Obesity and knee osteoarthritis: The Framingham Study. Ann Intern Med 109:18, 1988
11. Anderson JJ, Felson DT: Factors associated with osteoarthritis of the knee in the first National Health and Nutrition Examination Survey (NHANES I): Evidence for an association with overweight, race, and physical demands of work. Am J Epidemiol 128:179, 1988
12. Bergstrom G, Bjelle A, Sundh VM et al: Joint disorders at ages 70, 75 and 79 years: A cross-sectional comparison. Br J Rheumatol 25:333, 1986
13. Aro S, Leino P: Overweight and musculoskeletal morbidity: A ten-year follow-up. Int J Obes 9:267, 1985
14. Greenblatt DJ, Abernethy DR, Boxenbaum HG et al: Influence of age, gender, and obesity on salicylate kinetics following single doses of aspirin. Arthritis Rheum 29:971, 1986

15. Abernethy DR, Greenblatt DJ: Ibuprofen disposition in obese individuals. Arthritis Rheum 28: 1117, 1985

16. Tauber C, Bar-On EB, Ganel A et al: The total condylar knee prosthesis: A review of 71 operations. Arch Orthop Trauma Surg 104:352, 1986

17. Dicken CH: Bowel-associated dermatosis-arthritis syndrome: Bowel bypass syndrome without bowel bypass. J Am Acad Dermatol 14:792, 1986

18. Parfitt AM, Pdenphant J, Villanueva AR et al: Metabolic bone disease with and without osteomalacia after intestinal bypass surgery: A bone histomorphometric study. Bone 6:211, 1985

19. Kelley WN: In Kelly WN, Harris ED, Ruddy S et al (eds): Textbook of Rheumatology, p 1397. Philadelphia, WB Saunders, 1981

20. Liel Y, Edwards J, Shary J et al: The effects of race and body habitus on bone mineral density of the radius, hip, and spine in premenopausal women. J Clin Endocrinol Metab 66:1247, 1988

21. Ribot C, Tremollieres F, Pouilles JM et al: Obesity and postmenopausal bone loss: The influence of obesity on vertebral density and bone turnover in postmenopausal women. Bone 8:327, 1987

22. Dawson HB, Shipp C, Sadowski L et al: Bone density of the radius, spine, and hip in relation to percent of ideal body weight in postmenopausal women. Calcif Tissue Int 40:310, 1987

23. Seeman E, Melton LJ III, O'Fallon WM et al: Risk factors for spinal osteoporosis in men. Am J Med 75:977, 1983

Altered Respiratory Function in Obesity: Sleep-Disordered Breathing and the Pickwickian Syndrome

P. G. KOPELMAN

The observation that obesity affects respiratory and cardiac function is not new, nor is the general advice to such patients to lose weight irrespective of whether their breathlessness is secondary to lung disease or cardiac failure or is the result of obesity itself.[8] Investigations show that there are many ways in which obesity may affect the function of the lungs. The majority of obese persons with normal results on respiratory function tests and arterial carbon dioxide concentrations may, nevertheless, have subtle abnormalities of ventilatory mechanics, circulating blood volume, and the energy cost of breathing. Such abnormalities may become prominent and clinically important during sleep. Moreover, an important minority of obese patients will present to their physician with clinically obvious hypoventilation, hypercapnia, hypersomnolence, and right-sided cardiac failure, a situation recognized as the obesity-hypoventilation syndrome (OHS) and often referred to as the *pickwickian syndrome*, in honor of the fat boy Joe in Charles Dickens' *Pickwick Papers*.[4] No close correlation exists between body weight and impaired ventilatory function, and it remains unclear why most obese individuals show only minor abnormalities of respiratory function whereas a minority develop respiratory failure. The purpose of this chapter is to present information obtained from studies of the effect of adiposity on the mechanical function of breathing and control of respira-

tion (when awake and asleep) in order to discuss those factors that may predispose individuals to develop OHS and to give guidance to clinicians for the investigation and management of obesity-related disorders of respiration.

PATHOGENESIS OF THE RESPIRATORY COMPLICATIONS OF OBESITY

Effects of Obesity on Respiratory Mechanics and Lung Volumes

An increased amount of fat in the chest wall and abdomen has a predictable effect on the mechanical properties of the chest and diaphragm and leads to an alteration of respiratory excursions during inspiration and expiration, reducing lung volume and altering the pattern of ventilation to each region. Furthermore, the increased mass of fat leads to a decrease in compliance of the respiratory system as a whole (i.e., change of volume per unit change of pressure), with a greater reduction being noted in the chest wall rather than the lungs.[23] A further significant reduction in total compliance occurs when an obese person lies flat, a similar situation being observed in normal-weight volunteers when weights are attached to their chests.[27] The mass loading effect of fat increases both the elasticity and inertia of the respiratory system and requires increased respiratory muscle force to overcome the excessive elastic recoil and an associated increase in the elastic work of breathing.[5,28] The mechanical work of breathing is increased by 30% in simple obesity and by three times normal in OHS.[29]

The muscular activity of the diaphragm estimated from diaphragmatic electromyogram (EMG) readings is increased in extremely overweight subjects,[21,25] and the diaphragmatic response to carbon dioxide stimulation is nearly four times that in normal-weight subjects and in patients with OHS. This observation suggests that the majority of obese persons are in this way able to overcome the excessive respiratory impedance exerted by the obese thorax, whereas patients with OHS for some reason cannot or do not.[20]

Most studies of lung volume in obesity are difficult to interpret because the subjects are compared with predictions based on normal populations, which may or may not be representative for obese individuals. Nevertheless, characteristic changes are noted in the respiratory system mechanics: The compressive effect of adipose tissue on the thorax reduces the resting end-expiratory lung volume, principally because of a reduction in the expiratory reserve volume (ERV).[7] Vital capacity (VC) and total lung capacity are frequently decreased. In normal-weight individuals, a change from the sitting to lying position is accompanied by a decrease of ERV, a situation accentuated by obesity.[33] The changes in obese persons tend to be more marked in those who are the most overweight and are of greatest severity in patients with OHS.

Effects of Obesity on Total Blood Volume and Gas Exchange

An increase in total blood volume is found in obese persons with normal arterial blood gases. This increase is directly related to increased body weight, and a linear relationship exists between the total blood volume and body weight in excess of ideal weight.[25] Cardiac output is also increased in obesity, and a close relationship exists between an increase in cardiac output and total blood volume.[25] Because the increased blood flow, which is largely distributed to fat depots, must be accommodated as augmented venous return by the lungs, it is not surprising that pulmonary blood volume is increased in obesity in proportion to increased total blood volume.

A ventilation-perfusion disturbance is the most striking abnormality of gas exchange found in extreme obesity.[1] It is manifested by various degrees of hypoxia but normal arterial carbon dioxide values. The decrease in arterial oxygen tension is usually magnified when an obese patient lies flat, presumably as a result of shallower breathing and further compression of the lungs; abdominal distribution of fat (central obesity) particularly impedes the mechanical movement of the chest wall in the supine position.[2] The most convincing demonstration of the mechanisms underlying hypoxia of extreme obesity has come from radioisotope examination of the regional distribution of pulmonary ventilation and perfusion using xenon-133.[14] These studies show less ventilation to the well-perfused lower lobes in obese patients compared with normal-weight subjects, and this abnormality is most marked in patients with the greatest decrease in ERV. The ventilation-perfusion abnormality in extreme obesity is a regional one, with the lower portions of the lungs being relatively underventilated but overperfused. Pulmonary arterial hypoxia further expands the pulmonary blood volume, which in turn leads to additional strain on both right and left ventricles.

The subtle changes in respiratory function are generally of little significance in an awake obese person, but it is with the onset of sleep that they may become physiologically important.

NORMAL NOCTURNAL RESPIRATION

Respiration during sleep is dependent on sleep stage, ventilatory drives, and the presence or absence of pulmonary pathology. While a person is awake, respiration is under both voluntary and automatic control, whereas during sleep, automatic mechanisms are of greater importance.[24] Because level of consciousness varies between waking and light sleep, irregularity of respiration is often accompanied by a small decrease in arterial oxygen, ventilation, pharyngeal muscle tone, and the response to hypoxia and hypercapnia.[5,10] Short apneic episodes (periodic respiration) may also occur. As sleep becomes deeper, the breathing pattern becomes more regular. In deep sleep (slow-wave sleep), respiration is regular, oxygen saturation and carbon dioxide tension are generally similar to those in the awake state, and apneic episodes are rare. Periods of sleep characterized by rapid eye movements (REM) with a fast desynchronized electroencephalogram (EEG) and reduced muscle tone correspond to dreaming. In REM sleep, there are decreases in voluntary muscle tone and in the responses to hypoxia, hypercapnia, and airway obstruction; oxygen saturation is reduced, and carbon dioxide tension rises. Irregular respiration and occasional apneic episodes often occur in normal persons during REM sleep; an increase in body weight, with its influence on respiratory mechanics, increases their frequency and may cause significant alveolar hypoventilation. Definitions of characteristic sleep abnormalities are outlined in Table 48-1.

SLEEP-DISORDERED BREATHING AND ABNORMALITIES OF RESPIRATORY CONTROL IN OBESITY

Alveolar hypoventilation is associated with obesity, but obesity alone does not necessarily lead to hypoventilation unless there are associated abnormalities of the respiratory center, respiratory muscles, or lungs.[2,6] Investigations have shown hypercapnic ventilatory drive to be decreased in some obese patients but normal in others,[35] and it seems likely that a combination of obesity, impaired neuromuscular function, and diminished respiratory center response to hypoxia or hypercapnia predetermine the development of severe hypoventilation.[9,35] Nevertheless, studies now

suggest that abnormal nocturnal respiration in obesity occurs more commonly than previously suspected.

Obese Men

Extremely obese men show a profound decrement in oxygen saturation during sleep ($> 15\%$) that is accompanied by sleep apnea, which is central or obstructive in origin (Fig. 48-1). In addition, obese men generally sleep less well than their lean counterparts. They commonly snore, and their sleep is disturbed by frequent waking. When normal-weight and obese men are examined together, increasing fatness (estimated by body mass index: weight in kilograms divided by height in m^2) is associated with a greater reduction in oxygen saturation independent of age.[19] Indeed, some obese men demonstrate saturation values as low as 65% during REM sleep (6.5 kpA) but have normal arterial blood gases when awake. On the other hand, obese hypogonadal men may not show nocturnal oxygen desaturation until they are treated with testosterone as replacement therapy, indicating a detrimental action of androgens on respiratory control.[31]

Obese Women

In obese women with regular menstrual cycles, episodes of hypoventilation but not apnea may occur during sleep, with a mean decrease in oxygen saturation of 7%. Normal-weight premenopausal women have normal nocturnal respiration.[16] After menopause, both nonobese and

TABLE 48-1

Definitions of the Different Types of Nocturnal Irregular Breathing Demonstrable During a Sleep Study

Significant nocturnal hypoventilation: decrease in oxygen saturation of more than 4% (as measured by an earlobe oximeter) during sleep

Sleep apnea: pause of airflow for more than 10 seconds

Obstructive apnea: characterized by increased respiratory effort with paradoxical collapse of the chest during inspiration, with no airflow as a result of obstruction at the pharynx or larynx

Central apnea: absence of airflow with no abdominal or chest movements

Mixed apnea: no chest movement early in the episode and unsuccessful movement later in the episode

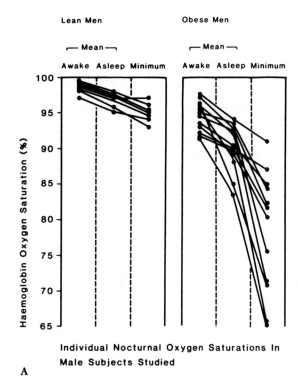

FIGURE 48-1

Individual nocturnal oxygen saturation values in obese men and women and normal-weight controls. **(A)** Results in men. **(B)** Results in postmenopausal women including obese, amenorrhoeic women with a documented hypothalamic-pituitary disorder.

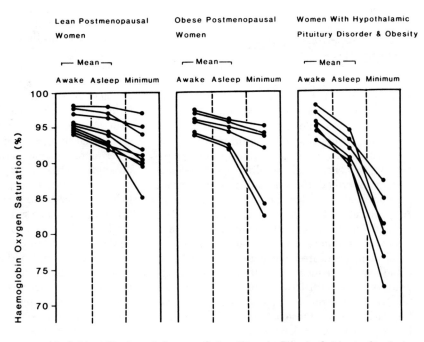

obese women show significant oxygen desaturation during sleep (mean decrease in oxygen saturation of 7%). This finding suggests that increasing age and plasma sex hormone concentrations in women are additionally important determinants of normal nocturnal respiration (see Fig. 48-1).[18] In support of this idea is the finding that obese women who are amenorrhoeic, have hypopituitarism, and are under 45 years of age show profound oxygen desaturation (> 15%) and frequent apneic episodes despite replacement treatment with hydrocortisone and thyroxine.

Investigation of obese and normal-weight men and women who display obstructive sleep apnea has shown that the obstruction occurs in the larynx and is associated with a loss of tone of the pharyngeal and glossal muscles, in particular the genioglossus muscle.[12] Relaxation of the genioglossus allows the base of the tongue to fall back against the posterior pharyngeal wall, occluding the pharynx. Not uncommonly, a central abnormality is associated with obstructive apnea and may be unmasked after treatment of the apnea by a permanent tracheostomy.[22] Thus, there exists a complex interaction between the respiratory centers and the effects of intermittent airways obstruction.

OBESITY-HYPOVENTILATION SYNDROME

In simple, uncomplicated obesity, the ventilation-perfusion disturbance in gas exchange is counteracted by augmented ventilation, which restores blood composition toward normal.

If transient hypercapnia should occur in persons with intrinsic weakness in respiratory muscles and low chest wall compliance, then (as previously described) the ventilatory response may be inadequate to restore blood gas composition. A universal finding in patients with OHS is a marked depression in both the hypercapnic and hypoxic respiratory drives,[9,25] accompanied by an abnormal and irregular pattern of breathing, usually with frequent and often prolonged apneic episodes (obstructive, central, or mixed pattern) occurring both during sleep and in the waking state.[9] Sleep in these patients is characterized by frequent awakening, which follows apneic episodes and is temporally related to the resump-

tion of effective breathing.[11] As the obesity worsens, so does the apnea, and with time, sleep deprivation presents as daytime hypersomnolence. Persistent hypoxia, if profound, blunts the hypoxic ventilatory drive. Evidence suggests that this situation creates a further vicious circle of events, with less and less responsiveness of the respiratory centers, pulmonary hypertension, and right-sided cardiac failure, the clinical manifestations of OHS.[27,34] Patients with OHS and sleep apnea show a remarkable improvement with weight loss. Apneic episodes become shorter, esophageal pressures required to overcome pharyngeal obstruction are reduced, the hypoxia becomes less profound, and the daytime somnolence improves or disappears.[13]

INVESTIGATION AND MANAGEMENT OF RESPIRATORY DISORDERS IN OBESITY

A diagnosis of sleep-disordered breathing can often be made from a history of sleeping habits taken from the patient or a close relative, but the symptoms frequently are nonspecific. Most patients who have central apnea are asymptomatic, but if the apneic episodes are frequent or prolonged, patients may frequently awaken in a panic attack, unaware that they were not breathing. In contrast, patients with obstructive sleep apnea characteristically snore loudly, have disturbed sleep, and experience daytime hypersomnolence. A relative usually can confirm these findings and may have observed episodes of obstruction during snoring; the snoring may be so severe that the spouse has begun sleeping in another room. In some patients, the history may be unhelpful. These patients, in whom significant hypoventilation is suspected, require admission to hospital for 24-hour monitoring of arterial oxygen saturation using an earlobe oximeter. Only rarely is it necessary to perform a complete sleep study with additional measurements of nasal airflow, chest and abdominal movements, and EMG, EEG, and eye movement recordings.[17] Nevertheless, the dangers of hypoxia are exacerbated by cigarette smoking, which should be the first problem to address in any overweight patient. The subsequent weight gain after stopping smoking is a lesser risk than its continuation.[26] In the

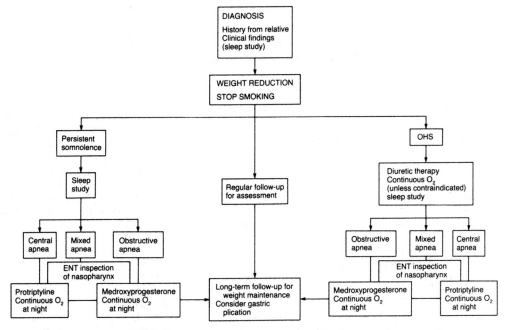

FIGURE 48-2

Flowchart for the management of an obese patient with nocturnal hypoventilation and sleep apnea.

majority of patients, weight loss is accompanied by a significant improvement in sleep, fewer periods of disordered breathing, and a reduction in the severity of oxygen desaturation.[13] An outline for treatment of sleep-disordered breathing is shown in Fig. 48-2. In patients with obstructive apnea, treatment is directed at removing any obstruction to the nasopharynx, such as adenoids or retropharyngeal masses, and alteration of sleep patterns. To obviate the need for a tracheostomy in some patients, a nasopharyngeal tube has been developed to deliver pressurized air into the pharynx, raising the intrapharyngeal pressure and reducing the number of sleep apneic episodes.[32] Drugs that alter the tone of the pharyngeal muscles, the respiratory drive, or the quantity and quality of sleep have been used with some success for patients with sleep apnea. Protriptyline reduces the amount of REM sleep and thereby restricts the amount of time during which obstruction may occur.[3] Medroxyprogesterone acts as a respiratory stimulant and may be

useful in patients with either central or obstructive sleep apnea. The response of patients to medroxyprogesterone is somewhat variable, and the 60 mg daily (in divided doses) that is usually required may occasionally result in undesirable fluid retention.[30]

CONCLUSION

Altered respiratory function in obesity results from a combination of mechanical impedance to breathing exerted by thoracic and abdominal fat and a ventilation-perfusion mismatch. Sleep-disordered breathing with periods of hypoventilation, with or without apneic episodes, may commonly occur in patients with extreme obesity. The ensuing nocturnal hypercapnia and hypoxia may lead to a decrease in ventilatory drive, abnormal central respiratory control, and in some obese persons the development of OHS. Respiratory abnormalities should be suspected in obese patients with a history of restlessness at night, loud snoring, and daytime somnolence. Treatment is substantial weight reduction, but short-term measures include the use of compressed air by way of nasal cannulas for obstructive apnea and drugs that alter sleep pattern or stimulate respiration.

Acknowledgment: I thank M. Apps for his enthusiastic help with the nocturnal respiratory studies and Beryl Winehouse for her secretarial assistance.

References

1. Barrera F, Hillyer P, Ascanio G et al: The distribution of ventilation, diffusion and blood flow in obese patients with normal and abnormal blood gases. Am Rev Respir Dis 108:819, 1973
2. Bedell GN, Wilson WR, Seebohm PM: Pulmonary function in obese persons. J Clin Invest 37:1049, 1958
3. Brownell LG, West P, Sweatman P et al: Protriptyline in obstructive sleep apnoea: A double blind trial. N Engl J Med 307:1037, 1982
4. Burwell CS, Robin ED, Whaley RD et al: Extreme obesity associated with alveolar hypoventilation: Pickwickian syndrome. Am J Med 21:81, 1956
5. Douglas NJ, Leggett RJE, Calverley PMA et al: Transient hypoxaemia during sleep in chronic bronchitis and emphysema. Lancet 1:1, 1979
6. Emirgil C, Sobol BJ: The effects of weight reduction on pulmonary function and the sensitivity of the respiratory centre in obesity. Am Rev Respir Dis 108:831, 1973
7. Farebrother MJB: Respiratory function and cardiorespiratory response to exercise in obesity. Br J Dis Chest 73:211, 1979
8. Fothergill J: A Complete Collection of the Medical and Philosophical Works of John Fothergill MD, FRS & SA, pp 525–527. Elliott J (ed). London, John Walker, 1781
9. Garay SM, Rapoport D, Sorkin B et al: Regulation of ventilation in the obstructive sleep apnea syndrome. Am Rev Respir Dis 124:451, 1981
10. Gothe B, Altose MD, Goldman MD et al: Effect of quiet sleep on resting and CO_2-stimulated breathing in humans. J Appl Physiol 50:724, 1981
11. Guilleminault C, Tilkian A, Dement WC: The sleep apnoea syndromes. Annu Rev Med 27:465, 1976
12. Guilleminault C, Hill MW, Simmons FB et al: Obstructive sleep apnoea: Electromyographic and fibreoptic studies. Exp Neurol 62:48, 1978
13. Harman EM, Wynne JW, Block AJ: The effect of weight loss on sleep-disordered breathing and oxygen desaturation in morbidly obese men. Chest 82:291, 1982
14. Holley MS, Milic-Emili J, Becklake MR et al: Regional distribution of pulmonary ventilation and perfusion in obesity. J Clin Invest 46:475, 1967
15. Kaufman BJ, Ferguson MH, Cherniack RM: Hypoventilation in obesity. J Clin Invest 38:500, 1959
16. Kopelman PG, Apps MCP, Cope T et al: Nocturnal hypoxia and prolactin secretion in obese women. Br Med J 287:859, 1983
17. Kopelman PG: Clinical complications of obesity. Clin Endocrinol Metab 13:613, 1984
18. Kopelman PG, Apps MCP, Cope T et al: The influence of menstrual status, body weight and hypothalamic function on nocturnal respiration in women. J R Coll Physicians Lond 19:243, 1985
19. Kopelman PG, Apps MCP, Cope T et al: Nocturnal hypoxia and sleep apnoea in asymptomatic obese men. Int J Obes 10:211, 1986
20. Lopata M, Onal E: Mass loading, sleep apnoea and the pathogenesis of obesity hypoventilation. Am Rev Respir Dis 126:640, 1982
21. Lourenco RV: Diaphragm activity in obesity. J Clin Invest 48:1609, 1969
22. Lugaresi E, Coccagna G, Mentovani M: Hypersomnia with periodic apnoeas. Jamaica, NY, Spectrum Publications, 1978
23. Naimark A, Cherniack RM: Compliance of the respiratory system and its components in health and obesity. J Appl Physiol 15:377, 1960
24. Phillipson EA: Control of breathing. Am Rev Respir Dis 118:909, 1978
25. Rochester DF, Enson Y: Current concepts in the pathogenesis of the obesity-hypoventilation syndrome: Mechanical and circulatory factors. Am J Med 57:402, 1974
26. Royal College of Physicians, London: Report on obesity. J R Coll Physicians 17:5, 1983
27. Sharpe JT, Barrocas M, Chokroverty S: The cardiorespiratory effects of obesity. Clin Chest Med 1:103, 1980
28. Sharpe JT, Henry JP, Sweany SK et al: Effects of mass loading on the respiratory system in man. J Appl Physiol 19:959, 1964
29. Sharpe JT, Henry JP, Sweany SK et al: The total work of breathing in normal and obese men. J Clin Invest 43:728, 1964
30. Strohl KP, Hensley MJ, Saunders NA et al: Progesterone and progressive sleep apnoeas. JAMA 245:1230, 1981
31. Stumpf IJ, Reynolds SF, Vash P et al: A possible relationship between testosterone, central control

of ventilation and the pickwickian syndrome. Am Rev Respir Dis (Suppl 2) 117:183, 1978

32. Sullivan CE, Issa FG, Berthon-Jones M et al: Reversal of obstructive sleep apnoea by continuous positive airway pressure applied through the nares. Lancet 1:862, 1981

33. Tucker DH, Sicker HO: The effect of change in body position on lung volumes and interpulmonary gas mixing in patients with obesity, heart fail-

ure and emphysema. Am Rev Respir Dis 82:787, 1960

34. Weil JV, Byrne-Quinn E, Sodal IE et al: Acquired attenuation of chemoreceptor function in chronically hypoxic man at high altitude. J Clin Invest 50:186, 1971

35. Zwillich CW, Sutton FD, Pierson DJ et al: Decreased hypoxic ventilatory drive in the obese-hypoventilation syndrome. Am J Med 59:343, 1975

PART EIGHT

HEALTH IMPAIRMENTS ASSOCIATED WITH ABDOMINAL DISTRIBUTION OF ADIPOSE TISSUE

CHAPTER 49

Regional Obesity

PER BJÖRNTORP

Recognition of the marked differences between adiposity localized to different parts of the body has clearly improved our understanding of the syndrome of human obesity, which is a heterogenous group of conditions with wide variations in risk for complicating diseases. This field has been the subject of several symposia that have been published.[1-4]

In this summary of findings, reference is mainly given to these and other reviews in which further detailed information and references are found.

BACKGROUND

The knowledge of differences in risk with various types of obesity is old and described in the history of royal families in which the stout, choleric, pyknic type of person is known to be prone to sudden death, stroke, and gout. Another historical note is found in Shakespeare's *Julius Caesar*, in which a sleek-headed, socially well-adapted obese person is described, showing the other, more benign type of obesity. Anthropometrists in the 1920s described body types in systematized studies in which not only adipose tissue distribution but other bodily characteristics were associated with disease. Vague[5] is the founder of research focusing on adipose tissue distribution, described in great detail, with correlations with disease. Vague's system also has a component of muscle tissue mass. In the decades that followed, this phenomenon was described by a number of laboratories but had not attracted much attention until the 1980s.

EPIDEMIOLOGY

The renewed interest in this field seems to have arisen from population studies in which large materials cross-sectional observations seemed to clearly point out the hazards of abdominal male-type obesity, whereas gluteofemoral female-type obesity seemed to be more benign. In prospective studies, this observation could be demonstrated in a more conclusive way. Abdominal obesity, or localization of an increased proportion of body fat to abdominal regions, has been found to be an independent risk factor for myocardial infarction, angina pectoris, stroke, and non–insulin-dependent diabetes mellitus (NIDDM). It increases the risk of premature mortality in both men and women. Preliminary data also suggest an association with carcinoma in women. Statistical correlations have been found between abdominal obesity and most of the established other risk factors for these diseases. (For further review of epidemiologic studies, see reference 6.)

An analysis of two population studies in Gothenburg, Sweden, including both men and women, has shown that the well-known difference in incidence of myocardial infarction between the sexes disappears when the sex-linked difference in the waist:hip circumference (W:H) ratio is adjusted for.[7] This finding probably means that either the W:H ratio is closely linked to a sex-related factor associated with myocardial infarction or that a component of the W:H ratio is actually causing myocardial infarction, perhaps through a generation of risk factors triggering the disease.[8] This observation illustrates the fundamental importance of the W:H ratio in the association with myocardial infarction.

CLINICAL CHARACTERISTICS

Abdominal obesity is a typical male characteristic. Men seem to have two to three times more visceral fat than women, whether obese or not.[9] Men and women with an enlarged proportion of abdominal fat often have hypertension; elevated concentrations of blood glucose, plasma insulin, and very low density lipoproteins (VLDL); and low concentrations of high-density lipoproteins (HDL). They smoke more and use more alcoholic beverages than average. Interestingly, men and women with this type of fat distribution also often have socioeconomic disadvantages, psychosomatic diseases, and psychological and psychiatric problems, including depressive and anxiety states. Endocrine abnormalities are also often found, including low testosterone in men and lack of ovulation in women, who are often hyperandrogenic. Indications of increased secretion of cortisol are also noted, although these reports so far are inconsistent. Taken together, the endocrinologic aberrations suggest a dominance of the hypophysis-adrenal cortex axis and a disturbed or low activity in the gonadotropic-gonadal axis. There may well be other disturbances of similar character, including hyperactivity of the hypothalamic-sympathetic nervous system axis, although this is not well established. Observations also suggest low thyroid-stimulating hormone values with normal thyroid hormone concentrations (unpublished). It should be noted that many of these endocrine abnormalities follow alcohol consumption, smoking, and some of the psychological-psychiatric conditions mentioned.

In contrast, gluteofemoral obesity is associated with fewer problems. Hyperinsulinemia and deranged glucose tolerance are less pronounced. Hypertension is found but seems to be followed less frequently by vascular catastrophes in vital organs than when present in persons with abdominal obesity. Specific abnormalities that accompany this syndrome seem to be varicose veins and problems in the weight-carrying joints. In terms of sociopsychological variables, the picture is totally different from that noted in abdominal obesity. Both men and women who are obese but who do not have prominent abdominal localization of excess body fat seem robust. They are less susceptible to alcohol problems and smoke less often than average. The endocrine pattern of steroid hormones seems to be normal. This syndrome seems to be an expression only of a positive energy balance, with excess fat deposited harmonically in proportion to a normal adipose tissue distribution. The typical female depot in the gluteofemoral region has been suggested to be a reserve depot for the augmented needs of childbearing and lactation, and an enlargement of this depot might thus be an expression of a physiological phenomenon. (For a more detailed review of this field and references, see references 6, 10-12.)

Taken together, these observations suggest that obesity with abdominal fat distribution is a more hazardous type of obesity. It should be noted that the epidemiologic observations here have been based on anthropometric measurements, mainly the W:H ratio. In cross-sectional studies, however, it has been shown repeatedly that the crucial factor seems to be the amount of visceral fat, which is strongly associated with the risk factors for the diseases in question. (For review, see references 8, 11, 12.) It should be noted, however, that several observations show or suggest that a small hip circumference is also contributing to a high W:H ratio. Either the skeletal frame or, more likely, the muscle girth of the pelvic region, mainly the gluteal muscles, might be a factor. It has been shown in men[13,14] that this anatomy specifically correlates with alcohol consumption.[15] Hip size is of particular interest in terms of regulation of insulin sensitivity, in which muscle tissue is a major contributor. Qualitative muscle changes have also been demonstrated, suggesting involvement of muscle tissue in the marked insulin resistance in persons with a high W:H ratio.[11]

REGULATION OF REGIONAL DEPOT FAT ACCUMULATION

With some simplification, it thus seems that visceral depot fat is the adipose tissue of main interest in abdominal obesity whereas the gluteofemoral adipose tissue is the major adipose tissue in peripheral, benign obesity. Functionally these depots are quite different. Visceral fat seems to have a much more rapid turnover than the sluggish gluteofemoral fat depot. The subcutaneous abdominal, mammary, and retroperitoneal adipose tissues seem to have an intermediary position in this respect. (For review, see reference 16.)

Examining the regulation of the metabolism of the adipocytes in these regions may allow elucidation of the mechanisms involved in excess accumulation of fat in one or the other of these depots. Such studies have therefore attracted considerable interest and are reviewed briefly here. The information is still far from complete, but some key observations deserve mention.

The gluteofemoral depot is characterized mainly by a sluggish lipid mobilization in both men and women. The depot is larger in women. During late pregnancy and lactation, changes take place to allow an excess of this triglyceride for mobilization and utilization. The lipid uptake seems to be slower also. In other words, the turnover of this fat is apparently rather slow under ordinary conditions. The factors regulating lipid mobilization here are largely unknown. The main regulating enzyme for lipid uptake, lipoprotein lipase (LPL), seems to be dependent on cortisol and female sex steroid hormones, particularly progesterone. There is an apparent absence of specific receptors for the sex steroid hormones in human adipose tissue. Therefore, it is speculated that interactions with the glucocorticoid activity by way of the glucocorticoid receptor, present in abundance, may be likely, and it may well be that progesterone enhances LPL activity through this receptor.

The reason for accumulation of fat in gluteofemoral obesity then may only be a normal traffic of circulating lipid, trapped in these regions by high LPL activity and slow lipid mobilization, all normally regulated.

Several discrete intra-abdominal adipose tissues exist. The visceral fat depots of specific interest here seem to be those drained by the portal vein (portal adipose tissues), the mesenteric and omental adipose tissues. Both are highly sensitive to lipolytic stimuli, apparently with an exception in normal women. Lipid uptake also

seems to be high, suggesting a rapid turnover of this fat. Regulation of these processes is most likely also occurring by means of an interaction between cortisol and the sex steroid hormones, a statement based on the following observations. The density of glucocorticoid receptors seems to be particularly high in these adipose tissue depots, subjecting them to more pronounced cortisol effects than other adipose tissues. Presumably, this density would induce more LPL activity here, explaining a high lipid uptake. The interactions by the sex steroid hormones here are unclear. Testosterone effects might, however, *a priori* be suspected to be of importance because the abdomen is a typical male depot. Androgen receptors are present, but the relative density is so far unknown. Testosterone seems to inhibit LPL activity induced by cortisol, but apparently not through competition at the hormonal receptor level, and might instead be regulated at the level of the gene expression of LPL activity.

The regulation of lipid mobilization is also only partially known. Testosterone causes an expression of β-adrenergic receptors, found in abundance in male portal adipose tissue. Cortisol also seems to be lipolytically active. Again, the interactions of these hormones are not occurring at the receptor level but may well be found at later steps of interactions, such as when the receptor-hormone complexes interact with the gene for the expression of β-adrenergic receptors, in this case apparently causing an amplification of the basic glucocorticoid signal. Again, this is mainly speculation. The interactions, if any, of the female sex hormones at this level are so far unknown.

What mechanisms then would promote accumulation of depot fat in visceral adipose tissue? In principle, this would occur by either stimulation of the uptake mechanisms, inhibition of the lipolytic mechanisms, or both in combination. Stimulation of LPL by the high density of glucocorticoid receptors seems to be a likely mechanism; high cortisol secretion then would be expected to be followed by visceral lipid accumulation. This response is also noted in Cushing's syndrome and might be a consequence of the potentially elevated cortisol secretion in abdominal obesity. Low testosterone secretion would also give this final result because of a smaller than normal lipid mobilization potential. Low testosterone values have indeed been observed in abdominally obese men. This might in addition release a relative inhibition of the cortisol-induced LPL induction. As mentioned earlier, women with abdominal obesity often do not ovulate and therefore secrete abnormally small amounts of progesterone. The effects of progesterone on the regulation of the metabolism of visceral adipocytes are not known. It should be noted, however, that a lack of progesterone effects on the gluteofemoral adipocytes might mean a passive, compensatory accumulation of excess lipid in all depots, including visceral fat depots.

These attempts at synthesis of available incomplete data might serve as a working hypothesis for further studies (Fig. 49-1). (For a detailed review and references, see references 16, 17.)

Taken together, these data suggest different populations of adipocytes in different regions of human adipose tissue. The principal differences in characteristics might well be found in the expression of different densities of steroid hormone receptors, as exemplified by the high density of glucocorticoid receptors in visceral adipose tissue. The high density of β-adrenergic receptors in these tissues might be expressed by cortisol action or might be a consequence of a putative high density of androgen receptors. Steroid hormone interactions may also well be different in adipocytes from different regions. For example, interactions between cortisol and progesterone at the level of the glucocorticoid receptor might vary. It is also an interesting possibility that certain of these hormones may interact at the genomic level. Particularly strong candidates for such synergistic or antagonistic effects are cortisol and testosterone, as mentioned earlier. Also, such interactions might be regionally specific. In short, various adipocytes may well be genetically different in expressing steroid hormone receptors or in the synergistic-antagonistic receptor hormone complex interactions. If this is so, then adipose tissue becomes an organ with a varying population of different cells, such as muscle tissue and brain, for example. The genetic predisposition to different types of fat distribution and obesity may well be at least partly found at this level. Molecular genetics may thus be a fruitful field for studies of these problems.

MECHANISMS FOR THE ASSOCIATIONS BETWEEN ABDOMINAL OBESITY AND DISEASE

In principle, abdominal obesity might be a causative factor in the statistically associated diseases or might be a parallel phenomenon. Both these alternatives are discussed next.

Direct Cause-and-Effect Relationship

As mentioned earlier, visceral fat is most probably the critical part of adipose tissue enlargement. The specific function of this adipose tissue may well be considered to be the direct cause of the abnormalities and diseases associated with abdominal obesity, as considered first here.

As mentioned previously, portal adipose tissue is highly sensitive to stimulation of lipid mobilization, particularly in abdominal obesity in men and women. This fact in combination with the increased mass of these adipose tissues in abdominal obesity most likely results in large elevations of free fatty acid (FFA) concentrations in the portal vein. Several consequences may then follow.

A first metabolic consequence is stimulation of gluconeogenesis. This has been shown to occur in several experimental systems including iso-

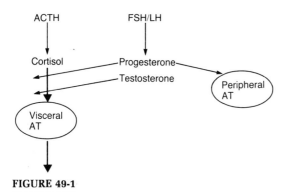

FIGURE 49-1

The interactions of steroid hormones to direct excess fat for storage in different adipose tissue regions. (Visceral AT, visceral adipose tissue; Peripheral AT, peripheral adipose tissue; FSH, follicle-stimulating hormone; LH, luteinizing hormone)

lated hepatocytes in intact rats and humans, and the mechanisms at the enzyme level have been described. Fatty acid oxidation seems to be a prerequisite for this stimulation.

Portal FFA stimulates the secretion of VLDL from the liver. This stimulation seems to occur by means of delivery of triglyceride to an assembly site of the VLDL in the liver, where the other VLDL constituents, including the protein moitey, apo B-100, are present in excess. Therefore, the concentrations of FFA determine the synthesis and secretion of VLDL, as well as apo B-100. Low-density lipoproteins (LDL) are a product of VLDL through triglyceride removal; therefore, increased VLDL production implies an increased risk for retention also of LDL in the circulation.

Finally FFA may well interact with hepatic clearance of insulin. Insulin is produced by the pancreatic beta cells and secreted into the portal vein. A large part is then directly taken up by the liver. It is known that this hepatic clearance of insulin is diminished in obesity, particularly with abdominal localization. In isolated liver cells, fatty acids in physiologic concentrations cause a decreased binding, degradation, and effect of insulin. These effects seem to be dependent on fatty acid oxidation. In the perfused rat liver, fatty acids seem to have similar effects. Livers from overfed rats, with elevated portal FFA concentrations and increased liver triglyceride contents, also clear insulin in an abnormally inefficient way. It thus seems that the decreased liver clearance of insulin in abdominal obesity might be an additional effect of portal FFA. The consequence would be peripheral hyperinsulinemia, which is further amplified by increased insulin production, known to occur in obesity in general. (For review, see reference 8.)

The consequences of the effects on liver metabolism of portal FFA would then be, in summary, that gluconeogenesis is triggered and insulin shunted away from the liver, both apparently consequences of fatty acid oxidation. Excess fatty acids are then secreted from the liver as VLDL. This may well be a physiological regulatory mechanism of importance when absorbtive metabolism is shifted to postabsorbtive, at which point fatty acids are mobilized for energy purposes. In this situation, liver gluconeogenesis is needed for brain metabolism. The lipolytically

sensitive portal adipose depots will presumably mobilize FFA into the portal vein early in the postabsorbtive phase and might then be an important regulatory mechanism to trigger hepatic gluconeogenesis. Insulin would counteract hepatic glucose production, and it is therefore meaningful that insulin is removed from the scene by the same mechanism that starts gluconeogenesis—namely, fatty acid oxidation.[8,18]

Although probably a useful regulatory mechanism under physiological conditions, it is apparent that the consequences of increased FFA mobilization into the portal circulation might be exaggerated, particularly in visceral obesity. Glucose and VLDL production would increase and insulin clearance decrease, with a resulting risk of hyperglycemia, hyperlipidemia, and hyperinsulinemia. These are all established risk factors for cardiovascular disease, stroke, and NIDDM. Information now also suggests that hyperinsulinemia produces hypertension, another strong risk factor for the diseases mentioned.

In summary, then, there is now evidence that the increased mass of portal adipose tissue in abdominal obesity may, through increased concentrations of portal FFA, generate most of the established risk factors for cardiovascular disease, stroke, and NIDDM. If this is correct, then there would be a direct cause-and-effect relationship between increased visceral fat masses in abdominal obesity and the diseases for which abdominal obesity is a risk factor in prospective studies. (For a more detailed review and references, see references 8, 18.)

Parallel Phenomenon to a Disease-Causing Factor

A central phenomenon in abdominal obesity is insulin resistance. When the cause of this insulin resistance is elucidated, then many of the secrets of the pathogenesis of the complications of abdominal obesity will be known. This possibility is considered next.

Insulin resistance is found in most insulin-responsive tissues in obese persons. A major tissue determining total body insulin sensitivity is muscle. Therefore, the cause of insulin resistance in muscle is of considerable interest.

In addition to severe insulin resistance in muscle, abdominal obesity is characterized by a specific muscle morphology with a diminished number of type 1, slow-twitch, insulin-sensitive fibers and an increase in type 2, fast-twitch, less insulin-sensitive fibers.

The insulin sensitivity of these muscle fibers in a steady-state, resting situation is probably determined by the number of insulin receptors, which is higher in type 1 than type 2 fibers. This is, however, unlikely to be the only factor determining insulin sensitivity of muscles. Capillary density has been repeatedly shown to be inversely correlated with insulin sensitivity in obesity, particularly of the abdominal type. This is also the case in individual muscles in insulin-resistant rats. Studies now indicate that it is not only the capillary density but actually capillary blood flow that is associated with insulin sensitivity. Kinetic studies suggest that insulin is bound to capillary endothelium, which acts as an intermediary reservoir for the diffusion of insulin out to its active site on the muscle cells. Low capillary blood flow then results in a smaller reservoir of insulin and therefore perhaps is followed by less insulin action, observed as insulin insensitivity of muscle with low capillary blood flow.

One might then ask why muscle in abdominal obesity has a low degree of capillarization and a preponderance of less insulin-sensitive muscle fibers. Muscle fiber composition has been suggested to be to a large extent genetically determined, but environmental factors clearly have an at least equally important role. For example, physical training is known to shift muscle morphology toward a picture with more capillarization and more insulin-sensitive type 1 muscle fibers. In ordinary training programs, this change is not very impressive, but in extreme cases of maximal recruitment of fibers versus total inactivity, type 1 fibers have been shown to vary in proportion from almost 100% to absence, respectively.

The endocrine status is of major importance here also. Administration of corticosteroids or endogenous overproduction of cortisol as in Cushing's syndrome is associated with a low number of insulin-sensitive muscle fibers. Sex steroids are also of importance. Estrogen seems to diminish muscle fiber diameter and increase the number of insulin-sensitive fibers, a typical female characteristic. Testosterone clearly has the opposite effect. Administration of testosterone in moderate doses to female rats is followed by dramatic insulin resistance in the total animal, caused by insulin resistance in muscle, which changes to fewer type 1 fibers and less capillarization. (For review of this topic and references, see references 11, 19.)

These endocrine modifications are of interest in abdominal obesity, when increased secretion of cortisol and, in women, of testosterone probably is an established abnormality (see above). The question is then whether the endocrine aberrations in steroid hormone secretion might be the cause of muscular insulin resistance in abdominal obesity. In women, cortisol plus testosterone would be responsible, whereas in men, only cortisol hypersecretion might be a causative factor because abdominally obese men have lower testosterone concentration than normal (see above).

The next question is, How do these endocrine aberrations change muscle insulin sensitivity and morphology? At first glance it would seem most plausible to believe that cortisol or, in women, testosterone changes muscle fiber composition and capillarization so that less insulin-responsive tissue is developing. This seems not to be the case, however. It is well known that cortisol has an immediate (hours to days) effect on insulin sensitivity in various tissues, including muscle. This also seems to be the case with testosterone, which produces marked insulin resistance, localized primarily in muscle, after only 2 days of administration, before muscle morphology has changed (Holmäng et al, unpublished). This observation then suggests that insulin resistance is a primary feature whereas the morphology changes might be secondary.

After considering these observations, it seems possible that the insulin resistance in abdominal obesity is primary to the endocrine aberration(s) and, in analogy with the rat experiments referred to earlier, that the muscle morphology changes are secondary. As suggested previously, the distribution of fat primarily to the abdominal regions might also be a consequence of the endocrine aberration, which then becomes a primary factor for the whole syndrome of abdominal obesity. This is depicted schematically in Figure 49-2.

A remaining problem is to try to understand

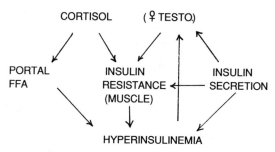

FIGURE 49-2

Interactions between steroid hormones and portal FFA on insulin homeostasis.

how the increased testosterone secretion is brought about in women with abdominal obesity. There is evidence that hyperinsulinemia might act as a gonadotropic factor, causing increased testosterone secretion.[20] This then would mean a vicious cycle with hyperinsulinemia, insulin resistance, and testosterone secretion as participants.

Peripheral FFA concentrations have been reported to be elevated in abdominal obesity, being most pronounced in the late night and early morning.[21] Also, at normal FFA concentrations, the turnover rate has been reported to be ele-

vated.[22] The consequence of such aberrations would also be expected to cause insulin resistance in muscle, according to the so-called Randle's hypothesis.[23]

Attempt at a Synthesis of Pathogenetic Factors

It thus seems apparent that most of the abnormalities in anthropometry, adipose tissue, muscle and liver metabolism, as well as the secondary consequences of these aberrations in central energy metabolism with associated risk for disease, might possibly be explained by the endocrine perturbations. These then seem to be an increased secretion of cortisol in combination with abnormalities in other hypothalamic-pituitary axes, including low sex steroid hormone secretions, increased central sympathetic nervous system activity, and possibly a poorly defined aberration in the thyroid axis, as mentioned earlier.

The background for these aberrations in turn might be a combination of factors in an arousal syndrome caused by factors such as stress, alcohol ingestion, and smoking. The role of these factors in the pathogenesis of the consequences of abdominal obesity, cardiovascular disease,

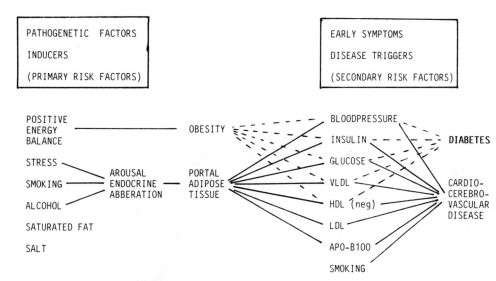

FIGURE 49-3

Hypothetical scheme of the role of primary and secondary risk factors in the pathogenesis of cardiovascular disease, stroke, and diabetes. (Björntorp P: "Portal" adipose tissue as a generator of risk factors for cardiovascular disease and diabetes. Arteriosclerosis [in press])

stroke, and NIDDM is not clear. Smoking is of course a well-known strong risk factor for cardiovascular disease and might have direct effects on the vascular endothelium. Stress and alcohol are less well established factors, however, and reports suggesting their importance have competed with investigations showing no associations. One might consider the situation as depicted schematically in Figure 49-3. Primary risk factors might generate secondary risk factors, which in turn might act as direct triggers at the diseased locus, such as the arterial wall. These risk factors are well established and are consistently found just because of their proximity to their consequences. The primary factors are, in contrast, more "distant" from the disease process and might therefore more easily be confounded by various other factors. These viewpoints have now been developed in more detail.[8] Such primary risk factors might be mediated or paralleled by abdominal obesity. This possibility should generate more studies along these lines.

References

1. Vague J, Björntorp P, Guy-Grand B et al (eds): Metabolic Complications of Human Obesities. Amsterdam, Elsevier Science Publishers, 1985
2. Björntorp P, Smith U, Lönnroth P (eds): Health Implications of Regional Obesities. Stockholm, Almqvist & Wiksell, 1988
3. Bouchard C, Johnson FE (eds): Fat Distribution During Growth and Later Health Outcomes. New York, Alan R Liss, 1988
4. Bouchard C, Bray GA, Hubbard VS: Basic and clinical aspects of regional fat distribution. Am J Clin Nutr 52:946, 1990
5. Vague J: La différenciation sexuelle, facteur déterminant des formes de l'obésité. Presse Méd 30:339, 1947
6. Björntorp P: The associations between obesity, adipose tissue distribution and disease. Acta Med Scand (Suppl) 723:121, 1988
7. Larsson B, Lapidus L, Bengtsson C et al: Is body fat distribution a main explanation for the male/female difference in the risk of myocardial infarction? Am J Epid (in press)
8. Björntorp P: "Portal" adipose tissue as a generator of risk factors for cardiovascular disease and diabetes. Arteriosclerosis 10:493, 1990
9. Kvist H, Chowdhury G, Grangård U et al: Predictive equations of total and visceral adipose tissue volumes derived from measurements with computed tomography in adult men and women. Am J Clin Nutr 48:1351, 1988
10. Björntorp P: Possible mechanisms relating fat distribution and metabolism. In Bouchard C, Johnson FE (eds): Fat Distribution During Growth and Later Health Outcomes, pp 175–191. New York, Alan R Liss, 1988
11. Björntorp P: Abdominal obesity and the development of noninsulin-dependent diabetes mellitus. Diabetes Metab Rev 4:6:615, 1988
12. Kissebah AH, Peiris AN: Biology of regional body fat distribution: Relationship to non-insulin dependent diabetes mellitus. Diabetes Metab Rev 5: 83, 1989
13. Larsson B, Seidell J, Svärdsudd K et al: Obesity, adipose tissue distribution and health in men: The study of men born in 1913. Appetite 13:37, 1989
14. Seidell J, Björntorp P, Sjöström L et al: Regional distribution of muscle and fat mass in men: New insight into the risk of abdominal obesity using computed tomography. Int J Obes 13:289, 1989
15. Pettersson P, Hallgren P, Sjöberg C et al: Muscle and adipose tissue mass and distribution in alcoholic men. (in press)
16. Rebuffé-Scrive M, Björntorp P: Regional adipose tissue metabolism in man. In Vague J et al (eds): Metabolic Complications of Human Obesities, pp 149–159. Amsterdam, Elsevier Science Publishers, 1985
17. Björntorp P, Ottosson M, Rebuffé-Scrive M et al: Regional obesity and steroid hormone interactions in human adipose tissue. In Bray G, Ricquier D, Spiegelman B (eds): Obesity: Towards a Molecular Approach" UCLA Symposia. New York, Alan R Liss, 1990
18. Björntorp P: Abdominal obesity and risk. Clinical and Experimental Hypertension. A12:783, 1990
19. Holmäng A, Svedberg J, Jennische E et al: The effects of testosterone on muscle insulin sensitivity and morphology of female rats. Am J Physiol E555, 1990
20. Poretsky L, Carlin MF: The gonadotropic function of insulin. Endocrinol Rev 8:132, 1987
21. Kissebah AH, Evans DJ, Peiris A et al: Endocrine characteristics in regional obesities: Role of sex steroids. In Vague J, Björntorp P, Guy-Grand B et al (eds): Metabolic Complications of Human Obesities, pp 115–130. Amsterdam, Elsevier Science Publishers, 1985
22. Jensen MD, Haymond MW, Rizza RA et al: Influence of body fat distribution on free fatty acid metabolism in obesity. J Clin Invest 83:1168, 1989
23. Randle PJ, Garland PB, Hales CN et al: The glucose fatty acid cycle: Its role in insulin sensitivity and the metabolic disturbances of diabetes mellitus. Lancet 1:785, 1963

PART NINE

SPECIAL FORMS OF OBESITY

CHAPTER 50

Genetic Syndromes

WILLIAM H. DIETZ

PRADER-WILLI SYNDROME

The Prader-Labhart-Willi syndrome was first described in Germany in 1956.[1] As originally described, the syndrome consisted of obesity, short stature, hypogonadism, mental retardation, and a history of hypotonia and failure to thrive in infancy. The syndrome, now more commonly known as Prader-Willi syndrome, is associated with a partial deletion of the long arm of chromosome 15 (q11–13).[2-4] The syndrome occurs with a prevalence of approximately one per 5000 to 10,000 live births[5,6] and has occasionally been described in siblings[7] and twins.[2]

More recent information indicates that the deletion is not specific for Prader-Willi syndrome but has also been found in the Angelman syndrome and the Williams syndrome.[8] Hypotonia, infant feeding difficulties, and developmental delay are common to all of these syndromes, but obesity appears limited to patients with Prader-Willi syndrome. Not all patients with clinical Prader-Willi syndrome have the characteristic chromosomal deletion. However, those who have the deletion do not differ in any significant way from those without this finding.

Growth, Development, and Behavior

The early history of patients with the syndrome is characteristic. Infants are born at term, usually following an uncomplicated pregnancy in which mothers may report reduced fetal activity. Approximately 40% have a breech presentation, and

20% have a birth weight of less than 5 pounds.[9] At birth, affected infants are markedly hypotonic and suck so poorly that gavage, nasogastric, or gastrostomy feeding may be required.

In the first and second years of life, both major and minor motor milestones are delayed. Hypotonia gradually improves near the end of the first year of life. However, sitting is delayed until 12 months and walking until 30 months.[4,9] Speech may not occur until well after the second birthday, and often children are unable to speak in short sentences until 42 months of age.[9] Mental retardation is commonplace, but some patients may have normal intelligence.[10,11]

Because of the hypotonia and poor suck, feeding and failure to thrive in infancy pose major difficulties for parents and pediatricians. However, after age two or three years, affected children commonly develop a ravenous appetite and a variety of food-seeking behaviors. These may include eating out of the garbage bin, eating the dog's food, or foraging in the refrigerator at night when other family members are asleep. Before the diagnosis was widely recognized, a family with a lock on the refrigerator typically had a child with Prader-Willi syndrome. This practice was and often still is the inevitable result of a protracted, losing battle with the child over the control of food intake.

Behavioral problems, particularly stubbornness and impulsivity, are the most intractable problems for patients with Prader-Willi syndrome and their families.[11] Children and more often adolescents will often act impulsively, occasionally in destructive or aggressive ways. Disagreements about rules frequently provoke confrontations. Affected children doggedly pursue their goals, continue to voice their requests, or refuse distraction, long after other children have moved onto other concerns. If they are unsuccessful in their quest, they may have a major temper tantrum that requires considerable restraint. Because many of these children are both short and obese, containing their tantrums requires considerable effort.

Self-mutilation is another persistent difficulty that occurs in a majority of patients[11] and may reflect an insensitivity to pain. Patients may pick repeatedly at small skin lesions until they bleed, and continue to do so despite every effort to convince them to stop. This behavior appears to be cyclic and rarely correlates with any obvious alteration in either mood or environment.

Food-Seeking Behaviors

The persistence and resourcefulness of patients with Prader-Willi syndrome in their search to obtain food is deservedly legendary. Although the characteristic is not universal, many patients with Prader-Willi syndrome are obsessed with food. Even in residential settings, where access to food is restricted, eating is a major preoccupation. The level of caloric intake is a constant subject of discussion and debate. Exercise programs that allow for some flexibility in dietary intake are avidly pursued, and many residential institutions find it necessary to introduce programs of food restriction, fixed to weight goals, that are implemented following weekend passes to settings like the home, where access to food is less carefully regulated.

Clinical Findings

The major characteristics of the Prader-Willi syndrome are short stature, obesity, hypogonadism, and mild to moderate mental retardation. Affected patients are usually below the fifth percentile for height.[12] Obesity has its onset in early childhood and may be severe. Frequently, untreated patients are in excess of 200% of their ideal body weight. The body fat is centrally distributed but ends abruptly at the wrist and ankle,

and may account for the prevalence of type II diabetes mellitus in 20% of patients.[11,12] Obesity has also been linked to the age-related decline in intelligence in patients with the syndrome,[13] although the mechanism by which this effect is mediated is unclear. The respiratory complications of obesity, such as pickwickian syndrome, that may accompany Prader-Willi syndrome are reportedly responsible for a mortality of 30% by the third decade of life.[14]

Few female patients have regular menstrual cycles, and those that do probably have anovulatory cycles. Pregnancy is rare.[6] Cryptorchidism occurs in over 80% of males; the testicles, when present, are infantile.[6,11] The penis is also infantile in size and is often obscured by the prepubertal fat pad. Both sexes may develop pubic hair, but in general, secondary sexual characteristics are lacking. Although patients are characteristically viewed as retarded, they are clearly trainable, and many are capable of holding a job in a tightly structured setting.

The syndrome is also accompanied by a variety of minor characteristics.[6,9,10] These include a narrow bifrontal diameter, a bow-shaped mouth, almond-shaped eyes, and small hands and feet. Scoliosis is found in over 50% and may have its onset in early childhood.[15] Approximately 40% of patients have strabismus.[9] Impaired development of tooth enamel occurs in 10% of patients. Speech is delayed, and impaired articulation makes speech difficult to understand.

Although the hypogonadism, hypotonia, mental retardation, and persistent food-seeking behaviors suggest that the syndrome is associated with abnormalities of the central nervous system, particularly the hypothalamus, autopsy data have failed to reveal any abnormalities.[7,12]

Body Composition and Energy Metabolism

Although many of the characteristics of Prader-Willi syndrome are consistent with a hypothalamic origin, the apparent genetic origin of obesity makes studies of body composition and energy metabolism of considerable interest. Patients with Prader-Willi syndrome appear to have a fat-free mass that is considerably lower than that expected for age- and sex-matched controls.[16,17] Such reductions may in part account for the reduced in utero activity and for the hypotonia present at birth.

Both basal metabolic rate (BMR) and total daily energy expenditure (TEE) of subjects with Prader-Willi syndrome are reduced.[17] The low metabolic rate is consistent with the reduction in fat-free mass, but when expressed per kg of fat-free mass, metabolic rate does not appear to differ substantially from control values. The reduction in TEE reflects the reduction in BMR. The energy spent on activity appears significantly lower than that observed in controls.[17] Other observations, based on measurements obtained with actometers and pedometers, have failed to demonstrate differences in activity,[18] suggesting that the energy associated with movement may be lower in patients with the syndrome.

These data, in conjunction with the behavioral data reviewed above, suggest that the genesis of obesity probably involves central regulatory mechanisms controlling food intake rather than alterations in one or more components of energy expenditure.

Treatment

Because of the diversity of physical, developmental, and behavioral abnormalities that occur in Prader-Willi syndrome, treatment entails a multidisciplinary approach. Here we will focus on the treatment of feeding difficulties and the prevention and treatment of obesity. Therapeutic approaches to other problems have been extensively reviewed elsewhere.[5,6,19]

In infancy, the feeding difficulties that accompany the syndrome often require aggressive interventions, such as gavage feeding, nasogastric intubation, or the early use of a gastrostomy. Continued efforts are required to promote oral intake, regardless of the approach that is elected, in order to maintain the oral reflexes necessary to a successful transition from enteral to oral intake. The gradual resolution of hypotonia near the end of the first year of life makes the transition to oral intake possible.

As the child begins to develop autonomous

feeding behavior, the introduction of controls on meal content, size, and the frequency of snacks becomes essential to prevent the development of obesity. Such measures usually avert the use of low-fat diets, which should be avoided until after the second year of life. Our experience suggests that a concrete plan that offers few choices is the most effective approach to limiting the conflicts that arise over feeding. Anticipation of the potential for variations that exist in visits to family or friends and attention to diet at school may reduce the likelihood of binges when parental attention is directed elsewhere and may help avoid the circumstances that precipitate a tantrum.

Although control of obesity is clearly necessary to limit the potential developmental, metabolic, and respiratory consequences of Prader-Willi syndrome, the problems that preoccupy parents in the first decade of life are primarily behavioral rather than food-related. Early recognition of the syndrome makes possible referral to early intervention programs that can assist parents with early feeding and treatment of hypotonia. Such programs also offer speech therapy, which may be necessary to improve articulation.

Several reports have emphasized the effectiveness of the protein-sparing modified fast in the treatment of established obesity.[16,20] Although such diets are clearly effective in weight reduction for this population, the use of ketones to monitor adherence and the limited choices available may be more important to success than the composition of the diet.

The role of surgery remains controversial. Although at least one report has recommended gastric bypass surgery,[21] few five-year follow-up data are available. Of the three patients on whom we have performed gastric bypass surgery, all three returned to their preoperative weights within three years of the operation, despite substantial losses immediately after the operation. Weight regain and the need for operative revisions have also been noted in other published reports.[21] Because of these observations, we no longer recommend bypass surgery for the treatment of obesity.

In our experience, the optimum setting for long-term weight reduction and management is a residential setting. Weight and dietary intake can be rigorously monitored and controlled. Additional advantages of this setting are that parents are relieved of the constant and tedious task of dietary oversight and the behavioral difficulties that attend the syndrome. Patients are generally relieved by being in a setting where they can live in relative autonomy with others who share their problems.

BARDET-BIEDL SYNDROME

The Bardet-Biedl syndrome, formerly known as the Laurence-Moon-Bardet-Biedl syndrome, is characterized by mental retardation, pigmentary retinopathy, polydactyly, obesity, and hypogenitalism.[22-24] Patients with the Laurence-Moon syndrome appear to differ because they lack polydactyly and obesity, but are paraplegic.[24] The disorder appears to occur with a prevalence of one per 17,500 live births[25] and is transmitted as an autosomal recessive trait. Although one kindred has been described with both Prader-Willi syndrome and Laurence-Moon-Biedl syndrome,[26] the two syndromes are sufficiently different in onset and appearance that they should not be confused. Nonetheless, the association suggests that they may partly share a common genetic defect.

The characteristics of the syndrome were recently revised.[25] It now appears that the syndrome is accompanied by severe retinal dystrophy, dysmorphic extremities (polydactyly, syndactyly, or brachydactyly), obesity, renal abnormalities, and male hypogonadism. Mental retardation appears to be a function of blindness rather than a characteristic of the syndrome. Half of affected patients are hypertensive,[27] and 30% die of renal failure.[28,29]

Obesity occurs in over 80% of cases[23] and increased birth weight in 70% of cases,[23] suggesting that the predisposition to obesity may begin in utero. Most obesity is said to begin in childhood,[23] and anecdotal descriptions suggest that the obesity is truncal.[30] In our experience, the childhood obesity is rarely as pronounced as that in Prader-Willi syndrome, and the fat distribution is not as characteristic. The eating behaviors that occur in Prader-Willi syndrome rarely occur in Bardet-Biedl syndrome. Approximately half of all patients have type II diabetes, but

whether the diabetes is a consequence of obesity remains unclear.

References

1. Prader A, Labhart A, Willi H: Ein Syndrome von Adipositas, Kleinwuchs, Kryptorchismus, and Oligophrenie nach myotonieartigem Zustand im Neugeborenenalter. Schweiz Med Wochenschr 86:1260, 1956
2. Ledbetter DH, Riccardi VM, Airhart SD et al: Deletions of chromosome 15 as a cause of the Prader Willi syndrome. N Engl J Med 304:325, 1981
3. Ledbetter DH, Mascarello JT, Riccardi VM et al: Chromosome 15 abnormalities and the Prader Willi syndrome: A follow-up report of 40 cases. Am J Hum Genet 34:278, 1982
4. Cassidy SB, Thulin HC, Holm VA: Deletion of chromosome 15 (q11–13) in a Prader-Labhart-Willi syndrome clinic population. Am J Med Genet 17: 485, 1984
5. Holm VA, Sulzbacher SJ, Pipes PL: Prader-Willi Syndrome. Baltimore, University Park Press, 1981
6. Cassidy SB: Prader-Willi syndrome. Curr Prob Pediatr 14:1, 1984
7. Alexander RC, Hanson JW: Overview. In Greenswag LR, Alexander RC (eds): Management of Prader-Willi Syndrome, p 3. New York, Springer-Verlag, 1988
8. Kaplan LC, Wharton R, Elias E et al: Clinical heterogeneity associated with deletions in the long arm of chromosome 15: Report of 3 new cases and their possible genetic significance. Am J Med Genet 28:45, 1987
9. Hall BD, Smith DW: Prader Willi syndrome. J Pediatr 81:286, 1972
10. Holm VA: The diagnosis of Prader-Willi syndrome. In Holm VA, Sulzbacher S, Pipes PL (eds): Prader-Willi Syndrome, p 27. Baltimore, University Park Press, 1981
11. Greenswag LR: Adults with Prader-Willi syndrome: A survey of 232 cases. Dev Med Child Neurol 29:145, 1987
12. Bray GA, Dahms WT, Swerdloff RS et al: The Prader-Willi syndrome: A study of 40 patients and a review of the literature. Medicine 62:59, 1983
13. Crnic KA, Sulzbacher S, Snow J et al: Preventing mental retardation associated with gross obesity in the Prader-Willi syndrome. J Pediatr 66:787, 1980
14. Laurence BM, Brito A, Wilkinson J: Prader-Willi syndrome after age 15 years. Arch Dis Child 56:181, 1981
15. Holm VA, Lauman EL: Prader-Willi syndrome and scoliosis. Dev Med Child Neurol 23:192, 1981

16. Nelson RA, Huse DM, Holman RT et al: Nutrition, metabolism, body composition and the response to the ketogenic diet in Prader-Willi syndrome. In Holm VA, Sulzbacher SJ, Pipes PL (eds): Prader-Willi Syndrome, p 105. Baltimore, University Park Press, 1981

17. Schoeller DA, Levitsky LL, Bandini LG et al: Energy expenditure and body composition in Prader-Willi syndrome. Metabolism 37:115, 1988

18. Nardella MT, Sulzbacher SI, Worthington-Roberts BS: Activity levels of persons with Prader-Willi syndrome. Am J Ment Defic 87:498, 1983

19. Greenswag LR, Alexander RC: Management of Prader-Willi Syndrome. New York, Springer-Verlag, 1988

20. Bistrian BR, Blackburn GL, Stanbury JB: Metabolic aspects of a protein sparing modified fast in the dietary management of Prader-Willi obesity. N Engl J Med 296:774, 1977

21. Soper RT, Mason EE, Printen KJ et al: Surgical treatment of morbid obesity in Prader-Willi syndrome. In Holm VA, Sulzbacher SJ, Pipes PL (eds): Prader-Willi syndrome, p 121. Baltimore, University Park Press, 1981

22. Klein D, Ammann F: The syndrome of Laurence-Moon-Bardet-Biedl and allied diseases in Switzerland. J Neurol Sci 9:479, 1969

23. Bauman ML, Hogan GR: Laurence-Moon-Biedl syndrome. Am J Dis Child 126:119, 1973

24. McKusick VA: Mendelian Inheritance in Man: Catalogs of Autosomal Dominant, Autosomal Recessive and X-linked Phenotypes, 8th ed, p 834. Baltimore, Johns Hopkins University Press, 1988

25. Green JS, Parfrey JS, Harnett JD et al: The cardinal manifestations of Bardet-Biedl syndrome, a form of the Laurence-Moon-Biedl syndrome. N Engl J Med 321:1002, 1989

26. Endo M, Tasaka N, Matsuura N et al: Laurence-Moon-Biedl syndrome and Prader-Willi syndrome in a single family. Eur J Pediatr 123:269, 1976

27. Harnett JD, Green JS, Cramer BC et al: The spectrum of renal disease in Laurence-Moon-Biedl syndrome. N Engl J Med 319:615, 1988

28. Hurley RM, Dery P, Nogrady MB et al: The renal lesion of the Laurence-Moon-Biedl syndrome. J Pediatr 87:206, 1975

29. Alton DJ, McDonald P: Urographic findings in the Bardet-Biedl syndrome, formerly the Laurence-Moon-Biedl syndrome. Radiology 109:659, 1973

30. Bowen P, Ferguson-Smith MA, Mosier D et al: The Laurence-Moon syndrome. Association with hypogonadotrophic hypogonadism and sex chromosome aneuploidy. Arch Intern Med 116:598, 1965

CHAPTER 51

Polycystic Ovary Syndrome and Obesity

ANDREA DUNAIF

Polycystic ovary syndrome (PCOS) is probably the most common endocrine disorder of reproductive-age women, affecting 1.5% to 6% of this population.[1] Moderate obesity (about 50% above ideal body weight) is frequently found in the syndrome.[2] Thus, obese women with PCOS form one of the most prevalent subgroups of obesity. Moreover, this association has led to speculation that obesity and PCOS may be causally related. This chapter reviews the features of PCOS, the impact of obesity on PCOS, and the possible mechanisms underlying the association of PCOS and obesity.

DEFINITION OF PCOS

Stein and Leventhal first designated the constellation of hirsutism, obesity, menstrual irregularity, and infertility associated with enlarged sclerocystic ovaries as a discrete syndrome, amenable to the surgical intervention of ovarian wedge resection.[3] With the advent of urinary and plasma reproductive hormone determinations, a characteristic biochemical profile for this syndrome was defined.[4,5] This consisted of disordered gonadotropin release with elevated luteinizing hormone (LH) relative to follicle-stimulating hormone (FSH) secretion, hyperandrogenism, and constant, noncyclic (i.e., tonic) estrogen production. The diversity of clinical features associated with the ovarian morphology was emphasized in the classic literature review of Goldzieher and Green.[2] It was evident from this work that none

of the characteristics initially reported by Stein and Leventhal were consistent features of the syndrome (Table 51-1).

Subsequently, it became evident that the clinical and biochemical features of PCOS could occur in the presence of ovaries that appeared normal on laparoscopy.[6] Conversely, enlarged polycystic ovaries could be detected by laparoscopy or by ultrasonography (US) in otherwise reproductively normal women.[7] Moreover, a variety of causes of hyperandrogenism such as nonclassic congenital adrenal hyperplasia, androgen-secreting neoplasms, and Cushing's syndrome could be associated with polycystic ovaries.[8]

It was thus clear that the signs and symptoms reported by Stein and Leventhal[3] were not adequate for diagnosing all cases of the syndrome. The syndrome is now known as the polycystic ovary syndrome. It remains controversial whether documentation of polycystic ovaries (usually by vaginal US) is a requisite for diagnosing the syndrome. Indeed, many authors define PCOS as the association of hyperandrogenism and chronic anovulation when secondary causes (e.g., nonclassic congenital adrenal hyperplasia, androgen-secreting neoplasms) have been specifically excluded.[9]

OVARIAN MORPHOLOGY

The ovary in PCOS is usually enlarged. The ovarian cortex is thickened. Subcapsularly, there are

TABLE 51-1

Frequency of Clinical Symptoms in PCOS (1,079 cases)

Symptom	Mean (%)	Range (%)
Obesity	41	16–49
Hirsutism	69	17–83
Virilization	21	9–28
Amenorrhea	51	15–77
Infertility	74	35–94
Functional Bleeding	29	6–65
Dysmenorrhea	23	–
Biphasic Basal Body Temperature	15	12–40
Corpus Luteum at Operation	22	0–75

Data from Goldzieher and Green.[2]

multiple ovarian follicles and an increased number of atretic follicles.[10] The theca cells, which are the androgen-producing cells of the ovary, lining the follicles are hyperplastic.[10] The granulosa cells of the follicles are immature and thus are unable to perform their normal function of converting the thecal androgens into estrogens via aromatization.[9]

The ovarian stroma, which is formed largely from atretic follicles, is also androgen secreting and is usually hyperplastic in PCOS.[9] Islands of thecal cells can also be found within the ovarian stroma.[10] This finding, known as stromal hyperthecosis, is frequently but not consistently associated with more profound hyperandrogenism.[11] Finally, corpora lutea, the morphological result of recent ovulation, are an infrequent finding in PCOS because of the chronic anovulatory state.[10]

GONADOTROPIN SECRETION

The most distinctive feature of PCOS is a characteristic disorder of gonadotropin release resulting in increased LH secretion relative to FSH secretion.[12] An increased LH:FSH ratio, however, can escape detection on a random blood sample because of the pulsatile nature of gonadotropin secretion. Detailed frequent blood sampling studies of gonadotropin secretion (which reflects hypothalamic release of gonadotropin-releasing hormone [GnRH]) in PCOS have demonstrated that elevated LH levels are the result

of an increased amplitude of LH pulses.[12-14] The frequency of LH pulses may also be increased.[14] The increased LH pulse amplitude results primarily from increased pituitary sensitivity to GnRH.[12] It remains possible that an increased amount of GnRH may be secreted per pulse. FSH release is in the normal range for women in the follicular phase of the menstrual cycle; it is not suppressed.[15]

STEROIDOGENESIS IN PCOS

The ovaries are the major source of androgens in PCOS. However, even in the absence of identifiable adrenal enzyme deficiencies, the adrenals contribute to the androgen excess in a substantial minority of patients.[16] The ovarian androgen production in PCOS is LH-dependent, whereas that of the adrenal is ACTH-dependent. Androstenedione (A) and testosterone (T) are secreted by the ovaries.[8] The adrenals secrete these androgens as well as dehydroepiandrosterone (DHEA) and its sulfate (DHEAS). T is also formed in the periphery from prehormones such as A, DHEA, and DHEAS. There is continued estradiol secretion by the ovary.[9] Estrone is both gonadally secreted in PCOS and derived from extragonadal aromatization of A.[9] Both fat and muscle contain the aromatase enzyme system, and aromatization rates of A to estrone are positively correlated with body weight.[17,18]

The major gonadal steroids, T and estradiol,

as well as the peripherally produced potent T metabolite, dihydrotestosterone, circulate bound to a specific serum transport protein sex hormone–binding globulin (SHBG).[19] Only the steroids that are not specifically bound to SHBG (i.e., those that are free or are loosely associated with albumin) are biologically available to enter target cells. SHBG is synthesized by the liver; estrogens and thyroid hormone increase its production, whereas androgens and insulin suppress production.[19,20] Obesity is associated with decreased SHBG levels,[21] probably as a result of the hyperinsulinemia of obesity. Thus, in PCOS, SHBG levels are decreased secondary to hyperandrogenism and hyperinsulinemia.

PATHOPHYSIOLOGY OF PCOS

The increased LH release relative to FSH release results in arrested folliculogenesis and increased ovarian androgen production. This is secondary to LH-dependent thecal androgen secretion and insufficient granulosa cell estrogen production because of relative FSH deficiency.[8,9] Increased LH release produces thecal and stromal hyperplasia. There is anovulation because of the disordered gonadotropin release. This results in the formation of subcapsular follicular cysts. Androgens directly cause thickening of the ovarian cortex and increased rates of follicular atresia.[9] The androgens also feed back on the hypothalamic-pituitary axis by their conversion to estrogens in the periphery and in the hypothalamus.[8,9] This tonic estrogen feedback, primarily of estradiol, enhances pituitary sensitivity to GnRH, resulting in an increased amplitude of LH pulses.[8,9] This feedback may also result in alterations in the frequency or amount of hypothalamic GnRH secretion. Androgens do not appear to directly (independent of conversion to estrogens) modulate gonadotropin release in PCOS.[22]

When polycystic ovaries are placed in a normal hormonal environment, they function normally.[9] This has led to the hypothesis that the ovarian abnormalities are secondary to the abnormal hormonal milieu. It remains possible that there are subtle intrinsic ovarian abnormalities in PCOS.[8,9] These could result in cyst formation or in abnormal steroidogenesis.

The primary etiologic event in PCOS is unknown. Increased ovarian or adrenal androgen secretion[23] can cause the syndrome, as can increased hypothalamic GnRH secretion.[9] To date, no intrinsic ovarian, adrenal, or hypothalamic-pituitary abnormalities have been identified in the majority of women with PCOS. Hyperinsulinemia secondary to insulin resistance has recently been recognized as a common feature in PCOS (see below). It has been postulated that insulin may initiate the syndrome by directly stimulating ovarian androgen secretion.[9] Although this hypothesis is appealing, we have shown[15] that obese and lean women with PCOS have similar patterns of gonadotropin release and gonadal steroids, despite significantly different degrees of chronic hyperinsulinemia. Moreover, the primary drive to androgen production, even in hyperinsulinemic women with PCOS, is LH.[24] Thus, the role of hyperinsulinemia in the pathogenesis of PCOS remains unknown.

INSULIN ACTION IN PCOS

The observation that a disorder of insulin action is associated with hyperandrogenism is not new. In 1921 Achard and Thiers[25] reported "le diabete des femmes a barbe" (the diabetes of bearded women). In the mid-1970s Kahn and co-workers[26] described a distinct syndrome in adolescent girls of insulin-resistant diabetes mellitus and hyperandrogenism associated with the dermatologic lesion acanthosis nigricans. They named this constellation the type A syndrome of insulin resistance. Recent studies[27,28] have identified several mutations in the insulin receptor gene as causal of the insulin resistance in a few individuals affected with this rare disorder.

Several rare syndromes of extreme insulin resistance and acanthosis nigricans, often with hyperandrogenism, were identified (e.g., type B, lipoatrophic diabetes, Rabson-Mendenhall syndrome, leprechaunism).[29] Burghen, Givens, and Kitabchi were the first to report[30] that a disorder of insulin action might be associated with PCOS. They found that women with PCOS had basal and glucose-stimulated hyperinsulinemia compared to obese weight-matched normal women. Further, they noted significant positive linear correlations between insulin and androgen levels and suggested that this might have etiologic significance.

It was also noted[31-33] that acanthosis nigricans occurred more commonly than previously appreciated in hyperandrogenic women. Further, these women had a distinct disorder of insulin action, compared to women with the rare syndromes of extreme insulin resistance. Indeed, these women had typical PCOS, although on histologic examination of their ovaries, an increase in stromal hyperthecosis was found, suggesting that the insulin-resistant state modified ovarian function. At the same time, a number of investigators[35-37] were confirming and extending the original observation that women with PCOS had hyperinsulinemia independent of obesity and secondary to some degree of insulin resistance. Thus, it was evident that PCOS represented a new and uncharacterized disorder of insulin action.

Hyperinsulinemia and Hyperandrogenism

To determine the prevalence of hyperinsulinemia in hyperandrogenic women, we prospectively evaluated 62 such women, stratified on the basis of weight and ovulatory status, for basal and glucose-stimulated insulin secretion and glucose tolerance.[38] The presence of acanthosis nigricans on clinical examination was noted, and since approximately 50% of the obese women with PCOS also had acanthosis nigricans, it was also used to stratify this group. We found that only anovulatory hyperandrogenic women whom we diagnosed as having PCOS had basal or glucose-stimulated hyperinsulinemia independent of obesity. Ovulatory hyperandrogenic women were not hyperinsulinemic. These findings strongly suggested that hyperinsulinemia was a unique feature of PCOS and not of hyperandrogenic states in general.

The women with PCOS and acanthosis nigricans had significantly higher insulin responses than those without this skin change on clinical examination. Otherwise, the sex hormone and gonadotropin levels were identical in these two subgroups of women with PCOS. Most impor-

tant, 20% of the obese women with PCOS had previously undiagnosed frank diabetes mellitus or impaired glucose tolerance, independent of the presence of acanthosis nigricans. The mean age of these women was 27 years. Thus, PCOS represented a previously unappreciated risk factor for the development of non-insulin-dependent diabetes mellitus (NIDDM) at an extremely early age.

Insulin Resistance in PCOS

Except in rare instances of mutant insulins, hyperinsulinemia results from target tissue insulin resistance.[39] To determine the magnitude of this defect in insulin action in PCOS, we performed euglycemic glucose clamp studies in lean and obese women with PCOS.[40] Muscle is the major site of insulin-mediated glucose disposal,[41,42] whereas fat mass independently decreases insulin-mediated glucose disposal.[43] Since there is an increased prevalence of obesity in women with PCOS,[2] it had been argued that the insulin resistance was secondary to obesity,[44] rather than an independent defect. It was also possible that women with PCOS might have increased muscle mass because of elevated plasma androgen levels.[45] To control for these potentially confounding factors, we matched lean and obese normal control women to women with PCOS on the basis of fat and fat-free mass determined by hydrostatic weighing.

The euglycemic glucose clamp is the most accurate and widely accepted method for assessing insulin resistance in vivo.[46] This technique permits the measurement not only of peripheral (primarily muscle) insulin sensitivity but also the sensitivity of hepatic glucose production to insulin suppression (with the addition of an isotope-labeled glucose infusion) and of the metabolic clearance rate of insulin. A fixed dose of insulin is infused to produce the desired ambient insulin concentration. A variable infusion of glucose is administered to maintain euglycemia. The amount of glucose infused at steady state is equal to the peripheral glucose utilization (insulin-mediated glucose disposal) and is reported as the index of insulin action in these studies.

Even though none of the women with PCOS

had a previous history of abnormalities in glucose tolerance, as a group the obese women with PCOS had significantly increased basal and two-hour post-glucose load glucose levels, compared to findings in controls matched for body composition.[40] This was the result of significantly increased rates of basal hepatic glucose production. Further, PCOS and obesity had synergistic and deleterious effects on glucose tolerance. Glucose tolerance and basal hepatic glucose production were completely normal in the lean women with PCOS.

Peripheral insulin action was significantly and substantially decreased in lean and in obese women with PCOS compared to control groups matched for body composition.[40] The magnitude of the insulin resistance in PCOS was similar in severity to that reported for NIDDM.[46] This is even more striking, since age independently decreases insulin action,[47] because women with PCOS are much younger (third and fourth decades) than individuals with NIDDM (sixth and seventh decades). Insulin also failed to suppress hepatic glucose production in some women with PCOS, whereas hepatic glucose production was completely suppressed in all normal subjects, although the magnitude of this change did not achieve statistical significance. This observation strongly suggested the presence of hepatic as well as peripheral insulin resistance. There was no significant difference in the metabolic clearance rate of insulin in PCOS, suggesting that decreased insulin clearance did not contribute to the hyperinsulinemia. Thus, this study[40] found that women with PCOS had a unique disorder of insulin action that was independent of obesity or glucose tolerance impairment.

Acanthosis Nigricans, Insulin Action, and Hyperandrogenism

There has been a tendency in the field to use the clinical finding of acanthosis nigricans to subgroup hyperandrogenic women (Figs. 51-1 and 51-2).[31-33,38] The only reported biochemical difference is that acanthotic women have higher insulin levels than women without this skin lesion.[33,38] We found no differences in sex hormone levels or the pattern of pulsatile gonad-

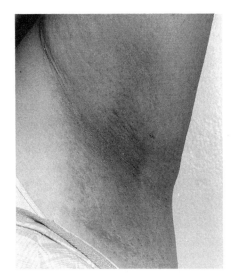

FIGURE 51-1

Axilla of a woman with PCOS and clinically obvious acanthosis nigricans. Note the papillomatous hyperpigmented area.

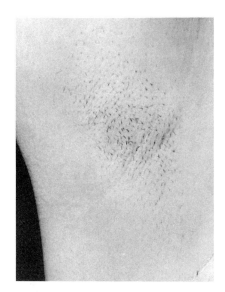

FIGURE 51-2

Axilla of a woman with PCOS without clinically identifiable nigricans.

otropin release in women with PCOS with and without this lesion.[15,38]

Acanthosis nigricans is diagnosed from pathognomonic histologic changes (Fig. 51-3): dermal thickening and papillomatosis, hyperkeratosis, and occasionally increased melanin.[48] To determine the sensitivity of clinical skin examination for diagnosing acanthosis nigricans as well as the best biochemical correlates of this lesion, we obtained skin biopsy specimens from unselected women with PCOS and from age- and weight-matched normal women.[49] The specimens were taken from the neck or the axilla and were evaluated blindly by a dermatopathologist. Acanthosis nigricans was identified on clinical examination in 11 of 13 obese women with PCOS, three of six lean women with PCOS, four of 14 normal obese women, and none of four normal lean women. Acanthosis nigricans was diagnosed his-

tologically in 13 of 13 obese women with PCOS, five of six lean women with PCOS, 13 of 14 normal obese women, and one of four normal lean women. The lesion occurred in women of all ethnic groups and skin types.

Clinical examination of the skin proved quite insensitive for detecting acanthosis nigricans (see Fig. 51-2). Thus, acanthosis nigricans was more frequently detected on microscopic examination of skin biopsy specimens than clinically (see Fig. 51-3). The presence of this dermatologic change correlated better with the magnitude of peripheral insulin resistance (i.e., decreased insulin-mediated glucose disposal) than with basal or glucose challenge–induced hyperinsulinemia. The only sex steroid associated with acanthosis nigricans was DHEAS. The lesion occurred in normal women and in women with PCOS. This study indicates that acanthosis nigricans is an epiphenomenon of insulin resistance, and that subgrouping subjects on the basis of clinical identification of the lesion is not valid.

Androgens and Insulin Resistance

Because of the significant positive correlations noted between androgen and insulin levels in PCOS, it has been postulated that androgens may directly decrease insulin action.[30] Evidence to support this hypothesis comes from studies demonstrating that persons receiving anabolic steroids become hyperinsulinemic.[50,51] Conversely, natural androgen administration to men[52] and to female nonhuman primates[53] has not altered insulin levels or glucose tolerance. Studies altering androgen levels in PCOS have been conflicting[54,55] and have been constrained by small sample sizes.

To investigate the causal role of endogenous hyperandrogenism in the insulin resistance of PCOS, we suppressed gonadal steroid production for 12 weeks with a long-acting analogue of GnRH, GnRHa.[56] Despite suppressing androgen levels into the normal range for ten weeks, there was no significant change in plasma insulin levels, hepatic glucose production, or insulin-mediated glucose disposal as determined by the euglycemic clamp technique. The sample size ($n = 9$) was adequate to detect a clinically sig-

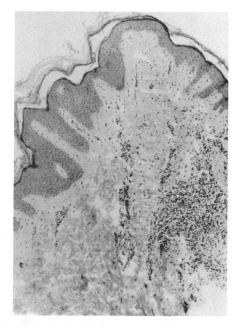

FIGURE 51-3

Histologic section of a skin biopsy specimen taken from the axilla of the woman shown in Figure 51-2. The specimen shows acanthosis nigricans, characterized by dermal papillomatosis. Acanthosis nigricans can escape detection on clinical examination.

nificant change in insulin action (*i.e.*, an improvement in insulin-mediated glucose disposal of ≥ 0.6 mg/kg/min).

This study indicated that plasma androgen elevations do not actively sustain insulin resistance in PCOS. We cannot exclude, however, that the hyperandrogenic state caused an irreversible change in target tissue insulin sensitivity. If this were the case, then altering androgen levels would not have an effect on insulin action. Previous studies that suggested a direct action of androgens on insulin action[50,51] used orally active 17-alkylated synthetic androgens, and these compounds may have different effects on glucose tolerance than natural androgens. Finally, suppressing androgen levels cannot be used as a therapeutic modality to improve insulin sensitivity and thereby decrease the risk of NIDDM in PCOS.

OBESITY, HYPERANDROGENISM, AND ANOVULATION

Obesity and PCOS

Obesity occurs in only 35% to 60%[2,15,57] of women with PCOS, and clearly, not all obese women have hormonal disturbances. There are several mechanisms by which obesity might be involved in the development of the chronic hyperandrogenic anovulation characteristic of PCOS. First, gonadal steroid feedback changes could result from obesity because of increased extraglandular (fat and muscle) aromatization of androgen to estrogen[17] and decreased SHBG levels.[21] Second, neuroendocrine abnormalities, such as a central lesion involving the putative feeding center of the ventromedial hypothalamus and the anatomically closely related neurons in the arcuate nucleus involved in pulsatile GnRH secretion, might explain the association of PCOS and obesity.[29] Alternatively, insulin might alter gonadotropin secretion and ovarian steroidogenesis to produce PCOS.[58,59] A correlation between hyperinsulinemia and hyperandrogenism has been shown in PCOS,[30] and obese women with PCOS are significantly more hyperinsulinemic than nonobese women with PCOS.[38] Finally, obesity might be secondary to metabolic changes such as androgen-mediated increases in body weight,[60] or a decrease in energy expenditure.[61,62]

Impact of Obesity on Gonadal Steroids

Obesity is associated with increased extragonadal aromatization of androgens to estrogens,[17] decreased SHBG production, and increased androgen production.[21,63,64] These changes may play a role in the development of PCOS by causing chronic inappropriate estrogen feedback on the hypothalamic-pituitary axis, leading to distorted gonadotropin release and anovulation,[12] and by increasing androgen production, which may directly inhibit follicular maturation.[65]

However, decreased SHBG and increased androgen production occur in obese women with and without reproductive dysfunction.[21,66-68] Only the anovulatory obese women had increased serum androgen levels, suggesting that obesity is not the only factor contributing to chronic anovulation. These findings suggest that the putative servo-control mechanism[67] that adjusts the production rate of steroids to maintain constant plasma levels despite an increased metabolic clearance rate is not operative in obese noncycling women.

Recent studies have shown that the plasma levels of androgens and estrogens are similar in lean and obese women with PCOS.[15,69] These findings indicate that hyperandrogenism and anovulation can occur independent of obesity. However, there is evidence that obesity has some impact on the clinical and endocrinologic abnormalities characteristic of PCOS. Obese women with PCOS have a greater prevalence of anovulation and hirsutism than nonobese women with PCOS.[69] The increased incidence of hirsutism appears related to a greater activity of the 5α-reductase enzyme system in peripheral androgen-sensitive tissues in obese women compared to lean women with PCOS.[69] Moreover, a number of studies have shown that weight reduction can improve hormonal abnormalities and restore ovulation in obese women with PCOS.[70-73] There was a significant decrease in mean LH levels and a return of ovulation in some women with PCOS after weight loss.[72] Similarly, significant decreases in T and mean LH levels and improved cyclicity without changes in A or DHEAS levels were found in obese anovulatory hyperandrogenic women.[70] No hormonal differences were identified between women who responded to weight reduction and those who did not. Therefore, although obesity may contribute to anovulation in some women with PCOS, the mechanism of this action remains unknown. Moreover, it is not possible to predict which patients will benefit from weight loss.

Impact of Obesity on the Metabolic Consequences of PCOS

We have clearly demonstrated that insulin resistance in PCOS is independent of obesity.[40] However, obesity and PCOS interact such that insulin resistance is significantly worse in obese women with PCOS[40] and, to date, only such obese women have developed impaired glucose tolerance leading to NIDDM.[38] Similarly, PCOS in lean women results in decreased insulin action comparable to that seen in age-matched normal obese women (≥ 28 kg/m^2).

It has been suggested that the hyperandrogenism associated with PCOS may be an independent risk factor for the development of cardiovascular disease because of the direct negative impact of androgens on high-density lipoprotein (HDL) metabolism.[74,75] The independent effects of obesity and hyperinsulinemia were not adequately controlled for in these studies. When we matched obese and lean women with PCOS with age- and weight-matched normal ovulatory women and adjusted statistically for hyperinsulinemia, we found that obesity rather than PCOS was the major factor associated with lowered HDL levels.[76] PCOS abolished the protective effect of leanness on triglyceride levels such that total triglyceride levels were similar in lean and obese women with PCOS and in obese normal women.[76] Thus obesity rather than PCOS or the hyperandrogenism associated with it was the major potential cause of an increased risk for cardiovascular disease in PCOS.

The impact of obesity on the metabolic complications of PCOS was therefore either synergistic or of primary pathogenic importance.[40,76] Lean women with PCOS, however, lose the protective effect of leanness on carbohydrate and lipid metabolism. These women have similar degrees of hyperinsulinemia, insulin resistance, and total triglycerides as normal obese women.[38,40,76]

ETIOLOGY OF OBESITY IN PCOS

Distinct Neuroendocrine Disorder

PCOS could result from a primary central disorder of GnRH release that leads to disrupted pulsatile gonadotropin secretion, producing anovulation and hyperandrogenism.[29] We have recently shown, however, that obese and nonobese women with PCOS have similar patterns of pulsatile gonadotropin release.[15] This finding strongly suggests that obese women with PCOS do not have a distinct neuroendocrine disorder.

Lesions of the ventromedial hypothalamus (VMH) in animals can lead to obesity and hyperinsulinemia.[77] Hence, the association of hyperinsulinemia and obesity in PCOS might be secondary to an abnormality in the VMH. Nonobese women with PCOS are hyperinsulinemic, but less so than their obese counterparts.[38] Obesity and insulin resistance do occur without PCOS,[78] and nonobese women with PCOS usually have no history of obesity (Dunaif, unpublished observations). Thus it remains possible that the gonadotropin abnormalities of PCOS, the obesity that can be associated with PCOS, and insulin resistance could represent defects at different but anatomically close loci that overlap to result in a heterogeneous disorder.

Alternatively, it is possible that other hormonal abnormalities that occur in obese women with PCOS, such as hyperinsulinemia, could produce neuroendocrine changes. Indeed, obese women with PCOS have significantly increased fasting and glucose-stimulated plasma insulin levels compared to nonobese women with PCOS and normal obese women.[15] Positive linear correlations have been found between hyperinsulinemia and hyperandrogenism, leading to speculation that increased insulin levels cause PCOS.[30] Insulin can alter steroidogenesis in human and animal ovarian tissue,[58,59] and supraphysiological doses of insulin can increase androgen production in vivo,[79,80] but high doses of exogenous insulin have no effect on gonadotropin release in women with PCOS.[79] Moreover, we have shown that obese and nonobese women with PCOS have similar patterns of gonadotropin release and reproductive hormone levels despite significant differences in their degree of endogenous hyperinsulinemia.[15] These results suggest that physiological hyperinsulinemia does not play a major role in sustaining the hormonal abnormalities characteristic of PCOS.

Metabolic Defect

It is also possible that hyperandrogenism could cause alterations in body composition by directly increasing muscle mass or by stimulating food intake.[60] However, we found no differences in either muscle or fat mass in obese women with PCOS as compared with normal obese women.[40] Further, not all hyperandrogenic women are obese; some nonobese women have PCOS.

Alternatively, obesity may be related to a primary deficit in energy expenditure, increased energy intake, or both.[81,82] Decreased total energy expenditure predicted the development of obesity in a prospective familial study.[81] These subjects had low baseline resting metabolic rates (RMR), which after weight gain became similar to that in nonobese subjects. This suggests that weight gain is a way of correcting an abnormal RMR. Similarly, decreased total energy expenditure in infants of obese women compared to infants of nonobese women has been found[82] and was related to rapid weight gain in the first year of life. A low energy expenditure in some infants who did not develop obesity implies the existence of additional factors contributing to eventual weight gain.

The decreased energy expenditure in obese subjects may be secondary to insulin resistance. A defect in postprandial thermogenesis has been found in insulin-resistant obese subjects; this was related to a decrease in glucose uptake and storage.[83] Thus, impaired glucose tolerance may be the mechanism responsible for the reduced thermic effect of a meal that is seen in obese subjects. This defect could be corrected by restoring normal glucose uptake using increasing doses of insulin in a euglycemic glucose clamp.[84]

Obesity is associated with significantly greater insulin resistance in PCOS.[38,40] It is possible that

obesity in PCOS may result from a deficit in energy expenditure. We demonstrated, however, that both normal obese women and obese women with PCOS had similarly blunted postprandial thermogenesis.[85] Thus, women with PCOS did not have altered energy expenditure when compared with normal women of similar weight and body composition, despite significantly higher basal and post-glucose load glucose levels and decreased insulin-stimulated glucose utilization. Thus, impaired thermogenesis may reflect a defect intrinsic to the obese state, independent of insulin resistance. Taken together, these studies suggest that a defect in this component of energy expenditure, i.e., postprandial thermogenesis, is a result of obesity rather than a cause. Finally, there is little evidence that hyperandrogenism or a defect in energy expenditure, is the primary cause of obesity in PCOS.

SUMMARY

Obesity is common in PCOS but is not associated with discernible changes in gonadotropin release or gonadal steroid levels. Despite significant insulin resistance in obese women with PCOS, there is no additional defect in energy expenditure. Weight reduction can improve menstrual function in some obese women with PCOS. Thus, by an unknown mechanism obesity may contribute to the hormonal abnormalities of PCOS. A common neuroendocrine change, closely linked genetic abnormalities, or obesity unmasking an underlying predisposition to anovulation could explain the association of obesity and PCOS.

References

1. Futterweit W: Polycystic Ovarian Disease. New York, Springer-Verlag, 1984
2. Goldzieher JW, Green JA: The polycystic ovary. I. Clinical and histologic features. J Clin Endocrinol Metab 22:325, 1962
3. Stein IF, Leventhal ML: Amenorrhea associated with bilateral polycystic ovaries. Am J Obstet Gynecol 29:181, 1935
4. Keettel WC, Brodbury JT, Stodard FJ: Observations on the PCO syndrome. Am J Obstet Gynecol 73: 954, 1957
5. DeVane GW, Czekala NM, Judd HL et al: Circulating gonadotropins, estrogens, and androgens in

polycystic ovarian disease. Am J Obstet Gynecol 121:496, 1975

6. Kim MH, Rosenfield RL, Hosseinian AH et al: Ovarian hyperandrogenism with normal and abnormal histologic findings of the ovaries. Am J Obstet Gynecol 134:445, 1979

7. Polson DW, Adams J, Wadsworth J et al: Polycystic ovaries: A common finding in normal women. Lancet 1:870, 1988

8. Mechanick JI, Dunaif A: Masculinization: A clinical approach to the diagnosis and treatment of hyperandrogenic women. Adv Endocrinol Metab 1:129, 1990

9. Dunaif A, Givens JR, Haseltine F et al: The Polycystic Ovary Syndrome. Cambridge, Mass., Blackwell Scientific Publishers, 1991

10. Hughesdon PE: Morphology and morphogenesis of the Stein-Leventhal ovary and of so-called "hyperthecosis." Obstet Gynecol 37:59, 1982

11. Geist SH, Gaines JA: Diffuse luteinization of the ovaries associated with the masculinization syndrome. Am J Obstet Gynecol 43:975, 1942

12. Rebar R, Judd HL, Yen SSC et al: Characterization of the inappropriate gonadotropin secretion in polycystic ovary syndrome. J Clin Invest 57:1320, 1976

13. Kazer RR, Kessel B, Yen SSC: Circulating luteinizing hormone pulse frequency in women with polycystic ovary syndrome. J Clin Endocrinol Metab 65:233, 1987

14. Waldstreicher J, Santoro N, Hall JE et al: Hyperfunction of the hypothalamic-pituitary axis in women with polycystic ovarian disease: Indirect evidence for partial gonadotroph desensitization. J Clin Endocrinol Metab 66:165, 1988

15. Dunaif A, Mandeli J, Fluhr H et al: The impact of obesity and chronic hyperinsulinemia on gonadotropin release and gonadal steroid secretion in the polycystic ovary syndrome. J Clin Endocrinol Metab 66:131, 1988

16. Siegel SF, Finegold DN, Lanes R et al: ACTH stimulation tests and plasma dehydroepiandrosterone sulfate levels in women with hirsutism. N Engl J Med 323:849, 1990

17. Edman CD, MacDonald PC: Effect of obesity on conversion of plasma androstenedione to estrone in ovulatory and anovulatory young women. Am J Obstet Gynecol 130:456, 1978

18. Segal KR, Dunaif A, Gutin B et al: Body composition, not body weight, is related to cardiovascular disease risk factors and sex hormone levels in men. J Clin Invest 80:1050, 1987

19. Anderson DC: Sex hormone-binding globulin. Clin Endocrinol (Oxf) 3:69, 1974

20. Plymate SR, Matej LA, Jones RE et al: Inhibition of

sex hormone-binding globulin production in the human hepatoma (Hep G2) cell line by insulin and prolactin. J Clin Endocrinol Metab 67:460, 1988

21. Plymate SR, Fariss BL, Bassett ML et al: Obesity and its role in polycystic ovary syndrome. J Clin Endocrinol Metab 52:1246, 1981

22. Dunaif A: Do androgens directly regulate gonadotropin secretion in the polycystic ovary syndrome? J Clin Endocrinol Metab 63:215, 1986

23. Dunaif A, Scully RE, Andersen RN et al: The effects of continuous androgen secretion on the hypothalamic-pituitary axis in women: Evidence from a luteinized thecoma of the ovary. J Clin Endocrinol Metab 59:389, 1984

24. Dunaif A, Green G, Futterweit W et al: Suppression of hyperandrogenism does not improve peripheral or hepatic insulin resistance in the polycystic ovary syndrome. J Clin Endocrinol Metab 70:699, 1990

25. Achard C, Thiers J: Le virilisme pilaire et son association à l'insuffisance glycolytique (diabetete des femmes à barbe). Bull Acad Natl Med (Paris) 86:51, 1921

26. Kahn CR, Flier JS, Bar RS et al: The syndromes of insulin resistance and acanthosis nigricans. N Engl J Med 294:739, 1976

27. Yoshimosa Y, Seino S, Whittaker J et al: Insulin-resistant diabetes due to a point mutation that prevents insulin proreceptor processing. Science 240:784, 1988

28. Kadowaki T, Kadowaki H, Rechler MM et al: Five mutant alleles of the insulin receptor gene in patients with genetic forms of insulin resistance. J Clin Invest 86:254, 1990

29. Dunaif A, Hoffman AR: Insulin resistance and hyperandrogenism: Clinical syndromes and possible mechanisms. In Pancheri P, Zihella L (eds): Biorhythms and Stress in the Physiopathology of Reproduction. Hemisphere Publishing Corp, 1988

30. Burghen GA, Givens JR, Kitabchi AE: Correlations of hyperandrogenism with hyperinsulinemia in polycystic ovarian disease. J Clin Endocrinol Metab 50:113, 1980

31. Flier JS, Eastman RC, Minaker KL et al: Acanthosis nigricans in obese women with hyperandrogenism: Characterization of an insulin-resistant state distinct from the type A and B syndromes. Diabetes 34:101, 1985

32. Dunaif A, Hoffman AR, Scully RE et al: Clinical, biochemical, and ovarian morphologic features in women with acanthosis nigricans and masculinization. Obstet Gynecol 66:545, 1985

33. Stuart CA, Peters JE, Prince MJ et al: Insulin resistance with acanthosis nigricans: The roles of obesity and androgen excess. Metabolism 35:197, 1986

34. Pasquali R, Casimirri F, Venturoli S et al: Insulin resistance in patients with polycystic ovaries: Its relationship to body weight and androgen levels. Acta Endocrinol 104:110, 1983

35. Pasquali R, Venturoli S, Paradis R et al: Insulin and C-peptide levels in obese patients with polycystic ovaries. Horm Metab Res 14:284, 1982

36. Chang RJ, Nakamura RM, Judd HL et al: Insulin resistance in nonobese patients with polycystic ovarian disease. J Clin Endocrinol Metab 57:356, 1983

37. Shoupe D, Kumar D, Lobo RA: Insulin resistance in polycystic ovary syndrome. Am J Obstet Gynecol 147:588, 1983

38. Dunaif A, Graf M, Mandeli J et al: Characterization of groups of hyperandrogenic women with acanthosis nigricans, impaired glucose tolerance, and/ or hyperinsulinemia. J Clin Endocrinol Metab 65:499, 1987

39. Defronzo RA: The triumvirate: Beta-cell, muscle, liver. A collusion responsible for NIDDM. Diabetes 37:667, 1988

40. Dunaif A, Segal KR, Futterweit W et al: Profound peripheral insulin resistance, independent of obesity, in the polycystic ovary syndrome. Diabetes 38:1165, 1989

41. Yki-Jarvinen H, Koivisto VA: Effects of body composition on insulin sensitivity. Diabetes 32:965, 1983

42. Defronzo RA, Jacot E, Jequier E et al: The effect of insulin on the disposal of intravenous glucose. Diabetes 30:1000, 1981

43. Bogardus C, Lillioja S, Mott DM et al: Relationship between degree of obesity and in vivo insulin action in man. Am J Physiol 248:E286, 1985

44. Sathanadan M, Mortola J, Kolterman OG et al: Characterization of insulin resistance in polycystic ovary syndrome using hyperinsulinemic euglycemic clamp (abstr 176). Proceedings of the 43rd Annual Meeting American Fertility Society, Reno, Nevada, 1987

45. Wade GN, Gray JM: Gonadal effects on food intake and adiposity: A metabolic hypothesis. Physiol Behav 22:583, 1979

46. Bergman RN, Finegood DT, Ader M: Assessment of insulin sensitivity in vivo. Endocr Rev 6:45, 1985

47. Rowe JW, Minaker KL, Pallota JA et al: Characterization of the insulin resistance of aging. J Clin Invest 71:1581, 1983

48. Brown J, Winklemann RK: Acanthosis nigricans: A study of 90 cases. Medicine 47:33, 1968

49. Dunaif A, Green G, Phelps RG et al: Acanthosis nigricans, insulin action, and hyperandrogenism: Clinical, histologic and biochemical findings. J Clin Endocrinol Metab (in press) 1990

50. Woodard TL, Burghen GA, Kitabchi AE et al: Glucose intolerance and insulin resistance in aplastic anemia treated with oxymetholone. J Clin Endocrinol Metab 53:905, 1981

51. Cohen JC, Hickman R: Insulin resistance and diminished glucose tolerance in powerlifters ingesting anabolic steroids. J Clin Endocrinol Metab 64:960, 1987

52. Friedl KE, Jones RE, Hannan CJ Jr et al: The administration of pharmacological doses of testosterone or 19-nortestosterone to normal men is not associated with increased insulin secretion or impaired glucose tolerance. J Clin Endocrinol Metab 68:971, 1989

53. Billiar RB, Richardson D, Schwartz R et al: Effect of chronically elevated androgen or estrogen on the glucose tolerance test and insulin response in female rhesus monkeys. Am J Obstet Gynecol 157:1297, 1987

54. Shoupe D, Lobo RA: The influence of androgens on insulin resistance. Fertil Steril 41:385, 1984

55. Geffner ME, Kaplan SA, Bersch N et al: Persistence of insulin resistance in polycystic ovarian disease after inhibition of ovarian steroid secretion. Fertil Steril 45:327, 1986

56. Dunaif A, Green G, Futterweit W et al: Suppression of hyperandrogenism does not improve peripheral or hepatic insulin resistance in the polycystic ovary syndrome. J Clin Endocrinol Metab 70:699, 1990

57. Franks S: Polycystic ovarian syndrome: A changing perspective. Clin Endocrinol 31:87, 1989

58. Barbieri RL, Markris A, Randal RW et al: Insulin stimulates androgen accumulation in incubations of ovarian stroma obtained from women with hyperandrogenism. J Clin Endocrinol Metab 62:904, 1986

59. Poretsky L, Kalin MF: The gonadotropic function of insulin. Endocr Rev 8:132, 1987

60. Rowland DL, Perrings TS, Thomas JA: Comparison of androgenic effects on food intake and body weight in adult rats. Physiol Behav 24:205, 1980

61. James WPT, Trayhurn P: Thermogenesis and obesity. Br Med Bull 37:43, 1981

62. Jung RT, Setty PS, James WTT: Reduced thermogenesis in obesity. Nature 279:322, 1979

63. Kirschner MA, Samjolik E, Silber D: A comparison of androgen production and clearance in hirsute and obese women. J Steroid Biochem 19:607, 1983

64. Samjolik E, Kirschner MA, Siber D et al: Elevated production and metabolic clearance rates of androgens in morbidly obese women. J Clin Endocrinol Metab 59:949, 1984

65. Louvet JP, Harman SM, Schreiber JR et al: Evidence for a role of androgens in follicular maturation. Endocrinology 97:366, 1975

66. Zhang Y, Ster B, Rebar RW: Endocrine comparison

of obese menstruating and amenorrheic women. J Clin Endocrinol Metab 58:1077, 1984

67. Kurtz BR, Givens JR, Kamidr S et al: Maintenance of normal circulating levels of androstenedione and dehydroepiandrosterone in simple obesity despite increased metabolic clearance rates: Evidence for a servo-control mechanism. J Clin Endocrinol Metab 64:1261, 1987

68. Hossenian AH, Kim MH, Rosenfield RL: Obesity and oligomenorrhea are associated with hyperandrogenism independent of hirsutism. J Clin Endocrinol Metab 42:765, 1976

69. Kiddy DS, Sharp PS, White DM et al: Differences in clinical and endocrine features between obese and nonobese subjects with polycystic ovary syndrome: An analysis of 263 consecutive cases. Clin Endocrinol (in press)

70. Pasquali R, Antemucci D, Casimirri F et al: Clinical and hormonal characteristics of obese amenorrheic hyperandrogenic women before and after weight loss. J Clin Endocrinol Metab 68:173, 1989

71. Bates GW, Whitworth NS: Effect of body weight reduction on plasma androgens in obese, infertile women. Fert Steril 38:406, 1984

72. Harlass FE, Plymate SR, Fariss BL et al: Weight loss is associated with correction of gonadotropin and sex steroid abnormalities in the obese anovulatory female. Fert Steril 42:649, 1984

73. Mitchell GW, Rogers J: The influence of weight reduction on amenorrhea in obese women. N Engl J Med 249:835, 1953

74. Wild RA, Painter PC, Coulson PB et al: Lipoprotein lipid concentrations and cardiovascular risk in women with polycystic ovary syndrome. J Clin Endocrinol Metab 61:946, 1985

75. Mattsson L, Cullberg G, Hamberger L et al: Lipid metabolism in women with polycystic ovary syndrome: Possible implications for an increased risk of coronary heart disease. Fertil Steril 42:579, 1984

76. Graf MJ, Richards CJ, Brown V et al: The independent effects of hyperandrogenaemia, hyperinsulinaemia, and obesity on lipid and lipoprotein profiles in women. Clin Endocrinol 33:119, 1990

77. Bray GA, York DA: Hypothalamic and genetic obesity in experimental animals: An autonomic and endocrine hypothesis. Physiol Rev 59:719, 1979

78. Bar RS, Gorden P, Roth J et al: Fluctuations in the affinity and concentrations of insulin receptors on circulating monocytes of obese patients: Effects of starvation, refeeding, and dieting. J Clin Invest 58:1123, 1976

79. Dunaif A, Graf M: Insulin administration alters gonadal steroid metabolism independent of changes in gonadotropin secretion in insulin-resistant women with polycystic ovary syndrome. J Clin Invest 83:23, 1989

80. Stuart GA, Prince MJ, Peters EJ et al: Hyperinsulinemia and hyperandrogemia: In vivo androgen response to insulin infusion. Obstet Gynecol 699: 921, 1987

81. Ravussin E, Lillioja S, Knowler WC et al: Reduced rate of energy expenditure as a risk factor for body-weight gain. N Engl J Med 318:467, 1988

82. Roberts SB, Savage J, Coward WA et al: Energy expenditure and intake in infants born to lean and overweight mothers. N Engl J Med 318:461, 1988

83. Ravussin E, Bogardus C, Schwartz RS et al: Thermic effect of infused glucose and insulin in man. J Clin Invest 72:893, 1983

84. Ravussin E, Acheson KJ, Vernet O et al: Evidence that insulin resistance is responsible for the decreased thermic effect of glucose in human obesity. J Clin Invest 76:1268, 1985

85. Segal KR, Dunaif A: Resting metabolic rate and postprandial thermogenesis in polycystic ovary syndrome. Int J Obes 14:559, 1990

CHAPTER 52

Childhood Obesity

WILLIAM H. DIETZ

Pediatric obesity is among the most prevalent nutritional problems in the United States. Recent data indicate that the prevalence of childhood obesity, defined as a triceps skin-fold thickness above the 85th percentile, has increased by over 40% in the period from 1965 to 1980 in both children and adolescents.[1] This chapter summarizes the salient differences between children and adults with respect to the natural history, morbidity, and treatment of obesity.

NATURAL HISTORY

In contrast to adults, the onset of obesity in children occurs in the context of complex and interrelated physical, physiological, and psychosocial growth patterns. Factors that affect the onset of obesity probably operate in all of these domains, although few have been clearly specified. Further, because of the time, expense, and difficulties inherent in longitudinal studies, few studies have encompassed the entire period of childhood. Nonetheless, several observations become apparent from a review of the literature on this disorder.

With the exception of adolescence, childhood obesity appears to have a uniform onset throughout childhood.[2] Among adolescent girls, the onset of obesity appears increased. This observation is consistent with the increased deposition of fat that occurs in adolescence, and suggests that this process may pose an increased physiological risk.

The age at onset appears to affect the likelihood of persistence. Among children with later onset of obesity, persistence appears to increase, consistent with the canalization of growth and fatness[3] with age. The only exception has been a report indicating that approximately one third of all children with increased rates of growth in the first year of life went on to develop adult obesity.[4] The second major factor that appears to affect the risk of persistence is severity. Among Swedish boys, the risk of persistence after seven years was directly proportional to the degree of severity of the obesity.[5]

An earlier study of English children hospitalized or seen for pediatric obesity indicated an approximately 20% chance of remission in adulthood.[6] However, in a complete follow-up study of over 500 overweight children ages 0 to 16 years who were admitted to the hospital as children and restudied after 40 years,[7] there was a 34% remission rate for subjects more than 5 SD from mean weight for height in childhood. Some 47% of those with a weight for height more than 5 SD above mean weight for height were still obese 40 years later.

These data emphasize that childhood obesity is a significant risk factor for obesity in adulthood and that the risk of persistence may rise with age. Because the severity of adult obesity may be greater in adults who had adolescent-onset obesity,[8] treatment and prevention of childhood- and adolescent-onset obesity may have a major impact on adult disease.

AFTEREFFECTS

Because children and adolescents grow rapidly, it is not surprising that childhood obesity has a major impact on several different but related aspects of growth. Obese children tend to be taller than their nonobese peers.[9] This consequence may be of some benefit to boys in a society where height is valued; it also serves as a screen to rule out endogenous causes of obesity. Most endocrinologic causes of obesity such as hypothyroidism, hypercortisolism, and genetic syndromes are associated with short stature.

A second major consequence of obesity is that the increase in fatness is accompanied by an increase in fat-free mass (FFM).[10] The increase in FFM may promote increased frame size. In addition, increases in FFM increase resting metabolic rate and, as a consequence, total energy expenditure.[11] The increase in FFM may also become a significant source of morbidity. At least one report has found that the association of FFM with blood pressure is greater than the association of fat with blood pressure.[12]

Bone age is advanced in obese children and adolescents. Whether advanced bone age reduces adult stature because of early epiphysial closure is not clear. Nonetheless, the advanced bone age is consistent with the increase in height. Whether the effects of obesity on height, FFM, and bone age are consequent on the trophic effects of overnutrition or result from the adaptation to increased to the trophic weight-bearing remains unclear. A final consequence of childhood obesity in females is early menarche.[13] This problem may make it difficult to differentiate an endocrinopathy from exogenous obesity.

Because bone in early childhood is predominantly cartilaginous, weight-bearing in obese children may be associated with several adverse orthopedic consequences. Among these is Blount's disease, a condition caused by a condition of bowed tibia associated with medial beaking. Although Blount's disease appears to have a genetic basis, approximately 80% of all children with Blount's disease are obese.[14] The degree of adiposity appears to have a direct and significant effect on the severity of the bowing. A second major problem is the slipped capital femoral epiphysis in adolescents.[15] Slippage probably results from increased stress across the growth plate.

The most prevalent consequences of childhood obesity are psychosocial. Few problems in childhood have as significant an impact on growth and development and psychosocial functioning as obesity in a child. Early studies demonstrated that children as young as five years of age had learned to associate obesity with a variety of negative characteristics.[16] The images of ideal weight are probably reinforced by images of thinness on television. The virtual absence of overweight characters on television may also contribute to the image of what constitutes an ideal weight and appearance for adolescent girls.

The major health consequences of obesity in adolescents are related to the adverse cardiovascular effects of the disease. In contrast to adults, fat distribution in children may not have as significant an impact on the development of cardiovascular complications. In part this may be due to the normal central distribution of fat that occurs with adolescence.[17] In addition, because the cardiovascular effects occur with lower prevalence in adolescents than in adults, the sample size in which these effects must be studied must be considerably larger.

Hyperlipidemia occurs in approximately one third of all adolescents, and there is some suggestion that the prevalence of hyperlipidemia is increased in obese adolescents.[18] Consistent with findings in adults, levels of low-density lipoprotein are increased and levels of high-density lipoprotein are decreased. Whether this pattern reflects decreased fitness, an increase in fatness, or both remains unclear.

Although hypertension occurs with a prevalence of approximately 1% to 2% in adolescents, obese adolescents account for approximately 50% of all cases of adolescent hypertension.[19] Although substantial follow-up data on obese adolescents are lacking, at least one group has described a significant prevalence of adverse cardiovascular consequences in a group of obese hypertensive adolescents.[20]

The prevalence of glucose intolerance is unclear. Diabetes mellitus is clearly a risk in patients with Prader-Willi syndrome. In addition, we have observed four cases of type II diabetes mellitus in massively obese adolescents with a very strong family history of diabetes. Attempts to link fat distribution to abnormal glucose tolerance have been confounded by the absence of controls for body fat.

TREATMENT

In childhood obesity, both the focus and approach to treatment are probably age dependent. For example, in the family of a young child, the most appropriate focus is parental food purchasing, food preparation, and food availability. However, focusing on the parents may be counterproductive if the adolescent is in the process of achieving autonomy. Therefore, it is essential at the outset of therapy to consider a broader system that surrounds the obese pediatric patient rather than the individual.

Because of the long-term nature of weight reduction, it is appropriate to focus dietary therapy on the family rather than on the individual. Appropriate techniques would include the elimination of high caloric density foods as well as attention to portion sizes for the entire family rather than for just the obese child or adolescent. Such an approach may help to reduce the possibility that the child or adolescent will become the family's scapegoat and be blamed for the family's inability to consume highly desirable foods. In this context, the elimination of high caloric density foods may be more appropriate than the use of a balanced calorie deficit diet focused on the child. Changes in life-style, including permanent alterations in diet, represent a more appropriate target than short-term behavior changes.

A large body of experimental data produced by Epstein and his co-workers at the University of Pittsburgh has demonstrated clearly the utility of behavior modification that focuses on both parent and child.[21] In multiple studies conducted over a number of years, programs that incorporated diet, exercise, and life-style counseling had a significant impact on long-term weight reduction. In the short term, no apparent differences existed with any of these therapeutic modalities.

In our experience, highly restrictive diets must be used with extreme caution. Little is known regarding the cardiovascular response to hypocaloric dietary therapy. Furthermore, the importance of an adequate diet during weight reduction in adolescents who are in a phase of rapid growth is preeminent. Very restrictive hypocaloric diets probably should be used only experimentally or to redress conditions in which rapid weight reduction is essential. Such conditions include massive obesity with either sleep apnea, primary alveolar hypoventilation, or hypertension.

Finally, surgery plays only a limited role in the management of such patients. On long-term follow-up of nine adolescent patients with exogenous obesity who underwent gastric bypass surgery, four maintained their weight reduction after five years; one of the four became anorectic. Three subjects regained their weight, and one was lost to further follow-up. No major complications of surgery were observed. Nonetheless, we approach surgical management of such patients with extreme caution.

References

1. Gortmaker SL, Dietz WH, Sobol AM et al: Increasing pediatric obesity in the United States. Am J Dis Child 141:535, 1987
2. Dietz WH Jr: Obesity in infants, children and adolescents in the United States. I. Identification, natural history and aftereffects. Nutr Res 1:117, 1981
3. Zack PM, Harlan WR, Leaverton PE et al: A longitudinal study of body fatness in childhood and adolescence. J Pediatr 95:126, 1979
4. Charney E, Goodman HC, McBride M et al: Childhood antecedents of adult obesity. N Engl J Med 295:6, 1976
5. Borjeson M: Overweight children. Acta Paediatr 51(suppl 132), 1962
6. Lloyd JL, Wolff OH, Whelan WS: Childhood obesity. Br Med J 2:145, 1961
7. Mossberg HO: 40-year follow-up of overweight children. Lancet 2:491, 1989
8. Rimm IJ, Rimm AA: Association between juvenile onset obesity and severe adult obesity in 73,532 women. Am J Public Health 66:479, 1976
9. Forbes GB: Nutrition and growth. J Pediatr 91:40, 1977
10. Forbes GB: Lean body mass and fat in obese children. Pediatrics 34:308, 1964
11. Bandini LG, Schoeller DA, Dietz WH: Energy expenditure in obese and nonobese adolescents. Pediatr Res 27:198, 1990
12. Weinsier RL, Norrs DJ, Barch R et al: Obesity and hypertension. Hypertension 7:578, 1985
13. Ellison PT: Skeletal growth, fatness, and menarcheal age: A comparison of two hypotheses. Hum Biol 54:269, 1982
14. Dietz WH Jr, Gross WL, Kirkpatrick JA Jr: Blount disease (tibia vara): Another skeletal disorder asso-

ciated with childhood obesity. J Pediatr 101:735, 1982

15. Cheung S: Diseases of the developing hip joint. Pediatr Clin North Am 24:857, 1977

16. Goodman N, Dornbusch SM, Richardson SA et al: Variant reactions to physical disabilities. Am Soc Rev 28:429, 1963

17. Mueller WH: Changes with age of the anatomical distribution of fat. Soc Sci Med 16:191, 1982

18. Laskarzewski P, Morrison JA, Mellies MJ et al: Relationships of measurements of body mass to plasma lipoproteins in school children and adults. Am J Epidemiol 111:395, 1980

19. Rames LK, Clarke WR, Cannon WE et al: Normal blood pressures and the evaluation of sustained blood pressure elevation in childhood: The Muscatine study. Pediatrics 61:245, 1978

20. Heyden S, Bertel AG, Hames CG et al: Elevated blood pressure levels in adolescents: Evans County, Georgia. JAMA 209:1683, 1969

21. Epstein LH, Wing RR, Valaski A: Childhood obesity. Pediatr Clin North Am 32:363, 1985

CHAPTER 53

Obesity Among
North American Indians

GAIL G. HARRISON and CHERYL K. RITENBAUGH

Native peoples in North America constitute more than 500 politically distinct tribes that can be grouped into a smaller number of linguistically or culturally related groups. They are relatively small populations, ranging from 900 for the Hualapai of northwestern Arizona to more than 190,000 for the Navajo nation of Arizona, Utah, and New Mexico.[1,2] Among North American native tribes and individuals one can find the full range of modernization or distance from the traditional way of life. Shared characteristics, particularly among reservation-dwelling people, are a generally low economic status, including high rates of unemployment and low per-capita incomes; the persistence of marginal to moderate nutritional deficiency conditions along with high rates of obesity and diabetes; and rapid changes in life-style over the last several decades and continuing through the present.

Obesity among North American native populations is an epidemiologically unique phenomenon characterized by relatively recent onset and variable but generally very high prevalence. In most tribes for which sufficient data are available, the onset of obesity as a common phenomenon has occurred in the last 40 to 50 years, accompanied by increased incidences of obesity-related morbidity.[3-7] Similar patterns of type II diabetes (adult-onset, non–insulin-dependent diabetes mellitus; NIDDM) in many of the same tribes has led some to assume a causal link.[5] Recent work indicates, however, that obesity is not the only antecedent to insulin

resistance and the development of NIDDM in Indian populations[7-9]; insulin resistance appears to characterize all Indians, independently of adiposity, and it is likely that the insulin resistance contributes to the development of obesity rather than the other way around. There is increasing evidence that despite the efforts of some health professionals and some tribes to institute preventive programs, obesity and its complications are increasing and occurring at younger ages.

HISTORY OF NORTH AMERICAN NATIVE PEOPLES

Ancestors of today's American Indian people appear to have entered North America in three distinct waves between 20,000 and 4000 years ago.[9] All had to enter across the Bering land bridge from northeastern Asia. Laughlin and Wolf,[10] using archaeological and ecological evidence, suggest that each of these founding populations consisted of only 60 to 200 individuals. Studies on mitochondrial DNA (mtDNA), which is inherited solely through the mother, show close associations between American Indian and Asian mtDNA and a high prevalence of rare Asian mtDNA in American Indian populations, supporting the conclusions that American Indians are direct descendants of a small number of female lineages from Asian aboriginal populations.[11]

The life-style of the original small groups of American Indians would necessarily have been

610

high in energy cost and based on nomadic hunting and gathering. In the far northern regions of the continent, diets would have been similar to the traditional diets of today's less acculturated far northern tribes, i.e., very high in animal protein, moderate in fat, and relatively lacking in carbohydrates.[12,13] Food availability would have been variable, with both seasonal and cyclic severe dietary stress, including periods (late winter and early spring) during which lean meat may have been virtually the only food available.[11] Young[14] speculates that the diet of sub-Arctic Canadian Indians up until European contact was probably very high in meat and fish, and that they likely did not suffer from chronic malnutrition, although acute starvation was intermittent.

By the early 18th century, traders' and explorers' journals began to provide some account of the health of American Indian peoples.[14,15] The picture that emerges with near unanimity is one of robust health with a relatively low burden of infectious illness; this conclusion is supported by Hrdlička's findings that thousands of pre-Columbian American Indian skeletons were apparently disease-free.[16] There is little doubt that the peoples of North America were spared the ravages of the epidemics that swept Europe during the Middle Ages. Parasitic diseases were likely present but not at high levels, with lack of concentrations of either favorable conditions or intermediate animal hosts. Mortality was not necessarily low or life expectancy high, but violence and accidents played major roles in mortality.[17]

The introduction of infectious illnesses by European contact had devastating effects on Native American populations, often reducing tribes to a fraction of their size in a short period of time and providing a repetitive cycle over several centuries of potential rapid genetic change. Smallpox was the first of these diseases to appear, and it behaved in a typical "virgin soil" epidemic fashion, producing a very high mortality in young, productive adults as well as in traditionally vulnerable groups such as children and the elderly. The first historically recorded smallpox epidemics in eastern Canada were in the 17th century,[18] but there may have been major epidemics prior to this.[19] Efforts to curb the spread of smallpox in the American Southwestern Territories in the

early 1800s by U.S. military physicians eventually resulted in the 1832 treaty which formed the basis for the administration of medical care for Native American peoples by the U.S. federal government.[20] During the 19th century, many more documented epidemics occurred as measles, influenza, pertussis, and scarlet fever in addition to smallpox took regular toll of the Indians and substantially reduced population numbers.[14] These diseases may have been spread widely in the New World by indirect contact among tribes after initial European contact. That is, it was possible for a tribe to experience a devastating epidemic of a disease introduced to the continent by Europeans long before coming face to face with a European. Tuberculosis and sexually transmitted diseases took their place in the repertoire of infectious burden on American Indian peoples somewhat later.

By the beginning of the 20th century, accounts of the health of Native American peoples were dismal indeed. Settled communities living in very poor sanitary conditions, with a high incidence of tuberculosis, skin infections, and gastrointestinal and respiratory illnesses, are described repeatedly. Nutritional status, when mentioned, appeared to be compromised. An early account of northern Ontario Indians described individuals "far below the average size and weight of the white man, their muscles and bones undeveloped . . . ."[15] Obesity is largely absent from travelers' descriptions, paintings, and early photographs of American Indians during the 19th and early 20th centuries,[21] although Hrdlička does document some obesity among Ute and Pima in the early 20th century.[16]

Joslin in 1940 studied the "Arizona Indian" population (Pima and Papago) and concluded that diabetes was no more prevalent among them than in the rest of the American people; he did not remark either on any unusual prevalence of obesity.[22] As recently as the 1950s, Darby et al noted an obesity prevalence of less than 5% among Navajo men and only about 15% in women.[23] Undernutrition among American Indian groups received some attention in the 1960s and early 1970s; frank malnutrition in the form of kwashiorkor and marasmus was reported in Navajo children in alarming proportions.[24-26] Butte et al studied the nutritional status and diets of pregnant and lactating Navajo women in 1976–1977 and found a high prevalence of mild nutrient deficiencies, notably in iron, vitamin A, folic acid, and zinc.[27] A study of White Mountain Apache preschool children in eastern Arizona in 1979 showed low biochemical indices of nutrient status in 15% to 25% of children for one or more micronutrients and an apparently stunted population, with one third of children below the 10th percentile of U.S. standards for height for age.[28]

By the mid- to late 1980s, a number of improvements in health care and health status among American Indians were evident. Infant and maternal mortality now approximate the national averages, reflecting major improvements in the delivery of primary health care and in the availability of clean water and adequate housing for most reservation-dwelling people. Injuries, substance abuse, and chronic disease are now the major Indian health problems; obesity and diabetes lead the list of health problems, with diabetes and hypertension the leading reasons for outpatient visits to Indian Health Service facilities.[29]

PREVALENCE OF OBESITY IN CONTEMPORARY AMERICAN INDIANS

Although there has been no general survey of obesity in U.S. and Canadian native peoples, there is an abundant literature on prevalence levels in different groups. By the standards traditionally used in the epidemiologic study of obesity, a majority of adults in most tribes are obese. Between 1972 and 1979, 2095 adults representing more than 15 tribes in Oklahoma were screened for diabetes[30]; 77% were obese. The average weight for height was 145% of the reference standard. Rates were slightly higher in diabetic than nondiabetic individuals and higher in women than in men. A community health screening among the Zuni in 1988 found that 55% of women ages 21 to 40 years and 29% of men of the same age were obese; among adults over age 40, two thirds of women and 35% of men were obese. Among young Zuni Indians ages 11 to 20, more than half of girls and more than one third of boys were obese.[31] Other studies have noted prevalences of obesity higher than

50% in adults among Seminoles,[32] Canadian Cree and Ojibwa,[6] Cocopah,[33] and Pima.[34] The latter group, the Pima of Arizona, have the highest known rate of NIDDM of any group in the world.

When body fat patterning has been studied, it has been clear that most American Indian adiposity is of the central or abdominal type. Two investigators have studied fat patterning in relation to differential outcomes. Teufel and Dufour[2] studied dietary patterns among obese Hualapai women compared with nonobese controls matched for age and percentage of Hualapai ancestry; they found that the obese women had higher waist-to-hip ratios than the nonobese. Szathmary and Holt[12] found that among the Dogrib of the Northwest Territories of Canada, a group that has only recently begun incorporating nontraditional elements into its diet and still has low levels of obesity and almost no diabetes, subjects with fasting hyperglycemia had a more centripetal distribution of body fat than did normoglycemic subjects.

Obesity is a well-identified problem among children and adolescents in many Indian groups. Story et al[35] found that half of Cherokee boys and one third of girls ages 13 to 17 years had triceps skin-fold measurements above the 85th percentile of the reference population. Pettitt et al[36] identified a strongly increased risk of obesity in Pima children whose mothers were diabetic prior to pregnancy, indicating that the cycle of diabetes and obesity may be perpetuated intergenerationally. Nutrition surveillance data from the federal Women, Infants and Children (WIC) supplementary feeding program, instituted in the mid-1970s, and other public health programs substantiate that Native American children are, in general, shorter than the general U.S. population of children and prone to be relatively heavy for height and length, and that these differences are evident from very early life.[37] We found among Arizona infants between one and two years of age in 1978 and 1979 that the prevalence of short stature and high weight for length was greater for American Indian than for Hispanic or Anglo infants, even when birth weight (which is high in American Indians) was controlled for.[38] As might be expected if there were a strong genetic component to body size and proportion variability in children, Hispanic children in the Southwest tended to show intermediate prevalences of both short stature and heaviness for height.[37,38] Navajo infants studied between 1975 and 1980 had low length for age and high weight for length relative to the reference population.[39] The data on changes over time are much more sparse, but a follow-up survey in 1976 of White Mountain Apache, after the 1969 survey cited earlier,[28] found that nutritional status had generally improved in the intervening years, along with improvements in health care, housing, and general conditions on the reservation; but that age-adjusted stature remained identical, and short relative to U.S. reference standards. Skin-fold thicknesses were greater among preschool children than they had been seven years earlier.[40]

DIETARY PATTERNS IN AMERICAN INDIAN POPULATIONS

Dietary information on American Indian populations is relatively limited, since Native Americans are not adequately represented in national surveys and our information depends entirely on published studies in particular groups. A small number of relatively thorough studies on dietary intake in different reservation-dwelling groups in the last two decades have been published, and a few of these have specifically compared obese and nonobese individuals. In general, energy intakes are unremarkable and fat intakes are either similar to or lower than those in the general U.S. population.

Story et al[35] compared intakes of obese and nonobese Cherokee adolescents in North Carolina and found no differences between the two groups in energy intake or proximate composition of the diet. Butte et al[27] and Wolfe and Sanjur[41] independently studied the food and nutrient intakes of reservation-dwelling Navajo women. Butte et al studied pregnant and lactating women and found median energy intakes of 2406 kilocalories at term and 1911 kcal/day at one month post partum (100% of the RDA for pregnancy, and 82% for lactation). Diets averaged 16% of energy from protein, 37% from fat, and 47% from carbohydrate.[27] Wolfe and Sanjur found a median energy intake of 1542 kilocalo-

ries among 107 nonpregnant Navajo women, comparable with median energy intakes among U.S. women in national samples and also comparable with the data reported by Bass and Wakefield on women on the Standing Rock Reservation in North Dakota.[42]

Among the Dogrib Indians of the Northwest Territories of Canada, where there is still relatively little obesity, Szathmary et al[13] observed energy intakes of 2528 kcal/day and 1843 kcal/day respectively among adult men and women in the summer; proximate composition was more unusual, with 31% of energy from protein, 33% from fat, and 36% from carbohydrate. Dietary acculturation among the Dogrib was associated with increased caloric intake, as Western foods supplemented rather than replaced the traditional diet.

Teufel and Dufour,[2] in a careful study of dietary intakes of obese and nonobese Hualapai women, found significantly higher intakes among obese women (median, 2866 kcal/day, vs. 2367 kcal/day for nonobese women). Energy intake per unit of lean body mass was similar for the two groups. The difference in energy intake between the obese and nonobese women was accounted for by higher consumption of both nonalcoholic and alcoholic beverages by the former group.

EVOLUTIONARY CONSIDERATIONS

That there is a genetic susceptibility to obesity among American Indians is well accepted; the origins of this susceptibility and plausible explanations for its recent expression are becoming increasingly clear. In populations that undergo periodic food stresses, the individuals who are best able to increase adipose stores during times of high energy availability will have a selective advantage. In 1962, J.V. Neel theorized that American Indian populations were characterized by a "thrifty gene," a rapid-storage metabolic genotype that would have had a marked selective advantage for early aboriginal populations.[43] His concept has been more recently updated[44] and is routinely cited in the literature on American Indian obesity and diabetes. However, a specific biochemical variant deriving from this hypothesized genotype has not yet been described.

Weiss et al[8] put the hypothesis in broader context when they described the "New World syndrome," a complex of conditions with unusually high prevalence among American Indians. The conditions that make up the New World syndrome include obesity, gallstones, gallbladder cancer, abnormalities of cholesterol metabolism, and NIDDM; Weiss et al hypothesized that these co-occurring conditions increase together in prevalence in Native American peoples in proportion to the degree of modernization of lifestyle and suggested that some underlying abnormality in lipid metabolism must be responsible for the syndrome, in interaction with modern diet and exercise patterns.

Most theorists attempting to explain the particular morbidity and obesity patterns among modern American Indians have focused on these populations in their relatively recent agriculture-based settings and even more recent cash economies. Szathmary[45] has pointed out the need to take into account that founder effects would also have occurred during a much earlier period, and the specific selective pressures would have been those of the northern hunting adaptation, namely the extreme and chronic shortage of dietary carbohydrate in conjunction with intermittent total energy shortage. And Weiss et al[8] have described well the evolutionary setting which existed prior to and early in the history of human habitation of the New World, which were ideal for rapid evolutionary change based on founder effect, genetic drift, and selection: small, isolated populations; a population bottleneck with migration to the new continent; and environmental conditions characterized by seasonal or sporadic availability of food sources and the harsh Arctic climate.

Ritenbaugh and Goodby[46] have further elucidated possible mechanisms by which an adaptation favoring the storage of fat could have failed to express itself as obesity in noticeable proportions through the transition to agriculture, only to become manifest in the permissive environment of the sedentary, modern life-styles that characterize modern-day American Indian peoples. Basically, their hypothesis is that high energy demands suppressed the expression of obesity until very recently. Indeed, Amerindian

groups that maintain relatively traditional life-styles, such as the Dogrib, maintain low prevalences of both obesity and diabetes. The Navajo, which have the lowest prevalences in the Southwest, continue a tradition of scattered housing on a large and remote reservation. Accepted aspects of life for many still include hauling water and fuel, splitting wood, herding sheep and goats, weaving, and small-scale agriculture. Among the Hopi, it is anecdotally reported that the least obese and most healthy elders are those pursuing a traditional life-style, including farming and walking, and a traditional diet.[47] Movement into the modern life-style is associated with creeping obesity and failing health.[48] Even the northernmost tribes (Aleuts, Eskimos, Northern Athabaskans) are now showing evidence of this pattern.[49]

RELATION OF NIDDM TO OBESITY IN AMERICAN INDIANS

Table 53-1 shows the rates of NIDDM estimated in the 1980s across a range of American Indian populations. Except where noted, these prevalence rates (per 100) are based on clinical diagnoses rather than population screening. Considerable effort has focused on determining the mechanisms underlying the broad range of prevalences still observable, especially since the rates seem to be rising in all but the most severely affected populations. In nearly all situations, NIDDM is associated with obesity, but the correlation is not perfect; where studied, NIDDM has also been found to be strongly associated with centripetal fat patterning.

The search for a genetic mechanism has been a continuing focus of effort. Szathmary[53] investigated the Gc locus which regulates the binding of dihydroxycholecalciferol to insulin receptors and which was hypothesized to affect carbohydrate metabolism. She showed that, among the Dogrib, the lowest fasting insulin levels were found in individuals homozygous for Gc1F. However, a study in the San Luis Valley of Colorado of Anglos and Mexican-Americans with Indian admixture showed that subjects with the Gc1F homozygote had the highest fasting glucose levels, and no difference in insulin.[54] Aside from

TABLE 53-1

Prevalence of Noninsulin-Dependent Diabetes Mellitus Among American Indian Adults, Based on Clinical Diagnosis (Percent of Population Over 35 Years)

Pueblos[50,*]		Pima[50,*]	49.5
Cochiti	25.0		
Isleta	17.8	Athabaskans	
Jemez	13.8	Jicarilla Apache[50,*]	9.8
Nambe	14.7	Mescalero Apache[50,*]	16.4
Picuris	17.0	Alamo Navajo[50,*]	16.5
Pojoaque	14.6	Navajo (Navajo Nation)[51,*,†]	16.9
San Felipe	22.8	Alaska Indians[49,*]	4.0
San Ildefonso	13.8	Dogrib (NWT)[13,*]	5.1
San Juan	17.1		
Sandia	31.5	Cree-Ojibwa (Canada)[52,†,‡]	11.6
Santa Ana	31.4		
Santa Clara	30.7	Eskimos (Alaska)[49,*]	1.7
Santo Domingo	22.6		
Taos	27.6	Aleuts (Alaska)[49,*]	4.8
Tesuque	31.2		
Zia	23.4		
Zuni	28.2		

*Crude rates.
†Over 45 years of age.
‡Age-adjusted rates.

this locus, no standard genetic variant has been shown to be associated with NIDDM in American Indians.[55]

Recently, attention has turned to investigating variations in energy expenditure that may be associated with increased obesity and NIDDM. Ravussin et al showed that lowered resting metabolic rates clustered in Pima families,[56] and that rates lower than the population norms were predictive of weight gain in the subsequent five years.[57] In a study of the thermic effect of glucose and insulin infusion, healthy Pima Indians had a lower thermic response to low-dose insulin infusion than Anglos (when matched exactly on body mass factors), suggesting possible lower thermic response within the dietary range.[58] This would also tend to lower metabolic requirements. Few studies have examined exercise-related responses in energy expenditure or metabolism. A tribal exercise project was begun at Zuni in 1985 with strikingly positive results in terms of decreasing fasting glucose and medica-

tion requirements among participants, despite an average weight loss of only 4 kg.[31,59] Recent studies of Anglos with NIDDM suggest impaired muscle glycogen synthesis in comparison to normal controls[60]; a similar pattern was suggested in Pima Indians after overfeeding.[61] Together these studies suggest that an important component of the obesity-NIDDM picture may be mediated through energy expenditure, both resting and related to skeletal muscle activity.

Metabolic responses associated with different dietary patterns have been evaluated in terms of their relationship to obesity and NIDDM. Among the Pima, acute overfeeding led to elevated fasting insulin levels with no changes in glucose levels, perhaps due to decreased activity of glycogen synthetase.[61] When Pima Indians with and without NIDDM were given high-carbohydrate (65% of energy) or high-fat (42% of energy) diets, no differences in 24-hour energy expenditures were observed.[62] However, in another study comparing healthy Indians to healthy Anglos, there was

a lower thermic response to low-dose insulin infusion, suggesting a blunted thermic effect of
food and perhaps accounting for the lack of difference seen in response to the diets.[58] A recent
evaluation of the glycemic effect of traditional
Pima foods compared to the current Western diet
showed that the traditional diet had a far lower
glycemic index, due particularly to a higher
quantity of soluble fiber, slowing glucose absorption.[63] This suggests that, for Indians, part of the
acculturation stress of the modern U.S. diet may
be related to its rapid absorbability.

In summary, more than 20 years of research
have failed to show a single major difference in
metabolic processes between Indians and Anglos
that alone would account for the greatly elevated
rates of obesity and NIDDM in these populations.
However, a combination of factors, each contributing smaller amounts of variance, is beginning
to emerge. These factors include lowered energy
expenditure in resting and postprandial states;
recent increases in sedentariness and greater sensitivity to the effects of sedentariness, perhaps
due to decreased glycogen synthetase activity;
and higher energy intakes, especially of rapidly
absorbed carbohydrate sources (soft drinks,
snacks) and fats. Population prevalence rates appear to be highest in settings where exposure to
these factors has been longest, especially where
the current adults were exposed in childhood.
Children born of diabetic mothers (gestational or
NIDDM) in these environments seem to have
even greater risks of developing NIDDM.

The picture that is appearing seems to be a
positive feedback loop, with intergenerational effects magnifying intragenerational ones. Although exact biochemical mechanisms are not
clear, consensus is growing among tribal leaders,
IHS directors, and diabetes researchers that the
time has come for designing and testing prevention strategies that focus on life-style and obesity
factors. Such studies will contribute much to elu-
cidating the biochemical bases of American Indian obesity and NIDDM.

References

1. Jackson MY, Broussard BA: Cultural challenges in
   nutrition education among American Indians. Diabetes Educator 13:46, 1987

2. Teufel NI, Dufour DL: Patterns of food use and nutrient intake of obese and non-obese Hualapai Indian women of Arizona. J Am Diet Assoc 90:1229,
   1990
3. Sievers ML, Fisher JR: Diseases of North American
   Indians. In Rothschild HR (ed): Biocultural Aspects of Disease. New York, Academic Press, 1981
4. Jackson MY: Nutrition in American Indian health:
   Past, present, and future. J Am Diet Assoc 86:1561,
   1986
5. West KM: Diabetes in American Indians and other
   native populations. Diabetes 23:841, 1974
6. Young T, Sevenheysen G: Obesity in northern Canadian Indians: Patterns, determinants, and consequences. Am J Clin Nutr 49:789, 1989
7. Saad MF, Knowler WC, Pettitt DJ et al: The natural
   history of impaired glucose tolerance in the Pima
   Indians. N Engl J Med 319:1500, 1988
8. Weiss KM, Ferrell RE, Hanis CL: A New World
   syndrome of metabolic diseases with a genetic and
   evolutionary basis. Yearbook Phys Anthropol 27:
   153, 1984
9. Wendorf M: Diabetes, the ice-free corridor, and paleoindian settlements of North America. Am J Phys
   Anthropol 79:503, 1989
10. Laughlin WS, Wolf SI: The first Americans: Ori-
    gins, affinities and adaptations. In Laughlin WS,
    Harper AB (eds): The First Americans: Origins,
    Affinities and Adaptations. New York, Gustav
    Fischer, 1979
11. Wallace DC, Garrison K, Knowler WC: Dramatic
    founder effects in Amerindian mitochondrial
    DNAs. Am J Phys Anthropol 63:149, 1985
12. Szathmary EJE, Holt N: Hyperglycemia in Dogrib
    Indians of the Northwest Territories, Canada: As-
    sociation with age and a centripetal distribution of
    body fat. Hum Biol 55:493, 1983
13. Szathmary EJE, Ritenbaugh C, Goodby CS: Dietary
    change and plasma glucose levels in an American
    population undergoing cultural transition. Soc Sci
    Med 24:791, 1987
14. Young TK: Are subarctic Indians undergoing the
    epidemiologic transition? Soc Sci Med 26:659,
    1988
15. Young TK: Changing patterns of health and sick-
    ness among the Cree-Ojibwa of northwestern On-
    tario. Med Anthropol 3:191, 1979
16. Hrdlička A: Disease, medicine and surgery among
    the American aborigines. JAMA 99:1661, 1932
17. Johansson SR: The demographic history of the Na-
    tive Peoples of North America: A selective bibliog-
    raphy. Yearbook Phys Anthropol 25:133, 1982
18. Dobyns HF: Their Number Become Thinned.
    Knoxville, Tenn., University of Tennessee Press,
    1983

19. Martin C: Keepers of the Game: Indian-Animal Relationships and the Fur Trade. Berkeley, University of California Press, 1978

20. Hoffman BH, Haskell AJ: The Papago Indians: Historical, social and medical perspectives. Mt Sinai J Med 51:707, 1984

21. West KM: Diabetes in American Indians. Adv Metab Dis 9:29, 1978

22. Joslin EP: The universality of diabetes: A survey of diabetic mortality in Arizona. JAMA 115:2033, 1940

23. Darby WJ et al: A study of the dietary background and nutriture of the Navajo Indian. J Nutr 60(suppl 2):3, 1956

24. Wolfe CB: Kwashiorkor on the Navajo Indian reservation. Henry Ford Hosp Med Bull 9:566, 1961

25. Van Duzen J, Carter JP, Zwagg RV: Protein and calorie malnutrition among Navajo Indian children. Am J Clin Nutr 29:657, 1976

26. Van Duzen J, Carter MP, Secondi J et al: Protein and calorie malnutrition among preschool Navajo Indian children. Am J Clin Nutr 22:1362, 1969

27. Butte NF, Calloway DH, Van Duzen JL: Nutritional assessment of pregnant and lactating Navajo women. Am J Clin Nutr 34:2216, 1981

28. Owen GM, Nelsen CE, Kram KM et al: Nutrition survey of White Mountain Apache preschool children. In Moore WM, Silverberg MM, Read MS (eds): Nutrition, Growth and Development of North American Indian Children. DHEW publication No. NIH-72-26. Washington, DC, 1972

29. Rhoades ER, Hammond J, Welty TK et al: The Indian burden of illness and future health interventions. Public Health Rep 102:361, 1987

30. Lee ET, Anderson PS, Bryan J et al: Diabetes, parental diabetes, and obesity in Oklahoma Indians. Diabetes Care 8:107, 1985

31. Leonard B, Wilson R, Leonard C: Zuni diabetes project. Public Health Rep 101:282, 1986

32. Mayberry RH, Lindemann RD: A survey of chronic disease in Seminole Indians in Oklahoma. Am J Clin Nutr 13:127, 1963

33. Henry RE, Burch TA, Bennett PH et al: Diabetes in the Cocopah Indians. Diabetes 18:33, 1969

34. Knowler WC, Pettitt DJ, Bennett PH et al: Diabetes mellitus in the Pima Indians: Genetic and evolutionary considerations. Am J Phys Anthropol 62:107, 1983

35. Story M, Tompkins RA, Bass MA et al: Anthropometric measurements and dietary intakes of Cherokee Indian teenagers in North Carolina. J Am Diet Assoc 86:1555, 1986

36. Pettitt DJ, Baird R, Aleck KA et al: Excessive obesity in offspring of Pima Indian women with diabetes during pregnancy. N Engl J Med 308:242, 1983

37. Trowbridge FL: Prevalence of growth stunting and obesity: Pediatric nutrition surveillance system, 1982. MMWR 32:23SS, 1986

38. Harrison GG, White M: Overweight in Arizona infants: Association with birthweight and ethnic background. In Green L, Johnston FE (eds): Biological and Social Predictors of Growth, Development and Nutritional Status. New York, Academic Press, 1980

39. Peck RE, Marks JS, Dibley MJ et al: Birthweight and subsequent growth among Navajo children. Public Health Rep 102:500, 1987

40. Owen GM, Garry PJ, Seymoure RD et al: Nutrition studies with White Mountain Apache preschool children in 1976 and 1969. Am J Clin Nutr 34:266, 1981

41. Wolfe WA, Sanjur D: Contemporary diet and body weight of Navajo women receiving food assistance: An ethnographic and nutritional investigation. J Am Diet Assoc 88:822, 1988

42. Bass MA, Wakefield LM: Nutrient intake and food patterns of Indians on Standing Rock Reservation. J Am Diet Assoc 64:36, 1974

43. Neel JV: Diabetes mellitus: A "thrifty" genotype rendered detrimental by "progress." Am J Hum Genet 14:353, 1962

44. Neel JV: The thrifty genotype revisited. In Kobberling J, Tattersall R (eds): The Genetics of Diabetes Mellitus. Serono Symposium. New York, Academic Press, 1982

45. Szathmary EJE: The search for genetic factors controlling plasma glucose levels in Dogrib Indians. In Chakraborty R, Szathmary EJE (eds): Diseases of Complex Etiology in Small Populations: Ethnic Differences and Research Approaches. New York, Alan R Liss, 1985

46. Ritenbaugh C, Goodby CS: Beyond the thrifty gene: Metabolic implications of prehistoric migration routes into the New World. Med Anthropol 11:227, 1989

47. Ritenbaugh C: Use of clines in the analysis of diabetes. In Mai LL, Shanklin E, Sussman RW (eds): The Perception of Evolution. Los Angeles, UCLA Publications, 1981

48. Mohs ME, Leonard TK, Watson RR: Selected risk factors for diabetes in Native Americans. Nutr Res 5:1035, 1985

49. Schraer CD, Lanier AP, Boyko EJ et al: Prevalence of diabetes mellitus in Alaskan Eskimos, Indians and Aleuts. Diabetes Care 11(9):693, 1988

50. Carter J, Horowitz R, Wilson R et al: Tribal differences in diabetes: Prevalence among American Indians in New Mexico. Public Health Rep 104:665, 1989

51. Sugarman JR, Hickey M, Hall T et al: The changing

epidemiology of diabetes mellitus among Navajo Indians. West J Med 153:140, 1990

52. Young TK, McIntyre LL, Dooley J et al: Epidemiologic features of diabetes mellitus among Indians in northwestern Ontario and northeastern Manitoba. Can Med Assoc J 132:793, 1985

53. Szathmary EJE: The effect of Gc genotype on fasting insulin level in Dogrib Indians. Hum Genet 75:368, 1987

54. Iyengar S, Jamman RF, Marshall JA et al: On the role of vitamin D binding globulin in glucose homeostasis: Results from the San Luis Valley diabetes study. Genet Epidemiol 6:691, 1989

55. Iyengar S, Jamman RF, Marshall JA et al: Genetic studies of type 2 (non-insulin-dependent) diabetes mellitus: Lack of association with seven genetic markers. Diabetologia 32:690, 1989

56. Bogardus C, Lillioja S, Ravussin E et al: Familial dependence of the resting metabolic rate. N Engl J Med 315:96, 1986

57. Ravussin E, Lillioja S, Knowler WC et al: Reduced rate of energy expenditure as a risk factor for body-weight gain. N Engl J Med 318:467, 1988

58. Bogardus C, Lillioja S, Mott D et al: Evidence for reduced thermic effect of insulin and glucose infusions in Pima Indians. J Clin Invest 75:1264, 1985

59. Heath GW, Leonard BE, Wilson RH et al: Community-based exercise intervention: Zuni diabetes project. Diabetes Care 10:579, 1987

60. Shulman GI, Rothman DL, Jue T et al: Quantitation of muscle glycogen synthesis in normal subjects and subjects with non-insulin-dependent diabetes by ^{13}C nuclear magnetic resonance spectroscopy. N Engl J Med 322:223, 1990

61. Mott DM, Lillioja S, Bogardus C: Overnutrition induced decrease in insulin action for glucose storage: In vivo and in vitro in man. Metabolism 35:160, 1986

62. Abbott WGH, Howard BV, Ruotolo G et al: Energy expenditure in humans: Effects of dietary fat and carbohydrate. Am J Physiol 258 (Endocrinol Metab 21):E347, 1990

63. Brand JC, Snow BJ, Nabham G et al: Plasma glucose and insulin responses to traditional Pima Indian meals. Am J Clin Nutr 51:416, 1990

CHAPTER 54

Obesity in Pacific Populations

GARY DOWSE, PAUL ZIMMET, VERONICA COLLINS, and
CAROLINE FINCH

Obesity is not a new phenomenon in Pacific populations. For many centuries, Polynesian and Micronesian societies of this region have valued obesity as a symbol of high social status and prosperity.[1,2] However, obesity now occurs much more commonly in Pacific peoples as a result of rapid change from a traditional to a more modernized life-style. Therefore, any discussion of obesity in the Pacific must take into account the importance of social, cultural, and possibly genetic factors determining body size in these populations.

This review is largely confined to a consideration of the health ramifications of obesity in the indigenous inhabitants of the island states of the Western Pacific region. Ethnically and geographically, these people can be broadly divided into three major groups—Polynesians, Micronesians, and Melanesians (Fig. 54-1). They populated the region via South East Asia over several thousand years by a series of harrowing island-hopping canoe voyages.[3,4] Within each of these three groups, particularly the Melanesians, there is considerable genetic and cultural heterogeneity.

Contacts between Pacific islanders and European explorers were initially only transitory, but European settlement took place throughout the 19th and early 20th centuries, spurred by political and economic opportunism and missionary zeal. Early descriptions of islanders invariably referred to their good state of health and fine physiques.[2,5] Obesity of the order seen today would appear not to have been a problem.

More contemporary evidence, such as the paintings by Gauguin[6] of French Polynesians and early photographic records (Fig. 54-2), indicate that while people were not uniformly lean, neither were they as grossly obese as is now commonly seen. Even today, the more traditional rural inhabitants of a number of Pacific nations remain leaner than their relatively modernized peers.[7-12] Certainly the levels of obesity now observed in populations such as the Polynesians of Samoa,[7,8] Wallis Island,[11] and Rarotonga[12] and the Micronesians of Nauru[13] and Kiribati[9] are substantially higher than those seen in the Caucasian inhabitants of Australia[14,15] and the United States.[15]

To illustrate this, Figure 54-3 compares the mean body mass index (BMI) levels according to age decade and gender in four Pacific population samples with those of European-origin Australians from the Busselton community study. At all ages, each Pacific population is considerably more obese than the Australians. Levels in Nauruans, particularly the younger individuals, are especially extreme. In all but the Australians, the degree of obesity is more marked in females than in males.

The increase in the frequency and extent of obesity in the Pacific must be viewed in the context of the epidemic of noncommunicable diseases that has accompanied the modernization of life-style and development of cash economies in most countries in the region. Non-insulin-dependent diabetes mellitus (NIDDM), coronary

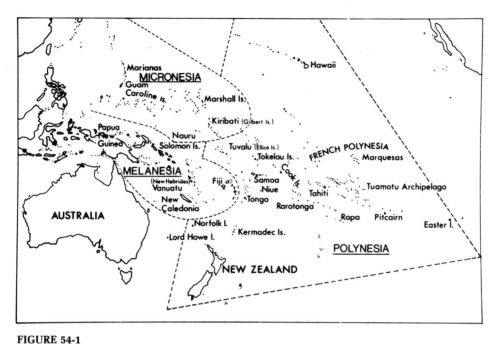

FIGURE 54-1

Map of the Pacific region showing major geographic and ethnic divisions.

heart disease (CHD), hypertension, stroke, and cancer (such as carcinomas of the cervix and lung), once unknown or rare, are now major causes of morbidity and mortality.[17-20] These diseases have now supplanted infectious diseases as the major causes of mortality in most Pacific populations. This change has profound social and economic implications for these fledgling nations, quite apart from the obvious health consequences. There is evidence that gains in life expectancy anticipated as a consequence of infectious disease control have not occurred in some countries because of the rising epidemic of life-style–related noncommunicable diseases.[18-20]

PREVALENCE OF OBESITY IN PACIFIC ISLANDERS

The recommended standards for obesity in European communities, themselves subject to debate,[21] may not be applicable to Pacific islanders. It has been suggested that a BMI of at least 30 kg/m^2 may most clearly define people with a high risk

of disease.[15] However, without more extensive research, it is difficult to determine appropriate standards for obesity in Pacific populations. Prospective studies should investigate the risk of premature mortality and other adverse health outcomes in relation to various measures and degrees of obesity. Comparison of such data with data already available for Europeans may yield a clearer picture of the significance of obesity in Pacific islanders. Some preliminary data from longitudinal studies in Nauru and Fiji are discussed later.

The prevalence data shown in Table 54-1 are from our studies conducted in the Pacific during the period 1976–1985 and are based on conventional obesity standards of a BMI of 27 kg/m^2 or higher in males and 25 kg/m^2 or higher in females, which approximate 120% of "desirable" weight as derived for Caucasians.[22] In nearly all the Pacific groups, the prevalence of obesity is substantially higher than in Caucasian communities, particularly in females. Notable exceptions include the highlanders of Papua New Guinea, whose life-style remains largely traditional and involves considerable habitual exertion.

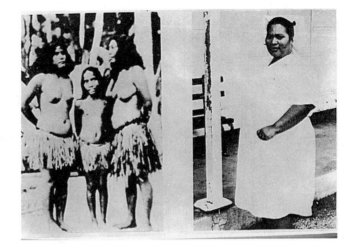

FIGURE 54-2

Nauruan women in 1925 (left) and 1979 (right). (From Zimmet P, Whitehouse S: Pacific islands of Nauru, Tuvalu and Western Samoa. In Trowell HC, Burkitt DP (eds): Western Diseases: Their Emergence and Prevention, p 204. London, Edward Arnold, 1981. Reproduced by permission.)

ANTECEDENTS OF OBESITY IN THE PACIFIC

Neel[23] hypothesized that the marked tendency to obesity observed in Pacific islanders and other traditional populations experiencing modernization represented the effect of a "thrifty genotype." This genotype would promote efficient storage of fat in times of plenty and afford a survival advantage in periods of hardship such as droughts, following hurricanes, and during long migratory canoe voyages. This hypothesis has neither been refuted nor proved, and the nature of the responsible gene(s) remains obscure. Nonetheless, the consistency with which obesity and associated metabolic abnormalities are observed in developing Pacific populations argues strongly for some genetic basis to the susceptibility.

The proposed genetic susceptibility interacts

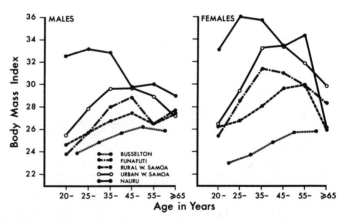

FIGURE 54-3

Mean body mass index (kg/m^2) by age group for males and females in Funafuti and Western Samoa (Polynesian), Nauru (Micronesian) and Busselton, Australia (caucasian). (From Zimmet P, Whitehouse S: Pacific islands of Nauru, Tuvalu and Western Samoa. In Trowell HC, Burkitt DP (eds): Western Diseases: Their Emergence and Prevention, p 204. London, Edward Arnold, 1981. Reproduced by permission.)

TABLE 54-1

Age-Standardized* Prevalence of Obesity in Pacific Populations
(Age ≥ 20 years)

Population		Males (BMI ≥ 27 kg/m²)		Females (BMI ≥ 25 kg/m²)	
		No.	Prevalence (%)	No.	Prevalence (%)
Micronesians					
Nauru		667	84.7	680	92.8
Kiribati	Urban	886	52.8	849	70.2
	Rural	465	24.4	515	41.5
Polynesians					
Western Samoa	Urban	324	48.6	396	78.9
	Rural	358	28.1	361	60.8
Cook Islands—Rarotonga		534	56.0	544	74.5
Niue		529	39.4	559	69.4
Loyalty Islands—Ouvea (part-Polynesians)		164	20.8	217	55.9
Wallis Islanders					
Noumea	Urban	253†	78.5	297	88.6
Wallis	Rural	261	36.0	255	77.0
Melanesians					
Fiji	Urban	399	30.7	442	65.2
	Rural	238	21.7	212	51.5
Loyalty Islands—Ouvea		228	20.6	285	58.2
New Caledonia					
Noumea	Urban	71†	46.5	81	69.8
Touho	Rural	90	9.8	81	36.9
PNG highlands	Periurban	118	18.0	139	23.5
	Rural	144	1.9	163	14.2
PNG coastal (Tolai)	Periurban	126	17.5	147	39.4
	Rural	126	12.1	143	34.8
Migrant Asian Indians					
Fiji	Urban	384	12.0	440	35.8
	Rural	213	7.0	223	31.6
Caucasians					
Australia (NHF)‡		2765	38.8	2838	26.8

*Standardized to Nauru Survey population.
†Ages 25 to 64 years only.
‡Based on a BMI ≥ 26 in both sexes, for ages 25 to 64 years. Data from NHF study.[14]

with diet and levels of physical activity, both of which are determined by cultural and socioeconomic factors. Anthropological evidence suggests that the Polynesians of Samoa do not in fact view obesity as desirable or healthy except in people of high status, in whom it is traditionally the norm.[24] This implies that the widespread obesity observed in Samoans is unlikely to result from commoners seeking status, as the community perception is that obesity should follow the attainment of status rather than precede it.[24]

Feasting and complex customary obligations regarding food and its consumption remain important in Pacific cultures, and these traditional practices may play a large role in the excess caloric intake observed in some populations. Hanna et al[25] suggested that the Samoan pattern of Sunday feasting was probably responsible for a continuing accumulation of excess calories, particularly in sedentary workers. In Micronesian Nauruans, a 24-hour dietary recall study found mean daily energy intakes of 7191 kcal in men and 5223 kcal in women.[26] Coupled with an extremely sedentary life-style made possible by wealth from phosphate mining,[26] it is not difficult to understand the extremely high prevalence of obesity in Nauruans, irrespective of any genetic predisposition.

Dietary studies in populations such as the Micronesians of Nauru[26] and Kiribati,[9] the Polynesians of Tuvalu[27] and Samoa,[25,28] and the Melanesians of Fiji[29] have highlighted the change from high-fiber traditional diets comprised of foods such as breadfruit, taro, yams, coconut, and fish to modern diets characterized by low-fiber processed foods such as polished rice, sugar, white flour, beer, and canned fish and beef. Large quantities of these manufactured foods must be eaten to achieve the same feeling of satiety associated with the traditional foods. It is likely, therefore, given the rapid change in diets experienced in Pacific populations, that individuals have not had time to adjust their pattern of eating to reflect the higher caloric density of the modern processed foods.

Although a number of studies have found total energy intakes to be higher in rural (traditional) than urban (modernized) sections of the population,[9,25,29] energy expenditures are certainly higher in the relatively traditional populations that still engage in agriculture and hunting.[9,25] Moreover, a much higher proportion of total energy consumption in modernized populations is derived from readily metabolized processed foods.[9,28]

It is generally assumed that decreased levels of physical activity in modernized Pacific populations have played a large part in the overall positive energy balance and promotion of obesity. To date there is little direct evidence of decreased levels of energy expenditure in modernized groups, but the likelihood that this is the case is very strong. Support is provided by the finding of lower levels of habitual physical activity in urban compared to rural communities of Micronesians in Kiribati[9,10] and Melanesians and Asian Indians in Fiji,[10] even though the index of activity was crude. Using more elaborate methods, Greska et al[30] found reduced levels of energy expenditure, fitness, and work capability in Samoans living less traditional life-styles.

The available evidence, therefore, generally supports the hypothesis that obesity in Pacific populations results from an interplay of cultural and socioeconomic determinants of both the quantitative and qualitative composition of the diet and levels of physical activity. These factors interact in turn with a probable genetic susceptibility to the development of obesity.

RECENT SECULAR CHANGES IN OBESITY IN THE PACIFIC

There are few published studies on secular changes in obesity in the Pacific. Our research group has studied this phenomenon in recent years in adults of the Micronesian population of Nauru, and a summary of our findings is shown in Figure 54-4. Despite an increasing awareness of the adverse health consequences of obesity, mean BMI basically remained unchanged over the period 1975–1987 in Nauruans. If anything, there seemed to be a trend toward increasing levels in males in all but the oldest age group. A longitudinal study in the Polynesian population of Rarotonga also found an increase in obesity in nearly all age groups of both sexes for the period 1980–1987.[31]

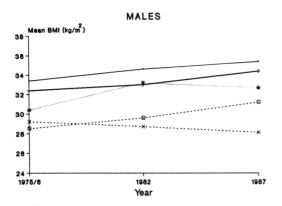
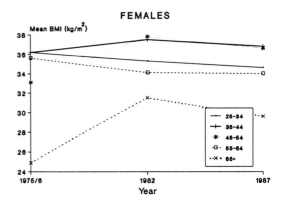

FIGURE 54-4

Secular changes in age-specific mean body mass index in Nauruans, 1975–1976 to 1987.

In our Nauru study we also assessed changes in BMI in the same individuals followed over a 6.5-year period.[13] The mean BMI increased in nearly all baseline age groups. Nauruans aged less than 20 years initially were only mildly obese in 1975–1976 (mean BMI, 25.5 kg/m^2), with a low prevalence of abnormal glucose tolerance. However, this group gained the most weight on average and at follow-up had a mean BMI of 33.1 kg/m^2 (Table 54-2). The magnitude of the weight gain in such a short period in these young Nauruans was remarkable, especially because they were already relatively obese.

As is also the case in the Pima Indians of Arizona, the prevalence of NIDDM in Nauruan teenagers and young adults is much higher than in comparable Caucasian populations in both sexes.[32,33] It has been suggested that the earlier onset of NIDDM in these high-prevalence groups may be related to the rapid increase in weight as these young people enter adulthood.[32] An increase in the prevalence of obesity has been documented in Tokelauan (Polynesian) children who migrated to New Zealand from their native country,[34] suggesting that the weight gain is modulated by life-style change.

In our study of Nauruans,[13] weight loss was more frequent than weight gain only in the oldest individuals, and the weight loss was most commonly seen in diabetic subjects. Because weight loss may be a consequence of untreated or inadequately controlled NIDDM, and because over 50% of Nauruans more than 50 years old have diabetes,[33] this finding was not surprising.

DISTRIBUTION OF BODY FAT

The heterogeneous nature of the association between overall obesity, as indicated by crude measures such as BMI, and disease outcome has sparked renewed interest in the importance of distribution of body fat as a risk factor. There is now evidence that "central" or "android" obesity, most usually measured as waist-to-hip-circumference ratio (WHR), is positively associated with CHD, stroke, and NIDDM, as well as with metabolic risk factors for these diseases, such as glucose intolerance, hyperinsulinemia, and hypertension.[35-37] In general, central obesity appears to act independently of overall body mass in conferring risk for these parameters.[35,36]

Until recently, there was little information on the importance of fat distribution in the pathogenesis of chronic disease in Pacific populations. New cross-sectional data from Micronesian Nauruans indicate that abdominally distributed fat is at least as significant in this population as in Europeans in whom it has been most studied, despite the marked differences in overall body mass. Interestingly, percentile levels for WHR in the obese Nauruan population were remarkably similar to those seen in much leaner groups.

TABLE 54-2

Obesity Levels and Weight Change Over 6.5 Years in Nauruans Followed From Baseline

BASELINE AGE GROUP (years)	n	Mean BMI (kg/m²)		BMI CHANGE (kg/m²)
		1975–76	1982	
Males				
0–19	28	25.5 (0.9)	33.1 (1.0)	7.6 (0.8)
20–29	47	32.3 (0.7)	37.1 (0.9)	4.8 (0.5)
30–39	29	33.1 (0.9)	34.1 (1.0)	1.2 (0.6)
40–49	35	31.6 (1.1)	33.1 (1.3)	1.6 (0.4)
50–59	17	30.2 (1.3)	30.5 (1.6)	0.4 (0.6)
60+	6	31.3 (1.4)	30.1 (1.8)	− 1.3 (1.0)
Total	162	30.8 (0.5)	34.1 (0.5)	3.4 (0.3)
Females				
0–19	45	27.2 (0.9)	34.1 (1.3)	7.0 (0.6)
20–29	66	34.4 (1.0)	38.3 (1.0)	4.0 (0.5)
30–39	31	35.6 (1.0)	38.2 (1.3)	2.5 (0.7)
40–49	35	35.7 (1.0)	36.7 (1.0)	1.0 (0.5)
50–59	23	33.8 (1.3)	35.2 (1.5)	1.4 (0.6)
60+	4	29.7 (2.3)	29.0 (2.2)	− 0.7 (1.3)
Total	204	33.0 (0.5)	36.6 (0.5)	3.6 (0.3)

Modified from Sicree RA, Zimmet PZ, King H et al: Weight change amongst Nauruans over 6.5 years: Extent and association with glucose intolerance. Diabetes Res Clin Pract 3:327, 1987. Reproduced by permission.
Results are expressed as means (SE).

As summarized in Table 54-3, WHR in Nauruans was more strongly associated with fasting plasma glucose and lipid levels in both sexes, and with mean arterial blood pressure (MAP) in males, than was BMI. Only serum insulin levels in both sexes and MAP in females seemed to be more strongly influenced by BMI. In both sexes the age-standardized prevalence of diabetes was much more clearly influenced by WHR than by BMI, increasing across tertiles of WHR from 14.3% to 39.8% in males and from 16.8% to 43.2% in females. In contrast, there was no trend across tertiles of BMI: in males the prevalence ranged from 28.9% to 29.7%, and in females the prevalence actually decreased from 31.9% to 25.0% (unpublished data).

The findings in Nauruans may well be applicable to other Pacific populations. O'Dea[38] has suggested that a propensity to fat deposition in the abdominal area may be of profound importance in determining the high ethnic susceptibility of Australian Aborigines to metabolic and cardiovascular diseases. Future cross-sectional and prospective studies should clarify the significance of adverse fat distribution in conferring risk of chronic disease in Pacific populations. The early data discussed above indicate a major role of adverse fat deposition patterns in conferring risk for NIDDM. It is possible that the thrifty genotype[23] that has been invoked to explain the high levels of obesity and NIDDM in developing Pacific populations may act in part by controlling the distribution and type of fat deposited. In support of this possibility, data from the Tokelauan (Polynesian) migrant study[39] and from longitudinal observations in Melanesians of Papua New Guinea[40] have suggested that acculturation is associated not only with increasing obesity but also, and perhaps to a larger extent, with a shift to a more truncal pattern of fat distribution.

TABLE 54-3

Significance of Differences in Means of Various Physiological
and Biochemical Parameters Across Tertiles of Body Mass
Index (BMI) and Waist-Hip Circumference Ratio (WHR) in
Nauruan Adults

	Significance of Association			
	Males		Females	
Parameter	BMI	WHR	BMI	WHR
Fasting plasma glucose	NS	***	NS	***
2-hour plasma glucose	***	**	***	***
Fasting serum insulin	***	NS	***	***
2-hour serum insulin	***	NS	***	*
Mean arterial blood pressure	*	***	***	*
Plasma triglycerides	**	***	**	***
Plasma cholesterol	**	***	NS	*
Plasma HDL cholesterol	***	***	NS	***

Differences were tested using analysis of variance. Variables with nonnormal distributions were
log-transformed prior to analysis. Mean levels increased across tertiles of obesity indices for
all variables excepting HDL cholesterol, where the association was in a negative direction.
NS = not significant, $*P < .05$, $**P < .01$, $***P < .001$.

Preliminary studies of adipose tissue cellularity in Tuvaluan men suggested that their obesity was of adult onset and predominantly due to fat cell hypertrophy rather than hyperplasia.[41] With increasing acculturation, obesity may occur at younger ages and may tend toward a more mixed hypertrophic/hyperplastic variety. Such a pattern may have different metabolic and health consequences than the adult-onset obesity observed today.[8]

Further studies of fat distribution, adipose tissue morphology, and associated metabolic parameters in Pacific populations should help to clarify whether their obesity has features that make it distinct from that observed in other populations. It seems likely, however, that the difference is more one of degree (susceptibility) than of biologic distinctiveness.

OBESITY AND HEALTH OUTCOMES IN PACIFIC POPULATIONS

Obesity and NIDDM

Although there appears to be some ecological correlation between the prevalence of obesity and that of NIDDM in the Pacific region (Fig. 54-5), the association is not clear-cut, especially when the somewhat unique Nauruan population is excluded from consideration.

West[42] noted that obesity had been considered to be of etiological importance for diabetes since the earliest times, and the World Health Organization Expert Committee on Diabetes Mellitus considered obesity to be the most powerful known risk factor for the development of NIDDM.[43]

Recently, however, as the heterogeneity of these two conditions has become more evident, the role of obesity in the pathogenesis of NIDDM has been placed in clearer perspective. Identical twin studies suggest that the genetic component of NIDDM acts independently of obesity.[44] Similarly, data from the Pima Indians show that obesity may act more as a potentiator of NIDDM in persons who already possess a genetic susceptibility.[32]

Results from Pacific studies, although largely based on cross-sectional surveys, indicate that the effect of obesity, both within and between populations, may be heterogeneous.[10] At least part of this finding may, however, be related to

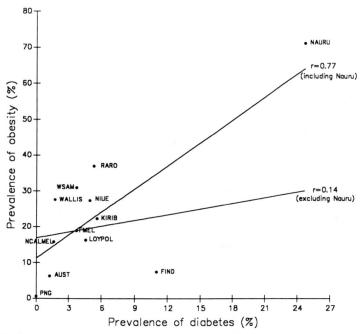

FIGURE 54-5

Ecological comparison of age-standardized prevalence of obesity (BMI ≥ 30 kg/m²) and prevalence of diabetes (WHO criteria, 1985) as determined in community samples of adults in various Pacific populations. (Aust, Australia; Raro, Rarotonga; Fmel, Fiji Melanesians; Find, Fiji Indians; Kirib, Kiribati; Niue, Niue Island; Loypol, Loyalty Islands Polynesians; Ncalmel, New Caledonia Melanesians; PNG, Papua New Guinea; Wsam, Western Samoa; Wallis, Wallis Island)

weight loss associated with onset of disease or therapeutic intervention. In Melanesians of Fiji, increasing BMI had little effect on diabetes prevalence, particularly in urban males. By contrast, in Fijian Indians the prevalence of diabetes increased with obesity in both sexes, and there was no striking difference in this trend between rural and urban groups. Yet another pattern was evident in Micronesians from Kiribati: diabetes prevalence increased with BMI in both sexes, and the prevalence was consistently higher in urban dwellers than in rural dwellers.[10] These data suggest that obesity and other factors associated with life-style modernization may interact, resulting in the high diabetes prevalence exhibited by many of these populations.

A longitudinal study in Nauruans has shown obesity to be a significant predictor of NIDDM in women, although it had only marginal predictive power in men, perhaps reflecting a gender differential in the pathogenesis of NIDDM.[45] In other analyses, BMI was an independent predictor of progression from impaired glucose tolerance to NIDDM, but not from normal glucose tolerance to NIDDM.[46] Longitudinal studies in other populations have examined the role of obesity in the development of NIDDM, and associations between the two have varied. In Nauruans,[46] Caucasians,[47] and Japanese[48] it appears that BMI acts independently of insulin resistance in conferring risk of NIDDM, but in Pima Indians[49] the effect of obesity seems to be explained by insulin resistance.

Furthermore, as indicated in Figure 54-5, prevalence studies suggest that while differences in obesity between populations can explain some of the variation in diabetes prevalence, obesity is not the only or even the main factor responsible for such differences. Supporting this, Kawate et al[50] found that the prevalence of diabetes was higher in migrant Japanese in Hawaii and mainland United States than in Hiroshima, and this difference was independent of weight.

Other studies of Pacific migration in Polynesians of Tokelau[51] and Wallis Island[11] have also revealed that differences in obesity do not account for all of the variation in diabetes prevalence between migrants and sedentees. Similarly, apparent differences in the prevalence of diabetes between migrant Asian Indians in Fiji and the indigenous peoples of India cannot be explained by changes in obesity, since levels of obesity in these groups are not very different.[52] Supporting evidence also comes from rural–urban comparisons of diabetes prevalence within the same country. The marked difference in prevalence of abnormal glucose tolerance between rural and urban Polynesians from Western Samoa persisted even after age and weight standardization.[7] Moreover, obesity did not account for the sex difference in NIDDM prevalence.

Obesity and Hypertension

The association between body weight and blood pressure has long been known and has been demonstrated in both cross-sectional and longitudinal epidemiologic studies, using a variety of indices of obesity.[53] This relationship has been observed in both adults and children and in studies of Western populations as well as those of less industrialized nations.

The link between obesity and hypertension is unclear, but it has been variously suggested that increased sodium intake, increased cardiac output, neuroendocrine disturbances, and hyperinsulinemia with an associated increase in renal tubular resorption of sodium may be responsible.[54,55]

The relationship between the prevalence of obesity (BMI $\geq$ 30) and the prevalence of hypertension (WHO criteria[56]) determined in community samples in a number of Pacific island countries is shown in Figure 54-6. There is a moderate correlation between the two conditions, even when the unusual population of Nauru is excluded ($r = 0.41$), although it is clear that other factors must be important in determining popu-

lation differences in the prevalence of hypertension.

A number of studies in the Pacific region have demonstrated differences in mean blood pressure and the prevalence of hypertension between persons residing in rural areas and those of similar ethnicity who either live in urban areas or have migrated to developed countries. Prior et al[57,58] found increases in blood pressure in Tokelauans who had migrated to New Zealand, and McGarvey and Baker[59] reported similar trends in American Samoans who had migrated to Hawaii. These differences appear to be related to changing life-style factors, including increased body mass in urban dwellers.

Comparisons of rural and urban populations of Melanesians and migrant Indians in Fiji, Micronesians in Kiribati, and Polynesians in New Caledonia, Niue, and Rarotonga showed a lower prevalence of hypertension and generally lower mean blood pressures in the rural groups than in their urban counterparts. In addition, rural residents were slimmer than urban residents, as judged from mean BMI or triceps skin-fold thickness.[60] However, this study, along with others from the Pacific region,[61-64] concluded that rural–urban variations in adiposity did not fully explain the observed differences in blood pressure and that other environmental factors such as salt intake might be important.

Interestingly, a study in Solomon Islands communities found that the increase in blood pressure following acculturation preceded any observed increases in body weight.[63] The authors felt that dietary changes, and specifically increased salt intake, might explain much of this early increase in blood pressure. A cross-sectional study of rural and urban Western Samoans found that approximately half of the rural–urban differences in mean blood pressure and the prevalence of hypertension could be attributed to BMI differences.[64] Moreover, within both the rural and the urban groups, the age-standardized prevalence of hypertension clearly increased with increasing BMI.

However, a recent study of relatively traditional rural villagers in the Papua New Guinea highlands found no relationship between age and blood pressure and only a very weak association with indices of obesity.[65] The subjects were generally very lean, and the results may indicate

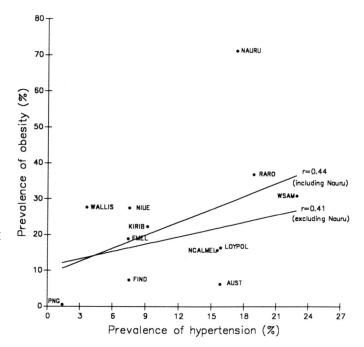

FIGURE 54-6

Ecological comparison of age-standardized prevalence of obesity (BMI ≥ 30 kg/m²) and prevalence of hypertension (systolic BP ≥ 160 and/or diastollic BP ≥ 95 mm Hg, or on oral therapy) as determined in community samples of adults in various Pacific populations. (For abbreviations, see Fig. 54-5).

that a threshold level of adiposity is required before a clear association between obesity and blood pressure is observed within populations (Fig. 54-7).

Data from studies in 11 Pacific populations were pooled in an ecological analysis of blood pressure and its determinants.[66] MAP increased across quantiles of BMI in both sexes within each of these populations. In a linear regression model, BMI explained 24% of the interpopulation variation in age-adjusted MAP, and it was concluded that dietary factors that determined differences in body mass, plasma cholesterol, and glucose intolerance contributed much to the observed population differences in blood pressure.

In Nauruans, a longitudinal study has shown

a somewhat inconsistent rise in the cumulative incidence of hypertension across quartiles of BMI over a five-year follow-up period, 1982–1987 (Fig. 54-8). The age-adjusted relative risk of hypertension for subjects in the upper quartile of obesity was twice that of subjects in the lower quartile. However, the cumulative incidence was still over 10% in subjects in the lowest quartile. As 70% of these subjects had BMIs above 25 kg/m², it is possible that a more dramatic effect of obesity on incidence of hypertension may have been masked by the generally high frequency of obesity in this population. Of three obesity indices (BMI, triceps skin-fold thickness, midarm circumference) that were measured in the 1982 baseline survey, none was a significant predictor in a multiple logistic regression analy-

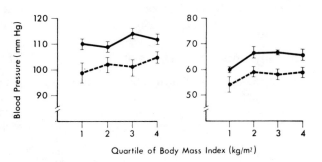

FIGURE 54-7

Mean systolic (left) and diastolic (right) blood pressure by quartiles of body mass index in adults of two villages of the Papau New Guinea highlands (Q1 = 20.5, Q2 = 21.8, Q3 = 23.5 kg/m²).

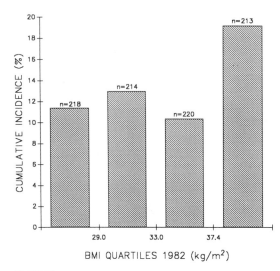

FIGURE 54-8

Age-standardized cumulative incidence (1982–1987) of hypertension by quartiles of baseline body mass index in adult Nauruans. RR = relative risk compared to lowest quartile.

sis of incident hypertension in 1987, after accounting for baseline age, systolic blood pressure, two-hour postload plasma glucose, and sex. Conversely, when a similar analysis was done to assess factors associated with prevalent hypertension in 1987, both indices of obesity (WHR and BMI) were independently important.

These results may indicate that an inherent susceptibility to hypertension (as indicated by higher baseline blood pressure) is a more important predictor of future hypertension than is obesity, even though obesity may have had a modulating influence on the initial blood pressure level. Alternatively, obesity may indeed exert its effects on blood pressure in the short term rather than through longer acting mechanisms. This view is supported by studies that have demonstrated relatively rapid responses of blood pressure to changes in body weight.[67]

Obesity and Coronary Heart Disease

Obesity has not been shown to have a consistent, independent association with CHD.[21,68-70] In the Framingham Heart Study, however, over a 26-year follow-up, obesity was found to be an inde-

pendent predictor of the incidence of and mortality from CHD.[71] It has been suggested that such long follow-up periods may be necessary to show the association.[70]

As argued by Tuomilehto et al,[70] it is not surprising that an independent effect of obesity on CHD is lost when blood pressure and blood lipid values are controlled, because these factors may well represent a substantial component of the biologic pathway through which obesity acts. Nonetheless, evidence such as that from the Framingham study[71] does suggest that obesity may operate through other mechanisms as well.

A possible explanation for some of the reported differences in the association between obesity and CHD is suggested by recent prospective studies demonstrating that it is probably the subgroup of obese persons with a predominantly abdominal or truncal distribution of body fat that is at greatest risk for CHD.[36,72] A 12-year follow-up study of men in the Honolulu Heart Program used subscapular skin-fold thickness as a measure of central obesity and found that the risk of incident coronary events was directly related to this measure, independent of age, cholesterol, glucose, triglyceride levels, hypertension, and cigarette smoking.[36]

There is a paucity of data on the relationship between obesity and cardiovascular disease endpoints in Pacific populations. The susceptibility of these populations to CHD is indicated by rising mortality rates, such as have been documented in Fijians[17] and Nauruans,[18,20] and by the higher CHD mortality in New Zealand Maoris than in their European-origin compatriots.[73] The published studies are mostly of a cross-sectional nature and use electrocardiographic (ECG) abnormalities (Minnesota Code[74]) as an indicator of CHD. Figure 54-9 shows the relationship between the prevalence of possible or probable CHD, as indicated by ECG codes, and the prevalence of obesity (BMI ≥ 30) in several Pacific populations. A negative association is evident (r = −0.50), perhaps reflecting the complexity of the relationship between obesity and CHD and the variability of other risk factor levels in the populations under study.

In a cross-sectional study of Melanesians and Asian Indians in Fiji, BMI was significantly higher in both men and women with ECG abnor-

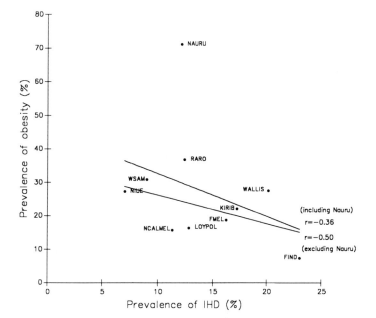

FIGURE 54-9

Ecological comparison of age-standardized prevalence of obesity (BMI ≥ 30 kg/m²) and prevalence of ECG abnormalities suggesting ischemic heart disease (IHD) (Q waves, ST-depression or T-wave changes) as determined in community samples of adults in various Pacific populations. (For abbreviations, see Fig. 54-5.)

malities indicative of CHD than in subjects with normal ECGs, regardless of glucose tolerance status.[75] Multivariate analysis of the data on men demonstrated that BMI was independent of plasma cholesterol, blood pressure, plasma glucose, and other factors in determining ECG abnormalities in Indians, while in Melanesians there was some evidence that BMI had an effect, although this was not statistically significant.[76]

Similarly, an urban–rural comparison of Polynesians from Wallis Island identified a trend toward a higher prevalence of ECG Q-wave changes in migrant urbanized Wallisians than in those with a rural life-style.[77] However, while the urban group was more obese than the rural dwellers, this geographic variation could be due to the confounding effects of other risk factors, such as hypertension and diabetes, which were also more common in the urbanized population.

In our prospective study in Nauru, the incidence of ECG-indicated CHD over five years of follow-up (1982–1987) did not appear to be related to baseline obesity. Figure 54-10 shows the cumulative incidence of CHD by tertiles of baseline BMI. A multiple logistic regression analysis revealed that baseline age, systolic blood pres-

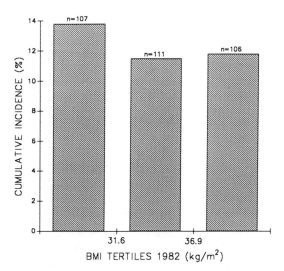

FIGURE 54-10

Age-standardized cumulative incidence (1982–1987) of ECG abnormalities suggesting coronary heart disease (Q waves, ST-depression or T-wave changes) by tertiles of baseline body mass index in adult Nauruans.

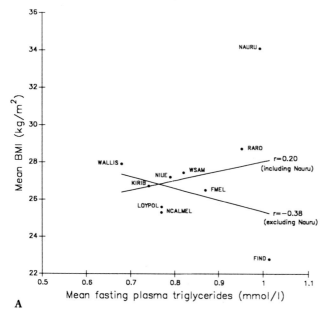

A

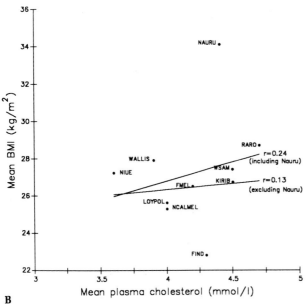

B

FIGURE 54-11

Ecological comparison of age-adjusted mean body mass index and mean levels of fasting plasma triglycerides **(A)**, plasma cholesterol **(B)**, and plasma uric acid **(C)** as determined in community samples of adults in various Pacific populations. (For abbreviations, see Fig. 54-5.)

sure, and blood cholesterol level were important independent predictors of incident CHD. Neither BMI, triceps skin-fold thickness, nor midarm circumference contributed significantly to the model. However, obesity may still be operating as an indirect risk factor for CHD in Nauruans

through its effect on blood pressure and blood lipid levels.

Obesity and Other CHD Risk Factors

Considerable evidence implicates obesity in the pathogenesis of both glucose intolerance and hy-

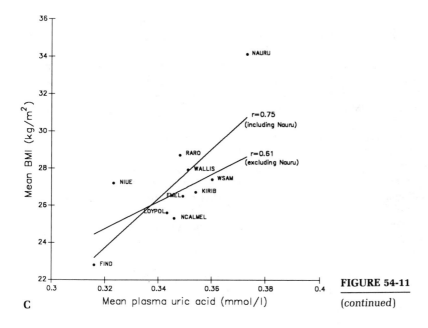

FIGURE 54-11

(continued)

C

pertension in Pacific populations, and both the latter conditions have been related to CHD in these populations. However, the relationship between obesity and other known correlates of CHD has been less frequently studied.

On an ecological basis, the relationship between population mean BMI and mean plasma cholesterol and triglyceride levels does not appear convincing (Fig. 54-11). In contrast, there is a strong positive correlation (r = 0.75) between obesity and mean plasma uric acid levels across populations. Uric acid was the only significant factor independently associated with prevalent ECG abnormalities in Melanesian males in Fiji.[76] Elevated uric acid levels have been reported in a number of Polynesian[78] and Micronesian[78,79] communities, and a strong association with obesity within populations seems clear.[78,80]

There have been few published analyses of the link between obesity and lipid levels within Pacific populations. Egusa et al[81] found that in Polynesians of Rarotonga, obesity was positively associated with elevated triglyceride levels in both sexes and with total cholesterol levels in males only, and was negatively associated with HDL cholesterol levels in females. In Fijians, obesity was not an independent predictor of apolipoprotein A1 levels.[82] In Nauruan men,

plasma triglycerides and total cholesterol levels increased significantly across tertiles of both BMI and WHR, whereas there was a negative association with HDL cholesterol (see Table 54-3). In women, the positive association with cholesterol and the negative relationship with HDL cholesterol were significant across tertiles of WHR but not BMI.

Obesity and Mortality

The current evidence from population-based studies regarding the relative impact of obesity on premature mortality is both controversial and confusing. In some studies obesity has been found to act independently of other traditional cardiovascular risk factors (such as serum lipid levels, blood pressure, blood glucose values, and smoking habits).[71] However, there are just as many studies negating these findings.[21,68,70] For the Pacific region, very little has been published on the association of obesity with premature mortality.

Nauru

Obesity, as measured by BMI, was not found to be independently associated with all-cause mortality in Nauruans during the period 1982–

1985.[83] However, since these analyses controlled for glucose tolerance status, itself closely associated with obesity in this population, and since diabetes is a major cause of mortality, the link between obesity and mortality may have been obscured. New data presented in Table 54-4 explore this possibility for the period 1982–1987. The age-adjusted relative risk of mortality has been calculated for the upper two tertiles of BMI (compared to the lowest tertile) measured at baseline, before and after controlling for plasma glucose levels and cigarette smoking.

In Nauruan males BMI values in the mid and upper tertiles appear to confer a lesser risk of death than do the lower index levels, in disagree-

ment with the J- or U-shaped trends in mortality risk observed in some other populations.[21,70] Adjustment for fasting glucose levels or cigarette smoking had little effect. In females, however, there did appear to be a J-shaped association of obesity with risk of mortality. Adjustment for fasting plasma glucose led to increased estimates of relative risk, whereas cigarette smoking had little effect, in contrast to findings in other populations.[70]

The unconvincing association of obesity with mortality in Nauru is not surprising, in that the majority of this population is obese by conventional standards (see Table 54-1). The boundary between low and mid tertiles was 30.1 kg/m^2 in

TABLE 54-4

Cox Relative Risks* of Mortality in Nauruans (1982–87) and Melanesian and Indian Fijians (1980–85), by Tertiles of Baseline Body Mass Index

Ethnic Group	Tertile of BMI (kg/m^2)	Adjusted for Age: RR (95% CI)	Adjusted for Age and Fasting Glucose: RR (95% CI)	Adjusted for Age and Cigarette Consumption: RR (95% CI)
Males				
Nauruans (n = 660, deaths = 67)				
Mid	(30.2–35.0)	0.69 (0.38, 1.23)	0.65 (0.36, 1.16)	0.70 (0.39, 1.25)
High	(35.1+)	0.82 (0.44, 1.54)	0.81 (0.43, 1.52)	0.84 (0.45, 1.58)
Melanesians (n = 398, deaths = 31)				
Mid	(24.2–27.1)	1.01 (0.40, 2.54)	1.01 (0.40, 2.54)	1.02 (0.40, 2.57)
High	(27.2+)	0.99 (0.40, 2.51)	0.99 (0.43, 2.27)	1.00 (0.43, 2.31)
Asian Indians (n = 383, deaths = 25)				
Mid	(21.1–24.6)	1.01 (0.32, 3.14)	1.16 (0.36, 3.67)	1.02 (0.33, 3.18)
High	(24.7+)	1.77 (0.67, 1.54)	1.91 (0.71, 5.09)	1.84 (0.69, 4.94)
Females				
Nauruans (n = 653, deaths = 35)				
Mid	(31.5–37.8)	0.74 (0.31, 1.76)	0.78 (0.33, 1.87)	0.74 (0.31, 1.75)
High	(37.9+)	1.54 (0.70, 3.39)	1.89 (0.84, 4.27)	1.51 (0.68, 3.32)
Melanesians (n = 463, deaths = 21)				
Mid	(25.3–30.3)	0.95 (0.36, 2.53)	0.94 (0.35, 2.52)	0.93 (0.35, 2.51)
High	(30.4+)	0.55 (0.18, 1.69)	0.54 (0.18, 1.66)	0.54 (0.18, 1.67)
Asian Indians (n = 463, deaths = 14)				
Mid	(21.0–26.0)	0.21 (0.02, 1.90)	0.18 (0.02, 1.65)	0.21 (0.02, 1.88)
High	(26.1+)	1.30 (0.40, 4.22)	0.99 (0.28, 3.54)	1.25 (0.38, 4.09)

*Comparison is against the lowest tertile of BMI. Tertiles were determined separately for each sex and ethnic group.

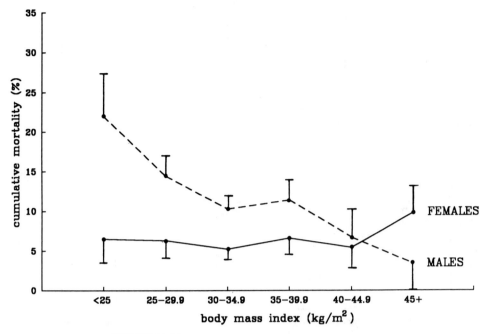

FIGURE 54-12

Cumulative all-cause mortality in adult Nauruans according to baseline body mass index for the period 1982–1987. Bars represent 1 SE.

males and 31.4 kg/m² in females. Even in the lowest tertile a large proportion of individuals (54.7% of males and 77.0% of females) had BMIs exceeding 27 and 25 kg/m², respectively. As shown in Figure 54-12, however, there was no clear association with all-cause mortality in Nauruans, even when the full range of BMI was considered. If anything, there was a trend toward declining mortality with increasing BMI in males.

Fiji

Mortality surveillance was carried out for a cohort of 861 Melanesian and 846 migrant Asian Indian residents of an urban area of Fiji who participated in a survey of metabolic and cardiovascular diseases in 1980.[84] For the five-year period 1980–1985, there was evidence for some heterogeneity in the effect of obesity on mortality between these populations and between the sexes (see Table 54-4). In Melanesians of both sexes, increasing BMI was not associated with increas-ing risk of mortality, whereas in Indian males a BMI in the upper tertile did elevate mortality risk (albeit not significantly).

Cumulative mortality for the period 1980–1985 across the spectrum of BMI for Melanesian and Indian Fijians is compared in Figure 54-13. There is no clear association of obesity with mortality in Melanesians of either sex. In Indians there is some support for a positive association in men only.

The lack of a convincing association between obesity and mortality in Nauruans and in Melanesian and Indian Fijians is similar to that reported for Pima Indians, another group with a high NIDDM prevalence.[85] As suggested by Pettitt et al,[85] this may reflect the survival advantage afforded by the thrifty genotype. It is possible that the type of obesity seen in Pacific and other modernizing populations differs in some fundamental way from that of Caucasian populations, with less grave implications for mortality. Further study may help elucidate the reasons, which

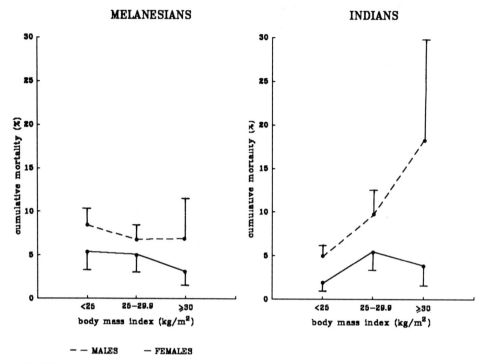

FIGURER 54-13

Cumulative mortality in adult Melanesian and Indian Fijians according to
baseline body mass index for the period 1980–1985. Bars represent 1 SE.

might relate to other intermediate risk factors,
such as cholesterol levels. These have been
found to be surprisingly low in many Pacific
populations, considering their degree of
obesity.[86]

CONCLUSIONS

Available data suggest that obesity adversely influences a variety of known and putative risk factors for CHD and other cardiovascular disease
end points in Pacific populations. It remains
somewhat curious, therefore, that in longitudinal
cohort studies in Nauru and Fiji, there does not
appear to be a convincing relationship between
obesity and overall mortality, even though results from other populations have been similarly
equivocal.[21,68] It seems unlikely that the lack of
effect can be explained by weight loss associated
with pre-existing chronic disease prior to death.
The lack of association between obesity and

mortality in these populations might be explained in terms of the selective advantage offered by obesity as a product of the thrifty genotype.[85] However, given the obvious adverse
effects of acculturation on risk factor and chronic
disease levels in the Pacific, presumed to be a
product of the same thrifty genotype, it is difficult to reconcile this view. It may yet be too early
to observe a major effect of obesity on mortality
in the Nauruan and Fijian populations, where a
significant proportion of deaths is still attributable to infectious diseases. Continuing longitudinal studies may clarify the role of obesity in determining total mortality in developing Pacific
populations.

Nevertheless, the evidence that obesity plays a
major role in determining the risk of diabetes and
hypertension in these populations seems irrefut-
able. The development of obesity may well be
partly a consequence of a thrifty genotype, but
cultural factors that favor feasting and a liking

for readily available high-calorie processed foods interact with an increasingly sedentary life-style to produce large positive energy balances.

Attempts have been made in a number of Pacific island states to develop life-style intervention programs aimed at reducing obesity, increasing physical activity, and improving diet. Such programs face enormous financial, logistic, and cultural barriers. Longitudinal studies in Nauru (see Fig. 54-4) and Rarotonga[31] have shown continuing increases in obesity, despite much awareness of the problem and of the need for prevention. The considerable ethnic and cultural diversity of Pacific populations may mean that a number of different responses to the problem of obesity will need to be developed. Unless workable prevention strategies are implemented quickly, the noncommunicable disease problem is likely to worsen considerably in the Pacific, particularly in some of the Melanesian populations that have not yet experienced the degree of modernization of their Polynesian and Micronesian neighbors.

Acknowledgment: These studies were supported by NIH grant DK 25446.

References

1. Coates A: Western Pacific Islands. London, Her Majesty's Stationery Office, 1970
2. Langdon R: The Lost Caravel. Sydney, Pacific Publications, 1975
3. Serjeantson SW, Ryan DP, Thompson AR: The colonization of the Pacific: The story according to human leukocyte antigens. Am J Hum Genet 34:904, 1982
4. Bellwood PS: The peopling of the Pacific. Sci Am 243:138, 1980
5. Cooper HS: Coral Lands, vols I and II. London, Bentley, 1880
6. Brettell R, Cachin R, Freches-Thory C et al: The Art of Gauguin. Washington, DC, National Gallery of Art, 1988
7. Zimmet P, Faaiuso S, Ainuu J et al: The prevalence of diabetes in the rural and urban Polynesian population of Western Samoa. Diabetes 30:45, 1981
8. Pawson IG: The morphological characteristics of Samoan adults. In Baker PT, Hanna JM, Baker TS (eds): The Changing Samoans: Behaviour and Health in Transition, p 254. New York, Oxford University Press, 1986
9. King H, Taylor R, Zimmet P et al: Non-insulin-dependent diabetes (NIDDM) in a newly independent Pacific nation: The Republic of Kiribati. Diabetes Care 7:409, 1984
10. King H, Zimmet P, Raper LR et al: Risk factors for diabetes in three Pacific populations. Am J Epidemiol 119:396, 1984
11. Taylor R, Bennett P, Uili R et al: Diabetes in Wallis Polynesians: A comparison of residents of Wallis Island and first generation migrants to Noumea, New Caledonia. Diabetes Res Clin Pract 1:169, 1985
12. Taylor R, Zimmet P, Levy S et al: Group comparisons of blood pressure and indices of obesity and salt intake in Pacific populations. Med J Aust 142:499, 1985
13. Sicree RA, Zimmet PZ, King H et al: Weight change amongst Nauruans over 6.5 years: Extent, and association with glucose intolerance. Diabetes Res Clin Pract 3:327, 1987
14. National Heart Foundation of Australia: Risk factor prevalence study. Report No. 1. Canberra, National Heart Foundation, 1980
15. Gurney M, Gorstein J: The global prevalence of obesity: An initial overview of available data. World Health Stat Q 41:251, 1988
16. Zimmet P, Whitehouse S: Pacific islands of Nauru, Tuvalu and Western Samoa. In Trowell HC, Burkitt DP (eds): Western Diseases: Their Emergence and Prevention, p 204. London, Edward Arnold, 1981
17. Tuomilehto J, Ram P, Eseroma R et al: Cardiovascular diseases and diabetes mellitus in Fiji: Analysis of mortality, morbidity and risk factors. Bull WHO 62:133, 1984
18. Taylor R, Thoma K: Mortality patterns in the modernized Pacific island nation of Nauru. Am J Public Health 75:149, 1985
19. Taylor R, Lewis N, Levy S: Mortality in Pacific island countries, circa 1980. Noumea, South Pacific Commission, 1987
20. Schooneveldt M, Songer T, Zimmet P et al: Changing mortality patterns in Nauruans: An example of epidemiological transition. J Epidemiol Commun Health 42:89, 1988
21. Jarrett RJ: Is there an ideal body weight? Br Med J 293:493, 1986
22. Bennett PH: Recommendations on the standardization of methods and reporting of tests for diabetes and its microvascular complications in epidemiological studies. Diabetes Care 2:98, 1979
23. Neel JV: Diabetes mellitus: A thrifty genotype rendered detrimental by "progress"? Am J Hum Genet 14:353, 1962
24. Howard A: Questions and answers: Samoans talk about happiness, distress and other life experi-

ences. In Baker PT, Hanna JM, Baker TS (eds): The Changing Samoans: Behaviour and Health in Transition, p 174. New York, Oxford University Press, 1986

25. Hanna JM, Pelletier DL, Brown VJ: The diet and nutrition of contemporary Samoans. In Baker PT, Hanna JM, Baker TS (eds): The Changing Samoans: Behaviour and Health in Transition, p 275. New York, Oxford University Press, 1986

26. Ringrose H, Zimmet P: Nutrient intakes in an urbanized Micronesian population with a high diabetes prevalence. Am J Clin Nutr 32:1334, 1979

27. Wicking J, Ringrose H, Whitehouse S et al: Nutrient intake in a partly westernized isolated Polynesian population: The Funafuti survey. Diabetes Care 4:92, 1981

28. Bindon JR: Breadfruit, banana, beef, and beer: Modernization of the Samoan diet. Ecol Food Nutr 12:49, 1982

29. Ringrose H, Ram P, Mollard C et al: Energy intakes and diabetes prevalence of rural and urban Melanesian and Indian populations in Fiji. Fiji Med J 13:250, 1985

30. Greska LP, Pelletier DL, Gage TB: Work in contemporary and traditional Samoa. In Baker PT, Hanna JM, Baker TS (eds): The Changing Samoans: Behaviour and Health in Transition, p 297. New York, Oxford University Press, 1986

31. Taylor R, Bach F, Teariki T et al: Preliminary report: Rarotonga non-communicable disease evaluation survey. Noumea, South Pacific Commission, 1987

32. Knowler WC, Pettitt DJ, Savage PJ et al: Diabetes incidence in Pima Indians: Contributions of obesity and parental diabetes. Am J Epidemiol 113:144, 1981

33. Zimmet P, King H, Taylor R et al: The high prevalence of diabetes mellitus, impaired glucose tolerance and diabetic retinopathy in Nauru: The 1982 survey. Diabetes Res 1:13, 1984

34. Prior I, Tasman-Jones C: New Zealand Maori and Pacific Polynesians. In Trowell HC, Burkitt DP (eds): Western Diseases: Their Emergence and Prevention, p 227. London, Edward Arnold, 1981

35. Ohlsson LO, Larsson B, Svardsudd K et al: The influence of body fat distribution on the incidence of diabetes mellitus: A 13.5 years follow-up of the participants in the study of men born in 1913. Diabetes 35:1055, 1985

36. Donahue RP, Bloom E, Abbott RD et al: Central obesity and coronary heart disease in men. Lancet 1:821, 1987

37. Björntorp P: The associations between obesity, adipose tissue distribution and disease. Acta Med Scand Suppl 723:121, 1988

38. O'Dea K: Body fat distribution and health outcome in Australian Aborigines. Proc Nutr Soc Aust 12:56, 1987

39. Ramirez ME, Mueller WH: The development of obesity and fat patterning in Tokelau children. Hum Biol 52:675, 1980

40. Norgan NG: Fat patterning in Papua New Guineans: Effects of age, sex and acculturation. Am J Phys Anthropol 74:385, 1987

41. Zimmet P, Björntorp P: Adipose tissue cellularity in obese non-diabetic men in an urbanized Pacific island (Polynesian) population. Am J Clin Nutr 32:1788, 1979

42. West KM: Epidemiology of Diabetes and Its Vascular Lesions. New York, Elsevier, 1978

43. World Health Organization Expert Committee on Diabetes Mellitus: Second report. Technical report series 646. Geneva, WHO, 1980

44. Barnett AH, Eff C, Leslie RDG et al: Diabetes in identical twins: A study of 200 pairs. Diabetologia 20:87, 1981

45. Balkau B, King H, Zimmet P et al: Factors associated with the development of diabetes in the Micronesian population of Nauru. Am J Epidemiol 122:594, 1985

46. Sicree RA, Zimmet PZ, King HOM et al: Plasma insulin response among Nauruans: Prediction of deterioration in glucose tolerance over 6 yr. Diabetes 36:179, 1987

47. Keen H, Jarrett RJ, McCartney P: The ten-year follow-up of the Bedford Survey (1962–1972): Glucose tolerance and diabetes. Diabetologia 22:73, 1982

48. Kadowaki T, Miyake Y, Hagura R et al: Risk factors for worsening to diabetes in subjects with impaired glucose tolerance. Diabetologia 26:44, 1984

49. Saad MF, Knowler WC, Pettitt DJ et al: The natural history of impaired glucose tolerance in the Pima Indians. N Engl J Med 319:1500, 1988

50. Kawate R, Yamakido M, Nishimoto Y et al: Diabetes mellitus and its vascular complications in Japanese migrants on the island of Hawaii. Diabetes Care 2:161, 1979

51. Stanhope JM, Prior IAM: The Tokelau island migrant study: Prevalence and incidence of diabetes mellitus. NZ Med J 92:417, 1980

52. Zimmet P, Taylor R, Ram P et al: The prevalence of diabetes and impaired glucose tolerance in the biracial (Melanesian and Indian) population of Fiji: A rural-urban comparison. Am J Epidemiol 118:673, 1983

53. Berchtold P, Juergens V, Finke C et al: Epidemiology of obesity and hypertension. Int J Obes 5:1, 1981

54. Messerli FH, Christie B, DeCarvalho JGR et al: Obesity and essential hypertension: Hemodynamics, intravascular volume, sodium excretion and

plasma renin activity. Arch Intern Med 141:81, 1981

55. Dustan HP: Mechanisms of hypertension associated with obesity. Ann Intern Med 98:860, 1983

56. WHO Technical Report Series, No. 628. Arterial hypertension: Report of a WHO Expert Committee. Geneva, World Health Organization, 1978

57. Prior IAM, Stanhope JM, Evans JG et al: The Tokelau island migrant study. Int J Epidemiol 3:225, 1974

58. Beaglehole R, Salmond CE, Hooper A et al: Blood pressure and social interaction in Tokelauan migrants in New Zealand. J Chronic Dis 30:803, 1977

59. McGarvey ST, Baker PT: The effect of modernization and migration on Samoan blood pressures. Hum Biol 51:461, 1979

60. Taylor R, Zimmet P, Levy S et al: Group comparisons of blood pressure and indices of obesity and salt intake in Pacific populations. Med J Aust 142:499, 1985

61. Prior I, Evans JG: Sodium intake and blood pressure in Pacific populations. Isr J Med Sci 5:608, 1969

62. Prior I, Evans JG, Harvey HPB et al: Sodium intake and blood pressure in two Polynesian populations. N Engl J Med 279:515, 1968

63. Page LB, Damon A, Moellering RC: Antecedents of cardiovascular disease in six Solomon Islands societies. Circulation 49:1132, 1974

64. Zimmet PZ, Taylor R, Jackson L et al: Blood pressure studies in rural and urban Western Samoa. Med J Aust 2:202, 1980

65. King H, Collins A, King LF et al: Blood pressure in Papua New Guinea: A survey of two highland villages in the Asaro Valley. J Epidemiol Commun Health 39:215, 1985

66. Tuomilehto J, Zimmet P, Taylor R et al: A cross-sectional ecological analysis of blood pressure and its determinants in eleven Pacific populations. J Am Coll Nutr 7:132, 1988

67. Reisen E, Abel R, Modan M et al: Effect of weight loss without salt restriction on the reduction of blood pressure in overweight hypertensive patients. N Engl J Med 298:1, 1978

68. Keys A, Menotti A, Aravanis C et al: The Seven Countries Study: 2289 deaths in 15 years. Prev Med 13:141, 1984

69. Hubert HB: The importance of obesity in the development of coronary risk factors and disease. Annu Rev Public Health 7:493, 1986

70. Tuomilehto J, Salonen JT, Marti B et al: Body weight and risk of myocardial infarction and death in the adult population of eastern Finland. Br Med J 295:623, 1987

71. Hubert HB, Feinleib M, McNamara PM et al: Obesity as an independent risk factor for cardiovascular disease: A 26-year follow-up of participants in the Framingham Heart Study. Circulation 67:968, 1983

72. Larsson B, Svardsudd K, Welin L et al: Abdominal adipose tissue distribution, obesity, and risk of cardiovascular disease and death: A 13 year follow-up of participants in the study of men born in 1913. Br Med J 288:1401, 1984

73. Prior IAM: Cardiovascular epidemiology in New Zealand and the Pacific. NZ Med J 80:245, 1974

74. Rose GA, Blackburn H, Gillum RF et al: Cardiovascular Survey Methods, 2nd ed, p 123. Geneva, World Health Organization, 1982

75. Tuomilehto J, Zimmet P, Kankaanpaa J et al: Prevalence of ischaemic ECG abnormalities according to the diabetes status in the population of Fiji and their associations with other risk factors. Diabetes Res Clin Pract 5:205, 1988

76. Sicree RA, Tuomilehto J, Zimmet P et al: Electrocardiographic abnormalities amongst Melanesian & Indian men of Fiji: Prevalence and associated factors. Int J Cardiol 19:27, 1988

77. Taylor R, Bennett P, Uili R et al: Hypertension and indicators of coronary heart disease in Wallis Polynesians: An urban-rural comparison. Eur J Epidemiol 3:247, 1987

78. Jackson L, Taylor R, Faaiuso S et al: Hyperuricaemia and gout in Western Samoans. J Chronic Dis 34:65, 1981

79. Zimmet P, Whitehouse S, Jackson L et al: High prevalence of hyperuricaemia and gout in an urbanized Micronesian population. 1:1237, 1978

80. Tuomilehto J, Zimmet P, Wolf E et al: Plasma uric acid level and its association with diabetes mellitus and some biologic parameters in a biracial population of Fiji. Am J Epidemiol 127:321, 1988

81. Egusa G, Bennett PH, Aleck K et al: Hyperlipidemia and arteriosclerotic cardiovascular disease in the Polynesian population of Rarotonga. Atherosclerosis 53:241, 1984

82. Nestel P, Ringrose R, Taylor R et al: High density lipoprotein apoprotein variability in a biracial population. Arteriosclerosis 3:132, 1983

83. Zimmet P, Finch C, Schooneveldt M et al: Mortality from diabetes in Nauru: Results of a 4-yr follow-up. Diabetes Care 11:305, 1988

84. Sicree RA, Ram P, Zimmet P et al: Mortality and health service utilization amongst Melanesian and Indian diabetics in Fiji. Diabetes Res Clin Pract 1:227, 1985

85. Pettitt DJ, Lisse JR, Knowler WC et al: Mortality as a function of obesity and diabetes mellitus. Am J Epidemiol 115:359, 1982

86. Pelletier DL, Hornick CA: Blood lipid studies. In Baker PT, Hanna JM, Baker TS (eds): The Changing Samoans: Behaviour and Health in Transition, p 327. New York, Oxford University Press, 1986

PART TEN

TREATMENT— NONPHARMACOLOGIC

CHAPTER 55

Indications for Treatment

J. F. MUNRO and I. H. STOLAREK

In general terms, any condition warrants treatment only if each of three prerequisites are satisfied. These are (1) The condition itself has the potential to cause harm. (2) An effective treatment exists. (3) The risks of the condition outweigh the hazards of the therapy. Within these constraints, the management of any condition can be considered under various headings (Table 55-1).

Most obese subjects, and indeed many therapists, would probably argue that weight loss is by far the most important, perhaps the only criterion, by which to judge the effectiveness of a management regimen. However, this presupposes that the only indication for initiating therapy in the overweight is to promote weight reduction. Indications clearly depend on the management objectives. Although weight loss may be an important objective, it is by no means the only one.

TREATMENT OF THE CAUSE

The fundamental cause of obesity is the sustained imbalance between energy intake and expenditure. Influencing factors are often multifactorial. Although there is accumulating evidence that a genetic component may increase the propensity to obesity,[1,2] other factors include the subject's age, sex, height, marital status,[3] and psychological aspects. Although the prevalence of psychological disorders is no greater in the obese than in the general population,[4] this finding may simply indicate that the response to various stresses by different subjects produces different patterns of eating behavior. The behavioral factors involved in the development of obesity are complex and have been extensively reviewed elsewhere.[5]

There are, however, a few specific conditions that predispose to obesity (Table 55-2). For some of these situations treatment is directed toward the underlying cause, particularly in the case of Cushing's disease or hypothyroidism. In the vast majority of obese subjects, however, it is not possible to effect a cure by identifying and treating the underlying cause. In these subjects treatment is at best palliative and is inevitably directed toward the obesity problem itself.

THE CONDITION ITSELF

The primary purpose of any management plan must be to improve the present health of the subject, both medically and psychologically, and to ensure that this well-being does not deteriorate in the future. The principal treatment objectives in the management of obesity are the following:

1. The promotion of weight loss.
2. The prevention of weight gain.
3. The amelioration or prevention of associated medical complications.
4. The promotion of psychological well-being.

PROMOTION OF WEIGHT LOSS

Any therapeutic decision must take into consideration four interrelated factors: the inherent risks of obesity, the presence or absence of other

TABLE 55-1

Principles of Obesity Management Programme

1. Treat the cause
2. Treat the aggravating and precipitating factors
3. Treat the condition itself
   General principles
   Specific measures
     Medical
     Surgical
4. Treat the complications of the condition
5. Treat the complications of the management of the condition

risk factors, the probable efficacy of the treatment plan, and the safety of the treatment regimen. It follows that each subject poses a unique management problem in which various considerations must be assessed before a particular plan of action is selected. The risk of obesity influences the extent to which interventional treatment may or may not be justified. The 20-year-old woman with a body mass index (BMI) of 25 kg/m² who wishes to lose 2 to 4 kg before a holiday, represents a completely different problem from the 50-year-old man with a BMI above 45 kg/m² who

TABLE 55-2

Specific Conditions Associated with Obesity

Excessive corticosteroids
  Steroid therapy
  Cushing's disease
  Cushing's syndrome
Hypothalamic obesity
  Frohlich's syndrome
  Inflammatory, traumatic, or neoplastic lesions
Hypothyroidism
Drug-associated
  Psychotherapeutic drugs
  Anabolic steroids
Genetically associated obesity
  Laurence-Moon Biedl syndrome
  Prader-Willi syndrome
  Alstrom syndrome
  Glycogen storage disease
Polycystic ovary disease

presents with a sleep apnea syndrome. Paradoxically, it may be the former subject who appears to be most anxious and determined to reduce. This illustrates two points. First, the indications for weight reduction are not only medical but also psychological. Second, the subject's desire to lose weight is not always an indication of the medical need to do so, as is clearly exemplified by anorexia nervosa. Some factors that influence the medical grounds for advising weight loss are listed in Table 55-3.

Degree of Obesity

The relationship between the degree of obesity and life expectancy is well established.[6-8] The excess mortality reaches clinical significance when the BMI is in excess of 30 and increases progressively thereafter with increasing BMI (Fig. 55-1). The excess mortality is most marked in young people.[9] Moreover, it may correct to normal in subjects who subsequently reduce to a normal weight,[10] though this is an area in which further epidemiological studies are urgently required.

From such crude data, it could be concluded that the health risk of all subjects with grade 2 or grade 3 obesity mandates treatment of the obe-

TABLE 55-3

Factors Influencing the Medical Need to Treat Obesity

Degree of obesity
Regional distribution of adiposity
Associated medical conditions
  Diabetes
  Hypertension
  Ischemic heart disease
  Hyperlipidemia
  Cholelithiasis
  Sleep apnea syndrome
  Osteoarthrosis of weight-bearing joint
Family history of medical conditions, especially diabetes
Age and sex of patient
Pregnancy
Presence of unrelated risk factor (e.g., smoking)
Presence of unrelated diseases influencing life expectancy (e.g., neoplasia, dementia)

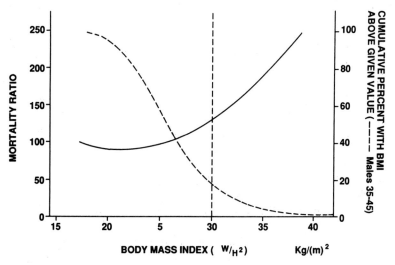

FIGURE 55-1

Relationship of cumulative percentage of males aged 35 to 45 years above a given body mass index (BMI) and the mortality ratio for males the same BMI. Approximately 20% of men in this age group are above the BMI at which excess mortality becomes medically significant (30 kg/m²). (From Bray GA: To treat or not to treat. In Bray GA (ed): Recent Advances in Obesity Research; vol 11, 2nd International Congress on Obesity. London, Neuman Publishing, 1978. Reproduced by permission.)

sity. Subjects in this category make up some 12% of the adult U.S. population and a slightly lower proportion in the United Kingdom and Australia.[11] A much smaller proportion of subjects have a BMI in excess of 40; the risk in this group is especially high. The greater the obesity risk, the more valid is the reason to undertake extensive or hazardous therapy (Table 55-4).

Regional Distribution of Obesity

Much of the available data on the effect of obesity on longevity fails to take into consideration the independent influence of regional fat distribution on excess mortality. This aspect constitutes an independent risk factor for vascular complications such as coronary heart disease and adverse metabolic effects, particularly type II diabetes mellitus, both in men[12] and in women.[13] The influence of waist–hip circumference ratio (WHR) on mortality explains why men appear to be at greater risk than women for any degree of overall obesity. The full significance of the influence of

regional fat distribution on life expectancy and mortality has yet to be established. It is, however, noteworthy that men at highest risk of dying from any cause, of suffering from ischemic heart disease and from stroke, have a relatively low BMI with a high WHR.[14] The immediate inference is that such subjects are most in need of treatment. It remains to be established whether or not weight loss will favorably affect WHR and whether a reduction in WHR will improve life expectancy. Nevertheless, it is clear that the unqualified use of BMI to categorize risk from obesity is a serious oversimplification.

Complications and Other Risk Factors

Another important risk factor is the relationship between diabetes mellitus and increasing magnitude of obesity.[15] This relationship carries particular significance because many insulin-independent diabetics will best improve their carbohydrate tolerance and thereby control their

TABLE 55-4

Relation of Treatment Regimens to Degree of Obesity

	Grade 0	Grade 1	Grade 2 (Uncomplicated)	Grade 2 (Complicated)	Grade 3
Health promotion	X	X	X	X	X
Behavioral modification*	0	X	X	X	X
Pharmacotherapy	0	0	X	X	X
Very low-calorie diets	0	0	0	X	X
Dental splinting	0	0	0	X	X
Gastric surgery	0	0	0	X	X

*Includes dietary restraint and exercise.

symptoms by losing weight. Moreover, the familial predisposition of type II diabetes mellitus[16] suggests that close relatives of known diabetics are at high risk for obesity.

Conventionally, a history of angina or the finding of hypertension in the setting of hyperlipidemia is an additional indication for weight reduction. However, obesity is only one of many factors that may predispose to the development of vascular disease, and others may demand a higher priority. Before a weight reduction program is initiated, subject and therapist must assess the medical problems in relation to the various risk factors. Such assessment may confirm the need to reduce or may have the opposite effect. For example, if the purpose of weight loss is to reduce the risk of sudden death in a subject with a family history of ischemic heart disease, or to ease the breathlessness of a patient with chronic bronchitis, it may be much more appropriate to concentrate on smoking cessation than on weight reduction.

Efficacy of Treatment

The efficacy of weight reduction programs is often assessed in the short term rather than the longer term. However, obesity is a chronic disorder, and the indications for weight loss are usually lifelong.

Short-Term Indications

The vast majority of obese subjects have little or no difficulty in losing weight in the short term. If there is a clearly defined, short-term justifica-

tion for weight reduction, any treatment regimen that can achieve the necessary degree of weight loss is relatively easy to justify. Such short-term indications are listed in Table 55-5. They account for a small minority of cases, but in some instances the indication for treatment may be particularly clear-cut.

Long-Term Indications

Although there is some evidence to suggest that the long-term results of various treatment stratagems, used separately or in combination, are improving,[17-24] during prolonged follow-up weight regain is common. Common treatment options include behavioral modification, drug treatment, very low-calorie diets, dental splinting, intragastric balloons, and surgery. With the notable exception of gastric surgery, which replaces the problems of obesity with those of a small stomach, weight regain is a major problem. One might argue that treatment is always indicated because only through trial and error can subjects be identified in whom a reasonable long-term benefit might be achieved. Nonetheless, certain prerequisites exist that influence the prospect of long-term success.

Motivation. Although groups of subjects can be identified who should be encouraged to reduce weight for medical reasons, many others, especially those under the age of 40, are motivated psychologically. Social pressures induce many subjects to feel inadequate unless they achieve their concept of "ideal" body weight, whatever that might mean. Subjects who wish to reduce place themselves in a sacrifice situation.

TABLE 55-5

Short-Term Indications for Weight Reduction

Medical

Prior to elective surgery

To facilitate conception and successful pregnancy

To enhance the technical value of various investigations (e.g., coronary angiography)

For various medical reasons (e.g., to promote healing of gravitational ulcers)

Personal

For life insurance purposes

To increase the prospects of obtaining employment or as a prerequisite to employment (e.g., the armed forces)

Psychological

Prior to an important social event (e.g., wedding, holiday)

Either they must do without the pleasure, satisfaction, and comfort they obtain from their present eating habits and life-style or they must forgo the advantages, as they conceive them, of weight reduction. Sometimes the preconceived benefit of weight loss is an illusion. For example, although low back pain, infertility, feelings of personal inadequacy, difficulties in obtaining employment, or marital disharmony may sometimes be improved by weight reduction, these problems may in fact be unrelated to the obesity. It is the responsibility of the therapist to provide the individual subject with sufficient information to permit the subject to make an informed decision. An essential prerequisite to any weight reduction program is that the subject be aware of the realistic benefits that might accrue from weight reduction, the health risks involved in remaining obese, and the hazards of the various treatment options. If the subject elects nontreatment, then active treatment is hard to justify.

Realistic Anticipated Rate of Weight Loss. A further prerequisite to successful weight reduction is that the subject have a realistic target weight and concept of the anticipated rate of weight loss (AROWL),[25] although it has been suggested that those with unrealistically optimistic expectations may fare better in the short term.[26]

The energy value of 1 kg of adipose tissue is 9,000 kcal. Any weight reducing stratagem will result in loss not only of fat, but also of fat-free mass (FFM). It follows that an energy deficit of 1,000 kcal/day or of 7,000 kcal/week will produce a "fat" loss of about 1 kg/week. If this degree of energy deficit produces a greater magnitude of weight loss, then the reduction has been achieved at the expense of an increased proportion of FFM—a counterproductive effort. Few subjects adhering to any form of dietary restriction, with or without behavioral modification, can expect to sustain an energy deficit in excess of 1,000 kcal/day. In practice, however, many expect to achieve a much higher AROWL. Often the most overweight subjects tend to have the least realistic concepts. Such subjects run the risk of becoming disillusioned and giving up while in fact making satisfactory progress. It is worth reminding the obese subject that a modest weight reduction of 0.5 kcal/week will result in an annual weight loss of 26 kg.

Realistic Goal Weight. Even the most severely obese subjects may equate target weight with "ideal weight," though to achieve such a goal they might need to halve their total body weight. This expectation is unrealistic. A weight loss of 15% of total body weight involves a considerable achievement, and individual weight losses of more than 20% are relatively exceptional (Fig. 55-2).[27,28] By aiming at an improbable target weight, many subjects set themselves up for failures from the start of treatment. It is much better to aim at a target weight that can be realistically achieved; any additional weight loss that occurs thereafter can be considered a bonus.

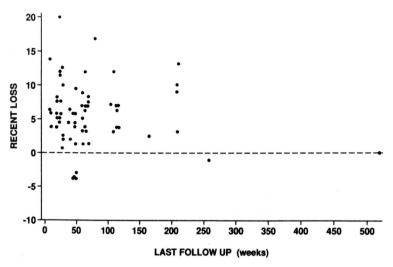

FIGURE 55-2

Dietary treatment of obesity from 1977 to 1985 in 1861 subjects. In most cases, the maximum weight loss achieved was 15%. The loss decayed toward zero with the passage of time. (From Bennett W: Dietary treatment of obesity. In Human Obesity. Reproduced by permission.)

Indications for Specific Treatment Regimens

Indications for specific management programs are discussed elsewhere in this book. Only a few comments will be made here.

Behavioral Modification

In theory, there are methods of producing weight loss without altering behavioral pattern; e.g., by using thermogenic agents or drugs that impair absorption. In practice, all the currently available options involve the structured or unstructured use of a behavioral modification program. Such an approach may be especially important for the long-term efficacy of other treatment strategies. Indeed, if weight loss is indicated at all, a very strong case can be advanced for including behavioral modification.

Exercise

Exercise training has numerous benefits in the obese. Exercise alone is a very poor method of promoting weight loss.[29,30] Some subjects, either because of the magnitude of their adiposity, or because of physical disability such as os-teoarthrosis, cannot significantly increase their level of exercise. All others should be encouraged to do so in combination with dietary restraint. Exercise is best incorporated into a behavioral modification program.

Pharmacotherapy

The mean additional weight loss that can be attributed to pharmacotherapy is about 0.25 kg/week, but once therapy is discontinued, weight regain is common.[31] It follows that drug treatment is best used to meet a medical need for short-term weight loss. Alternatively, drugs may be prescribed indefinitely, for continuous or intermittent use. Such an approach increases the hazards of possible adverse effects. It may be justified if the drug not only produced weight loss but also had an additional beneficial effect, perhaps as a hypoglycemic or hypotensive agent or as an antidepressant. For example, if its efficacy as an antiobesity agent is confirmed,[32] fluoxetine may have a useful therapeutic role in the management of the depressed subject with obesity.

Very Low-Calorie Diets

Used appropriately, very low-calorie diets are a reasonably safe method of promoting weight loss. By and large, however, the longer the follow-up, the more disappointing the mean end result. Current indications for this approach are limited.[33] The two major therapeutic challenges of the future are to identify prospectively those subjects most likely to benefit from very low-calorie diets and to develop strategies that reduce the likelihood of weight regain.

Dental Splinting

Dental splinting adds a mechanical restraint that promotes adherence to a liquid diet. It is not without risk, and the end results are uncertain.[34,35] The indications for treatment should be clearly defined. Subjects should have a BMI in excess of 40 kg/m^2, although this value might be reduced to 35 if the obesity is medically complicated. The procedure should be restricted to those between the ages of 18 and 50 or 60. All subjects should have attempted to reduce with a less radical approach or should have attended a special clinic that will accept responsibility for their supervision not less than three months prior to the proposed dental splinting. During this time the subject must have experienced the proposed weight maintenance program without gaining weight and must also have lost weight with the jaw wiring regimen prior to dental splinting. The need for long-term supervision following dental splinting must be emphasized as part of a patient contract. This should include willingness to accept a nylon waist cord when the splints are removed and, if all else fails, to undergo a gastric reduction procedure.

Surgery

Surgery probably offers the best prospects of permanent weight loss. However, it has major disadvantages and is not without risk. The need for caution is reflected in the guidelines laid down by the task force of the American Society for Clinical Nutrition.[36] Surgery should only be performed in subjects who are at least 100 pounds (45 kg) or 100% in excess of their ideal, or who have a significant but less severe degree of obesity in combination with one or more serious medical conditions. In addition, subjects should have been substantially overweight for at least three years despite repeated attempts at nonsurgical weight loss. Contraindications include serious underlying medical problems such as severe cardiorespiratory disease or malignancy. The task force emphasized the importance of explaining the full implications of surgery and the need for long-term postoperative follow-up. An alternative approach is to apply the same criteria but to offer gastric surgery as part of a comprehensive program intended to minimize weight regain following substantial weight loss achieved by nonsurgical means such as very low-calorie diets or dental splinting.

Patient Selection

High levels of unexplained variance are common in the outcome of weight loss attempts. Regardless of the treatment modality, some subjects do well and others fail to reduce. It follows that the ability to prospectively select subjects likely to benefit from a particular treatment would considerably increase the therapeutic indications for that treatment. Ideally, weight loss is most strongly indicated if the individual subject *needs* and *wants* to lose weight and is *capable* of achieving and maintaining weight reduction. Various personal characteristics have been identified retrospectively that may influence specific outcomes. These include a strong desire for social acceptance[37] and strong feelings of self-efficacy,[38] but not self-motivation.[39] Outcome correlates negatively with ego weakness and impulsiveness.[40] At present, however, the ability to prospectively identify subjects likely to succeed is daunting, though this may be partly resolved with the further refinement of objective questionnaires.[41] When radical options are being considered, an overriding factor is the subject's grasp of the possible hazards of the treatment. Otherwise, at present, the therapist's subjective assessment of outcome should not overly influence management decisions.

WEIGHT MAINTENANCE— AN INDICATION FOR TREATMENT

Weight maintenance is an important treatment objective in the nonobese, the postobese, and the obese.

Weight Maintenance in the Nonobese

Although a high proportion of the population is overweight, every year an even higher proportion will attempt to diet. Some of these subjects are dieting either because they have a misconception of body image or are intermittently dieting as a method of maintaining body weight. Prevention of inappropriate weight gain is an important aspect of health promotion and should be encouraged both nationally and individually.

Weight Maintenance Following Weight Loss

The prevention of weight regain following weight loss is an essential component of successful treatment. Any substantial weight loss becomes an important indication for developing a weight maintenance program.[42,43]

Weight Maintenance in the Obese

A substantial number of obese subjects are unable to lose significant amounts of weight. For such subjects, it is important to review the management objectives and to adopt a realistic approach. If a more radical treatment is not justified, management should not be abandoned but the emphasis should shift from weight loss to weight maintenance. If progressive weight gain produces increasing morbidity and mortality,[44] prevention of weight gain is an important indication for treatment whether or not such weight change may be attributed to normal weight fluctuations.[45]

TREATMENT OF COMPLICATIONS

In clinical terms, management always is directed toward the obese subject rather than the obesity *per se*. Superseding any need to achieve weight loss or prevent weight regain, there may be indications to treat either presymptomatic complications, such as significant hypertension, or the symptoms of obesity-related conditions, such as type II diabetes mellitus, angina of effort, or coexisting osteoarthrosis. All too often, obese subjects meet with medical intolerance when they present with specific symptoms. For example, patients with low back ache may receive gratuitous and unhelpful advice about weight loss when the primary need is for an appropriate analgesic.

CONCLUSIONS

At first glance, the indications for the treatment of obesity appear to be straightforward. It is widely held that "obesity is a hazard to health and a deterrent to well-being. It is common enough to constitute one of the most important medical and public health problems of our time, whether we judge its importance by a shorter expectation of life, increased morbidity or cost to the community in terms both of money and anxiety."[46] This assessment provides grounds for recommending that all obese subjects should lose weight; and the greater the degree of obesity, the greater the indication. Such a simplistic view, however, fails to take into consideration the practical realities. Some subjects who wish to reduce do not need to lose weight. Many who need to reduce either do not wish to or are unable to achieve weight reduction. This clinical paradox may promote an inappropriate negative approach toward treatment.[47]

Obesity is a significant health hazard. Sometimes, however, its therapeutic importance should take second place to the need to treat other risk factors, including smoking.

Because of the unpredictability of the outcome of therapy, the specific indications for the treatment of any given individual are often difficult to define and will remain so until the method of selection can be improved or more effective therapies become available.

Weight loss is only one indication for treatment. Other indications are the symptomatic improvement of obesity-associated conditions and the maintenance of a stable weight.

Obesity prevention is an important component of health promotion.

References

1. Brook CGD, Huntley RMC, Slack J: Influence of hereditary and environment in the determination of skin fold thickness in children. Br Med J 2:719, 1975
2. Stunkard AJ, Sorensen TIA, Hanis C et al: An adoption study of human obesity. N Engl J Med 314:193, 1986

3. Jeffrey RW, Forster JL, Folsom AR et al: The relationship between social status and body mass index in the Minnesota Heart Health program. Int J Obes 13:59, 1989

4. Silverstone JT: Obesity. Proc R Soc Med 61:371, 1968

5 Rodin J, Wing RR: Behavioural factors in obesity. Diabetes Metab Rev 4:701, 1988

6. Seltzer CC: Some re-evaluation of the build and blood pressure study 1959 as related to ponderal index, somatotype and mortality. N Engl J Med 274:254, 1966

7. Lew EA, Garfinkel L: Variations in mortality by weight among 750,000 men and women. J Chronic Dis 32:563, 1979

8. Cochrane AL, Moore F, Baker IA et al: Mortality in two random samples of women aged 55–64 followed up for 20 years. Br Med J 280:1131, 1980

9. Blair BF, Haines LW: Mortality experience according to build at higher durations. Trans Actuar Soc Am 18:35, 1966

10. Dublin LI: Relation of obesity to longevity. N Engl J Med 248:971, 1953

11. Bray GA: Obesity: Definition, diagnosis and disadvantages. Aust J Med 142(suppl 7):S2, 1985

12. Larsson BO: Regional obesity as a health hazard in men: Prospective studies. Acta Med Scand Suppl 723:45, 1988

13. Lapidus L, Bengtsson C: Regional obesity as a health hazard in women: A prospective study. Acta Med Scand Suppl 723:53, 1988

14. Larsson B, Svardsudd K, Welin L et al: Abdominal adipose tissue distribution, obesity and risk of cardiovascular disease and death. Br Med J 288:14011, 1984

15. Cahill GF: Obesity and diabetes. In Bray GA (ed): Recent Advances in Obesity Research, vol 11, 2nd International Congress on Obesity, p 101. Newman Publishing, 1978

16. Baird JD: The role of obesity in the development of clinical diabetes. In Robertson RF (ed): Anorexia and Obesity. Royal College of Physicians, publication 42, p 83. Edinburgh, Royal College of Physicians, 1973

17. Douglas JG, Preston PG, Haslett C et al: Long term efficacy of fenfluramine in the treatment of obesity. Lancet 1:384, 1983

18. Kirschner MA, Schneider G, Ertel NH et al: An eight-year experience with a very-low-calorie formula diet for control of major obesity. Int J Obes 12:69, 1988

19. Griffiths RA, Holliday J: An evaluation and follow-up investigation of a behavioural group treatment programme for obesity. Psychother Psychosom 48:157, 1987

20. Garrow JS, Webster JD: Long term results of treatment of severe obesity with jaw wiring and waist cord. Proc Nutr Soc 45:119a, 1986

21. Simpson GK, Farquhar DL, Carr P et al: Intermittent protein-sparing fasting with abdominal belting. Int J Obes 10:247, 1986

22. Bjorvell H, Rossner S: Long term treatment of severe obesity: Four year follow up of results of combined behavioural modification programme. Br Med J 291:379, 1985

23. Brownell KD, Kramer FM: Behavioral management of obesity. Med Clin North Am 73:185, 1989

24. Wadden TA, Sternberg JA, Letizia KA et al: Treatment of obesity by very-low-calorie diet, behavior therapy and their combination: A five-year perspective. Int J Obes 13(suppl 1), 1989

25. Ford MJ, Scorgie RE, Munro JF: Anticipated rate of weight loss during dieting. Int J Obes 1:239, 1977

26. Bradley I, Poser EG, Johnson JA: Outcome expectation ratings as predictors of success in weight reduction. J Clin Psychol 36:500, 1980

27. Wing RR, Jeffrey RW: Outpatient treatments of obesity: A comparison of methodology and clinical results. Int J Obes 3:261, 1979

28. Bennett W: Dietary treatments of obesity. In Wurtman RJ, Wurtmann JJ (eds): The Treatment of Obesity. Ann NY Acad Sci 499:250, 1987

29. Pacy PJ, Webster J, Garrow JS: Exercise and obesity. Sports Med 3:89, 1986

30. Segal KR, Pi-Sunyer FX: Exercise and obesity. Med Clin North Am 73:217, 1989

31. Douglas JG, Munro JF: Drug treatment and obesity. Pharmacol Ther 18:351, 1982

32. Ferguson JM, Feighner JP: Fluoxetine induced weight loss in non-depressed overweight humans. Aliment Nutr Metab 7:19, 1986

33. Department of Health and Social Security: Report on Health & Social Subjects. The use of very low calorie diets in obesity. London, Her Majesty's Stationery Office, 1987

34. Tedesco C, Buchanan PDC, Hall HD: Jaw wiring for obesity. Gen Hosp Psychiatry 2:156, 1980

35. Drenick EJ, Hargis HW: Jaw wiring for weight reduction. Obes Bariatr Med 7:210, 1978

36. Task Force of the American Society for Clinical Nutrition: Guidelines for surgery for morbid obesity. Am J Clin Nutr 42:904, 1985

37. Rodin J, Bray GA, Atkinson RL et al: Predictors of successful weight loss in an outpatient obesity clinic. Int J Obes 1:79, 1977

38. Rodin J, Elias M, Silberstein LR et al: Combined behavioral and pharmacologic treatment of obesity: Predictors of successful weight maintenance. J Consult Clin Psychol 56:399, 1988

39. Edell BH, Edington S, Herd B et al: Self-efficacy and self-motivation as predictors of weight loss. Addict Behav 12:63, 1987

40. Jonsson B, Bjorvell H, Levander S et al: Personality traits predicting weight loss outcome in obese patients. Acta Psychiatry Scand 74:384, 1986

41. Straw MT, Straw RB, Mahoney ML et al: The master questionnaire: Preliminary report on an obesity assessment device. Addict Behav 9:1, 1984

42. Marston AR, Criss J: Maintenance of successful weight loss: Incidence and prediction. Int J Obes 8:435, 1984

43. Forster JL, Jeffrey RW, Schmid TL et al: Preventing weight gain in adults: A pound of prevention. Health Psychol 7:515, 1988

44. Gray GA, Gray DS: Treatment of obesity: An overview. Diabetes Metab Rev 4:653, 1988

45. Williamson PS, Levy BT: Long-term body weight fluctuation in an overweight population. Int J Obes 12:579, 1988

46. Department of Health and Social Security: Recommended Daily Amounts of Food Energy and Nutrients for Groups of People in the United Kingdom. London, Her Majesty's Stationery Office, 1979

47. Hall A, Franz CP: Obesity: Time for sanity and humanity. NZ Med J 102:134, 1989

Weight Cycling, Mortality, and Cardiovascular Disease: A Review of Epidemiologic Findings

LAUREN LISSNER and KELLY D. BROWNELL

The high prevalence of obesity in affluent societies, coupled with an increasingly lean aesthetic ideal, has resulted in unprecedented rates of dieting. For instance, the 1985 Health Interview Survey revealed that 27% of American men and 46% of women questioned were trying to lose weight.[1] Among participants in the Framingham Offspring/Spouse study, 21.5% reported annual weight fluctuations of 10 to 20 pounds at least once a year, and another 2.4% reported yearly fluctuations that were even larger (pers. commun., B. Posner). High recidivism rates following weight loss may contribute to this epidemic of dieting,[2,3] and many individuals engage in repeated attempts at weight loss in pursuit of their ideal body weights. We refer to this pattern of weight loss and subsequent regain as "weight cycling."

Dieting to control body weight is not confined to overweight individuals or to adults. In one metropolitan, adult population, dieting was widely reported among men and women who had never been overweight.[4] The pressure to be thin occurs even in children; a survey of girls ages 9 to 18 in California found that 70% were restricting their eating.[5] Although adherence to weight reduction diets is often assumed to be beneficial to health, the high rates of dieting have created some concern regarding potential negative health consequences.

OVERVIEW OF WEIGHT CYCLING IN EPIDEMIOLOGIC STUDIES

A number of investigators have examined relationships between weight fluctuation on one hand and health and longevity on the other. It has been speculated that variability in body weight might be a useful indicator of weight cycling, which could be used in prospective studies to predict chronic disease. In the first section of this review, we describe various data bases and analytic methods that have been used for this purpose; these are summarized in Table 56-1. The following section describes associations that have been observed between weight fluctuation and all-cause mortality. Next, we describe studies that have examined weight fluctuation in relation to cardiovascular disease. Finally, we present data from one paper that related weight fluctuation to simultaneous changes in cardiovascular disease risk factors. We conclude with a discussion of methodological issues inherent to this type of analysis and possible interpretations of the findings to date.

The Gothenburg Prospective Study of Women

This cohort consists of a random sample of 1462 women born between 1908 and 1930 in Gothen-

TABLE 56-1

Description of Studies

Investigators	Study	N	Indicator
Lissner, Bengtsson, Lapidus et al	Gothenburg Prospective Studies		CV of BMI
	Men	855	
	Women	1462	
Hamm, Shekelle, Stamler	Western Electric Study (men)	2107	10% gain and 10% loss
Blair, Collins, Brownell et al	MRFIT†		SD of BMI
	SI men	5393	
	UC men	5295	
Lissner, Andres, Muller et al	Baltimore Longitudinal Study of Aging (men)	846	Residual variability*
Lissner, Odell, D'Agostino et al	Framingham Heart Study		CV of BMI
	Men	1351	
	Women	1779	
Stevens	Charleston Heart Study		CV of BMI
	White males	291	
	White females	300	
	Black males	153	
	Black females	184	
Hoffmans, Kromhout	Zutphen Study (men)	630	Residual variability*

CV = coefficient of variation, BMI = body mass index (weight/height^2), SD = standard deviation.

*Residual variability = variability about time-dependent regression line.

†SI = special intervention, UC = control.

burg, Sweden.[6,7] Weight fluctuation patterns were studied in relation to several health end points.[8] Intraindividual body weight variability was the independent variable of interest and was defined as the within-subject coefficient of variation of an individual's body mass index (BMI = wt/ht^2) at three points in time. The two key covariates in this analysis were also within-person variables. The first was a woman's mean BMI across the same three observations. The second covariate represented the direction and magnitude of her change in BMI and was calculated as the third weight minus the first. The rationale for including these two covariates was the following. By including the change in BMI over time as an independent variable, it was possible to distinguish effects of linear trend in body weight from effects of random or periodic fluc-

tuation. This was done because the variability in BMI and the slope of BMI are likely to be correlated. Similarly, correcting for a subject's mean BMI enables one to separate any effects of obesity from effects of weight cycling. This may be important because obesity is in itself a risk factor, and obese individuals are likely to exhibit more dieting-induced weight fluctuation than nonobese subjects. An additional covariate was age group, which referred to the five birth cohorts in this study. The independent and dependent variables considered in this analysis were separated chronologically by placing a time interval of at least seven months between the last body weight and the first end point. The purpose of excluding the earlier end points was to remove variability in body weight, which were likely to reflect prior or concurrent disease.

The Gothenburg Prospective Study of Men

A random sample of 855 men born in Gothenburg, Sweden, in 1913 underwent a series of medical examinations between 1963 and 1988.[9] Weight fluctuations in this population were also studied in relation to chronic disease.[8] As in the women's study, body weight variability was calculated as the coefficient of variation of a subject's first three BMI values. The covariates included in the analysis included his average BMI on exams one through three (an index of obesity) and the difference between the third and first BMI measured (direction and magnitude of the trend). It was not necessary to include age as a covariate in this analysis because all of the men were born in the same year.

The Western Electric Study

Researchers from the Western Electric Study used another approach in evaluating weight fluctuation in relation to all-cause and coronary heart disease mortality.[10] This analysis was based on a sample of 2107 men aged 40 to 56 years who were questioned on their weight history and were studied prospectively between 1957 and 1983.[11] Self-reported body weight reflecting five-year intervals between ages 20 to 40 were used to compare a group of middle-aged men who had gained and lost 10% of their body weight with another group whose weight had remained stable.

The Framingham Heart Study

The Framingham Heart Study, initiated in 1948, has been monitoring the health status of 5127 male and female residents of Framingham, Massachusetts, who were initially free of coronary heart disease. The subjects' ages at entry were between 30 and 62 years, and body weight was subsequently measured every two years.[12] Weight fluctuation has been studied in this population, again using a design based on a chronological separation of weight change and health outcomes.[13] All body weights measured during the first 14 years (eight examinations) of the project, along with recalled body weight at the age of 25, were used to construct independent variables representing body weight and its fluctuation. The dependent variables were various end points occurring at least two years after the last observed body weight. Weight cycling was defined as the intraindividual coefficient of variation in BMI during the initial observation period. Covariates were age, mean BMI, and the time-dependent slope in BMI across the observations. Separate analyses were done for men and women. Three proportional hazards regression models were used in the analysis of these data: the first including age and variability in BMI as independent variables, the second adding mean and slope of BMI (analogous to the Gothenburg studies), and finally, five baseline cardiovascular risk factors.

The Baltimore Longitudinal Study of Aging

This study[14] provided an opportunity to examine weight fluctuation and concurrent changes in a wide range of cardiovascular risk factors, including lipid profiles, adipose distribution, glucose tolerance, and blood pressure. The cohort consists of 846 Baltimore–Washington area males, ages 20 to 92 years, who have undergone physical examinations every 12 to 24 months. In a recent study,[15] changes in cardiovascular risk factors were assessed in relation to concurrent changes in body weight. Weight cycling was defined here as the intraindividual variability in body weight about a time-dependent regression slope, in contrast to the Gothenburg and Framingham analyses, which calculated variability about an individual's mean. The end points in this analysis were changes in a subject's cardiovascular risk factors over the same time period. Linear regression was used to evaluate changes in a risk factor relative to variability in body weight after correction for age, mean BMI, and linear trend in body weight. "Hard" end points such as mortality and coronary heart disease were also evaluated using proportional hazards regression if these events occurred after the fourth observed body weight.

The Multiple Risk Factor Intervention Trial

The Multiple Risk Factor Intervention Trial (MRFIT) was a randomized clinical primary prevention trial designed to test the effect of a multifactor intervention program on mortality from coronary heart disease in 12,866 high-risk men aged 35 to 57 years.[16] Half of the subjects were randomized to a special intervention group and the others received usual medical care and served as controls. In a recent analysis of the 10-year follow-up data,[17,18] the intraperson standard deviation of BMI was used as an indicator of weight fluctuation. This index was calculated from body weights measured at annual examinations for the control group and every four months for the special intervention group. Proportional hazards regression was used to relate body weight variability to cardiovascular and all-cause mortality during follow-up. In the analysis of total mortality, all men who were hospitalized or diagnosed with cancer during the trial were excluded[18]; in the analysis of cardiovascular disease mortality, development of cancer was an exclusion criterion.[17]

The Charleston Heart Study

The effects of body weight fluctuation on mortality were examined using data from the Charleston Heart Study. The Charleston study began in 1960 with the examination of a random sample of 2182 residents of Charleston County, South Carolina.[19] Approximately one third of the sample was black. A subset of the cohort was reexamined in 1963–1964 and 1973–1974, during which time body weight and height were remeasured. The vital status of over 95% of the members of the cohort has been ascertained through 1986. Body weight variability was calculated as the coefficient of variation of body weights measured at three points in time between age 25 and the year 1963 in 932 subjects. Body weight variability and covariates age, mean BMI, and change in BMI were examined as predictors of subsequent mortality (1965–1986) in four race and sex groups: white males, white females, black males, and black females (pers. commun., J. Stevens).

The Zutphen Study

The Zutphen Study is a population-based prospective study of 40- to 59-year-old Dutch men with a complete 25-year morbidity and mortality

follow-up.[20] Body weight variability was calculated in 630 men who had remained free of cardiovascular disease during the first ten years of the study.[21] All cases of fatal and nonfatal myocardial infarction that occurred during the following 15 years were evaluated in relation to mean BMI, the linear trend in BMI, and intraperson variability in BMI, which was calculated as the residual fluctuation. Using proportional hazards regression, residual fluctuation was appointed as the exposure variable, after adjustment for other BMI variables and for age and smoking status.

WEIGHT CYCLING AND MORTALITY

Positive associations have been consistently observed between body weight fluctuation and all-cause mortality in the studies described in Table 56-2, with the exception of nonsmokers in MRFIT. The results are statistically significant in five of the analyses reported here; these associations were independent of obesity and systematic weight change. It is important to note that when the MRFIT participants were stratified by smoking status, the association was not present in nonsmokers from either intervention group. In the special intervention group, the association remained highly significant in individuals who were smokers both at the beginning and the end of the trial.

Several of these studies calculated risk estimates of body weight variability relative to stability in body weight. In the Western Electric Study, the 95% confidence interval was 1.0–2.3. In the Framingham Heart Study the point estimates of the risk associated with being in the most weight-variable group ranged from 1.3 to 1.7 in men and from 1.2 to 1.3 in women, the higher estimates reflecting the adjustment for BMI and linear trend. Among men who smoked cigarettes at the beginning and end of the MRFIT trial, the relative risks posed by weight fluctuation were 1.7 for the special intervention group and 1.2 in the control group.

WEIGHT CYCLING AND CARDIOVASCULAR DISEASE

A number of studies have examined weight fluctuation in relation to cardiovascular and coronary heart disease. As shown in Table 56-3, the majority have observed significant, positive associations between weight fluctuation and these end points. Specifically, the male cohorts from the Gothenburg and Western Electric studies, the men and women in the Framingham Heart Study, and men who smoked at the beginning and the end of the MRFIT trial all had an elevated cardiovascular risk associated with large fluctuations in body weight. In contrast, the male cohorts of the Baltimore and Zutphen studies displayed no association between weight fluctuation and coronary heart disease. In MRFIT, the association was strongest in leaner men but was not significant in nonsmokers.

WEIGHT CYCLING AND CHANGES IN RISK FACTORS FOR CARDIOVASCULAR DISEASE

In the Baltimore Longitudinal Study of Aging (BLSA), body weight variability was evaluated in relation to concomitant changes in the following dependent variables: glucose tolerance, ratio of subscapular to triceps skin folds, ratio of waist circumference to hip circumference, systolic blood pressure, serum cholesterol levels, and triglyceride levels. It was hypothesized that some of the associations that have been found between weight fluctuation and cardiovascular disease might be explained by changes in cardiovascular risk factors during weight gain that are not fully reversible with weight loss.

Body weight variability was not significantly associated with rates of change in systolic blood pressure, serum triglycerides, total cholesterol, or waist–hip circumference ratio after controlling for age, obesity, and linear trend in body weight. There was no evidence that the low-density or high-density lipoprotein fractions were differentially affected. However, significant, positive associations were observed between body weight variability and changes in serum glucose concentration following an oral glucose challenge ($P < .05$), suggesting that individuals with the most variable weights had greater decreases in glucose tolerance over time. The magnitude of this association was roughly half of the effect of 1 kg weight gain on glucose tolerance.

TABLE 56-2

Review of Studies Describing Associations Between Body Weight Fluctuation and All-Cause Mortality

Study	Association	Significance
Gothenburg Prospective Studies		
Men	Positive	$P = .003$
Women	Positive	$P = .03$
Western Electric Study	Higher in gain–loss group	NS
Framingham Heart Study		
Men	Positive	$P = .0001$
Women	Positive	$P = .0001$
MRFIT*		
SI smokers	Positive	$P = .01$
UC smokers	Positive	NS
Nonsmokers (SI and UC)	Negative	NS
Baltimore Longitudinal Study of Aging	Positive	NS
Charleston Heart Study	Positive (all groups)	NS (all groups)

*SI = special intervention, UC = control.

The other statistically significant correlate of body weight variability in this analysis was in the change in the ratio of subscapular to triceps skin folds ($P < .02$), suggesting that individuals with the most weight fluctuation had the greatest increases in truncal adiposity. This could be indicative of an increased centralization of body fat during the process of body weight fluctuation. However, as mentioned previously, this effect was not manifested in any changes in the waist–hip circumference ratio.

DISCUSSION

One limitation of epidemiologic analyses is that the associations cannot be considered causal, in part because of the difficulty in ascertaining that

TABLE 56-3

Studies Describing Associations Between Body Weight Fluctuation and Cardiovascular Disease

Study	End point	Association	Significance
Gothenburg prospective study Men†	All CHD	Positive	P = .02
Western Electric study‡	CHD death	Higher in gain–loss group	P < .05
Framingham Heart study†			
Men	All CHD	Positive	P = .0001
	CHD death	Positive	P = .0001
Women	All CHD	Positive	P = .05
	CHD death	Positive	P = .005
MRFIT§	CVD death		
All		Positive	P = .001
Nonsmokers		Positive	NS (SI); NS (UC)
Smokers		Positive	P = .001 (SI)
			P = .02 (UC)
Baltimore Longitudinal study of Aging†	All CHD	Negative	NS
Zutphen study‖	All MI	Negative	NS

CHD = Coronary heart disease, CVD = cardiovascular disease, MI = myocardial infarction.
*Only 10 cases in women's cohort.
†Adjusted for age, BMI, weight change.
‡Adjusted for age, cholesterol, systolic blood pressure, smoking, alcohol intake.
§Adjusted for age; baseline weight, cholesterol, smoking status, diastolic blood pressure, total cholesterol; final weight; smoking status; study group; incidence of nonfatal events.
‖Adjusted for age, BMI, weight change, smoking.

a large, free-living cohort is initially free of disease. However, data from several independent population studies have shown elevated rates of mortality and cardiovascular disease in subjects with large body weight fluctuations. The methods that were used in these positive studies varied, including identification of individuals who gain and lose weight[10] and calculation of the intraindividual standard deviation,[17,18] coefficient of variation,[8,13] or residual variability[13] in BMI over time. Although other populations did not display these associations,[15,21] it seems unlikely that the inconsistencies can be attributed to different definitions of weight fluctuation, for the following reasons. First, the use of residual variability in the Framingham analysis as an alternative to the coefficient of variation[13] yielded similar positive associations with the same end points. Conversely, use of the coefficient of variation rather than residual variability in the BLSA population[15] did not produce an association where there was none before. Finally, a categorical indicator of weight fluctuation that was not based on statistical definitions of variation also produced suggestive findings.[10] Therefore, differences in population characteristics rather than in computational methods used probably account for the lack of agreement across studies with respect to the association between weight fluctuation and hard end points.

We will present four possible interpretations for the positive associations that have been observed between weight fluctuation and disease. First, preclinical illness may have been present in some subjects during the observation periods, when they were assumed to be disease-free. In such a case, the weight fluctuation would be a likely consequence rather than a cause of the end points. In a number of studies, the "windows" of time that were placed between each subject's last observed body weight and follow-up were meant to remove serious pre-existing illnesses that might have been affecting weight, although the time intervals may not have been sufficiently long enough to remove subclinical illness. In addition, many of the multivariate analyses also controlled for linear trends in body weight in order to decrease the influence of systematic weight loss (presumably associated with chronic illness) on the findings. Although this precaution allows one to conclude with some degree of confidence that subjects were generally healthy during the initial observation period, underlying illness remains one viable explanation for these observations.

It is also possible that some subjects intentionally lost weight because of certain indicators of disease (e.g., elevated serum glucose, cholesterol, blood pressure) that placed them at increased risk. These individuals may have been advised to reduce their weight for health reasons, and may have subsequently regained the lost weight or experienced disease in spite of the weight loss. For this reason, several of the studies included baseline cardiovascular risk factors as background variables in the regression models. The independence of many of the results from these covariates decreases the plausibility of this second potential explanation.

The MRFIT data provide another perspective on these combined findings. The increased risk of CVD and all-cause mortality among weight-variable men was largely confined to those who smoked cigarettes at the beginning and end of the trial. Many of the subjects in both intervention groups attempted to quit smoking during the trial, and weight gain is a known consequence of smoking cessation.[22] It is likely that many of these individuals experienced weight loss and regain as they tried to reduce their cigarette consumption. These data raise the possibility that weight fluctuation may often reflect unsuccessful attempts at smoking cessation, and that the associated health outcomes may be a consequence of past and current smoking habits.

Alternatively, these associations might reflect an adverse effect of single or repeated cycles of weight loss and regain. Although one might question the assumption that body weight variability is a valid indicator of weight cycling, most of the studies have not provided direct information on voluntary weight reduction. An exception is the Gothenburg Women's Study, which did document adherence to weight loss diets; as expected, dieting history was found to be significantly correlated with variability in body weight. In addition, a review of a selection of Framingham Heart Study medical records indicated that weight reduction dieting occurred in 50% of the most weight-variable individuals, which is likely to be an underestimate, insofar as information on dieting was not recorded consistently during the examinations. Therefore, one cannot exclude the possibility that weight reduction dieting is a promoter of disease; however, its specific role can only be elucidated by future prospective studies that are designed to collect this type of information.

Two suggestive findings that emerged from the BLSA study involved changes in glucose tolerance and changes in the ratio of subscapular to triceps skin-fold measurements. A redistribution of body fat to more malignant locations or a change in insulin resistance might play a role in the adverse cardiovascular outcomes that have been observed among weight-variable individuals in other studies. However, the fact that the same study detected no associations between body weight variability and the hard end points such as congestive heart disease and mortality indicates that other methodologies will be required in order to understand the role of weight loss and regain in health and longevity.

Although different individuals may experience large body weight fluctuations for a variety of reasons, the data presented here suggest that as a group, they are at greater risk of coronary heart disease and mortality than individuals with stable body weights. The relative risks described here are comparable in magnitude to the risks posed by being overweight in relation to total mortality,[23] cardiovascular disease,[24] and coronary heart disease.[12] Therefore, it appears that weight fluctuation is a useful indicator, together with obesity and other known disease risk factors, in the prediction of mortality and coronary heart disease. While these findings are consistent with the possibility that weight cycling by dietary means may play a role in the development of chronic disease, there are other plausible explanations. The specific impact of weight reduction dieting will require further investigation, including long-term follow-up studies of dieters who undergo repeated weight loss and gain cycles. Another important avenue for epidemiologic research will be to further examine relationships between body weight variability and the standard cardiovascular risk factors, particularly cigarette smoking. Finally, clearer understanding of the dynamics of weight change and atherogenesis could provide insight into the increased incidence of cardiovascular disease in individuals with high body weight variability.

References

1. National Center for Health Statistics: Provisional data from the Health Promotion and Disease Prevention Supplement to the National Health Interview Survey, Jan–March 1985. Advance data, November 1985, 2–5

2. Stunkard AJ, Penick SB: Behavior modification in the treatment of obesity: The problem of maintaining weight loss. Arch Gen Psychiatry 36:801, 1979

3. Sohar E, Sneh E: Follow-up of obese patients: 14 years after a successful reducing diet. Am J Clin Nutr 26:845, 1973

4. Jeffrey RW, Folsom AR, Luepker RV et al: Prevalance of overweight and weight loss behavior in a metropolitan adult population: The Minnesota Heart Survey experience. Am J Public Health 74:349, 1984

5. Mellin LM, Scully S, Irwin CE: Disordered eating characteristics in preadolescent girls. Presented at the annual meeting of the American Dietetic Association, Las Vegas, 1986

6. Bengtsson C, Blohmé G, Hallberg L et al: The study of women in Gothenburg 1968–1969: A population study. General design, purpose and sampling results. Acta Med Scand 193:311, 1973

7. Lapidus L, Bengtsson C, Larsson B et al: Distribution of adipose tissue and risk of cardiovascular disease and death: A 12-year follow-up of participants in the population study of women in Gothenburg, Sweden. Br Med J 289:1257, 1984

8. Lissner L, Bengtsson C, Lapidus L et al: Body weight variability and mortality in the Gothenburg prospective studies of men and women (55–60). In Björntorp P, Rossner S (eds): Obesity in Europe 88. London, Libbey, 1989

9. Larsson B, Svardsudd K, Welin W et al: Abdominal adipose tissue distribution, obesity, and risk of cardiovascular disease and death: 13-year follow-up of participants in the study of men born in 1913. Br Med J 288:1410, 1984

10. Hamm PB, Shekelle RB, Stamler J: Large fluctuations in body weight during young adulthood and 25-year risk of coronary death in men. Am J Epidemiol 129:312, 1989

11. Paul O, Leper M, Phelan WH et al: A longitudinal study of coronary heart disease. Circulation 28:20, 1963

12. Dawber T: The Framingham Study: The Epidemiology of Atherosclerotic Disease. Cambridge, Mass, Harvard University Press, 1980

13. Lissner L, Odell P, D'Agostino R et al: Variability of body weight and health outcomes in the Framingham population. N Engl J Med (in press)

14. Shock NW, Greulich RC, Andres R et al: Normal Human Aging: The Baltimore Longitudinal Study of Aging. NIH publication No. 84-2450. Washington, DC, National Institutes of Health, 1984

15. Lissner L, Andres R, Muller DC et al: Body weight variability in men: Metabolic rate, health and longevity. Int J Obes 14:373, 1990

16. Multiple Risk Factor Intervention Trial Research Group: Multiple Risk Factor Intervention Trial: Risk factor changes and mortality results. JAMA 248:1465, 1982

17. Blair S, Collins G, Brownell K et al: Weight cycling and increased risk of cardiovascular disease death in men (abstr). Presented at the 29th annual meeting of the AHA Council on Epidemiology, Washington, DC, June 19–22, 1989

18. Lissner L, Collins G, Blair S et al: Weight fluctuation in the Multiple Risk Factor Intervention Trial Population (abstr). Am J Epidemiol 130:845, 1989

19. Keil JE, Loadholt CB, Weinrich MC et al: Incidence of coronary heart disease in blacks in Charleston, South Carolina. Am Heart J 108:779, 1984

20. Kromhout D: Changes in energy and macronutrients in 871 middle-aged men during 10 years of follow-up (the Zutphen Study). Am J Clin Nutr 37:287, 1983

21. Hoffmans MDAF, Kromhout D: Changes in body

mass index in relation to myocardial infarction incidence and mortality (abstr). Int J Obes 13:25, 1989

22. Shimokata S, Muller DC, Andres R: Studies in the distribution of body fat. III. Effects of cigarette smoking. JAMA 261:1169, 1989

23. Lew EA: Mortality and weight: Insured lives and the American Cancer Society studies. Ann Intern Med 103:1024, 1985

24. Hubert HB, Feinleib M, McNamara PM et al: Obesity as an independent risk factor for cardiovascular disease: A 21-year follow-up of participants in the Framingham Heart Study. Circulation 67:968, 1983

CHAPTER 57

Treatment of Obesity: Conventional Programs and Fad Diets

JOHANNA T. DWYER

Conventional dietary treatment for obesity consists of a hypocaloric diet. However, most obese people do not have grossly elevated caloric intakes over those of nonobese people. Obesity is fostered by low energy needs, especially low energy outputs because of low physical activity, and psychological and social factors, which may influence both energy intakes and energy outputs. For obesity treatment to be successful over the long term, these other issues must also be addressed. Therefore the hypocaloric diet is usually accompanied by nutrition education, emphasis on increased physical activity and exercise, behavior modification, and psychological and social support. This chapter discusses the characteristics of conventional reducing diets that are suitable for use with modest amounts of medical supervision. Examples of questionable and unreasonable popular diets are mentioned. Very low calorie diets of less than 800 calories, which require greater amounts of medical supervision, are discussed in another chapter in this volume.[5]

PREVALENCE OF OBESITY AND ITS ASSOCIATION WITH ENERGY INTAKES

The prevalence of obesity is high and increasing in the United States despite indications that energy intakes have decreased in the past three decades.[10] The association between calorie intake in excess of energy needs and obesity has been obscured by many confounding variables. These include difficulties in assessing energy intakes, demographic changes in the age and sex structure of the population, and changes in life-styles and behaviors that influence the expression of obesity, such as physical activity, smoking, and alcohol use.[34]

PREVALENCE OF DIETING AND WEIGHT CONTROL EFFORTS

Dieting prevalence is high, ranging from 45% to 47% among women and 24% to 30% among men, depending on age. The highest dieting rates occur in young women, many of whom are virtually perpetual dieters.[11] Obese young women of high socioeconomic status are especially likely to be dieting. In a recent National Health Interview survey, over half of all overweight adults reported that they were trying to lose weight by dieting, physical activity, or both. Even lean young women were attempting to lose weight.[11] The quest for slimness is reflected in the large and rapidly expanding sales volume in the industry. Table 57-1 shows that current spending for weight loss products and services is well over $29 billion per year. The projected growth in spending is 15% to 19% per year until at least 1995.[30]

Most dieters fail to achieve and maintain their desired weights. The failure rates of obesity treatment approach 60% to 90% over five years, so that many individuals are constantly searching for a new diet or weight control program that will provide lasting relief from their problem.[11]

Some weight control products and services are

TABLE 57-1

The Diet and Weight Loss Market 1988

Method	Estimated Sales, 1988 ($ Billions)
Programs for weight loss	
Hospital weight loss clinics and programs	4.5
Other weight loss programs and clinics	1.5
Exercise clubs and health clubs	8.0
Residential spas	1.4
Diet foods	
Diet soft drinks	10.0
Low-calorie foods and entrees	1.5
Artificial sweeteners	1.0
Diet books	0.382
Appetite suppressants	0.314
Surgery (liposuction, stomach reduction, jaw wiring)	0.455 (estimated)
Mail-order diet and weight remedies	NA*
Total	$29.07

Source: Market Data Enterprises.[30]

*Mail order diet and weight loss estimates are fragmentary and less reliable, but probably total $5.8 billion per year.

effective. Others are inefficacious, costly, promoted in a false or misleading manner, and pose risks to health. Health professionals must be able to distinguish between reasonable and unreasonable regimens themselves and help patients to do so. Reliable sources of information include the Food and Drug Administration, nutrition units of state health departments, the American Dietetic Association, occasional reviews in professional journals, and some recent publications.[16,22,31]

CHARACTERISTICS OF REASONABLE REDUCING DIETS

Several characteristics of a reasonable, sound reducing diet are easily enumerated. Calorie deficits and levels must be safe, the composition of the diet must be appropriate, components of the program other than diet must be complete, and costs must be economical.

Table 57-2 lists recent examples of popular diets promoted in books, magazines, or the mass media. The particular diets are reviewed in depth elsewhere.[6,31] Based on the characteristics of a sound reducing diet, the diets are grouped into two categories: reasonable and questionable.

Diets considered reasonable meet the four criteria enumerated above, diets considered questionable fail in one or more areas, and additionally may present health hazards. The remainder of this chapter considers the reasonable reducing diets and questionable diets, with some of the diets listed in Table 57-2 used to illustrate general principles.

Calories

Current Energy Intakes

Adult energy intakes in the United States are approximately 1600 calories for women and 2400 calories for men per day.[4] Obese people frequently do not have higher calorie intakes than nonobese people and do not necessarily underreport their calorie intakes to a greater extent than nonobese individuals.[10]

As a rule of thumb, the energy density of fat lost is taken to be the constant quantity of 3500 calories per pound of fat lost (equivalent to 7780 cal/kg, or 32.30 MJ/kg).[22] It follows that to lose a pound a week, an individual must subtract 500 cal/day from current intake, and to lose two pounds a week must subtract 1000 cal/day.

If usual energy intakes are known or can be

TABLE 57-2

Some Reasonable, Questionable, and Unreasonable Diets for the Treatment of Obesity

1200 calories per day or more

Reasonable diets
   I Don't Eat (But I Can't Lose) Weight Control
     Program
   Harvard Square Diet
   Red Book Wise Women's Diet
   Doctor's Calorie Plus
   Behavioral Control Diet
   California Nutrition Book
   California Diet
   LEARN Program for Weight Control
   Complete University Medical Diet
Questionable diets
   Oat and Wheat Bran Health Plan
   New Canadian Fiber Diet (DePrey)
   Women's Advantage Diet (Mallek)
   The 35 Plus Diet for Women
   Bad Back Diet Book (Green and Ceresa)
   "T" Factor Diet
   The Mediterranean Diet
   Atkin's Diet Revolution
   Nutrition Breakthrough
   Dr. Abravanel's Body Type Diet
   Doctor's Quick Weight Loss
   Pritikin Program Diet
   Craig Claibourne's Gourmet Diet
   Rechtschaffen Diet
   Orthocarbohydrate Diet
   Easy No Risk Diet
   Slender Now
   Never Say Diet
   F Plan Diet
   Carbohydrate Craver's Diet
   Dr. Atkin's Health Revolution
   Immune Power
   What Your Doctor Didn't Learn in Medical School

800 to 1199 calories per day

Reasonable diets
   Lean and Green Diet
   Hilton Head Metabolism Diet
   Weight Watcher's Quick Start Program
   Diet Workshop Lo Carbo and Beacon Hill Diets
Questionable diets
   Two Day Diet
   Rotation Diet
   Diet Workshop Wild Weekend
   The Hilton Head Over 35 Diet
   L.A. Diet
   Doctor's Metabolic Diet
   No Choice Diet
   Woman Doctor's Diet
   Southhampton Diet
   Bloomingdale Diet
   Snowbird Diet
   Herbalife Slim Trim Diet
   Fit for Life
   Thin So Fast (Eades)
   The Rice Diet
   Beverly Hills Diet

800 calories or less

Reasonable diets (only if administered under medical
  supervision)
   HMR (Health Management Resources)
   Optifast
   United Weight Control
   New Directions (Ross Laboratories)
   Nutrisystem
Questionable diets
   Herbalife
   Last Chance Diet
   Fasting Is A Way of Life

estimated, it is possible to design a diet that will produce the weight loss desired by simply building in a caloric deficit of appropriate size. This is perhaps the commonest and simplest method for devising the caloric level of a conventional reducing diet. From what is assumed to be the usual energy intake, food items, especially high-calorie, low-nutrient density items such as fats, sweets, and oils are removed. Although the method is fairly imprecise, some weight loss is usually achieved, and at the follow-up visit energy intakes can be increased or decreased as needed to achieve the desired degree of weight loss.

The major difficulty with this method is that it requires a knowledgeable counselor. In addition, it relies on memory or reports of food intakes. Some people are unable or unwilling to

TABLE 57-3

**Percent of Usual Calorie Intakes and Energy Deficits
with Different Reducing Diets from Mean Caloric Intakes
of American Adults**

Diet	Males: Mean Intake, 2350 cal/day*		Females: Mean Intake, 1640 cal/day*	
	% Mean Intake	% Energy Deficit	% Mean Intake	% Energy Deficit
Difference between usual intakes and reducing diet				
−500 calories	79	21	70	30
−1000 calories	57	43	39	61
Effect of standard reducing diets				
1800-calorie diet, males†	77	23	110	+10
1200-calorie diet, females†	51	49	73	27
800	34	66	49	51
500	21	79	30	70
300	13	87	18	82

*Data from Braitman et al.[4]
†Estimated resting calorie need of reference individual for the recommended dietary allowances most closely approximates this energy level.

remember or report their usual energy intakes; others, including some of the obese, have such wide swings in their energy intakes due to binging that they cannot report,[25] and thus it may be difficult to provide useful counseling suggestions.

A second and more common way to select caloric levels for reducing diets is to choose from a variety of standardized low-calorie diets with a fixed caloric level. Fixed menus specifying every food or variable menus that incorporate a system of exchanging food choices in different categories are available. These low-calorie diets have the seeming advantage of being prepackaged; the dieter need not rely on a health care counselor to devise the diet. However, such diets frequently are not sufficiently individualized to encourage compliance. Also, reducing diets of a predetermined, fixed calorie level, such as 1200 calories, generate very different weight losses and percentages of fat and lean weight lost in one individual than they do in another, if the consumers differ in the calories they require for energy balance and hence in the size of their en-

ergy deficits on the hypocaloric diet. For example, a teenager with high energy needs would lose more weight on a 1200-calorie diet than an obese middle-aged woman with low energy needs.

The various diets in Table 57-2 are categorized into those of approximately 1200 calories or more, which would generate a weight loss of one pound or greater a week, and those of 800 calories or slightly more, which would induce slightly more rapid weight losses for reference individuals. All reducing diets are designed to be hypocaloric. The diet programs claiming that the dieter can eat as much as desired also limit energy intakes, but indirectly by limiting the intake of specific nutrients such as fat or sugar or by limiting the kinds of food a dieter may eat. If the rules are followed, it is virtually impossible for the dieter to avoid eating less than before.

Table 57-3 provides estimates of the energy deficits from usual intakes created by several standard low-calorie reducing diets of the type used in many physicians' offices and by some commercial weight loss firms. Although the estimates of deficits are only approximations derived from usual energy intakes for the entire population, these calculations do illustrate why most conventional reducing diets are approximately 1200 calories for females (which would generate losses of slightly less than a pound a week) and 1800 calories for males. Diets that promise losses of two pounds per week are even lower in calories—800 calories or less.

Resting energy needs range from about 1100 to 1500 calories for females of various ages, weights, and body compositions and from about 1100 to 2000 calories for males.[36] As shown in Table 57-3, 800-calorie diets provide only one-half or less of usual intakes for both sexes and two-thirds or less of usual estimated resting metabolic rates.[36] Thus it is not surprising that as reducing diets dip below 800 cal/day, decrements in resting metabolism become more pronounced, the metabolic changes become more profound, and medical supervision becomes increasingly important.

Table 57-3 gives estimates of the percent of usual intakes and the percent energy deficits resulting from subtracting 500 and 1000 calories from usual intakes. Because most Americans are extremely sedentary, an energy deficit of 500 calories is enough to result in a reducing diet that barely covers the resting energy needs of the reference man and woman. A 1000-calorie deficit is considerably below resting metabolic rate for virtually all individuals.

Some considerations should be kept in mind when selecting appropriate calorie levels for reducing diets:

1. The deficit should not exceed 500 to 1000 cal/day unless the subject is under medical supervision.
2. The calorie level (explicit or implied) should be 800 cal/day or more unless the subject is under medical supervision.
3. Medical advice should be sought for attempted weight loss in certain situations (growth in childhood and adolescence, pregnancy and lactation, chronic illness, emotional difficulties) or for adverse reactions to the reducing program.

Patients can often apply these principles on their own. Periodic reviews of currently popular re-

ducing diets are also available in the popular literature and may be helpful in evaluating specific diets.[6]

Both the use of fixed deficits from presumed energy intakes and the use of standard low-calorie diets of fixed caloric levels have disadvantages. They fail to take into account body composition, which determines in part the resting metabolic rate, the availability of lean body mass, the proportions of fat and lean most likely to be lost at a fixed energy intake, and the point at which metabolic adaptations such as ketosis ensue.[18] The two methods of fixing calorie intakes during reducing also neglect weight, which is associated with both the absolute and the proportional amount of lean body mass and thus with resting metabolic rates, and is also important in determining the caloric costs of movement.[18]

Another way of determining energy levels for a reducing diet is to calculate the two major components of energy need (resting energy needs and physical activity) in the individual case and to prescribe a diet that is slightly lower in calories than this. However, resting energy needs may vary by 30% or more for persons of the same age and sex. Thus nomograms for estimating resting energy needs are relatively inaccurate, and unless a metabolic cart is available for measuring resting energy expenditure directly, errors are large.[36] Estimates of energy needed for physical activity are even more imprecise. So, for the extra calculation necessary, little is gained over the previous methods. However, if there were an easier way to take body composition into account by some simple index which reflected it, it might be easier to select appropriate energy intakes for reducing diets.

Resting energy needs depend in part on body weight and body composition.[18] Lean body mass, which consists of actively metabolizing tissue (total weight minus fat), accounts for much of this association. Individuals with a high lean body mass have higher resting metabolic rates than those who have lower endowments. Among adults, lean body mass is higher in males than in females, higher in younger than in older adults, and higher in obese than in leaner people.[17,20]

The use of body mass index (BMI) to estimate

body composition, coupled with estimates of energy intakes and outputs due to physical activity, permits the selection of a reducing diet that will avoid undue stimulation of counterproductive metabolic adaptations such as the starvation response, or drops in resting metabolism and discretionary physical activity when extremely hypocaloric diets are employed. The BMI (weight (kg)/height (m²)) is a simple index that takes into account the greater weight and lean body mass and greater tolerance of obese persons to hypocaloric diets from the metabolic standpoint. Obese dieters are less likely to become ketotic, they lose relatively more fat to lean than do nonobese subjects on reducing diets of fixed calorie levels, and they have relatively larger amounts of lean body mass, which may permit them to tolerate more rapid and prolonged periods of weight loss than leaner individuals.

The appropriate energy deficit for a mildly overweight (BMI = 25 to 27.9) individual is 50%. For a moderately overweight person (BMI = 28 to 31.9) it is 60%. It is these individuals who do the best on conventional diets. Such energy deficits are normally achieved by diets of 800 calories or more for most individuals (see Table 57-3).

The deficit for the severely overweight person with a BMI of 32 to 41.9 kg/m² is 70% to 80%. Energy deficits over 70% should not be imposed without medical monitoring and guidance, since the rate of weight loss and the metabolic alterations are considerable.

The deficit for the morbidly obese person (BMI of 42 kg/m² or more) is 80% to 85%. These individuals sometimes succeed with conventional diets but usually fare better with more intensive programs incorporating very low calorie diets and medical supervision. In general, severely and morbidly obese individuals are not candidates for conventional diets.

Causes of Variation in Weight Lost on Reducing Diets

Differences in adherence to the diet, differences in energy deficits imposed by the diet and by increased physical activity, the composition of the reducing diet (which may alter losses of lean body mass or water balance), body composition, and other aspects of the reducing program all contribute to differences between predicted and actual losses on weight loss regimens. The commonly used rule of thumb, that the energy cost of a pound lost on reducing diets is 3500 calories, is only an approximation. It does not apply in unusual situations in which the tissue of loss is not what is expected—15% to 20% or less lean tissue and the rest fat. The energy density of weight lost increases as metabolic adaptations occur that permit the dieter to lose more fat than lean weight. Very fat subjects lose relatively more fat on hypocaloric diets than do very lean subjects, so the energy density of weight lost is quite high for them. Those who are already nearly normal in their body composition have a lower energy density of weight lost since lean tissue is being depleted. For example, among relatively normal weight men on a reducing diet, the energy density of weight lost was only 2000 calories per pound, suggesting that a great deal of lean body mass was being lost.[1]

Composition

In addition to being hypocaloric, reducing diets must be of appropriate composition to ensure nutritional adequacy and to promote health. This is done by avoiding imbalances and excesses of dietary constituents that may have adverse effects on health. Table 57-4 summarizes these considerations.

Carbohydrate

Approximately 100 g of carbohydrate per day is recommended to spare protein and avoid large shifts in weight due to changes in water balance. When carbohydrate levels are lower than 100 g, insulin levels fall and protein is catabolized to provide glucogenic amino acids that can be converted to glucose to feed the brain and other tissues that use glucose as a fuel. The protein-sparing effect of carbohydrate is greatest in the early days on a reducing diet; as time goes on, other metabolic adaptations occur and help to spare protein to some extent.

Diets that provide less than 100 g of carbohydrate or less than 800 calories stimulate ketosis, which induces diuresis and loss of fluid weight in the first few days on the diet. Diuresis is rapid

TABLE 57-4

Characteristics of Reasonable Reducing Diets: Composition

Carbohydrate: 100 g or more to spare protein, prevent ketosis, and avoid large weight shifts due to changes in water balance

Protein: At least 0.8 g/kg/day, plus at least 1.75 g high-quality mixed protein per 100-calorie deficit (or 44 g for women and 56 g for men, plus calorie deficit adjustment for reference individuals)

Fat: 30% of calories or less

Alcohol: Low or none

Vitamins, minerals, and electrolytes: At least levels specific in recommended dietary allowances

Dietary fiber: 20–30 g/day dietary fiber from food sources

Cholesterol: 200 mg/day or less

Water: At least 1 liter/day or 1 ml/cal/day, whichever is more

---

initially on diets that are very low in carbohydrate.[39] In general, for every gram of protein or glycogen that is broken down, 3 g of water is released. Fat losses are no greater on ketogenic diets than on other diets at the same calorie level. Nor do differences in appetite or mood seem to be improved on low-carbohydrate, ketogenic diets, although claims are frequently made that this is the case.[35] Nevertheless, such diets are extremely popular. Current examples include Weight Watcher's Quick Start, the Diet Workshop Beacon Hill and Lo-Carbo Diet, the Over 30 All Natural Health and Beauty Plan Basic Weight Loss Diet, and Dr. Atkin's Health Revolution. Protein-supplemented modified fasts that are very low in calories and carbohydrate also induce a ketosis-related diuresis, and the individual remains relatively dehydrated for as long as the regimen continues.[27,38]

Another reason for the popularity of low-carbohydrate diets is that if carbohydrate restrictions are very severe, even if the dieter is permitted to eat as much of other foods as desired, an automatic caloric deficit will ensue, since at present the usual American diet provides 42% of calories or nearly 200 g from carbohydrate. Thus the dieter has the temporary illusion that energy intakes are irrelevant. Examples include the Calories Don't Count diet popularized by Herman

Taller, the Stillman Diet, the Doctor's Quick Weight Loss Diet, and the Scarsdale Diet. The same fat losses can be achieved by lowering energy intakes in other ways with less discomfort to the dieter.

The adverse effects of ketogenic diets are fatigue, postural hypotension, elevated serum uric acid levels, and a stale, fetid taste in the mouth.[38] There is little evidence that ketogenic diets spare protein by inhibiting the release of amino acids from muscle, so that a protein-sparing advantage does not appear to exist.[33] Low-carbohydrate diets also tend to be very high in fat as well as being ketogenic. Thus their caloric density is high, and they may also be high in saturated fatty acids, which increases the risks for coronary artery disease. Finally, water balance is eventually restored, and the resulting refeeding edema that ensues when an individual has been maintained on a very low carbohydrate intake that is suddenly increased can increase weight by several pounds in a day.[7]

Carbohydrate intakes also affect catecholamines, and they in turn may have effects on fluids and electrolytes, the sympathetic nervous system, and the cardiovascular system. Very low carbohydrate diets low in sugar decrease blood pressure and heart rates to a greater extent than very high carbohydrate diets equal in calories, but these effects seemed to depend more on differences in electrolyte status resulting from the two regimens than on carbohydrate level.[16] Therefore there seems to be little advantage gained over the long run from low-carbohydrate diets.

High-carbohydrate, hypocaloric diets are often low in fat, which in itself may promote health. If they are relatively limited in concentrated and refined sugars and sweets they also have the advantage of being high in bulk while low in caloric density, permitting the dieter to consume a fairly large amount of food without going off the diet. This is because naturally occurring foods that are high in carbohydrate such as fruits, vegetables, and cereals tend to be high in water or are consumed with liquids. These are also the foods highest in dietary fiber, which further increases bulk. These diets appear to provide satisfactory satiety even though they are low in fat.

High-carbohydrate, high-fiber diets are especially popular today. Among the popular diets of this type are the Kempner Rice Diet, the Duke University Rice Diet, the Oat and Wheat Bran Health Plan, the F Plan, the California Diet, and the New Canadian Fiber Diet.

High-carbohydrate, high-sugar diets are not popular today but were in the past. One example of such a regimen was the Fabulous Fructose Diet, which claimed special virtues for fructose. The Carbohydrate Craver's Diet, which is still popular, includes a modest sweet reward but is actually not high in sugars. High-sugar reducing diets promote dental caries if the sugar is in a form that sticks to the teeth.

Whether high-carbohydrate diets are actually more efficient in assisting weight loss is still undemonstrated. Theoretically, the energy cost of storing dietary fat as triglyceride is close to 9 cal/g, whereas of the 4 cal/g provided by carbohydrates, only 3.27 calories are available when they are subsequently oxidized for energy. That is, the conversion of dietary fat to body fat may be more efficient than the conversion of carbohydrate or protein.[13] Thus high-carbohydrate diets should provide an advantage, making it slightly more difficult to gain weight. When diets high in complex carbohydrates are also very high in fiber, absorption may also be slightly less than is usually assumed. Although such slight differences may in fact be present, in clinical practice it is the energy deficit and not the composition of the reducing diet that correlates most closely with fat loss.

Protein

Protein is particularly important because it is necessary for maintaining lean body mass and other essential functions. A rule of thumb is to allow at least 1.5 g/kg ideal body weight/day, which will provide generous amounts of protein on most conventional reducing diets. This amounts to as much as 50% of total calories on very low calorie diets and nearly 20% of total calories on conventional 800-calorie diets. The rationale for such a recommendation is as follows. At least 0.8 g/kg of high-quality mixed protein is needed per day by healthy adults who are not dieting. Additional amounts are needed for pregnant (+30 g) or lactating (+20 g) women. Further adjustments are necessary on reducing

diets.[9] When energy intakes fall below the level needed for energy balance, the requirement for protein rises, since some of the amino acids that could have been used for gluconeogenesis or other functions are diverted into energy-yielding catabolic pathways. The magnitude of the loss in lean body mass depends on the magnitude of the energy deficit, regardless of whether this deficit comes from decreased intake or increased energy output. In general, for every 100-calorie deficit, 0.2 to 0.3 g of additional nitrogen is required to maintain nitrogen balance.[8] This amounts to an additional 1.75 g of high-quality mixed protein per 100-calorie deficit. Although some lean body mass is always lost when fat tissue is lost, assuring that protein intakes are satisfactory can minimize these losses.

Total fasts completely devoid of protein or very low-calorie, low-protein diets may deplete lean body mass rapidly and have other untoward effects as well, such as hair loss.[19] If continued long enough they may have serious, even fatal consequences. Low-calorie liquid protein formula diets that were inadequate in the quantity and quality of protein, and possibly in other respects as well increased the risks of cardiac irregularities and of sudden death.[28] Diets low in protein include Fit for Life, popularized by the Diamond couple, which provides only 23 g/day, and the Beverly Hills diet, which was popular a few years ago.

The amount of lean body mass lost on reducing diets depends on four factors: dietary composition with respect to protein and carbohydrate level, time, initial body fat content, and the energy deficit.[17,18,22] The shifts engendered by alterations in dietary composition with respect to protein and carbohydrate relate to the need to maintain blood sugar levels; these have already been discussed. *Time* is important because the amount of lean body mass as a percentage of total weight lost is greatest initially, in the first several days on the diet, with lesser amounts lost thereafter as metabolic adaptations take place.[17] These adaptations include a greater reliance on fat oxidation as a source of energy, and sparing of protein and carbohydrate, which is achieved by hormonal shifts and by downward alterations in resting metabolism and discretionary physical activity.[22] The losses of lean body mass resulting from a constant hypocaloric diet may be less than from brief bouts of dieting, which require new metabolic adaptations on each occasion before protein begins to be spared. Also, "yo-yo" dieting that combines a hypocaloric regimen on some days with usual intakes or binges on others may be difficult to adapt to psychologically. This is of some practical significance, since in the past few years "rotation" diets that vary the calorie levels every few days, every few weeks, between weekdays and weekends, or between dieting days and "binge" or "out of control" days have become popular. These diets include such favorites as the "I Love New York" Diet, the Rotation Diet, the Wild Weekend Diet, and the Two-Day diet. In addition to possible effects on lean body mass, there is the inevitable tendency of most humans to avoid the hypocaloric periods and to lengthen the periods when calories are relatively unrestricted, with resulting nonadherence. Finally, since many obese individuals have difficulties in controlling food intake when they do not consciously restrain themselves, and since some suffer from bulimia or other eating disorders, such schemes decrease the risks of excess. Rotation or yo-yo dieting patterns are to be discouraged on many counts; such regimens are classified as questionable in Table 57-2.

Body composition also affects how much lean body mass is lost. The fatter the individual, the smaller is the proportion of lean body mass to pound of weight lost. Obese subjects usually have more lean body mass initially than lean subjects and thus higher resting metabolic rates. They are also better able to conserve lean body mass and protein on hypocaloric diets than leaner individuals. For example, obese subjects lose only about a third as much nitrogen and lean body mass per day as do nonobese subjects on total fasts.[17]

The greater the *energy deficit* or the lower the energy intake, the greater is the lean body mass loss to total weight which is lost. Thus losses of lean body mass as a percentage of weight lost are most profound on total fasts, but greater on 500-calorie diets than on 1200-calorie diets.[17,19] At approximately 1100 calories the composition of weight loss is roughly equivalent to the body composition of the slightly leaner normal individual.[17]

Intakes of roughly 1000 calories and above give rise to declines in lean body mass among the mildly obese that could be predicted from the body compositions of the slightly leaner individuals they wish to become. Very fat people lose more fat than expected and very lean people lose less. However, there is no level of reduced energy intake that completely spares lean body mass when significant amounts of weight are lost. Diets allowing only 500 calories generate losses of about 20% lean tissue, and 1000-calorie deficit diets somewhat less lean tissue.[17] But even mildly hypocaloric diets (e.g., 500-calorie deficits) with modest weight losses of 15 pounds over several months result in the loss of several pounds of lean tissue.[40]

Total fasts result in very large losses of lean body mass, often as much as 50% or 60% weight lost, especially in leaner individuals. These losses of lean body mass continue over time and are often accompanied by adverse effects on bodily functioning.[19] Total fasts are an unreasonable and dangerous means to lose weight, and diets that suggest medically unsupervised fasts are classified as unreasonable in Table 57-2. Very low calorie diets without medical supervision also pose risks of excessive losses of lean body mass and jeopardize other aspects of health. They are unreasonable for dieters to undertake on their own, based on the frightening problems that resulted from the sales of certain brands of liquid protein and other extremely low calorie diets in the 1970s. However, for the very obese, who have greater lean body mass to begin with and who lose proportionately more less lean tissue per pound of weight, very low calorie diets may be a suitable option if they are undertaken under medical guidance and monitoring.

Fat

Fat generally should not exceed 30% of calories. Diets high in fat are also often high in saturated fat and cholesterol, which in turn increases the diet-related risks of coronary artery disease.[11] There is increasing evidence that diets high in fat are associated with undesirably high levels of body fatness. Diets high in fat are highly palatable. Some experts postulate that a "fat tooth" is present in humans as well as in experimental animals.[14] There is some evidence that obese people prefer fat, rich foods. Fatter people often report eating diets higher in fat and lower in sugar than nonobese people, even when their caloric intakes are similar.[15] Also, when an individual is attempting to control food intake, errors in estimation of portion size result in more calories with high-fat, high-caloric density foods than with lower caloric density foods. Errors in portion size estimation are large in any case. Although some of these findings may be explained by the tendency of the obese to underreport consumption of sweets and other foods they regard as fattening, it is also possible that diets high in complex carbohydrates may in fact be less fattening than was previously assumed, so that there is actually a metabolic advantage to eating diets lower in fat.[13]

Regardless of whether high-fat diets are adipogenic or not, low-fat diets do appear to have an advantage in producing weight loss. When individuals who usually consume diets relatively high in fat are provided with low-fat (e.g., 15% to 23% of calories), high–complex carbohydrate diets, even if energy intakes are not explicitly restricted, weight and fat will be lost over the short term. This has long been known, and a recent study has confirmed the finding.[24] Therefore, over the short term, decreasing the fat content of the diet causes a spontaneous decrease in energy intakes. If the diet is further restricted to 800 calories, even more fat, lean body mass, and weight will be lost, although hunger also increases.[24]

Low-fat diets are currently very popular. Examples include the California Diet and the Pritikin Diet.

One good effect of the recent attention devoted to disease prevention has been that previously popular high-fat, high–saturated fat, high-cholesterol reducing diets have gone out of style. Examples from the past included the Over 30 All Natural Health and Beauty Plan's Basic Weight Loss Diet, which is a low-carbohydrate, high-fat, ketogenic diet; Calories Don't Count, popularized by Herman Taller; and the Drinking Man's Diet. However, even diets relatively low in fat can be atherogenic if they are high in saturated fat and cholesterol. Therefore, in addition to being low in fat, intakes should consist of 10% of calories from saturates, not more than 10% from

polyunsaturated fats, and the remainder from monounsaturates. There is no particular advantage from diets high in omega 3 fatty acids, the so-called fish oils, in weight reduction. Although diets high in these oils do appear to have favorable serum lipid-lowering effects, the effects of adding fish oil capsules to reducing diets or to any diet are dubious.

Alcohol

Since alcohol is energy dense, providing 7 cal/g, and usually low or devoid of other nutrients, there is little reason for including it on reducing diets. Years ago a high-fat, high-alcohol diet called the Drinking Man's Diet which advocated eating steak and drinking alcohol to the exclusion of practically all other foods was popular. The more current version is the Mediterranean Diet, which stresses several glasses of wine a day and a diet high in monounsaturated fats similar to that eaten by the Italians. This is far more wine than anyone needs. The claimed good effect of raising high-density lipoprotein cholesterol levels is suspect; the dangers of excessive consumption of alcohol and calories on this regimen are clear. Therefore they are both questionable diets.

Vitamins, Minerals, and Electrolytes

Vitamins, minerals, and electrolytes must be supplied in levels that meet recommended levels.[9] This is difficult to do while relying on normal food sources on diets that provide less than about 1000 calories. It may be necessary to have recourse to a vitamin-mineral supplement if energy intakes are very low. Electrolytes are usually not included in such supplements, and vitamin pills do not contain minerals. Therefore various supplements must be considered and prescribed separately. The inclusion of lean meats, poultry, and low-fat dairy products, ascorbic acid–rich fruits and vegetables, and iron-fortified cereals can help ensure that iron needs are met, but supplemental iron may be necessary in some cases. Examples of diets that fall short in iron include Dr. Abravanel's Body Type Diet, Aerobic Nutrition, the Delicious Quick Trim Diet, and Fasting: the Ultimate Diet, none of which recommend supplements.

Chronic ketosis can wash out bone, and low-calorie reducing diets that are restricted in calcium-rich milk products, such as Fit For Life Nutraerobics, and Fasting: The Ultimate Diet, are examples of diets that are deficient in calcium. Ill-advised dieting efforts can adversely affect bone, and therefore it is especially important for chronic dieters to pay attention to their intakes of calcium, phosphorus, and other minerals.[12]

Dietary Fiber

Current recommendations for dietary fiber are for 20 to 30 g/day. These amounts are desirable to promote laxation by providing dietary bulk. Since constipation is often a problem on diets, there is every reason to recommend intakes of this level from food sources. The water-soluble fibers may also have positive effects on serum lipids and blood glucose levels.

Cholesterol

Current recommendations for dietary cholesterol intakes are that no more than 300 mg/day should be consumed on the average.[10]

Water

At least one liter of water, which may be obtained from foods containing water, is necessary even on normal diets.[9] On ketogenic reducing diets additional water is necessary because of the obligatory osmotic diuresis that ensues. On all hypocaloric diets protein catabolism is elevated, and so the amount of nitrogenous waste that must be eliminated in the urine is also increased. Therefore at least one liter of water per day or more than 1 ml water per calorie should be provided on reducing diets. Many noncaloric beverages are now available. The dieter should be encouraged to use them ad libitum.

Components

The third requirement of a sound reducing program is that it provide other necessary components in addition to a reasonably low-calorie diet. These other components are summarized in Table 57-5.

Food and nutrition information, common sense in weight reduction, and skill in buying, preparing, and choosing food are essential. Dieters should be informed consumers. Before they embark on a reducing diet, they should ask the questions posed in Table 57-6 to make sure that the regimen they select is reasonable.

Behavioral modification is also essential. Among the techniques the dieter needs to learn are self-motivation, means of identifying problem areas in eating patterns, and altering the physical, social, psychological microenvironment to control eating cues. Self-monitoring techniques, patience, and knowledge that gradual incremental changes are sufficient are salient components of a reducing program.

The psychological and social support of the dieter can take a variety of forms. They include realistic goals, means of reinforcing adherence to the diet by finding and using meaningful non-food rewards, and developing ways of coping with lapses and limiting them. Some dieters are "joiners" who do best with the support of a dieting group. Others are "loners," unable or unwilling to join dieting-specific groups but still benefiting from the support of other persons in their lives for their dieting efforts.

Increased physical activity and exercise are also essential components of reducing diets. Physical activity levels influence energy outputs. Most nonobese individuals in the United States who engage in light physical activity need only about 11 calories per pound per day to maintain their weights, and obese people usually need less.[18] The obese tend to be more sedentary than the nonobese, and therefore their energy outputs in the form of physical activity are lower. Energy outputs are also low in formerly obese individuals who have lost weight, in part because of reduced body mass and in part because of very low physical activity levels.[29] Therefore, low energy outputs are a part of the problem and high energy outputs are part of the solution.

The physical activity prescription includes two major components, which should be specified. First is encouraging the dieter to move more in the activities of daily living: walking instead of driving, climbing stairs instead of using elevator, and the like. There is an unconscious tendency to restrict discretionary physical activity when on a hypocaloric diet, so a prescription is necessary; exhortations and vague encouragement are not likely to bring about desired results.

Second is the inclusion of regular aerobic exercise that involves vigorous physical activity.

TABLE 57-5

Characteristics of Reasonable Reducing Diets: Components

Nutrition education
  Information (label reading, information on calories in foods)
  Skills for buying, preparing, and choosing food
Physical activity and exercise
  More movement in daily life (e.g., walking, climbing stairs, lifting)
  Regular aerobic exercise (at least 30 minutes at 60% maximal vital capacity three times a
    week, such as speed walking, jogging, swimming, biking, volleyball, basketball, exercise
    cycling, rowing and skiing machines, or actual sports)
Behavior modification
  Motivational aids
  Identification of problem areas in eating patterns
  Environmental manipulation (cue control)
  Self-monitoring (eating diaries, diaries of lapses, food records, pulse monitoring for fit-
    ness, etc.)
  Reinforcement of positive behavior
  Successive approximations with incremental changes
Psychological support
  Realistic goals
  Assistance in overcoming barriers to reducing
  Coping with lapses
  Finding alternative gratifications
Social support
  Group support provided or suggestions of means to obtain social support and to deal with
    social situations
Medically sound
  Meets special life-cycle needs, both biological and psychological
  Conforms to current scientific knowledge
  Supports good general health
  Physician consultation prior to dieting for high-risk individuals (very young, old, those
    with chronic physical or emotional ailments, those easily depressed)
  Warnings of potential health risks requiring physician consultation arising during diet
    (depression, dizziness, fainting, nausea, nervousness)
  Periodic checks with physician after losses of more than 20 pounds
Provision for long-term maintenance of weight loss
Consumer friendly
  Ethical marketing (no false or misleading claims, pyramid marketing structures, or client
    hectoring)
  Avoids berating or stigmatizing dieter

Health permitting, at least 30 minutes of aerobic physical activity at 60% of maximal vital capacity three times a week should be included, more if it is tolerated. Such a regimen, coupled with a 1200-calorie diet, increases cardiorespiratory functional capacity, retards the loss of lean body mass, improves serum lipid levels, and in moderately obese individuals increases fat loss.[23] Rates of weight loss may also improve with physical activity,[26] and physical fitness may improve.[32,37]

If energy deficits are relatively modest, these effects seem to be achieved without large compensatory decreases in resting metabolism.[2,3,26] In contrast, very vigorous physical activity coupled with very low calorie diets may trigger decreases of 4% or more over the 6% to 8% decreases in resting metabolism that are usually reported on diet alone.[32] Even on a diet of 800 to 900 calories, resting metabolism falls more when dieting is coupled with exercise.[26] However, this compen-

TABLE 57-6

Criteria Consumers Can Use in Judging Weight Loss Programs

1. Is the program safe? Is there medical supervision or are periodic physical checks by physicians required?
2. Does the plan include aerobic and other physical activity and exercise?
3. Is the rate of weight loss reasonable (4 to 8 pounds/month)?
4. Is the diet too restrictive?
5. Is the diet nutritionally balanced?
6. Does the diet use liquid formulas rather than foods, and if so are suitable precautions taken and is the formula nutritionally adequate?
7. Does the program prescribe appetite suppressants of unproven efficacy?
8. Can the diet be followed?
9. Does the program make scientific and common sense?
10. Does it suit the dieter's particular psychological, social, and physiological needs? Does it deal with emotional adjustments to weight loss? Does it include behavioral and environmental modification techniques?
11. Is individual or group motivation and support provided to help the dieter assume responsibility for weight loss?
12. Is the cost reasonable? Are special foods, special devices, books, or fees required?
13. Will provision be made for weight maintenance and keeping weight off after the program ends?
14. Does the diet permit the dieter to monitor the program?

Recommendations reproduced by permission of the Frances Stern Nutrition Center of the New England Medical Center Hospitals.

sation does not eradicate the positive effects of exercise. Also, long-term maintenance of weight loss is usually better among those who combined very low calorie diets with exercise as opposed to diet alone.[37]

A good reducing diet also provides for medically sound supervision. In addition to ensuring that the diet, exercise, and psychological needs of the patient are met, the health professional must ensure that special life cycle needs, both biological (as in adolescence) and psychological, are met.[38] The program must conform to general medical recommendations for health promotion and disease prevention, such as cessation of smoking. Physician consultation is encouraged prior to entry and periodically during the program; constant monitoring is recommended if the diet is below 800 calories or if the individual falls in a high-risk group. The patient must be alerted to the signs and symptoms of dieting-related problems such as depression, dizziness, fainting, nausea, nervousness, hair loss, dry skin, and the like, and what to do about them.

Reasonable reducing programs provide the dieter with a plan for long-term maintenance of weight loss, perhaps by continuing on a somewhat liberalized reducing diet or by switching to an entirely new diet. In any event, the lifelong program must be based on ordinary foods available to the eater, not on special products or formulas.

Finally, a good reducing program is consumer friendly. It is marketed in an ethical manner, without gimmicks such as pyramid sales schemes in which every customer becomes a potential salesman. This form of marketing rapidly leads to oversaturation of the market and the inevitable recruitment of some individuals who should not be on reducing diets. Programs that insist on unbreakable contracts for large amounts of diet formulas, foods, or exercise sessions are questionable in their marketing practices. Most harmful are programs that berate or stigmatize the dieter, who already may suffer from low levels of self-esteem. Lapses in dieting are common if not inevitable.[25] Lapses and relapses should not be regarded as signs of moral turpitude but as problems to be avoided by planning whenever possible, and to be learned from when they do occur. Programs that shame dieters into compliance may leave the dieter worse off psychologically, regardless of whether weight is lost or gained.

Cost

Last but not least, the cost of reducing programs must be considered. Obesity uncomplicated by other medical problems is rarely reimbursible by third-party insurance. Many health maintenance organizations and prepaid health insurance plans do not provide comprehensive weight-reducing programs. Therefore the treatment of obesity is an out-of-pocket expense to most patients. The costs of conventional dietary treatment range from a few hundred dollars a year for some clinic or commercial diet groups to several thousand dollars a year for the more luxurious residential programs. The cost-effectiveness of various conventional dietary treatments or, for that matter, of more drastic procedures such as surgery or protein-sparing fasts has rarely been studied in a rigorous fashion, nor are five-year outcomes available for most treatments. In the absence of such information, little can be said except to warn the dieter not to expect or spend too much for any obesity treatment, or to mistakenly assume that cost is synonymous with effectiveness.

CONCLUSION

Reducing diets and reducing programs, whether administered under a doctor's direction or attempted by the dieter without expert assistance, have health effects. Some potentially harmful and many ineffective diets are currently available. Federal and other regulatory efforts are insufficient to ensure that all such products are identified and removed from the market in a timely fashion. Potential dieters will do well to remember the ancient warning: "Let the buyer beware." Health services providers can help their patients select reducing programs that are appropriate for their condition. A health coun-

selor's support and monitoring of the program is valuable to the dieter.

References

1. Alpert SS: The energy density of weight loss in semistarvation. Int J Obes 12:533, 1988
2. Ballor DL, Katch VL, Becquie MD et al: Resistance weight training during calorie restriction enhances lean body mass maintenance. Am J Clin Nutr 47:19, 1988
3. Belko AZ, Van Loan M, Barbieri TF et al: Diet, exercise, weight loss and energy expenditure in moderately overweight women. Int J Obes 11(2):93, 1987
4. Braitman LE, Adler EV, Stanton JL: Obesity and calorie intake: The NHANES survey of 1971–75 (NHANES I). J Chronic Dis 38:727, 1985
5. Brodoff BN: Very low calorie diets. In Björntorp P, Brodoff BN (eds): Obesity. Philadelphia, JB Lippincott, 1990
6. Burland T: Rating the Diets. New York, Signet Books, 1986
7. Calloway CW: Unproven, but popular approaches in treating obesity: Metabolic consequences. In Frankle RT, Dwyer J, Moragne L et al (eds): Dietary Treatment and Prevention of Obesity, p 11. London, John Libbey, 1983
8. Calloway DH, Spector H: Nitrogen balance as related to calorie and protein intake in active young men. Am J Clin Nutr 2:405, 1954
9. Committee on Dietary Allowances, Food and Nutrition Board: Recommended Dietary Allowances, 9th rev. ed. Washington, DC, National Academy of Sciences, 1980
10. Committee on Diet and Health, Food and Nutrition Board, Institute of Medicine: Diet and Health: Implications for Decreasing Chronic Disease Risk, p 144. Washington, DC, National Academy Press, 1989
11. Committee on Diet and Health, Food and Nutrition Board, Institute of Medicine: Diet and Health: Implications for Decreasing Chronic Disease Risk, p 576. Washington, DC, National Academy Press, 1989
12. Davie MW, Abraham RR, Hewins B et al: Changes in bone and muscle constituents during diets for obesity. Clin Sci 70:285, 1986
13. Donato K, Hegsted DM: Efficiency of utilization of various sources of energy for growth. Proc Natl Acad Sci USA 82:4866, 1985
14. Drewnowski A, Brunzell JB, Sande K et al: Sweet tooth reconsidered: Taste responsiveness in human obesity. Physiol Behav 35:617, 1985

15. Drewnowski A, Greenwood MRC: Cream and sugar: Human preferences for high fat foods. Physiol Behav 30:629, 1983

16. Fagerberg B, Andersson O, Nilsson U et al: Weight reducing diets: Role of carbohydrates on sympathetic nervous activity and hypotensive response. Int J Obes 8:237, 1984

17. Forbes GB: Human Body Composition: Growth, Aging, Nutrition and Activity, p 237. New York, Springer Verlag, 1987

18. Forbes GB, Brown MR: Energy need for weight maintenance in human beings: Effect of body size and composition. J Am Dietet Assoc 89:499, 1989

19. Forbes GB, Drenick EJ: Loss of body nitrogen on fasting. Am J Clin Nutr 32:1570, 1979

20. Forbes GB, Welle SL: Lean body mass in obesity. Int J Obes 7:99, 1983

21. Frances Stern Nutrition Center and Massachusetts Department of Public Health: Criteria consumers can use in judging weight loss programs. Boston, New England Medical Center Hospitals, 1987

22. Garrow JS: Physiological aspects of obesity. In Brownell KD, Foreyt JP (eds): Handbook of Eating Disorders: Physiology, Psychology, and Treatment of Obesity, Anorexia, and Bulimia, p 45. New York, Basic Books, 1986

23. Hagan RD: Benefits of aerobic conditioning and diet for overweight adults. Sports Med 5:144, 1988

24. Hammer RL, Barrier CA, Roundy ES et al: Calorie restricted low fat diet and exercise in obese women. Am J Clin Nutr 49:77, 1989

25. Herman CP, Polivy J: A boundary model for the regulation of eating. In Stunkard AJ, Stellar E (eds): Eating and Its Disorders, p 171. New York, Raven Press, 1984

26. Heymsfield SB, Casper K, Heam J et al: Rate of weight loss during underfeeding: Relation to level of physical activity. Metabolism 38:215, 1989

27. Howard AN, Baird IM: Physiopathology of protein metabolism in relation to very low calorie regimens. In Björntorp P, Cairella M, Howard AN (eds): Recent Advances in Obesity Research III, p 124. London, John Libbey, 1981

28. Lantigua RA, Amatruda JM, Biddle TL et al: Cardiac arrhythmias associated with a liquid protein diet for the treatment of obesity. N Engl J Med 303:735, 1980

29. Leibel RL, Hirsch J: Diminished energy requirements of reduced obese patients. Metabolism 33:164, 1984

30. Market Data Enterprises: U.S. Weight Loss and Diet Control Market. Lynbrook, New York, Market Data Enterprises, 1989

31. Nicholas P, Dwyer J: Diets for weight reduction: Nutritional considerations. In Brownell KD, Foreyt JP (eds): Handbook of Eating Disorders: Physiology, Psychology, and Treatment of Obesity, Anorexia, and Bulimia, p 122. New York, Basic Books, 1986

32. Phinney SD, LaGrange BM, O'Connell M et al: Effects of aerobic exercise on energy expenditure and nitrogen balance during very low calorie dieting. Metabolism 37:758, 1988

33. Pi-Sunyer FX: Obesity. In Shils ME, Young VR (eds): Modern Nutrition in Health and Disease. Philadelphia, Lea & Febiger, 1988

34. Romieau I, Willett WC, Stampfer MJ et al: Energy intake and other determinants of relative weight. Am J Clin Nutr 47:406, 1988

35. Rosen JC, Hunt DA, Sims EA et al: Comparison of carbohydrate containing and carbohydrate restricted hypocaloric diets in the treatment of obesity: Effects on appetite and mood. Am J Clin Nutr 36:464, 1982

36. Shils ME, Young VR: Modern Nutrition in Health and Disease, 7th ed, p 1535. Philadelphia, Lea & Febiger, 1988

37. Sikland G, Kando A, Foreyt JP et al: Two year followup of patients treated with a very low calorie diet and exercise training. J Am Diet Assoc 88:487, 1988

38. VanItallie TB: Diets for weight reduction: Mechanisms of action and physiological effects. In Bray G (ed): Obesity: Comparative Methods of Weight Control, p 15. London, John Libbey, 1980

39. VanItallie TB, Yang MU: Current concepts in nutrition: Diet and weight loss. N Engl J Med 297:1158, 1977

40. Welman A, Matter S, Stamford BA: Caloric restriction and/or mild exercise: Effects on serum lipids and body composition. Am J Clin Nutr 33:1002, 1980

CHAPTER 58

Dietary Fiber and Obesity

ANTHONY R. LEEDS

According to popular belief, dietary fiber helps overweight and obese people lose weight. Does available evidence support the prescription of high-fiber diets or fiber products to achieve weight loss? Is there reason to believe that dietary fiber may help reduce food intake or cause energy malabsorption, thereby contributing to weight loss? Does fiber play a role in weight maintenance?

Fiber was defined in 1976 by the late Hugh Trowell and colleagues as "plant polysaccharides and lignin resistant to digestion by the small intestinal enzymes of man."[1] The term has since been superseded by "nonstarch polysaccharides" (NSP).[2] This term is more concise and self-explanatory but is not the same thing as dietary fiber. Fiber and NSP have multiple chemical components that can be broadly grouped into cellulosic and noncellulosic polysaccharides; the latter can be divided into non-water-soluble and water-soluble noncellulosic polysaccharides. Thus the term "soluble fiber" (water-soluble NSP) has entered the literature and proves to be useful as a label for some materials with marked physiologic effects. However, the physical nature as well as the chemical composition of the material must be considered. Solid tablets of guar gum (a form of soluble fiber) may behave differently in the gut than fine granules of the same material. Breads made from flours of different particle sizes may have different textures and mouth feel and may affect energy intake to different degrees.

MECHANISMS OF ACTION*

To facilitate weight loss, dietary fiber must act in one of three ways (Fig. 58-1). Weight loss will occur if absorbed energy falls sufficiently below energy utilization. Thus, any action of fiber that results in reduced energy intake or reduced energy absorption may be beneficial. It is important to distinguish between the effects of dietary fiber in its own right and, in foods, secondary effects of fiber on other variables. For example, by comparison with a low-fiber diet, a high-fiber diet tends to be higher in total carbohydrate, lower in total and saturated fat, higher in potassium, lower in sodium, higher in plant proteins, lower in "energy density," and so on. Some of these variables in themselves have effects on energy intake. The range within which the variable is changed may also be important. Some experiments may have failed to demonstrate any effect because of insufficient differences in fiber intake. Certainly in the study by Russ and Atkinson, described below, the target fiber intake was not achieved.[3] Time scales also matter. Short studies may fail to show the effect of adaptation or a decrease in dietary compliance with time. Longer studies that address long-term outcome may give false negative results if lack of compliance is great.

---

*The section on mechanisms of action was presented at the 6th International Congress on Obesity (Japan) and published in Progress in Obesity Research 1990, London: John Libbey and Co. Ltd. 1991.

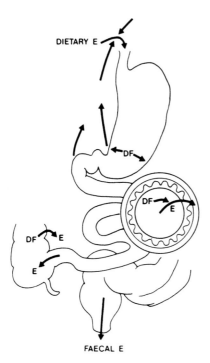

FIGURE 58-1

Mechanisms of action of dietary fiber in obesity. Dietary fiber may modify dietary energy intake, reduce energy absorption, or have secondary metabolic effects that may influence lipolysis and lipogenesis. A role for fiber in modifying food intake, perhaps by an association with the bulk of the food, is portrayed, moving distally down the gut. In the stomach, fiber may influence gastric emptying, which along with changes in small intestinal motility may signal higher centers. The digestibility of energy may be affected in the small gut, thus influencing fecal energy. However, potentially available food energy, and fiber itself, may be fermented in the colon and be absorbed to some extent as short chain fatty acids. (Reproduced by permission.)

ENERGY INTAKE

Apart from direct measurement of energy intake, subjective variables that relate to food intake can be measured by visual analogue tracking. Satiety (the inhibition of food consumption resulting from the consequences of ingestion), satiation (the process that brings eating to a close), hunger (the urge to begin eating), and appetite (the per-

ceived pleasantness of food) can be assessed by asking the subject to mark lines on a graded scale or to respond to a checklist of food preferences.[4,5] Experimental evidence is available for studies on purified and isolated fiber materials, on fiber-supplemented foods, and on foods naturally high in fiber. Blundell and Burley, who tabulated this evidence,[4] found marked differences in the reported effects of fiber on hunger. For example, in the study by Mickelson et al,[6] ingestion of a fiber-supplemented bread compared to a "regular" control product resulted in fewer subjects reporting hunger at night and at the end of the study period. By contrast, Burley and colleagues[7] failed to demonstrate an effect of a 12-g dietary fiber breakfast (guar bread and wheat bran cereal) in comparison with a 3-g dietary fiber breakfast (white wheat bread and corn flakes) on hunger ratings and lunchtime food intake in nonobese women. Studies with fiber isolates or supplements have similarly yielded varying results. Krotkiewsky reported reduced hunger when gum was alternated weekly with wheat bran,[8] but Rossner and colleagues were unable to demonstrate an effect of cereal grain and citrus fiber tablets on hunger in obese women.[9] An effect may thus be very dependent on the design of the study, particularly the dose of fiber used. Where evidence for an effect on hunger was adduced, it often was not substantiated by measurement of energy intake. There is also little evidence to show that any effect demonstrated in acute single-meal studies or even for up to five days[10] is maintained or whether compensation in energy intake occurs in the long term. Study designs also must take into account differences in eating behavior between individuals: those who consciously restrain or limit their food intake may respond differently than those who do not. Those who eat large numbers of small meals may respond to a strengthening of satiety by reducing energy intake, while those who eat small numbers of large meals may not. Intensification of satiation may facilitate weight loss in those who eat small numbers of large meals but not in those who eat large numbers of small meals. Different treatments can affect satiety and not satiation, and therefore distinguishing between different types of eating behavior is important. Although considerably more work remains to be done, there is sufficient evidence to conclude that fiber may, though not always, exert some control over food consumption in the short term.

ENERGY ABSORPTION AND EXCRETION

Twofold or threefold increases in fiber in the diet can decrease energy digestibility by 2% (from 95%).[11] Fecal energy losses can be doubled (from 50 to 100 kcal/day) and energy digestibility reduced by 2%[12] to 4%[13] by changing to high-fiber diets. Table 58-1 shows that within reasonable ranges of changes of fiber intake, fecal energy increases by no more than 100 kcal. However, in many of these studies subjects were not recruited on the basis of following low-fiber diets before entry into the study, and it is possible that response to a high-fiber diet may depend on initial levels. To address this question, Rigaud et al[24] randomly allocated 20 young volunteers who ate less than 18 g dietary fiber daily to fiber or placebo supplements. Fecal energy losses, while significantly different, were small (153 kcal/day on placebo, 173 kcal/day on fiber supplement). It thus seems possible that increasing fecal energy loss is not important as a mechanism of action. On the other hand, in studies where significant weight loss is achieved, additional energy deficits achieved by fiber administration may be in the range of only 30 to 180 kcal/day, so it may be incorrect to dismiss small increases in fecal energy losses as insignificant. It is also possible that specific formulations of dietary fiber may result in greater fecal energy loss.

SECONDARY METABOLIC EFFECTS

The effects of dietary fiber on absorption of glucose and insulin responses[25] may have important consequences for fat deposition and lipolysis. A reduction in prevailing insulin levels presumably shifts peripheral fat metabolism toward lipolysis. Other metabolic effects of fiber, namely reducing low-density lipoprotein (LDL) cholesterol levels[26] and reducing fluctuations of blood glucose, may be of benefit in obese individuals with hyperlipidemia or diabetes. In recently published studies, appreciable reductions in blood pressure have been obtained.[27,28]

TABLE 58-1

Mean Daily Loss of Energy in the Feces in Subjects on Lower and Higher Fiber Intakes

Means Used to Raise Fiber Intake (Ref.)	Daily Fecal Energy (kcal)	
	Diet Lower in Fiber	Diet Higher in Fiber
Whole meal bread, fruit, vegetables[11]	83	210
Whole meal bread (diet mainly of bread)[14]	99	321
Whole meal bread, bran[12]	151	241
Whole meal bread, bran[15]	199	279
Bran bread[16]	178	263
Bran crispbread[17]	108	166
Bran biscuits[18]	96	160
Bran[19]	296	352
Bran[20]	179	211
Oat bran[21]	98	189
Oat bran[22]	230	354
Cellulose[23]	103	189
Cellulose-enriched bread[6]	124	195
Fruit and vegetables[13]	117	255
Ispaghula biscuits[18]	96	161
Mean	144	236

Table prepared by K. W. Heaton, Department of Medicine, Bristol Royal Infirmary, England, and reproduced with permission.

EVIDENCE FOR EFFICACY

The evidence for weight loss can be divided into controlled and uncontrolled studies, and into studies using high-fiber diets, high-fiber foods, and fiber supplements. It is almost impossible to design a double-blind, placebo-controlled study comparing high-fiber food products and low-fiber food products[29,30] or high-fiber diets and low-fiber diets. Where fiber materials can be pressed into tablets, double-blind, placebo-controlled studies are possible. In such studies it is possible to feel confident that placebo effects have been eliminated. Table 58-2 lists the results of some recent studies which showed that generally, the weight losses achieved in three months can be 2 kg greater on fiber tablet doses of 5 to

TABLE 58-2

**Double-Blind, Placebo-Controlled Weight Reduction Trials
With Dietary Fiber Supplements**

Study	N	Fiber Dose (g)	Observation Period (wks)	Weight Loss (kg)	
				Fiber	Placebo
Rossner et al[28]	60	5	8	7.0	6.0
Rossner et al[28]	45	7	12	6.2	4.1
Solum et al[27]	60	6	12	8.5	6.4
Walsh et al[31]	20	3	8	2.5	+0.7
Ryttig et al[32]	90	10	11	6.3	4.2
Solum[33]	53	5	8	3.0	1.5
Ryttig et al[34]	97	7	11	4.9	3.3
Ryttig et al[35]	53	6/4	26	6.7	5.7
Ryttig et al[36]	60	7	26	5.3	2.9

Modified from Ryttig KR et al: In Leeds AR (ed): Dietary Fibre Perspectives, Vol 2. London, John Libbey & Co, 1990. Reproduced by permission.

10 g/day than on placebo tablets. The additional weight loss occurring as a result of the fiber tablet treatment is thus about 180 g/week more than with placebo administration. Assuming that 1 kg of body weight as lost is 75% adipose and 25% lean tissue and has an energy content of 7000 kcal, the additional weight loss of 180 g/week represents an addition to the energy deficit of 1260 kcal/week, or 180 kcal/day. In studies run over 26 or 52 weeks, the additional weight loss falls to between 30 and 90 g/week, that is, an additional energy deficit of 30 to 90 kcal/day. These figures are not very different from those for increases in fecal energy losses, which suggests that it may be wrong to totally dismiss increased fecal energy losses as a mechanism of action. The studies in Table 58-2 also show quite clearly that statistically significant weight losses can be demonstrated in well-designed studies. Unfortunately, however, good-quality dietary data was not collected in all of those studies, and it is not possible to comment on whether fiber-treated patients adhered more closely to their prescribed reduced-energy diets. However, in the study by Rossner et al,[28] when energy intake before and after treatment was calculated, no significant difference emerged between the treatment groups. The question of adherence to diet was addressed by Beattie et al,[37] who placed three groups of eight newly diagnosed over-

weight non-insulin-dependent diabetics on low-fiber reducing diets for four weeks and then treated the groups with 15 g/day of guar gum granules, 10 to 15 g/day of cereal fiber, or no additional treatment. Subsequent weight losses over 16 weeks showed that no additional benefit in terms of weight loss was conferred by fiber administration. However, Beattie's study on small numbers of subjects may not have been powerful enough to detect the small differences in weight loss often seen in fiber/weight loss studies.

Weight reduction with high-fiber diets was investigated by Russ and Atkinson,[3] who compared the effects of a high-fiber diet (35 to 40 g/day) and a low-fiber diet (12 to 14 g/day) in 32 obese subjects. All subjects were also taught an exercise program and behavioral modifications to maintain lower weight. Mean weight loss was 3.7 kg in the low-fiber group and 3.1 kg in the high-fiber group, but the fiber intake in the high-fiber group was about 24 g/day—well short of the intended 35 to 40 g. The subjects were compliant in other aspects of the program, and it was concluded that there were practical difficulties in achieving high-fiber intake by food selection. The solution may be to use specially prepared fiber-fortified food products. Mickelson et al[6] reported one such study in which eight overweight men (initial weight, 91 ± 4.5 kg) ate 12 slices of regular bread each day for eight weeks and eight overweight men (initial weight, 94 ± 5.8 kg) ate 12 slices of reduced-calorie, high-fiber bread per day for the same period. Daily energy intakes were 2350 and 1975 kcal and weight losses were 6.3 and 8.8 kg for regular and reduced-calorie groups, respectively. The bread to which cellulose had been added (providing 26 g of crude fiber per day) resulted in a significantly greater weight loss than regular bread (providing 1 g of crude fiber per day).

WEIGHT MAINTENANCE

Since weight maintenance demands less restriction of energy intake than weight reduction, it follows that if dietary fiber has a role in facilitating energy intake reduction, that role may be more easily demonstrated in weight maintenance than during weight reduction. Only one good study in the literature has reported on weight maintenance. Ryttig et al[34] reported that 97 overweight women were prescribed a 1200-kcal diet and randomly allocated to either 7-g fiber tablets per day or placebo tablets for 11 weeks. During this time the mean weight loss was 4.9 kg in the fiber-treated group and 3.3 kg in the placebo-treated group ($P < .05$). The subjects were then switched to a 1600-kcal diet, but the fiber (at a slightly reduced dose of 6 g/day) or placebo treatment was continued for an additional 16 weeks. Weight losses during this period amounted to 3.8 kg in the fiber-treated group and 2.8 kg in the placebo-treated group. At this point placebo treatment was stopped and all adhering subjects were given fiber tablets. At 52 weeks weight loss in the group originally treated with fiber was 6.7 kg. Other studies also show that differences in weight lost between subjects given fiber tablets and those given placebo can persist to 26 weeks,[33,34] supporting the view that dietary fiber preparations may have a role in weight maintenance.

CONCLUSION

Dietary fiber does influence some of the variables related to energy intake in the short term, but what happens beyond five days or so is uncertain. Dietary fiber slightly increases fecal energy losses to an extent that could account for some of the weight loss demonstrated in some studies. Dietary fiber reduces energy intake and causes greater weight loss than placebo treatment under some circumstances. Dietary fiber can be shown to cause greater weight losses than placebo treatment up to 26 weeks. However, the outcome of any intervention depends on the characteristics of the subject population, the study design, and the physical and chemical nature of the dietary fiber foods or material used. It is thus more difficult to determine whether prescribing high-fiber diets or fiber products for weight loss is warranted. A cautiously qualified positive response is probably indicated, but evidence for real effects is limited to specific products and materials. These products may thus be used confidently in the type of situation in which they have been tested.

References

1. Trowell H, Southgate DAT, Wolever TMS et al: Dietary fiber redefined. Lancet 1:967, 1976
2. Englyst H, Cummings JH: Dietary fibre and starch: Definition, classification and measurement. In Leeds AR (ed): Dietary Fibre Perspectives, vol 2. London, John Libbey & Co., 1990
3. Russ CS, Atkinson RL: Use of high fibre diets for the outpatient treatment of obesity. Nutr Rep Int 32:193, 1985
4. Blundell JE, Burley VJ: Satiation, satiety and the action of fibre on food intake. Int J Obes 11(suppl 1): 9, 1987
5. Hill AJ, Magson LD, Blundell JE: Hunger and palatability: Tracking ratings of subjective experience before, during and after the consumption of preferred and less preferred food. Appetite 5:361, 1984
6. Mickelson O, Makdani DD, Cotton RH et al: Effects of a high fiber bread diet on weight loss in college-age males. Am J Clin Nutr 32:1703, 1979
7. Burley VJ, Leeds AR, Blundell JE: The effect of high and low-fibre breakfasts on hunger, satiety and food intake in a subsequent meal. Int J Obes 11(suppl 1): 87, 1987
8. Krotkiewski M: Effect of guar on body-weight, hunger ratings and metabolism in obese subjects. Br J Nutr 52:97, 1984
9. Rossner S, von Zweigberk D, Ohlin A: Effects of dietary fiber in treatment of overweight outpatients. In Björntorp P, Vahouny GV, Kritchevsky D (eds): Dietary Fiber and Obesity, p 69. New York, Alan R Liss, 1985

10. Duncan K, Bacon JA, Weinsier RL: The effects of high and low energy density diets on satiety, energy intake, and eating time of obese and non-obese subjects. Am J Clin Nutr 37:763, 1983

11. Southgate DAT, Durnin JVGA: Conversion factors: An experimental reassessment of the factors used in the calculation of the energy value of human diets. Br J Nutr 24:517, 1970

12. Farrell DJ, Girle L, Arthur J: Effects of dietary fibre on the apparent digestibility of major food components and on blood lipids in men. Aust J Exp Biol Med Sci 56:469, 1978

13. Kelsay JL, Behall KM, Prather ES: Effects of fiber from fruits and vegetables on metabolic responses of human subjects. Am J Clin Nutr 31:1149, 1978

14. Macrae TF, Hutchinson JCD, Irwin JO et al: Comparative digestibility of wholemeal and white breads and the effect of the degree of fineness of grinding on the former. J Hyg 423, 1942

15. Cummings JH, Hill MJ, Jenkins DJA et al: Changes in fecal composition and colonic function due to cereal fiber. Am J Clin Nutr 29:1468, 1976

16. Stephen AM, Wiggins HS, Englyst HN et al: The effect of age, sex and level of intake of dietary fibre from wheat on large bowel function in thirty healthy subjects. Br J Nutr 56:349, 1986

17. Southgate DAT, Branch WJ, Hill MJ et al: Metabolic responses to dietary supplements of bran. Metabolism 25:1129, 1976

18. Stevens J, Levitsky DA, van Soest PJ et al: Effect of psyllium gum and wheat bran on spontaneous energy intake. Am J Clin Nutr 46:812, 1988

19. Findlay JM, Smith AN, Mitchell WD et al: Effects of unprocessed bran on colon function in normal subjects and in diverticular disease. Lancet 1:146, 1974

20. Yu MHM, Miller LT: Influence of cooked wheat bran on bowel function and fecal excretion of nutrients. J Food Sci 46:720, 1981

21. Calloway DH, Kretsch MJ: Protein and energy utilization in men given a rural Guatemalan diet and egg formulas with and without added oat bran. Am J Clin Nutr 31:1118, 1987

22. Kirby RW, Anderson JW, Sieling B et al: Oat bran intake selectively lowers serum low-density lipoprotein cholesterol concentrations of hypercholesterolemic men. Am J Clin Nutr 34:824, 1981

23. Slavin JC, Marlett JA: Effect of refined cellulose on apparent energy, fat and nitrogen digestibilities. J Nutr 110:2020, 1980

24. Rigaud D, Ryttig KR, Leeds AR et al: Effects of a moderate dietary fibre supplement on hunger rating, energy input and faecal energy output in young, healthy volunteers. Int J Obes 11(suppl 1): 73, 1987

25. Jenkins DJA, Wolever TMS, Jenkins AL et al: Dietary fiber, gastrointestinal, endocrine, and metabolic effects: Lente carbohydrate. In Vahouny GV, Kritchevsky D (eds): Dietary Fiber: Basic and Clinical Aspects, p 69. New York, Plenum Press, 1986

26. Leeds AR: Dietary fat, dietary fibre, blood lipids. In Cambie RC (ed): Fats for the Future, p 87. Chichester, England, Ellis Horwood, 1989

27. Solum TT, Ryttig KR, Solum E et al: The influence of a high fibre diet on body weight, serum lipids and blood pressure in slightly overweight persons: A randomized, double blind, placebo-controlled investigation with diet and fibre tablets (DumoVital). Int J Obes 11(suppl 1):67, 1987

28. Rossner S, von Zweigbergk D, Ohlin A et al: Weight reduction with dietary fibre supplements: Results of two double-blind randomized studies. Acta Med Scand 222:83, 1987

29. Leeds AR: Treatment of obesity with dietary fibre: Present position and potential developments, and following discussion. Scand J Gastroenterol 22 (suppl 129):156, 1987

30. Leeds AR: Conclusion [Symposium on Dietary Fibre and Obesity]. Int J Obes 11(suppl 1):107, 1987

31. Walsh DE, Yaghoubian V, Behforooz A: Effect of glucomannan on obese patients: A clinical study. Int J Obes 8:289, 1984

32. Ryttig K, Larsen S, Haegh L: Treatment of slightly to moderately overweight persons: A double-blind placebo-controlled investigation with diet and fiber tablets (DumoVital). Tidsskr Nor Laegefor 104: 989, 1984

33. Solum TT: Dumovital, as a means to achieve weight reduction. Tidsskr Nor Laegefor 103:1707, 1983

34. Ryttig KR, Tellnes G, Haegh L et al: A dietary fibre supplement and weight maintenance after weight reduction: A randomized, double-blind, placebo-controlled long-term trial. Int J Obes 13:165, 1989

35. Ryttig KR, Birketvedt GS: The effect of a combination of fibre tablets and reduced energy intake in the treatment of overweight, and on maintenance of an achieved weight reduction. Abstracts of the First European Congress on Obesity, Stockholm, 1988

36. Rigaud D, Ryttig KR, Angel LA et al: Mild overweight treated with energy restriction and a dietary fibre supplement: A 6-month randomized, double-blind, placebo-controlled trial. Int J Obes 14:763, 1990

37. Beattie VA, Edwards CA, Hosker JP et al: Does adding fibre to a low energy, high carbohydrate, low fat diet confer any benefit to the management of newly diagnosed overweight type II diabetics? Br Med J 296:1147, 198

CHAPTER 59

Very Low Calorie Diets

BERNARD N. BRODOFF and ROSA HENDLER

At present, there is general agreement among investigators that the term "very low calorie diet" (VLCD) or "supplemental fasts" should be reserved for commercially prepared liquid formulations providing less than about 600 kcal/day and taken for seven days or longer. When conventional food of high protein content (1.5 g/kg ideal body weight) is used, these diets are referred to as protein-sparing modified fasts (PSMF). Aside from calorie restrictions, modern VLCDs contain high-grade protein, sufficient carbohydrate to reduce ketonemia and nitrogen and electrolyte wasting, minimal amounts of fat but with essential fatty acids, and all essential vitamins and minerals to conform to recommended daily allowances. While the critical importance of high-grade protein from milk and eggs in restricted-diet formulations has been known for decades by the medical and scientific communities, this requirement was brought forcefully to the public's eye by the liquid protein diet scandal in the United States in the late 1970s.[131,132,193] This diet, which used hydrolyzed collagen and gelatin from animal hide and other sources, had a high mortality rate attributed to myocardial atrophy and arrhythmias caused by the poor-quality protein, lack of vitamins and minerals, and possibly some other undetermined toxic element. Since then there have been some 10 to 15 million users of modern VLCDs in the United States, Western Europe, and Japan.[214]

The popularity of VLCDs for weight loss may be attributable to two factors. One is the aggressive marketing of these products to both the lay public and the medical profession by commercial interests. Equally important may have been the 1985 report of the National Institutes of Health (NIH) Consensus Development Conference on Obesity.[145] This comprehensive statement received wide publicity in the lay press. Among other things it concluded that studies of large populations showed a continuous relationship between indices of body fat like relative weight or body mass index and morbidity and mortality. Relative weight is defined as measured body weight divided by the midpoint of medium frame desirable weight recommended in the 1959 or 1983[140] Metropolitan Life Insurance tables. Body mass index (BMI) is defined as weight (kg) divided by height (m²). Furthermore, the panelists agreed that an increase in body weight of 20% or more above desirable body weight (Metropolitan Life Insurance tables) constituted an established health hazard.

HISTORICAL PERSPECTIVES

The development of VLCDs in the past 60 years has recently been reviewed by Howard.[106] As early as 1924, Mason used diets of 500 kcal for as long as 100 days and achieved weight losses of 31 to 43 kg, but without specific metabolic measurements.[136] In 1929 Evans and Strang published the first of their scientific papers on diets of very low energy content containing about 400 kcal and 50 g protein. Three hundred eight outpatients studied for up to six months lost an average of 1.2 kg/week, with nitrogen losses over an eight-week period averaging less than 4% of total body nitrogen.[66] Despite the success of this treatment in promoting rapid and apparently safe weight loss, this work was largely ignored for several decades. Research on fasting in the 1950s renewed interest in VLCDs as a method of weight loss. The original papers on total starvation were published in 1915 by Folin and Dennis,[72] who studied two obese females, and by Benedict,[21] who studied a single normal-weight man who fasted for one month. In 1959 Bloom reported on nine obese subjects who fasted for a week and lost a mean of 8.4 kg with no ill effects.[35] Subsequently large numbers of patients were treated in the 1960s for periods of two weeks to 76 days, with mean weight losses ranging from about 10 kg in the shorter time period to about 23 kg in the longer studies.[36,60,61,188] Anorexia, which develops within 48 to 72 hours, makes fasting acceptable and permits dramatic weight losses. However, the appearance in some subjects of severe side-effects such as gouty arthritis, postural hypotension and syncope, and abdominal cramps,[63] and a number of deaths reported by 1970, led to the abandonment of fasting as a viable therapeutic option for the treatment of obesity.[163] Loss of lean body mass was a source of serious concern, and long-term maintenance of weight loss was disappointing.[61] In 1966–1967, Bollinger et al[37] in the United States and Apfelbaum[7] in France experimented with a supplement of egg albumin to stem nitrogen losses, achieving approximate nitrogen equilibrium with 40 to 60 g/day. In 1973 Blackburn and associates[32,33] used a supplement of lean meat and egg albumin and coined the term "protein-sparing" to describe this regimen.

The prototype of the modern VLCD was Metrocal, marketed by Mead Johnson in 1962 and sold over the counter.[106] This was a canned liquid diet of 900 kcal containing 70 g protein, 100 g carbohydrate, and 20 g fat. In 1974 Genuth and Vertes in the United States[89,90] and Howard and Baird in the United Kingdom[16,105,107] restricted carbohydrate intake, the latter group to 30 to 45 g/day. The most comprehensive critique on the use of VLCDs is the publication, "The Use of Very Low Calorie Diets in Obesity," issued in 1987 by the United Kingdom Department of Health and Social Security and known as the COMA Report.[58] This report issued guidelines for the composition of VLCDs and suggested

minimal daily protein and caloric intakes for most women of 40 g and 400 kcal, respectively; for tall women and men the values were increased to 50 g/day and 500 kcal/day. Partially as a result of this report, present-day commercial products have changed their composition by increasing energy content from 400 to 600 kcal/day and protein to 40 to 70 g/day. Debate continues over the optimal proportions of carbohydrate and protein needed to maximize weight loss and preserve body mass. Whether or not these restrictive diets can spare body protein remains an important question and will be discussed in a later section.

In France and Australia medical supervision of subjects on VLCDs is mandatory. In the United Kingdom, some of the Scandinavian countries, and some states in the United States, VLCDs are distributed by lay counselors who are involved in marketing the product. Other methods of sale, depending on the product and country, are exclusively by physicians or hospital-based plans, in pharmacies, or in supermarkets.[214]

PATIENT SELECTION AND INDICATIONS

The COMA Report in its guidelines suggested that VLCDs should be considered only after conventional diets have failed and only in individuals with a BMI above 30 kg/m^2 (classes 2 and 3, Fig. 59-1), in whom obesity carries clear health risks that might be reduced with weight reduction.[58] In the past, investigators limited the use of VLCDs to adults aged 18 to 70 who were moderately (60% to 99%) or morbidly (100% or more) overweight.[206] With the proliferation and widespread use of these diets, however, they are now frequently used for overweight of lesser degree and for cosmetic reduction. In a recent discussion of VLCDs, Munro and Stolarek defined short-term (up to 14 days) indications for the use of these diets.[143] Among these indications are (1) the demonstration to an individual that she or he is not metabolically unique and can lose weight at a predictable rate on a hypocaloric regimen, (2) as a means of assessing the suitability of a patient for a more radical form of treatment such as jaw wiring, (3) for psychological reasons, as for an important social event, (4) for financial

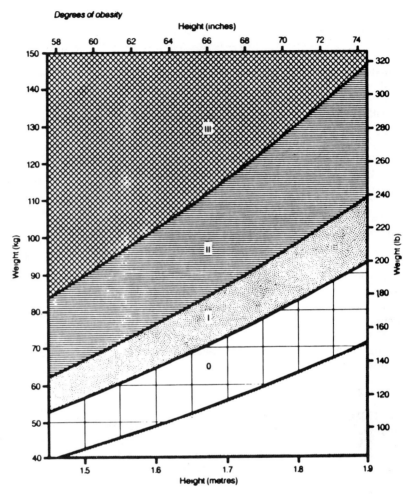

FIGURE 59-1

Relation of weight to height defining the desirable range (○), and grades I, II, and III obesity, marked by the boundaries of Body Mass Index (W/H²) = 25–29.9, 30–40, and over 40, respectively. I = overweight; II = moderately overweight; III = severely overweight. (From Garrow JS: Obesity and Related Diseases. London, Churchill Livingstone, 1988. Reproduced by permission.)

reasons, such as to gain employment, and (5) for medical reasons, as before elective surgery.

The COMA Report suggested that the longer term (up to 30 days) use of VLCDs would be justified only if they resulted in a sustained weight loss.[58] Unfortunately, as Munro and Stolarek point out, it is impossible at this time to predict with accuracy those individuals who will have a successful outcome on VLCDs.[143]

Although the strongest indication for a long-term VLCD is in the morbidly obese, such a diet may also be indicated for those with a complication of obesity that places them at substantial risk of increased morbidity and mortality, such as maturity-onset diabetes and sleep apnea. In the case of maturity-onset diabetes, reduction to lean body weight may be the only effective treatment or means of delaying the onset of this disease. The devastating effects of morbid obesity are well known. Drenick and associates reported a 12-fold increase in mortality in men aged 25 to 34 years who were 125% over ideal weight and a sixfold increase in mortality in those aged 35 to 44 years when compared with normal-weight men.[60] In life-threatening conditions, therefore, in which rapid and drastic weight loss is beneficial, long-term use of VLCDs appears to be indicated. Since fasting for up to four weeks under close supervision carries no major mortality risk, the COMA Report suggested that manufacturers recommend that the diet be used for no longer than four weeks at a time.[58]

Not all recognized authorities in the field agree on the use of VLCDs for the treatment of obesity. Garrow, for example, is firmly opposed to their use, with the possible exception of the obese patient who is more likely to lose weight if removed entirely from conventional food and transferred to a bland diet of known composition. For this type of patient Garrow suggests a self-produced VLCD of 1200 ml of milk, with iron and vitamin supplements, as a safer and less expensive alternative.[78,79,81,82]

CONTRAINDICATIONS

The COMA Report also enumerated several contraindications to VLCDs[58]:

1. Physiologic states such as infancy, childhood, pregnancy and lactation, and advanced age.
2. Nonobesity, particularly if the subject is attempting to reach an unrealistically low target weight. Typical subjects in whom VLCDs are contraindicated for this reason are young women at risk for or who have a history of anorexia nervosa, ballet dancers, jockeys, and athletes.
3. A history of severe psychological disturbance or severe behavior disorder, especially disorders involving eating, alcoholism, or drug abuse.
4. Serious medical conditions in which food restriction may precipitate severe metabolic dysfunction. These conditions include porphyria, in which restriction of food energy intake may precipitate acute attacks; and serious cardiac disorders, unstable angina, re-

cent myocardial infarction, cerebrovascular disease, hepatic or renal disease, type I diabetes mellitus, and malignant disease.
5. Conditions in which medication may have to be adjusted in response to the low caloric intake. Patients to whom this relative contraindication applies include hypertensive patients, in whom syncope may appear, and type II diabetics taking either insulin or oral agents, in whom hypoglycemic episodes may occur.

The clinical dilemma of the grossly obese patient with ischemic heart disease facing bypass surgery has been discussed by Munro and Stolarek,[143] who pose the question of whether the risk-reward ratio might not be improved in some of these patients by using a radical approach to weight loss, such as a VLCD, before surgery. Furthermore, although the Food and Drug Administration (FDA)[234] in its 1979 guidelines considered heart disease a contraindication to VLCDs, Vertes[198] has recently suggested that stable angina in the severely obese patient may still permit treatment with a VLCD.

COURSE OF THE DIET

Some physicians have used a low-calorie diet of conventional food for several weeks to evaluate the suitability of subjects for a course of a VLCD. In actual practice today subjects are usually started on a VLCD immediately or in some cases on a liquid formulation and a single low-calorie meal during an adaptation period of several days to a week or less before beginning the diet. The VLCD comes in powdered form, is mixed with water, and is consumed three to five times daily. The patient is required to drink a minimum of two liters of noncaloric fluid daily.

Workup should include a history and physical examination, complete blood cell count, blood chemistry screen, complete urinalysis, and electrocardiogram (ECG). The subject should be seen by a member of the ancillary staff and a physician weekly, with blood tests repeated biweekly. Because of the potentially malignant nature of arrhythmias, ECG rhythm strips should be done every one to two weeks, but as Lantigua and associates have pointed out, arrhythmias may be missed. Holter monitoring is indicated in any patient with symptoms suggestive of an arrhythmia; if arrhythmia is present, the VLCD should be discontinued immediately.

The standard length of time for the full supplemental fast is about 16 weeks. Weight loss is rapid, up to 5 kg during the first week, with subsequent losses averaging 1.5 to 2.5 kg/week in men and 1 to 2 kg in women.[206] Use of individual counseling, nutritional education, behavior modification, exercise guidance and overall supervision varies with the quality of the program. In subjects with relative contraindications to a VLCD or a personal preference for some food, a low-calorie meal is included in the regimen.

The efficacy and risks of a single long-term VLCD versus several shorter treatment periods are unknown. Adaptive reduction in nitrogen wasting favors a single long-term course of the diet, as protein loss diminishes with duration of therapy.[28,64,69,104,135,219] Proponents of interrupted therapy point out the opportunity for nutrition education and behavior modification with regular food, and the opportunity to achieve a permanent change in eating habits.

Alimentation after the conclusion of a supplemental fast is introduced slowly over several weeks with the partial or complete elimination of the liquid formula diet and the gradual addition of lean meat, fish, and fowl, salad, cooked vegetables, fruit, and milk. Simple sugars and salt are added gradually to prevent fluid accumulation. This gradual reintroduction of food to a contracted and relatively dormant gastrointestinal (GI) tract is done to prevent unpleasant side-effects. Large increases in food intake (binging) after severe dietary restriction can induce electrolyte imbalances and an increase in metabolic rate, resulting in cardiac arrhythmias,[93,119] and may also precipitate attacks of acute cholecystitis and pancreatitis.[208] A number of deaths attributed to the liquid protein diet occurred within the two-week period after the dieters returned to conventional food.[178,193] Follow-up care with either individual counseling or group therapy is a crucial factor in successful weight loss maintenance. Instruction by a behavioral psychologist and dietician is recommended for a minimum of three to 4 months after rapid weight loss[203] and ideally should be continued for an additional six to 12 months.[153]

COMPLICATIONS

Sudden Death

The most serious complication with the use of VLCDs has been sudden death. All of the deaths reported thus far that were attributable directly to the use of VLCDs and not to a pre-existing illness were associated with the liquid protein diet. By 1978 reports of over 60 deaths had been received by the FDA[132] and the Centers for Disease Control (CDC).[50] About 98,000 American women between the ages of 25 and 52 had used the liquid protein diet without supplemental food for one month or longer and about one third of them had used this diet for over two months. The relative risk of death in this group was calculated to be 37 times that of women in the general population. Seventeen of the cases were reviewed by Sours, Isner and their co-workers in two separate reports,[108,178] and an additional 36 deaths were reviewed by Frank et al.[76] The 17 patients described by Sours and Isner were young (median age, 35 years), and morbidly obese (median weight, 106.5 kg). They stayed on the diet for two to eight months and lost a substantial amount of weight (median, 39 kg) at a rapid rate (2.1 kg/week). While 13 subjects received their entire caloric intake from the liquid protein diet (aqueous solutions of collagen or gelatin hydrolysate to which tryptophan preservatives and artificial flavor had been added and containing 300 to 400 kcal/day), two subjects supplemented the liquid protein once daily with protein food of high biological value, and two others used powdered products based on lactalbumin or casein and containing carbohydrate and, in one case, mineral supplements. None of these 17 patients had a pre-existing illness. In the series reported by Frank and associates, the patients were all somewhat older (average age, 45), morbidly obese (average weight, 108 kg), had dieted for an average of four months, and lost 29 kg. No deaths occurred in any subject who dieted for less than two months. In this series 30 of 36 patients had a pre-existing illness. In the series by Isner and co-workers histologic study of the left ventricular myocardium revealed attenuated myocardial fibers in 12 of 14 patients, lipofuscin pigment in 11 of 14, and mononuclear cell myocarditis in one subject. The ECGs of 10 patients were available. All had normal sinus rhythm with recorded episodes of ventricular tachycardia, and nine had prolongation of the QT interval as well as low-voltage QRS complexes. The proximal cause of death was attributed to an acquired and unexplained QT prolongation and associated ventricular tachydysrhythmias. Electrolyte disturbances or a toxin associated with the liquid protein were ruled out as factors in precipitating sudden death in these patients. In contrast, Frank and colleagues in their study of 36 patients found hypokalemia in 14 subjects and inadequate supplementation of calcium, magnesium, sodium, and other minerals in most of the patients studied. Although the exact cause of death was unclear, some of the deaths were attributed to electrolyte abnormalities and ensuing lethal cardiac arrhythmias. Lantigua and associates using Holter monitoring also reported the presence of cardiac arrhythmias in patients on the liquid protein diet.[124] In reviewing the available data on these deaths, Van Itallie and Yang concluded that the ability to defer the lethal effects of severe caloric restriction might be a function of the proportion of body fat at the start of dieting.[194] Not only do obese subjects have an enlarged lean body mass, but during weight loss the ratio of nitrogen loss to weight loss varies inversely with the body fat content.[74] In their view, the most likely underlying cause of death was protein depletion with resulting myocardial atrophy.

What stands out in this unfortunate medical episode are the dietary deficiencies, the absence of competent medical supervision in many cases, the presence of pre-existing illness in some, and finally, and probably most important, obsessive adherence to the diet, resulting in massive and precipitous weight loss.

Other Side-Effects

Numerous side-effects of VLCDs have been reported, and while most are not serious, they can be unpleasant and, for the most part, are identical to the side-effects seen in total starvation. These are discussed in the COMA Report and in recent reviews.[11,58,206,208] Bloating, nausea, vomiting, and abdominal cramping and diarrhea have been attributed to the high osmolar content of the liquid formulation. These symptoms usu-

ally abate or disappear but can make the diet unacceptable to some patients. Constipation and exacerbation of hemorrhoids can be controlled by a bulk-forming fiber additive. Biliary sludge, the precursor to cholesterol gallstones, may be formed, and there is a possibility of exacerbating pre-existing gallbladder disease in obese subjects, already at high risk for cholesterol gallstone formation.[11,22] Whereas an earlier study demonstrated no significant change in the lithogenic index of bile in obese patients on a 600-kcal diet,[167] two recent studies have shown an incidence of clinical gallbladder disease during VLCDs of 4.4% and 5.8%.[41,128] Aspirin and ursodeoxycholic acid (Actigall) have been recommended as prophylactic agents for decreasing biliary cholesterol saturation in obese dieters.[41] Elevated plasma uric acid levels, which usually peak in one to two weeks,[13,121] can be attenuated by a high fluid intake. Exacerbation of pre-existing gout has been reported and the precipitation of uric acid renal stones is a potentially serious complication. If extreme hyperuricemia or symptoms of gout develop, a less radical approach to weight loss or pharmacologic intervention for the hyperuricemia is indicated. Other side-effects that have been reported are menstrual irregularity, loss of libido, dry skin, hair loss, and cold intolerance.[58] Any of these, but particularly the rare and troublesome appearance of hair loss, may be an indication to abort the diet. Headaches, difficulty in concentrating, lethargy, fatigue, weakness, postural hypotension, restlessness, and muscle cramps may appear at times early in the diet and have been attributed to a diuresis and salt depletion secondary to the low carbohydrate intake and the appearance of ketonemia and base wasting.[31,68,176] Although these symptoms are usually transitory, hypotension and syncopal episodes, particularly in patients with prior hypertension or a history of ischemic heart disease, are potentially serious. Patients should be cautioned about rising abruptly, exposure to heat, and taking hot baths.

The psychological hazards of dieting have been reviewed by Stunkard and Rush.[184] Serious emotional disturbance does not appear to be a factor with VLCDs, at least in reported studies, in which professional guidance is the rule.[20,52] Moreover, subjects with serious psychological disorders are usually screened out, and either behavior therapy or the opportunity for discussion with ancillary staff serves as an additional screen for mood disorders. Finally, the state of semi-starvation and the sense of accomplishment and recognition that accrue with rapid and major weight reduction may both induce a feeling of well-being.

Cardiac arrhythmias, a lethal complication on the liquid protein diet, have not been a problem with modern VLCDs containing high-quality protein and mineral supplementation. A number of studies using ECGs, Holter monitoring, and exercise testing have found no increase in cardiac arrhythmias or ECG abnormalities on the modified fast.[15,42,47,69,130,141,154,172,177,226] Repeated 12-lead ECGs are not sufficiently sensitive, however, to detect an increase in ectopic rhythms, and periodic Holter monitoring is recommended during long-term weight reduction on a VLCD.[124]

Myocardial Function

The presence of overt and subclinical left ventricular failure at rest or after exercise and the presence of myocardial hypertrophy at autopsy have been reported in the morbidly obese.[2,3,4,60,113] Some of the cardiovascular changes reversed after weight reduction.[4] In a recent study using noninvasive techniques, Ramhamadany et al[157] studied 34 obese subjects (mean weight, 105.8 kg) before and after four weeks on a VLCD containing 330 kcal/day. Intra-arterial ambulatory blood pressure fell in all subjects and an improvement in left ventricular function after exercise occurred in the hypertensive and control (uncomplicated obesity) groups, but not in those with ischemic heart disease. In another study, Stokholm and co-workers[181] studied cardiac contractility in seven obese subjects before and during a two-week period of treatment with a VLCD. There was a minor diminution in contractility, within the normal range. There is little or no information available at this time on the long-term effect of VLCDs on myocardial function.

Liver Pathology

Anderson et al recently studied liver morphology in 41 morbidly obese subjects before and after VLCDs.[6] The subjects were young (median age,

34), mostly female (35 of 41), and overweight by 89%. A relative reduction in overweight of 56% was achieved (median weight, 123 kg; weight loss, 34 kg). All subjects were healthy apart from their obesity. None was diabetic or taking medications influencing the liver, and alcohol abuse was excluded. The VLCD provided 388 kcal/day with 56 g of high-quality protein and contained all the required dietary supplements. Histologic studies showed regression of fatty changes, lipogranulomas, and areas of focal necrosis, findings previously noted in morbid obesity. At the same time, however, the prevalence of portal inflammation increased significantly, and portal fibrosis, absent in all of the control studies, appeared in five subjects. Regarding chemistries, there was a significant reduction in alkaline phosphatase, aspartate aminotransferase, and lactic dehydrogenase levels, with an elevation in serum bilirubin levels (within the normal range). There were no significant associations between liver biochemistry and histologic pathology. Whether the appearance of portal inflammation and fibrosis is an effect of drastic weight loss, progression of pre-existing liver disease associated with morbid obesity, or some other undetermined factor is unclear.

METABOLIC ADAPTATION DURING SEVERE ENERGY RESTRICTION

A major source of concern during rapid weight reduction by radical means is the loss of lean body mass and the potential effect of this on vital organs, such as the heart, liver, and kidneys. Considerable study has been devoted to finding the optimal dietary approach that would promote rapid weight loss while maximizing the depletion of adipose tissue and conserving body protein.

Protein Metabolism

After an overnight fast, glucose is produced exclusively in the liver and utilized primarily to meet the obligate metabolic needs of the brain. This requirement (about 125 g/day) exceeds the entire store of liver glycogen (70 to 90 g), and if the fasting state exceeds 12 to 14 hours, fasting euglycemia is maintained by a progressive increase in hepatic glucose production from alanine and other amino acids from muscle.[47] Loss of body protein is inexorable but exhibits a time-dependent decline over several weeks and stabilizes at about 3 to 6 g of nitrogen per day in prolonged starvation.[62,68,149,150] This represents a loss of 20 to 40 g of protein per day (1 g N = 6.25 g protein), or 100 to 200 g of lean body mass (20% protein by weight), and correlates well with the figures of Forbes and Drenick, who established that fasting obese humans lose about 10 g of nitrogen for each kg of body weight loss.[74] Nitrogen wasting may be two to three times greater early in the fast and, coupled with the diuresis seen with carbohydrate lack, results in a dramatic weight loss.[92] This stabilizes to about 0.3 to 0.5 kg body weight per day in the obese.[62,68] While absolute weight loss is greater in the obese during starvation because of a higher metabolic rate, nitrogen wasting relative to total body weight is less, as the obese are more efficient in conserving protein than their lean counterparts.[74]

Since protein malnutrition was considered to be the cause of death after therapeutic starvation,[9,17] the addition of small amounts of high-quality protein to the fast was recommended to conserve body protein sources, leading to evolution of the modern VLCD. The critical questions in the use of these diets are (1) to what extent VLCDs are effective in sparing protein,[58,78-80] and (2) what effect altering the ratio of protein and carbohydrate has on the long-term composition of weight loss. A major problem in obtaining answers has been the methodological uncertainties in the nitrogen balance and turnover studies used to measure changes in lean body mass.

In the balance method, nitrogen intake in food and nitrogen loss from all sources must be accurately calculated—not an easy task. The sources of loss include primarily urine and stool but also skin, menstrual flow, seminal fluids, nasal secretions, and unmeasured expired gaseous nitrogen. Diarrhea and constipation are sources of error in fecal measurements, and nitrogen losses from secondary sources are difficult to assess.[9] Apfelbaum et al[9] for example, tried to measure skin losses by taping nitrogen-free gauze on the skin of the thorax, and Bell et al searched for nitrogen in menstrual tampons. Results were poorly re-producible in both cases.[20] As a result, most investigators either overlook or estimate these secondary nitrogen losses. In addition, nitrogen intake may be overestimated by including unconsumed foods in the calculations.[210] For these reasons nitrogen losses tend to be underestimated and nitrogen intake overestimated, leading to a built-in bias toward positive nitrogen balance.[24,73,84,96,97,148,170,224] Other factors that influence balance studies and can lead to errors in interpretation are initial body weight and composition,[218] age, hormonal status,[28,29] sex (females may conserve nitrogen more efficiently than males), micronutrient balance (especially phosphorus, potassium, and sodium), prior dietary history, and meal frequency.[25,133,142,162] Also, obese subjects conserve nitrogen more efficiently with caloric deprivation than do the nonobese,[74,91] and nitrogen balance may therefore be altered by drastic weight reduction. Finally, any errors in aliquot analysis of nitrogen in urine are multiplied by total urine volumes and may result in a substantial laboratory error in nitrogen determination.[122]

Turnover studies also have methodological limitations. Leucine flux is measured in the fasting state, which makes extrapolation to overall protein metabolism difficult, since the effects of meal ingestion are excluded,[104] and the N-glycine technique is flawed by the requirement to measure nitrogen intake and excretion.

Nitrogen wasting and the loss of lean body mass are significantly less with VLCDs than in total starvation but exhibit the same time-dependent course, gradually declining over a two- to three-week period before stabilizing. The weight loss mirrors nitrogen excretion and is also, as in starvation, most rapid during the first few weeks of the diet.[28,64,69,104,135,219] It is for this reason that prior dietary status is important in evaluating balance studies. Subjects who have adapted to starvation may show a positive nitrogen balance after the introduction of a VLCD.[16,29,135] The effect of varying protein intake and energy content of VLCDs on nitrogen balances is shown in Table 59-1. The most important determinant of nitrogen retention appears to be the level of protein intake, with nitrogen balance achieved in a number of studies at protein intakes over 60 to 70 g/day. This is not univer-

TABLE 59-1

Representative Nitrogen Balance Results in Obese Patients Consuming Very Low Calorie Diets

			Final Daily Nitrogen Balance	
Reference	Protein Intake (g/day)	Energy Intake (kcal/day)	Negative Balance*	Nitrogen Equilibrium†
229	30	300	(−4.4)	
218	33	320	(−1.3)	
104	44	500	(−2)	
228	45	660	(−3)	
89	45	300	(−2.5)	
57	50	400	(−1.6)	
233	50	700	(−2.3)	
28	50	440	(−2.1)	
69	55	400	(−3)	
197	60	500	(−1)	
227	65	200		×
228	70	760		×
232	75	300		×
30	80	320		×
29	80	320		×
25	80	320		×
135	83	400		×
26	85	340		×
104	86	500		×
155	90	720		×
69	100	500	(−1.5)	
98	104	440		×
114	100	400	(−2.5)	
223	120	700	(−1.7)	
231	125	500		×

From Gelfand RA, Hendler R: Diabetes Metab Rev 5:17, 1989. Reproduced by permission. Studies in the table are listed in order of increasing dietary protein content.

*Persistent daily nitrogen loss (≥1 g/day) after three or more weeks on the diet (g/day).

†Final daily nitrogen balance was not significantly less than zero, designated by ×.

sally the case, however; negative mean nitrogen balances have been reported on protein intakes over 100 g/day in several studies. Adding to the difficulty in interpreting this data is the fact that individual patients can show markedly different nitrogen balance under identical conditions.[69,70,206,211,217] These studies, therefore, do not answer the question as to whether nitrogen equilibrium can be achieved with VLCDs containing 70 g or more of high-quality protein.

There is substantial evidence from body composition studies that fat accumulation is accompanied by an increase in lean body mass in approximate proportions of 65% to 70% fat, 25% lean body mass, and the remainder extracellular fluid.[109,112,117,118,159] Furthermore, measurement of body composition before and after substantial weight loss has demonstrated a loss of lean body mass in the range of 25% to 35%, very close to the figure cited for nitrogen loss during starvation.[19,23,56,68,80,103,158,212] As suggested in the recent review by Gelfand and Hendler,[86] VLCDs may modulate degradation of protein but do not appear to change the composition of body constituents lost during prolonged dieting. Since lean body mass increases with obesity, it is not unexpected that it is lost with weight reduction. What is unknown, however, is the specific organ and tissue origin of the protein lost and whether the protein supplementation of the VLCD is incorporated into organs and tissues that have been depleted.[58,78,79] More specifically, are vital organs such as the heart, liver, and kidneys depleted preferentially, or is the protein loss identical to that associated with the accumulation of adipose tissue?

It is apparently much harder to replace body protein than fat during weight regain. In the classic study by Keys and co-workers on a group of 12 young normal-weight male volunteers, it took 58 weeks to regain the lean body mass lost during a 24-week period of food deprivation (1600 kcal/day).[119] The average proportion of fat-free mass (FFM) lost during the first 12 weeks was 60.8%; during the next 12 weeks it was 71%. During refeeding of 7,000 to 10,000 kcal/day for 2 weeks and about 4,000 kcal/day thereafter, FFM was restored by only 42.4% after 12 weeks and by 50% in the next 8 weeks. After weight loss and regain, therefore, body composition changed, with less fat-free tissues and a larger fat mass. Repeated bouts of weight loss and regain (weight cycling) have been reported to be associated with changes in body fat distribution and decreased lean body mass, as well as with an increased efficiency of weight gain during refeeding and a resistance to weight loss during food restriction.[34,85,119,125,126,192] This has been disputed in a recent report on four subjects studied after an 18-month hiatus between diets.[235]

Experimental results in animal models are conflicting. A recent study of ovariectomized female rats demonstrated no effect on body weight or composition,[94] whereas an earlier study on male rats showed an increased metabolic efficiency after repeated bouts of weight loss and regain.[43] There were, however, important metabolic differences between these two models, and the relevance of these studies to the problem of weight loss and regain and effects on body composition in humans requires further study. Factors such as age, sex, hormonal status, and genetic background, among others, may play a role.[94]

Except for clinically supervised trials, VLCD users are self-selected for the most part and many do not suffer from major degrees of obesity.[58] It is possible, therefore, that the loss of lean tissue may be proportionately greater in these subjects, and there may be greater risks for them when exposed to severe, prolonged or repeated episodes of negative nitrogen balance.

Carbohydrate Intake and Electrolytes

The use of carbohydrate in VLCDs has been a matter of controversy, with some favoring the complete exclusion of carbohydrates to maintain low plasma insulin levels and a high degree of ketosis, with ketones replacing glucose as fuel for the brain, thereby sparing protein.[32,33,71] Commercial products today, however, provide about 50 to 60 g of carbohydrate on the assumption that this will promote maximal protein conservation, retention of electrolytes, a moderate ketosis, and inhibition of hyperuricemia.[107,138] Reduced carbohydrate during caloric restriction augments the use of fat as a metabolic fuel, leading to the increased production of the ketoacids β-hydroxybutyrate and acetoacetate, as well as acetonuria with associated excretion of cations and water. The decline in circulating insulin and the increasing glucagon levels promote glycogen breakdown, gluconeogenesis from protein with nitrogen wasting, diminished sodium reabsorption, and electrolyte losses in the urine.[38,57,165,166] These factors explain the diuresis and rapid weight loss seen during the first week on VLCDs, with energy deficit determining the rate of weight loss subsequently. The addition of sufficient carbohydrate with its stimulating effect on insulin secretion not only has a direct protein-sparing effect[48] but also diminishes the loss of electrolytes, calcium, magnesium, and zinc.[55] Preservation of bone calcium is especially important in women, zinc deficiency can impair protein synthesis, and potassium supplementation diminishes ammoniagenesis, thereby decreasing nitrogen losses.[68] Although the daily requirements for vitamins and minerals are unknown, it is unlikely that the requirement for the B vitamins in intermediary metabolism is reduced proportionately to the reduced energy intakes on

VLCDs.[58,79] The present-day VLCD, therefore, either includes or adds as a supplement the recommended daily allowances of all the essential micronutrients.

Whether ketosis produces the anorexia associated with starvation and drastic energy restriction, as has long been thought, is controversial. This subjective effect has been studied in two control studies which found no relationship between hunger and ketosis.[160,175]

Energy Expenditure

The magnitude of weight loss on any diet depends on the caloric deficit, specifically the difference between energy intake and energy expenditure. VLCDs minimize intake but also produce hormonal and metabolic adjustments that tend to conserve energy.[8,18,40,83,158,215] To better understand the changes associated with caloric restriction, a brief description of the components of energy expenditure follows.

Resting metabolic rate (RMR) accounts for 65% to 75% of daily energy expenditure and represents the minimum energy needed to maintain all physiological cell functions in the resting state. The principal determinant of RMR is lean body mass (LBM).[158] Obese subjects have a higher RMR (in absolute terms) than lean individuals, an equivalent RMR when corrected for LBM and per unit surface area, and a lower RMR when expressed per kg body weight.[110,159] Physical activity accounts for about 15% to 20% of daily energy expenditure in sedentary individuals. The obese require more energy for any given activity because of a larger mass,[110,111,158] but they tend to be more sedentary than lean subjects. Thermogenesis is the increase in RMR due to the calorigenic effect of food (also called dietary-induced thermogenesis), physiological stress, and cold exposure, and also accounts for about 15% to 20% of daily energy expenditure. Ravussin et al demonstrated a blunted thermogenic response to food in some obese subjects, in particular those with marked insulin resistance.[158] The diminution in energy expenditure seen with restricted calorie intake[40,119] has obvious survival advantages but is one factor interfering with weight loss in the obese subject on a diet. This phenomenon is demonstrable within three days of starvation,[144] and its mechanism was recently discussed by Apfelbaum et al.[9] A number of factors may be operative in this effect as body weight diminishes: A smaller cell mass will require less maintenance energy, less energy will be required for work, reduced food intake will lower dietary-induced thermogenesis, and there may be an adaptive reduction of the basal metabolic needs of the LBM above and beyond its diminished size. This latter concept has been challenged,[23,158] but there is substantial evidence for a disproportionate fall in metabolic rate when compared with body weight. With caloric restriction, metabolic rate falls by 15% in three weeks, whereas the decline in body weight is about half of this; and in starvation, resting metabolism falls by 8% by the third day.[144] It is unlikely that a reduction in LBM alone can account for this early fall in energy expenditure. When caloric restriction extends beyond five to six weeks, this discrepancy between the decline in RMR and the decline in body weight tends to disappear.[86] As suggested by Keys et al in earlier studies on caloric deprivation in nonobese volunteers,[119] after an early adaptive reduction of cellular metabolism, tissue losses accounted for a progressively larger share of the continuing gradual fall in RMR.[93,119,186,211] This adaptive reduction in metabolic rate apparently persists in the obese on weight maintenance regimens without caloric deficit[85,125] and predisposes these individuals to rapid postreduction weight gain.

Hormonal Changes

The importance of thyroid hormone in regulating metabolic rate has long been appreciated. This effect is mediated by triiodothyronine (T_3), which falls during fasting and hypocaloric carbohydrate-restricted diets. Table 59-2 summarizes different studies showing the fall in circulating T_3 levels during VLCDs. During starvation T_3 falls more than 40% during the first week.[86] This decline can be attenuated by macronutrients, mainly carbohydrates,[99] and is most apparent during the first two weeks of caloric restriction. This effect of carbohydrates on circulating T_3 requires a minimal caloric intake of about 600 kcal.[98] The fall in T_3 parallels the fall in RMR.[99,155] It is tempting to speculate that T_3 may

TABLE 59-2

Decline in Serum Triiodothyronine (T₃) During Severe Caloric Restriction: Summary of 23 Studies in Humans*

Diet	Time		
	1 wk	2 wks	>3–4 wks
Starvation	42% (8)†		54% (1)
All VLCD (200–800 kcal)	15% (15)	25% (19)	29% (22)
VLCD by energy content			
200–400 kcal/day	16% (9)	25% (8)	31% (13)
400–800 kcal	15% (6)	25% (11)	27% (9)
VLCD by carbohydrate content			
<75 g	19% (9)	30% (14)	31% (18)
75–200 g	11% (6)	10% ((5)	20% (4)

From Gelfand RA, Hendler R: Diabetes Metab Rev 5:17, 1989. Reproduced by permission.

*References 14, 45, 46, 70, 77, 88, 99, 100, 114, 116, 137, 144, 146, 155, 163, 171, 179, 191, 197, 201, 215, 216, and 230.

†Figure in parentheses indicates number of studies whose results were averaged.

mediate the adaptive metabolic decline in RMR during severe caloric restriction. In fact, exogenous T₃ administration is able to prevent the decline in RMR[161,216] while at the same time increasing the loss of LBM during rapid weight loss.[77] One problem with these studies, however, was a rise of T₃ plasma levels above pretreatment levels. Furthermore, other studies with VLCDs showed no relationship between T₃ levels and changes in RMR, body weight, or nitrogen balance.[1,18,137,223] Since thyroid hormones stimulate whole body and muscle protein breakdown,[49,65,87,189] the fall in T₃ may play an important role in conserving LBM during fasting and very low calorie dieting.

Other humoral factors may play important roles in regulating RMR. Shetty et al have maintained RMR during low-calorie diets,[174] despite diminished plasma levels of T₃, with supplements of L-dopa. The role of the sympathetic nervous system in energy metabolism has been demonstrated in humans in overfeeding studies,[115] in which overall norepinephrine turnover is increased, and conversely in hypocaloric dieting, in which a decrease in norepinephrine turnover has been reported.[123,147] It is noteworthy that insulin has been reported to stimulate both T₃ pro-

duction and sympathetic nervous system activity.[164]

RESULTS OF TREATMENT

A number of studies on small numbers of subjects have been published.* The results of eight major studies are presented in Table 59-3, adapted from the review by Wadden et al, in which five of these studies are summarized. As discussed by Wadden, control studies were not performed, and the subjects were, for the most part, of middle to high income because of the fees involved. Further, these were closely supervised studies, with the advantage of professional follow-up and behavior modification therapy in some, and the results therefore may not be representative of the VLCD dieting population at large. The relationship of weight loss to duration of time on the VLCD in these studies was essentially linear, with short-term treatments of four weeks producing substantial losses of about 9 kg, ranging up to 21 to 31 kg, with diets lasting 14 to 24 weeks. Palgi and associates found that

*References 26, 27, 30, 31, 51, 53, 89, 102, 134, 139, 156, and 221.

TABLE 59-3

Results of Treatment From Eight Major Studies on Obese Patients Consuming Very Low Calorie Diets

Study	N	Sex	Mean Baseline Weight (kg)	Mean Age (yr)	Diet Regimen		Mean Treatment Duration (wk)	Mean Weight Loss (kg)
Howard et al[107]	22	19 F 3 M	107.8	—	Protein CHO	31 g 44 g	4	9.6
Tuck et al[190]	25	14 F 11 M	103.9	40.7	Protein CHO	70 g 30 g	12	20.2
Atkinson and Kaiser[13]	234	200 F 34 M	104.5	37.9	Protein IBW CHO IBW	1 g/kg 0.5 g/kg	12	18.7
Palgi et al[151]	668	564 F 104 M	98.0	38.0	Protein IBW CHO	1.5 g/kg —	17.4	21.4
Vertes et al[199]	530	411 F 119 M	109.6 136.6	40.0 40.0	Protein CHO	45 g 30 g	23.8 19.9	31.2 37.6
Kirschner et al[120]	4,026	3,060 F 966 M	111.3	40.0	Protein CHO	70 g 30 g	13.7	24.5
Kreitzman[121]	27	— —	110.4	—	Protein CHO	30 g 40 g	4	8.6
Van Gaal and De Leeuw[195]	15	13 F 2 M	110.4	39.5	Protein CHO	60 g 54 g	6	14.4

Modified from Wadden et al: Ann Intern Med 99:675, 1983. Reproduced by permission.

weight loss on VLCDs corresponded significantly with percentage overweight, length of time on the diet, and rate of weight loss—identical, therefore, to predictors of short-term weight loss with other treatments.[151] In those studies in which weight loss was analyzed by sex, men achieved larger weight losses, but percentage reduction from original weight was the same in men and women.[89,151,199]

Weight Maintenance and Compliance

In a 1958 review of the literature and report on a series of 100 patients, Stunkard and McLaren-Hume documented the dismal results of weight reduction programs at that time.[183] Although the subjects of these reports were grossly overweight, only 25% were able to lose as much as 20 pounds, and only 5% lost 40 pounds. Of the 100 consecutive patients treated at the nutrition clinic of a large teaching hospital, only 12% were able to lose 20 pounds, and only one patient lost 40 pounds. The dropout rate after only one visit was 28%, and after two years only two patients had maintained their weight loss. In a survey of more recent results with conventional diet therapy, including anorectic drugs and behavior modification in some subjects, weight losses averaged less than 5.4 kg.[182,219]

From this point of view, VLCDs represent an advance in the treatment of significantly overweight individuals. There is concern, however, that many of these patients regain substantial amounts of weight when treatment is ended. In a large series reported by Genuth et al,[90] 56% of patients regained more than half of the lost weight by 22 months follow-up. In the series reported by Palgi et al, more than two thirds of the weight lost had been regained by 4.5 years, and Anderson et al reported that only 17% of patients maintained 10 kg or more of a 22-kg weight loss at a five-year follow-up.[5] Furthermore, subject attrition on VLCDs is substantial, and many are lost to long-term follow-up. Dropout rates of as much as one third to 50% have been reported.[59,138,199] Neither the overall attrition rate, the dropout time after initiation of the VLCD, or long-term weight maintenance is quantifiable, however, since this issue is not addressed in most reports.

Rapid Versus Gradual Weight Loss

In a recent study, Foster and associates[75] have compared effects of a VLCD and a 1,000- to 1200-kcal balanced deficit diet containing 60% carbohydrate, 30% fat, and 10% protein in a group of 16 obese women with uncomplicated obesity (173% recommended weight) during a 24-week study. Both groups began and finished the study period on the balanced deficit diet. One group then received a 500-kcal VLCD for eight weeks after the initial four-week adaptational period on the BDD. After just two weeks on the 500-kcal VLCD, patients showed a reduction in resting energy expenditure of 17.3% with a weight loss of only 5.8%. At the end of treatment these figures were 11% and 12%, respectively. By comparison, patients who remained on the balanced deficit diet for the entire study period of 24 weeks showed an 11% weight loss with only a 2% reduction in resting energy expenditure. Loss of FFM was comparable in the two groups, 2.1 kg in the patients on VLCD and 2.4 kg in the group on the balanced deficit diet. This pilot study showed a possible metabolic advantage for those who lose weight by a more conservative dietary approach.

In another study reported by Stock,[180] however, weight-matched obese Zucker rats were placed on either 3 g/day of a formula diet (VLCD, equivalent to 330 kcal/day in a 90-kg human) or 11 g/day of a stock diet (LCD, 1400 kcal/day) un-til their body weights had fallen to that of an age-matched group of lean Zucker rats. Percentage of fat and FFM were unchanged in the VLCD rats, whereas the LCD group showed, if anything, a relative increase in percentage fat. At the end of treatment, when the final body weights of the obese group and their lean littermates were identical, the genetically obese animals were still considerably fatter on body composition analysis. Of particular interest was the finding that daily energy expenditure and RMR were reduced equally (55% to 60%) in both the VLCD and LCD groups even though the rate of weight loss in the VLCD group was twice that of the LCD group. Stock has suggested that in this genetic form of obesity, maximal increases in energetic efficiency occur at relatively modest levels of energy restriction and that further restriction has no additional effect on metabolic rate; more specifically, that gradual weight loss has no metabolic advantage over rapid weight reduction. Prospective studies and elucidation of the genetics of human obesity may shed some light on which individuals respond best to rapid and drastic weight loss.

ANCILLARY MODALITIES

Because of the high attrition rate and mediocre long-term results, a number of ancillary modalities are currently being tested in conjunction with VLCD therapy.

Behavior Modification

Wadden et al,[202] in an important long-term study of 76 obese women, compared VLCD alone, behavior therapy alone, and their combination in the treatment of obesity and reported changes in weight at the end of a six-month treatment period (four months in the VLCD alone group) and then at one- and five-year follow-up periods. These are illustrated in Figure 59-2[182] taken from an earlier study done by the same group on 59 women,[203] with results essentially the same as those outlined below. Weight losses for the three conditions at the end of treatment in the current report were 13.1, 13.0, and 16.8 kg respectively, with losses for the combined-treatment group significantly greater than in the VLCD-alone

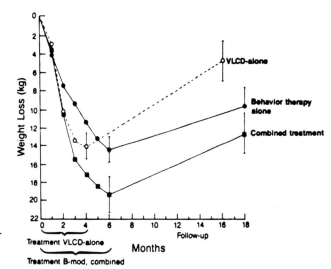

FIGURE 59-2

Weight changes during treatment and at 12-month follow-up. (From Stunkard AS: Conservative treatments for obesity. Am J Clin Nutr 45:1142, 1987. Reproduced by permission. Data originally published by Wadden and Stunkard.[203])

group and behavior therapy–alone group. Weight losses one year after treatment were 4.7, 6.6, and 10.6 kg, respectively, with approximately one third of the patients in the behavior therapy–alone and combined-treatment groups maintaining their full end-of-treatment weight losses, compared to 5% in the VLCD-alone group. Five years after treatment a majority of subjects in all three conditions had returned to their pretreatment weight and 55% of all patients had received additional weight reduction treatment. This is the first study of weight reduction to correct for the effects of additional therapy after completion of the diet treatment program.[202,204] What stands out in this report is the success of all three modalities in the short term, the success of behavior therapy alone, and the long-term failure of all three weight reduction modalities.

Protein-Sparing Modified Fast

In an attempt to diminish attrition rates and improve long-term results when subjects either find the formula diets unpalatable or complain of hunger, some investigators have used the protein-sparing modified fast. Wadden and coworkers[205,207] have reported that subjects on a protein-sparing modified fast (developed by Blackburn, Bistrian, and colleagues and containing 1.5 g of protein per kg ideal body weight,

derived from lean meat, fish, and fowl, with no carbohydrate and with fat limited to the protein sources)[30-32] exhibited significantly less hunger and preoccupation with eating than did subjects on liquid formula diets. Van Gaal and De Leeuw[195] have also shown substantial weight losses on the protein-sparing modified fast in morbidly obese subjects, comparable to those achieved on a VLCD, with stabilization of weight loss after switching to a maintenance diet in the 12% of patients who were followed for two years.

Fiber

Astrup and Quaade[10] have reported that 30 gm of dietary fiber per day added to the VLCD improved compliance by overcoming constipation and hunger without affecting absorption of divalent cations (a nongelling fiber without phytate was used).

Hospital-Based Programs

The need for treatment and long-term follow-up, although obvious in the obese with associated serious medical conditions, has a low priority at hospitals and in practice. Shapiro et al[173] reported improved long-term compliance in a group of 408 patients with serious concurrent medical conditions who failed to lose weight with conventional treatment prescribed by their own physicians and who were then treated at a hospital-based referral clinic. Patients were treated with a VLCD and followed up for three years, with reported improved long-term compliance and overall amelioration of hypertensive disease, anginal syndrome, pulmonary function, gastroesophageal reflux, and maturity-onset diabetes mellitus.

Group Settings

In a recent report Cox et al[54] discussed a pilot project in which seriously overweight subjects were brought together in a self-help group after a one- to two-week introductory period in a halfway house. Apart from the obvious advantages of group therapy, this approach appears to offer promise in situations where financial resources for support services are limited and extended periods on a VLCD are necessary for health reasons.

Exercise

The thermic effect of exercise is about 15% to 20% of total daily expenditure in the sedentary individual and is the only factor in the energy equation that can be increased voluntarily.[111,192] The exercise capacity of many obese individuals is limited, however, and life-style activities (walking, using the stairs) rather than programmed sports activities are preferred early in a training program.[182] Recent studies of the combined effects of exercise and energy restriction have been reviewed by Van Dale[192] and Kreitzman[122] and support the idea that exercise may make a marginal contribution, if any, to weight loss in subjects on VLCDs. Lemons et al[127] compared the effect of two distinct exercise regimens, isotonic resistance (Universal machines) and aerobic (bicycle ergometer training), in a controlled study during a period of weight reduction on a VLCD. While weight loss was not significantly improved, the efficiency of the residual FFM (RMR/FFM [%]) and strength per kg body weight were improved in the isotonic training groups. Furthermore, a subjective improvement in mood and motivation was noted in the diet and exercise groups.

Pharmacologic

Heraief et al[101] have presented evidence that carbohydrate deprivation in weight-reducing regimens suppresses plasma tryptophan levels. For this reason Finer and associates[67] used dexfenfluramine, a serotonin agonist, in conjunction with VLCD in treating patients with refractory morbid obesity. In a controlled study of 45 patients on a VLCD, some subjects were better able to maintain or improve their weight loss during a 26-week follow-up period with the concurrent use of dexfenfluramine and a VLCD. Combined therapy with this anorexigenic agent may therefore be useful in the treatment of refractory obesity, and long-term studies with larger numbers of patients are currently in progress to evaluate this possibility.

MEDICAL BENEFITS

Since improvement in a number of medical conditions has been reported after substantive weight loss by conventional dieting, it is not surprising that medical benefits have been reported after the use of VLCDs and the associated rapid and significant weight loss. These have been summarized in reviews by Wadden et al[206] and Atkinson.[11] There are now numerous reports of improvement in several conditions, described below.

Hypertension

Large reductions in both systolic and diastolic blood pressure are associated with the use of VLCDs[13,89,102.129,190,225] and are attributable in part to the rapid reduction in body mass and profound diuresis of salt, water, and other electrolytes during the first week of dieting. Reduction or even elimination of antihypertensive medication has been possible in some cases, and necessary in others, to prevent postural hypotension.

Maturity-Onset Diabetes Mellitus

Here also, rapid and dramatic improvement may be seen.[12,25,59,90,129] The association of overweight with type II diabetes has been known for decades, and a very high percentage of these patients are obese and insulin resistant, while many obese subjects without overt glucose intolerance also manifest insulin resistance. Over 30 years ago, Yalow and co-workers[220] demonstrated that weight reduction improved glucose tolerance, lowered plasma insulin levels, and improved sensitivity to insulin. If weight reduction is maintained, patients are frequently able to dispense with antidiabetic medication; in fact this may be mandatory in some cases to prevent hypoglycemia.

Lipids

Several studies have shown significant decreases in serum cholesterol of up to 20% to 25%[59,129,168,213,218] with an associated fall in low-density lipoprotein cholesterol[213] and reductions in triglyceride levels of as much as 38%.[129] The effect on high-density lipoprotein cholesterol fraction may vary with the sex of the patient and other factors such as exercise, but a fall from the already lower levels seen in obese subjects has been reported in women and a rise reported in men.[44,187] In a recent report, however, Waggonner and associates noted a marked elevation in serum cholesterol, after an initial fall, in subjects who remained on a VLCD or a protein-sparing modified fast for over two months.[209] The increase in some cases over baseline levels was attributed to adipose cholesterol mobilization (biopsy data) and resolved after weight loss stopped.

Other Conditions

There have also been reports of improvement in respiratory function and sleep apnea,[185] anginal syndrome, and mild congestive heart failure[173] in morbidly obese subjects who lost significant amounts of weight.

Whether or not improvement in these serious conditions can be sustained with maintenance of weight loss undoubtedly depends on the severity of the illness and other factors, in particular the mechanism of the disease process and its relationship to overweight. Long-term follow-up studies are needed to identify those individuals who respond to the rapid and drastic weight re-

duction on VLCDs with a lasting improvement in their medical condition.

SAFETY

Although there have been several deaths among several thousand patients followed in closely supervised studies, none of these have been attributable to the modern VLCD. As discussed by Wadden and associates,[206] no deaths were reported by Apfelbaum in a series of 4000 patients or by Bistrian and Blackburn in a series of 1200 patients. Although Vertes and Genuth reported six deaths in 3000 patients (where 12 might have been expected); all were accounted for by pre-existing illness.[206] Palgi and associates[151] reported no deaths in 668 obese subjects on a protein-sparing modified fast during treatment and only five deaths subsequently, at least one year after subjects had left the program. These results attest to the safety of VLCDs in medically controlled programs, especially since many of the subjects treated were high risk because of associated serious medical conditions. On the other hand, the COMA Report[58] states that fewer than half of all prospective users of VLCDs in the United Kingdom sought medical advice before commencing self-dieting with a VLCD, and these figures may apply generally. Furthermore, one quarter of consumers admitted to VLCD use for longer than three to four weeks, in some cases as a nutritional supplement, without medical supervision. The potential for abuse and adverse risk therefore does exist for the nonobese, mildly obese, and those with medical contraindications to a VLCD.

FUTURE PERSPECTIVES

The development of the modern VLCD represents an advance in the treatment of moderate to severe obesity and associated medical conditions. These diets appear to be safe when used for limited time periods under careful medical supervision, but a number of unresolved problems relating to their use remain. Chief among these problems is the question of nitrogen balance. Is the protein loss during weight reduction greater than that associated with the excess adipose tissue? Does any of it come from vital organs? With prolonged or repeated use, what is the effect of a VLCD on myocardial function? Are there any long-term effects on hepatic, gastrointestinal, or renal function and structure?

Who is most likely to benefit from a VLCD as a means of weight reduction? Obesity has many causes, and there are different types of obesity. Prospective studies and clarification of the genetics of human obesity may help identify those most likely to succeed on this regimen.

Should VLCDs be used in a single long treatment period or intermittently, until satisfactory weight goals are achieved?

What is the effect on resting energy expenditure of prolonged and drastic energy restriction? Is there a maximal increase in energetic efficiency, and if so, at what level of energy restriction does this occur?

The results of VCLD treatment using the ancillary modalities of exercise and behavior modification are encouraging. Even under the best of circumstances, however, the relapse rate is high and additional strategies are needed to improve the success rate in the long term.

References

1. Adami S, Ferrari M, Golranini G et al: Serum thyroid hormone concentrations and weight loss relationships in eight obese women during semistarvation. J Endocrinol Invest 2:271, 1979
2. Alexander JK: Obesity and the heart. Curr Prob Cardiol 5(3):1, 1980
3. Alexander JK, Amad KH, Cole VW: Observations on some clinical features of extreme obesity with particular reference to cardiorespiratory effects. Am J Med 32:512, 1962
4. Alexander JK, Peterson KL: Cardiovascular effects of weight reduction. Circulation 45:310, 1972
5. Andersen T, Backer OG, Stokholm KH et al: Randomized trial of diet and gastroplasty compared with diet alone in morbid obesity. N Engl J Med 310:352, 1984
6. Andersen T, Gluud C, Christoffersen P: The effect of very-low-calorie diet on liver morphology. Int J Obes 13(suppl 2):153, 1989
7. Apfelbaum M: Traitment de l'obesite par la diete protidique. Entriens de Biachat 1:62, 1967
8. Apfelbaum M, Bostsarron J, Lactis D: Effect of caloric restriction and excessive caloric intake on energy expenditure. Am J Clin Nutr 24:1405, 1971
9. Apfelbaum M, Fricker J, Igoin-Apfelbaum L: Low-

10. Astrup A, Quaade F: VLCD compliance and lean body mass. Int J Obes 13(suppl 2):27, 1989
11. Atkinson RL: Low and very low calorie diets. Med Clin North Am 73:203, 1989
12. Atkinson RL, Kaiser DL: Effects of calorie restriction and weight loss on glucose and insulin levels in obese humans. J Am Coll Nutr 4:411, 1985
13. Atkinson RL, Kaiser DL: Nonphysician supervision of a very low calorie diet: Results in over 200 cases. Int J Obes 5:237, 1981
14. Azizi F: Effect of dietary composition on fasting-induced changes in serum thyroid hormones and thyrotropin metabolism. Metabolism 27:935, 1978
15. Baird IM: Ambulatory monitoring of obese subjects on normal and very low calorie diets. In Blackburn GL, Bray GA (eds): Management of Obesity by Severe Caloric Restriction, p 215. Littleton, Mass, PSG Publishing, 1985
16. Baird IM, Parsons RL, Howard AN: Clinical and metabolic studies of chemically defined diets in the management of obesity. Metabolism 23:645, 1974
17. Ball MF, Canary JJ, Kyle LH: Comparative effects of caloric restriction and total starvation on body composition in obesity. Ann Intern Med 67:60, 1967
18. Barrows K, Snook JT: Effect of a high-protein, very-low-calorie diet on resting metabolism, thyroid hormones, and energy expenditure of obese middle-aged women. Am J Clin Nutr 45:391, 1987
19. Barrows K, Snook JT: Effect of a high-protein, very-low-calorie diet on body composition and anthropometric parameters of obese middle-aged women. Am J Clin Nutr 45:381, 1987
20. Bell JD, Margen S, Calloway DH: Ketosis, weight loss, uric acid and nitrogen balance in obese women fed single nutrients at low calorie levels. Metabolism 18:193, 1969
21. Benedict FG: A study of prolonged fasting. Carnegie Institute publication No. 203. Washington, DC, Carnegie Institute, 1915
22. Bennion LG, Grundy S: Effects of obesity and caloric intake on biliary lipid metabolism in man. J Clin Invest 56:996, 1975
23. Bessard T, Schutz Y, Jequier E: Energy expenditure and post-prandial thermogenesis in obese women before and after weight loss. Am J Clin Nutr 38:680, 1983
24. Bier DM, Motil KJ, Matthews DE et al: Energy intake and whole body protein dynamics in man. In Nutrition and Child Health: Perspectives for the 1980s, p 161. New York, Alan R Liss, 1981

25. Bistrian BR, Blackburn GL, Flatt JP et al: Nitrogen metabolism and insulin requirements in obese diabetic adults on a protein sparing modified fast. Diabetes 25:494, 1976

26. Bistrian BR, Blackburn GL, Stanbury JB: Metabolic aspects of protein sparing modified fast in the dietary management of Prader-Willi obesity. N Engl J Med 296:774, 1977

27. Bistrian BR, Sherman M: Results of the treatment of obesity with a protein-sparing fast. Int J Obes 2:143, 1978

28. Bistrian BR, Sherman M, Young VR: The mechanisms of nitrogen sparing in fasting supplemented by protein and carbohydrate. J Clin Endocrinol Metab 53:874, 1981

29. Bistrian BR, Winterer J, Blackburn GL et al: Effect of a protein-sparing diet and brief fast on nitrogen metabolism in mildly obese subjects. J Lab Clin Med 89:1030, 1977

30. Blackburn GL, Bistrian BR, Flatt JP: Role of a protein-sparing modified fast in a comprehensive weight reduction program. In Howard AN (ed): Recent Advances in Obesity Research, Vol I, p 279. London, Newman Publishing, 1975

31. Blackburn GL, Bray GA (eds): Management of Obesity by Severe Caloric Restriction. Littleton, Mass, PSG Publishing, 1985

32. Blackburn GL, Flatt MP, Cloves GHA et al: Protein sparing therapy during periods of starvation with sepsis of trauma. Ann Surg 177:588, 1973

33. Blackburn GL, Flatt JP, Cloves GH et al: Peripheral intravenous feeding with isotonic amino acid solutions. Am J Surg 125:447, 1973

34. Blackburn G, Kanders B, Brownell K et al: The effects of weight cycling on the rate of weight loss in man (abstr). Int J Obes 11:84, 1987

35. Bloom WL: Fasting as an introduction to the treatment of obesity. Metabolism 8:214, 1959

36. Bloom WL, Azar G, Clark J et al: Comparison of metabolic changes in fasting obese and lean patients. In Brodoff BN (Conf Chair): Adipose Tissue Metabolism and Obesity. Ann NY Acad Sci 131:632, 1965

37. Bollinger RE, Lukert BD, Brown RV et al: Metabolic balance of obese subjects during fasting. Arch Intern Med 118:3, 1966

38. Boulter PR, Hoffman RS, Arky RA: Pattern of sodium excretion accompanying starvation. Metabolism 22:675, 1973

39. Boyle PC, Storlien LH, Keesey RE: Increased efficiency of food utilization following weight loss. Physiol Behav 21:261, 1978

40. Bray GA: Effect of caloric restriction on energy expenditure in obese patients. Lancet 2:397, 1969

41. Broomfield PH, Chopra R, Scheinbaum RC et al: Effects of ursodeoxycholic acid and aspirin on the formation of lithogenic bile and gallstones during loss of weight. N Engl J Med 319:1567, 1988

42. Brown MR, Forbes GB, Klish WJ et al: Protein sparing modified fast in obese adolescents: Long-term effects on lean body mass (abstr). J Am Coll Nutr 1:127, 1982

43. Brownell KD, Greenwood MRC, Stellar E et al: The effects of repeated cycles of weight loss and regain in rats. Physiol Behav 38:459, 1986

44. Brownell KD, Stunkard AJ: Differential changes in plasma high-density lipoprotein-cholesterol levels in obese men and women during weight reduction. Arch Intern Med 141:1142, 1981

45. Burman KD, Dimond RC, Harvey GS et al: Glucose modulation of alterations in serum iodothyronine concentrations induced by fasting. Metabolism 28:291, 1979

46. Burman KD, Wartofsky L, Dinterman RE et al: The effect of T_3 and reverse T_3 administration on muscle protein catabolism during fasting as measured by 3-methylhistidine excretion. Metabolism 28:805, 1979

47. Cahill GF Jr: Starvation in man. N Engl J Med 282:668, 1970

48. Calloway DH, Spector H: Nitrogen balance as related to calories and protein intake in active young men. Am J Clin Nutr 2:405, 1954

49. Carter WJ, Benjamin WSVD, Faas FH: Effect of experimental hyperthyroidism on protein turnover in skeletal and cardiac muscle. Metabolism 29:910, 1980

50. Centers for Disease Control: Liquid protein diets. US Public Health Service Publication EPI-78-11-2. Atlanta, US Public Health Service, 1979

51. Contaldo F, DiBiase G, Fischetti A et al: Evaluation of the safety of very-low-calorie diets in the treatment of severely obese patients in a metabolic ward. Int J Obes 5:221, 1981

52. Cook RF, Howard AN, Mills IH: Low dose mianserin as adjunctant therapy in obese patients treated by a very-low-calorie diet. Int J Obes 5:267, 1981

53. Cormillot A, Zukerfeld R, Olkies A et al: A multiple approach to the treatment of obesity using total fasting on a very low-calorie diet. Int J Obes 5:297, 1981

54. Cox J, Kreitzman S, Coxon A et al: A model for group therapy in major obesity using VLCD. Int J Obes 13(suppl 2):197, 1980

55. Davie MWJ, Abraham RR, Hewins B et al: Changes in bone and muscle constituents during dieting for obesity. Clin Sci 70:285, 1986

56. De Boer JO, Van Es AJH, Roovers LA et al: Adaptation of energy metabolism of overweight

women to low-energy intake, studied with whole-body calorimeters. Am J Clin Nutr 44:585, 1986

57. DeHaven I, Sherwin R, Hendler R et al: Nitrogen and sodium balance and sympathetic nervous system activity in obese subjects treated with a low-calorie protein or mixed diet. N Engl J Med 302:477, 1982

58. Department of Health and Social Security: The Use of Very Low Calorie Diets in Obesity. Report on Health and Social Subjects No. 31. London, Her Majesty's Stationery Office, 1987

59. DiBiase G, Mattioli PL, Contaldo F et al: A very-low-calorie formula diet (Cambridge diet) for the treatment of diabetic-obese patients. Int J Obes 5:319, 1981

60. Drenick EJ, Bale GS, Setzer F et al: Excessive mortality and causes of death in morbidly obese men. JAMA 243:443, 1980

61. Drenick EJ, Johnson D: Weight reduction by fasting and semistarvation in morbid obesity: Long term followup. Int J Obes 2:123, 1978

62. Drenick EJ, Swendseid ME, Blahd WH et al: Prolonged starvation as treatment for severe obesity. JAMA 187:100, 1964

63. Duncan GG, Duncan TG, Schless GL et al: Contraindications and therapeutic results of fasting in obese patients. In Brodoff BN (Conf Chair): Adipose Tissue Metabolism and Obesity. Ann NY Acad Sci 131:632, 1965

64. Durrant ML, Garrow JS, Royston P et al: Factors influencing the composition of the weight lost by obese patients on a reducing diet. Br J Nutr 44:275, 1980.

65. Elia M, Carter A, Bacon S et al: Clinical usefulness of urinary 3-methylhistidine excretion in indicating muscle protein breakdown. Br Med J 282:351, 1981

66. Evans FA, Strang JM: A departure from the usual methods of treating obesity. Am J Med Sci 177:339, 1929

67. Finer N, Finer S, Naoumova RP: Prolonged use of a very low calorie diet (Cambridge diet) in massively obese patients attending an obesity clinic: Safety, efficacy and additional benefit from dexfenfluramine. Int J Obes 13(suppl 2):91, 1989

68. Fisler JS, Drenick EJ: Starvation and semistarvation diets in the management of obesity. Ann Rev Nutr 7:465, 1987

69. Fisler JS, Drenick EJ, Blumfield DE et al: Nitrogen economy during very low calorie reducing diets: Quality and quantity of dietary protein. Am J Clin Nutr 35:471, 1982

70. Fisler JS, Kaptein EM, Drenick EJ et al: Metabolic and hormonal factors as predictors of nitrogen re-

tention in obese men consuming very low calorie diets. Metabolism 34:101, 1985

71. Flatt JP, Blackburn FL: The metabolic fuel regulatory system: Implications for protein-sparing therapies during caloric deprivation and disease. Am J Clin Nutr 27:175, 1974

72. Folin O, Dennis W: On starvation and obesity with special reference to acidosis. J Biol Chem 21:183, 1915

73. Forbes GB: Another source of error in the metabolic balance method. Nutr Rev 31:297, 1973

74. Forbes GB, Drenick EJ: Loss of body nitrogen on fasting. Am J Clin Nutr 32:1570, 1979

75. Foster GD, Wadden TA, Feurer ID et al: Controlled trial of the metabolic effects of a very-low-calorie diet: Short and long term effects. Am J Clin Nutr 51:167, 1990

76. Frank A, Graham C, Frank S: Fatalities on the liquid protein diet: An analysis of possible causes. Int J Obes 5:243, 1981

77. Gardner DF, Kaplan MM, Stanley CA et al: Effect of tri-iodothyronine replacement on the metabolic and pituitary responses to starvation. N Engl J Med 300:579, 1970

78. Garrow J: Are liquid diets safe or necessary? In Berry EM, Blondheim SH, Eliahou HE (eds): Recent Advances in Obesity Research, Vol V, p 327. London, John Libbey & Co, 1986

79. Garrow JS: Very low calorie diets should not be used. Int J Obes 13(suppl 2):145, 1989

80. Garrow JS: Is there a body protein reserve? Proc Nutr Soc 41:373, 1982

81. Garrow JS: Obesity and Related Diseases. London, Churchill Livingstone, 1988

82. Garrow JS, Webster JS, Pearson M et al: Inpatient-outpatient randomized comparison of Cambridge diet versus milk diet in 17 obese women over 24 weeks. Int J Obes 13:521, 1989

83. Garrow JS, Durrant ML, Mann S et al: Factors determining weight loss in obese patients in a metabolic ward. Int J Obes 2:441, 1978

84. Garza C, Scrimshaw NS, Young VR: Human protein requirements: Long-term metabolic nitrogen balance studies in young men to evaluate the 1973 FAO/WHO safe level of egg protein intake. J Nutr 107:335, 1977

85. Geissler CA, Miller DS, Shah M: The daily metabolic rate of the post-obese and the lean. Am J Clin Nutr 45:914, 1987

86. Gelfand RA, Hendler R: Effect of nutrient composition on the metabolic response to very low calorie diets: Learning more and more about less and less. Diabetes Metab Rev 5:17, 1989

87. Gelfand RA, Hutchinson-Williams KA, Bonde AA et al: Catabolic mechanism in thyroid hormone

excess: The contribution of adrenergic activity to hypermetabolism and protein breakdown. Metabolism 36:562, 1987

88. Gelfand RA, Sherwin RS: Nitrogen conservation in starvation revisited: Protein sparing with intravenous fructose. Metabolism 35:37, 1986

89. Genuth SM, Castro JH, Vertes V: Weight reduction in obesity by outpatient semistarvation. JAMA 230:987, 1974

90. Genuth SM, Vertes V, Hazelton J: Supplemental fasting in the treatment of obesity. In Bray G (ed): Recent Advances in Obesity Research, p 370. London, Newman, 1978

91. Goodman MN, Lowell B, Belur E et al: Sites of protein conservation and loss during starvation: Influence of adiposity. Am J Physiol 246:383, 1984

92. Grande F: Energy balance and body composition changes: A critical study of three recent publications. Ann Intern Med 68:467, 1968

93. Grande F, Anderson JT, Keys A: Changes of basal metabolic rate in man in semistarvation and refeeding. J Appl Physiol 12:230, 1968

94. Gray DS, Fisler JS, Bray GA: Effects of repeated weight loss and regain on body composition in obese rats. Am J Clin Nutr 47:393, 1988

95. Hanefeld M, Weck M: Very low calorie diet therapy in obese non insulin dependent diabetes patients. Int J Obes 13(suppl 2):33, 1989

96. Hegsted DM: Balance studies. J Nutr 106:307, 1976

97. Hegsted DM: Assessment of nitrogen requirements. Am J Clin Nutr 31:1669, 1978

98. Hendler R, Bonde AA: Very low calorie diets with high and low protein content: Impact on triiodothyronine, energy expenditure and nitrogen balance. Am J Clin Nutr 48:1, 1988

99. Hendler RA, Walesky M, Sherwin RS: Sucrose substitution in prevention and reversal of the fall in metabolic rate accompanying hypocaloric diets. Am J Med 81:280, 1986

100. Henson LC, Heber D: Whole body protein breakdown rates and hormonal adaptation in fasted obese subjects. J Clin Endocrinol Metab 57:316, 1983

101. Heraief E, Burckhardt P, Mauron C et al: Treatment of obesity by carbohydrate deprivation suppresses plasma tryptophan and its ratio to other large neutral amino acids. J Neural Transm 57:187, 1983

102. Hickey N, Daly L, Bourke G et al: Outpatient treatment of obesity with a very-low calorie formula diet. Int J Obes 5:227, 1981

103. Hill JO, Sparling PB, Shields TW et al: Effects of exercise and food restriction on body composition and metabolic rate in obese women. Am J Clin Nutr 46:622, 1987

104. Hoffer LJ, Bistrian BR, Young VR et al: Metabolic effects of very low calorie weight reduction diets. J Clin Invest 73:750, 1984

105. Howard AN: Dietary treatment of obesity. In Silverstone T (ed): Obesity: Its Pathogenesis and Management, p 123. Lancaster, England, MTP Press, 1975

106. Howard AN: The historical development of very low calorie diets. Int J Obes 13(suppl 2):1, 1989

107. Howard AN, Grant A, Edwards O et al: The treatment of obesity with a very-low-calorie liquid formula diet: An inpatient/outpatient comparison using skimmed milk as the chief protein source. Int J Obes 2:321, 1978

108. Isner JM, Sours HE, Paris AL et al: Sudden unexpected death in avid dieters using the liquid protein modified fast diet: Observations in 17 patients and the role of the prolonged QT interval. Circulation 60:1401, 1979

109. James WPT, Davies HL, Bailes J et al: Elevated metabolic rates in obesity. Lancet 1:1122, 1978

110. Jecquier E: Energy expenditures in obesity. Clin Endocrinol Metab 13:563, 1984

111. Jecquier E: Energy utilization in human obesity. Ann NY Acad Sci 499:73, 1987

112. Johnston LC, Bernstein LM: Body composition and oxygen consumption of overweight, normal and underweight women. J Lab Clin Med 45:109, 1955

113. Kaltman AJ, Goldring RM: Role of circulatory congestion in the cardiorespiratory failure of obesity. Am J Med 60:645, 1976

114. Kaptein EM, Fisler JS, Duda MJ et al: Relationship between the changes in serum thyroid hormone levels and protein status during prolonged protein supplemented caloric deprivation. Clin Endocrinol 22:1, 1985

115. Katzeff HL, Danforth E Jr: The thermogenic response to norepinephrine, food and exercise in lean man during overfeeding. Clin Res 29:663A, 1981

116. Katzeff, HL, O'Connell M, Horton ES et al: Metabolic studies in human obesity during overnutrition and undernutrition: Thermogenic and hormonal responses to norepinephrine. Metabolism 35:166, 1986

117. Keys A, Anderson JT, Brozek J: Weight gain from simple overeating: I. Character of the tissue gained. Metabolism 4:427, 1955

118. Keys A, Brozek J: Body fat in adult man. Physiol Rev 33:245, 1953

119. Keys A, Brozek J, Henschel A et al: The Biology of Human Starvation. Minneapolis, University of Minnesota Press, 1950

120. Kirschner MA, Schneider G, Ertel NH et al: An eight-year experience with a very-low-calorie formula diet for control of major obesity. Int J Obes 12:69, 1988

121. Kreitzman SN: Clinical experience with a very low calorie diet. In Blackburn GL, Bray GA (eds): Management of Obesity by Severe Caloric Restriction, p 359. Littleton, Mass, PSG Publishing, 1985

122. Kreitzman SN: Lean body mass, exercise, and VLCDs. Int J Obes 13(suppl 2):17, 1989

123. Landsberg L and Young JB: The role of the sympatho-adrenal system in modulating energy expenditure. Alberti KGMM et al (eds): In Clinics in Endocrinology and Metabolism, Chapter 3, 475, 1984.

124. Lantigua RA, Amatruda JM, Biddle TL et al: Cardiac arrhythmias associated with a liquid protein diet for the treatment of obesity. N Engl J Med 303:735, 1980

125. Leibel RL, Hirsch J: Diminished energy requirements in reduced-obese patients. Metabolism 33:164, 1984

126. Leibel RL, Hirsch J, Berry EM et al: Alterations in adipocyte free fatty acid reesterification associated with obesity and weight reduction in man. Am J Clin Nutr 42:198, 1985

127. Lemons AD, Kreitzman SN, Coxon A et al: Selection of appropriate exercise regimes for weight reduction during VLCD and maintenance. Int J Obes 13(suppl 2):119, 1989

128. Liddle RA, Goldstein RB, Saxon J: Gallstone formation during weight-reduction dieting. Arch Intern Med 149:1750, 1989

129. Lindner PG, Blackburn GL: Multidisciplinary approach to obesity utilizing fasting modified by protein-sparing therapy. Obes Bariatr Med 5:198, 1976

130. Linet OI, Butler D, Caswell K et al: Absence of cardiac arrhythmias during a very low calorie diet with high biological-quality protein. Int J Obes 7:313, 1983

131. Linn R, Stuart SL: The Last Chance Diet. Secaucus, NJ, Lyle Stuart, 1976

132. Liquid protein and sudden death: an update. FDA Drug Bull 8:18, 1978

133. Lubin M: Intracellular potassium and macromolecular synthesis in mammalian cells. Nature 213:451, 1967

134. Mancini M, Contaldo F, Fivellese A et al: A practical and safe programme of calorie restriction for the treatment of massive obesity. In Howard AN (ed): Recent Advances in Obesity Research, Vol I, p 273. London, 1975

135. Marliss EB, Murray FT, Nakhooda AF: The metabolic response to hypocaloric protein diets in obese man. J Clin Invest 62:468, 1978

136. Mason EH: The treatment of obesity. Can Med Assoc J 14:1052, 1924

137. Mathieson RA, Walberg JL, Gwazdauskas FC et al: The effect of varying carbohydrate content of a very low calorie diet on resting metabolic rate and thyroid hormones. Metabolism 35:394, 1986

138. McLean Baird I, Howard AN: A double-blind trial of mazindol using a very low calorie formula diet. Int J Obes 1:271, 1977

139. McLean Baird I, Parsons RL, Howard AN: Clinical and metabolic studies of chemically defined diets in the study of obesity. Metabolism 23:645, 1974

140. Metropolitan Life Insurance Company: 1983 Metropolitan Height and Weight Tables: Stat Bull Metropol Life Ins Co 64:2, 1984

141. Moyer CL, Holly RG, Atkinson RL: Effects of cardiac stress tests during very low calorie diets. Fed Proc 44:1502, 1985

142. Munro HN, Crim MC: The proteins and amino acids. In Goodhard RS, Shils ME (eds): Modern Nutrition in Health and Disease. Philadelphia, Lea & Febiger, 1980

143. Munro JF, Stolarek: VLCD: Future perspectives. Int J Obes 13(suppl 2):11, 1989

144. Nair KS, Woolf PD, Welle SL et al: Leucine, glucose, and energy metabolism after 3 days of fasting in healthy human subjects. Am J Clin Nutr 46:557, 1987

145. National Institutes of Health: Consensus Development Conference Statement: Health Implications of Obesity. Bethesda, Md, NIH, 1985

146. O'Brian JT, Bybee DE, Burman KD et al: Thyroid hormone homeostasis in states of relative caloric deprivation. Metabolism 29:721, 1980

147. O'dea K, Esler M, Leonard P et al: Noradrenaline turnover during under and overeating in normal weight subjects. Metabolism 31:896, 1982

148. Oddoye EA, Margen S: Nitrogen balance studies in humans: Long-term effect of high nitrogen intake on nitrogen accretion. J Nutr 109:363, 1979

149. Owen OE, Felig P, Morgan AP et al: Liver and kidney metabolism during prolonged starvation. J Clin Invest 48:574, 1969

150. Owen OE, Morgan AP, Kemp HG et al: Brain metabolism during fasting. J Clin Invest 46:1589, 1967

151. Palgi A, Read JL, Greenberg I et al: Multidisciplinary treatment of obesity with a protein-sparing modified fast: Results in 668 outpatients. Am J Public Health 75:1190, 1985

152. Patton ML, Amatruda JM, Biddle TL et al: Prevention of life-threatening cardiac arrhythmias associated with a modified fast by dietary supplementation with trace metals and fatty acids. Clin Res 29:663A, 1981

153. Perri MG, McAllister DA, Garge JJ et al: Effects

of four maintenance programs on the long term management of obesity. J Consult Clin Psychol 56:529, 1988

154. Phinney SD, Bistrian BR, Kosinski E et al: Normal cardiac rhythm observed during hypocaloric diets of varying carbohydrate content. Arch Intern Med 143:2258, 1983

155. Phinney SD, LaGrange BM, O'Connell M et al: Effects of aerobic exercise on energy expenditure and nitrogen balance during very low calorie dieting. Metabolism 37:758, 1988

156. Quaade F, Backer O, Stokholm KH et al: The Copenhagen PLAFA project: A randomized trial of gastroplasty versus very-low-calorie diet in the treatment of severe obesity (preliminary results). Int J Obes 5:257, 1981

157. Ramhamadany E, Dasgupta P, Brigden G et al: Cardiovascular changes in obese subjects on very low calorie diet. Int J Obes 13(suppl 2):95, 1989

158. Ravussin E, Burnand B, Schutz Y et al: Energy expenditure before and during energy restriction in obese patients. Am J Clin Nutr 41:753, 1985

159. Ravussin E, Burnand B, Schutz Y et al: Twenty-four hour energy expenditure and resting metabolic rate in obese, moderately obese, and control subjects. Am J Clin Nutr 35:566, 1982

160. Rosen JC, Hunt DA, Sims EAH et al: Comparison of carbohydrate-containing and carbohydrate-restricted hypocaloric diets in the treatment of obesity: Effects on appetite and mood. Am J Clin Nutr 36:463, 1982

161. Rozen R, Abraham G, Falcon R et al: Effect of physiological dose of T_3 on obese subjects during a protein sparing diet. Int J Obes 10:303, 1986

162. Rudman D, Millikan WJ, Richardson TJ et al: Elemental balances during intravenous hyperalimentation of underweight adult subjects. J Clin Invest 55:94, 1975

163. Runcie J, Thomson TJ: Prolonged starvation: Dangerous procedure? Br Med J 3:432, 1970

164. Sato K, Robbins J: Thyroid hormone metabolism in primary cultured rat hepatocytes: Effects of glucose, glucagon and insulin. J Clin Invest 68:475, 1970

165. Saudek CD, Boulter PR, Arky AR: The natriuretic effect of glucagon and its role in starvation. J Clin Endocrinol Metab 36:761, 1973

166. Scheen AJ, Luyckx AS, Fossion A et al: Effect of protein-supplemented fasting on the fuel-hormone response to prolonged exercise in obese subjects. Int J Obes 7:327, 1983

167. Schlierf G, Schellenberg B, Stiehl A et al: Biliary cholesterol saturation and weight reduction: Effects of fasting and low calorie diet. Digestion 21:44, 1981

168. Schouten JA, Van Gent CM, Popp-Snijders C et

al: The influence of low calorie (240 kcal/day) protein-carbohydrate diet on serum lipid levels in obese subjects. Int J Obes 5:333, 1981

169. Schroeder LA: Weight control: Fad, fact, or fiction? Popular approaches to weight control. Nutr Int 2:281, 1986

170. Scrimshaw NS: Through a glass darkly: Discerning the practical implications of human dietary protein-energy inter-relationships. Nutr Rev 35:321, 1977

171. Serog P, Apfelbaum M, Ourtissier N et al: Effects of slimming and composition of diets on VO_2 and thyroid hormones in healthy subjects. Am J Clin Nutr 35:24, 1982

172. Shalom FM, Santora LJ, Iseri LT et al: Electrocardiogram observations before, during and after rapid weight loss in morbidly obese subjects (abstr). Circulation 64:81, 1981

173. Shapiro H, Weinkove C, Coxon A et al: Three year hospital experience with control of major obesity by VLCD in medically compromised individuals. Int J Obes 13(suppl 2):123, 1989

174. Shetty PS, Jung RT, James WPT: Effect of catecholamine replacement with levodopa on the metabolic response to semi-starvation. Lancet 1:773, 1979

175. Silverstone jT, Stark JE, Buckle RM: Hunger during total starvation. Lancet 1:343, 1966

176. Sims EAH, Danforth E Jr, Horton ES: Endocrine and metabolic effects of experimental obesity in man. Recent Prog Horm Res 29:457, 1973

177. Singer DL: Twenty-four hour Holter monitoring fails to diagnose significant cardiac arrhythmias in six patients on prolonged protein-sparing modified fast. Obes Metab 1:159, 1981

178. Sours HE, Frattali VP, Brand CD et al: Sudden death associated with very low calorie weight reduction regimens. Am J Clin Nutr 34:453, 1981

179. Spaulding SW, Chopra IJ, Sherwin RS et al: Effect of caloric restriction and dietary composition on serum T_3 and reverse T_3 in man. J Clin Endocrinol Metab 42:197, 1976

180. Stock MJ: Effects of low (LCD) and very low (VLCD) energy diets on metabolic rate and body composition in obese (fa/fa) zucker rats. Int J Obes 13(suppl 2):61, 1989

181. Stokholm KH, Astrup A, Breum L et al: Cardiac stroke work output during a short-term very-low-calorie diet, noradrenaline-induced thermogenesis and T_3 supplementation. Int J Obes 13(suppl 2):151, 1989

182. Stunkard AJ: Conservative treatments for obesity. Am J Clin Nutr 45:1142, 1987

183. Stunkard AJ, McLaren-Hume M: The results of treatment for obesity. Arch Intern Med 103:79, 1959

184. Stunkard AJ, Rush J: Dieting and depression reexamined: A critical review of reports of untoward responses during weight reduction for obesity. Ann Intern Med 81:526, 1974

185. Suratt PM, McTier RF, Findley LJ et al: Changes in breathing and the pharynx after weight loss in obstructive sleep apnea. Chest 92:631, 1987

186. Taylor HL, Keys A: Adaptation to caloric restriction. Science 112:215, 1950

187. Thompson PD, Jeffery RW, Wing RR et al: Unexpected decrease in plasma high density lipoprotein cholesterol with weight loss. Am J Clin Nutr 32:2016, 1979

188. Thomson TJ, Runcie J, Miller V: Treatment of obesity by total fasting for up to 249 days. Lancet 2:992, 1966

189. Tischler ME: Hormonal regulation of protein degradation in skeletal and cardiac muscle. Life Sci 28:2569, 1981

190. Tuck ML, Sowers J, Dornfeld L et al: The effect of weight reduction on blood pressure, plasma renin activity, and plasma aldosterone levels in obese patients. N Engl J Med 304:930, 1981

191. Vagenakis AF, Burger A, Portnay GI et al: Diversion of peripheral thyroxine metabolism from activating to inactivating pathways during complete fasting. J Clin Endocrinol Metab 41:191, 1981

192. Van Dale: Diet and exercise in the treatment of obesity, thesis, University of Limburg, 1984

193. VanItallie TB: Liquid protein mayhem (editorial). JAMA 240:140, 1978

194. Van Itallie TB, Yang MU: Cardiac dysfunction in obese dieters: A potentially lethal complication of rapid, massive weight loss. Am J Clin Nutr 39:695, 1984

195. Van Gaal LF, De Leeuw IH: Short and long-term effects of protein-sparing very-low-calorie diets. In Berry EM, Blondheim SH, Eliahou HE et al (eds): Recent Advances of Obesity Research, vol V, p 347. London, John Libbey, 1987

196. Van Gaal L, Vansant G, Van Acker K et al: Effect of a long term very low calorie diet on glucose/insulin metabolism in obesity: Influence of fat distribution on hepatic insulin extraction. Int J Obes 13(suppl 2):47, 1989

197. Van Gaal LF, Snyders D, De Leeuw IH et al: Anthropometric and calorimetric evidence for the protein sparing effects of a new protein supplemented low calorie preparation. Am J Clin Nutr 41:540, 1985

198. Vertes V: In Blackburn GL, Bray GA (eds): Management of Obesity by Severe Caloric Restriction, p 243. Littleton, Mass, PSG Publishing, 1985

199. Vertes V, Genuth SM, Hazelton IM: Supplemented fasting as a large scale outpatient program. JAMA 238:2151, 1977

200. Vertes V, Hazelton IM: The massively obese hypertensive patient: An analysis of blood pressure response to weight reduction with supplemented fasting. Angiology 30:793, 1979

201. Visser TJ, Lamberts SWJ, Wilson JHP et al: Serum thyroid hormone concentrations during prolonged reduction of dietary intake. Metabolism 27:405, 1979

202. Wadden TA, Sternberg JA, Letizia KA et al: Treatment of obesity by very-low-calorie diet, behavior therapy, and their combination: A five-year perspective. Int J Obes 13 (suppl 2):39, 1989

203. Wadden TA, Stunkard AJ: Controlled trial of very-low-calorie diet, behavior therapy, and their combination in the treatment of obesity. J Consult Clin Psychol 54:482, 1986

204. Wadden TA, Stunkard AJ: Three-year follow-up of the treatment of obesity by very low calorie diet, behavior therapy, and their combination. J Consult Clin Psychol 54:925, 1988

205. Wadden TA, Stunkard AJ, Brownell KD et al: A comparison of two very-low-calorie diets: Protein-sparing modified fast versus protein-formula liquid diet. Am J Clin Nutr 41:533, 1985

206. Wadden TA, Stunkard AJ, Brownell KD: Very low calorie diets: Their efficacy, safety, and future. Ann Intern Med 99:675, 1983

207. Wadden TA, Stunkard AJ, Day SC et al: Less food, less hunger: Reports of appetite and symptoms in a controlled study of a protein-sparing modified fast. Int J Obes 11:239, 1987

208. Wadden TA, Van Itallie TB, Blackburn GL: Responsible and irresponsible use of very-low calorie diets in the treatment of obesity. JAMA 263:83, 1990

209. Waggonner CR, Tang AB, Davis PA et al: Adipose cholesterol mobilization contributes to hypercholesterolemia with very low calorie diets. Presented at the sixth annual meeting of the NASSO, 1989, p A82

210. Wallace WM: Nitrogen content of the body and its relation to retention and loss of nitrogen. Fed Proc 18:1125, 1959

211. Waterlow JC: Metabolic adaptation to low intakes of energy and protein. Annu Rev Nutr 6:495, 1986

212. Webster JD, Hesp R, Garrow JS: The composition of excess weight in obese women estimated by body density, total body water and total body potassium. Hum Nutr Clin Nutr 38:299, 1984

213. Wechsler JG, Hutt V, Wenzel H et al: Lipids and lipoproteins during a very-low-calorie diet. Int J Obes 5:325, 1981

214. Welborn T, Wahlquist ML: Scientific Conference on "Very Low Calorie Diets." Med J Aust 151:457, 1989

215. Welle SL, Amatruda JM, Forbes GB et al: Resting metabolic rates of obese women after rapid weight loss. J Clin Endocrinol Metab 59:41, 1984

216. Welle SL, Campbell RG: Decrease in resting metabolic rate during rapid weight loss is reversed by low dose thyroid hormone treatment. Metabolism 35:289, 1986

217. Williams HH: Amino acid requirements. J Am Diet Assoc 35:929, 1959

218. Wilson JH, Lamberts SWJ: Nitrogen balance in obese patients receiving a very low caloric liquid formula diet. Am J Clin Nutr 32:1612, 1979

219. Wing RR, Jeffery RW: Outpatient treatments of obesity: A comparison of methodology and clinical results. Int J Obes 3:261, 1979

220. Yalow RS, Glick SM, Roth J et al: Plasma insulin and growth hormone levels in obesity and diabetes. In Brodoff BN (Conf Chair): Adipose Tissue Metabolism and Obesity. Ann NY Acad Sci 131:632, 1965

221. Yang M-U, Barbosa-Saldivar JL, Pi-Sunyer FX et al: Metabolic effects of substituting carbohydrate for protein in a low-calorie diet: A prolonged study in obese outpatients. Int J Obes 5:231, 1981

222. Yang M-U, Van Itallie TB: Composition of weight lost during short-term weight reduction: Metabolic responses of obese subjects to starvation and low-calorie ketogenic and nonketogenic diets. J Clin Invest 58:722, 1976

223. Yang M-U, Van Itallie TB: Variability in body protein loss during protracted, severe caloric restriction: Role of triiodothyronine and other possible determinants. Am J Clin Nutr 40:611, 1984

224. Young VR, Scrimshaw NS, Bier DM: Whole body protein and amino acid metabolism: Relation to protein quality evaluation in human nutrition. J Agric Food Chem 29:440, 1981

225. Zollner N, Keller C: A 300 kcal (1.2 MJ) diet using conventional food. Int J Obes 5:217, 1981

226. Zwiauer K, Schmidinger H, Klicpera M et al: 24 hours electrocardiographic monitoring in obese children and adolescents during a 3 week low calorie diet (500 kcal). Int J Obes 13(suppl 2):101, 1989

227. Apfelbaum M, Bostsarron J, Brigant L et al: La composition du poids perdu au cours de la diete hydrique: Effets de la supplementation protidique. Gastroenterologia 108:121, 1967

228. Genuth S: Supplemented fasting in the treatment of obesity and diabetes. Am J Clin Nutr 32:2579, 1979

229. Henry RR, Weist-Kent TA, Scheaffer L et al: Metabolic consequences of very-low-calorie diet therapy in obese non-insulin-dependent diabetic and nondiabetic subjects. Diabetes 35:155, 1986

230. Van Der Heyden JTM, Docter JR, Van Torr H et al: Effect of caloric deprivation on thyroid hormone tissue uptake and generation of low T_3 syndrome. Am J Physiol 251:E156, 1986

231. Vasquez JA, Morse EL, Adibi SA: Effect of dietary fat, carbohydrate, and protein on branched-chain amino acid catabolism during caloric restriction. J Clin Invest 76:737, 1985

232. Winterer J, Bistrian BR, Bilmazes C et al: Whole body protein turnover, studied with ^{15}N-glycine, and muscle protein breakdown in mildly obese subjects during a protein-sparing diet and a brief total fast. Metabolism 29:575, 1980

233. Wynn V, Abraham RR, Densem JW: Method for estimating rate of fat loss during treatment of obesity by calorie restriction. Lancet 1:482, 1985

234. Life Sciences Research Office: Research Needs in Management of Obesity by Severe Caloric Restriction. Washington, DC, Federation of American Societies for Experimental Biology. Contract No. FDA 223-75-2090, 1979

235. Beeson V, Ray C, Coxon A et al: The myth of the yo-yo: Consistent rate of weight loss with successive dieting by VLCD. Int J Obes 13(suppl 2):135, 1989

CHAPTER 60

Physical Exercise in the Treatment of Obesity

PER BJÖRNTORP

Well-trained athletes in endurance sports are lean. It might be argued that this is an effect of selection, that lean subjects become better endurance athletes simply because they have less weight to carry. On the other hand, athletes not in training do show increases in body weight and skin-fold thickness.[1] Such observations indicate that regular exercise is followed by a decrease in body fat.

It does not necessarily follow that exercise is an important ingredient in the treatment of obesity. For example, the mechanism leading to a diminution of body fat in athletes might not operate in all obese subjects. In addition, the intensity and duration of exercise needed to lose weight might not be feasible for therapeutic purposes in obese subjects. These alternate possibilities are partially correct, as will be discussed later. It is also clear, however, that in most cases physical exercise is a useful adjunct to other obesity treatment. This field has been reviewed previously with this conclusion.[2-6]

The quantitative aspects of exercise treatment in relation to dietary treatment are often not realized. The principle of obesity treatment is to create a negative energy balance. By diet, a daily energy deficiency of, for example, 1500 kcal is easily achieved by decreasing the daily energy intake from 2500 to 1000 kcal. A feasible exercise program, on the other hand, produces a much smaller energy loss, perhaps in the order of a few hundred kcal/day. Clearly, exercise is much less

effective in obesity treatment than diet. Although not definitely proved, and probably varying among subjects, some unknown signals likely balance energy intake during exercise periods, adding to the effectiveness of exercise in obesity treatment. This possibility will also be examined in the discussion.

The main question, then, seems to be settled: in general, exercise programs are beneficial in the treatment of obesity. But questions of considerable importance remain. Who are the obese subjects who do not seem to benefit from exercise as much as obese people do in general? What other effects does exercise have in addition to creating a negative energy balance? How can recidivism in exercise programs for obese subjects be reduced? These questions will be addressed in the following discussion.

WHO ARE THE OBESE SUBJECTS WHO DO NOT LOSE BODY FAT IN EXERCISE PROGRAMS?

In the early 1970s we observed marked differences in decreases in body fat among different groups of people following similar exercise programs. The training program was standardized to incorporate an equal number of exercise sessions per week at similar duration and at the same relative intensity in relation to the maximal working capacity of each subject. Subjects were instructed not to deliberately decrease their energy intake, in an attempt to exclude effects other than those of exercise. This was an uncontrolled trial, but long-term exercise studies under conditions of fully controlled energy intake are not feasible in large groups. Such studies have been performed in smaller groups but are marred by a separate problem: the limited representation of the studied group restricts the application of results to the obese population in general. Extrapolation of results is easier in the design where only exercise sessions are fully controlled.

Using this approach, we noted that in general, men who had suffered a myocardial infarction and who were in such a training program on average and on an individual basis lost significant masses of body fat over a period of some months.[7] Severely obese women, by contrast, lost body fat much more slowly or not at all.[8] There are two obvious differences between these two groups, sex and degree of obesity. Recent studies using the same design have again shown a probable sex difference among obese subjects, with men losing body fat more readily than women.[9] A report suggests that this difference exists among nonobese subjects as well,[10] but it might be a question of what body fat mass should be considered normal in men and women. Women with the same body fat mass as men are leaner, because women constitutionally have more adipose tissue than men.[11] Such leaner women may have more difficulty losing weight than men with the same body fat mass. When losses are compared at body fat masses more representative for the sex in question, the difference is not that marked.[12]

Obese women thus seem to lose less body fat during exercise than equally obese men.[9] Differences among women have also been noted. Women with an abdominal fat distribution seem to lose body weight and body fat more easily during exercise programs than women with a femoral-gluteal distribution of body fat.[9] This information in aggregate suggests that men lose body fat more easily during exercise programs than women do, particularly women with gluteal-femoral obesity, who seem to be least successful.

The explanation for this apparent difference is not known. One obvious reason might be a difference in exercise intensity in absolute terms. Men have a higher maximal working capacity and may therefore lose more fat just by performing more exercise during a training program. However, obese women, who often have an enlargement of lean body mass, may have as great a working capacity as nonobese men.[9] Furthermore, the rather pronounced differences in body fat loss are not explainable by fairly limited differences in the quantity of work performed. For the same reason, differences in exercise habits in intervals between regularly scheduled exercise sessions would have to be of such magnitude that they should have been readily detectable. Although these alternatives cannot be definitely excluded, because they were not measured, they are rather unlikely causes of the differences noted.

Other possibilities appear more plausible. The thermogenic response to exercise before, during, or after exercise might have been different. Further, the effects of exercise on food intake might vary characteristically between these groups. Some observations support the latter possibility. For example, there are interesting differences in food intake between the sexes during exercise experiments in rats. Female rats seem to "defend" their body fat stores by compensatory eating during exercise, while male rats do not.[13] Similarly, nonobese young women also seem to consume relatively more energy during exercise training programs than men, apparently "protecting" their adipose stores, possibly with a regional preference.[14] It may not be irrelevant that the same phenomenon seems to occur during another means of creating a negative energy balance, namely energy intake restriction.[15] Although only suggestive evidence is available, the regulation of energy intake in relation to sex and perhaps in relation to different regional adipose depots seems to be an interesting area for further research. This would have practical implications for therapy by defining groups of responders and nonresponders to exercise treatment in terms of the efficacy of body fat loss. Exercise is not an easy way to create a negative energy balance, and if the prognosis for treatment is not favorable, other means of weight loss should be given higher priority.

WHAT ARE THE BENEFICIAL EFFECTS OF EXERCISE?

Obesity is followed by a number of perturbations in energy balance in terms of hyperinsulinemia, hyperlipidemia, and glucose intolerance or overt diabetes. Hypertension has recently been included among these metabolic aberrations as it is suspected to be associated with hyperinsulinemia.[16,17] By analogy, weight loss should be followed by improvements in these variables. Indeed, body weight and body fat loss in exercise programs is associated with a more favorable metabolic profile. Exercise by itself, without a decrease in body fat, is also followed by pronounced metabolic improvements. We observed that insulin concentrations during fasting and after a glucose load were dramatically lowered by exercise in obese subjects who did not decrease their body fat.[8] In later studies other variables, including blood lipids and blood pressure, were also decreased by exercise without a concomitant decrease in body fat.[2,3,5] These observations suggest effects of exercise itself, without a body weight or body fat decrease. Other work has shown that such phenomena might be temporary, lasting for only a day or two.[18] From a practical viewpoint, this means that exercise therapy needs regular, repeated "dosing," analogous to drug therapy for hypertension, diabetes, or hyperlipidemia.

What is the mechanism of this effect? The insulin resistance of obesity is at least partly localized to muscle tissue.[19] It is also clear that exercise improves insulin sensitivity of muscle.[20] It seems reasonable to conclude that insulin resistance is improved by exercise through an effect exerted on the muscle. There is considerable evidence that insulin resistance is associated with several of the other aberrations of metabolism as well as hypertension in obesity.[3,5] Improved insulin resistance, by making muscle tissue more insulin sensitive by exercise, might therefore be expected to result in a more favorable metabolic profile and may decrease the propensity for hypertension. This has also been observed (for reviews, see references 3, 5, and 6).

In the treatment of obesity, these effects of exercise may be considered at least equally as important as a decrease in body weight. If body fat loss also results from the exercise program, the beneficial effects are even more pronounced.

PROBLEMS OF FEASIBILITY WITH EXERCISE PROGRAMS

Exercise is considered by many to be inconvenient, time-consuming, and painful. Several studies have shown a considerable dropout rate from exercise programs. For example, many men participating in an exercise program after sustaining a myocardial infarction dropped out; only a minority remained after a few years, despite considerable psychological, functional, and metabolic improvements.[21] Similarly, in men with decreased glucose tolerance, almost none remained in an exercise program after a year.[22]

The reasons for the high recidivism in exercise programs are not known. Some problems have been identified. In the study that enrolled men who had sustained a myocardial infarction, the exercise sessions took place in a gymnasium at the hospital where the men had been admitted for treatment of the myocardial infarction. Although they felt that they improved physically and became stronger, the milieu reminded them of their disease, and this was an important reason for not wanting to continue. In several other studies time is reported to be a severely limiting factor, and therefore exercise programs far from home might not be feasible. Practical problems with availability of equipment, running paths, or tracks play a role. Weather and light conditions in northern parts of Europe and the United States might preclude outdoor activities for large parts of the year. In short, various aspects of the milieu contribute to subjects' inability or reluctance to continue an exercise program.

The groups most in need of exercise to prevent or cure obesity are middle-aged subjects. Work with exercise teaching or programs has shown that the difficulties might be different for middle-aged men and women. Obese, middle-aged women are more difficult to motivate than men. Both sexes may have little time for exercise because of work and other duties. In practice, an exercise program expected to produce useful weight loss entails three one-hour sessions a week. For each session, at least another hour is spent in transport, preparations, showering, and so forth. It may be difficult to find time and motivation for exercise during the work week. Trials that include physical exercise during the working hours in sedentary workers may be more promising because they may circumvent the problems of time and motivation.

Medical problems encountered during exercise programs are of varying significance. Vascular catastrophes such as cardiac arrest or myocardial infarction occur but are not frequent.[23] Their occurrence can be minimized with appropriate medical examinations before a regular exercise program is initiated. Other types of complications are less serious but much more frequent. Locomotor trauma often is not serious but may prevent further exercising for some time, and may prevent the subject from performing adequately at work. Locomotor trauma can be minimized with a warm-up period, the use of appropriate shoes and equipment, and so forth.

In practice, the usual exercise activities such as jogging, bicycling, and ballgames of various sorts are not feasible above a certain body weight. The risk of joint and back damage is much greater in such subjects. Swimming might be an alternative to be tried.

References

1. Parizkova J: Impact of age, diet, and exercise on man's body composition. Ann NY Acad Sci 110:661, 1963
2. Björntorp P: Interrelation of physical activity and nutrition on obesity. In White PL, Mondeika T (eds): Diet and Exercise: Synergism in Health Maintenance, p 91. Chicago, American Medical Association, 1981
3. Björntorp P: The effects of exercise on plasma insulin. Int J Sports Med 2:125, 1981
4. Oscai L: The role of exercise in weight control. Exerc Sport Sci Rev 1:103, 1973
5. Björntorp P: Physiological and clinical aspects of exercise in obese persons. Exerc Sports Sci Rev 11:159, 1983
6. Krotkiewski M: Physical training in obesity with varying degree of glucose intolerance. J Obes Weight Regul 4:179, 1985
7. Björntorp P, Berchtold P, Grimby G et al: Effects of physical training on glucose tolerance, plasma insulin and lipids and on body composition in men after myocardial infarction. Acta Med Scand 192:439, 1972
8. Björntorp P, de Jounge K, Sjöström L et al: The effect of physical training on insulin production in obesity. Metabolism 19:631, 1970
9. Krotkiewski M, Björntorp P: Muscle tissue in obesity with different distribution of adipose tissue: Effects of physical training. Int J Obes 10:331, 1986
10. Despres JP, Bouchard C, Savard R et al: The effect of a 20 week endurance training program on adipose tissue morphology and lipolysis in men and women. Metabolism 33:235, 1984
11. Sjöström L, Smith U, Krotkiewski M et al: Cellularity in different regions of adipose tissue in young men and women. Metabolism 21:1143, 1972
12. Andersson BU, Rebuffé-Scrive M, Terning K et al: The effects of exercise training on body composition and metabolism in men and women. Int J Obesity 15:75, 1991
13. Applegate E, Upton D, Stern J: Food intake, body composition and blood lipids following treadmill exercise in male and female rats. Physiol Behav 28:917, 1982
14. Tremblay A, Després JP, Leblanc C et al: Sex dimorphism in fat loss in response to exercise training. J Obes Weight Regul 3:193, 1984
15. Andersson B, Seidell J, Terning K et al: Influence on menopause on dietary treatment of obesity. J Intern Med 227:173, 1990
16. Björntorp P: Hypertension in obesity. Acta Med Scand 211:241, 1982
17. Reaven GR, Hoffman BB: A role for insulin in the aetiology of hypertension? Lancet 2:435, 1987
18. Fahlén M, Stenberg J, Björntorp P: Insulin secretion in obesity after exercise. Diabetologia 8:141, 1972
19. Bogardus C, Lillioja S, Mott DM et al: Relationships between obesity and maximal insulin-stimulated glucose uptake in vivo and in vitro in Pima Indians. J Clin Invest 73:800, 1989
20. Devlin JT, Horton SE: Effects of prior high-intensity exercise on glucose metabolism in normal and insulin-resistant men. Diabetes 34:973, 1985
21. Wilhelmsen L, Sanne H, Elmfeldt D et al: A controlled study of physical training after myocardial infarction. Prev Med 4:491, 1975
22. Skarfors ET, Wegener TA, Lithell H et al: Physical training as treatment for type 2 (non-insulin-dependent) diabetes in elderly men: A feasibility study over 2 years. Diabetologia 30:930, 1987
23. Haskell WL: Sudden cardiac death during vigorous exercise. Int J Sports Med 3:45, 1982

CHAPTER 61

Factors Determining the Long-Term Outcome of Obesity Treatment

STEPHAN RÖSSNER

TREATMENT PRINCIPLES

Whereas most studies on weight loss generally have concerned short-term effects, there is an increasing awareness that a long-term perspective is necessary if obese subjects are to lose weight and to maintain a lower body weight. The change in attitude was reflected in the criteria recently suggested for the presentation of weight loss programs in scientific literature.[1] This review deals with long-term treatment programs for individuals with moderate overweight and obesity. Severe obesity, defined as a body mass index (BMI) in excess of 40 kg/m^2 (corresponding to obesity Grade III in Garrow's terminology[2]), is comparatively rare but carries severe risks. Thus, in grade III obesity, radical treatments such as surgery may be justified. For most patients, however, the long-term treatment of overweight and obesity entails a combination of the standard nonsurgical treatment modalities that are available today.

There is general agreement that energy restriction will always be a cornerstone in all types of treatment for obesity. Whereas the basic principle—to induce a negative energy balance by reducing energy intake—is extremely simple conceptually, a large number of different dietary programs have been developed over the years, from total starvation to very low calorie diets to extremely complex diets, including (or excluding) components supposed to affect weight loss.

Although a number of studies have demonstrated that various types of food items may have different effects on diet-induced thermogenesis[3] there is still doubt whether the composition of the diets will prove to be of critical importance for long-term treatment outcome as long as the diet is "safe, sound and practical."[4] The treatment of overweight will follow a standard pattern for a great majority of individuals. After a phase of enthusiasm, when the obese patient is willing to submit to almost any type of program, most subjects drop out of treatment programs. The effect of expectation, known as the Hawthorne effect, will operate in favor of any weight loss program for some time.[5] Also, the placebo effect has been shown to be important in weight reduction.[2]

There is general agreement that behavior modification must be part of the treatment program if long-term effects are to be achieved. The exceptional early results reported by Stuart in 1967[6] using behavior modification have never been surpassed, but as a tool to be used in combination with others, behavior modification has become a standard component of most balanced long-term programs.

The integration of different treatment strategies has led to difficulties in determining the efficacy of the individual components. In the past, most reports on the effects of therapeutical intervention were published by specialists in discrete areas of treatment. In the literature on behavior modification, for example, the results presented basically concerned that treatment modality. In practice, it is reasonable to believe that most obese patients will benefit from long-term treatment with combined programs, even programs that are changed from time to time. The low self-esteem that follows after a relapse makes it less attractive to revert to the identical program once again.

COMPOUND TREATMENT PROGRAMS

Even minor program modifications may be seen by patients as a new tool in the treatment of obesity. It is quite possible that a patient may derive most benefit from a long-term program that includes the following components, for example: initial behavior modification with dietary advice and exercise, a period of waist cord maintenance treatment, intermittent use of dietary fiber preparation to prevent loss of control, a short and controlled treatment program with an anorexic drug during a problem phase, and so forth. Although such a combined approach is logical from a clinical point of view, it is impossible to segment and evaluate the contribution of each component. Indeed, there has been little effort to design and evaluate complex treatment programs of this type.

Table 61-1 describes the long-term outcome of four different review series of weight loss programs, published in the last ten years. The reviews show a change in treatment emphasis in that decade. The reviews concentrate on basic long-term nonsurgical treatment methods. Each summarizes findings from a number of background studies available at the time of review.

TABLE 61-1

Long-Term Outpatient Treatment of Obesity: A Comparison of Strategies in Four Reviews

Component	Wing and Jeffery, 1979[8]	Weinsier et al, 1984[4]	Bennett, 1987[9]	AMA Council on Scientific Affairs, 1988[10]
Diet	Results in greatest weight loss	Diet should improve health, not only lead to weight loss; any diet if, safe, sound, and practical, can be used	Long-term effect of diets minimal, micronutrients or dietary composition more promising	Mainstay of weight loss is restriction of energy intake
Behavior modification	Best maintenance results	Emphasis shifted from weight loss induction to weight loss maintenance	Doubtful long-term results	Long-term results not impressive; combination with diet and exercise suggested
Exercise	Difficult to evaluate	May accelerate fat loss		Exercise alone may decrease weight without alterations in diet
Long-term follow-up	>6 months recommended	Posttreatment follow-up, on stabilization at annual evaluation	Follow-up >3 years	Successful outcome: weight maintenance at least one year following treatment

The scope of these four reviews is not identical, as they were published under varying conditions. Also notable in the table is the scant attention paid to drug treatment as an element of long-term obesity therapy. Since studies concerning anorectic drugs generally have been carried out over shorter periods of time, few comprehensive studies are available demonstrating the value of anorectic drugs in a comprehensive long-term treatment program.[7]

Diet is clearly the backbone of any long-term treatment program, but interpretation of the results achieved with diet varies. Wing and Jeffery[8] in 1979 found that dietary intervention resulted in the greatest weight loss. Weinsier et al[4] in 1984 regarded the diet in obesity treatment as not only a factor leading to weight loss but also as a tool to promote health. Bennet[9] in 1987 was much more pessimistic, expressing doubt that hypocaloric diets would be helpful in the long term. He advocated an emphasis on micronutrients or dietary composition as targets for future research.

Whereas the studies reviewed by Wing and Jeffery support the concept that behavior modification will lead to the best maintenance results, Bennet was not impressed by these long-term results eight years later, and the Council of Scientific Affairs of the American Medical Association in 1988[10] indicated that behavioral modification on its own had not led to impressive long-term results but should be combined with dietary advice and exercise as well.

The definition of a long-term treatment program has also varied over the years. Whereas Wing and Jeffery suggested a long-term follow-up of more than six months, the AMA's Council on Scientific Affairs defined successful weight loss as maintenance of weight loss for at least one year following initial treatment. Bennet required at least a three-year follow-up. Weinsier et al suggested that once body weight had stabilized at a lower level, an evaluation should be carried out annually.

SEX DIFFERENCES

In most studies on long-term effects meeting reasonable standards with regard to program de-scription, attrition analysis, and follow-up time, women have constituted the main proportion of participants. It is generally assumed that 80% to 90% of participants in weight reducing clubs are women.[2,8] In the vast majority of women the excess body fat is in the thighs and buttocks. This gynoid type of obesity is not associated with cardiovascular complications and increased risk for cancer to the extent that has been described in abdominal obesity.[11] It thus seems clear that a great proportion of those who wish to lose weight may not be at high risk for severe complications of their increased body weight. Although overweight women may understandably be unhappy with their situation, it seems that gynoid obesity should mainly increase the risk for orthopedic problems of the weight-bearing joints and psychological problems. Krotkiewski's studies demonstrated that weight loss after six months correlates positively with a reduction in waist-hip circumference ratio and that weight loss is easier to achieve in individuals with initially high waist-hip circumference ratios.[12]

These data do not indicate that overweight in women may be neglected. Rather they suggest that one reason for the unsatisfactory weight reduction results frequently reported is that serious treatment programs for men have not been developed.

Comparatively few studies of the results of weight loss programs for men have been reported in the literature. It is important that such a distinction be made, since it is likely that in an integrated treatment program for obesity, the program for males and females should be different in several respects.[9]

Attrition in Men and Women

Dropout rates are generally high in all types of long-term treatment programs for obesity. Although some individuals may leave the program when they have reached a target weight, this is unlikely to apply to the majority of dropouts.

Our studies in subjects with severe obesity, who were initially treated at a day care unit for six weeks and then monitored for at least four years, demonstrated that it is possible to keep most patients in the program.[13] The dropout rate in our study was about 30% after four years.

In a study by Björvell and Langius, this program, initially developed in a day care hospital unit for grossly obese patients, was evaluated in a primary health care setting in a less obese population.[14] Of the 558 overweight and obese patients recruited into the study, only 9% were men. In this program the dropout rate was only 24% after two years, and the men had achieved an average sustained weight loss of 4.8 kg. Early weight loss was an important predictor of subsequent success.

New strategies must be developed to improve the long-term results for obese men. It is possible that closer feedback concerning improvement in obesity-related risk factors, such as blood pressure reduction, serum lipid normalization, and declines in blood sugar levels, may improve adherence.

For many men the alternative to weight reduction may be drug treatment. Although it has been difficult to demonstrate that long-term treatment with nonpharmacologic tools such as weight reduction will be an acceptable alternative for conditions such as hypertension, it is possible that these results can be improved with better techniques. Today there is a clear trend in many educated men to avoid long-term drug therapy, and here weight reduction could be perceived as a realistic alternative to drugs.

We recently initiated a few pilot studies to develop weight reduction programs for men only.[15] Forty-nine men (mean initial BMI 37.2 kg/m²) re-ferred to our obesity unit because of obesity with medical complications were monitored over a one-year period. The program was a conventional combined weight-losing program consisting of a diet plan, behavior modification, exercise, and continuous feedback from the group leader, who monitored the men throughout the program. Despite efforts to facilitate participation, to find suitable hours for weigh-in sessions, and to give the men all reports on weight-associated complications that diminished with weight loss, 42% of the men left the program after one year, the median weight loss being 6 kg. There was a significant correlation between weight loss and session adherence ($r = .51$, $P < .01$). Often these men reported work-related problems as a cause for leaving the program. These findings prompted a modified program for men, where all efforts were made to facilitate adherence. The results were encouraging: In the next group of similar men, only 9% had left after 1 year, and weight loss was similar.

We further analyzed data provided by the Swedish Weight Watchers, who treated 204 overweight men, all working at a work site in southern Sweden. The weight program was provided free of charge by the employer, and efforts were made to motivate the men to participate.[15] Over an eight-week period the mean weight loss was 7.4 kg in those who adhered to the program (Fig. 61-1), but about 50% of the men dropped out even during this short period of time.

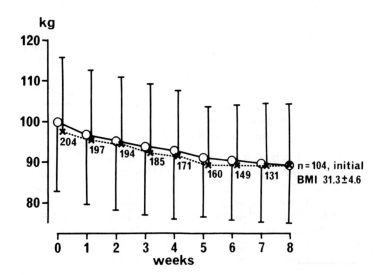

FIGURE 61-1

Weight loss (mean ± SD) in a Weight Watchers program for Swedish males. *Open circles* denote data from the 104 men who participated in the whole program, x denotes mean value for men coming to the respective weekly weigh-in session.

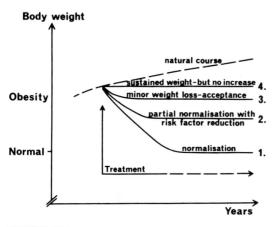

FIGURE 61-2

Indicators of success in long-term weight reduction programs.

INDICATORS OF SUCCESS OF OVERWEIGHT TREATMENT

Although the ultimate goal of treatment for overweight and obesity is to normalize body weight and keep it at the desired level, this does not happen very often in reality. It has become increasingly important to individualize treatment. A mean weight reduction of 5 ± 4 (SD) kg in a group of participants may not seem impressive but indicates that for some individuals the treatment clearly was of great value.[17] The participants that did not lose weight in such a program should have been shifted into other programs until they began to lose weight as well. Thus, mean weight loss values obtained in formalized trials may underestimate the true value of a treatment that is helpful to a subpopulation of the participants.[17,18]

The success of a certain treatment program could be defined in several ways (Fig. 61-2), any of which may be appropriate for a given patient:

1. Sustained weight normalization will occur (but only occasionally) as the result of treatment for obesity.

2. Maintenance of weight loss, particularly of a target weight, is often considered a very good result. Such a weight loss will affect obesity-related risk factors favorably, even if body weight is not completely normalized. A weight loss in

the range of 5 to 10 kg will significantly reduce elevated blood pressure in about two thirds of overweight men.[19] Likewise, blood sugar values will fall toward normal, serum triglyceride levels will drop, and high-density lipoprotein cholesterol levels will increase.[20,21]

3. Minor weight loss but increased ability to cope may be regarded as a very valuable result. In some cases a seemingly modest weight change may conceal the fact that adipose tissue has been lost and muscular mass gained as a result of increased physical activity, which also will affect carbohydrate and lipid metabolism favorably.[22] An unchanged body weight may also be the end result of fruitless weight-losing attempts, by which the patient may have learned to accept his or her situation and decided not to attempt further weight loss.

4. Sustained body weight at an obesity level may still represent an achievement. Few data are available on the longitudinal development of body weight over a long time, but cross-sectional data do emphasize that body weight increases considerably with age. Such data, from a large Swedish representative sample (Fig. 61-3), illustrate that particularly in women there is a pronounced increased in BMI with age.[23] A weight reduction program that results in a body weight kept constant in ensuing decades may actually represent a certain degree of success.

5. A lowered dropout rate from obesity treatment programs represents a different form of success. Since few studies have succeeded in keeping more than 20% to 30% of the original patients in the program after two or three years,[7] any program that can achieve lower dropout rates will be successful. Even if weight loss does not occur, the fact that obese individuals have stayed with the program means that one program can be developed further while retaining the core aspects that promoted adherence.

The effect of dietary fiber supplementation, known to be of some help in reducing body weight and maintaining that weight loss,[24,25] has been suggested to function in this way. The participants in some fiber programs have chosen to remain on fiber treatment instead of switching to other alternatives, not because of further weight loss but because fiber supplementation facilitated adherence to the basic program.

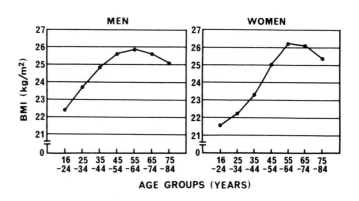

FIGURE 61-3

Body weight development in Sweden. Cross-sectional data obtained from the study on living conditions in Sweden (ULF) and corrected to represent recorded anthropometric values according to Kuskowska-Wolk and Rössner.[23]

RELAPSE PREVENTION

Relapse prevention has been considered a helpful tool in the treatment of addictive behaviors.[26] But in a comparison between such behaviors as smoking, alcoholism, and drug addiction, it is obvious that in long-term treatment of obesity, control rather than abstinence is the ultimate goal. Sternberg[27] pointed out that whereas abstinence is a discrete variable, "controlled eating" is continuous and difficult to measure. In contrast to other addictive behaviors, where definitions of compliance are simple, body weight may fluctuate spontaneously for physiological reasons. This may give the erroneous impression of inappropriate adherence or of overadjustment to a program and may thus result in inappropriate eating responses. Whereas maintenance refers to a weight loss that has been sustained over time, relapse indicates the subsequent regain of lost weight. This definition may be parsed more finely according to the amount of weight lost and the percentage regained.[27] Factors that seem to increase the likelihood of maintaining weight loss include:

1. A change in snacking behavior and eating-related activities.[28]
2. Close monitoring of weight and modification of food intake.[29]
3. Development of greater confidence in control abilities, adherence to a self-nominated diet, and increased frequency of exercise.[30]

Other strategies that have occasionally proved of value include booster sessions[31] and involvement of significant others, generally a spouse.[32]

A number of studies have focused on the role of cognition in the process of behavioral change to reduce weight and maintain weight loss. The belief of an individual about the value of his or her weight-losing efforts may be more important than the methods of weight loss and maintenance actually selected.[33] Likewise, Sjöberg and Persson reported that successful long-term weight losers have a high degree of self-efficacy in relation to their efforts to lose weight.[34]

Most standard weight reduction programs make little mention of the fact that a relapse may occur. Since it is overwhelmingly likely that relapses will occur during the weight loss and maintenance periods, the development of skills to cope with risk situations should be included in long-term treatment programs. In a weight relapse study two groups of obese individuals were restudied two months after a program that included relapse prevention techniques for one group but not for the other.[27] Although the mean weight loss immediately after initial treatment was similar in both groups, at later follow-up patients in the relapse prevention arm had lost 9% of their body weight, in comparison to 5% in the standard care group (P < .05). Similar results, causing cautious optimism, have been published by others.[35] There still is a need to further analyze the role of relapse prevention in the long-term treatment of obesity. It is not yet clear whether relapse prevention should be included in the initial behavioral treatment program or should be taught later in booster sessions.

Relapse prevention, which has shown to be of value in the treatment of several addictive behaviors, is more difficult to apply in the long-term

term results is individualization of treatment. Methods must still be developed and improved to enhance selection and to facilitate patient adjustment and relapse prevention.

Acknowledgment: Work was supported by the Swedish Council for Forestry and Agricultural Research, grant No. 867:88L.100:1.

TABLE 61-2

Strategies to Improve Long-Term Weight Control

Strategies	Problems
1. Develop selection and screening procedures	Method still to be developed
2. Ensure optimal timing for weight loss	Unwillingness to postpone treatment
3. Consider alternative treatment methods	Patient may be unwilling
4. Improve initial weight loss program	May not fit with patient expectations
5. Tailor initial treatment to patient needs	May not fit with patient expectations
6. Develop flexible long-term programs with multiple components tailored to needs	Evaluation difficult
7. Develop better relapse prevention techniques	Methods still to be developed

Strategies suggested from references 2, 9, 14, 18, 36, and author's experience.

treatment of obesity. Definitions are vague, and weight control is a much more complex situation than the either/or situation in other behaviors. However, relapse prevention holds some promise as an important tool in the development of a long-term treatment modality.

SUMMARY

Table 61-2 summarizes some possible strategies to enhance long-term weight control. The table is a condensed version of recommendations recently made by Brownell and Jeffery and suggestions summarized in this review.[36]

It is important not to embark on a treatment program unless the auspices are favorable (strategies 1 and 2 in Table 61-2). Strategies 3, 4, and 5 concern the need to improve the initial phase of the treatment period. Once this has been achieved, strategies 6 and 7 will address the overall long-term results.

Implementation of such methods is not without obstacles. Key to achieving optimal long-

References

1. Apfelbaum M, Björntorp B, Garrow J et al: Standards for reporting the results of treatment for obesity. Am J Clin Nutr 45:1035, 1987
2. Garrow JS: Treat Obesity Seriously: A Clinical Manual. London, Churchill Livingstone, 1981
3. Zed C, James WPT: Dietary thermogenesis in obesity: Response to carbohydrate and protein meals. The effect of beta-adrenergic blockade and semistarvation. Int J Obes 10:391, 1986
4. Weinsier RL, Wadden TA, Ritenbaugh C et al: Recommended therapeutic guidelines for professional weight control programs. Am J Clin Nutr 40:865, 1984
5. Mayo E: The Social Problems of an Industrial Civilization. London, Routledge, 1949
6. Stuart RB: Behavior control of overeating. Behav Res Ther 5:357, 1967
7. Brownell KD, Kramer FM: Behavioral management of obesity. Med Clin North Am 73:185, 1989
8. Wing RR, Jeffery RW: Outpatient treatment of obesity: A comparison of methodology and clinical results. Int J Obes 3:261, 1979
9. Bennett W: Dietary Treatment of Obesity. In Wurtman RJ, Wurtman JJ (eds): Human Obesity. Ann NY Acad Sci 499:250, 1987
10. Council on Scientific Affairs: Treatment of obesity in adults. JAMA 260:2547, 1988
11. Björntorp P, Smith N, Lönnroth P (eds): Health Implications of Regional Obesity. Acta Med Scand Suppl 723, 1988
12. Krotkiewski M: Can body fat patterning be changed? Acta Med Scand Suppl 723:213, 1988
13. Björvell H, Rössner S: Long term treatment of severe obesity: Four year follow-up of results of combined behavioral modification program. Br Med J 291:379, 1985
14. Björvell H, Langius A: Weight reduction in a primary health care setting—the results of a two-year follow-up.
15. Rössner S: Towards a new policy for obesity treatment. In Björntorp P, Rössner S (eds): Obesity in Europe. London, John Libbey, 1989
16. Andersson IL, Rössner S: A weight reduction pro-

gram for middle-aged overweight men (abstr 200). First European Congress on Obesity, Stockholm, 1988

17. Garrow JS: Criteria of success of weight reduction. In Björntorp P, Rössner S (eds): Obesity in Europe 88. London, John Libbey, 1989

18. Guy-Grand BJP: A new approach to the treatment of obesity. In Wurtman RJ, Wurtman JJ (eds): Human Obesity. Ann NY Acad Sci 499:313, 1987

19. Reisen E: Obesity and hypertension: Effect of weight reduction. In Robertson JIS (ed): Handbook of Hypertension 1, p 30. New York, Elsevier Science Publishers, 1983

20. Liu GC, Coulston AM, Lardinois CK et al: Moderate weight loss and sulfonylurea treatment of non-insulin-dependent diabetes mellitus. Arch Intern Med 145:665, 1985

21. Rössner S, Björvell H: Early and late effects of weight loss on lipoprotein metabolism in severe obesity. Atherosclerosis 64:125, 1987

22. Krotkiewski M, Björntorp P: Muscle tissue in obesity with different distribution of adipose tissue: Effects of physical training. Int J Obes 10:331, 1986

23. Kuskowska-Wolk A, Rössner S: Prevalence of obesity in Sweden. Int J Med 227:241, 1990

24. Krotkiewski M: Effect of guar-gum on body weight, hunger ratings and metabolism in obese subjects. Br J Nutr 52:97, 1984

25. Rössner S, van Zweigberg D, Öhlin A et al: Weight reduction with dietary fibre supplements: Results of two double-blind randomized studies. Acta Med Scand 222:83, 1987

26. Marlatt GA, Gordon JR (eds): Relapse Prevention: Maintenance Strategies in Addictive Behavior Change. New York, Guilford Press, 1985

27. Sternberg B: Relapse in weight control: Definitions, processes and strategies. In Marlett GA, Gordon JR (eds): Relapse Prevention. New York, Guilford Press, 1985

28. Leon G, Chamberlain K: Emotional arousal, eating patterns and body images as differential factors associated with varying success in maintaining a weight loss. J Consult Clin Psychol 40:474, 1973

29. Wing RR, Jeffery R: Successful losers: A descriptive analysis of the process of weight reduction. Obes Bariatr Med 7:190, 1978

30. Gormally J, Rardin D, Black S: Correlates of successful response to a behavioral weight control clinic. J Counsel Psychol 27:179, 1980

31. O'Leary KD, Wilson GT: Behavior Therapy: Application and Outcome. Englewood Cliffs, NJ, Prentice-Hall, 1975

32. Brownell KD, Heckerman C, Westlake R: The behavior control of obesity: A descriptive analysis of a large-scale program. J Clin Psychol 35:864, 1979

33. Bandura A: Self-efficacy: Toward a unifying theory of behavioral change. Psychol Rev 84:191, 1977

34. Sjöberg L, Persson L: A study of attempts by obese patients to regulate eating. Goteborg Psychol Rep 7:12, 1977

35. Perri MG, Shapiro RM, Ludwig WW et al: Maintenance strategies for the treatment of obesity: An evaluation of relapse prevention training and post treatment contact by mail and telephone. J Consult Clin Psychol 52:404, 1984

36. Brownell KD, Jeffery RW: Improving long-term weight loss: Pushing the limits of treatment. Behav Ther 18:353, 1987

CHAPTER 62

Anesthesia and Morbid Obesity

ROBERT W. VAUGHAN

Anesthesia management of the morbidly obese patient does not engender enthusiasm from most anesthesiologists. Such reluctance is not without good reason. Obese patients presenting for perioperative care can never be considered routine by anesthesiologists, even for minor surgery. Each severely obese patient requires major anesthetic preparation to optimize operative safety. Frustrations abound not only in the technical and mechanical aspects of care but also because of the presence of unique major organ system dysfunctions. Challenges to safe perioperative care are ever present, from anesthesia induction to postanesthetic care unit discharge. As examples of potential problems, one need only consider transport to and from the operating room, placement of intravenous and arterial catheters, problems in positioning massively obese patients on the operating table, and risks in the airway management of supine subjects. Rendering a morbidly obese patient unconscious and securing a guaranteed airway in the supine position can result in respiratory and cardiac arrest.[18]

Consequently, anesthetic management has been addressed specifically for this subset of the adult obese population. Approximately 40,000 patients undergo obesity operations in the United States each year. This chapter considers definitions of obesity, physiologic consequences of severe obesity, and the clinical implications of obesity in the operative population.

DEFINITION AND RISK ASSESSMENT

In industrialized countries, overweight adults are quite frequently encountered in clinical med-

icine. For example, 26% of civilian noninstitutionalized Americans ages 20 to 75 years are so classified by life insurance tables. Thirty-four million Americans have a body mass index (BMI; weight [kg]/height [m]^2) that would qualify them as 20% or more in excess of ideal body weight.[6] The prevalence of overweight increases with advancing age regardless of gender but is generally much higher among black than caucasian women. Also, women ages 25 to 55 years who live below the poverty line have a higher prevalence of overweight. Thus, both weight and poverty status become independent predictors of overweight in women. Moreover, the most important health risks of obesity—noninsulin-dependent-diabetes mellitus, hypertension, coronary artery disease, cancer, and sudden death—are curvilinearly related to overweight. Prevalences increase progressively and disproportionately with increasing weight (Fig. 62-1). At the weight level of 60% above American insurance standards of weight for height, there is a doubling of prevalences of all morbidity and mortality compared with prevalences in the general population.[8]

In addition, exponential increases in mortality and serious morbidity compared with normal-weight persons occur at weights 100 pounds (45.4 kg) or more above desirable weight for height. Such individuals are termed morbidly obese. They represent a specific subset of the total American obese population. Within the morbidly obese group there are two additional subgroups (Fig. 62-2). Subjects with normal levels of arterial carbon dioxide tension are referred to as having simple obesity, while those with hypo-

720

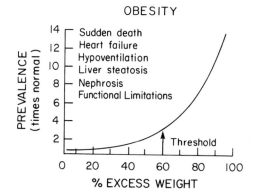

FIGURE 62-1

Health risks (prevalence times normal) as percent of
excess weight increases above ideal weight for
height. At 60% excess weight, mortality and morbidity become exponential. (Redrawn from Kral JG: Ann
Intern Med 103:1043, 1985, by permission.)

ventilation and hypercarbia at rest are referred to
as having obesity-hypoventilation syndrome.[11]
Fortunately, these latter pickwickian patients are
rare (5% to 10%) in the morbidly obese subset.

Severe obesity is causally related to a variety
of chronic diseases, including cerebral vascular
accidents, diabetes mellitus, cholelithiasis, hypercholesterolemia, cirrhosis, and cardiac disease. While all these diseases contribute to morbidity, the principal physiologic derangements
most important to consider in perioperative man-

agement are those of the cardiopulmonary system. The heart and lungs must function opti-
mally and in concert to facilitate oxygen
transport to tissues to avoid hypoxia and subsequent cardiovascular dysfunction.

DERANGED PHYSIOLOGY

Excess adipose tissue requires an increased
blood volume for adequate profusion. There is a
direct correlation between total blood volume
and body weight in excess of ideal weight, and
between cardiac output and total blood volume.[1]
The increased blood volume in obesity is distributed principally to fat depots. That "fat organ"
can weigh over 100 kg. The cardiac chambers
and pulmonary vasculature must accommodate
the entire augmented venous return. Pulmonary
blood volume increases in obesity in proportion
to the increase in total blood volume.[7] The volume of blood distending the left and right ventricles is also increased in proportion to the increase in total blood volume. Both ventricles are
distended by an increased blood volume at dias-
tole. Paul et al have shown that the average resting left ventricular end-diastolic pressure lies at
the upper limits of normal in severely obese
patients.[10]

The cardiovascular consequences of obesity
are best considered in terms of the effects on the
left and right sides of the heart. Over time, such
volume and pressure work loads produce biven-

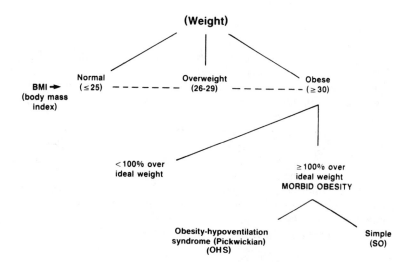

FIGURE 62-2

American population morphology in terms of body mass index (kg/m²).

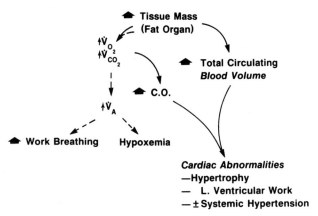

FIGURE 62-3

Cardiac dysfunction in morbid obesity. An increase in tissue mass leads to changes in alveolar ventilation ($\dot{V}_A$), cardiac output (CO), and total circulating blood volume, affecting principally the left ventricle. ($\dot{V}_{O_2}$, oxygen consumption; $\dot{V}_{CO_2}$, carbon dioxide production.) (From Vaughan RW: Anesthetic management of the morbidly obese patient. International Anesthesia Research Society, 1987 Review Course Lectures, p 12. Reproduced by permission.)

tricular dysfunction. As previously noted, the excess mass of fat requires an increased total circulating blood volume (Fig. 62-3). The combination of an increased cardiac output with increased total circulating blood volume leads to cardiac abnormalities on the left side of the heart, manifested by hypertrophy and increased left ventricular work. What results is an increase in cardiac size and weight, an increase in transverse cardiac diameter, increased left ventricular stroke work, and usually elevated systemic arterial pressure.[1] Arteriolar resistance can be influenced by elements of central hypertension as well as by the hydraulic load on the left ventricle.[9] The aggregate effects of premature airway closure and alveolar hypoxia on the right side of the heart can produce hypoxic pulmonary vasoconstriction (Fig. 62-4). Sustained pulmonary vasoconstriction accelerates right ventricular failure. With increasing degrees of obesity, the cardiovascular consequences of obesity become hypertension, hypercholesterolemia, and dyslipoproteinemia. Other circulatory abnormalities include increased total, central, and pulmonary blood volumes. When morbid obesity coexists with advanced age, the heart is at particular risk

for biventricular dysfunction (Fig. 62-5). Moreover, biventricular dysfunction results when the increased pulmonary blood flow is combined with decreased lung volume, alveolar hypoxia, hypoxic pulmonary vasoconstriction leading to pulmonary hypertension, and right ventricular compromise. These severe reductions in cardiopulmonary reserve can adversely affect anesthetic care in the intraoperative and postoperative period.

Because of its enormous size, maintenance of the "fat organ" in severely obese subjects requires increased oxygen consumption ($\dot{V}_{O_2}$) and results in increased carbon dioxide production ($\dot{V}_{CO_2}$) (Fig. 62-6). Added cardiorespiratory stress (e.g., increased cardiac output and elevated alveolar ventilation at rest) is necessary to sustain tissue needs of excess adiposity, in addition to transporting oxygen and carbon dioxide toward and away from the "fat organ." Pulmonary compensation attempts to balance the demand for increased alveolar ventilation despite the existence of a ventilatory system mechanically encumbered by excessive adipose tissue. Deleterious effects on mechanical and circulatory function of the lung can result. For example, functional re-

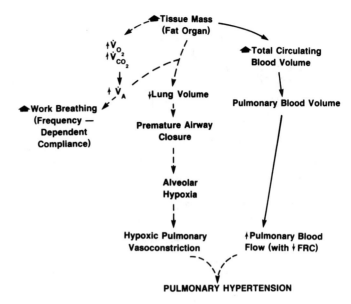

FIGURE 62-4

Changes in pulmonary vascular tone in morbid obesity. An increase in tissue mass leads to alterations in lung volume, producing the potential for hypoxic pulmonary vasoconstriction. Changes in circulating blood volume in the pulmonary circuit can further accentuate pulmonary hypertension. ($\dot{V}o_2$, oxygen consumption; $\dot{V}co_2$, carbon dioxide production; $\dot{V}_A$, alveolar ventilation; FRC, functional residual capacity.) (From Vaughan RW: Anesthetic management of the morbidly obese patient. International Anesthesia Research Society, 1987 Review Course Lectures, p 12. Reproduced by permission.)

sidual capacity (FRC) diminishes at the expense of expiratory reserve volume (ERV) without a change in residual volume.[14] This decrease in resting lung volume compromises the FRC minus closing capacity relationship and enhances premature airway closure during normal tidal ventilation. Profusion of pulmonary alveoli continues, resulting in blood flow to nonventilated and intermittently ventilated lung units. Consequently, resting arterial oxygenation predicted for age is reduced, especially in the supine, morbidly obese subjects (Fig. 62-7).[16]

In addition to cardiopulmonary derangements are biochemical (hepatic, renal, endocrine) derangements. Severely obese patients commonly manifest fatty infiltration of the liver. Accumulation of intracellular lipid (triglyceride) disrupts the cellular integrity of the hepatocyte, releasing

hepatic enzymes that are detectable in serum (SGOT, SGPT, and other intracellular enzymes).[13] Extruded lipid can obstruct bile canaliculi, increasing the serum alkaline phosphatase level and eventually disrupting the whole hepatic lobule. Necrosis, inflammatory changes, and collagen accumulation result. The amount of fatty infiltration seems more related to the duration than to the degree of obesity. Nevertheless, the etiology of the obesity-related hepatic lesion still remains obscure. Irrespective of the cause of hepatic triglyceride infiltration, the consequences are not in question. Mortality from hepatic cirrhosis in morbidly obesity subjects is 1.5 to 2.5 times the rate expected for their nonobese counterparts. Besides this derangement, obesity-related hepatic dysfunction can coexist with other hepatic diseases (diabetes mellitus, alco-

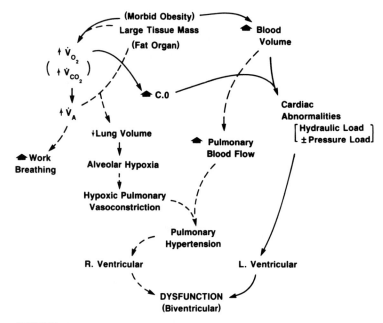

FIGURE 62-5

Effects of obesity-related cardiac dysfunction on the left and right sides of the heart. ($\dot{V}_{O_2}$, oxygen consumption; $\dot{V}_{CO_2}$, carbon dioxide production; $\dot{V}_A$, alveolar ventilation; CO = cardiac output.) (From Vaughan RW: Anesthetic management of the morbidly obese patient. International Anesthesia Research Society, 1987 Review Course Lectures, p 13. Reproduced by permission.)

holism, cirrhosis, jaundice, cholelithiasis). Each aberration contributes individually or synergistically to overall hepatic dysfunction. Such hepatic changes must be considered when anesthetic management is planned preoperatively.[13]

GENERAL ANESTHESIA AND THE METABOLISM OF INHALATION AGENTS

Inhalation anesthetic drugs have become the mainstay of modern general anesthesia. The selection of such agents for obese patients should take into consideration recent information concerning altered anesthetic biotransformation in obesity. Certain halogenated anesthetics (methoxyflurane, halothane, enflurane, and isoflurane) do undergo biotransformation in man. For example, anesthetic agent biotransformation and renal function were studied in 31 chronically

obese patients (148 ± 8 kg, mean ± SE) anesthetized for three hours with 60% nitrous oxide plus methoxyflurane or halothane for elective jejunoileal small bowel bypass operation.[20] During methoxyflurane anesthesia, serum ionic fluoride increased more rapidly, peak concentrations were greater, and the peak concentrations occurred sooner after discontinuation of methoxyflurane in obese adult patients than in nonobese subjects (Fig. 62-8). Previously it had been reported that the extent of renal dysfunction following methoxyflurane anesthesia in any patient was directly related to the peak measured serum ionic fluoride concentration. The average value for peak serum ionic fluoride concentration (55.8 μmol/liter) in obese subjects after three hours of methoxyflurane anesthesia was in the range associated with subclinical renal toxicity (e.g., increased serum uric acid and impaired urine concentrating ability). Further, four of the reported

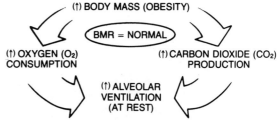

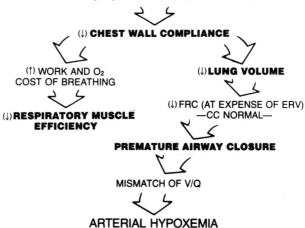

FIGURE 62-6

Pulmonary dysfunction in morbid obesity represented as an imbalance in supply and demand, leading to arterial hypoxemia in a patient at rest breathing room air. (Redrawn from Vaughan RW: Pulmonary and cardiovascular derangements in the obese patient. In Brown BR Jr (ed): Anesthesia and the Obese Patient: Contemporary Anesthesia Practice, Vol V, p 21. Philadelphia, FA Davis Co, 1982. Reproduced by permission.)

FIGURE 62-7

Effect of age (years) on Pa_{O_2}, in nonobese versus morbidly obese patients (awake, supine, breathing room air). *Dashed* line (nonobese subjects) represents data from Sorbini. (From Vaughan RW, et al: Ann Surg 180:879, 1974. Reproduced by permission.)

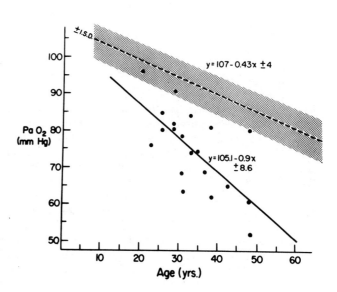

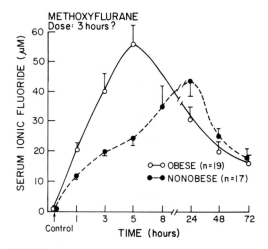

FIGURE 62-8

Serum ionic fluoride (μmol/liter) as a function of time (hours) after approximately three hours of methoxyflurane anesthesia. Comparisons are drawn between 19 obese (*solid line*) and 17 nonobese (*broken line*) patients from two different nonconcurrent studies. (Redrawn from Vaughan RW: Biochemical and biotransformation alterations in the obese. In Brown Br Jr (ed): Anesthesia and the Obese Patient. Philadelphia, FA Davis Co, 1982. Reproduced by permission.)

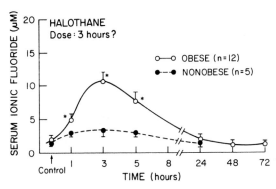

FIGURE 62-9

Serum ionic fluoride (μmol/liter) as a function of time (hours) after approximately three hours of halothane anesthesia. Data were drawn from two noncurrent studies of obese (*solid line*) and nonobese (*broken line*) patients. Asterisks represent obese patients who were statistically significantly different ($P < .05$) from control value. (Redrawn from Vaughan RW: Biochemical and biotransformation alterations in the obese. In Brown Br Jr (ed): Anesthesia and the Obese Patient. Philadelphia, FA Davis Co, 1982. Reproduced by permission.)

patients had peak serum ionic fluoride concentrations of 90 μmol/liter or more. At that level, slight clinical toxicity (serum hyperosmolality and hypernatremia, low urinary osmolality, and polyuria) would be predicted. Most anesthesiologists now would question the use of methoxyflurane for any intra-abdominal operations in morbidly obese patients.

With regard to halothane, a more commonly used volatile anesthetic, studies have demonstrated small but significant increases in serum ionic fluoride concentrations (e.g., mean, 10.4 μmol/liter) during and following halothane anesthesia in obese but not in nonobese subjects. (Fig. 62-9).[3,13] These serum ionic fluoride data would suggest altered halothane biotransformation in obese patients. Biodegradation of halothane does not produce levels of ionic fluoride causing renal toxicity, as previously discussed for methoxyflurane. There is concern, however, that altered biotransformation could be related to unex-

plained jaundice following halothane anesthesia.[2] Epidemiologically, obese subjects have been shown to be at greater risk for liver dysfunction than nonobese subjects.

Besides the earlier data on the biotransformation of methoxyflurane and halothane, recent data have confirmed that use of another inhalation anesthetic agent, enflurane, results in higher concentrations of serum ionic fluoride in morbidly obese subjects than in matched nonobese counterparts.[4] At equivalent end-tidal levels of volatile drug, obese patients metabolized enflurane at twice the rate of the nonobese group (5.5 vs 2.5 μmol/hour). Maximum serum ionic fluoride concentrations occurred two hours after enflurane anesthesia in both groups. The obese group had a 60% higher concentration (28 ± 2 vs 17 ± 3 μmol) (Fig. 62-10). Although these levels of serum ionic fluoride are not in the range associated with clinical renal toxicity, sustained exposure to such fluoride levels could produce subclinical dysfunction. Therefore, in current practice the least metabolized inhalation anesthetic (isoflurane) is used and combined with

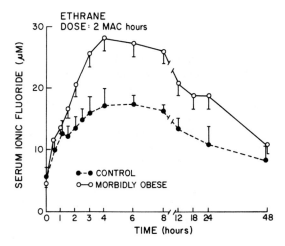

FIGURE 62-10

Serum ionic fluoride concentrations (μmol/liter) during and after two hours of enflurane anesthesia in obese (*open circles*, n = 24) and nonobese (*closed circles*, n = 7) patients (mean ± SE). (Redrawn from Bentley et al: Anesth Analg 58:409, 1979. Reproduced by permission.)

fixed drugs (sedatives, thiobarbiturates, narcotics, skeletal muscle relaxants) to produce balanced general anesthesia.

The respiratory system is of primary importance in general or regional anesthesia. Regardless of the regional anesthetic technique, consideration should be given to supplemental oxygen administration intraoperatively because of the adverse effect of reduced lung volumes in supine, morbidly obese patients. With this caveat, conduction anesthesia (spinal or epidural nerve blocks) may be an appropriate choice for selected peripheral operative procedures. When intra-abdominal surgery is contemplated, serious consideration must be given to a secured airway (e.g., by endotracheal intubation) and controlled mechanical ventilation.

Since inhalation anesthetics are metabolized differently, both quantitatively and qualitatively, in severely obese patients, one might select newer short-acting narcotics and sedatives for intraoperative anesthesia. However, because of the increased body mass and the differences in compartmental distribution of parenteral drugs in morbidly obese patients, the pharmacokinetics

and pharmacodynamics are likely to be different as well. Most anesthesiologists have found as a reasonable alternative to pure inhalation or a pure narcotic technique the selection of a combination of agents for specific desirable anesthetic effects. Such a general anesthetic technique would employ a short-acting narcotic given within the first 15 minutes of induction combined with nitrous oxide and minimal doses of isoflurane to adjust the depth of anesthesia to match the episodic nature of the surgical stimulus. This technique would produce modest cardiac depression from a volatile agent, minimal dose of inhalation anesthetic for biodegradation, and increased flexibility to permit a higher inspired oxygen concentration without concern for patient recall. Nondepolarizing skeletal muscle relaxants would be ideal because a peripheral nerve stimulator could be used to monitor adequate skeletal muscle relaxation during the operative procedure. Such a mixed technique affords optimal muscle relaxation to facilitate operative exposure while allowing a more alert patient at the conclusion of the operative procedure. Perioperative pain relief could include parenteral analgesics, intrathecal and epidural opioids, and patient-demand analgesia.[17]

The pulmonary consequences of morbid obesity must be taken into consideration during the operative procedure. Pulmonary changes in the awake obese patient include a reduction in FRC at the expense of ERV. Lying down results in a further decrease of about 25% in FRC in both nonobese and obese subjects. However, in the morbidly obese patient the reduced lung volume often places FRC below closing capacity so that during normal tidal ventilation premature airway closure occurs (Fig. 62-11). Hypoxia results from increased venous admixture. In such obese patients, the added effect of general anesthesia (e.g., reduced FRC) increases the likelihood of premature airway closure and exaggerates arterial hypoxemia.

When anesthesia for intra-abdominal surgery is planned in a morbidly obese patient, the combined effects of anesthesia, obesity, and the surgical procedure on cardiorespiratory function must be anticipated. Preoperatively, in the awake state, obese patients have reduced lung volume with mismatched ventilation and perfusion, in-

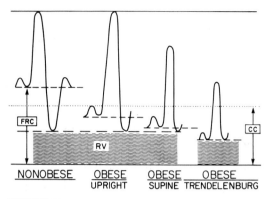

FIGURE 62-11

Effect of position on various lung volumes in non-obese compared to morbidly obese subjects. (FRC, functional residual capacity; RV, residual volume; CC, closing capacity.) (Redrawn from Vaughan RW: Pulmonary and cardiovascular derangements in the obese patient. In Brown BR Jr (ed): Anesthesia and the Obese Patient. Philadelphia, FA Davis Co, 1982. Reproduced by permission.)

creased pulmonary venous admixture, and lower arterial oxygen tension than predicted for age.[16] The combined effect of the supine operative posture and anesthetic induction further reduces FRC. Pulmonary venous admixture is accentuated, as many alveolar units are overperfused in relation to ventilation. During induction, certain fixed agents like sodium thiopental and potent inhalation anesthetics (isoflurane), used for maintenance of anesthesia, reduce cardiac output by combining vasodilation with a negative cardiac ionotropic effect to decrease mixed venous oxygen tension. Both arterial oxygenation and mixed venous oxygenation may subsequently be dangerously reduced. As the surgical procedure continues with the placement of laparotomy packs and retractors to achieve better exposure, lung volume and impaired venous return can further compromise cardiac output.[12] The need to measure intraoperative oxygenation during such procedures becomes evident.

POSTOPERATIVE PHASE

Emergence from anesthesia is a particularly crucial time for morbidly obese patients. Ventilatory capability postoperatively must be established

by objective criteria. The latter include sustained tetanus at 50 Hz for five seconds by a peripheral nerve stimulator, sustained head raising, and a level of consciousness that allows the patient to open the eye on command.[5] Arterial blood gases should be monitored to guide oxygenation or postoperative mechanical ventilation as necessary.

We evaluated postoperative hypoxemia in 20 morbidly obese adults after intra-abdominal operations. Preoperatively a significant reduction in supine arterial oxygen tension was present compared to nonobese patients matched for age. Some of these patients on postoperative days 1 and 2 had arterial oxygen values associated with a dangerous reduction in arterial oxygen content (Fig. 62-12).[16] Because oxygen tension is reduced, hemoglobin saturation functions on the more vertical portion of the oxyhemoglobin dissociation curve, and modest reductions in oxygen tension produce dramatic falls in arterial oxygen content. In additional studies we examined the effect of a change in body position in the postoperative period on the arterial oxygen tension in morbidly obese patients. In markedly obese women, position had a significant effect on arterial oxygen tension for 48 hours postoperatively.[19] Placing the patient in a semirecumbent rather than supine position early in the postoperative period was a valuable therapeutic maneuver that improved arterial oxygenation (Fig. 62-13).

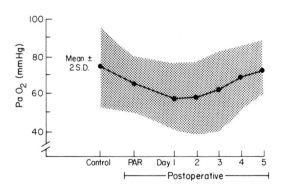

FIGURE 62-12

Fall in Pao_2 (mm Hg) with time postoperatively. *Solid line* represents the mean; *stippled area* represents ±2 SD. (Redrawn from Vaughan RW et al: Ann Surg 43:877, 1974. Reproduced by permission.)

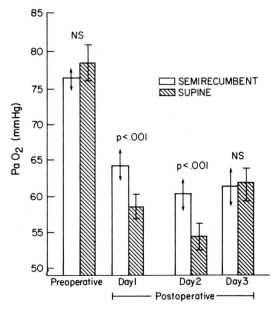

FIGURE 62-13

Arterial oxygen tension (PaO$_2$, mm Hg) in 22 morbidly obese female subjects in the semirecumbent position (*open bars*) and the supine position (*shaded bar*) preoperatively and on postoperative days 1 through 3. All values were obtained with the patient at rest and breathing room air. NS, not significant. (Redrawn from Vaughan RW, et al: Ann Surg 1982:705, 1975. Reproduced by permission.)

These data, obtained in young, nonsmoking, obese patients, demonstrate the sicker, morbidly obese patient's vulnerability to hypoxia. Each of the subjects studied was an otherwise healthy individual without evidence of cardiorespiratory disease. Age, weight (especially abdominal obesity), smoking habits, and position each independently alters gas exchange adversely by accentuating airway closure. Older morbidly obese patients undergoing intra-abdominal surgery would be at high risk for postoperative hypoxemia. Careful monitoring of oxygenation and titration of oxygen become essential for safe perioperative anesthesia care. An older morbidly obese patient with coexisting cardiovascular disease (e.g., coronary, valvular, or hypertensive cardiac disease) has minimal cardiac reserves. Previously, when operative procedures were performed in such severely obese patients, unex-

plained sudden death sometimes occurred in the immediate postoperative period. One can never assume that hypoxemia is not a problem unless arterial oxygenation is monitored. Pulse oximetry with continuous readout of oxygen saturation coupled with arterial blood gas analysis has served well as an early warning system for hypoxemia. Such monitoring of oxygenation for the first several days after intra-abdominal surgery has become accepted practice.

This discussion has focused on oxygenation because of the priority of the adverse impact of the cardiopulmonary system on tissue oxygenation. An association also exists between obesity and increased risk for coronary artery disease, hypertension, pulmonary vascular disease, noninsulin-dependent diabetes mellitus, and abnormalities of lipoprotein and cholesterol metabolism (Table 62-1). For example, if obesity and hypertension coexist, the left ventricle must support the elevated preload produced by obesity and work against the high afterload resulting from the central hypertension.[9] Obesity-related disturbances in lipid metabolism and perhaps physical inactivity may act through the common pathway of atherosclerosis to narrow the coronary arteries that supply oxygen to an excessively worked and inadequately nourished myocardium. Clinical signs of coronary artery disease (angina pectoris and sudden death) may appear when oxygen demand outstrips supply.[15] For such morbidly obese patients, it is important to minimize perioperative risks. Such a strategy entails a careful prospective plan, appropriate monitoring (anesthetic circuit, pulmonary ventilation, circulation, blood gas exchange), and a team approach. The latter includes extended educa-

TABLE 62-1

Clinical Problems Associated With Obesity

Coronary artery disease
Hypertension
Cerebrovascular disease and stroke
Diabetes mellitus
Dyslipoproteinemia
Cholelithiasis
Abnormal liver function

tion of various members of the anesthesia care team, surgical team, and nursing personnel (e.g., operating room nurses, postoperative recovery nurses, intensive care nurses, and unit nurses). Vigilance and timely communication can favorably influence the perioperative care of morbidly obese patients who present for anesthesia and surgery.

References

1. Alexander JK: The cardiomyopathy of obesity. Prog Cardiovasc Dis 27:325, 1985

2. Bentley JB, Vaughan RW, Corke RC et al: Does evidence of reductive halothane biotransformation correlate with hepatic binding of metabolites in obese patients? Anesth Anal 60:548, 1981

3. Bentley JB, Vaughan RW, Gandolfi AJ et al: Halothane biotransformation in obese and nonobese patients. Anesthesiology 57:94, 1982

4. Bentley JB, Vaughan RW, Miller MS et al: Serum inorganic fluoride levels in obese patients during and after enflurane anesthesia. Anesth Anal 58:409, 1979

5. Cork RC, Vaughan RW, Bentley JB: General anesthesia for morbidly obese patients: An examination of postoperative outcomes. Anesthesiology 54:310, 1981

6. Fankel HM: Determination of body mass index. JAMA 255:1292, 1986

7. Kannel WB, Gordon T: Obesity and cardiovascular disease: The Framingham Study. In Burland WL, Samuel PD, Yudkin J (eds): Obesity Symposium: Proceedings of the Research Institute Symposium, p 24. Edinburgh, Churchill Livingston, 1974

8. Kral JG: Morbid obesity and related health risks. Ann Intern Med 103:1043, 1974

9. Messerli FH: Cardiomyopathy of obesity: A not so Victorian disease. N Engl J Med 314:378, 1986

10. Paul DR, Hoyt JL, Boutras AR: Cardiovascular and respiratory changes in response to change of position in the very obese. Anesthesiology 45:73, 1976

11. Rochester DF, Enson Y: Current concepts in the pathogenesis of obesity-hypoventilation syndrome: Mechanical and circulatory factors. Am J Med 57:402, 1974

12. Vaughan RW: Anesthetic management of the morbidly obese patient. International Anesthesia Research Society, Review Course, 1987, pp 11–18

13. Vaughan RW: Biochemical and biotransformation alterations in the obese. In Brown BR Jr (ed): Anesthesia and the Obese Patient, p 55. Philadelphia, FA Davis Co, 1982

14. Vaughan RW: Pulmonary and cardiovascular derangements in the obese patient. In Brown BR Jr (ed): Anesthesia and the Obese Patient, p 19. Philadelphia, FA Davis Co, 1982

15. Vaughan RW, Conahan TJ: Cardiopulmonary consequences of morbid obesity. Life Sci 26:2119, 1980

16. Vaughan RW, Engelhardt RC, Wise L: Postoperative hypoxemia in obese patients. Ann Surg 180:877, 1974

17. Vaughan RW, Maccioli GA: Perioperative analgesia in obese patients. Prob Anesth 2:435, 1988

18. Vaughan RW, Vaughan MS: Morbid obesity: Implications for anesthetic care. Semin Anesth 3:218, 1984

19. Vaughan RW, Wise L: Postoperative arterial blood gas measurement: Effect of position on gas exchange. Ann Surg 182:705, 1975

20. Young SR, Stoelting RK, Peterson C: Anesthetic biotransformation and renal function in obese patients during and after methoxyflurane or halothane anesthesia. Anesthesiology 42:451, 1975

CHAPTER 63

Surgical Treatment of Obesity

JOHN G. KRAL

The term "morbid obesity" was originally used to describe the obesity of patients of twice-normal weight, or 100 pounds or more above the Metropolitan Life Insurance Company standards of weight for height. The original definition did not take into account whether manifest comorbid conditions in fact were present. Obviously, morbidity can appear at lower levels of weight and, conversely, can be absent at or above this index weight level. Surgical treatment can cure most of the obesity-related comorbidity and under proper circumstances can do so with an acceptable rate of complications and side-effects. Nonoperative treatment has been discouragingly ineffective in maintaining clinically significant weight loss in patients sufficiently obese to warrant surgical intervention. These patients are so heavy and have such a high prevalence of silent, functional, and clinical symptoms that there should be no controversy that their obesity truly is a disease and is worthy of treatment.

HISTORY AND OVERVIEW

Lipectomy, the surgical removal of excess skin and adipose tissue, was described in 1918, mainly as a cosmetic procedure to correct a pendulous abdomen.[48] It has never seriously been suggested as a legitimate treatment for morbid obesity but rather as an adjunct to other, intra-abdominal procedures, or as a method for treating sequelae of extreme weight loss.[24]

The first published account of an operation expressly performed to cause gradual weight loss was by Victor Henriksson in Swedish in 1952.[19]

Henriksson had excised a substantial portion of the small bowel in three obese women in 1950–1951 to produce controlled malabsorption. Around the same time, Kremen, Linner, and Nelson published their experiences with small bowel bypass in dogs, with an account of jejunoileal bypass in a patient.[26] After anecdotal reports of jejunocolic bypass,[41] Payne et al published the first results in a large series of patients who had undergone jejunoileal bypass (Fig. 63-1).[40] Numerous technical modifications of the jejunoileal bypass, mainly directed toward achieving greater weight loss by preventing reflux into the bypassed loop by creating an end-to-end anastomosis,[47,50] appeared during the 1970s. Other substantial modifications of jejunoileal bypass were developed, such as bilio-intestinal bypass,[8] biliopancreatic diversion,[49] and jejunoileostomy with ileogastrostomy,[15] although generally there was a strong trend toward abandoning the intestinal procedures[17] in favor of the gastric operations in the late 1970s and early 1980s.

The first account of a gastric operation for morbid obesity was published by Mason and Ito in 1967.[32] It was the first gastric bypass performed for morbid obesity and entailed the creation of a small (10% of gastric volume) fundic pouch, excluding the remaining 90% of the stomach. A loop of small bowel (jejunum) was attached to the small pouch, creating a loop gastrojejunostomy (Fig. 63-2). This operation was gastric restrictive and caused some malabsorption. Pure gastric restriction was attempted and quickly abandoned by Mason in 1971, when he intro-

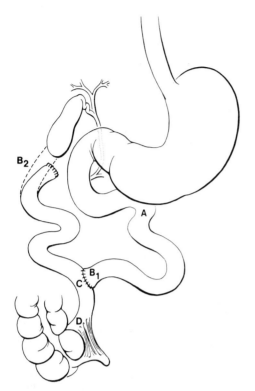

FIGURE 63-1

Intestinal bypass. In jejunoileal bypass (end-to-side), segment A-B_1 is 35 cm and segment C-D is 10 cm. In biliointestinal bypass, the "blind" stump B_2 is attached to the gallbladder. In duodenoileal bypass, A-B_1 is only 5 cm and C-D is 50 cm. Furthermore, an antireflux nipple valve is created just above C in the blind loop. Reprinted from Obesity and Weight Control: The Health Professional's Guide to Understanding and Treatment by R.T. Frankle and M. Yang (Eds.), with permission of Aspen Publishers, Inc., © 1988.

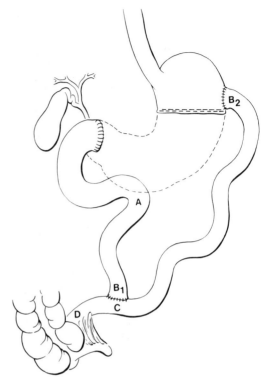

FIGURE 63-2

Gastric bypass–biliopancreatic bypass. In gastric bypass a stapled stomach pouch is attached to a loop of small bowel (B_2-C = 40 cm) so that food never enters the rest of the stomach. In biliopancreatic bypass a two-thirds gastrectomy (*dotted line*) is performed. A-B_1 diverts bile and pancreatic secretions to the terminal ileum (C-D = 50 cm). Reprinted from Obesity and Weight Control: The Health Professional's Guide to Understanding and Treatment by R.T. Frankle and M. Yang (Eds.), with permission of Aspen Publishers, Inc., © 1988.

duced horizontal gastroplasty in a small series of patients. The procedure was revived by Gomez in 1976[13] and has subsequently undergone numerous modifications leading to the present two variants of gastric restriction: (1) vertical gastroplasty with external stomal support (Fig. 63-3) and (2) gastric banding. Gastric restriction can also be achieved (temporarily) by space-occupying intragastric devices such as balloons or "bubbles," but these devices have largely been abandoned for lack of effectiveness.[22,28]

All of the surgical methods listed above were performed clinically without animal experimentation documenting weight loss in obese animal models. In contrast, early animal experiments laid the foundation for regulatory methods, *i.e.*, operations directly influencing appetite regulation. In 1974, Danish neurosurgeons prompted by F. Quaade performed stereotactic electrocoagulation of the putative hunger or feeding centers in the hypothalamus of morbidly obese patients.[42] Other such trials have never been re-

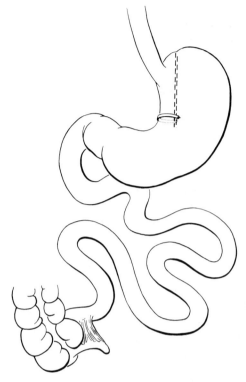

FIGURE 63-3

Vertical stapled gastroplasty with band. A 20-ml pouch with a band or ring to maintain outlet inner diameter at approximately 1 cm. Reprinted from Obesity and Weight Control: The Health Professional's Guide to Understanding and Treatment by R.T. Frankle and M. Yang (Eds.), with permission of Aspen Publishers, Inc., © 1988.

ported. A less dramatic regulatory method, truncal vagotomy, was first reported in 1978 in a small clinical series.[25] Vagotomy as a sole procedure has been abandoned, but it is still being used in combination with vertical gastroplasty.[14] Intestinal interposition, transposing a segment of terminal ileum, was attempted in a total of five patients, with grossly unsatisfactory weight loss, resulting in discontinuation of this procedure.

Table 63-1 summarizes the methods and principles reported up to 1989. The routine methods most widely used currently for treating obesity are vertical gastroplasty[7,31] (see Fig. 63-3) and gastric bypass[10,29] (see Fig. 63-2). Other methods performed on a more limited scale are different

TABLE 63-1

Surgical Methods for Treating Obesity

I. Physical methods
  A. Lipectomy*: surgical removal of adipose tissue
    1. Formal dermolipectomy
    2. Suction-assisted lipectomy
  B. Restriction
    1. Jaw wiring
    2. Esophageal banding
    3. Gastric restriction
      a. Gastroplasty (gastric banding)
      b. Gastric wrapping
      c. Intragastric balloon
  C. Malabsorption
    1. Small bowel resection
    2. Intestinal bypass
      a. Jejunoileal bypass: end-to-side (duodenoileal)
      b. Jejunoileal bypass: end-to-end (ileogastrostomy)
      c. Biliointestinal bypass
      d. Biliopancreatic diversion
  D. Combination of restriction and malabsorption
    1. Gastric bypass: loop
    2. Gastric bypass: Roux-Y
      a. "Distal" gastric bypass
      b. Biliopancreatic diversion
II. Regulatory methods
  A. Stereotactic lesions
  B. Truncal vagotomy
  C. Intestinal interposition
III. Combination of physical and regulatory methods
  A. Malabsorption
    1. Intestinal bypass
    2. Gastric bypass
  B. Gastric restriction
    1. Gastroplasty alone?
    2. Gastroplasty with vagotomy

*An adjunct. Lipectomy is *not* a treatment for obesity.

variants of distal gastric bypass (biliopancreatic diversion), gastric banding (with diminishing frequency), and, rarely, intestinal bypass (see Fig. 63-1).

PHYSIOLOGY

Only in rare exceptions is the etiology of obesity known, although it is clear that all obese patients

TABLE 63-2

Caloric Intake by Recall, Diary or Actual Measurement in Morbidly Obese Patients: NHANES I Study[1] Used as Reference

Study	Sex	n	Weight (kg)	Caloric Intake	
				kcal/24 hr	kcal/kg
Heshka et al[20]	M	6	117	3860	33.1
NHANES I[1]	M	79	(105)	2400	22.8
NHANES I[1]	M	2700	76.7	2350	30.7
Bray et al[2]	F	14	160	4810	30.1
Brown et al[3]	F	12	132	2820	21.4
Miskowiak et al[37]	F	11	116	2260	19.5
Naslund et al[38]	F	26	116	2300	19.8
NHANES I[1]	F	245	(75)	1500	20
NHANES I[1]	F	3519	63.2	1610	25.5
Condon et al[4]	M	17	?	3260	(25.1)*
	F	48			
Coughlin et al[5]	M	4	132	3980	30.1
	F	21			
Graney et al[16]	?	12	119	2480	20.9
McFarland et al[35]	M	2	125	3100	24.8
	F	16			
Raymond et al[43]	F	9	?	2590	(19.9)*
	M	4			
Rogus et al[44]	?	11	150	6830	45.5
	?	8	132	6010	45.5
Updegraff et al[56]	?	12	?	2730	(21.0)*

*Estimated weight = 130 kg.

ingest, assimilate, and store too many calories to allow maintenance of a healthy weight. Food intake has been measured in massively obese patients before and after intestinal bypass and gastric procedures.[4,5,37,38] Great differences between studies in baseline measurements can be explained by variations in sex distribution, age, weight, range, and socioeconomic, ethnic, and cultural factors of the patient population, as well as techniques of assessment (Table 63-2). Measurements of oxygen consumption in the massively obese have determined resting metabolic rates (RMR) around 1800 kcal/24 hours for women[55] and 2300 for men,[9] compared to Harris-Benedict standards of 1345 kcal/24 hours in women and 2180 in men of normal weight but similar age and height. Several investigators have claimed that obese people in fact have reduced RMR per unit body weight, but normalization to lean body mass demonstrated a relative elevation in metabolic rate in morbidly obese patients.[55]

Unexpectedly, it was revealed that intestinal bypass reduces food intake significantly[4] and does not solely rely on the graded or controlled malabsorption of calories that was originally the rationale for performing these operations.[26] The mechanisms for reducing ingestion are not known, although numerous good candidates have been proposed, based on animal and clinical studies (Table 63-3). Patients who have undergone reversal of jejunoileal bypass have often anecdotally reported feeling "healthier" after reversal of the operation, not having noted any difference relative to the prebypass state during several years with the operation. This would support the notion that malaise or aversion has a significant role in reducing food intake.

Gastric restriction works by causing nausea,

TABLE 63-3

Candidate Mechanisms Causing Reduced Food Intake After Malabsorptive Operations

I. Gastrointestinal peptide release
   A. "Satiety"
      1. Central: neurohumoral signals (e.g., cholecystokinin)
      2. Peripheral:
         (a) Gastric (delayed emptying) (e.g., neurotensin)
         (b) Hepatic receptors (e.g., glucagon)
   B. Aversion
      1. Dumping (e.g., gastrointestinal polypeptide)
      2. "Fullness" (= distention via delayed emptying)
II. Toxin production in blind loop
   A. "Malaise" (via liver)
      1. Bacterial decomposition
      2. Toxic bile acid production
III. Substrate mobilization
   A. Satiety or malaise from the liver (via portal circulation)
      1. Free fatty acids from adipose tissue

pain, discomfort, and potentially vomiting if the patient breaks the rules of the "gastroplasty diet" by not chewing well, eating too rapidly, or ingesting liquids after solids, all of which simply overdistend the gastric pouch. Ideally in gastroplasty, a small amount of food should elicit satiety, leading to early termination of the meal, but the degree to which satiety contributes to weight loss after gastroplasty has not been determined. Weight loss and weight maintenance after gastroplasty depend on the time it takes for the patient to develop maladaptive eating or distention of the gastric pouch. The smaller the pouch, the longer it will take for significant (and permanent) enlargement, thus overriding the effects of the operation.

Gastric bypass has been shown repeatedly to achieve greater and more sustained weight loss than simple gastric restriction.[57] This is attributed to the aversive effect of "dumping" into the loop of small intestine as well as to some malabsorption and maldigestion caused by exclusion of most of the stomach and the restriction

achieved by the small pouch of a gastroplasty. The recent trend to increase the length of the bypassed small intestine and to divert biliopancreatic and gastric secretions distally has introduced a greater element of malabsorption into the gastric bypass procedures.

Vagotomy potentiates weight loss from gastroplasty[14] through several mechanisms whose relative importance has not been delineated. Vagotomy delays emptying of solids, yet speeds transit of liquids in intact stomachs. In gastroplasty, vagotomy does not consistently slow emptying of a mixed meal.[14] Animal and clinical studies have shown that vagotomy reduces fluid intake and indeed decreases caloric intake.[21]

The causes of obesity and overeating are not known, so treatment is symptomatic at best. Greater knowledge of the pathogenesis of the syndromes of obesity may facilitate selection of surgical procedures in individual patients and introduce new principles for determining which patients are eligible for surgical treatment of obesity. For now, however, gastric restriction with or without a malabsorptive component is the mainstay of obesity surgery. After failure of gastric restriction alone, reoperation adding malabsorption has the greater likelihood of achieving sustained, clinically significant weight loss.[54]

PATIENT SELECTION

Patients with serious obesity-related morbidity (malignant obesity) that has improved with weight loss but who are unable to maintain the reduced weight are candidates for surgical treatment. Furthermore, patients who are 45 kg (100 pounds) above life insurance weight-for-height standards, whether or not they have manifest comorbidity, are candidates, since silent pathology is prevalent at this weight level and the likelihood of developing clinically significant symptoms is very great.

Patient cooperation is as essential for the successful outcome of antiobesity surgery as it is for any obesity treatment modality. Both motivational and cognitive factors probably influence outcome, though there are no published studies to prove it. No patient should be referred for surgery without a full understanding of the rationale for surgical treatment, including awareness of the health hazards of obesity. Denial is common in this population, as is the case with many addictive behaviors, and it will jeopardize the patient's ability to cooperate with follow-up care.

A thorough evaluation of candidates for surgical treatment of morbid obesity should include (1) analysis of health beliefs, (2) assessment of quality of life, (3) investigation of the patient's social environment with respect to mechanisms of secondary gain and codependency, and (4) analysis of eating behavior, particularly fondness for calorically dense sweet foods. During the workup there should be some tests of compliance such as appointment-keeping behavior, dieting, smoking cessation, and participation in group meetings.

CLINICAL RESULTS

The results of antiobesity surgery have traditionally been framed in terms of weight loss, which superficially might seem reasonable. However, there is no evidence that greater weight loss is beneficial from the perspective of health or longevity, although most patients aggressively want greater losses of weight. The high prevalence of comorbid conditions in obesity suggests use of a different method to evaluate clinical results of antiobesity operations. Improvement and even cure of these often life-threatening conditions can be quantitated relatively easily, although prospective, randomized trials ascertaining the natural history of untreated obesity are not feasible or ethical in this setting. Increasingly, papers are addressing this important aspect of evaluating results. Diabetes, hypertension, hypoventilation, and dyslipoproteinemia are significantly reduced postoperatively, even before substantial losses of weight occur (Table 63-4). It follows that with this reduction in important morbidity, there will be a reduction in mortality, although it is difficult to prove.

Weight loss results in several large series are presented in Table 63-5. Variations in population factors such as race,[52] socioeconomic background,[30] sex distribution, preoperative weight, duration and percentage of follow-up, and other factors probably contribute as much to variability of results as do variations in surgical technique.

Weight loss is characteristically on the order of

TABLE 63-4

Amelioration or Cure of Comorbid Conditions After Antiobesity Surgery (Pooled From Published Operative Series on More Than 1000 Patients)

Comorbid Condition	Prevalence (%)	Cured* (%)	Improved* (%)
Hypertension	30–60	60–65	90
Dyslipoproteinemia	15–25	70	85
Diabetes	15–20	90–95	100
Asthma	10–15	>95	100
Heart failure	10	60	90
Sleep apnea	2–5	100	100

*Cure denotes absence of need for medication or treatment; improved denotes reduced dosage of medication.

one third of preoperative weight. Thus, a 120-kg patient loses 40 kg. This corresponds to 55% to 65% of excess weight, the preoperative weight in excess of ideal or desirable body weight. For example, excess weight is 65 kg in a 120-kg woman whose ideal weight is 55 kg at 154 cm of height. A loss of 40 kg represents 61.5% of excess weight.

As Table 63-5 demonstrates, excess loss is greater after gastric bypass than after simple gastroplasty. More malabsorptive operations, such as biliopancreatic bypass, distal gastric bypass, and intestinal bypass operations, occasionally result in losses of 80% of excess weight. Furthermore, weight loss is achieved more consistently

TABLE 63-5

Long-Term Weight Loss After Antiobesity Surgery

Operation	n	Time (Months)	Excess weight lost (%)
Gastric bypass[10]	57	60	68
Gastric bypass[57]	225	60	68
Gastric bypass[36]	183	72	61
Banded gastroplasty[33]	139	60	53

with such operations, with less than 20% of patients typically failing to lose significant amounts of weight or to maintain that weight loss, compared with a 30% to 40% failure rate after gastric restriction.

An actuarial analysis would require a control population of untreated morbidly obese subjects, representing the natural history of the disease. Such data cannot be obtained ethically. Also, obese people are reclusive, by choice or through their inability to attend screening examinations. The vast majority do not even have scales for their weight level, preventing them from accurately responding to questionnaires, which further limits the feasibility of collecting appropriate reference data.

With the substantial amelioration of comorbid conditions and the significant reduction of excess weight, surgical treatment is far more successful than any nonsurgical modality described in the literature so far. In terms of improvement in quality of life, whether systematically evaluated by validated questionnaires[53] or through the testimonial of increasing numbers of self-referred patients requesting surgery, the results are extremely encouraging. Thus, it behooves us to take a close look at the liabilities of the surgical treatment of obesity.

COMPLICATIONS AND SIDE-EFFECTS

The perioperative morbidity and mortality improved significantly in the 1980s,[39] although it must be recognized that some patients with exceedingly poor prognoses without surgery are at great risk for perioperative complications as well. Addictive behavior is common among the obese, and particularly smoking is a significant risk factor for developing perioperative complications. Some of the well-known comorbid conditions of obesity are important independent risk factors for operative complications and ideally should be treated prior to surgery.

The number of complications of jejunoileal bypass is as great as that of complications of obesity itself, and new complications continue to surface, though conventional jejunoileal bypass has largely been abandoned for ten years. One difficulty in interpreting the complication rate lies in the inability to know if patients with complications have followed treatment plans recommended to prevent the complications. Often the patients have not returned for follow-up and have independently elected to discontinue prescribed supplements. It is true that large numbers of patients were not treated prophylactically starting immediately postoperatively because of lack of understanding on the part of the medical profession, but noncompliance is also very common among the obese.

Although fairly uncommon, liver cirrhosis can be fatal unless recognized in time. Such recognition requires serial needle biopsies of the liver, since blood tests can be normal in the context of morphological deterioration, ultimately leading to manifest failure.

The syndrome of bacterial overgrowth of the blind loop, causing enteritis ("gas bloat"), arthritis, dermatitis, and contributing to vitamin and mineral deficiencies, is treatable by antibiotics, dietary changes, surgical revision of the operation, or, as a last resort, complete reversal.[23] The percentage of patients requiring reversal varies in different series and may well be a function of the quality of follow-up care of the patients. Outcome analysis of patients who have had reversal has been anecdotal and related to specific symptoms such as arthritis[27] or hepatic failure.[12] In a comprehensive analysis of 43 patients who underwent reversal among approximately 800 who underwent jejunoileal bypass procedures between 1971 and 1978, the main indication for reversal was electrolyte imbalance or malnutrition or diarrhea (n = 16); nine patients had cirrhosis and nine had nephrolithiasis.[6] The majority of these patients were cured or improved, although two patients with cirrhosis complicated by ascites died.

Complications are less prevalent after gastric bypass and even rarer after gastroplasty. However, as might be anticipated intuitively, the frequency of long-term nutritional side-effects is inversely related to the efficacy of the operation.[46] Deficiencies occur much as they do with dieting and fasting and similarly require supervision and monitoring.

Perioperative morbidity and mortality have steadily decreased over the last ten years as protocols for risk reduction have been developed for patients with intrinsic cardiac and respiratory

TABLE 63-6

**Procedure-Related Complications
of Antiobesity Surgery**

Malabsorptive Operations

Operative
  Wound infection
Uncontrolled diarrhea
  Deficiencies
    Fat-soluble vitamins and electrolytes: K, Mg, Ca
"Blind loop" syndrome
  Enteritis
  Arthropathy
  Liver cirrhosis
  Dermatitis
Metabolic problems
  Gallstones
  Urolithiasis
  "Encephalopathy"

Gastric Operations

Operative
  Leaks
  Splenectomy
Uncontrolled vomiting
  Deficiencies
    Thiamine
    Alkalosis
  Esophagitis
Inadequate diet
  Iron
  Ca
  B_{12}
Erosions/ulcers
Strictures
Weight loss failure

compromise. Specific procedure-related complications are listed in Table 63-6. Long-term complications are predictably more prevalent after gastric bypass than after gastroplasty, but significantly less prevalent than after conventional intestinal bypass. Deficiencies in iron, vitamin B_{12}, and calcium are the most common in uncomplicated cases without vigorous attention to supplementation. In respect to excessive vomiting, rare case reports have documented thiamine deficiency with neurologic sequelae.[18]

Because of difficulties in obtaining comprehensive follow-up and the relatively high rate of spontaneous reversal of gastric restrictive proce-

dures, there is no information on the development of esophageal pathology in these patients, with a remarkably high frequency of preoperative morbidity.[45] It has been suggested that gastroplasty might even have a beneficial effect on reflux esophagitis,[51] although the data are equivocal.

Reasons for reoperation after gastroplasty are stomal stenosis, staple line disruption, pouch enlargement, erosion of the band, and weight loss failure. Stomal stenosis is treatable by endoscopic balloon dilation, although a subset of patients do indeed require reoperation to prevent excessive vomiting and weight loss.

WEIGHT LOSS FAILURE

It is difficult to agree on a definition of successful weight loss. On medical grounds, success might be defined as maintenance and loss of sufficient weight to ameliorate manifest complications of obesity or to prevent the development of such complications. On a humane level, success might be indicated by any improvement in quality of life, which can only be evaluated by the individual patient.

The most common adverse effect of all gastric operations and particularly gastroplasty is failure to lose weight or maintain weight loss. The main reason is not technical or organic but behavioral: the "soft calorie syndrome" or maladaptive eating contributes to the majority of these failures.

If failure is arbitrarily defined as inability to lose or maintain a loss of 20% of preoperative body weight, vertical banded gastroplasty has "failed" in about 40% of patients in several series (including my own) with five-year or longer follow-up. It is true that the "success" rate of 60% is far superior to that of any nonoperative treatment and that patients in whom the operation "fails" according to this definition are satisfied with the results, but there is nevertheless a demand for reoperation. The largest series of gastroplasty patients (1169 patients), with follow-up for a maximum of five years, reported a 7% mean revision rate, though the rate for patients with the longest follow-up has not been presented, and approximately 25% of patients are lost to follow-up.

Very little data has been published on weight loss failure after gastric bypass, particularly after the more aggressive malabsorptive, distal gastric or biliopancreatic bypass operations. The intestinal bypass operations (jejunoileal bypass) were associated with long-term failure of weight loss maintenance in 10% to 20% of cases.[34] It stands to reason that similar or greater failure rates are to be expected after gastric bypass; indeed, early modifications required revision in about 50% of cases.

Reoperations for failed gastric operations are associated with higher complication rates than are primary procedures,[11] as is the case with all reoperative surgery. This raises the question of developing criteria for reoperation based on weight alone. An argument could be made for only performing reoperations for manifest complications of the primary surgery or (relapse of) obesity-related complications. However, even in this setting quality-of-life aspects must be considered and weighed against the risk-benefit analysis of the informed patient.

OUTLOOK

It is clear that severe obesity is hazardous and limits quality of life. It is also clear that surgical techniques for treating obesity provide the only reasonably effective treatment to date. However, surgical procedures carry immediate and long-term risks, yet almost universally improve quality of life, according to the patients.

The severity of obesity is not necessarily linearly related to weight. It is true that serious comorbidity increases in prevalence with increasing weight, but typically there are thresholds for the clinical appearance of symptoms, and the index weight for height of 45 kg (100 pounds) above desirable (defined as morbid obesity) does not obligate manifest morbidity. It is important to find methods to identify patients at risk for developing malignant obesity. Since the safest operations are the least effective, a risk-benefit analysis must be based on identification of candidates in whom the performance of the riskier (more effective) operations is justifiable.

Serious comorbidity can often be cured by a very modest postoperative weight loss. It remains to be determined how much weight loss is enough and how long the salutary effects are sustained. So far there is no evidence that reduction of comorbidity differs among operations sufficiently to justify choosing riskier operations. The most important problem yet to be solved is how to identify preoperatively patients who will not benefit from the safer, purely gastric restrictive procedures and who thus might be candidates for increasingly malabsorptive operations. Should this not prove feasible, it might be necessary to accept the premise that a proportion of patients undergoing gastric restrictive operations as the primary procedure will need additional surgery to sustain an adequate weight loss. In essence, this means adopting a staged approach in antiobesity surgery. A further risk-benefit analysis will be needed for choosing the second procedure and weighing the risks of a second operation in this setting against the risks of performing a more effective but riskier operation primarily. There is no doubt that the informed patient will choose the approach leading to the most rapid weight loss. Who is better suited to make the choice?

References

1. Braitman LE, Adlin EV, Stanton JL Jr: Obesity and caloric intake: The National Health and Nutrition Examination Study of 1971–1975 (HANES I). J Chronic Dis 38:727, 1985
2. Bray GA, Zachary B, Dahms WT et al: Eating patterns of massively obese individuals. J Am Diet Assoc 72:24, 1978
3. Brown EK, Settle EA, Van Rij AM: Food intake patterns of gastric bypass patients. J Am Diet Assoc 80:437, 1982
4. Condon SC, Janes NJ, Wise L et al: Role of caloric intake in the weight loss after jejunoileal bypass for obesity. Gastroenterology 74:34, 1978
5. Coughlin K, Bell RM, Bivins BA et al: Preoperative and postoperative assessment of nutrient intakes in patients who have undergone gastric bypass surgery. Arch Surg 118:813, 1983
6. Dean P, Joshi S, Kaminski D: Long-term outcome of reversal of small intestinal bypass operations. Am J Surg 159:118, 1990
7. Eckout GV, Willbanks OL, Moore JT: Vertical-ring gastroplasty for morbid obesity: Five-year experience with 1463 patients. Am J Surg 152:713, 1986
8. Eriksson J: Biliointestinal bypass. Int J Obes 5:437, 1981

9. Feurer ID, Crosby LO, Buzby GP et al: Resting energy expenditure in morbid obesity. Ann Surg 197:17, 1983

10. Flickinger EG, Sinar DR, Swanson M: Gastric bypass. Gastroenterol Clin North Am 16:283, 1987

11. Forse RA, Deitel M, MacLean LD: Revision of failed horizontal gastroplasty by vertical banded gastroplasty. Can J Surg 31:118, 1988

12. Geiss DM, Shields S, Watts JD: Reversibility of hepatic failure following jejunoileal bypass. Arch Surg 111:1362, 1976

13. Gomez CA: Gastroplasty in the surgical treatment of morbid obesity. Am J Clin Nutr 33:406, 1980.

14. Gortz L, Wallin S, Kral JG: Truncal vagotomy improves weight loss after vertical banded gastroplasty. Int J Obes 11(suppl 2):116, 1987

15. Gourlay RH, Cleator IGM: jejunoileal bypass with drainage of the bypassed small bowel into stomach. In Deitel M (ed): Surgery for the Morbidly Obese Patient, p 91. Philadelphia, Lea & Febiger, 1989

16. Graney AS, Smith LB, Hammer KA: Gastric partitioning for morbid obesity: Postoperative weight loss, technical complications, and protein status. J Am Diet Assoc 86:630, 1986

17. Griffen WO Jr, Bivins BA, Bell RM: The decline and fall of the jejunoileal bypass. Surg Gynecol Obstet 157:301, 1983

18. Halverson JD: Vitamin and mineral deficiencies following obesity surgery. Gastroenterol Clin North Am 16:307, 1987

19. Henriksson V: [Is small bowel resection justified as treatment for obesity?] Nordisk Med 47:744, 1952

20. Heshka S, Karol-Nauss C, Nyman K et al: Effects of chlorocitrate on body weight in obese men on a metabolic ward. Nutr Behav 2:233, 1985

21. Kral JG: Behavioral effects of vagotomy in humans. J Autonom Nerv Syst 9:273, 1983

22. Kral JG: Gastric balloons: A plea for sanity in the midst of balloonacy. Gastroenterology 95:213, 1988

23. Kral JG: Malabsorptive procedures in surgical treatment of morbid obesity. Gastroenterol Clin North Am 2:293, 1987

24. Kral JG: Surgical treatment of regional adiposity: Lipectomy versus surgically induced weight loss. Acta Med Scand Suppl 723:225, 1988

25. Kral JG: Vagotomy for treatment of severe obesity. Lancet 1:307, 1978

26. Kremen AJ, Linner JH, Nelson CH: An experimental evaluation of the nutritional importance of proximal and distal small intestine. Ann Surg 140:439, 1954

27. Leff RD, Aldo-Benson MA, Madura JA: The effect of revision of the intestinal bypass on post-

28. Lindor KD, Hughes RW, Ilstrup DM et al: Intragastric balloons in comparison with standard therapy for obesity: A randomized double-blind trial. Mayo Clin Proc 62:992, 1987

29. Linner JH: Surgery for Morbid Obesity. New York, Springer Verlag, 1984

30. Martin LF: Is the risk/benefit ratio for bariatric operation different for patients dependent on public assistance than for the privately insured? Int J Obes 12:602, 1988

31. Mason EE: Vertical banded gastroplasty. Arch Surg 117:701, 1982

32. Mason EE, Ito C: Gastric bypass and obesity. Surg Clin North Am 47:1355, 1967

33. Mason EE, Scott DH, Maher MD et al: Vertical banded gastroplasty: Sixth year results. Int J Obes 12:605, 1988

34. McFarland RJ, Gazet J-C, Pilkington TRE: A 13-year review of jejunoileal bypass. Br J Surg 72:81, 1985

35. McFarland RJ, Ang L, Parker W et al: The dynamics of weight loss after gastric partition for gross obesity. Int J Obes 13:81, 1988

36. Miller DK, Gordon GN: Gastric bypass procedures. In Deitel M (ed): Surgery for the Morbidly Obese Patient, p 113. Philadelphia, Lea & Febiger, 1989

37. Miskowiak KH, Larsen L, Andersen B: Food intake before and after gastroplasty for morbid obesity. Scand J Gastroenterol 20:925, 1985

38. Naslund I, Jarnmark I, Andersson H: Dietary intake before and after gastric bypass and gastroplasty for morbid obesity in women. Int J Obes 12:503, 1988

39. Pasulka PS, Bistrian BR, Benotti PN et al: The risks of surgery in obese patients. Ann Intern Med 104:540, 1986

40. Payne JH, DeWind LT: Surgical treatment of obesity. Am J Surg 118:141, 1969

41. Payne JH, DeWind LT, Commons RR: Metabolic observations in patients with jejuno-colic shunts. Am J Surg 106:273, 1963

42. Quaade F, Vaernet K, Larsson S: Stereotaxic stimulation and electrocoagulation of the lateral hypothalamus in obese humans. Acta Neurochir 30:111, 1974

43. Raymond JL, Schipke CA, Becker JM et al: Changes in body composition and dietary intake after gastric partitioning for morbid obesity. Surgery 99:15, 1986

44. Rogus J, Blumenthal SA: Variations in dietary intake after bypass surgery for obesity. J Am Diet Assoc 79:437, 1981

45. Rosensweig NS, Newman JH, Kral JG: Esophageal pathology in morbid obesity. Proc Am Soc Bariatric Surg, Nashville, 1989, p 22, 1990

46. Ryden O, Olsson S-A, Danielsson A et al: Weight loss after gastroplasty: Psychological sequelae in relation to clinical and metabolic observations. J Am Coll Nutr 9:15, 1989

47. Salmon PA: The results of small intestine bypass operations for the treatment of obesity. Surg Gynecol Obstet 132:965, 1971

48. Schepelmann E: Über Bauchdenkenplastik mit besonderer Berücksichtigung des Hängebauches. Beitr Z Klin Chir 111:372, 1918

49. Scopinaro N, Gianetta E, Civilleri D et al: Biliopancreatic bypass for surgery. II. Initial experience in man. Br J Surg 66:618, 1979

50. Scott HW Jr, Dean RH, Shull HJ et al: New considerations in use of jejunoileal bypass in patients with morbid obesity. Ann Surg 177:723, 1973

51. Siminowitz DA, Dellinger EP, Stothert JC Jr et al: Gastroplasty in patients with symptoms of reflux esophagitis. Surg Gynecol Obstet 154:235, 1982

52. Sugerman HJ, Londrey GL, Kellum JM et al: Weight loss with vertical banded gastroplasty and Roux-Y gastric bypass for morbid obesity with selective versus random assignment. Am J Surg 157:93, 1989

53. Sullivan MBE, Sullivan LGM, Kral JG: Quality of life assessment in obesity: Physical, psychological and social function. Gastrointest Clin North Am 16:433, 1987

54. Tang S, Kral JG: Malabsorptive procedures after failed gastroplasty. Int J Obes 12:608, 1989

55. Tang S, Yang MU, Wang J et al: Energy expenditure after massive weight loss. Int J Obes 13:408, 1989

56. Updegraff TA, Neufeld NJ: Protein, iron and folate status of patients prior to and following surgery for morbid obesity. J Am Diet Assoc 78:135, 1981

57. Yale CE: Gastric surgery for morbid obesity. Arch Surg 124:941, 1989

PART ELEVEN

TREATMENT— PHARMACOLOGIC

CHAPTER 64

Pharmacologic Treatment of Obesity

BERNARD N. BRODOFF and CHRISTINE NATHAN

Obesity has long been considered a major health hazard but has been officially designated so since 1985, when the National Institutes of Health Consensus Development Conference on the health implications of obesity recommended treatment of all individuals whose body weight exceeded desirable body weight (according to Metropolitan Life Insurance Company tables) by 20% or more.[1] This included over 35 million Americans as well as a substantial number of individuals in Western Europe and elsewhere around the world. Weight reduction in persons with lesser degrees of obesity was recommended if hypertension, diabetes, or a familial predilection for these illnesses coexisted with obesity.

Unfortunately, dietary therapy and more radical approaches to the treatment of obesity are largely ineffective in the long term. Moreover, many of the currently available prescription and anorectic drugs (Table 64-1) have unacceptable side-effects.[2] With the exception of the serotonergic agonist fenfluramine, these agents are thought to act by modulating central adrenergic and dopaminergic mechanisms and are mostly phenethylamine derivatives. Phenylpropanolamine (PPA) and its active enantiomer (l-norephedrine), while often considered to be members of the amphetamine class of anorexiants, appear to have an atypical adrenergic mechanism. PPA is available over the counter without a prescription. Although short-term use of these agents results in weight loss greater than that achieved by placebo, the long-term use of catecholaminergic compounds is restricted by potential addiction, tolerance, and the occurrence of catecholamine-

like side-effects. There is, therefore, a great need for the development of effective and safe pharmacologic agents for long-term use in the treatment of obesity. The next two chapters in this book are devoted to new classes of antiobesity drugs, the serotonergic appetite suppressants and the thermogenic agents. These agents are either in clinical use at the present time or in advanced clinical testing. Although this field is still in its infancy, numerous other agents are currently in various stages of development and there are many sites within the satiety cascade and in intermediary metabolism where pharmacologic intervention can be used to effect loss of body fat.

PHARMACOLOGIC AGENTS FOR THE TREATMENT OF OBESITY

Agents for the pharmacotherapy of obesity can be broadly divided into two categories: inhibitors of fat deposition (anorectic drugs, inhibitors of food absorption or of fatty acid synthesis) and stimulants of fat utilization (thermogenic or lipolytic agents). Table 64-2 lists some of the newer types of antiobesity drugs currently in development. Potential sites of pharmacologic intervention in obesity are shown in Figure 64-1, which is a simple scheme relating energy intake, energy storage, and energy expenditure. Any role for brown fat in human thermogenic mechanisms remains to be clarified. No fewer than 14 substrate cycles in other tissues, however, have been listed as potential sites of thermogenesis (futile cycles) in humans.[3] Figure 64-2 shows the numerous po-

TABLE 64-1

Prescription Anorectic Drugs Currently Available in the United States

Generic Name	Proprietary Name	US Drug Enforcement Administration Schedule*
Amphetamine	Dexedrine, Obetrol	II
Methamphetamine	Desoxyn	II
Phenmetrazine	Preludin	II
Benzphetamine	Didrex	III
Phendimetrazine	Plegine and others	III
Diethylpropion	Tenuate, Tepanil	IV
Fenfluramine	Pondimin	IV
Mazindol	Sanorex, Mazanor	IV
Phentermine	Fastin and others	IV
Phenylpropanolamine		Nonprescription

*Classification of degree of addiction, class I representing the most addictive drugs.

Adapted from Sullivan AC: Drug treatment of obesity: A perspective. In Berry EM, Blondheim SH, Eliahou E et al (eds.): Recent Advances in Obesity Research, vol. 5, p. 293. London, John Libbey, 1987. Reproduced by permission.

tential sites within the satiety cascade where food intake may be controlled pharmacologically. Table 64-3 lists a number of endogenous peptides that are involved in increasing satiety or hunger. Some of these peptides are also thought to modulate specific feeding, such as the type and amount of macronutrient intake and the feeding response to stress. By acting on the underlying neural organization of feeding in which messages are transmitted by the noradrenergic and serotonergic systems, peptide modulation of specific feeding may greatly enhance the sensitivity of and control over the entire satiety cascade.[4,5] As more is learned about these complex control mechanisms, the future role of analogues of these endogenous peptides in the treatment of obesity will be clarified.[6]

INDICATIONS FOR PHARMACOLOGIC THERAPY

Several questions regarding the pharmacotherapy of obesity remain unresolved:

1. When is drug therapy indicated?

2. How should pharmacologic agents be used?
3. Is there drug specificity for the treatment of different types of obesity?
4. Should obesity be viewed as a chronic disease?

Munro has discussed indications for short- and long-term drug therapy of obesity.[7] Mean additional weight loss in dieting patients that can be attributed to drug therapy is about 0.25 kg/week, but weight regain is common when therapy is discontinued. Some short-term indications are medical (preparation for elective surgery), economic (to pass an insurance examination, for a job interview), and psychological (to attend a social function such as a wedding). Longer term use of pharmacologic agents should be reserved for specific types of patients, for example those with a body mass index over 30 kg/m², a waist-hip circumference ratio over 0.9, or associated risk factors such as hypertension or type 2 diabetes mellitus. Furthermore, the risk-reward ratio must be favorable. The potential benefit of weight reduction achieved by pharmacologic intervention must clearly outweigh any possible

TABLE 64-2

Novel Antiobesity Drugs

Drug	Mechanism of Action
Inhibitors of Fat Deposition	
Serotonergic agents	Suppresses food intake, increases serotonin activity
Naltrexone	Suppresses food intake; an opioid antagonist
Chlorocitric acid	Suppresses food intake, inhibits gastric emptying
Cholecystokinin-octapeptide	Suppresses food intake, inhibits gastric emptying
Acarbose	Dietary carbohydrate absorption; α glucosidase inhibitor (nonabsorbable)
Bay O 1248	Dietary carbohydrate absorption; α glucosidase inhibitor (absorbable)
Tetrahydrolipstatin	Dietary fat absorption, pancreatic lipase inhibitor
RO22-0654	Stimulates lipid oxidation, inhibits lipid synthesis
Bay n 4605	Pancreatic lipase inhibitor
Sucrose polyester	Nonabsorbable fat
Bay n 2920	Inhibits dietary lipid and carbohydrate absorption
Stimulants of Fat Utilization	
Thermogenic agents	Increase metabolism, stimulate β-adrenoceptors (β_3)
α_2-Adrenergic receptor antagonists	Stimulate lipolysis
Yohimbine	
Idazoxon	
Rx 821002	
MK 912	
Atpamezole	
Phenoxybenzamine	

hazard of drug therapy: in potentially fatal conditions such as refractory obesity of severe degree, morbid obesity, or sleep apnea, long-term therapy would be indicated. Also, if pharmacologic therapy had an independent effect on conditions associated with obesity, such as type 2 diabetes mellitus, hypertension, or depression, or if there was a molecular basis for drug therapy in a specific form of obesity, the indication for long-term use would be even more firmly established.

If safe and effective agents were developed, drug therapy could be used not only for weight loss but also for weight maintenance following weight loss and for preventing weight gain in subjects with a predilection for obesity. Jequier believes that the best indication for the use of thermogenic agents, for example, may be in the postobese subject in whom resting energy expenditure and the thermic effect of food are less than in lean controls, leading to rapid regain of weight after successful weight loss regimens.[8] Finally, should drug therapy be used with a reducing

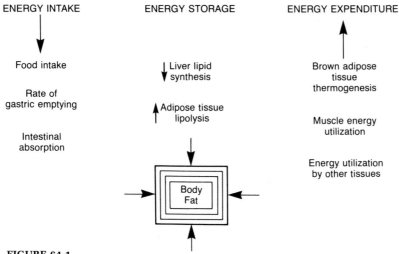

FIGURE 64-1

Potential sites of pharmacologic intervention in obesity. Adapted from Sullivan AC: Drug treatment of obesity: A perspective. In Berry EM, Blondheim SH, Eliahou E et al (eds): Recent Advances in Obesity Research, Vol. 5, p. 293. London, John Libbey, 1987. Reproduced by permission.

diet, before a diet is started, or after weight loss has been achieved? Should drug "holidays" be used in long-term treatment? After weight loss, multiple compensatory systems designed to maintain an elevated level of body fat in the obese subject come into play.[9] Should multiple pharmacologic interventions, either simultaneously or in series, be used in an attempt to overcome this problem? Partial or complete answers to these questions may be forthcoming with the continued use and clinical testing of these agents.

With regard to drug specificity, it is clear that obesity is multifactorial in its origin and manifestations, and different disorders of food intake and energy utilization may be involved in its development. Studies with the newer pharmacologic agents may shed light on the basic mechanisms of obesity and lead to a more specific classification of this disorder.

There is a growing perception among investigators that obesity should be treated as a chronic illness and subjected to long-term pharmacologic intervention, much as other chronic illnesses

such as hypertension and diabetes.[10,11] This will obviously require safe and effective drugs, as well as a reevaluation of the attitude toward treatment, not only on the part of the physician and patient, but also on the part of regulatory agencies like the Food and Drug Administration.

TABLE 64-3

Endogenous Peptides That Increase Satiety or Hunger

Stimulate hunger and food intake	Stimulate satiety, inhibit food intake
Opioids	Cholecystokinin
β-endorphin	Bombesin
Enkephalin	Neurotensin
Dynorphin	Calcitonin
Polypeptides	Glucagon
Neuropeptide Y	CRH
Peptide YY	Anorectin
Galanin	VPDPR
GRH	
Desacetyl MSH	

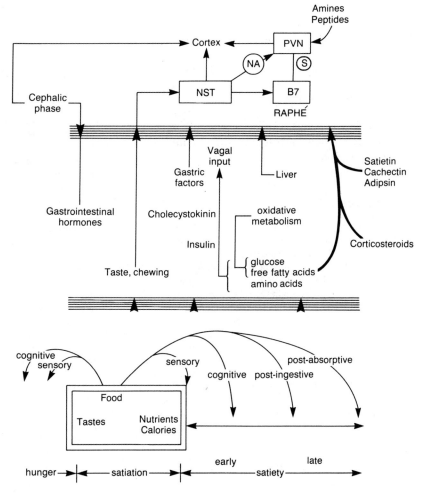

FIGURE 64-2

Contribution of different processes to the intensity and time course of satiety. The figure is read from left to right: hunger, feeding, and satiation through the early, mid and late stages of satiety leading to hunger and the next meal. Effects of food are read from bottom to top. Food has an anticipatory action to increase hunger before a meal by a cognitive process and also by its sensory properties. It acts after consumption to suppress hunger. This capacity is called satiating power or satiating efficiency. Satiety is the state of inhibition over further intake of food. Satiety can prolong the interval between meals or diminish intake at the next meal. The late stage can be extended by a diminished rate of digestion and absorption of food. The cephalic phase promotes intake and the response of the body to food. Sensory cues include taste, texture, and smell of food. Cognitive aspects refer to beliefs, for example, that food is high calorie or healthy. Postingestive effects denote gastric filling and emptying; distention of the gut. Postabsorptive effects denote the action of metabolic factors (e.g., volatile fatty acids in the large intestine). (NST, nucleus of the solitary tract, vagal input; PVN, paraventricular nucleus of the hypothalamus; NA, norepinephrine; S, serotonin; raphe nucleus, serotonin-containing cell bodies; T, tryptophan; LNAA, large neutral amino acids.) (Figure kindly supplied by Professor John E. Blundell, Biopsychology Group, Psychology Department, University of Leeds, Leeds, U.K.)

If an obese subject responds to pharmacologic therapy with weight loss, it is unrealistic to expect the weight loss to be maintained when the agent is stopped unless the drug has cured a disease process. Drug therapy may be useful in achieving and maintaining weight reduction to a greater degree than is currently possible with present-day methods, if this limitation is understood and accepted.

References

1. National Institute of Health Consensus Development Conference Statement: Health Implications of Obesity. Ann Intern Med 103:1073, 1985
2. Sullivan AC: Drug treatment of obesity: A perspective. In Berry EM, Blondheim SH, Eliahou E et al (eds): Recent Advances in Obesity Research, Vol 5, p 293. London, John Libbey, 1987
3. Newsholme RA, Challis RAJ, Leighton B et al: A possible common mechanism for defective thermogenesis and insulin resistance in obesity. In Berry EM, Blondheim SH, Eliahou HE et al (eds): Recent Advances in Obesity Research, Vol 5, p 144. London, John Libbey, 1987
4. Bray GA: Peptide control of food intake (abstr). Satellite Symposium to the 6th International Congress on Obesity: Pharmacological Treatment of Obesity, Yokohama, 1990
5. Smith GP, Gibbs J: Are gut peptides a new class of anorectic agents? (abstr). Satellite Symposium to the 6th International Congress on Obesity: Pharmacological Treatment of Obesity, Yokohama, 1990
6. Campfield AL: Pharmacology of CCK analogs for appetite suppression (abstr). Satellite Symposium to the 6th International Congress on Obesity: Pharmacological Treatment of Obesity, Yokohama, 1990
7. Munro JF: Clinical perspective on serotonin agents (abstr). Satellite Symposium to the 6th International Congress on Obesity: Pharmacological Treatment of Obesity, Yokohama, 1990
8. Jequier E, Munger R, Felber JP: Thermogenic effects of various β-agonists in humans (abstr). Satellite Symposium to the 6th International Congress on Obesity: Pharmacological Treatment of Obesity, Yokohama, 1990
9. Hirsch J: The present status of obesity research. In Hirsch J, Van Itallie TB (eds): Recent Advances in Obesity Research, Vol 4, p 374. London, John Libbey, 1990
10. Bray G: Round table discussion on clinical evaluation of antiobesity drugs: Issues and concerns. Satellite Symposium to the 6th International Congress on Obesity: Pharmacological Treatment of Obesity, Yokohama, 1990
11. Guy-Grand B, Apfelbaum M, Crepaldi G et al: Effect of withdrawal of dexfenfluramine on body weight and food intake after a one year's administration. Int J Obes 14(suppl 2):48, 1990

CHAPTER 65

Serotonin Agonists

CHRISTINE NATHAN

The use of serotoninergic drugs in the treatment of obesity has been the subject of growing research interest. In parallel with the interest in serotoninergic drugs, there is better understanding of the large variety of disorders of food intake and energy metabolism (or fuel utilization) that can cause or be associated with obesity. Recognition of this variety of phenomena (though not all present or present to the same degree in every subject) allows selection of specific treatment for the predominant aspect of obesity in individual patients.

Increasing evidence suggests distinct activities for some serotoninergic agents in obesity-related dysfunction. Serotoninergic drugs available for the treatment of human obesity have been limited to dl-fenfluramine and dexfenfluramine, and most of the data discussed here were obtained with the use of these two drugs. However, various other agents that may differ in their serotoninergic mechanisms of action are currently under evaluation. Some of them are listed in Table 65-1.

The assumption that experimental results in animals can predict the pharmacologic and therapeutic effects of a drug in humans is controversial. Differences exist between animal and human pathologies, especially in obesity. Another parameter that must be taken into account is the kinetics and metabolism of the drugs, which may vary with species, route of administration, dose, and several other factors. Nevertheless, animal data can be used to investigate the pharmacologic mechanisms underlying observed human behavior and the effects of drugs on it, even if such data are not primarily predictive.

SEROTONINERGIC DRUGS AND WEIGHT EVOLUTION

Animal Studies

Until recently, the effect of substances or drugs on the weight regulatory system was measured by weight changes in normal, young, nonobese, healthy animals. This does not reflect the situation obtaining human pathology and can lead to an erroneous determination of the active dose or of the potential clinical efficacy of the drugs under consideration. New models of animal obesity have been developed that more closely reflect the situation in humans. Such models include spontaneously obese old animals (rats, monkeys), obesity induced by a cafeteria-style diet (rats), and obesity in ovariectomized females (rats).

The efficacy of the serotoninergic drugs dl-fenfluramine and dexfenfluramine in inducing weight loss has been extensively demonstrated in different animal models and with various approaches. For dl-fenfluramine, active doses range from 1 mg/kg given orally (PO) to old rats up to 5 mg/kg given intraperitoneally (IP).[63,65] Dexfenfluramine is about twice as active in the same models.[65]

Other serotoninergic drugs have been less studied. Fluoxetine has been shown to induce weight loss in a few animal models. The daily doses were 10 mg/kg IP in rats and obese and

TABLE 65-1

Mode of Action of Various Compounds on the Serotoninergic System

Compounds	Serotoninergic Activity
Tryptophan, 5-hydroxytryptophan	Precursor
Fluoxetine (Fluvoxamine), Femoxetine (Sertraline), ORG 6582, RU 25591, LM 5008	Serotonin uptake inhibitors
dl-fenfluramine, dexfenfluramine, l-fenfluramine, CM 57373	Serotonin uptake inhibition and release
MCPP, CM57493, Quipazine, MK212	Postsynaptic 5-HT receptor agonists

nonobese mice, and 38 to 43 mg/kg PO in mice.[59,84,89]

Experimental Studies in Obese Patients

Weight-Lowering Effect of Serotonin Agonists in Obesity: Short-Term Studies

The weight-lowering effect of short-term administration of the racemic compound dl-fenfluramine is well documented.[63,73] With the selective serotonin agonist dexfenfluramine, several three-month double-blind placebo-controlled trials[17,22,23,45,53] have shown weight loss in unselected obesity,[17,53] refractory obesity,[22,53] and neuroleptic-induced obesity.[28] The products were given as the first treatment or after an initial trial of dietary treatment alone, permitting exclusion of patients that lost weight. The dose was 15 mg PO given twice daily. Whatever the methodological criteria, dexfenfluramine always resulted in a significantly greater weight loss than placebo. The mean difference between placebo and dexfenfluramine treatment was similar in the different studies; the absolute weight loss varied with selection criteria and study methodology.

The weight-lowering effects of several seroto-

nin reuptake blockers with antidepressant activity are currently being analyzed. A tendency to lose weight was reported in depressed patients treated with fluoxetine,[13,21] femoxetine,[74] and fluvoxamine.[30] By contrast, weight gain is often observed after treatment with nonserotoninergic antidepressants.

In double-blind, placebo-controlled studies, fluoxetine was reported to induce weight loss in obese patients treated for six to eight weeks,[41] with a statistically greater effect than was achieved with placebo. The effect depended on the doses used, with a maximal effect obtained with a daily dose of 60 mg PO. On the other hand, a 12-week controlled trial with fluvoxamine in patients with refractory obesity failed to demonstrate any significant effect compared to placebo, with both groups losing comparable amount of weight.[1] With femoxetine, a significantly larger weight loss was observed in the drug-treated obese patients in the first 16-week placebo-controlled study,[74] but this was not subsequently confirmed.[3] Finally, no significant effect was found for the serotonin precursor tryptophan in carbohydrate-craving obese subjects.[77] Therefore, although many drugs may modify serotonin metabolism or turnover in the brain, the effect on weight loss is not predictable.

Weight-Maintaining Effect of Serotonin Agonists in Obesity

The first goal in the treatment of obese patients with drugs may be to induce weight loss or to maintain (or increase) the weight loss previously achieved with other methods. If the limit of action of the first treatment has been reached, the metabolic and psychological counteracting factors typically become increasingly efficient, with a resulting weight gain.[31,33] In two six-month double-blind, placebo-controlled studies, dexfenfluramine further increased weight loss in patients who had already lost weight on a very low calorie diet[24] or any other conventional treatment.[54] Other serotonin agonists have not yet been tested.

Weight-Lowering Effect of Serotonin Agonists in Obesity: Long-Term Studies

The real goal of treating obesities is the long-term maintenance of a reduced body weight.[31] Until recently, metabolic disturbances leading to obesity were not therapeutically considered in the same way as other metabolic disturbances leading to hypertension, diabetes, hyperlipidemia, and so forth. In light of the long-term efficacy of drug treatment for obesity, new methodological problems have arisen that question existing pathophysiologic knowledge of human obesity. For instance, is a constant weekly decrement in weight to an ideal body weight not only utopian but physiologically impossible and psychologically risky? Which dynamic profile and what realistic amount of weight loss should be considered?

Another unresolved question is the homogeneity of patients entering a study (selection criteria). Can subjects with the indiscriminant diagnosis of obesity be enrolled without regard for the multifactorial origin of obesity?[31] As stated recently by Munroe, the major problem in long-term drug treatment is that it may require a change in the attitude on the part of health professionals as well as subjects, the latter often having unrealistic expectations of the target weight loss they hope to achieve.[51]

Very few studies have been carried out on the long-term effects of drugs in obesity. Munroe was an early pioneer in the analysis of long-term effects of a drug (fenfluramine) on weight loss. Patients who lost weight on a six-month drug treatment were enrolled in a further one-year placebo-controlled study. In the latter study the continuing drug treatment, unlike placebo, maintained the weight lost in a subgroup of patients.[16,52]

A one-year double-blind placebo-controlled trial was conducted with dexfenfluramine (15 mg twice daily) in 818 obese patients.[32] The study was conducted on an intention-to-treat basis. At the end of the trial, patients were subdivided into different groups according to weight lost, expressed as a percentage of initial body weight, whether they had been taking the drugs continuously or not. This led to an analysis of the result as the likelihood that a certain amount of weight loss would be achieved after one year of treatment. Results with dexfenfluramine were significantly and clinically better than with placebo. For example, after one year 34.9% of the initial cohort were 10% under their initial weight

in the dexfenfluramine group, compared to 17% in the placebo group. Analysis of weight evolution throughout the one-year study indicated that weight loss was achieved after six months and maintained for additional six months with dexfenfluramine. By contrast, a significant weight increase occurred in the placebo group. The dropout rate was higher in the placebo group, owing to significantly greater "dissatisfaction with treatment."

This study indicates that long-term drug therapy may be of therapeutic benefit in obesity, and that dexfenfluramine may be a good candidate for continuous use. Numerous questions remain, such as the appropriate duration of treatment (years? lifelong?) and the subgroup of obese patients (not all) who are most likely to benefit.

SEROTONINERGIC DRUGS AND EATING BEHAVIOR

Analysis of eating behavior should include measurement of various eating parameters, including total caloric intake, structure of eating throughout the day, food choice and macronutrient selection, eating sensation (hunger and satiety), environmental cues (e.g., hedonic value of food, including palatability and novelty), non-food-related stimulation of eating (stress or other stimuli), motivation to eat, and reward. Modification of the parameters will vary among subjects (animals or humans), but their evaluation should help clarify the different subgroups of obesity. Moreover, they can be specifically modified by certain categories of drugs. The effects of serotoninergic agonists on the different parameters have been studied.

Animal Studies and Clinical Pharmacology

Caloric Intake of a Test Meal

In classic models of nonobese, young, starved animals, most of the serotoninergic compounds decreased the caloric intake of a test meal, but with differences in the intensity of this effect (Table 65-2). The intensity of the effect for a given compound depends on the experimental paradigm. For example, the active dose of the only well-documented product, dexfenfluramine, ranges

TABLE 65-2

Caloric Intake at Meals in Nonobese, Young, Starved Rats Given Serotoninergic Compounds

Serotoninergic Compound	Mean Active Dose (mg/kg)
dl-fenfluramine	2.5
Dexfenfluramine	1–2
l-fenfluramine	>10
CM 57373	7.5
MCPP	2.5
CM 57493	10
Quipazine	5
MK 212	1.5–3
Tryptophan	50
5-HTP	37–50
5-HT	125
Fluoxetine	10–15
ORG 6582	20
RU 25591	20–40
LM 5008	No effect

from 0.06 mg/kg to 2 mg/kg, depending on the degree of obesity, the duration of pretest starvation, the quality of the meal, and other factors.[65] In humans, very few compounds have been studied. A single dose of dl-fenfluramine has a well-documented, dose-dependent effect.[53,73] A single dose of 60 mg given to human volunteers resulted in a 30% decrease in the amount of food eaten at a test meal. With dexfenfluramine, about the same effect was achieved with a dose of 30 mg.[53]

Structure of Eating Behavior: Eating Pattern Throughout the Day

The impact of serotoninergic drugs on feeding behavior throughout the day differs greatly from that seen with catecholaminergic compounds. Studies conducted with fenfluramine on the structure of eating behavior in rats indicate that the drug does not lead to a general inhibition of eating behavior, nor does it introduce abnormal patterns of behavior capable of interfering with the natural expression of eating.[7] The drug appears to produce a significant readjustment in the eating pattern by diminishing meal size and

slowing down the rate of eating, while having a negligible effect on meal initiation. By contrast, the amphetamines disrupt normal eating behavior. A similar effect on the pattern of eating has been observed with other serotonin agonists, including tryptophan, fluoxetine, and ORG 6582.[11,15] These findings are commonly referred to as the satieting effect of these drugs. The satiety system could be related to other aspects of eating behavior, including the motivational aspects of feeding, hoarding behavior, and food reward. Dexfenfluramine has been shown to have an effect on all these parameters, with a decrease in the motivational aspect of feeding as measured by runway performance,[65] a decrease in hoarding behavior as measured by the amount of food spared by deprived animals,[19,20] and a decrease in food reward as measured by self-stimulation.[36]

In humans, satiety can be analyzed through the effect of drugs on interprandial events. In humans, a meal decreases subsequent hunger, in lean as well as in obese subjects. Repeated administration of dexfenfluramine (15 mg twice a day for four days) to normal volunteers significantly prolonged the suppression of hunger and appetite after the meal and prevented the normal increase in eating motivation experienced two hours after a meal.[10]

In another study in which hunger and food intake were analyzed in obese and nonobese subjects, repeated administration (15 mg/kg twice a day for three to five days) of dexfenfluramine did not induce a significant premeal suppression of hunger but brought about a significant reduction of hunger and of meal size at a later test meal. It was concluded that in the long term, the drug may not lead to a tonic suppression of hunger, but may modulate the pattern of eating by intensifying the satieting effect of food.[6] This was confirmed by another study in which administration of dexfenfluramine (15 mg twice daily for four days) to normal volunteers decreased the number of small meals and snacks. These effects can be regarded as an inter-meal effect and are consistent with the drug's prolonged lowering of motivation to eat following a meal.[10]

Hedonic Value of Food

Overeating may result from the palatability or hedonic value of food, comprising different features such as taste, texture, sensory quality, novelty, and so forth.[8] Such an environmental cue could interfere with satiety or with satiation mechanisms.

The ventromedial area of the hypothalamus (VMH, paraventricular nucleus and medial region) involved in the regulation of the satiety processes integrates hedonic sensory outputs as well, and VMH-lesioned, obese rats are hyperreactive to hedonic factors.[29]

In animals, a decrease in ingestion linked to the palatability of food has been described with dexfenfluramine, using the dessert sucrose test, at a dose of 1.25 mg/kg,[12] and with fluoxetine, using a saccarine solution, at a dose of 10 mg/kg.[38] In humans, absorption of a standard meal significantly reduces the hedonic perception of highly preferred food (carbohydrate and protein). Administration of dexfenfluramine (15 mg twice daily) induced a further reduction in the preference for both carbohydrate and protein, with the effect particularly pronounced after the meal. Repeating the procedure for five days in the placebo group led to a decrease in hedonic perception of food (carbohydrate and protein) mainly after the meal, and no effect of dexfenfluramine was then observed.[34]

Stress-Induced Eating

The important role of emotional factors in overeating has long been recognized. Stress associated with traumatic emotional events has been held responsible for certain cases of obesity and implicated in the pathogenesis of eating disturbances such as night-eating syndrome and bulimia.[58,78] In animals, mild tail pressure induces eating and represents a model of stress eating in man. With this technique, considerable weight gain can be observed after repeated stimulation. Insulin-induced hypoglycemia, 2-deoxyglucose, and muscimol are also used in models of metabolic stress.

Fenfluramine, dexfenfluramine, quipazine, fluoxetine, and MK 212 reportedly reduce acute stress-induced eating at various doses, depending on the paradigms and the products.[2,66] Chronic administration of dexfenfluramine for 14 days (1.5 mg/kg/day IP) induced a sustained decrease in tail pinch–induced eating (Rowland, unpublished observations).

No well-established model of stress-induced eating is available in humans. Although bulimic episodes are linked to a stress situation, they correspond to a complex disease, which renders them an uncertain model of stress eating.

Macronutrient Selection

The involvement of various neurotransmitters, mainly the serotonin system, in macronutrient selection (protein and carbohydrate) is currently under study. It has been claimed that serotonin induces a selective depression of carbohydrate intake while sparing protein intake.[88] The mechanism described by Wurtman and Wurtman involves a complex loop in which modifications in the plasma ratio of tryptophan and neutral amino acids, triggered, for instance, by abnormality of insulin effect due to insulin resistance, play a major role through consequences on the serotonin system. The conditions under which this effect occurs are still under debate and may depend on the model and paradigm selected.

In animals, Wurtman's group has shown that fenfluramine and dexfenfluramine selectively inhibit high-carbohydrate diet of rats offered a two-choice diet (high protein, high carbohydrate).[85,86,88] This was recently confirmed by Li and Luo with dexfenfluramine at the same dose of 1 mg/kg IP.[44,49] The effect is shared by MK 212,[49] fluoxetine,[85] tryptophan,[85] and quipazine.[39]

Similarly, Leibowitz et al have demonstrated that the normally high intake of carbohydrates in early hours of dark cycle was selectively suppressed with dexfenfluramine in rats given 0.06 mg/kg of dexfenfluramine intraventricularly. At this dosage, no changes in protein and fat intake were observed.[37] Interestingly, chronic administration of dexfenfluramine (1 mg/kg IP once daily for five days) did not modify the selective effect of acute administration of the drug.[44]

In humans, studies were undertaken to determine if dexfenfluramine might selectively alter the disturbances in eating behavior manifested by carbohydrate-craving obese patients.[87] Patients, whose craving for carbohydrates in the form of snacks was established at the beginning of the study, were randomly allocated to dexfenfluramine (15 mg PO twice daily) or placebo for two eight-day periods in a double-blind, crossover design. They were given self-selected meals and had free access to a vending machine for snacks. The caloric and macronutrient content of the foods had been previously assessed in a way that allowed analysis of total food intake, macronutrient selection, and feeding pattern. After eight days of treatment, dexfenfluramine selectively decreased the abnormal pattern characterized by high-carbohydrate snacks, with no significant effect on protein consumption. The resultant drug effect was twice as great on the calories absorbed as snacks as on the calories absorbed at mealtimes.

A selective effect on carbohydrate-rich snacks has also been described with the parent drug dl-fenfluramine[86] and with the serotonin uptake inhibitor fluoxetine,[57] both given PO at a dosage of 60 mg/day in obese patients.

Therapeutic Applications

The specific effects of drugs on various parameters of feeding behavior open up a new field in the pharmacologic treatment of eating disorders in humans. The difficulties until now have been that eating behavior disturbances in man are far from being determined and that validated analytical rating scales have been available only for some eating parameters. Specific disorders of eating behavior in which the effect of serotoninergic drugs could be studied have therefore emerged only recently.

1. The effect of drugs on carbohydrate-craving obese patients was described in the previous section.

2. In patients with seasonal affective disorder, in which increased appetite, carbohydrate craving, and weight gain are associated with affective disturbances in the fall and winter, dexfenfluramine significantly reduced appetite disturbances, and improved affective disturbances.[55]

3. In patients with premenstrual syndrome, in which caloric, carbohydrate, and fat intake is significantly increased during the late luteal phase, accompanied by significant alterations in normal rating scales, the symptoms were reduced to their follicular-phase level with dexfenfluramine.[5,14]

The studies referred to in paragraphs 2 and 3

used a double-blind placebo-controlled crossover design, and results were taken into account only when statistically significant and clinically relevant.

4. Bulimia typically occurs in underweight or normal-weight subjects. In two separate double-blind placebo-controlled studies, Russell and Blouin have shown the effectiveness of dl-fenfluramine in alleviating acutely bulimic symptoms.[4,60] In a recent double-blind placebo-controlled study with dexfenfluramine, a tendency to reduce episodes of overeating and vomiting in the long term was reported.[68] The same was shown for fluoxetine in an open trial.[25]

These results are consistent with the mode of action of drugs on different components of the eating pattern. They also strongly suggest that decreased activity in some part of the serotonin system may be implicated in specific pathological disorders in humans.

SEROTONINERGIC DRUGS: METABOLIC EFFECTS

Thermogenic Effect

Numerous studies of dl-fenfluramine and dexfenfluramine indicate that these drugs also have a direct thermogenic effect in animals and humans. In rats, acute administration of the racemic compound dl-fenfluramine stimulated the activity of brown adipose tissue, measured by GDP binding to mitochondria in brown adipose tissue,[46,47,61] and enhanced metabolic rate.[61] This effect appeared to be at least partly dependent on the nutritional and metabolic status of the animals: Levitsky found no effect on metabolic rate in fasted animals, whereas the metabolic rate was enhanced in animals fed a large meal (thermic effect of food). This effect increased in animals fed a carbohydrate diet, disappeared in animals fed a lipid diet, and was significantly greater in diabetic than in nondiabetic animals.[42,43] The thermogenic effect persists after chronic treatment, as demonstrated by enhanced GDP binding in fenfluramine-treated rats compared with pair-fed controls[47] and by the maintenance of the pretreatment thermic effect of food in four-week-treated rats, despite weight loss.[43] However, the doses used in these animal studies were very high (20 mg/kg), much higher than usual pharmacologic doses.

Dexfenfluramine appears much more effective than the racemic compound. In rats, energy expenditure was significantly enhanced following acute administration of dexfenfluramine in dosages ranging from 0.5 mg/kg to 2 mg/kg, with different study paradigms. Results included an increase in metabolic rate and GDP binding in nondeprived animals,[61] an increase in basal metabolic rate and postprandial thermogenesis,[67] and enhanced energy expenditure after feeding, linked to the increased energy expenditure of the locomotor activity observed during the feeding period.[18] After chronic administration (1 to 3 mg/kg for four weeks) the brown adipose tissue thermogenic parameters were maintained at their pretreatment value, despite weight loss. By contrast, brown adipose tissue activity decreased in pair-fed control animals.[48]

Among the other serotoninergic compounds, a similar pattern (i.e., enhancement of the metabolic rate) was observed with 5-HT,[61] which confirms the involvement of the serotonin system in this effect. The effect of other serotoninergic agonists remains to be determined.

The enhancement of diet-induced thermogenesis after acute administration of dexfenfluramine (30 mg) has been confirmed in human, nonobese subjects[50] and obese patients.[71] Basal metabolic rate increased slightly or remained unchanged.

The importance of these effects in the weight-lowering efficacy of fenfluramine in obese patients must take into account several aspects:

1. In studies in humans, the quantitative importance of this effect in terms of number of extra calories burned after a caloric load is very low, compared with the total amount of energy expenditure. It is unlikely that this effect plays a noticeable role in the initial weight loss observed after treatment.

2. In animals or patients on restricted diets, weight loss is accompanied by a decrease in various thermogenic parameters, leading to an increase in metabolic efficiency. These effects have been said to counteract the weight-lowering efficacy of diet. The observed maintenance of normal thermogenesis by fenfluramine after weight

loss in animals, if confirmed in man, may partly explain the continuing efficacy of dexfenfluramine in long-term treatment or the additional weight loss in patients who have already lost weight on a very low calorie diet.

Glucose Metabolism

Glycemic parameters improve in obese diabetic patients who lose weight with the racemic compound dl-fenfluramine.[69] The same effect has recently been shown with fluoxetine.[83]

Diet and weight loss per se are well known to improve diabetic parameters in the obese. However, studies with dl-fenfluramine and dexfenfluramine suggest that an additional direct effect does occur. This effect is hypothesized to be peripheral. In man, dl-fenfluramine has been shown to improve glycemic control in obese, glucose-intolerant patients, independent of an effect on body weight and food intake.[79-81] In a recent double-blind placebo-controlled crossover study in patients with non-insulin-dependent diabetes mellitus treated with fenfluramine (60 mg daily) or placebo, a significant decrease in fasting blood glucose levels from baseline was observed after four weeks in the fenfluramine treatment group (13.0 vs. 8.4 mM), without any weight change (78.8 vs. 78.3 kg). Using the euglycemic hyperinsulinemic clamp technique, it was demonstrated that this effect was linked to enhanced insulin-induced peripheral glucose disposal. The metabolic clearance rate of insulin was increased.[56]

Comparable results have been obtained with dexfenfluramine. In a recent study in rats in which the euglycemic clamp was combined with the glucose-2-deoxyglucose technique, treatment with dexfenfluramine led to marked improvement in fat feeding insulin resistance, with effects on both liver and skeletal muscle.[76] In man, the effect of dexfenfluramine (30 mg PO) on glucose disposal was studied using the euglycemic hyperinsulinemic clamp technique, together with radiolabeled glucose infusion, in two double-blind placebo-controlled studies. To avoid weight change, short-term (1 week) treatment was given with a weight-maintaining diet. Obese diabetic (non-insulin-dependent diabetes mellitus) and nondiabetic (normal oral glucose tolerance) patients were included. In diabetic patients, dexfenfluramine significantly decreased fasting blood glucose (9.4 vs. 8.0 mM) and plasma free fatty acids without weight change. The glucose metabolic clearance rate was significantly enhanced during the glucose clamp. In contrast, no effect was observed in obese patients with normal oral glucose tolerance.[72]

The mechanism of action of these effects remains to be analyzed. Various hypotheses, mainly derived from in vitro experiments, include a direct inhibition of hepatic neoglucogenesis,[27] inhibition of lipogenesis in adipose tissue,[82] and increased glucose uptake by isolated skeletal muscle in some[37] but not all studies.[70] In the absence of studies of other serotoninergic agonists, an effect via the serotoninergic system remains to be determined.

CONCLUSION

The therapeutic benefit of a drug administered in the treatment of human obesity depends on its effects in three domains: weight, eating behavior, and fuel utilization. The recent interest in serotonin agonists in the treatment of human obesities focuses on the effects of one class of serotoninergic drug, the fenfluramines. The considerable number of studies now available allow one to hypothesize that the effects of dl-fenfluramine and dexfenfluramine are linked to their activity on the serotonin system and that the specific mechanism of action of the fenfluramines (i.e., inhibition of reuptake and enhancement of release) determine their therapeutic effects. A direct effect on glucose metabolism has also been implicated, although the specific mechanism has not been identified.

While the efficacy and profile of activity of the fenfluramines may serve as a model for serotoninergic drugs, we must be cautious about extrapolating data on the fenfluramines to any other agent that acts on the serotonin system. The effects of several serotonin agonists, all of whose mechanisms of action on the serotonin system differ from that of the fenfluramines, are currently under evaluation in humans. More data will help clarify the actions and effects of differ-

ent serotonin agonists as well as the serotonin system in general.

As a particular model for serotoninergic drugs, dexfenfluramine has two distinct kinds of effects. First is its effect on eating behavior, which is completely different from that of amphetamine-like compounds. Dexfenfluramine appears to enhance the satiating effect of a meal while decreasing interprandial food intake, the latter effect attributable to a decrease in patients' hyperreactivity to high-carbohydrate need, hedonic value of food, environmental stress, and so forth. Consequently, this effect may suggest a selective action on food intake triggered by nonenergetic needs.

Second is its effect on fuel utilization and glucose metabolism. Although more extensive analysis of this effect is needed, existing results suggest that fenfluramine decreases both the counterregulatory factors involved in weight regain and the insulin resistance often present in obese patients, for whom insulin resistance represents a cardiovascular risk factor.

Studies with other serotoninergic agonists, mainly fluoxetine, on eating parameters in animals reveal a similar pharmacologic profile of activity.

In aggregate, the data encourage continuing interest in serotoninergic drugs as promising agents in the treatment of human obesities.

References

1. Abell CA, Farquhar DL, Galloway SM et al: Placebo controlled double blind trial of fluvoxamine maleate in the obese. J Psychosom Res 30:143, 1986
2. Antelman SA, Rowland N, Kocan D: Anorectics: Lack of cross tolerance among serotonergic drugs and sensitization of amphetamine effect. In Garattini S, Samanin R (eds): Anorectic Agents. New York, Raven Press, 1981
3. Bitsh M, Skrumsager BK: Femoxetine in the treatment of obese patients in general practice. Int J Obes 11:183, 1987
4. Blouin A, Perez E, Blouin J et al: Bulimia treatment: Comparing desipramine to fenfluramine. Second International Conference on Eating Disorders. New York, April 19–20, 1986
5. Blundell J: Effect of dexfenfluramine on appetite in lean and obese human subjects and on changes

associated with premenstrual syndrome. In Paoletti R, Vanhoutte PM, Brunello N, Maggie FM (eds): Serotonin: From Cell Biology to Pharmacology and Therapeutics. Dordrecht, Kluwer Academic Publishers, 1990

6. Blundell J: Serotoninergic drug potentiates the satiating capacity of food: Action of dexfenfluramine in obese subjects. Ann NY Acad Sci 575:493. In Schneider LH, Cooper SJ, Halim KA (eds.): The psychology of human eating disorders, 1989

7. Blundell JE: Serotonin and appetite. Neuropharmacology 23:1537, 1984

8. Blundell JE: Systems and interactions: An approach to the pharmacology of eating and hunger. In Stunkard AJ, Stellar E (eds): Eating and Its Disorders. New York, Raven Press, 1984

9. Hill AJ, Blundell JE: Short-term effect of d-fenfluramine on hunger and food intake in obese women (abstr). 2nd European Congress on Obesity, Oxford, March-April, 1989

10. Blundell JE, Hill AJ: Serotoninergic modulation of the pattern of eating and the profile of hunger satiety in human. Int J Obes 11:141, 1987

11. Blundell JE, Latham CJ: Pharmacological manipulation of feeding behaviour: Possible influences of serotonin and dopamine on food intake. In Garattini S, Samanin R (eds): Central Mechanisms of Anorectic Drugs. New York, Raven Press, 1978

12. Borsini F, Bendotti C, Samanin R: Salbutamol, d-amphetamine and d-fenfluramine reduce sucrose intake in freely fed rats by acting on different neurochemical mechanisms. Int J Obes 9:277, 1985

13. Bremner JD: Fluoxetine in depressed patients: A comparison with imipramine. J Clin Psychiatry 45:414, 1984

14. Brzezinski A, Wurtman J, Wurtman R et al: Dexfenfluramine suppresses the increased calorie and carbohydrate intakes and improves the mood of women with premenstrual syndrome. Obstet Gynecol 76 (2):296, 1990

15. Clifton PG, Barnfield AMC, Philcox L: A behavioural profile of fluoxetine-induced anorexia. Psychopharmacology 97:89, 1989

16. Douglas JG, Gough J, Preston PG et al: Long term efficacy of fenfluramine in treatment of obesity. Lancet 1:384, 1987

17. Enzi G, Crepaldi G, Inelmen EM et al: Efficacy and safety of dexfenfluramine in obese patients: A multicenter study. Clin Neuropharmacol 11:173, 1988

18. Even P, Coulaud H, Aucouturier JL et al: Correlation between metabolic and behavioral effects of dexfenfluramine treatment. Clin Neuropharmacol 11:93, 1988

19. Fantino F, Faion F: Lowering body weight set point by dexfenfluramine. In Vague P, Björntorp P, Guy Grand B et al (eds): Metabolic Complications of Human Obesities. Amsterdam, Excerpta Medica, 1985

20. Fantino F, Faion F, Rolland Y: Effect of dexfenfluramine on body weight set-point: Study in the rat with hording behaviour. In Nicolaidis S (ed): Serotoninergic System, Feeding and Body Weight Regulation. London, Academic Press, 1986

21. Feighner JP: A comparative trial of fluoxetine and amitriptyline in patients with major depressive disorder. J Clin Psychiatry 46:369, 1985

22. Finer N, Craddock D, Lavielle R et al: Dextrofenfluramine in the treatment of refractory obesity. Curr Ther Res 38:847, 1987

23. Finer N, Craddock D, Lavielle R et al: Prolonged weight loss with dexfenfluramine treatment in obese patients. Diabetes Metabol 13:598, 1985

24. Finer N, Finer S: Dexfenfluramine after successful weight loss over 6 months (abstr). Int J Obes 13:130, 1989

25. Freeman CP: Fluoxetine treatment for bulimia. Second International Conference on Eating Disorders. New York, April 19–20, 1986

26. Garattini S, Borroni E, Mennini T et al: Differences and similarities among anorectic agents. In Garattini S, Samanin R (eds): Central Mechanisms of Anorectic Drugs. New York, Raven Press, 1978

27. Geelen MJH: Effects of fenfluramine on hepatic intermediary metabolism. Biochem Pharmacol 32:3321, 1983

28. Goodal E, Oxtoby C, Richards R et al: A clinical trial of the efficacy and acceptability of d-fenfluramine in the treatment of neuroleptic-induced obesity. Br J Psychiatry 153:208, 1988

29. Grossman SP: Contemporary problems concerning our understanding of brain mechanisms that regulate food intake and body weight. In Stunkard AJ, Stellar E (eds): Eating and Its Disorders. New York, Raven Press, 1984

30. Guy W, Wilson WH, Ba TA et al: Psychopharmacol Bull 20:73, 1984

31. Guy Grand B: Long-term pharmacotherapy in the management of obesity: From therapy to practice. In Björntorp P, Rossner S (eds): Obesity in Europe 88. London, John Libbey, 1989

32. Guy Grand B, Apfelbaum M, Crepaldi G et al: International trial of long-term dexfenfluramine in obesity. Lancet 2:1142, 1989

33. Guy Grand B, Waysfeld B, Le Barzic M: Resistances à l'amaigrissement. Rev Prat 34:3111, 1984

34. Hill AJ, Blundell JE: Model system for investigating the actions of anorectic drugs: Effect of dexfen-

fluramine. In Ferrari E, Brambilla F (eds): Disorders of Eating Behaviour. New York, Pergamon Press, 1986

35. Hill AJ, Blundell JE: Short-term effect of d-fenfluramine on hunger and food intake in obese women (abstr). Int J Obes 13:137, 1989

36. Hoebel BG, Hernandez L, McClelland RC et al: Dexfenfluramine and feeding reward. Clin Neuropharmacol 11:72, 1988

37. Kirby MJ: Dose related effect of fenfluramine and norfenfluramine on glucose uptake into human isolated skeletal muscle. Br J Clin Pharmacol 1:511, 1974

38. Leander JD: Fluoxetine suppresses palatability-induced ingestion. Psychopharmacology 91:285, 1987

39. Leibowitz SF, Shor-Posner G: Brain serotonin and eating behavior. In Nicolaidis S (ed): Serotoninergic System, Feeding and Body Weight Regulation. London, Academic Press, 1986

40. Leibowitz SF, Weiss GF, Shor-Posner G: Hypothalamic serotonine. Clin Neuropharmacol 11:51, 1988

41. Levine LR, Thompson RG, Bosomworth JC: Fluoxetine, a serotoninergic drug for obesity control. In Björntorp P, Rossner S (eds): Obesity in Europe 88. London, John Libbey, 1989

42. Levitsky AD, Schuster JA, Stallone D et al: Modulation of the thermic effect of food by fenfluramine. Int J Obes 10:169, 1986

43. Levitsky DA, Stallone D: Enhancement of the thermic effect of food by d-fenfluramine. Clin Neuropharmacol 11:90, 1988

44. Li ETS, Luo S: The effect of acute and daily administration of dexfenfluramine on food intake and choice of rats (abstr). Int J Obes 13:147, 1989

45. Louvet JP: Isomeride et traitement des surcharges pondérales. Ann Med Intern 140:17, 1989

46. Lupien JR, Bray GA: Effect of fenfluramine on GDP-binding to brown adipose tissue mitochondria. Pharmacol Biochem Behav 23:509, 1985

47. Lupien JR, Tokunaga K, Kemnitz JW et al: Lateral hypothalamic lesions and fenfluramine increase thermogenesis in brown adipose tissue. Physiol Behav 38:15, 1986

48. McCormarck JG, Dean HG, Midgley SE et al: Diet-induced obesity: The effects of long-term administration of d-fenfluramine (Isomeride) on weight gain and caloric-intake, brain neurotransmitter levels, and brown adipose tissue thermogenic parameters in the rat. 1st European Congress on Obesity, p 284. Stockholm, June 5–6, 1988

49. Moses PL, Wurtman RJ: The ability of certain anorexic drugs to suppress meal consumption depends on the nutrient content of the text diet. Life Sci 35:1297, 1984

50. Munger R, Lavielle R, Arnaud O et al: Enhanced diet induced thermogenesis in human after administration of dexfenfluramine. 1st European Congress on Obesity, p 283. Stockholm, June 5–6, 1988

51. Munro JF: Drug treatment of obesity: An overview. Int J Obes 11:13, 1987

52. Munro JF, Ford MJ: Drug treatment of obesity. In Silverstone T (ed): Drugs and Appetite. London, Academic Press, 1982

53. Nathan C, Rolland Y: Pharmacological treatments that affect CNS activity: Serotonin. Ann NY Acad Sci 499:272, 1986

54. Noble RE: A 6 month study of the effects of dexfenfluramine on partially successful dieters (abstr). Int J Obes 13:146, 1989

55. O'Rourke D, Wurtman JJ, Wurtman RJ: Serotonin implicated in the etiology of seasonal affective disorder with carbohydrate craving. In Pirke KM, Vandereycken W, Ploog D (eds): The Psychobiology of Bulimia Nervosa. Heidelberg, Springer-Verlag, 1988

56. Pestell RG, Crock PA, Ward GM et al: Fenfluramine increases insulin action in patients with NIDDM. Diabetes Care 12:252, 1989

57. Pijl H, Koppeschaar HPF, Meinders AE: Fluoxetine and dietary intake and composition (abstr). Int J Obes 13:131, 1989

58. Pyle RL, Mitchell JE, Eckert ED: Night eating syndrome. J Clin Psychiatry 42:60, 1981

59. Reid LR, Therelkeld PG, Wong DT: Reversible reduction of food intake and body weight by chronic administration of fluoxetine (abstr). Pharmacologist 26:184, 1984

60. Robinson PH, Checkley SA, Russell GMF: Suppression of eating by fenfluramine in patients with bulimia nervosa. Br J Psychiatry 146:169, 1985

61. Rotwell NJ, Lefeuve RA: Thermogenic effects of serotoninergic pathways and d-fenfluramine in the rat (abstr). Eighteenth Steenbock Symposium: Hormones, Thermogenesis, and Obesity, June 12–16, 1988

62. Rotwell NJ, Stock MJ: Effect of diet and fenfluramine on thermogenesis in the rat: Possible involvement of serotoninergic mechanisms. Int J Obes 11:319, 1987

63. Rowland N, Carlton J: Neurobiology of an anorectic drug: Fenfluramine. Prog Neurobiol 27:13, 1986

64. Rowland NE, Antelman SM, Bartness TJ: Comparison of the effect of fenfluramine and other anorectic agents in different feeding and drinking paradigms in rat. Life Sci 36:2295, 1985

65. Rowland NE, Carlton J: Dexfenfluramine: Effects

on food intake in various animal models. Clin Neuropharmacol 11:33, 1988

66. Rowland NE, Carlton J: Tolerance to the effects of d-fenfluramine in rats, hamsters and mice. In Ferrari E, Brambilla F (eds): Disorders of Eating Behavior. New York, Pergamon Press, 1986, pp 367–374

67. Rozen R, Fantino M, Mandenoff A et al: Thermogenic effects of d-fenfluramine in rat (abstr 144). 2nd European Congress on Obesity. Int J Obes 13, 1989

68. Russell GMF: Bulimia revisited. Second International Conference on Eating Disorders. New York, April 19–20, 1986

69. Salmela PJ, Sotaniemi EA, Viikari J: Fenfluramine therapy in non-insulin dependent diabetic patients. Diabetes Care 4:535, 1981

70. Sasson E, Cerasi E: Does dexfenfluramine reduce blood glucose by affecting skeletal muscle glucose transport (abstr 143). 2nd European Congress on Obesity, Oxford. Int J Obes 13, 1989

71. Scalfi L, D'Arrigo E, Carandente V et al: The effect of d-fenfluramine on BMR and postprandial thermogenesis in obese subjects (abstr 142). 2nd European Congress on Obesity. Int J Obes 13, 1989

72. Scheen AJ, Paolisso G, Lefebvre PJ: Dexfenfluramine improves insulin-induced glucose disposal in type-2 diabetic but not in non-diabetic obese subjects (abstr 286). 1st European Congress on Obesity, Stockholm, June 5–6, 1989

73. Silverstone T: Measurement of hunger and food intake. In Silverstone T (ed): Drugs and Appetite. London, Academic Press, 1982

74. Smedegaard J, Cristiansen P, Strumsager BK: Treatment of obesity by femoxetine, a selective 5-HT reuptake inhibitor. Int J Obes 5:377, 1981

75. Souquet AM, Rowland NE: Effect of chronic administration of dexfenfluramine on stress and palatability induced food intake in rats. Physiol Behav 46:145, 1989

76. Storlien AH, Thorburn AW, Smythe GA et al: Effect of d-fenfluramine on basal glucose turnover and fat feeding induced insulin resistance in rat. Diabetes 38:499, 1989

77. Strain GW, Strain JJ, Zumoff B: L-tryptophan does not increase weight loss in carbohydrate craving obese subjects. Int J Obes 9:375, 1985

78. Stunkard AJ: Obesity. In Freedman M, Kaplan L, Sadock J (eds): Comprehensive Textbook of Psychiatry, 2nd ed, p 1648. Baltimore, Williams & Wilkins, 1975

79. Turtle JR, Burgess JA: Hypoglycemic action of fenfluramine in diabetes mellitus. Diabetes 22:858, 1973

80. Verdy M, Charboneau L, Chiasson JL: Fenfluramine in the treatment of non-insulin dependent diabetics. Int J Obes 7:289, 1983

81. Wales JJ: The effect of fenfluramine on obese, maturity-onset diabetic patients. Curr Med Res Opinion 6:256, 1979

82. Wilson JPD, Galton DJ: The effect of drugs on lipogenesis from glucose and palmitate in human adipose tissue. Horm Metab Res 3:262, 1971

83. Wise S: Use of fluoxetine in obese diabetic patients (abstr). Int J Obes 13, 1989

84. Wong DT, Yen TT: Suppression of appetite and reduction of body weight in normal and obese mice by fluoxetine. Fed Proc 44:1162, 1985

85. Wurtman JJ, Wurtman RJ: Drugs that enhance central serotoninergic transmission diminish elective carbohydrate consumption by rats. Life Sci 24:895, 1979

86. Wurtman JJ, Wurtman RJ: Suppression of carbohydrate consumption as snacks and at mealtime by dl-fenfluramine or tryptophan. In Garattini S, Samanin R (eds): Anorectic Agents: Mechanisms of Action and Tolerance. New York, Raven Press, 1981

87. Wurtman JJ, Wurtman RJ, Mark S et al: d-Fenfluramine selectively suppresses carbohydrate snacking by obese subjects. Int J Eat Disord 4:89, 1985

88. Wurtman RJ, Wurtman JJ: Nutrients, neurotransmitter synthesis and the control of food intake. In Stunkard AJ, Stellar E (eds): Eating and Its Disorders, p 77. New York, Raven Press, 1984

89. Yen TT, Wong DT, Bemis KG: Reduction of food consumption and body weight of normal and obese mice by chronic treatment with fluoxetine. Drug Dev Res 10:37, 1987

CHAPTER 66

Thermogenic Drugs

M. A. CAWTHORNE

Body weight is maintained constant when energy intake in the form of nutrients is matched by energy expenditure. To lose weight, one must either reduce energy intake or increase energy expenditure. Traditionally, pharmacotherapy for obesity has focused on agents that affect appetite. Such agents lower food intake by modulating dopaminergic, adrenergic, or serotoninergic pathways in the brain. Careful analysis of 210 double-blind clinical trials by a Food and Drug Administration (FDA) working party showed that in 90% of the clinical studies, drugs produced a greater weight loss than placebo.[54] However, the overall weight loss attributable to drug therapy, 0.23 kg/week, was maintained for only four weeks. After this time, with the possible exception of fenfluramine, the rate of weight loss fell rapidly.[21] Chronic use of the currently available appetite suppressant drugs is restricted as a result of side effects, including potential addiction and the apparent development of tolerance. Most clinicians perceive the failure of phenylethylamine appetite suppressants to continue to cause significant weight loss after four weeks as reflecting pharmacologic tolerance, but this may not be the case.[15,48] Rather, since withdrawal of the therapy invariably results in rapid weight regain, it may indicate the achievement of a new steady state of energy balance.[15] New anorexic agents such as d-fenfluramine and fluoxetine, which modulate 5-hydroxtryptamine metabolism, are likely to be marketed in the near future. Although these agents have overcome the drug addiction liability, it remains to be established whether they will produce sustained weight loss.

Dietary restriction, with or without support from anorexic drug therapy, is likely to remain the cornerstone of obesity treatment for the foreseeable future. However, since nutrient intake is closely linked with metabolic rate, the effect of dietary restriction on body fat loss is limited invariably by a decline in the metabolic rate. Moreover, weight loss induced by dietary restriction in obese rodents,[69] and probably in man, results in a reduction in all body components.

Exercise is the most obvious way to increase energy expenditure, and there is much published work showing that exercise in rats has a marked antiobesity effect and that the tissue lost is principally fat. This effect of exercise on the composition of the weight loss contrasts with the effect of diet restriction (Fig. 66-1). In man, the value of exercise has been more difficult to substantiate, but it is likely that the energy cost of exercise extends well beyond the period of activity into the postexercise oxygen debt period. The available evidence suggests that the most successful form of exercise for weight reduction is aerobic daily exercise, such as running for substantial periods at 70% of Vo_2max. Unfortunately, in severely obese subjects, such exercise may be impossible because of cardiovascular or mechanical problems.

There is, therefore, a significant need for safe and efficacious agents that will complement dietary restriction to maintain or increase metabolic rate in subjects on a restricted diet. Such drugs should ideally mimic the metabolic effects of chronic exercise, and it is probable that they will be taken not only to lose weight but also

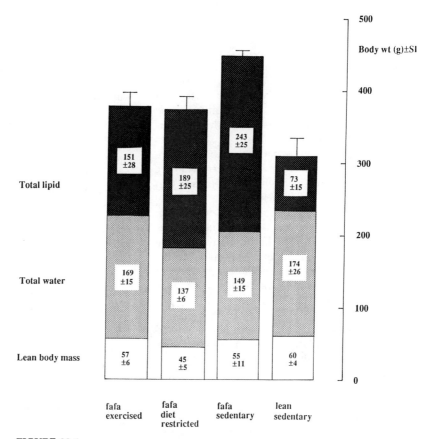

FIGURE 66-1

Effect of exercise and diet restriction on body composition in Zucker fa/fa rats. Six- to eight-week-old rats weighing 212 ± 34 g were allowed voluntary exercise in a wheel for 11 weeks. A sedentary group was diet-restricted by 34% (overall reduction in food intake), to maintain the same body weight as the exercised rats. (Data from Wilson et al.[69])

to prevent weight regain. Such agents should be regarded as weight-controlling rather than merely weight-reducing.

In trying to develop a new approach to the treatment of obesity, it is useful to define the properties of an ideal antiobesity agent. Sullivan[64] has suggested that the ideal treatment should achieve the following:

1. Produce a sustained reduction in body weight through a selective decrease in body fat stores, with a sparing of body protein,
2. Prevent weight regain once desirable body weight has been reached,

3. Improve compliance with a sound weight reduction program was based on a combination of diet and exercise,
4. Have no significant side effects or abuse potential when given chronically.

To this list one might add two more desirable properties. The agent should (1) have a greater effect in obese subjects than in lean subjects, and should not cause significant weight loss in lean subjects, and it should produce favorable alterations in the disturbed metabolic profile (e.g., lower plasma concentrations, triglycerides, free fatty acids, insulin, and glucose).

THYROID HORMONES

The prototype thermogenic drug is thyroid hormone, which was first used in the treatment of obesity in 1893.[12] Exogenous thyroid hormone administration suppresses endogenous thyroid hormone production. Since the majority of obese patients are euthyroid,[12] the use of thyroid hormone in the treatment of obesity is difficult to justify except in the few patients who are hypothyroid. It has been suggested that the metabolic rate falls during treatment with a low-calorie diet because of a fall in the plasma concentration of thyroid hormones,[36] and it may therefore be appropriate to provide triiodothyronine (T_3) together with a low-calorie diet to maintain metabolic rate. However, there are two further problems with thyroid hormone therapy. First, a substantial proportion of the weight lost is lean body mass rather than fat.[2] Indeed, the fall in thyroid hormone levels during dieting may be part of a mechanism to conserve lean body tissues rather than energy stores.[37] In experimental studies, negative nitrogen balance can be prevented with anabolic steroids and growth hormone administration without affecting oxygen consumption,[14] but these treatment adjuncts have not found clinical acceptability. The second problem with thyroid hormones is that they affect cardiac function.

Many mechanisms, by which thyroid hormones increase metabolic rate, have been postulated. These include uncoupling of oxidative phosphorylation,[31] enhancement of the activity of Na^+-K^+-ATPase thereby increasing Na^+ and K^+ pumping across cell membranes,[23] and enhanced activity of mitochondrial α-glycerophosphate dehydrogenase.[58] None of these mechanisms appears capable of explaining the thermogenic activity of thyroid hormones. Enhancement of the thermogenic action of noradrenaline and adrenaline in cardiac and skeletal muscle is a more plausible mechanism. This effect appears to be a consequence of increased β-adrenoceptor number or improved coupling of the receptor to adenylate cyclase activation by the guanosine triphosphate (GTP)-dependent protein, Gs.[11,40] However, such an effect is only important when sympathetic activity is increased and cannot account for thyroid hormone stimulation of basal metabolic rate, since in the latter case sympathetic activity is minimal. The most likely explanation for most of the increase in basal metabolic rate is that thyroid hormones increase the turnover rate of a number of cellular processes, including some in the glycolytic pathway, the Cori cycle, and protein turnover.[47]

DINITROPHENOL

Dinitrophenol was the first synthetic thermogenic drug used specifically for treating obesity. Its thermogenic action was noticed in workers in munitions plants during World War I, but it was not reported in the literature until 15 years later.[49] It was introduced for the treatment of obesity in 1933 and was very effective. However, side effects were common and serious, including rashes, neurologic defects, cataracts, and some deaths. Its use was discontinued in 1936,[57] although by this time it had been taken by 100,000 patients.

Dinitrophenol increases metabolic rate by uncoupling nicotinamide-adenine dinucleotide (reduced) (NADH) oxidation from adenosine triphosphate (ATP) production, resulting in unrestrained fuel combustion.[49] This action may be responsible for some of the serious side-effects. If so, it follows that uncontrolled uncoupling of NADH oxidation from ATP synthesis is an unacceptable mechanism for any thermogenic drug.

THERMOGENIC AGENTS IN EVERYDAY LIFE

Several agents commonly consumed by humans are known to increase metabolic rate.[45] Caffeine was first shown to increase the metabolic rate in 1914, but, despite the finding that the amount present in a cup of coffee will produce a significant thermogenic response,[32] there have been no reports of any antiobesity action in man, and mixed results have been obtained in animals.[22,67] This is probably because the metabolic stimulant effect is short-lived and followed by a period of depressed metabolic rate (see Fig. 66-2).[8] One would have to consume many cups of coffee in order to maintain the elevated metabolic rate throughout the day; such consumption would introduce both central nervous system and cardiovascular side-effects.

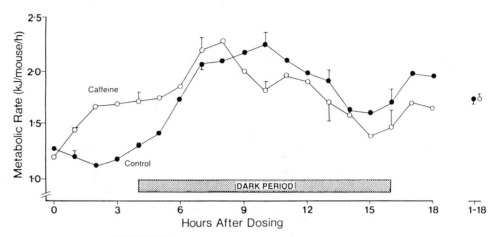

FIGURE 66-2

Effect of caffeine on metabolic rate in mice. CDI mice (23–26 g) were dosed with water and caffeine (50 mg/kg PO) and energy expenditure was measured by indirect calorimetry. (From Arch JRS et al: Recent Adv Obes Res 5:300, 1987. Reproduced by permission.)

The original proposal for the thermogenic action of caffeine was by increasing cAMP as a result of inhibition of cAMP phosphodiesterase. However, a concentration of caffeine in plasma of 30 μmol/liter increases metabolic rate markedly in man,[3] but the K_i of phosphodiesterase inhibition by caffeine is 600μM.[27] Furthermore, more potent phosphodiesterase inhibitors such as papaverine are less thermogenic than caffeine.[8] An alternative explanation is that caffeine blocks one of the actions of endogenous adenosine, but the more potent adenosine antagonist 8-phenyltheophylline has no thermogenic activity.[8] It seems likely that caffeine interacts selectively with either a currently undefined subtype of cAMP phosphodiesterase or with a subtype of the adenosine receptor.

The appetite-reducing effects of nicotine are well known and are generally thought to be responsible for the weight increase that often occurs on cessation of smoking.[20] It is also clear that in both animals and man, smoking has a thermogenic effect that is mainly due to nicotine, although smoking a denicotinized cigarette also increases metabolic rate.[25] It is likely that the effect of nicotine occurs via stimulation of nicotinic acetylcholine receptors, which are present in a wide range of tissues.

ETHICAL APPETITE SUPPRESSANTS

Some of the prescription anorectic drugs (phentermine, mazindol, diethylpropion) also increase sympathetic activity, and in rodents there is good evidence that much of their antiobesity activity is due to stimulation of metabolic rate (Fig. 66-3).[5,38] In the same studies,[5] it was not possible to demonstrate directly that dl-fenfluramine increased metabolic rate significantly; nevertheless, obese mice given fenfluramine had a lower body weight than pair-fed controls. In recent studies in normal rats,[13,41] fenfluramine significantly increased the binding of guanosine-5-diphosphate (an indicator of thermogenic activity) to mitochondria from brown adipose tissue,[41] the firing rate of efferent nerves to brown adipose tissue,[13] and oxygen consumption.[53] However, although fenfluramine has effects on brown adipose tissue in animals, there is no evidence that it stimulates thermogenesis in man.

SYMPATHOMIMETIC AGENTS

Phenylpropanolamines and N-methyl phenylpropanolamines such as ephedrine are sympathomimetic agents with known anorectic properties. In 1972, a Danish general practitioner in

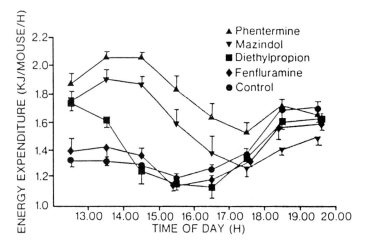

FIGURE 66-3

Acute thermogenic activity of anorexic drugs in mice. CFLP mice were
given anorexic drugs by oral gavage at
a dosage of 25 mg/kg. (From Arch JRS:
Am J Clin Nutr 34:2763, 1980. Reproduced by permission.)

Elsinore, Dr. Erikson, noted unintentional weight
loss in asthmatic patients for whom he had prescribed a mixture containing ephedrine, caffeine,
and phenobarbital.[42] He pursued this observation, and when sales culminated in 1979, more
than 70,000 people were taking the preparation.
At the same time, there were a disturbing number
of cutaneous reactions, some of them serious. It
is now realized that these were probably due to
the phenobarbital component.

More recently a controlled trial has been carried out using a barbiturate-free version of Erikson's preparation[42] in comparison with placebo
and a standard anorectic agent (diethylpropion)
in subjects instructed to take a 1200-kcal diet.
The ephedrine/caffeine pill and diethylpropion
were equally effective and significantly better
than placebo. Although the effects of ephedrine
were originally assumed to be due to its anorectic
action, it is now established that ephedrine is
thermogenic in man, and weight loss can be produced in animals independent of any effect on
food intake. A significant increase in metabolic
rate is produced in man[10] at dosages of 0.25 and
0.5 mg/kg (Fig. 66-4), and in subjects given 1 mg/
kg the effects can be detected by infrared thermography.[52] However, ephedrine given alone
has produced equivocal results with respect to
antiobesity effects, although it is effective in
combination with caffeine. The effect of ephedrine is believed to be a consequence of noradrenaline release, leading to thermogenesis in brown

adipose tissue and skeletal muscle. The release
of noradrenaline induced by sympathomimetics
occurs widely throughout the body and the endogenous noradrenaline can act at a wide variety
of adrenergic receptors. Thus, it would be surprising with this type of agent if thermogenesis
leading to weight loss could be achieved without
side-effects. A major site of these side-effects will
be the cardiovascular system, and studies using
1 mg/kg, which is two to four times the thermogenic dose, produced significant alterations in
diastolic and systolic blood pressure.

The ephedrine congeners dl-phenylpropanol-
amine and d-norpseudoephedrine are used in the
treatment of obesity in many parts of the world,
including the United States, Australia, and parts
of Europe, but serious reservations have been expressed concerning the safety of these compounds at the dose level employed for treating
obesity.

β-ADRENOCEPTOR AGONISTS

Sympathomimetic agents such as ephedrine
cause a nonselective stimulation of the sympathetic nervous system. It was first recognized by
Ahlquist[4] that adrenaline and noradrenaline
stimulate two types of adrenoceptor, α and β.
Later it was realized that both of these receptor
types could be further subdivided into at least
two subtypes, α_1, α_2 and β_1, β_2.

The development of thermogenic drugs for the

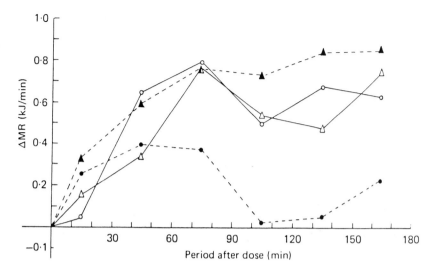

FIGURE 66-4

Thermic effect of ephedrine in man. Ephedrine hydrochloride, 0.50 mg/kg
($\triangle$-$\triangle$, $\bigcirc$-$\bigcirc$) or 0.25 mg/kg ($\blacktriangle$-$\blacktriangle$, $\bullet$-$\bullet$), was administered orally to men on
high energy intake ($\triangle$, $\blacktriangle$) or low energy intake ($\bigcirc$, $\bullet$). (From Morgan JB et al:
Br J Nutr 42:21, 1982. Reproduced by permission.)

potential treatment of obesity has been facilitated
by the development of rapid drug screening procedures based on the measurement of metabolic
rate in rodents.[16,62] The availability of such procedures allowed screening for the thermogenic
activity of pharmacologic tools. In our laboratory, in 1977, it was discovered that the partial
β-adrenoceptor agonist dichloroisoprenaline had
potent and long-lived thermogenic activity (Arch
and Cawthorne, unpublished findings). In contrast, α-adrenoceptor agonists had minimal or no
thermogenic activity. β-adrenoceptors are present in a wide range of tissues and are involved
in the stimulation of heart rate (β_1), contraction
of smooth muscle, and striatal muscle tremor
(β_2). The development of a β-adrenoceptor agonist as a thermogenic antiobesity agent is contingent on achieving selective stimulation of
thermogenesis rather than activation of β_1- and
β_2-adrenoceptors.

Most of the literature on the potential of β-
adrenoceptor agonists as antiobesity agents has
been published by four pharmaceutical companies: Beecham (now SmithKline Beecham) and
Imperial Chemical Industries in the United King-

dom, Eli Lilly in the United States, and Hoffman
LaRoche in Switzerland. The structures of the
key compounds, given in Figure 66-5, show a
remarkable similarity.

The first compounds to be designed using this
type of procedure included BRL 26830 and BRL
35135.[6,7] Both are potent stimulants of metabolic
rate but have little effect on heart rate, compared
with standard β-adrenoceptor agonists. When
given chronically to genetically obese (C57B1/6
ob/ob) mice, both compounds produce a significant reduction in body fat mass with no change
in body water or lean body mass (Figure 66-6).

BRL 26830 and BRL 35135 are methyl esters
and are rapidly converted to the free acids BRL
28410 and BRL 37344 in vivo. These latter compounds have generally been used in receptor selectivity studies in vitro. Studies by Foster and
Frydman[26] had demonstrated an important role
for brown adipose tissue in noradrenaline-
stimulated thermogenesis. In addition, two
groups in Great Britain,[52,66] stimulated by the
findings of Foster and Frydman and the pioneering studies of Hull on brown adipose tissue function in neonates, showed that brown adipose tis-

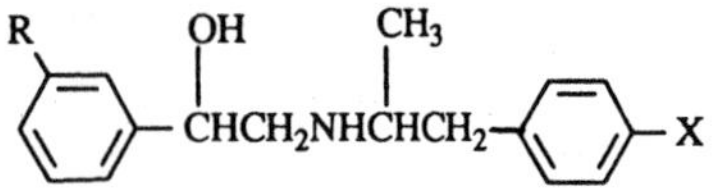

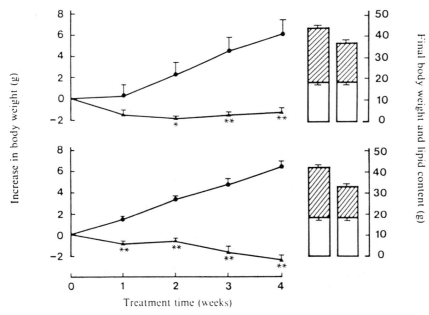

FIGURE 66-5

Structures of thermogenic β-adrenoceptor agonists.

BRL 26830 ; R = H , X = CO$_2$CH$_3$
BRL 35135 ; R = Cl , X = OCH$_2$CO$_2$CH$_3$

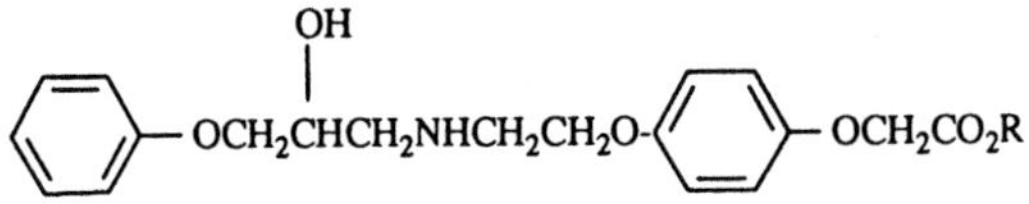

ICI 198157 ; R = CH$_3$
ICI 201651 ; R = H

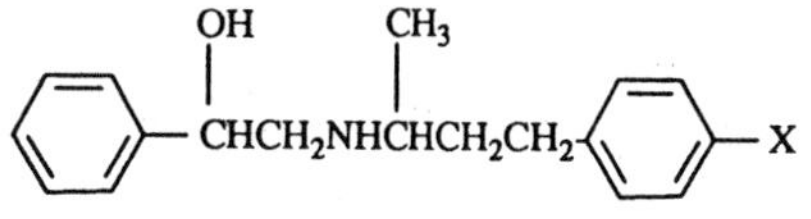

LY 79771 ; X = OH
LY 104119 ; X = CONH$_2$

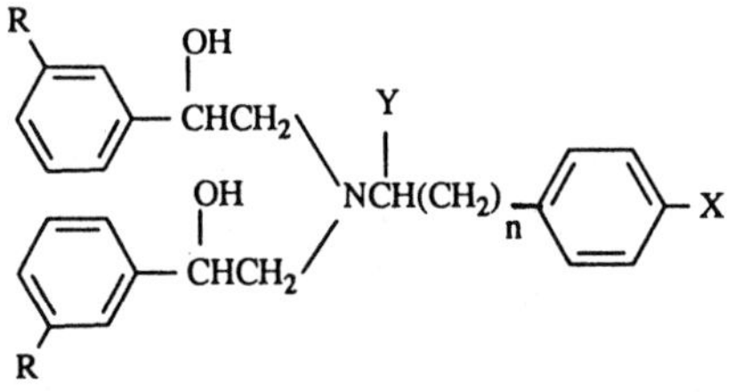

Ro 16-8714 ; R = H , Y = CH$_3$, n = 2 , X = CONH$_2$
Ro 40-2148 ; R = Cl , Y = H , n = 1 , X = O(CH$_2$)$_2$OCH$_2$CH$_3$

FIGURE 66-6

Effect of daily treatment with BRL 26830 (10.3 mg/kg PO; ▲ in upper panel),
BRL 35135 (0.64 mg/kg PO; ▲ in lower panel), or water (●) on body weight
and composition in female C57B1/6 ob/ob mice. Treatments were given daily
for four weeks. Body composition was determined gravimetrically. Final body
weight is shown in the histograms, with body lipid content indicated by
hatched area. (From Arch JRS et al: Nature 309:163, 1984. Reproduced by
permission.)

768

sue has an important role in energy balance. All of this work suggested that brown adipose tissue might be a site of the thermogenic response to compounds such as BRL 26830 and BRL 35135. Indeed, the metabolites BRL 28410 and BRL 37344 were found to stimulate selectively brown adipocyte lipolysis in vitro.[7] These compounds contrasted markedly with standard β-adrenoceptor agonists, which were more potent as stimulants of atrial rate and tension (β$_1$-adrenoceptor mediated) or as relaxants of tracheal or uterine tension (β$_2$-adrenoceptor mediated) (Table 66-1). This work strongly suggested that the β-adrenoceptor associated with lipolysis in brown[7] and white[68] adipose tissue was neither of the β$_1$- nor β$_2$-subtype. This conclusion was supported further by the finding that standard β-antagonists such as propranolol were less potent in blocking lipolysis than in antagonizing β$_1$ and β$_2$ effects[7,33] and led to the identification of this receptor as β$_3$. The pharmacologic identification of this subtype has been supported recently by the cloning of a gene for a β-adrenoceptor from a human cDNA library that shows homology with but is significantly different from human β$_1$ and turkey β$_2$ receptors. When expressed in Chinese hamster ovary cells, this adrenoceptor exhibits many features of the rat lipolytic receptor.[24]

The selectivity of β$_3$-adrenoceptor agonists has also been demonstrated in vivo by comparing the thermogenic activity of compounds with their effects on standard β$_1$- and β$_2$-mediated processes, such as changes in heart rate and in plasma K$^+$

concentration. All of the agents shown in Figure 66-5 demonstrate some selectivity for thermogenesis, which suggest that thermogenesis in vivo in rodents is activated by a non-β$_1$, non-β$_2$-adrenoceptor. Further support for this supposition is provided by the finding that propranolol (10 mg/kg PO) completely blocks the effect of BRL 26830 (10 mg/kg PO) on heart rate but has no effect on thermogenesis.[6] Similar findings have been obtained with LY 104119[71] and RO-40-2148.[44]

BROWN ADIPOSE TISSUE AS A THERMOGENIC SITE?

The pharmacology of brown adipocyte lipolysis in vitro and thermogenesis in vivo is consistent with brown adipose tissue being the major site of thermogenesis in rodents. The work of Foster and Frydman[26] suggested that this was likely. However, blood flow studies on the β$_3$-agonist BRL 26830 suggested that brown adipose tissue contributed only 8% of the acute thermogenic effect of BRL 26830 in mature rats.[65] This study suggested that skeletal muscle may be a quantitatively more important site when thermogenesis is stimulated by β$_3$-adrenoceptor agonists rather than by noradrenaline.

The possible role of brown adipose tissue in man as a potential site of thermogenesis has been debated over the last few years. Although its role in thermogenesis in the newborn is well established, there is no substantive evidence that it has a major role in the adult. Indeed, brown adipose tissue has often proved difficult to find in normal adults, but its presence has now been shown conclusively up to the sixth decade,[19,28,39] and significant quantities exist in subjects with pheochromocytoma.[50] Brown adipose tissue typically has multilocular fat droplets, in contrast to unilocular white adipose tissue. Its brown color results from the large number of mitochondria in the tissue. A possible reason for the apparent disappearance of brown adipose tissue in adult man is that a shift in the balance of lipogenesis and thermogenesis occurs, causing lipid accumulation, so that the brown cells take on the appearance of white adipose tissue. This has also been shown in the bladder fat pad of the dog. In the puppy, this is brown, but it becomes white in

TABLE 66-1

Selectivity of Various Agonists for Brown Adipose Tissue

| Agonist | Selectivity for Brown Adipocyte Lipolysis Over | |
	Atria (β$_1$)	Trachea (β$_2$)
Isoprenaline	0.14	0.23
Fenoterol	0.21	0.02
Salbutamol	0.35	0.01
BRL 37344	400	20.5
BRL 28410	20.6	8.3

Adapted from data reported by Arch et al.[7]

appearance in the adult dog, and mitochondrial uncoupling protein (a thermogenic marker) is undetectable.[9] These age-related biochemical and histologic changes were reversed by treatment with LY 79730 for only 12 days.[9] This finding presents the prospect that a similar situation might occur in adult man and that the age-related decrease in brown adipose tissue activity might be reversed by chronic treatment with thermogenic β-agonists. Nevertheless, it seems likely also that skeletal muscle will be quantitatively the major site of thermogenesis in man.

BRL 26830 AND BRL 35135

In animal studies, these two compounds (see Figure 66-5) fulfill much of the ideal profile for an antiobesity treatment. Chronic treatment of obese rodents produces a marked reduction in body weight or weight gain (see Figure 66-6), even though food intake is not decreased. Furthermore, these reductions are entirely due to reductions in body lipid content: lean tissue is either unaffected or may even increase slightly.[6,7] In contrast to obese animals, there is no reduction in body weight or lipid content in lean animals. In part this is because lean animals increase their food intake. However, the major effect is that the duration of the thermogenic response is reduced in chronically treated lean animals relative to that in obese animals.[6] In a wide range of animal studies, no behavioral effects have been seen that suggest any central stimulant activity, and thus it is unlikely that thermogenic β-agonists will have central addictive effects.

In chronic dosing studies in rodent models of non-insulin-dependent diabetes, both BRL 26830 and BRL 35135 improved glycemic control and lowered circulating insulin, triglyceride, and free fatty acid levels.[55,59,60] The effect on glycemic control arises from a body weight–independent improvement in insulin sensitivity, mediated in part by an increase in the insulin receptor tryosine kinase activity.[51] In fa/fa rats studied under euglycemic hyperinsulinemic clamp conditions to directly measure insulin sensitivity, chronic treatment with BRL 35135 produced a significant increase in the glucose infusion rate required to maintain euglycemia (Fig. 66-7).

Both BRL 26830 and BRL 35135 have pro-

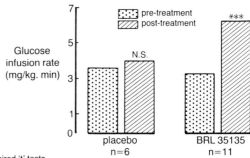

paired 't' tests
*** p<0.001 compared to pre-treatment
N.S. = not significant

FIGURE 66-7

Effect of BRL 35135 on whole body insulin-mediated glucose disposal in type II diabetics. Type II diabetic subjects received either BRL 35135 (2 mg/day for two days, 4 mg/day for four days, 6 mg/day for six days) or placebo. Following an overnight fast, they underwent a two-hour hyperglycemic euglycemic clamp (insulin, 40 mU/m[2], min) prior to treatment and 10 to 12 hours after the last dose of BRL 35135 or placebo. (Data from Smith SA et al, in preparation.)

gressed to human studies. In an 18-week antiobesity study, BRL 26830 produced a significantly greater antiobesity effect than placebo in patients given dietary advice.[18] However, in a second 12-week study BRL 26830 produced no significant effect.[17] Figure 66-8 provides pooled data from both studies on all patients who completed 12 weeks of treatment and shows that BRL 26830 had an appreciable antiobesity effect. Furthermore, BRL 26830 appeared to reduce the loss of body protein that accompanies an energy-restricted diet.[1,18]

BRL 35135 is more potent than BRL 26830 in animal studies, and its metabolite BRL 37344 is more selective for the β₃-receptor than the corresponding metabolite of BRL 26830.[7] In normal man, BRL 35135 at a dosage of 0.1 mg/kg PO increases thermogenesis in fasted subjects and increases glucose-induced thermogenesis.[61]

In two ten-day studies, evidence was obtained that BRL 35135 improves insulin sensitivity in man[46,60] by an action unrelated to weight reduction. Treatment of obese, glucose-intolerant patients for ten days (2 mg/day for five days, then 6 mg/day for five days) improved glucose tolerance while at the same time decreasing the postglu-

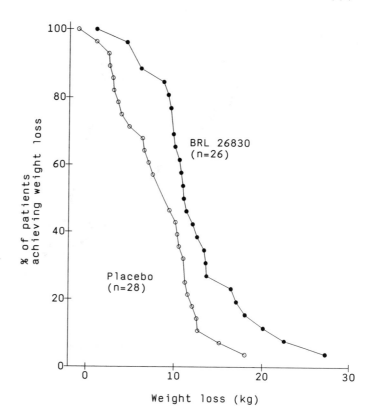

FIGURE 66-8

Effect of BRL 26830 (50 mg/day) or placebo on weight loss in obese patients treated for 12 weeks. Data are expressed as percentage of patients completing the study who achieved each stratum of weight loss at the end of the 12-week period. (Data from Chapman et al[17] and Connacher et al.[18])

cose load hyperinsulinemia. The improvement in glucose tolerance was due to improved glucose storage. In the second study in diabetic patients, which used the euglycemic hyperinsulinemic clamp technique to measure insulin sensitivity, a ten-day treatment with BRL 35135 (2 mg/day for two days, 4 mg/day for four days, 6 mg/day for six days) produced a twofold increase in glucose infusion rate required to maintain euglycemia.

LY 79771 AND LY 104119

In contrast to the direct approach taken by other pharmaceutical companies, these compounds appear to be spin-offs from a program on inotropic agents for congestive heart failure. Workers at Lilly found that LY 79771 (see Fig. 66-5 for structures) was a potent lipolytic agent in vitro and in vivo.[56] Unlike the Beecham compounds, its lipolytic activity may be blocked by propranolol,[73] which suggests that it might not be selec-

tive for the β_3-adrenoceptor. Nevertheless, when given by subcutaneous injection to genetically obese but not lean rodents,[56,70] LY 79771 exhibited significant antiobesity activity (Fig. 66-9). Later studies concentrated on the orally active compound, LY 104119,[73,74] but as yet there are no reports of human studies.

ICI 198157

The oxypropanolamine ICI 198157 is, like the Beecham compounds, a methyl ester and is rapidly metabolized in vivo to the free acid, ICI 201651 (see Fig. 66-5). Acute administration of ICI 198157 to conscious rats raises metabolic rate. The dose-response curve for increase in metabolic rate follows closely the dose-response for increase in GDP binding of brown adipose tissue mitochondria, whereas the dose-response effect on heart rate (mainly β_1 activity) is shifted markedly to the right (Fig. 66-10).[34] ICI 198157 has no β_2-adrenoceptor activity in a model of

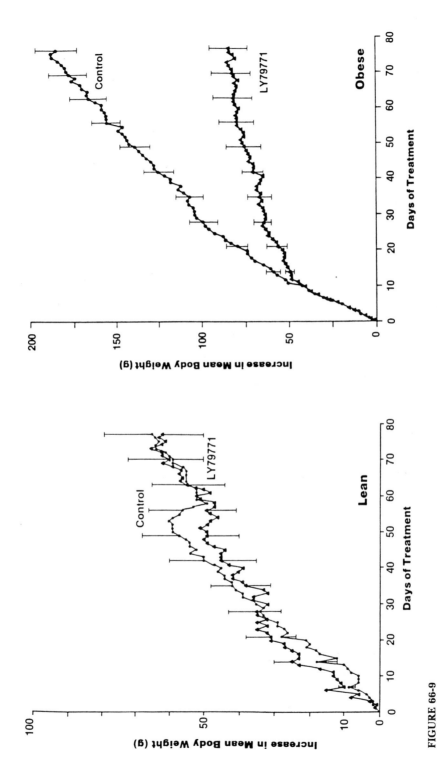

FIGURE 66-9

Effect of LY 79771 (10 mg/kg SC twice daily) or placebo (control) on the body weights of lean and obese Zucker rats. The initial mean body weights were: lean control, 259 g; lean treated, 248 g; obese control, 323 g; obese treated, 329 g. There was a significant difference ($P < .05$) between obese control and treated rats from the 21st day of treatment onward. (From Shaw WN et al: Life Sci 29:2091, 1981. Reproduced by permission.)

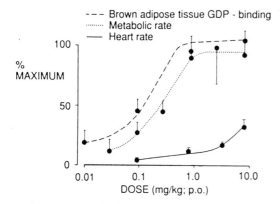

FIGURE 66-10

Effects of ICI 198157 in conscious rats. (From Holloway BR et al: ICI 198157: A novel selective agonist of brown fat and thermogenesis. In Björntorp P, Rössner S (eds): Obesity in Europe, p 323. London, John Libbey, 1989. Reproduced by permission.)

muscle tremor in the anesthetized cat, nor does it affect plasma potassium in the conscious dog at a dose level 100 times that producing half-maximal activation of GDP binding in brown adipose tissue in the rat. Chronic treatment of genetically obese Zucker rats by twice-daily oral gavage with ICI 198157 (5 mg/kg PO) resulted in a reduced rate of weight gain compared to controls, and the decreased weight gain was associated with a reduction in body fat.[35]

In vitro studies using ICI 201651 show that it is less potent than BRL 37344 (acid metabolite of BRL 35135) in stimulating rat brown adipose tissue respiration and lipolysis.[63] Antagonist studies suggest that both agents act on an identical receptor, which appears to be different from the receptor at which isoprenaline acts. In support of the *in vivo* data, ICI 201651 has little effect on either guinea pig atrial rate (β_1) or tracheal relaxation (β_2). Currently no reports of the effect of ICI 198157 in man are available.

RO 16-8714 AND RO 40-2148

Ro 16-8714 (see Fig. 66-5) selectively stimulates brown adipose tissue oxygen consumption (EC_{50} = 8µM), but unlike the other selective agents, it is not a full agonist, producing a maximum response 55% of that produced by noradrena-

line.[43] Chronic treatment of ob/ob mice with Ro 16-8714 (26 mg/kg/day in divided doses) resulted in marked hypertrophy of brown adipose tissue, a reduction in body fat content, and preservation of body protein. These changes were accompanied by normalization of the hyperglycemia that exists in these mice and a substantial reduction in the hyperinsulinemia (although insulin sensitivity was not improved).[43] However, it is not clear whether these metabolic effects are merely a consequence of the antiobesity action or an independent action of Ro 16-8714.

Dose-response studies show that Ro 16-8714 is more potent in increasing oxygen consumption in rats than in mice.[43] It also shows a similar potency but a lower maximum response in Zucker fa/fa rats than in lean. Nevertheless, Ro 16-8714 (3.9 mg/kg PO in divided doses) resulted in a marked antiobesity effect over a 68-day period in Zucker fa/fa rats. Body composition measurements showed that this weight reduction occurred via a selective effect on body lipid.

Two clinical studies have been reported on Ro 16-8714. In six normal volunteers given 5, 10, and 20 mg of Ro 16-8714, there was a dose-dependent increase in metabolic rate over a six-hour period (mean, 4%, 10%, and 21% increase, respectively) but there was also a dose-dependent increase in heart rate (mean, 2%, 22%, and 49%[30]) which was not directly related to the increase in metabolic rate. In a comparison of lean and obese subjects, similar increases in energy expenditure (mean, 12.2% and 14.4%) and heart rate (18% and 16%) were observed in the two groups. Ro 16-8714 also increased systolic blood pressure significantly.[29]

Ro 16-8714 appears to have insufficient separation of the thermogenic activity from the cardiostimulant effects to allow clinical development; however, Ro 40-2148 may hold more promise.[44] It enhances oxygen consumption in rats (EC_{50} = 0.45 mg/kg), cats (EC_{50} = 0.04 mg/kg), and dogs (EC_{50} = 0.06 mg/kg). In rats, the maximal increase in heart rate was only 16% greater than in controls, suggesting that if Ro 40-2148 is acting directly at cardiac β-adrenoceptors, it is only a partial agonist (Fig. 66-11). In fact, in the pithed rat, which lacks central autonomic cardiovascular regulation, there was no appreciable effect on heart rate or blood pressure. This suggests that

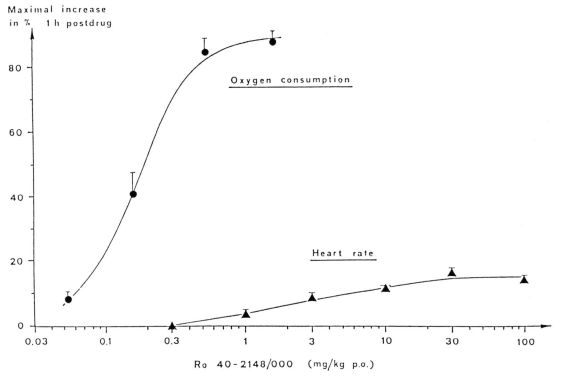

FIGURE 66-11

Maximum acute effects of RO 40-2148 on oxygen consumption and heart rate in conscious rats. (From Meier MK et al: RO 40-2148, a novel thermogenic β-agonist with anti-obesity activity. In Björntorp P, Rössner S (eds): Obesity in Europe, p 329. London, John Libbey, 1989. Reproduced by permission.)

Ro 40-2148 has no significant agonist properties at myocardial β_1- and vascular β_2-adrenoceptors and that the increase in heart rate in conscious animals may be a feedback response as a result of increased energy expenditure.

Ro 40-2148 (1.6 and 4.7 mg/kg PO) resulted in a dose-dependent antiobesity effect in Zucker fa/fa rats following an 11-week treatment period. The reduction in weight was accompanied by significant reductions in blood glucose, plasma insulin, triglycerides, and cholesterol and liver triglycerides. No clinical reports on this agent are available yet.

CONCLUSIONS

Of the available thermogenic agents, only the specifically designed β_3-adrenoceptor agonists

hold promise of being serious ethical treatments for obesity. To fulfill this promise, the agents will need to demonstrate in clinical studies consistent, additional weight reduction in obese patients over that produced by caloric restriction alone, and selectivity from β_1- and β_2-adrenoceptor-mediated actions. Furthermore, in line with the animal experiments, the body weight loss should be predominantly fat and should be associated ideally with additional clinical benefits on metabolic parameters.

References

1. Abraham R, Zed C, Mitchell T et al: The effect of a novel β-agonist BRL26830A on weight and protein loss in obese patients. Int J Obes 11:306A, 1987
2. Abraham RG, Denson JW, Davies P et al: The ef-

fects of triiodothyronine on energy expenditure, nitrogen balance and rates of weight and fat loss in obese patients during prolonged caloric restriction. Int J Obes 9:433, 1985

3. Acheson KJ, Zahorska-Markiewicz B, Pittet P et al: Caffeine and coffee: Their influence on metabolic rate and substrate utilization in normal weight and obese individuals. Am J Clin Nutr 33:989, 1980

4. Ahlquist RP: Historical perspective: Classification of adrenoreceptors. J Auton Pharmacol 1:101, 1980

5. Arch JRS: The contribution of increased thermogenesis to the effect of anorectic drugs on body composition in mice. Am J Clin Nutr 34:2763, 1981

6. Arch JRS, Ainsworth AT: Thermogenic and antiobesity activity of a novel β-adrenoceptor agonist (BRL 26830A) in mice and rats. Am J Clin Nutr 38:549, 1983

7. Arch JRS, Ainsworth AT, Cawthorne MA et al: Atypical β-adrenoceptor on brown adipocytes as a target for antiobesity drugs. Nature 309:163, 1984

8. Arch JRS, Piercy V, Thurlby PL et al: Thermogenic and lipolytic drugs for the treatment of obesity: Old ideas and new possibilities. Recent Adv Obes Res 5:300, 1987

9. Ashwell M, Stirling D, Freeman S et al: Immunological, histological and biochemical assessment of brown adipose tissue activity in neonatal control and β-stimulant treated adult dogs. Int J Obes 11:357, 1987

10. Astrup A, Lundgaard C, Madsen J et al: Enhanced thermogenic responsiveness during chronic l-ephedrine treatment in man. Am J Clin Nutr 42:83, 1985

11. Bilezikan IP, Loeb JN: The influence of hyperthyroidism and hypothyroidism on alpha- and beta-adrenergic systems and adrenergic responsiveness. Endocrine Rev 4:378, 1983

12. Bray GA: The Obese Patient, p 381. Philadelphia, WB Saunders, 1976

13. Bray GA: Fenfluramine: A thermogenic drug. Recent Adv Obes Res 5:290, 1987

14. Bray GA, Rabens MS, Londono J et al: Effects of triiodothyronine, growth hormone and anabolic steroids on nitrogen excretion and oxygen consumption in obese patients. J Clin Endocrinol 33:293, 1971

15. Cawthorne MA: Is tolerance to anorectic drugs a real phenomenon or an experimental artefact? In Garattini S, Samanin R (eds): Anorectic Agents: Mechanisms of Action and Tolerance, p 1. New York, Raven Press, 1981

16. Cawthorne MA: The use of animal models for detecting and evaluating compounds for the treatment of obesity. In Festing MFW (ed): Animal Models of Obesity. London, Macmillan Press, 1979

17. Chapman BJ, Farquahar DL, Galloway S McL et al:

The effects of a new β-adrenoceptor agonist BRL 26830A in refractory obesity. Int J Obes 12:119, 1988

18. Connacher AA, Jung RT, Mitchell PEG: Weight loss in obese subjects on a restricted diet given BRL 26830A, a new atypical β-adrenoceptor agonist. Br Med J 296:1217, 1988

19. Cunningham S, Leslie P, Hopwood D et al: The characterization and energetic potential of brown adipose tissue in man. Clin Sci 69:343, 1985

20. Dallosso HM, James WPT: The role of smoking in the regulation of energy balance. Int J Obes 8:365, 1984

21. Douglas JG, Munro JF: The role of drugs in the treatment of obesity. Drugs 21:362, 1981

22. Dulloo AG, Miller DS: Thermogenic drugs for the treatment of obesity: Sympathetic stimulants in animal models. Br J Nutr 52:179, 1984

23. Edelman IS, Ismail-Bergi F: Thyroid thermogenesis and active sodium transport. Recent Prog Horm Res 30:235, 1974

24. Emorine LJ, Marullo S, Briend-Sutren, MM et al: Molecular characterization of the human β₃-adrenergic receptor. Science 254:1118, 1989

25. Evans WF, Stewart HJ: Effects of smoking cigarettes on the peripheral blood flow. Am Heart J 26:78, 1943

26. Foster DO, Friedman ML: Non-shivering thermogenesis in the rat. II. Measurement of blood flow with microspheres points to brown adipose tissue as the dominant site of calorigenesis induced by noradrenaline. Can J Physiol Pharmacol 56:110, 1978

27. Fredholm BB: On the mechanism of action of theophylline and caffeine. Acta Med Scand 217:149, 1985

28. Heaton JM: The distribution of brown adipose tissue in the human. J Anat 112:35, 1972

29. Henny C, Bukert G, Schutz Y et al: Comparison of the thermogenic activity induced by the new sympathomimetic Ro 16-8714 between normal and obese subjects. Int J Obes 12:227, 1988

30. Henny C, Schutz Y, Bukert A et al: Thermogenic effect of the new β-adrenoceptor agonist Ro 16-8714 in healthy male volunteers. Int J Obes 11:473, 1987

31. Hoch FL: Thyrotoxicosis as a disease of mitochondria. N Engl J Med 266:446, 1962

32. Hollands MA, Arch JRS, Cawthorne MA: A simple apparatus for comparative measurements of energy expenditure in human subjects: The thermic effect of caffeine. Am J Clin Nutr 34:2291, 1981

33. Hollenga C, Zaagsma J: Direct evidence for the atypical nature of functional β-adrenoceptors in rat adipocytes. Br J Pharmacol 98:1420, 1989

34. Holloway BR: Selective β-agonists of brown fat and

thermogenesis. In Lardy H, Stratman F (eds): Hormones, Thermogenesis and Obesity. Amsterdam, Elsevier, 1989

35. Holloway BR, Howe R, Rao BS et al: ICI 198157: A novel selective agonist of brown fat and thermogenesis. In Björntorp P, Rössner S (eds): Obesity in Europe, p 323. London, John Libbey, 1989

36. Jung RT, Shetty PS, Barrand M et al: The role of catecholamines and thyroid hormones in the metabolic response to semi-starvation. Proc Nutr Soc 38:17A, 1979

37. Koppescharr HPF, Meinders AE, Schwartz F: Metabolic responses in grossly obese subjects treated with a very-low-calorie diet with and without triiodothyronine treatment. Int J Obes 7:133, 1983

38. Lang SS, Danforth E, Lien EL: Anorectic drugs which stimulate thermogenesis. Life Sci 33:1269, 1983

39. Lean MEJ, Trayhurn P, Murgatroyd PR et al: The case for brown adipose tissue function in humans: Biochemistry, physiology and computed tomography. Recent Adv Obes Res 5:109, 1986

40. Le Blanc J, Villemaire A: Thyroxine and noradrenaline on noradrenaline sensitivity, cold resistance and brown fat. Am J Physiol 218:1742, 1970

41. Lupien JR, Bray GA: Effect of fenfluramine on GDP-binding to brown adipose tissue mitochondria. Pharmacol Biochem Behav 23:509, 1985

42. Malchow-Moller A, Larsen S, Hey H et al: Ephedrine as an anorectic: The study of the Elsinore pill. Int J Obes 5:183, 1981

43. Meier MK, Alig L, Burgi-Saville ME et al: Phenethanolamine derivatives with calorigenic and antidiabetic qualities. Int J Obes 8(suppl 1):215, 1984

44. Meier MK, Blum-Kaelin D, Gerold M et al: Ro 40-2148, a novel thermogenic β-agonist with antiobesity activity. In Björntorp P, Rössner S (eds): Obesity in Europe, p 329. London, John Libbey, 1989

45. Miller DS: Thermogenesis in everyday life. In Jequier E (ed): 2nd International Conference on Regulation of Energy Balance, p 198. Geneva, Editions Medecine et Hygiene, 1975

46. Mitchell TH, Ellis RDM, Smith SA et al: Effects of BRL 35135, a β-adrenoceptor agonist with novel selectivity, on glucose tolerance and insulin sensitivity in obese subjects. Int J Obes 13:767, 1989

47. Muller MJ, Seitz HJ: Thyroid hormone action on intermediary metabolism. Part I. Respiration, thermogenesis and carbohydrate metabolism. Klin Wochenschr 62:11, 1984

48. Munro JF, Ford JE: Clinical trials of anorectic drugs. In Garattini S, Samanin R (eds): Central Mechanisms of Anorectic Drugs, p 419. New York, Raven Press, 1978

49. Parascandola J: Dinitrophenol and bioergetics: An historical perspective. Mol Cell Biochem 5:69, 1974

50. Ricquier D, Nechad M, Mory G: Ultrastructural and biochemical characterization of human brown adipose tissue in phaeochromocytoma. J Clin Endocrinol Metab 54:803, 1982

51. Rochet N, Tanti JF, Gremeaux T et al: Effect of a thermogenic agent, BRL 26830A, on insulin receptors in obese mice. Am J Physiol 255:E101, 1988

52. Rothwell NJ, Stock MJ: A role for brown adipose tissue in diet-induced thermogenesis. Nature 281: 31, 1979

53. Rothwell NJ, Stock MJ: Effect of diet and fenfluramine on thermogenesis in the rat: Possible involvement of serotonergic mechanisms. Int J Obes 11:319, 1987

54. Scoville BA: Review of amphetamine-like drugs by the Food and Drug Administration: Clinical data and value judgements. In Bray GA (ed): Obesity in Perspective. DHEW publication NIH-75-708, p 441. Washington, DC, p 441, DHEW, 1974

55. Sennitt MV, Arch JRS, Levy AL et al: Antihyperglycaemic action of BRL 26830, a novel β-adrenoceptor agonist, in mice and rats. Biochem Pharmacol 34:1279, 1985

56. Shaw WN, Schmiegel KK, Yen TT et al: LY 79771: A novel compound for weight control. Life Sci 29:2091, 1981

57. Simkins S: Dinitrophenol and desiccated thyroid in the treatment of obesity: A comprehensive clinical and laboratory study. JAMA 108:2100, 1973

58. Smith RE: Thermogenesis and thyroid action. Nature 204:1311, 1964

59. Smith SA, Levy AL, Sennitt MV et al: Effects of BRL 26830, a novel β-adrenoceptor agonist, on glucose tolerance, insulin sensitivity and glucose turnover in Zucker (fa/fa) rats. Biochem Pharmacol 34:2425, 1985

60. Smith SA, Sennitt MV, Cawthorne MA: BRL 35135: An orally active anti-hyperglycaemic agent with weight reducing effects. In Bailey CJ, Flatt PR (eds): New Anti-Diabetic Drugs, p 177. London, Smith-Gordon & Co, 1990

61. Smith SA, Zed C, McCullough D et al: Thermogenic activity in man of BRL 35135: A potent and selective atypical β-adrenoceptor agonist (abstr 133). Int J Obes 13(suppl 1), 1989

62. Stock MJ: Determination of the oxygen consumption and the carbon dioxide production of the rat. Proc Nutr Soc 25:xli, 1966

63. Sudera D: Thesis, University of London, 1989

64. Sullivan AC: Drug treatment of obesity: A perspective. Recent Adv Obes Res 5:293, 1986

65. Thurlby PL, Ellis RDM: Differences between the

effects of noradrenaline and the β-adrenoceptor agonist BRL 28410 in brown adipose tissue and hind limb of the anaesthetized rat. Can J Physiol Pharmacol 64:1111, 1986

66. Thurlby PL, Trayhurn P: Regional blood flow in genetically obese (ob/ob) mice: The importance of brown adipose tissue to the reduced energy expenditure of non-shivering thermogenesis. Pflugers Arch 385:193, 1980

67. Wilcox AR: The effects of caffeine and exercise on body weight, fat pad weight and fat cell size. Med Sci Sports Exerc 14:317, 1982

68. Wilson C, Wilson S, Piercy V et al: The rat lipolytic β-adrenoceptor: Studies using novel β-adrenoceptor agonists. Eur J Pharmacol 100:309, 1984

69. Wilson KL, Smith SA, Cawthorne MA: Comparative effects of voluntary exercise and caloric restriction on body composition and glucose tolerance in Zucker (fa/fa) rats. Int J Obes 8:381, 1984

70. Yen TT: The antiobesity and metabolic activities of LY 79771 in obese and normal mice. Int J Obes 8:69, 1984

71. Yen TT, Anderson DB, Veenhuizen EL: Phenethanolamines reduction of fat and increase of muscle, from mice to pigs. In Hardy HA et al (eds): Proceedings of the Eighteenth Steenbock Symposium: Hormones, Thermogenesis and Obesity, p 455. Amsterdam, Elsevier, 1989

72. Yen TT, Fuller RW, Hemrick-Luecke SK et al: Effects of LY 104119, a thermogenic weight-reducing compound, on norepinephrine concentrations and turnover in obese and lean mice. Int J Obes 12:59, 1988

73. Yen TT, McKee MM, Stamm NB: Thermogenesis and weight-control. Int J Obes 8(suppl 1):65, 1984

74. Yen TT, McKee MM, Stamm NB et al: Stimulation of cyclic AMP and lipolysis in adipose tissue of normal and obese A^{vy}/a mice by LY 79771, a phenethanolamine and stereo isomers. Life Sci 32:1515, 1983

Index

Page numbers in italics indicate figures; page numbers followed by a "t" indicate tables.

ISBN 0-397-50999-5

90000